# Practical Strategies in Obstetrics and Gynecology

# Practical Strategies in Obstetrics and Gynecology

EDITOR

**Scott B. Ransom, DO, MBA**

Vice President for Medical Affairs
Detroit Medical Center

Associate Professor and Director
Division of Community Programs and Health Effectiveness
Department of Obstetrics and Gynecology
Wayne State University School of Medicine

Chief, Section of Gynecology
John D. Dingell VA Medical Center
Detroit, Michigan

ASSOCIATE EDITORS

**Mitchell P. Dombrowski, MD**
Professor and Associate Chairman
Division of Maternal–Fetal Medicine
Department of Obstetrics and Gynecology
Wayne State University School of Medicine
Detroit, Michigan

**Kamran S. Moghissi, MD**
Professor
Division of Reproductive Endocrinology and Infertility
Department of Obstetrics and Gynecology
Wayne State University School of Medicine
Detroit, Michigan

**S. Gene McNeeley, Jr., MD**
Professor and Director
Division of Gynecology
Department of Obstetrics and Gynecology
Wayne State University School of Medicine
Director, Division of Gynecology
Detroit Receiving Hospital
Detroit, Michigan

**Adnan R. Munkarah, MD**
Assistant Professor
Division of Gynecologic Oncology
Department of Obstetrics and Gynecology
Wayne State University School of Medicine
Detroit, Michigan

**W.B. SAUNDERS COMPANY**
*A Division of Harcourt Brace & Company*
Philadelphia  London  Toronto  Montreal  Sydney  Tokyo

**W.B. SAUNDERS COMPANY**
*A Division of Harcourt Brace & Company*

The Curtis Center
Independence Square West
Philadelphia, Pennsylvania 19106

---

**Library of Congress Cataloging-in-Publication Data**

Practical strategies in obstetrics and gynecology / editor, Scott B. Ransom; section editors, Mitchell P. Dombrowski . . . [et al.]—1st ed.

p.   cm.

ISBN 0–7216–7854–8

1. Gynecology    2. Obstetrics    I. Ransom, Scott B.    I. Dombrowski, Mitchell P.    [DNLM: 1. Gynecology.    2. Obstetrics.    WQ 100 P8955 2000]

RG101.P887  2000    618—dc21

DNLM/DLC                                                                  99-33413

---

PRACTICAL STRATEGIES IN OBSTETRICS
AND GYNECOLOGY                                        ISBN 0–7216–7854–8

Copyright © 2000 by W.B. Saunders Company.

All rights reserved. No part of this publication may be reproduced or transmitted in any form or by any means, electronic or mechanical, including photocopy, recording, or any information storage and retrieval system, without permission in writing from the publisher.

Printed in the United States of America.

Last digit is the print number:     9    8    7    6    5    4    3    2    1

# CONTRIBUTORS

**Dorel Abramovici, MD**
Fellow, Division of Maternal–Fetal Medicine, University of Tennessee, Memphis College of Medicine, Memphis, Tennessee
Hypertensive Disorders in Pregnancy

**Aneel Advani, MD**
Department of Medical Information, Stanford University Medical School, Stanford, California
A Review of Medical Informatics

**Neil Athayde, MD**
Visiting Fellow, Perinatology Research Branch, National Institute of Child Health and Human Development, The National Institutes of Health, Bethesda, Maryland
Premature Rupture of Fetal Membranes (PROM)

**Nandalal Bagchi, MD, PhD**
Professor, Department of Internal Medicine, Division of Endocrinology and Metabolism, Wayne State University School of Medicine, Detroit, Michigan
Thyroid Disorders

**Ross Stuart Berkowitz, MD**
William H. Baker Professor of Gynecology, Harvard Medical School; Director of Gynecology and Gynecologic Oncology, Co-Director of New England Trophoblastic Disease Center, Co-Director of Gillette Center for Women's Cancer, Brigham and Women's Hospital and Dana Farber Cancer Institute, Boston, Massachusetts
Gestational Trophoblastic Disease

**Annette Bicher, MD**
Gynecologic Oncology, Northern Virginia Pelvic Surgery Associates, Annandale, Virginia
Epithelial Ovarian Carcinoma

**Charla M. Blacker, MD**
Assistant Professor of Obstetrics and Gynecology, Medical Director, Assisted Reproductive Technologies, Wayne State University School of Medicine; Hutzel Hospital, Detroit, Michigan
Assisted Reproductive Technologies

**Richard E. Blackwell, MD**
Professor of Obstetrics and Gynecology, Division of Reproductive Biology and Endocrinology, University of Alabama School of Medicine, Birmingham, Alabama
Amenorrhea

**Wendy R. Brewster, MD**
Clinical Instructor, Division of Gynecologic Oncology, University of California, Irvine College of Medicine, Orange, California
Cancer in Pregnancy

**Robert E. Bristow, MD**
Assistant Professor, Division of Gynecologic Oncology, Department of Gynecology and Obstetrics, Johns Hopkins University School of Medicine, Baltimore, Maryland
Cervical Cancer

**Thomas W. Burke, MD**
Associate Professor, Department of Gynecologic Oncology, University of Texas M.D. Anderson Cancer Center, Houston, Texas
Vulvar and Vaginal Cancers

**Lara J. Burrows, MD**
Resident, Department of Obstetrics and Gynecology, Johns Hopkins University School of Medicine; Johns Hopkins Hospital, Baltimore, Maryland
Leiomyoma; Pelvic Mass

**Steve Caritis, MD**
Professor, Maternal–Fetal Medicine, University of Pittsburgh School of Medicine, Magee Womens Hospital, Pittsburgh, Pennsylvania
Post-Term Pregnancy

**Sandra A. Carson, MD**
Professor of Obstetrics and Gynecology, Director, Baylor Assisted Reproductive Technology, Baylor College of Medicine, Houston, Texas
Spontaneous Abortion

**Annette Casoglos, MPH, RD**
Center for Healthcare Effectiveness Research,
Wayne State University, Detroit, Michigan
Clinical Epidemiology

**Kenneth Chang, MD**
Clinical Assistant Professor, Former USQA
Managed Care Fellow, Thomas Jefferson
University Hospital, Philadelphia, Pennsylvania
Managed Care

**David F. Colombo, MD**
Fellow, Maternal–Fetal Medicine, Department of
Obstetrics and Gynecology, The Ohio State
University Hospitals, Columbus, Ohio
Preterm Birth

**Chandice Y. Covington, PhD, RN**
Associate Professor, College of Nursing, Wayne
State University, Detroit, Michigan
Illicit Substance Abuse During Pregnancy

**Tracy Cowles, MD**
Associate Professor, Department of Obstetrics and
Gynecology, University of Kansas, Lawrence,
Kansas; University of Missouri, Kansas City,
Missouri
Infections in Pregnancy

**Kulmeet S. Dang, MS**
Project Manager and Epidemiologist, Center for
Healthcare Effectiveness and Research, Wayne
State University, Detroit, Michigan
Clinical Epidemiology

**Colleen Dargie, MD**
Anesthesiologist, Department of Anesthesiology,
Henry Ford Hospital, Detroit, Michigan
Obstetric Anesthesia

**Virginia Delaney-Black, MD, MPH**
Associate Professor of Pediatrics, Wayne State
University School of Medicine; Associate
Neonatologist, Children's Hospital of Michigan
and Hutzel Hospital, Detroit, Michigan
Illicit Substance Abuse During Pregnancy

**Gunter Deppe, MD**
Professor and Director, Division of Gynecologic
Oncology, Department of Obstetrics and
Gynecology, Wayne State University School of
Medicine, Hutzel Hospital, Detroit, Michigan
Uterine Cancers

**Sudipta Dhar, MBBS, DCH**
Research Associate, Wayne State University School
of Medicine, Detroit, Michigan
Illicit Substance Abuse During Pregnancy

**Michael P. Diamond, MD**
Kamran S. Moghissi Professor of Obstetrics and
Gynecology, Director, Division of Reproductive
Endocrinology and Infertility, Wayne State
University School of Medicine, The Detroit
Medical Center, Detroit, Michigan
Hyperandrogenism; Postoperative Adhesion Formation in
Gynecologic Surgery: Etiology and Treatment

**Roselyn M. Dinsay, MD**
Fellow, Division of Reproductive Endocrinology and
Infertility, Department of Obstetrics and
Gynecology, Wayne State University School of
Medicine, Detroit, Michigan
Premenstrual Syndrome

**Philip J. DiSaia, MD**
Professor, Dorothy Marsh Chair in Reproductive
Biology and Director, Division of Gynecologic
Oncology, University of California, Irvine College
of Medicine, Orange, California
Cancer in Pregnancy

**Michael Y. Divon, MD**
Professor of Obstetrics, Gynecology, and Women's
Health, Albert Einstein College of Medicine,
Bronx; Chairman of Obstetrics and Gynecology,
Lenox Hill Hospital, New York, New York
Fetal Growth Disorders: Diagnosis and Management

**Mitchell P. Dombrowski, MD**
Professor and Associate Chairman, Division of
Maternal–Fetal Medicine, Department of
Obstetrics and Gynecology, Wayne State
University School of Medicine, Detroit, Michigan
Vaginal Delivery, Operative and Breech; Asthma in
Pregnancy

**Thomas E. Elkin, MD**
Professor, Department of Obstetrics and
Gynecology, Johns Hopkins University School of
Medicine; Johns Hopkins Hospital, Baltimore,
Maryland
Leiomyoma; Pelvic Mass

**Philip N. Eskew, Jr., MD**
Clinical Associate Professor, Indiana University
School of Medicine; Medical Director, Women
and Infant Services, St. Vincent Hospital,
Indianapolis, Indiana
Current Procedural Terminology (CPT) and International
Classification of Diseases, Ninth Revision, Clinical
Modification (ICD-9-CM) Coding in Obstetrics and
Gynecology

**Mark I. Evans, MD**
Charlotte B. Failing Professor, Chairman and Chief
of Obstetrics and Gynecology, Professor and
Associate Director, Center for Molecular
Medicine and Genetics, Professor of Pathology,

Director of Human Genetics Program, Director of Division of Reproductive Genetics, Director of Center for Fetal Diagnosis and Therapy, Wayne State University School of Medicine, Detroit, Michigan
*Genetic Counseling, Screening, and Diagnosis*

**Lisa A. Farah, MD**
Division of Reproductive Endocrinology, University of Alabama School of Medicine, Birmingham, Alabama
*Amenorrhea*

**Dee Ellen Fenner, MD**
Associate Professor, Department of Obstetrics and Gynecology, Rush Medical College, Chicago, Illinois
*Genital Tract Prolapse*

**Jason O. Gardosi, MD**
Associate Professor, Consultant, and Director, Obstetrics and Gynecology, University Hospital, Queens Medical Center, Gestation Network, Nottingham, United Kingdom
*Multifetal Pregnancy*

**Melvin V. Gerbie, MD**
Professor, Department of Obstetrics and Gynecology, Northwestern University Medical School, Chicago, Illinois
*Hysterectomy*

**William E. Gibbons, MD**
Professor and Chairman, Department of Obstetrics and Gynecology, Eastern Virginia Medical School, Eastern Virginia University, Norfolk, Virginia
*Treatment of Anovulation*

**Kenneth A. Ginsburg, MD**
Associate Professor, Division of Reproductive Endocrinology and Infertility, Department of Obstetrics and Gynecology, Wayne State University School of Medicine, Detroit, Michigan
*Premenstrual Syndrome*

**Milton Goldrath, MD**
Assistant Professor, Department of Obstetrics and Gynecology, Wayne State University School of Medicine, Grace-Sinai Hospital, Detroit, Michigan
*Office Hysteroscopy and Suction Curettage in the Evaluation of Abnormal Uterine Bleeding*

**Donald Peter Goldstein, MD**
Clinical Professor of Obstetrics, Gynecology, and Reproductive Biology, Harvard Medical School; Co-Director, New England Trophoblastic Disease Center, Brigham and Women's Hospital and Dana Farber Cancer Institute, Boston, Massachusetts
*Gestational Trophoblastic Disease*

**Bernard Gonik, MD**
Professor and Chief, Obstetrics and Gynecology, Wayne State University School of Medicine, Northwest Region and Detroit Medical Center, Detroit, Michigan
*Infections in Pregnancy*

**Allen C. Goodman, PhD**
Professor of Economics, Wayne State University, Detroit, Michigan
*The Economics of Obstetrics and Gynecology*

**Carol Graham, MD**
Instructor, Women's Continence Center, Department of Obstetrics and Gynecology, Wayne State University School of Medicine; Hutzel Hospital, Detroit, Michigan
*Urinary Incontinence: Strategies for Evaluation and Nonsurgical Management*

**Victoria A. Gregonis**
Executive Director, Partners for Women's Health Care, an Affiliate of Fempartners, Houston, Texas
*Insurance Contracting for Obstetric–Gynecologic Services*

**Robert A. Hammer, MD**
Assistant Professor, Department of Obstetrics and Gynecology, Northwestern University Medical School, Chicago, Illinois
*Hysterectomy*

**Robert H. Hayashi, MD**
J. Robert Willson Professor of Obstetrics, Director, Division of Maternal–Fetal Medicine, University of Michigan School of Medicine; Director, Division of Maternal–Fetal Medicine, Department of Obstetrics and Gynecology, University of Michigan Medical Center, Ann Arbor, Michigan
*Postpartum Management*

**David L. Hemsell, MD**
Professor, Department of Obstetrics and Gynecology, University of Texas Southwestern Medical Center at Dallas; Director, Division of Gynecology, Parkland Health and Hospital System, Dallas, Texas
*Prevention and Treatment of Postoperative Infections*

**Susan L. Hendrix, DO**
Associate Professor and Director, Women's Health Initiative, Department of Obstetrics and Gynecology, Wayne State University School of Medicine; Hutzel Hospital, Detroit, Michigan
*Menopause*

**Jay D. Iams, MD**
Professor and Director, Division of Maternal–Fetal Medicine, The Ohio State University Hospitals, Columbus, Ohio
*Preterm Birth*

**Gail A. Jensen, PhD**
Professor of Economics and Gerontology, Wayne State University, Detroit, Michigan
*The Economics of Obstetrics and Gynecology*

**Donna D. Johnson, MD**
Assistant Professor, Department of Obstetrics and Gynecology, Medical University of South Carolina, Charleston, South Carolina
*Second-Trimester Ultrasonography*

**Mark Paul Johnson, MD**
Associate Professor, Department of Obstetrics and Gynecology, University of Pennsylvania, Philadelphia, Pennsylvania
*Genetic Counseling, Screening, and Diagnosis*

**Timothy R. B. Johnson, MD**
Bates Professor of the Diseases of Women and Children, Professor and Chair, Department of Obstetrics and Gynecology, Research Scientist, Center for Human Growth and Development, Professor of Women's Studies, University of Michigan, Ann Arbor, Michigan
*Fetal Assessment*

**Carolyn Johnston, MD**
Assistant Professor, Division of Gynecologic Oncology, University of Michigan, Ann Arbor, Michigan
*Diseases of the Breast*

**Theodore B. Jones, MD**
Assistant Professor and Residency Director, Department of Obstetrics and Gynecology, Wayne State University School of Medicine, Detroit, Michigan
*Human Immunodeficiency Virus Infection in Pregnancy*

**David E. Kauffman, MD**
Assistant Professor, Maternal–Fetal Medicine, University of Pittsburgh School of Medicine; Magee Womens Hospital, Pittsburgh, Pennsylvania
*Post-Term Pregnancy*

**David C. Kmak, MD**
Assistant Professor, Division of Gynecology, Department of Obstetrics and Gynecology, Wayne State University School of Medicine; Hutzel Hospital, Detroit, Michigan
*Early Pregnancy Loss*

**Peter N. Kolettis, MD**
Assistant Professor of Surgery, Division of Urology, University of Alabama, Birmingham School of Medicine, Birmingham, Alabama
*Andrology*

**Sally A. Kope, MSW**
Adjunct Lecturer, Department of Human Genetics, University of Michigan Medical School; Consultant, American Association of Sex Therapists, Counselors, and Educators, Ann Arbor, Michigan
*Sexuality*

**Jennifer Elston Lafata, PhD**
Interim Director, Center for Clinical Effectiveness, Henry Ford Health System, Detroit, Michigan
*Clinical Effectiveness: A New Set of Skills for Obstetrician–Gynecologists*

**Mark B. Landon, MD**
Associate Professor and Vice Chairman, Department of Obstetrics and Gynecology, The Ohio State University College of Medicine and Public Health, Columbus, Ohio
*Cesarean Section*

**Oded Langer, MD**
Blumberg Professor of Obstetrics, Professor of Obstetrics and Gynecology, Chief, Division of Obstetrics and Maternal–Fetal Medicine, University of Texas Health Science Center; University of Texas Hospital, San Antonio, Texas
*Diabetes in Pregnancy*

**Richard E. Leach, MD**
Associate Professor, Division of Reproductive Endocrinology and Infertility, Department of Obstetrics and Gynecology, Wayne State University School of Medicine; Director, Reproductive Endocrinology and Infertility, Grace–Sinai Hospital, Detroit, Michigan
*Postoperative Adhesion Formation in Gynecologic Surgery: Etiology and Treatment*

**Charles Levenback, MD**
Associate Professor of Gynecology and Medical Director for Quality Improvement, University of Texas M.D. Anderson Cancer Center, Houston, Texas
*Surgical Complications*

**Kenneth J. Leveno, MD**
Gillette Professor, Department of Obstetrics and Gynecology, University of Texas Southwestern at Dallas; Chief of Obstetrics, Parkland Health and Hospital System, Dallas, Texas
*Normal and Abnormal Labor*

**Gary H. Lipscomb, MD**
Associate Professor and Director, Division of Gynecology, Department of Obstetrics and Gynecology, University of Tennessee, Memphis, Tennessee
*Dysmenorrhea and Pelvic Pain*

**Veronica T. Mallett, MD**
Assistant Professor and Director, Women's Continence Center, Wayne State University School of Medicine; Hutzel Hospital, Department of Obstetrics and Gynecology, Detroit, Michigan
Urinary Incontinence: Strategies for Evaluation and Nonsurgical Management

**H. M. Marsh, MB**
Professor of Anesthesiology, Wayne State University School of Medicine; Specialist-in-Chief in Anesthesiology, Detroit Medical Center, Detroit, Michigan
Obstetric Anesthesia

**R. Michael Massanari, MD**
Professor of Internal Medicine, Director, Center for Healthcare Effectiveness Research, Wayne State University School of Medicine, Detroit, Michigan
Clinical Epidemiology

**Farid Mattar, MD**
Fellow, Department of Obstetrics and Gynecology, University of Tennessee, Memphis, Memphis, Tennessee
Hypertensive Disorders in Pregnancy

**Eli Maymon, MD**
Visiting Fellow, Perinatology Research Branch, National Institute of Child Health and Human Development, The National Institutes of Health, Bethesda, Maryland
Premature Rupture of Fetal Membranes (PROM)

**E. Trent McNeeley, MD**
Private Practice, Knoxville, Tennessee
Women's Preventive Care

**S. Gene McNeeley, MD**
Professor, Department of Obstetrics and Gynecology, Wayne State University School of Medicine; Director, Division of Gynecology, Hutzel Hospital; Chief, Department of Gynecology, Detroit Research Hospital, Detroit, Michigan
Women's Preventive Care; Early Pregnancy Loss; Lower Genital Tract Infection

**Jody L. Meinke, MS**
Center for Healthcare Effectiveness Research, Wayne State University, Detroit, Michigan
Clinical Epidemiology

**Michele Follen Mitchell, MD, MS**
Associate Professor, Department of Gynecologic Oncology, The University of Texas M.D. Anderson Cancer Center, Houston, Texas
Premalignant Disorders of the Lower Genital Tract

**Kamran S. Moghissi, MD**
Professor, Division of Reproductive Endocrinology and Infertility, Department of Obstetrics and Gynecology, Wayne State University School of Medicine, Detroit, Michigan
Contraception; Evaluation and Management of Infertility; Unexplained Infertility

**Frederick J. Montz, MD, KM**
Professor and Director, Division of Gynecologic Oncology, Department of Gynecology and Obstetrics, Johns Hopkins University School of Medicine; The Johns Hopkins Hospital and Medical Institutions, Baltimore, Maryland
Cervical Cancer

**Robert T. Morris, MD**
Assistant Professor, Division of Gynecology and Oncology, Department of Obstetrics and Gynecology, Wayne State University School of Medicine, Detroit, Michigan
Germ Cell and Stromal Ovarian Tumors

**Adnan R. Munkarah, MD**
Assistant Professor, Division of Gynecologic Oncology, Department of Obstetrics and Gynecology, Wayne State University School of Medicine; Hutzel Hospital, Detroit, Michigan
Uterine Cancers; Germ Cell and Stromal Ovarian Tumors

**David Muram, MD**
Professor of Obstetrics and Gynecology, State University of New York Health Sciences Center at Brooklyn, Brooklyn, New York
Pediatric and Adolescent Gynecology

**Ana A. Murphy, MD**
Associate Professor and Director of Reproductive Endocrinology and Infertility, Department of Gynecology and Obstetrics, Emory University School of Medicine, Atlanta, Georgia
Surgery of the Fallopian Tube

**David Nash, MD, MBA**
Associate Dean, Thomas Jefferson Medical College; Director, Office of Health Policy and Clinical Outcomes, Thomas Jefferson University Hospital, Philadelphia, Pennsylvania
Managed Care

**Chukwuma I. Onyeije, MD**
Assistant Professor of Obstetrics and Gynecology, Albert Einstein College of Medicine, Bronx; Director of Education, Department of Obstetrics and Gynecology, Lenox Hill Hospital, New York, New York
Fetal Growth Disorders: Diagnosis and Management

**Anthony W. Opipari, MD, PhD**
Lecturer, Department of Obstetrics and Gynecology, University of Michigan Medical School, Ann Arbor, Michigan
Fetal Assessment

**Steven J. Ory, MD**
Assistant Clinical Professor, Department of Obstetrics and Gynecology, University of Miami School of Medicine, Miami, Florida
Laparoscopy

**Percy Pacora, MD**
Visiting Fellow, Perinatology Research Branch, National Institute of Child Health and Human Development, The National Institutes of Health, Bethesda, Maryland
Premature Rupture of Fetal Membranes (PROM)

**John Y. Phelps, MD**
Fellow, Division of Reproductive Endocrinology, Department of Obstetrics and Gynecology, Johns Hopkins University School of Medicine, Baltimore, Maryland
Evaluation and Management of Infertility

**Karoline S. Puder, MD**
Assistant Professor of Obstetrics and Gynecology, Wayne State University School of Medicine; Attending Physician, Maternal–Fetal Medicine, Grace Hospital, Detroit, Michigan
Vaginal Delivery, Operative and Breech

**Scott B. Ransom, DO, MBA**
Vice President for Medical Affairs, Detroit Medical Center; Associate Professor and Director, Division of Community Programs and Health Effectiveness, Department of Obstetrics and Gynecology, Wayne State University School of Medicine; Chief, Section of Gynecology, John D. Dingell VA Medical Center, Detroit, Michigan
Clinical Pathways; Outcome Measurement: The Emerging Quality Barometer

**Emad Rizk, MD**
Senior Manager, Vice-Chairman, Clinical Advisory Board, Deloitte and Touche, LLP, Chicago, Illinois
Outcome Measurement: The Emerging Quality Barometer

**Carla P. Roberts, MD, PhD**
Clinical Fellow, Division of Reproductive Endocrinology and Infertility, Department of Gynecology and Obstetrics, Emory University School of Medicine, Atlanta, Georgia
Surgery of the Fallopian Tube; Endometriosis

**John A. Rock, MD**
James Robert McCord Professor and Chairman, Department of Gynecology and Obstetrics, Emory University School of Medicine, Atlanta, Georgia
Endometriosis

**Roberto Romero, MD**
Chief, Perinatology Research Branch, National Institute of Child Health and Human Development, The National Institutes of Health, Bethesda, Maryland
Premature Rupture of Fetal Membranes (PROM)

**Yuval Shahar, MD**
Associate Professor, Department of Medical Informatics, Stanford University Medical School, Stanford, California
A Review of Medical Informatics

**Baha M. Sibai, MD**
Professor and Chief, Division of Maternal–Fetal Medicine, Department of Obstetrics and Gynecology, University of Tennessee, Memphis College of Medicine, Memphis, Tennessee
Hypertensive Disorders in Pregnancy

**Lester Silberman, MD**
Associate Clinical Professor, Yale University School of Medicine, New Haven; Chairman, Department of Obstetrics and Gynecology, Danbury Hospital, Danbury, Connecticut
Clinical Integration and Quality Management

**Dean G. Smith, PhD**
Associate Professor, Department of Health Management and Policy, University of Michigan, Ann Arbor, Michigan
Business Principles in Obstetrics and Gynecology Financial Decision-Making

**Robert J. Sokol, MD**
Professor of Obstetrics and Gynecology, Dean, School of Medicine, Wayne State University School of Medicine, Detroit, Michigan
Illicit Substance Abuse During Pregnancy

**David E. Soper, MD**
Professor, Department of Obstetrics and Gynecology, Medical University of South Carolina, Charleston, South Carolina
Pelvic Inflammatory Disease

**Yoram Sorokin, MD**
Professor, Wayne State University School of Medicine; Director, Obstetrics and Maternal–Fetal Medicine Division, Hutzel Hospital, Detroit Medical Center, Detroit, Michigan
Obstetric Hemorrhage

**Leon Speroff, MD**
Professor of Obstetrics and Gynecology, Oregon Health Sciences University, Portland, Oregon
Dysfunctional Uterine Bleeding

**Thomas G. Stovall, MD**
Professor and Vice-Chair, University of Tennessee, Memphis College of Medicine; Clinical Chief of Women's Health Services, Executive Director, Center for Women's Health Improvement, Memphis, Tennessee
Ectopic Pregnancy

**Shannon Downing Striebich, MHA**
Clinical Operations Manager for Primary Care Services, Detroit Medical Center, Detroit, Michigan
Clinical Pathways

**Sam S. Thatcher, MD, PhD**
Director and Reproductive Endocrinologist, Center for Applied Reproductive Science, Johnson City, Tennessee
Hyperandrogenism

**Anthony J. Thomas, Jr., MD**
Head, Section of Male Infertility, Department of Urology, The Cleveland Clinic Foundation, Cleveland, Ohio
Andrology

**Mark W. Tomlinson, MD**
Assistant Professor, Department of Obstetrics and Gynecology, Wayne State University School of Medicine; Attending Physician, Division of Maternal–Fetal Medicine, Detroit, Michigan
Overview of Routine Prenatal Care

**Marjorie C. Treadwell, MD**
Associate Professor, Division of Maternal–Fetal Medicine, Department of Obstetrics and Gynecology, Wayne State University School of Medicine; Director, Obstetric Ultrasonography, Hutzel Hospital, Detroit, Michigan
First-Trimester Ultrasonography

**J. Peter VanDorsten, MD**
Professor and Vice Chairman, Department of Obstetrics and Gynecology, Medical University of South Carolina, Charleston, South Carolina
Second-Trimester Ultrasonography

**Ivana M. Vettraino, MD, FACOG**
Associate Professor and Chief, Department of Obstetrics and Gynecology, Providence Hospital, Southfield, Michigan
Drug Therapy in Pregnancy

**Edward E. Wallach, MD**
Professor, Department of Obstetrics and Gynecology, Johns Hopkins University School of Medicine, Baltimore, Maryland
Evaluation and Management of Infertility

**Richard E. Ward, MD, MBA**
Vice President and General Manager, Healthcare Organization Products, Oceania, Inc., Palo Alto California
Clinical Effectiveness: A New Set of Skills for Obstetrician-Gynecologists

**Louis Weinstein, MD**
Professor and Chair, Department of Obstetrics and Gynecology, Medical College of Ohio; Chief of Service, Obstetrics and Gynecology, Medical College Hospital; Attending Physician, Division of Maternal–Fetal Medicine, Grace–Sinai Hospital, Toledo, Ohio
Understanding Medical–Legal Issues in Obstetrics and Gynecology

**Robert A. Welch, MD**
Medical Director of Women's Services, Associate Professor of Obstetrics and Gynecology, Wayne State University School of Medicine, Detroit; Chairman, Department of Obstetrics and Gynecology, Providence Hospital, Southfield, Michigan
Drug Therapy in Pregnancy

**Judith K. Wolf, MD**
Assistant Professor, Department of Gynecologic Oncology, The University of Texas M.D. Anderson Cancer Center, Houston, Texas
Vulvar and Vaginal Cancers

**Mary Ann Zettelmaier, MSN, MS**
Clinical Nurse Specialist, Maternal–Newborn Services, University of Michigan Medical Center, Ann Arbor, Michigan
Postpartum Management

# PREFACE

*Practical Strategies in Obstetrics and Gynecology* was written to present a comprehensive yet concise overview of obstetrics and gynecology. As competition in the health-care markets escalates, physicians who manage their patients in the highest quality manner while reducing unnecessary resource consumption should prove to be in a superior competitive position. Although many of the basic concepts presented in this book have existed for many years, the practice of obstetrics and gynecology has dramatically changed from providing all possible diagnostic and treatment alternatives for the patient to a more thoughtful and efficient application of these principles with an eye to value. We are fortunate to have recruited top individuals to serve as contributors for each of the chapters in this book. Each chapter offers an evidence-based approach to the principles of obstetrics and gynecology. Thus, each chapter provides an efficient and cost-effective appraisal of the pathophysiology, diagnosis, and treatment of common obstetric and gynecologic disorders.

The editor appreciates the commitment to excellence provided by each of the contributors. I am indebted to all of the chapter contributors for taking time from their families, patients, research, teaching, and administrative tasks to contribute to this book. I am especially appreciative of the assistance, expertise, and guidance of the associate editors: Mitchell P. Dombrowski, MD; S. Gene McNeeley, Jr., MD; Kamran S. Moghissi, MD; and Adnan R. Munkarah, MD. The editorial support from W.B. Saunders was outstanding through all phases of this book. I would like to extend special thanks to William Schmitt, former editorial assistant Sunny Kim, Frank Polizzano, Susanna L. Leuci, and Mary Reinwald for their expertise in editing and publishing this book. Finally, I give my highest praise and thanks to my administrative assistant, Cydni Wills, for all her support, editorial comments, organizational skills, and valuable advice. This book could not have been produced with such quality in a timely fashion without the hard work and dedication of all those who contributed to this effort. Thanks to all of you.

Scott B. Ransom

## NOTICE

Obstetrics and Gynecology is an ever-changing field. Standard safety precautions must be followed, but as new research and clinical experience broaden our knowledge, changes in treatment and drug therapy become necessary or appropriate. The editors of this work have carefully checked the generic and trade drug names and verified drug dosages to ensure that the dosage information in this work is accurate and in accord with the standards accepted at the time of publication. Readers are advised, however, to check the product information currently provided by the manufacturer of each drug to be administered to be certain that changes have not been made in the recommended dose or in the contraindications for administration. This is of particular importance in regard to new or infrequently used drugs. It is the responsibility of the treating physician, relying on experience and knowledge of the patient, to determine dosages and the best treatment for the patient. The editors cannot be responsible for misuse or misapplication of the material in this work.

THE PUBLISHER

# CONTENTS

## GYNECOLOGY

**1** Contraception .......................... 3
KAMRAN S. MOGHISSI

**2** Women's Preventive Care ........... 15
S. GENE McNEELEY, JR. and
E. TRENT McNEELEY

**3** Early Pregnancy Loss ................ 20
DAVID C. KMAK and
S. GENE McNEELEY, JR.

**4** Ectopic Pregnancy .................... 27
THOMAS G. STOVALL

**5** Dysmenorrhea and Pelvic Pain ..... 40
GARY H. LIPSCOMB

**6** Leiomyoma ........................... 51
LARA J. BURROWS and
THOMAS E. ELKINS

**7** Lower Genital Tract Infection ....... 57
S. GENE McNEELEY, Jr.

**8** Pelvic Inflammatory Disease ........ 65
DAVID E. SOPER

**9** Pelvic Mass .......................... 75
LARA J. BURROWS and
THOMAS E. ELKINS

**10** Pediatric and Adolescent
Gynecology .......................... 82
DAVID MURAM

**11** Hysterectomy ...................... 107
ROBERT A. HAMMER and
MELVIN V. GERBIE

**12** Laparoscopy ....................... 122
STEVEN J. ORY

**13** Office Hysteroscopy and Suction
Curettage in the Evaluation of
Abnormal Uterine Bleeding ....... 129
MILTON GOLDRATH

**14** Genital Tract Prolapse ............. 134
DEE ELLEN FENNER

**15** Sexuality ........................... 141
SALLY A. KOPE

**16** Urinary Incontinence: Strategies
for Evaluation and Nonsurgical
Management ....................... 150
CAROL GRAHAM and
VERONICA T. MALLETT

**17** Diseases of the Breast ............. 170
CAROLYN JOHNSTON

**18** Prevention and Treatment of
Postoperative Infections ........... 187
DAVID L. HEMSELL

## OBSTETRICS

**19** Overview of Routine Prenatal
Care ................................. 199
MARK W. TOMLINSON

**20** Genetic Counseling, Screening,
and Diagnosis ..................... 213
MARK I. EVANS and
MARK PAUL JOHNSON

| | | | | | |
|---|---|---|---|---|---|
| 21 | Fetal Assessment .................... 224<br>ANTHONY W. OPIPARI and<br>TIMOTHY R. B. JOHNSON | | 35 | Diabetes in Pregnancy .............. 360<br>ODED LANGER | |
| 22 | First-Trimester Ultrasonography ... 234<br>MARJORIE C. TREADWELL | | 36 | Asthma in Pregnancy .............. 369<br>MITCHELL P. DOMBROWSKI | |
| 23 | Second-Trimester<br>Ultrasonography .................... 239<br>DONNA D. JOHNSON and<br>J. PETER VANDORSTEN | | 37 | Hypertensive Disorders<br>in Pregnancy ....................... 380<br>DOREL ABRAMOVICI<br>FARID MATTAR and<br>BAHA M. SIBAI | |
| 24 | Premature Rupture of Fetal<br>Membranes (PROM) ............... 249<br>NEIL ATHAYDE<br>ELI MAYMON<br>PERCY PACORA and<br>ROBERTO ROMERO | | 38 | Illicit Substance Abuse During<br>Pregnancy .......................... 390<br>VIRGINIA DELANEY-BLACK<br>CHANDICE Y. COVINGTON<br>SUDIPTA DHAR and<br>ROBERT J. SOKOL | |
| 25 | Normal and Abnormal Labor ..... 267<br>KENNETH J. LEVENO | | 39 | Infections in Pregnancy ............ 403<br>TRACY COWLES and<br>BERNARD GONIK | |
| 26 | Obstetric Anesthesia ............... 276<br>COLLEEN DARGIE and<br>H. M. MARSH | | 40 | Human Immunodeficiency Virus<br>Infection in Pregnancy ............ 413<br>THEODORE B. JONES | |
| 27 | Vaginal Delivery, Operative and<br>Breech ............................. 291<br>KAROLINE S. PUDER and<br>MITCHELL P. DOMBROWSKI | | 41 | Drug Therapy in Pregnancy ....... 424<br>IVANA M. VETTRAINO and<br>ROBERT A. WELCH | |
| 28 | Cesarean Section .................... 299<br>MARK B. LANDON | | | | |

## GYNECOLOGIC ONCOLOGY

| | | |
|---|---|---|
| 29 | Obstetric Hemorrhage .............. 311<br>YORAM SOROKIN | |
| 30 | Postpartum Management .......... 321<br>ROBERT H. HAYASHI and<br>MARY ANN ZETTELMAIER | |
| 42 | Premalignant Disorders of<br>the Lower Genital Tract .......... 439<br>MICHELE FOLLEN MITCHELL | |
| 31 | Fetal Growth Disorders:<br>Diagnosis and Management ...... 326<br>CHUKWUMA I. ONYEIJE and<br>MICHAEL Y. DIVON | |
| 43 | Vulvar and Vaginal Cancers ....... 449<br>JUDITH K. WOLF and<br>THOMAS W. BURKE | |
| 32 | Multifetal Pregnancy ............... 337<br>JASON O. GARDOSI | |
| 44 | Cervical Cancer .................... 458<br>ROBERT E. BRISTOW and<br>FREDRICK J. MONTZ | |
| 33 | Preterm Birth ....................... 344<br>DAVID F. COLOMBO and<br>JAY D. IAMS | |
| 45 | Uterine Cancers .................... 471<br>GUNTER DEPPE and<br>ADNAN R. MUNKARAH | |
| 34 | Post-Term Pregnancy .............. 353<br>DAVID E. KAUFFMAN and<br>STEVE CARITIS | |
| 46 | Epithelial Ovarian Carcinoma .... 479<br>ANNETTE BICHER | |

| 47 | Germ Cell and Stromal Ovarian Tumors ............................... 490
ROBERT T. MORRIS and
ADNAN R. MUNKARAH |
|---|---|
| 48 | Surgical Complications ............ 498
CHARLES LEVENBACK |
| 49 | Gestational Trophoblastic Disease ................................ 511
DONALD PETER GOLDSTEIN and
ROSS STUART BERKOWITZ |
| 50 | Cancer in Pregnancy ................ 519
WENDY R. BREWSTER and
PHILIP J. DiSAIA |

## REPRODUCTIVE ENDOCRINOLOGY AND INFERTILITY

| 51 | Spontaneous Abortion ............. 533
SANDRA A. CARSON |
|---|---|
| 52 | Treatment of Anovulation ......... 539
WILLIAM E. GIBBONS |
| 53 | Amenorrhea ........................ 551
RICHARD E. BLACKWELL and
LISA A. FARAH |
| 54 | Dysfunctional Uterine Bleeding ............................ 560
LEON SPEROFF |
| 55 | Hyperandrogenism ................ 570
SAM S. THATCHER and
MICHAEL P. DIAMOND |
| 56 | Thyroid Disorders .................. 581
NANDALAL BAGCHI |
| 57 | Menopause ......................... 593
SUSAN L. HENDRIX |
| 58 | Evaluation and Management of Infertility ........................... 609
JOHN Y. PHELPS
EDWARD E. WALLACH and
KAMRAN S. MOGHISSI |
| 59 | Andrology .......................... 629
PETER N. KOLETTIS and
ANTHONY J. THOMAS, JR. |

| 60 | Assisted Reproductive Technologies ....................... 641
CHARLA M. BLACKER |
|---|---|
| 61 | Unexplained Infertility ............. 657
KAMRAN S. MOGHISSI |
| 62 | Surgery of the Fallopian Tube ..... 673
CARLA P. ROBERTS and
ANA A. MURPHY |
| 63 | Premenstrual Syndrome ........... 684
KENNETH A. GINSBURG and
ROSELYN DINSAY |
| 64 | Endometriosis ...................... 695
CARLA P. ROBERTS and
JOHN A. ROCK |
| 65 | Postoperative Adhesion Formation in Gynecologic Surgery: Etiology and Treatment ..................... 709
RICHARD E. LEACH and
MICHAEL P. DIAMOND |

## BUSINESS PRINCIPLES IN OBSTETRICS AND GYNECOLOGY

| 66 | The Economics of Obstetrics and Gynecology .................... 719
GAIL A. JENSEN and
ALLEN C. GOODMAN |
|---|---|
| 67 | Managed Care ..................... 734
KENNETH CHANG and
DAVID NASH |
| 68 | Clinical Epidemiology ............. 744
ANNETTE CASOGLOS
KULMEET S. DANG
JODY L. MEINKE and
R. MICHAEL MASSANARI |
| 69 | Clinical Integration and Quality Management ...................... 760
LESTER SILBERMAN |

| | | | |
|---|---|---|---|
| 70 | Clinical Effectiveness: A New Set of Skills for Obstetrician–Gynecologists ....... 773<br>RICHARD E. WARD and<br>JENNIFER ELSTON LAFATA | 75 | Current Procedural Terminology (CPT) and International Classification of Diseases, Ninth Revision, Clinical Modification (ICD-9-CM) Coding in Obstetrics and Gynecology ........................ 826<br>PHILIP N. ESKEW, JR. |
| 71 | Understanding Medical–Legal Issues in Obstetrics and Gynecology ...................... 785<br>LOUIS WEINSTEIN | 76 | A Review of Medical Informatics .......................... 834<br>ANEEL ADVANI and<br>YUVAL SHAHAR |
| 72 | Clinical Pathways .................. 793<br>SHANNON DOWNING STRIEBICH and<br>SCOTT B. RANSOM | 77 | Outcome Measurement: The Emerging Quality Barometer .......................... 845<br>EMAD RIZK and<br>SCOTT B. RANSOM |
| 73 | Insurance Contracting for Obstetric-Gynecologic Services ............................ 809<br>VICTORIA A. GREGONIS | | Index .......................................... 861 |
| 74 | Business Principles in Obstetrics and Gynecology Financial Decision-Making .................. 816<br>DEAN G. SMITH | | |

# GYNECOLOGY

# 1

# Contraception

KAMRAN S. MOGHISSI

The desire for family planning dates back to antiquity. In early times, a combination of disease and a high mortality rate among the newborn, augmented by abortion, infanticide, and frequent wars, usually controlled population size. Within individual families, various measures to prevent conception, such as prolonged lactation, delayed marriage, coitus interruptus, or various substitutes for natural sexual intercourse, were developed. In addition, primitive societies often relied on the rites of medicine men or diets, potions, or crude devices to prevent conception.

In today's society, despite the availability of effective and safe methods of contraception, a high proportion of pregnancies are unplanned and frequently unwanted. In the United States, it is estimated that 56% of 6.4 million pregnancies each year are unplanned. Available data indicate that of the 39 million women in the United States who are at risk for unintended pregnancy, 90% use some form of contraception. The 10% of women who do not use contraception account for 53% of unintended pregnancies, half of which end in abortion. Younger women and teenagers are particularly at risk.

The degree of fertility varies with age. For some months or years after menarche, there is a relative degree of infertility. The fertility rate is highest between the ages of 20 and 30 and declines after the age of 35. In the first few weeks postpartum, pregnancy is unlikely. Similarly, the lactation period is associated with infertility. However, neither age-related infertility or lactation provides sufficient protection against unwanted pregnancies.

An ideal contraceptive has been defined as one that is safe, highly effective, inexpensive, unrelated to coitus, and requiring no motivation. Such a contraceptive is not yet available and probably will not be forthcoming in the foreseeable future. However, there is now available an array of contraceptive preparations and devices to suit the needs of almost any population group.

## Oral Contraceptives

The first generation of oral contraceptives (OCs) contained large amounts of estrogen and progestogens and was associated with a number of undesirable side effects. Currently available OCs contain lower doses of estrogen in the range of 20 to 35 mg of ethinyl estradiol and a reduced amount of progestins. Despite their lower doses, newer OCs approach 100% efficacy in preventing pregnancy. However, this estimate may be substantially diminished by failures in compliance.

### FORMULATION

Monophasic OCs deliver the same dose of estrogen and progestin throughout the cycle, whereas multiphasic OCs provide two or three different hormone doses throughout each cycle. The estrogen component in the majority of formulations available in the United States is ethinyl estradiol (EE), a synthetic estrogen. Mestranol is used in a few others. Progestogen components consist of seven different types of steroids, including norethindrone, ethynodiol diacetate, norgestrel, and three new progestin preparations: norgestimate, desogestrel, and gestodene. All these progestins are 19 norsteroids derived from testosterone.

Combination OCs are usually taken for 21 of every 28 days. In a 28-day regimen, the pills taken in the last 7 days are a placebo.

Progestin-only agents, known as minipills, contain only a low-dose progestin that is administered continuously.

## MECHANISM OF ACTION

For all OCs, the primary mechanism of action is the inhibition of ovulation. This is achieved by a synergistic action of estrogens and progestins on the hypothalamic-pituitary centers to eliminate luteinizing hormone (LH) surge and suppress the secretion of gonadotropins. In addition to ovulation suppression, contraceptive compounds affect several other target sites. These include the cervix, the endometrium, and the oviduct. All synthetic oral or parenteral progestogens, alone or in combination with estrogen, diminish mucorrhea, alter many physical and chemical properties of cervical secretion, and inhibit sperm migration through the cervical mucus to varying degrees.

OCs also affect endometrial morphology. Under the influence of combined preparations, there is rapid progression of the endometrium from the proliferative phase to early secretory changes. By midcycle, varying degrees of mixed hormonal effects are observed. Thereafter, the endometrium shows regressive change and appears to be thin, inactive, and unsuitable for implantation. Inhibition of sperm migration through the cervical mucus and endometrial changes provide additional efficacy for OC action should a breakthrough ovulation occur.

With continuous low-dose progestin therapy, most women exhibit suppression of midcycle LH and follicle-stimulating hormone (FSH). However, corpora lutea, presumably indicating ovulation, have been visualized in 85% of women who are treated with continuous daily minipills. Inhibition of sperm transport through the cervical mucus and endometrial changes appear to be primarily responsible for the contraceptive action of these agents.

# Risks and Benefits of Oral Contraceptives

## RISKS AND ADVERSE EFFECTS

Modern OCs are highly effective and safe. They are devoid of many side effects and complications associated with high-dose OCs of earlier years.

The most common adverse effects of OCs occur during the first few months of use and may include nausea, weight changes, headache, spotting, and breakthrough bleeding.

**Nausea.** This is caused by the estrogenic component of the OC and is dose related. It is a self-limited effect and usually disappears after the first 3 months. Selection of a pill with reduced estrogen content usually alleviates nausea and other gastrointestinal problems.

**Breakthrough Spotting and Bleeding.** These side effects are likely to occur within the first 3 to 6 months of use and are related to the dosage and type of progestogen. An important cause of breakthrough spotting and bleeding is missing a scheduled dose of the pill.

Taking the pill faithfully at approximately the same time each day is the best way of managing spotting and bleeding. Occasionally, it is advisable to change to another formulation to obviate these side effects.

**Weight Gain.** Several surveys have suggested that weight gain may be an important contributor to patient noncompliance. Managing diet appropriately and using pills containing newer progestins are tactics recommended to prevent excessive weight gain.

**Headache.** This is experienced by some women, but usually subsides within the first few months of OC use. Persistent headache may be an indication to switch to another OC preparation with a lower estrogenic or progestogenic content, or both. Severe headache or a history of migraine are considered to be a relative contraindication to OC use.

**Cardiovascular Diseases.** These diseases constitute the most important risks of combined OCs. They include thromboembolic diseases, myocardial infarction, thrombotic and hemorrhagic stroke, and hypertension. These risks assume greater magnitude among smokers and in women who are taking pills containing high doses of estrogen.

Older epidemiologic studies indicated a dose-related effect of estrogen on the increased incidence of venous thrombosis in current OC users, an increased risk of myocardial infarction in women over age 35, and an association between the use of higher dose oral contraceptives and neurovascular accidents in otherwise healthy young women. According to these retrospective studies, OC use increased the risk of thrombotic stroke three fold and that of hemorrhagic stroke two fold. Subsequent studies have demonstrated that increased risk of cardiovascular disease in OC users, particularly older women, is related to smoking and the dosage of estrogen. Women who have inherited plasma protein abnormalities of protein C or S, or antithrombin deficiencies and factor V Linden mutation (thrombophilia), may be at increased risk of thromboembolic disorder when exposed to OCs. Protein C is a vitamin K dependent anticoagulant, and its deficiency is an inherited autosomal dominant trait. Protein S is a vitamin K dependent cofactor of activated protein C (APC). Factor V Linden mutation is an autosomal dominant disorder characterized by a gene mutation of clotting Factor V (proaccelerin). Antithrombin III deficiency is inherited as an autosomal dominant trait. With the advent of low-dose, estrogen-containing OCs (20 to 35 mg ethinyl estradiol), the increased risk of thrombophilia in OC users is believed to be eliminated or negligible. Several recent epidemiologic studies have shown a twofold increase in the risk of deep venous thrombosis with the use of OCs containing desogestrel or gestodene. Careful analysis of these data, however, identified a number of biases. The general consensus is that OCs, when used as indicated, including those containing desogestrel, are still safe and highly effective method for preventing pregnancy.

A small percentage of patients who have borderline or established hypertension may show an idiosyncratic rise in blood pressure with use of OCs. High blood pressure should be controlled before prescribing OCs. If hypertension is uncontrolled, OCs should be avoided.

## CANCER RISKS

OC use protects against endometrial and ovarian cancers. However, there appears to be an increased risk of cervical dysplasia and carcinoma in situ in women receiving OCs. Invasive cervical cancer may be increased minimally after 5 years of use. Because of this concern, OC users should have at least a yearly pelvic examination and a Papanicolaou (Pap) smear.

The relationship between breast cancer and oral contraceptive use is more controversial. The results of a large number of epidemiologic studies indicate that in the middle of reproductive life (ages 25 to 39) the combination OCs have no effect on breast cancer risk. However, a few studies suggest that a subgroup of young women who use OCs early and for a long time (longer than 4 years) have a slightly increased risk of breast cancer before the age of 45. The risk of breast cancer in OC users does not appear to be related to the dose of estrogen in the OC formulation or the duration of use. Furthermore, it appears that among women who develop breast cancer, the survival rate is greater in OC users than it is in nonusers. Women who have benign breast disease do not have an increased risk of breast cancer if they use OCs.

## PREGNANCY AND LACTATION

The use of OCs during pregnancy is contraindicated. However, there is no evidence that OCs increase the risk of congenital anomalies if taken inadvertently during pregnancy. Combination OCs have been shown to diminish the quantity and alter the quality of milk in postpartum women. Therefore, they should not be used postparatum by lactating women. Progestogen-only contraception, administered orally (minipills) or parenterally (depot medroxyprogesterone acetate), does not interfere with lactation.

## OTHER RISKS AND CLINICAL EFFECTS

**Lipid, Lipoprotein, and Carbohydrate Effects.** OCs that were developed in the past contained relatively high doses of progestins with high androgenic activity. Their use was associated with a decrease in high-density lipoprotein (HDL) and an increase in low-density lipoprotein (LDL). In contrast, OCs containing lower doses of these compounds, as well as formulations with norgestimate or desogestrel, have the opposite effect, raising HDL and lowering LDL levels. All combinations OCs, including the newer low-dose preparations, increase the triglyceride level. A very high triglyceride level is a contraindication for combination OCs, but minipills are appropriate.

Similarly, the high doses of progestins in older OCs often had an adverse effect on testing of glucose tolerance. However, none of the current low-dose formulations appear to have a clinically significant effect on glucose tolerance.

## BENEFITS OF OCs

Health benefits of OCs have been well documented. The most important of these benefits is the high degree of efficacy in preventing pregnancy and the morbidity and mortality sometimes associated with pregnancy. Other noncontraceptive health benefits of OCs are shown in Table 1–1. Additionally, it is known that prolonged use of OCs is also effective in arresting the progression of endometriosis and preventing other disease processes. These include the

**Table 1–1**  Noncontraceptive Benefits of Oral Contraceptives

| Pregnancy Mortality | Reduction in Risk (%) |
|---|---|
| Ectopic pregnancy | 90 |
| Cancer | — |
|    Ovary | 40 |
|    Endometrium | 40 |
| Benign breast disease | 40 |
| Functional ovarian cysts | |
|    Luteal | 78 |
|    Follicular | 49 |
| Fibroids | 17 |
|    (5 yr combined oral contraceptives) | |
| Pelvic inflammatory disease | 50 |
| Menorrhagia | 50 |
| Iron deficiency anemia | 50 |
| Dysmenorrhea | 40 |

From Drife JO: The Benefits and Risks of Oral Contraceptives. New York, Parthenon Publishing Group, 1993, pp 1–31.

onset of rheumatoid arthritis, acne, hirsutism, and loss of bone mineral density. Continuous administration of OCs has been used for many years for medical therapy of endometriosis. Considering the risk-benefit ratio of OCs, it is clear that the benefits far outweigh the potential risk. In addition to reducing the risk of endometrial and ovarian malignancies, taking OCs can prevent many benign gynecologic disorders. Appropriate counseling of women regarding these issues goes a long way toward alleviating the fear of women who have been influenced by inappropriate advice and adverse publicity.

## Contraindications to OCs

Absolute contraindications to OCs are listed in Table 1–2. Table 1–3 shows relative contraindications for the use of these agents. Thus, clinical judgment and expertise are required when the use of OCs is considered in patients who have a history of gestational diabetes, leiomyoma of the uterus, elective uterine surgery, and sickle cell disease. Appropriate counseling and, possibly, a consent form may serve to avoid

**Table 1–2**  Absolute Contraindications to the Use of Oral Contraceptives

1. Thrombophlebitis and thromboembolic disorders or a past history of these conditions
2. Known or suspected breast cancer
3. Undiagnosed abnormal vaginal bleeding
4. Known or suspected pregnancy
5. Suspected estrogen-dependent neoplasia
6. Marked impairment of liver function
7. Smoker older than 35 yr of age

**Table 1–3**  Relative Contraindications to the Use of Oral Contraceptives

1. Migraine headache
2. Hypertension
3. Epilepsy
4. Gallbladder disease

future misunderstanding when the use of OCs is considered in patients with these disorders.

## Patient Selection and Evaluation

OCs may be offered to all premenopausal sexually active women who have no contraindication for their use. They are particularly indicated for use by adolescents, who have a high rate of unintended pregnancies. Nonsmoking women older than 35 years may also safely use these preparations. Women of all ages who smoke should be urged to stop. Cigarette smoking after the age of 35 is a contraindication to OC use, because smoking and OC use combined are associated with a high risk of myocardial infarction.

Other important indications for OC use include menstrual regulation and treatment of polycystic ovarian disease, hirsutism, acne, and dysmenorrhea.

Evaluation of the patient should include a history, a physical examination (including pelvic examination), cervical cytology, and screening for sexually transmitted diseases, as indicated. The history should ascertain any potential contraindication to use of OCs (see Tables 1–2 and 1–3).

All women who use OCs should be strongly advised not to smoke. A family history of breast cancer is not a contraindication to OC use. OCs may be used in women who have diabetes as long as they are free of retinopathy, nephropathy, hypertension, or other vascular complications.

## Selection of Appropriate OCs

A wide variety of OC formulations (Table 1–4) is available today, which permit the clinician to tailor therapy. In selecting the most suitable preparation, the physician should take into consideration the needs and characteristics of the individual patient as well as relying on his or her expertise.

OCs containing less than 50 μg-estrogen do not significantly increase the risk of myocardial infarction or stroke in normotensive nonsmoking women.

For the first time user, acceptance of OC therapy

Table 1–4 Composition of Combination Oral Contraceptives

| Type | Name | Estrogen | μg | Progestin | mg |
|---|---|---|---|---|---|
| **LOW ANDROGENIC ACTIVITY OF PROGESTIN COMPONENT** ||||||
| Monophasic | Modicon<br>Brevicon<br>Nelova 0.5/35 | EE | 35 | Norethindrone | 0.5 |
|  | Ovcon 35 | EE | 35 | Norethindrone | 0.4 |
|  | Ortho-Cyclen | EE | 35 | Norgestimate | 0.25 |
|  | Ortho-Cept<br>Desogen | EE | 30 | Desogestrel | 0.15 |
| Triphasic | Ortho Tri-Cyclen | EE | 35/35/35 | Norgestimate | 0.18/0.25/0.25 |
| **MEDIUM ANDROGENIC ACTIVITY OF PROGESTIN COMPONENT** ||||||
| Monophasic | Norlestrin 1/50 | EE | 50 | Norethindrone acetate | 1.0 |
|  | Ovcon 50<br>Genora 1/50<br>Norethin 1/50M | EE | 50 | Norethindrone | 1.0 |
|  | Ortho-Novum 1/50<br>Norinyl 1+50 | mestranol | 50 | Norethindrone | 1.0 |
|  | Demulen 1/50 | EE | 50 | Ethynodiol diacetate | 1.0 |
|  | Demulen 1/35 | EE | 35 | Ethynodiol diacetate | 1.0 |
|  | Ortho-Novum 1/35<br>Norinyl 1+35<br>Genora 1/35<br>Norethin 1/35E<br>Norcept-E 1/35<br>Nelova 1/35E<br>N.E.E. 1/35 | EE | 35 | Norethindrone | 1.0 |
|  | Loestrin 1/20 | EE | 20 | Norethindrone acetate | 1.0 |
| Biphasic | Ortho-Novum 10/11<br>N.E.E. 10/11<br>Jenest-28 | EE | 35/35 | Norethindrone | 0.5/1.0 |
| Triphasic | Ortho-Novum 7/7/7 | EE | 35/35/35 | Norethindrone | 0.5/0.75/1.0 |
|  | Tri-Norinyl | EE | 35/35/35 | Norethindrone | 0.5/1.0/0.5 |
|  | Triphasil<br>Tre-Levlen | EE | 30/40/30 | Levonorgestrel | 0.05/0.075/0.125 |
| **HIGH ANDROGENIC ACTIVITY OF PROGESTIN COMPONENT** ||||||
| Monophasic | Ovral | EE | 50 | Norgestrel | 0.5 |
|  | Norlestrin 2.5/50 | EE | 50 | Norethindrone acetate | 2.5 |
|  | Loestrin 1.5/30 | EE | 30 | Norethindrone acetate | 1.5 |
|  | Lo-Ovral | EE | 30 | Norgestrel | 0.3 |
|  | Nordette | EE | 30 | Levonorgestrel | 0.15 |
|  | Levlen | EE | 30 | Levonorgestrel | 0.15 |

EE = ethinyl estradiol.

is of utmost importance in ensuring compliance and continuation. It is, the therefore, recommended that a preparation containing 30 to 35 μg of estrogen be prescribed to minimize side effects. Common troublesome problems, such as gastrointestinal symptoms, breakthrough bleeding, spotting, and breast tenderness, should be discussed with the patient, and appropriate steps should be taken to address these side effects. An OC formulation with more than 35 μg of estrogen should be reserved for patients who have specific conditions, that require hepatic enzyme-inducing drugs (e.g., phenytoin, carbamazepine, rifampin). Use of 20 μg estrogen OCs or the progestin-only pill may be preferable for women who have persistant estrogen-related side effects, such as nausea and breast tenderness.

## PROGESTIN-ONLY CONTRACEPTIVES (MINIPILLS)

Several progestational steroids, when ingested continuously in small doses, exert a potent antifertility effect and are free of certain systemic and metabolic side effects characteristic of the estrogen-containing OCs. From the mid-1960s to the early 1970s, several progestin-only contraceptive pills were developed, but only two of these have actually been marketed and available date in the United States. Table 1–5 lists the so-called minipills, which are available worldwide. Minipill contraceptive pills exert their antifertility action in several ways:

1. An alteration of physical and chemical proper-

**Table 1–5** Progestin Only (Minipills)

| Progestin | Dose (μg) | Trade Name |
|---|---|---|
| Norethindrone | 350 | Micronol,* NOR-QD,* Norad |
| Norgestrel | 75 | Ovrette,* Norgest |
| Levonorgestrel | 35 | Microval, Norgeston, Microlut |
| Lynestrenol | 500 | Exluton |
| Ethynodiol diacetate | 500 | Femulen |

*Available in the United States.

ties of cervical mucus takes place along with the inhibition of sperm transport.
2. Subtle disturbances of hypothalamic pituitary function that are characterized by suppression or modification of the midcycle FSH and LH.
3. There is inhibition of ovulation in some cases and changes in the function of the morphologically normal corpus luteum.
4. Endometrial changes prevent implantation.

Minipills are taken daily and continuously, beginning on the first day of the menstrual cycle. Their failure rate ranges from 1.1 to 9.6 per 100 women in the first year of use. The average failure rate is about 3.1 per 100 women per year in younger women and 0.3 per 100 women per year in women over 40 years of age.

The major side effect of minipills is irregularity of menstrual bleeding, which is the result of the unpredictable effect of these preparations on ovulation and possibly endometrial development. Approximately 40% of women receiving minipills have normal ovulatory cycles, 40% have short, irregular cycles, and 20% have the acyclic pattern of anovulatory cycles. This is the major reason for discontinuation of these contraceptives despite their safety record.

Women who take minipills have a likelihood of developing functional follicular cysts of the ovary. However, these cysts resolve spontaneously. Progestin-only contraceptive pills are particularly useful for postpartum use, because they do not interfere with lactation.

## Injectables and Implants

Injectables and implants provide effective and continuous contraception for prolonged periods, extending from several months to several years.

Depot medroxyprogesterone acetate (DMPA) is the only injectable method of contraception available in the United States. DMPA, a 17-acetoxyprogesterone, is similar in structure to naturally occurring progesterone. It is administered by deep gluteal or deltoid intramuscular injection in a dose of 150 mg every three months. To ensure slow release of the drug, it is recommended that the injection site not be massaged. DMPA should be administered within 5 days of the onset of menses to ensure that the patient is not pregnant and that ovulation is inhibited to provide immediate contraception. DMPA acts primarily by inhibiting ovulation. There is also some effect on the endometrium and minor changes on the cervical mucus. During DMPA use, the ovary continues to secrete estradiol in amounts similar to those produced in the early follicular phase of a normal cycle. Clinically, therefore, signs and symptoms of estrogen deficiency do not develop in women using DMPA. The safety and efficacy of DPMA have been established by its use in over 90 countries by at least 30 million women. Most women using DMPA become amenorrheic. Breakthrough and unpredictable bleeding may occur during the first few months of use. However, irregular bleeding is usually not heavy and will eventually cease with continuous use. DMPA may be used safely during the postpartum period, because it does not interfere with lactation. The return of fertility is delayed in women using DMPA. However, approximately 70% of otherwise fertile women are expected to conceive within the first 12 months following discontinuation of the injections and the remaining group within 24 months. Early concerns about the potential for increased risk of breast cancer with use of DMPA have been largely refuted. The multicenter World Health Organization (WHO) collaborative study showed no significant increase in the overall relative risk of breast cancer in ever users of DMPA. In women under age 35, short-term exposure to DMPA was associated with a slight increase in relative risk (1.4) of the same magnitude as that for OCs. Use of DMPA is not associated with clinically significant changes in coagulation parameters. Minimal changes in serum lipids and lipoproteins have been observed in some studies. As with all progestins, evidence of impaired glucose tolerance is sometimes seen in users of DMPA. Thus, women who have a history of diabetes should be carefully monitored while using any hormonal contraceptive. On the positive side, a WHO study found that the use of DMPA was associated with a major (80%) reduction in the risk of endometrial cancer, with no significant impact on the risk of epithelial ovarian cancer or squamous cervical cancer.

### NORPLANT

Development of long-acting contraceptive implants that release progestogens has been in progress for many years. However, only two implants, both releasing levonorgestrel, have been released for general clinical use. Norplant System is the only contraceptive implant available in the United States. It consists of a set of six capsules, each 3.4 mm in length and 2.4 mm in diameter. The set contains a total of 216 mg of crystallized levonorgestrel. One third of the drug load is released in 5 years, the currently approved lifetime of the implant. Silicone rubber provides the encapsulating rate-metering membrane through which levonorgestrel diffuses into the body.

Norplant implants are inserted sequentially beneath the dermal layer of the arm through a 2- to 3 mm incision after a local anesthetic has been applied. A No. 10-gauge (G) trocar deposits the capsules in a superficial plane 5 to 6 mm above the incision. The recommended site of placement is in the inner aspect of the upper arm, contralateral to the handedness of the woman and well above the elbow.

Levonorgestrel is detectable in blood within 2 hours of placement. Maximum drug concentration of 1000 to 2000 pg/ml are found between 8 and 24 hours. Drug release and concentrations in the blood are maximal in the first month of use, when a set of six capsules releases approximately 85 mg/day of levonorgestrel. Release is 25 to 30 mg/day at 60 months.

Norplant System is a highly effective contraceptive with a failure rate below those of OCs. In large population studies, the pregnancy rate was .02 pregnancies per 100 women years of use.

Norplant exerts its contraceptive action in several ways. Ovulation is inhibited in many cycles. If ovulation occurs, the low level of progesterone renders the woman infertile. Marked alterations of cervical mucus make it impenetrable to spermatozoa. There is also a change in endometrial morphology.

Use of Norplant System is associated with marked changes in menstrual bleeding patterns. Most women, particularly those of low weight, tend to experience oligomenorrhea or amenorrhea, whereas women who weigh 60 kg or more are likely to experience irregular bleeding. Many of these episodes of bleeding, spotting, or both, occur during the first year of use, when 70 to 80% of women may experience disruption of their normal menstrual pattern. By the fifth year of use, approximately 62% of users have regular cycles, whereas 38% continue to have irregular cycles. Irregular bleeding and spotting is, in fact, the major reason for discontinuation of this form of contraception.

Candid comprehensive counseling about all aspects of Norplant implants before insertion, and appropriate support and reassurance during use, are essential and go a long way to encourage acceptance of this form of contraception. In the event of prolonged bleeding, a short course of EE (20 to 50 mg qd for 10 to 20 days) or ibuprofen (400 to 800 mg tid for 5 days) may be used. Menstrual blood loss is eventually decreased with continuous use of the implants and most women experience a modest increase in hemoglobin.

Other side effects include headache, acne or other skin problems, and changes of weight and mood. Despite these minor side effects, Norplant is highly acceptable for prolonged contraceptive use and as an alternative to sterilization for those women who wish to maintain their reproductive function.

## POSTCOITAL (EMERGENCY) CONTRACEPTION

These contraceptive methods are recommended when unprotected coitus has occurred that may result in an unwanted pregnancy. They should be considered and offered in all cases of rape.

In the past, the regimen included the use of large doses of estrogen, such as conjugated estrogen 15 mg bid for 5 days, or 50 mg administered intravenously on each of 2 consecutive days. Alternatively, EE 2.5 mg bid may be used for 5 days. More recently, the administration of a combination oral contraceptive (Ovral, 2 tablets initially and 2 tablets 12 hours later) has been found to be better tolerated and equally effective. The mechanism of action is believed to be caused by rapid endometrial changes that prevent implantation. The failure rate is reported to be approximately 1% with high doses of estrogen and 2% with combination OCs. For best results, these formulation should be given as soon as possible, and no later than, 72 hours after coitus. Because of the potential harmful effect of these agents, the presence of an existing pregnancy should be excluded by a sensitive assay. Furthermore, the patient should be offered therapeutic abortion if the method fails. The use of high-dose estrogen is frequently associated with nausea and sometimes with vomiting. Combination OCs are less likely to cause these side effects.

Another method of postcoital contraception is the insertion of a copper intrauterine device (IUD) (TCu-380) up to 5 days following unprotected intercourse. The reported failure rate is very low (0.1%). This method clearly interferes with implantation, and it is not recommended for nulliparous women or those at risk for pelvic infection.

## IUDs

Modern IUDs were introduced in the early 1960s. These devices were made of plastic (polyethylene) impregnated with barium sulfate for ready identification by radiograph. They performed well and were devoid of major complications. Another IUD, the Dalkon Shield, was introduced in 1970. Because of its defective construction and a multifilamented tail that allowed a pathway for bacteria to ascend into the uterine cavity, the use of this device was found to be associated with a high rate of pelvic infection. The Dalkon Shield was finally removed from use, in 1980. The incidence of pelvic infection resulting from use of the Dalkon Shield brought about a general decline in the use of all IUDs, even those that were believed to be perfectly safe.

A major innovation in IUD technology was the discovery that copper is spermicidal and acts on the endometrium in such a way as to create a hostile environment for sperm survival.

## Types of IUDs

The Lippes loop and other plastic IUDs are still used throughout the world, but they are no longer available in the United States. The only two types of IUDs available in the United States are the copper IUD and the progesterone-releasing IUD.

An early type of copper IUD, the Copper 7, was extensively used throughout the world, but sales were discontinued in 1986 in the United States because of the increasing cost of litigation.

Modern IUDs have more copper, which increases their efficiency and life span. Currently, only one copper IUD, the TCu-380A (Paragard), is available in the United States. This device has a T-shaped configuration and is made of polyethylene for holding 380 mm$^3$ of an exposed surface area of copper. The pure electrolytic copper wire wound around the stem weighs 176 mg, and copper sleeves on the horizontal arms weigh 66.5 mg. A polyethylene monofilament is tied through the ball of the stem, providing two white threads for detection and removal.

The contraceptive effect of copper IUDs, as with all IUDs, is caused by their action on the uterine cavity, creating a sterile inflammatory environment that is spermicidal. Ovulation is not affected, but there may be a cytotoxic effect on the ova. Additionally, copper IUDs release free copper and copper salts. These have biochemical and morphologic effects on the endometrium; in addition, they are spermicidal.

The progestogen released from the progestin-releasing IUDs also acts directly on the endometrium and brings about decidual and atrophic changes of the glands. Thus, these IUDs have an adverse effect on sperm survival and capacitation, and they inhibit implantation as well as sperm migration through the cervical mucus.

## Contraceptive Efficacy

In the United States, the TCu-380A is approved for use for 10 years. The Progestasert (progesterone-releasing IUD) must be replaced every year.

In large clinical studies, the cumulative pregnancy rates associated with the TCu-380A IUD have been reported to be between 0.5 and 1.6%. Cumulative ectopic pregnancy rates were 0.1%. IUDs do not increase the risk of ectopic pregnancy and may offer some protection from it.

In selecting an appropriate IUD, the needs of the individual patient must be considered. IUDs are appropriate for parous women who are at low risk of sexually transmitted diseases (STDs), who have no history of pelvic inflammatory disease (PID), and who are in a stable, mutually monogamous relationship.

IUDs are contraindicated in women who have small uterine size or shape incompatible with IUD use and in those who have medical conditions, such as valvular heart disease or suppression of the immune system that increases the risk of infection, known or suspected pregnancy, known or suspected PID, undiagnosed vaginal bleeding, or high risk for STDs. Additionally, copper IUDs should not be used in patients who have Wilson's disease.

Contrary to previously published data, the use of modern IUDs by women who have only one sexual partner has little appreciable effect on increasing risk of PID.

IUDs can be safely inserted during the menstrual cycle and after delivery or abortion. To reduce the rate of expulsion, it is suggested that copper IUDs not be inserted until 4 to 8 weeks after delivery. Insertion is somewhat easier during menstruation; thus many physicians prefer to insert the IUD at this time. In every case, the insertion technique recommended by the manufacturer should be followed.

Side effects and complications of IUDs include increased cramping and menstrual flow, pelvic infection, uterine perforation, and displacement and expulsion of the IUD.

Cramping and menorrhagia usually subside with use of nonsteroidal anti-inflammatory drugs. If perforation or displacement is suspected, a sonogram of the pelvis should be performed to diagnose the proper location of the IUD. Mild pelvic infection in IUD wearers may be treated with appropriate antibiotic therapy. However, persistent or severe infection should be vigorously treated and the IUD removed.

To remove the IUD, the cervix is exposed by a vaginal speculum and the string of the IUD is grasped with a dressing ring forceps. The string is then pulled with a firm traction until the device is extracted.

# Barrier Contraceptives

Barrier contraceptives are among the oldest and most widely used methods of birth control. Throughout history, a variety of barrier techniques have been devised for preventing deposition of semen in the vagina and interfering with survival of spermatozoa in the vagina or inhibiting their migration to the female upper reproductive tract. There has been a resurgence of interest in barrier contraceptives because of their ability to prevent STDs. Modern barrier methods and their efficacy relative to fertility control are listed in Table 1–6. Barrier contraceptives are very safe and have the great advantage of protecting against STDs and PIDs, including gonorrhea, chlamydia, herpes simplex, cytomegalovirus, human papillomavirus, and human immunodeficiency virus (HIV). Other benefits consist of lack of any effect on the menstrual cycle or on systemic and metabolic processes. The disadvantages of these techniques include a higher pregnancy rate relative to hormonal contraceptives and IUDs, involvement with coitus, and the motivation required to use them consistently and correctly. There is also an increased risk of toxic shock syndrome and an occasional allergic reaction to the spermicidal chemicals or rubber.

## VAGINAL DIAPHRAGM

The vaginal diaphragm is one of the earliest contraceptives used by women in the United States and throughout developed countries of the world. The efficacy of the diaphragm depends upon the key factors of correct selection of the correct type and size for the individual women and proper use of the device (Table 1–6).

The diaphragm is a shallow rubber cup with a metal rim. The device is inserted into the upper part of the vagina so that it covers the cervix. The rim must fit snugly behind the symphysis pubis and the posterior cul-de-sac behind the cervix. The diaphragms acts as a mechanical barrier that provides a receptacle for spermicidal agents. Diaphragms range in size from 50 to 105 mm in diameter, with a 2.5- to 5-mm gradation. The three types of diaphragms currently available are the coil spring, the flat spring, and arcing spring. Each design is appropriate for use in a specific case.

The coil spring diaphragm is commonly used when the vagina is of normal size and shape, with a deep arch behind the symphysis pubis and no uterine displacement. The flat spring diaphragm is preferred when there is a shallow arch behind the symphysis pubis and an anteflexed uterus. The arcing spring type diaphragm is selected for women who have poor vaginal muscle tone; moderate prolapse, anteflexion, or both, or retroversion of the uterus. The diaphragm must be fitted, and the correct size is selected by the use of fitting rings. The diaphragm should be covered with spermicidal preparation before use and left in the vagina for at least 8 hours after intercourse. If repeated coital activities are attempted, additional spermicidal creams should be inserted without removing the diaphragm before each intercourse. The patient must also be taught how to insert the diaphragm correctly and maintain it in place. Most diaphragm failures occur as a result of incorrect insertion or nonuse. Diaphragms should be changed at least yearly. After each pregnancy, the patient should be refitted for her diaphragm when postpartum changes have subsided.

## FEMALE CONDOM

The female condom is a thin, soft, loose-fitting pouch made of polyurethane plastic with two flexible rings at either end. One ring helps to hold the device in place inside the vagina over the cervix, whereas the other ring rests outside the vagina. The female condom covers the inside of the vagina, cervix, and perineum and may be construed as a combination of diaphragm and condom. The device acts as a barrier for preventing pregnancy and STDs. The failure rate of the female condom, according to data provided to the Food and Drug Administration (FDA), is 25% after 6 months of clinical trials, with a pregnancy rate of 12.4% with average use. When data were reanalyzed, it was estimated that with perfect use the estimated failure rate was only 5.1%. Protection against STD also depends on correct and consistent use. With perfect use, it is estimated that the device can afford 94% protection against HIV.

## CERVICAL CAP

The cervical cap was used extensively in Europe before it was reintroduced in the United States. A reason for its lack of popularity is difficulty of insertion and removal.

The cervical cap is similar to a diaphragm in structure, but it is made of much more rigid plastic and

Table 1–6  Barrier Contraceptives

| Method | Effectiveness (%) | Use Effectiveness (%) |
|---|---|---|
| Diaphragm and spermicide | 6 | 18 |
| Spermicide alone | 3 | 21 |
| Cervical cap | 6 | 18 |
| Sponge | | |
|   Parous women | 9 | 28 |
|   Nulliparous women | 6 | 18 |
| Condom | 2 | 12 |
| Female condom | 5 | 25 |
| No method | 85 | 85 |

requires deeper insertion into the vagina in a fashion to ensure a snug fit around the cervix without touching the cervical os. Most women can be fitted with a cap measuring 24, 30, or 36 mm in diameter.

The cervical cap has several advantages over the diaphragm. It can be left in place up to 36 hours. Also, it may be used by women who have a cystocele, a rectocele, or uterine prolapse. However, the cervical cap should not be used by women who have an abnormally long or short cervix, or by those who have cervicitis, cervical erosion, or lacerations. Just like the diaphragm, the cap should be properly fitted and the patient should receive appropriate instruction in its insertion and removal. The cervical cap is removed by pulling the rim away from the cervix to break the seal. The cervical cap has about the same degree of efficacy as the diaphragm (Table 1–7).

## CONTRACEPTIVE SPONGE

The vaginal contraceptive sponge is a dimpled disc made of polyurethane and impregnated with nonoxynol-9, a spermicide that is released from the sponge for 24 hours. The sponge must be thoroughly moistened with water before insertion to activate the spermicide. It provides continuous protection for up to 24 hours. In most studies, the failure rate of the sponge is lower than that of foam and jellies but higher than the failure rate of the diaphragm.

Side effects include vaginal irritation and allergic reaction in about 4% of users. The risk of toxic shock syndrome is not increased.

## SPERMICIDES

A large number of vaginal spermicidal preparations are currently in use. They can be categorized into five general groups: jellies, creams, aerosol foams, suppositories, and foaming tablets or films. These products contain a relatively inert base material that physically blocks the passage of sperm and simultaneously serves as a carrier for an effective spermicide. The majority of these preparations contain nonoxynol-9, a surfactant, as an active spermicide. Over 170 types of vaginal spermicidal products are being used throughout the world. In the United States, they are available without a prescription.

Vaginal spermicides must be used at the time of anticipated sexual intercourse. This is advantageous for women who have infrequent sexual relations, but it represents a disadvantage for women who engage in frequent sexual activity, because it requires the motivation to use them consistently. Additionally, some couples dislike the preparation required in the middle of lovemaking and the messiness of some of the products.

The contraceptive failure rate of these agents ranges from less than 1% to almost 30% in the first year of use, depending on the population studied and, to some extent, the product used. A 20% failure rate during the first year of use is frequently reported (see Table 1–7).

Vaginal spermicides provide protection against STDs. However, there is no evidence that these products can prevent HIV infection. Vaginal spermicides are safe, and their use has not been associated with any major side effect. Approximately 1 to 5% of users of either gender may exhibit minor allergic reactions; these resolve readily with discontinuation of the suspected product.

## CONDOMS

Condoms are by far the most used contraceptive product worldwide. In 1990, it was estimated that 6 billion condoms were used worldwide. The great advantage of the condom is that, if used continuously and correctly, it effectively prevents pregnancy as well as STDs, including HIV (see Table 1–7). However, in order to achieve these goals, condoms must be affordable and readily available. Almost all condoms are made of latex. The thickness of the condom is between 0.3 and 0.8 mm. This thickness makes the condom impermeable by sperms, which are 0.003 mm in diameter. The organisms that cause HIV or STDs are also unable to penetrate the latex condom. About 1% of condoms sold are made of natural skin (intestine).

Because spermicides also provide protection against pregnancy and STDs, condoms and spermicides used together offer greater protection than either method used alone. A large array of condoms have been developed to suit individual tastes and include those that are straight or tapered, smooth or ribbed, colored or clear, lubricated or nonlubricated, and with or without spermicide impregnation.

A concern expressed by some couples is the alleged reduction in penile sensitivity that accompanies condom use. This may be, however, more a matter of perception than reality. Condoms must be placed on

**Table 1–7** Median Times and Range of Ovulation Relative to Hormonal Events

| Hormone | Median Time (hr) | Ranges (hr) |
|---|---|---|
| LH Surge | 16 | 8–40 |
| Estradiol Peak | 24 | 17–32 |
| Progesterone Rise | 8 | −12.5 to +16 |

LH = luteinizing hormone.

the penis before it touches the partner. The tip of the condom should extend beyond the end of the penis to provide a reservoir for semen collection. Oil-based lubricants (e.g., petroleum jelly) should not be used because they weaken the condom. If spillage or breakage is evident, a spermicidal agent should be inserted quickly into vagina. Condoms should never be used more than once.

## Periodic Abstinence

Periodic abstinence, or natural family planning (NFP), is often used by couples who, because of their religious or moral beliefs, find hormonal or barrier contraceptives unacceptable.

These methods are based on the sperm's period of viability in the female reproductive tract (estimated at 2 to 7 days) and the life span of the ovum (1 to 3 days). The central issue in devising an effective method of NFP is accurate timing of ovulation. Achieving precise timing is difficult because ovulation patterns show considerable variation in the female populations (see Table 1–7).

This method requires a serious commitment from both partners and is more effective in women who have regular menstrual cycle. For best results, women who consider NFP should receive appropriate training before they use it. They must also be careful to practice the methods correctly and consistently. Current methods of NFP are based on the concept of fertility awareness; namely, the woman's ability to identify, on a day-to-day basis, certain physiologic changes that respond to hormonal changes associated with ovulation. These include the following methods:
- Calendar
- Basal body temperature (BBT)
- Ovulation or cervical mucus
- Symptothermal

Among these the two latter have proven to be more reliable and are commonly practiced.

### OVULATION (CERVICAL MUCUS) METHOD

The ovulation method was devised and popularized by Billings. It is based on periovulatory changes in characteristics of the cervical mucus, which have been shown to reflect hormonal events closely. To use the ovulation method, the woman needs to learn to recognize the sequence of changes in the quantity and quality of her mucus and the associated sensation at the vulva. These changes occur in the following context:

Dry days: These extend over several days; during this time, which corresponds to the early follicular phase, there is no mucus secretion.

End of dry sensation: This indicates that the production of cervical mucus has started. The infertile type of mucus is tacky, crumbly, and either white or yellow in color.

Preovulatory or fertile period: The mucus appears clear, thin, glistering and lubricative, similar to raw egg white. The last day of lubricative mucus is called the "Peak Day," which indicates the day of maximum fertility and coincides with ovulation.

Postovulation days: The mucus becomes thick, tacky, scanty, and opaque.

### SYMPTOTHERMAL METHOD

This method combines the cervical mucus method with the shift of BBT. Additionally, other symptoms and signs of ovulation, such as midcycle pain or bleeding and breast fullness and tenderness, may be used. These methods of NFP incorporate several markers of peripheral changes associated with cyclic hormonal alteration in ovulatory women.

### EFFICACY

Multicenter studies conducted by world health organizations revealed that among those who had learned the NFP method, the pregnancy rate was 22.5 per 100 women years. However, almost all failures could be attributed to a conscious departure from the method. Abstinence was necessary for 17 days in each cycle. For those who followed the method strictly, the actual method failure during the first year was only 3.1%, but imperfect use resulted in a pregnancy rate of 86.4%. Thus, if used correctly and consistently, the NFP method is highly effective, but imperfect use results in an unacceptably high pregnancy rate.

The efficacy of the cervical mucus method has also been compared with that of the symptothermal method. The two methods were found to be comparable, with pregnancy rates of 20 to 24%. Once again, most pregnancies resulted from imperfect use.

## How to Select a Contraceptive

Appropriate selection of a contraceptive for a couple depends on their preference, age, medical condition, parity, and other factors. Oral contraceptives are highly effective and safe. They may be used at any age unless there is a specific medical contraindication for their use. They should not be used by smokers after the age of 35. Steroidal injectables and implants are preferred for those who lack the motivation and discipline to take OCs and who plan a relatively long period of fertility control. IUDs are ideal contraceptives for parous women in a monogamous relationship. Barrier contraceptives are suitable for almost any couple at any age. They are particularly indicated for couples at risk of STD. Specifically, the use of condoms should be encouraged for all couples in a casual sexual relationship or for those who have multiple sexual partners. Female or male sterilization should be recommended to couples who have an absolute medical contraindication for pregnancy or to those who have had their family and who are not interested in future fertility.

## REFERENCES

Alvarez F, Brachi V, Fernandez E, et al: New insights on the mode of action of intrauterine contraceptive devices in women. Fertil Steril 49:768, 1988.

Bonnas J: Natural family planning including breast feeding. In Mishell DR (ed): Advances in Fertility, Vol 1. New York, Raven Press, 1982, pp 1–18.

Bottinger LE, Boman G, Eklund G, et al: Oral contraceptives and thromboembolic disease. Effects of lowering estrogen content. Lancet 1:1097, 1980.

Centers for Disease Control: Combination oral contraceptives and the risk of endometrial cancer. JAMA 257:796, 1987.

Centers for Disease Control: The reduction in risk of ovarian cancer associated with oral contraceptive use. N Engl J Med 316: 650, 1987.

Connell EB: Vaginal contraception; In Mishell DR (ed): Advances in Fertility Research, Vol 1. New York, Raven Press, 1982, pp. 19–38.

Darney PD, Klaisle CM: Management of menstrual changes in Norplant implant recipient. Dialogues Contracept 4:6, 1994.

Drife JO: The Benefits and Risks of Oral Contraceptives. New York, Parthenon Publishing Group, 1993, pp 1–31.

Fasoli M, Parazzini F, Cacchetti G, et al: Postcoital contraception: An overview of published studies. Contraception 39:459,1989.

Gerstman BB, Piper JM, Tomita DK, et al: Oral estrogen dose and the risk of deep venous thromboembolic disease. Am J Epidemiol 133:32, 1991.

Ginsburg K, Moghissi KS: Alternative delivery system for contraceptive progestogens. Fertil Steril (suppl 2) 49:165, 1988.

Goldziehier, JW: Hormonal Contraception; Pills, Injections and Implants, 3rd ed. Ontario, Canada, EMIS, 1994.

Kaunitz AM, Mishell DR: Progestin only contraceptives, current perspectives, and future directions. Dialogues Contracept 4:1, 1994.

Lee NC, Rubin GL, Borucki R: The intrauterine device and pelvic inflammatory disease revisited: New results from the women's health study. Obstet Gynecol 72:1, 1988.

McIntyre SL, Higgins JE: Parity and use effectiveness with the contraceptive sponge. Am J Obstet Gynecol 155:796, 1986.

Medina JE, Cifuentes A, Abernathy JR, et al: Comparative evaluation of two methods of natural family planning in Columbia. Am J Obstet Gynecol 138:1142, 1980.

Mills A: Combined oral contraception and the risk of venous thromboembolism. Hum Reprod 12:2595, 1997.

Mishell DR: Noncontraceptive benefits of oral steroidal contraceptives. Am J Obstet Gynecol 142:819, 1982.

Moghissi KS: Microdose progestogens for contraception. In Moghissi KS, Evans TN (eds): Regulation of Human Fertility. Detroit, Wayne State University Press, 1976, pp 57–84.

Mosher WD: Contraception practice in the United States, 1982–1988. Fam Plann Perspect 22:198, 1990.

Pabinger I, Schneider B, GTH Study Group: Thrombotic risk of women with hereditary antithrombin III, protein C and protein S deficiency taking oral contraceptive medication. Thromb Haemost 5:548, 1994.

Ross RK, Pike MC, Vessey MP, et al: Risk factors for uterine fibroids; Reduced risk associated with oral contraceptives. BMJ 293:359, 1986.

Schlesselman JJ: Cancer of the breast and reproductive tract in relation to use of oral contraceptives. Contraception 40:1, 1989.

Shervington DO: Female condom becomes available nationwide. Contracept Reprod 5:11, 1995.

Sivin I: Contraception with Norplant implant. Hum Reprod 9:1818, 1994.

Speroff L, DeCherney A: Evaluation of a new generation of oral contraceptives. Obstet Gynecol 81:1034, 1993.

Trussell J, Sturgen K, Strickler J, et al: Comparative contraceptive efficacy of female condom and other barrier methods. Fam Plann Perspect, 26:66, 1994.

Vessey MP: Oral contraception and cancer. In Filshie M, Guillebaud J (eds): Contraception: Science and Practice. London, Butterworths, 1989, pp 52–68.

Wade ME, McCarthy P, Braunstein GD, et al: A randomized perspective study of the use effectiveness of two methods of natural family planning. Am J Obstet Gynecol 141:368, 1981.

World Health Organization: A prospective multicenter trial of the ovulation method of natural family planning II. The effectiveness phase. Fertil Steril 36:591, 1981.

World Health Organization: Collaborative study of neoplasia and steroid contraceptives: Depomedroxyprogesterone acetate (DMPA) and risk of endometrial cancer. Int J Cancer 49:186, 1991.

World Health Organization Collaborative study of neoplasia and steroid contraceptives: Breast cancer and depomedroxyprogesterone acetate: A multi-national study. Lancet 338:833, 1991.

World Health Organization: The TCu-380A, TCu220C, multiload 250 and Nova T IUDs at 3.5 and 7 years of use—results from three randomized multicenter trials. Contraception 42:141, 1990.

Yuzpe AA, Smith RP, Rademaker AW: A multicenter clinical investigation employing ethinyl estradiol combined with dl-norgestrel as a postcoital contraceptive agent. Fertil Steril 37:508, 1982.

# 2

# Women's Preventive Care

S. GENE McNEELEY
E. TRENT McNEELEY

Over the past decade, women's health issues have received increased attention. It has been recognized that there are significant differences in the morbidity and mortality of women and men who have the same medical condition. Excluding routine gynecologic and obstetric care, women make more visits to healthcare providers than men and are more likely to be restricted in their activity due to illness.

The goals of preventive care are prolonging life, improving the quality of life and reducing the morbidity and mortality caused by disease or injury. It is important, therefore, that physicians who provide primary and preventive care know which interventions are valuable and cost effective. Prevention can be defined as primary or secondary. *Primary* prevention describes those actions that decrease the likelihood of acquiring a disease, such as providing counseling about sexually transmitted disease to reduce the risk of acquiring human immunodeficiency virus. *Secondary* prevention detects early disease, thus potentially reducing the morbidity or mortality rate attributed to a disease. An example of secondary prevention is testing for fecal occult blood in the hope of detecting early colon cancer.

## Primary Prevention

It is estimated that approximately 50% or half of all deaths occurring in the United States may be preventable. Eighty percent of preventable deaths are attributed to smoking, poor diet and lack of exercise, and alcohol abuse (Table 2–1). Smoking alone contributes to approximately one in five deaths in the United States. Although it is easy to focus on reproductive health during a comprehensive gynecologic exam, it is imperative that counseling regarding other health behaviors not be overlooked. Conditions causing illness and death change throughout a woman's life (Table 2–2). Screening, counseling, and other interventions should reflect these changes over time.

### SMOKING

The largest potentially modifiable health risk is smoking tobacco. It is estimated that over 50 billion dollars are spent annually in the United States in treating cardiovascular and pulmonary disease and cancer

**Table 2–1** Causes of Preventable Deaths in the United States in 1990

| | Deaths | |
|---|---|---|
| Cause | Estimated No. | Percentage of Total Deaths |
| Tobacco | 400,000 | 19 |
| Diet and activity patterns | 300,000 | 14 |
| Alcohol | 100,000 | 5 |
| Microbial agents | 90,000 | 4 |
| Toxic agents | 60,000 | 3 |
| Firearms | 35,000 | 2 |
| Sexual behavior | 30,000 | 1 |
| Motor vehicles | 25,000 | 1 |
| Illicit use of drugs | 20,000 | <1 |
| TOTAL | 1,060,000 | 50 |

From McGinnis JM, Foege WH: Actual causes of death in the United States. JAMA 270:2207–2212, 1993.

caused by tobacco smoking. Passive exposure to smoke is also associated with pulmonary disease and cancer. The majority of people who successfully quit smoking do so on their own. The treating physician should provide counseling and literature as needed and be knowledgeable about nicotine replacement. Bupropion hydrochloride (Zyban) (150 mg orally once daily for 3 days, followed by 150 mg twice daily) has also been shown to be an effective adjunct in smoking cessation.

## DIET AND ACTIVITY

Approximately 30% of adults in the United States are overweight. The incidence of obesity is higher in African-American and Mexican-American women. Physicians can play a critical role in effecting dietary change. A 1% reduction of cholesterol may reduce the risk of coronary heart disease by 2 to 3%. In addition to the cardiovascular benefits, dietary modification can reduce the morbidity and mortality of diabetes, cancer, and hypertension.

Increased physical activity goes hand in hand with dietary modification. Avoiding a sedentary lifestyle decreases the likelihood of developing coronary artery disease. A reasonable goal is moderate to vigorous physical activity (20 to 30 minutes of activity three to five times weekly).

## SEXUAL HEALTH

Many aspects of sexual health are discussed in this chapter. Contraceptive needs should be reviewed on an annual basis. All women who are not in a mutually monogamous relationship should be advised to use a barrier contraceptive for vaginal, oral, and anal intercourse.

**Table 2–2** Age-Related Morbidity and Mortality

| Age Group (yr) | Morbidity | Mortality |
|---|---|---|
| 13–18 | Nose, throat, and upper respiratory conditions<br>Viral, bacterial, and parasitic infections<br>Sexual abuse<br>Musculoskeletal and soft tissue injuries<br>Acute ear infections<br>Digestive system and acute urinary conditions | Motor vehicle accidents<br>Homicide<br>Suicide<br>Leukemia |
| 19–39 | Nose, throat, and upper respiratory conditions<br>Musculoskeletal and soft tissue (including back and upper and lower extremities) injuries<br>Viral, bacterial, and parasitic infections<br>Acute urinary problems<br>Sexually transmissible infections | Motor vehicle accidents<br>Cardiovascular disease<br>Homicide<br>Acquired immunodeficiency syndrome<br>Cerebrovascular disease<br>Cancer |
| 40–64 | Nose, throat, and upper respiratory conditions<br>Osteoporosis<br>Arthritis<br>Hypertension<br>Orthopedic deformities, including back and upper and lower extremities<br>Heart disease<br>Hearing and vision impairments | Coronary artery disease<br>Breast, lung, colorectal, and ovarian cancer<br>Cerebrovascular disease<br>Obstructive pulmonary disease |
| 65 years + | Nose, throat, and upper respiratory conditions<br>Osteoporosis<br>Arthritis<br>Hypertension<br>Urinary incontinence<br>Heart disease<br>Musculoskeletal and soft tissue injuries<br>Hearing and vision impairments | Cardiovascular disease<br>Coronary artery disease<br>Cerebrovascular disease<br>Pneumonia and influenza<br>Obstructive lung disease<br>Colorectal, lung, and breast cancer<br>Accidents |

## ALCOHOL AND DRUGS

Alcohol and illicit drug use account for approximately 120,000 deaths in the United States annually. Healthcare providers screen inadequately for alcohol and drug abuse. Screening tests, such as the CAGE (cut down; annoyed by criticism; guilty about drinking; eye-opener drinks) questionnaire, have been shown to be effective in detecting alcohol abuse. The annual gynecologic visit is an opportune time for assessing the patient's potential for substance abuse, for providing counsel, or for referring for treatment.

## SAFETY ISSUES

Motor vehicle accidents are the leading cause of death of women aged 24 to 34. Fifty percent of these victims were not using seat belts at the time of the accident. The most effective intervention for reducing morbidity and mortality in women 24 to 34 years of age is counseling regarding seat-belt use and avoidance of drinking and driving. Homicide is the second most common cause of death in this age group; this emphasizes the need for questioning women about the potential for domestic violence. If there is concern for personal safety, plans for evacuation from the household and referral to appropriate authorities can be made at the office visit.

In summary, a health-risk assessment should be performed on a regular basis. Counseling regarding diet, exercise, drug and alcohol abuse, smoking cessation, safe sexual practices, and seat-belt use is the most important preventive intervention available to health-care providers.

## IMMUNIZATION

Before 1970, rubella epidemics occurred every 6 to 10 years. The pandemic of 1964 resulted in 12 million rubella infections in the United States. It is estimated there were 11,000 fetal losses and 20,000 infants born with congenital rubella syndrome. Since the introduction of rubella vaccine, there has been a 99% reduction in the incidence of rubella infection. Although obstetrician-gynecologists have been strong advocates for rubella immunizations, physicians in this specialty have a poor track record for counseling their patients on receiving other adult immunizations for preventable disease. Forty percent or less of a target disease population is immunized. It has been estimated that 50,000 to 70,000 US adults die annually of vaccine-preventable diseases. Most of these deaths are caused by infection with influenza, hepatitis B, or pneumococcal pneumonia. Recommendations for adult vaccination are noted in Table 2–3.

# Secondary Prevention

Many physicians are surprised to learn that performing only an annual comprehensive physical examination, is not a cost-effective intervention. Significant benefit results only when the examination is combined with counseling, risk-behavior intervention, appropriate cancer screening, and immunization. Screening and intervention strategies are based on the opportunity to impact leading causes of morbidity and mortality. The leading causes of morbidity and mortality by age group are noted in Table 2–2.

There are few unanimous health-screening recommendations. This lack of consensus can be confusing to the practitioner. We will review the women's health-screening recommendations that appear in the second edition of the US Preventive Services Task Force (USPSTF) and the American College of Obstetricians and Gynecologists (ACOG). Recommendations of the American Cancer Society (ACS) and the American College of Physicians (ACP) will also be discussed.

# Screening Guidelines

## ANNUAL HISTORY AND PHYSICAL EXAMINATION

The annual comprehensive physical examination is not cost effective, does not reduce morbidity or mortality, and is not recommended by most authorities. It can be argued, however, that an annual examination allows health-risk assessment and intervention, cancer screening, and immunization as deemed appropriate.

## PELVIC EXAMINATION

The pelvic examination is not a sensitive or specific screening tool for detecting ovarian or uterine cancer and is not recommended by USPSTF. However, the ACOG, the American Medical Association, and the ACS recommend bimanual pelvic examination every 1 to 3 years for women between the ages of 18 and 40, and annually after age 40, because there is no other feasible, cost-effective screening test for ovarian cancer. It is reasonable to perform a bimanual pelvic examination as clinically indicated for other gynecologic reasons.

## THE PAPANICOLAOU SMEAR

Routine Papanicolaou (Pap) smear screening has significantly reduced the incidence and mortality rate for

### Table 2–3  Vaccines for Adults

| Vaccine | Indicated for | Dosage |
|---|---|---|
| Tetanus-diphtheria (toxoid) | All adults | Booster every 10 yr of 0.5 ml IM |
|  | Never immunized | Primary series of 3 doses: 0.5 ml IM at 0, 1–2, and 6–12 mo |
| Measles (live vaccine) | Unimmunized, born after 1956 | 2 doses 0.5 ml SC at least 1 mo apart |
|  | Previously immunized with one dose; for college entry, health-care workers, and foreign travel | 1 dose 0.5 ml SC |
| Rubella (attenuated live virus grown in human diploid cells) | Unimmunized young women and health-care workers | 1 dose 0.5 ml SC |
| Hepatitis B (noninfectious recombinant hepatitis B surface antigen) | High-risk patients and health-care workers | 3 doses 1 ml IM in the deltoid, second dose after 1 mo, third dose 6 mo after first dose; higher dose for immuno-compromised and dialysis patients |
| Influenza (inactivated whole or virus subunits, grown in chick embryo cells) | High-risk patients, health-care workers, and persons older than 65 years of age | 1 dose 0.5 ml IM annually |
| Pneumococcal (capsular polysaccharide from 23 types) | High-risk patients and persons older than 65 years of age | 1 dose 0.5 ml IM |

IM = intramuscular; SC = subcutaneous.

cervical cancer. The USPSTF recommends routine screening of cervical cancer beginning at age 18. In contrast, the ACOG and the ACS recommend routine Pap smears at the onset of sexual activity or age 18, whichever occurs first. There is little agreement as to the optimal frequency of performing the Pap smear in women at low risk for cervical cancer, that is, those who have at least two consecutive normal Pap smears and who have had mutually monogamous relationship. In this circumstance, screening every 3 years offers a cost-effective alternative to annual Pap smears. All groups recommend more frequent screening of women at high risk for cervical dysplasia and cancer, particularly those at risk for sexually transmitted diseases and women who have multiple partners. In women who have undergone total abdominal hysterectomy for disorders unrelated to cervical neoplasia, we do not recommend routine Pap smears of the vaginal cuff.

## SELF BREAST EXAMINATION

Self breast examination (SBE) is a free, convenient method of cancer screening. Unfortunately, SBE is not an effective screening tool. ACS and ACOG recommend monthly SBE; however, USPSTF has no mandate for or against this examination.

## CLINICIAN BREAST EXAMINATION

USPSTF does not have a mandate for or against clinician breast examination. All other groups recommend an annual clinician breast examination beginning at age 40. ACS recommends clinician breast examinations every 3 years in women 20 to 39 years of age, with more frequent examinations in women who have a family history of breast cancer. USPSTF recommends annual screening beginning at age 35 in women who have a family history of breast cancer.

## MAMMOGRAPHY

There is also a lack of a consensus regarding mammography. ACS and ACOG recommend initial screening at age 40, with additional screening every 1 to 2 years until age 50, when mammography should be performed annually. ACP recommends annual mammograms beginning at age 50. USPSTF takes a more conservative stance, recommending mammography every 1 to 2 years for women aged 50 to 69.

## DIGITAL RECTAL EXAMINATION

Opinions also vary as to the need for annual digital rectal examination (DRE). The majority of colorectal cancers are not palpable on rectal exam; therefore, the DRE is not a sensitive screening tool. The ACS and the ACOG recommend annual DREs beginning at age 50. USPSTF does not have a mandate for or against DRE.

## FECAL OCCULT BLOOD SCREENING

Recent studies suggest a reduction in mortality when annual screening for fecal occult blood is performed. The ACS and the ACP recommend annual fecal occult blood testing beginning at age 40, whereas

ACOG recommends routine testing beginning at age 50. USPSTF recommends annual screening for fecal occult blood *or* sigmoidoscopy on an annual basis.

## SIGMOIDOSCOPY

ACS, ASP, and ACOG are also in agreement in recommending annual screening by sigmoidoscopy. If two consecutive examinations are normal, subsequent exams can be performed every 3 to 5 years. The USPSTF recommendation was noted previously.

## SCREENING FOR MEDICAL CONDITIONS

Periodic screening for elevated blood cholesterol in women aged 45 to 65 is recommended by USPSTF. Screening for diabetes and thyroid disease in asymptomatic adults is not recommended.

## REFERENCES

American College of Obstetricians and Gynecologists: Guidelines for Women's Health Care. Washington, DC, ACOG, 1995.

American College of Obstetricians and Gynecologists. Routine Cancer Screenings. ACOG Committee Opinion 185. September 1997.

Canadian Task Force on the Periodic Health Examination: The periodic health examination. CMAJ 121:1193–1254, 1979.

Gall SA: Adult Immunization. ACOG Clin Rev 2:1–2; July/August 1997.

Hayward PS, Steinberg EP, Ford DE, et al: Preventive care guidelines: 1991. Ann Intern Med 114:758–783, 1991.

McGinnis JM, Foege WH: Actual causes of death in the United States. JAMA 270:2207–2212, 1993.

U.S. PREVENTIVE SERVICES TASK FORCE: Guide to Clinical Preventive Services, 2nd ed. Baltimore, Williams & Wilkins, 1995.

# 3

# Early Pregnancy Loss

DAVID C. KMAK
S. GENE McNEELEY, JR.

Early pregnancy loss and habitual abortion can be confusing subjects for clinicians to understand and treat. This confusion ranges from changes in etiologies, definitions, and understanding disease processes to debate on timing of proper evaluation and treatment.

This confusion is exemplified in the management of habitual abortion. Many conditions usually assumed to be associated with habitual abortion have never been demonstrated to have a cause and effect relationship. In addition, it is well documented that the overall live birth rate in women who have experienced three or more consecutive spontaneous abortions is 65 to 70% for the next pregnancy without any treatment. Although no statistical improvement has been shown over this baseline live birth rate of 65 to 70%, many old and new treatments for habitual abortion are still being advocated. An example of this is seen with luteal phase defect and progesterone supplementation.

## Definitions

The terminology regarding pregnancy loss has changed owing to the negative connotation associated with abortion (Table 3–1).

Spontaneous abortion is defined as a pregnancy loss at less than 20 weeks of gestation or the birth of a fetus weighing less than 500 g.

Habitual abortion is defined as three or more consecutive spontaneous abortions, usually during the first trimester. However, any loss occurring before 20 weeks of gestation is included in this definition so as not to exclude a number of potential etiologies.

## Background

Spontaneous abortion, or early pregnancy loss, occurs in 12 to 20% of all recognized clinical pregnancies. It is estimated that as many as 65% of all pregnancies result in spontaneous abortions if clinically unrecognized pregnancies, evidenced by a positive β-human chorionic gonadotropin (β-hCG), are included. Approximately 1% of women experience three or more consecutive pregnancy losses and thus are considered

Table 3–1 Terminology for Pregnancy Loss

| Old Terminology | New Terminology |
| --- | --- |
| Spontaneous abortion | Early pregnancy loss/miscarriage |
| Habitual abortion | Recurrent pregnancy loss |
| Recurrent abortion | Recurrent miscarriage |

to be suffering from recurrent pregnancy loss or habitual abortion. Potential factors associated with recurrent pregnancy loss are noted in Table 3–2.

At the present time, the reason for recurrent abortion can be determined in only 50% of women. The likelihood of a woman's having a miscarriage after experiencing one, two, or three consecutive miscarriages is 21%, 26%, and 35%, respectively. Thus, even with no treatment, 60 to 70% of women who have had recurrent pregnancy losses will successfully complete the subsequent pregnancy.

It is unclear whether to begin testing for recurrent pregnancy loss after two or three consecutive losses, and testing should be determined on an individual basis. It should be remembered that these definitions were present before ultrasonography and sensitive blood tests for β-hCG were available, so clinically unrecognized pregnancy losses were not recognized; therefore, nonviable pregnancies, such as a blighted ovum, were not detected. We recommend beginning a workup after two losses only if the previous pregnancies documented a viable pregnancy with cardiac activity. When counseling a couple regarding pregnancy loss, it is important to convey that in future pregnancies, if cardiac activity is detected by ultrasonography in the first trimester, they can be assured of having a greater than 95% likelihood of a successful outcome if the pregnancy is normal. The loss rate, however, may be as much as four or five times greater in women who experience recurrent pregnancy loss.

## Etiology of Spontaneous Abortion

### GENETIC

Genetic abnormalities are detected in 3 to 5% of couples who experience recurrent pregnancy loss. Chromosomal abnormalities account for at least 50% of clinically evident first-trimester losses. Because of the early detection of β-hCG, recent studies indicate that aneuploidy rates of over 70% are detected among all first-trimester losses. Chromosomal abnormalities have been detected in 80% of pregnancies diagnosed as blighted ova. Other genetic conditions include single gene defects and polygenic multifactorial syndrome.

**Table 3–2** Potential Causes of Recurrent Pregnancy Loss

| | |
|---|---|
| Genetic | Infection |
| Anatomic | Immunologic |
| Endocrine abnormalities | Unexplained |

**Table 3–3** Parental Chromosomal Abnormalities in Recurrent Pregnancy Loss

Reciprocal translocation, 50%
Robertsonian translocation, 24%
Sex chromosome mosaicism, 12.5%

Trisomies are the most commonly detected genetic abnormality. Monosomy X is the most common specific chromosomal abnormality. Most losses due to chromosomal abnormalities occur before 8 to 10 weeks' gestation.

Structural chromosomal rearrangements account for 1.5% of all spontaneous abortions. The most common structural parent rearrangement is a translocation (Table 3–3). Parents who have a balanced translocation are phenotypically normal, but their offspring may carry unbalanced arrangements, such as chromosomal duplications or deletions.

Parental karyotyping should be performed after three consecutive losses. Testing may be considered after two consecutive spontaneous abortions if a couple is particularly anxious or if maternal age is advanced. Obtaining a karyotype of the products of conception after two or more consecutive pregnancy losses may lead to detection of a genetic abnormality; however, parental karyotyping provides more useful information for couples who have recurrent pregnancy losses.

### ANATOMIC

Uterine anomalies are known to occur in 0.5% of all fertile women and up to 27% of women diagnosed as having recurrent pregnancy loss. The majority of women who have uterine anomalies have successful pregnancy outcomes; therefore, other causes of recurrent abortion should be excluded before a uterine anomaly is treated.

Uterine anomalies can be categorized as congenital or acquired and are listed in Table 3–4. Incompetent

**Table 3–4** Uterine Anomalies Associated With Recurrent Pregnancy Loss

| Congenital | Acquired |
|---|---|
| Unicornuate uterus | DES exposure |
| Didelphic uterus | Asherman's syndrome |
| Bicornuate uterus | Leiomyomas |
| Septate uterus | Incompetent cervix |
| Incompetent cervix | |

DES = diethylstilbestrol.

cervix has been defined as three consecutive second-trimester losses associated with painless cervical dilatation and bulging or ruptured membranes. The use of ultrasonography to check for cervical funneling and shortening enhances the ability to detect an incompetent cervix.

Cervical cerclage is recommended for women who have had a history of recurrent second-trimester losses in which signs and symptoms of labor were absent. Cerclage is also recommended if ultrasound scan shows cervical shortening or funneling regardless of the number of previous second-trimester losses. More difficulty is encountered in managing patients who have experienced a second-trimester pregnancy loss associated with signs of labor, inasmuch as the advanced dilatation may have preceded the onset of cramping. These patients can benefit from one or more second-trimester ultrasound examinations specifically aimed at assessing cervical length and funneling so that an incompetent cervix does not go undetected.

## CONGENITAL UTERINE ANOMALIES

As stated earlier, the majority of women who have uterine anomalies have successful pregnancy outcomes. Approximately 27% of women who suffer recurrent pregnancy loss have uterine anomalies. Women who have uterine anomalies have an increased incidence of spontaneous abortion and preterm labor.

The evaluation of a suspected uterine anomaly is straightforward. Acquired and congenital abnormalities of the uterine cavity and cervix can be diagnosed by hysterosalpingography. Magnetic resonance imaging (MRI) can distinguish between a bicornuate and a septate uterus if the hysterosalpingogram is inconclusive.

### Unicornuate Uterus

This anomaly is a consequence of inadequate fusion of the müllerian ducts. A rudimentary horn is present in up to 65% of the anomalies and may communicate with the main cavity. Pregnancy loss rates associated with the presence of a uterine horn approach 45% during the first and second trimesters and are thought to be caused by poor blood supply and an associated incompetent cervix. The uterine horn should be resected before any subsequent pregnancies. Frequent bimanual or pelvic ultrasonograms should be performed to allow early detection of an incompetent cervix. A cerclage should be placed in women suspected of having an incompetent cervix.

### Didelphic Uterus

Two endometrial cavities are present in this anomaly. Each cavity usually connects to its own uterine cervix; however, fusion of the distal uterine horn can occur, resulting in a single cervix. A longitudinal vaginal septum is frequently located at the midline of the vagina. Pregnancy outcomes in women who have a didelphic uterus are generally better than in women who have other congenital uterine anomalies.

Surgical correction of this condition is rarely indicated. In women who have recurrent pregnancy losses, a metroplasty that creates a single uterine cavity is the preferred method.

### Bicornuate Uterus

A bicornuate uterus is defined as a uterus with two separate but communicating cavities. Sixty percent of pregnancies that occur in women who have this uterine anomaly are successful. Approximately one third of women experience a spontaneous abortion, and 14% of women who have recurrent pregnancy loss have a bicornuate uterus. Compared with all other uterine anomalies, the bicornuate uterus has the strongest association with an incompetent cervix, occurring in approximately 40% of women who have bicornuate uterus.

As with most uterine anomalies, a hysterosalpingogram is the preferred initial test. A bicornuate uterus may not be easily differentiated from a septate uterus, and further testing by ultrasonography or MRI is recommended.

Surgery is reserved for women who have had multiple pregnancy losses. Following metroplasty, approximately 85% of pregnancies are successful. Women who have a bicornuate uterus should be followed closely for incompetent cervix with frequent pelvic or ultrasound examinations performed. There is no evidence that prophylactic cerclage improves outcome.

### Septate Uterus

The septum in a septate uterus is largely composed of fibrous tissue that can vary greatly in size. The incidence of septate uterus is approximately twice that of bicornuate uterus in women who have recurrent spontaneous abortions or preterm labor. Live birth rates as low as 15 to 28% are reported with this anomaly. The poor outcome is thought to be caused by the inadequate blood supply in the septum along with impaired implantation and fetal growth.

The septate uterus is usually diagnosed by hysterosalpingography. Hysteroscopic resection of the uterine septum has emerged as the procedure of choice. Surgery should be considered for repeated first-trimester losses, a single second-trimester loss, or a history of preterm labor.

## ACQUIRED ANOMALIES

### Diethylstilbestrol Exposure

This is a rare cause of uterine defects, which includes an abnormal endometrial cavity, and is likely to be associated with an incompetent cervix. Diethylstilbestrol (DES) exposure is also associated with a live birth rate of only 42%. Diagnosis is by history and hysterosalpingography, which shows uterine anomalies. A prophylactic cerclage was shown to be beneficial in one controlled study.

### Asherman's Syndrome

Intrauterine adhesions form after instrumentation of the uterine cavity. They are often associated with infection, resulting in altered menses (amenorrhea or hypomenorrhea). Pregnancy loss is thought to be due to impaired implantation.

Hysterosalpingography should be performed if this condition is suspected. Hysteroscopic resection is the treatment of choice. The patient should receive estrogen postoperatively, although there is no definitive evidence proving its efficacy in reducing the occurrence of intrauterine adhesions. Likewise, it has been recommended that an intrauterine device be placed to prevent reformation of intrauterine synechiae.

### Uterine Leiomyomas

The vast majority of uterine fibroids are asymptomatic and have no association with spontaneous abortion or recurrent pregnancy loss. Retrospective studies have suggested an association between leiomyomas and spontaneous abortion, recurrent pregnancy loss, preterm labor, or placental abruption. One prospective study has failed to demonstrate any association of fibroids with spontaneous abortion or preterm labor.

Transvaginal ultrasound is an excellent tool for determining the size and location of myomas. Encroachment of a myoma on the uterine cavity can be detected. In addition, hysterosalpingography can detect submucosal myomas and may detect the rare case of the tubal ostium obstructed by a fibroid.

Small submucosal fibroids can be removed by hysteroscopic resection. Larger myomas thought to be responsible for infertility or pregnancy loss can be removed laparoscopically or by laparotomy.

## ENDOCRINE CAUSES OF PREGNANCY LOSS

Endocrine conditions thought to be associated with pregnancy loss are noted in Table 3–5. Although thyroid disorders and diabetes were considered to be important causes of spontaneous abortion, in reality, they are rarely associated with pregnancy loss. Reports of women who have hypothyroidism have failed to find an association with spontaneous abortion. Likewise, only women who have uncontrolled diabetes mellitus appear to be at increased risk for abortion. Euglycemic women are not at significant risk for spontaneous abortion. Although this is controversial, luteal phase defect (LPD) and polycystic ovary syndrome (PCO) may be important endocrine causes of early pregnancy loss.

### Luteal Phase Defect

Luteal phase defect (LPD) is potentially the most common endocrine abnormality associated with pregnancy loss, and its role in recurrent abortion is controversial. Intact luteal phase function is needed until 7 weeks' gestation when the trophoblast is able to maintain progesterone production. Luteal phase abnormalities include inadequate progesterone production by the corpus luteum and inadequate secretory changes of the endometrium. While some investigators report that LPD is present in approximately one third of women who have recurrent abortion, others state it is an uncommon cause of abortion. The lack of controlled studies in this arena precludes drawing conclusions regarding the role of LPDs in pregnancy loss.

The diagnosis of LPD is most commonly made by performing an endometrial biopsy at the end of the luteal phase. Histologic dating is correlated with chronologic dating by comparing the day the sample was obtained with a corresponding day in a standardized 28-day cycle. An LPD is defined as the endometrial sample's being more than 2 days out of phase with the menstrual cycle. Whether the chronologic date is best assigned coming back from the start of

**Table 3–5** Endocrine Causes of Pregnancy Loss

| | |
|---|---|
| Luteal phase defect | Hyperthyroidism |
| Polycystic ovary syndrome | Diabetes mellitus |
| Hypothyroidism | |

the next menstrual cycle or prospectively from the date of the luteinizing hormone (LH). LH surge is a source of controversy. Evidence suggests benefits with the use of the LH surge rather than the onset of menses; however, LH indicator kits add an additional expense. A luteal phase of less than 10 days is abnormal. The variability of progesterone secretion limits the usefulness of serum progesterone levels in diagnosing LPD.

Treatment of LPD is also controversial. Indeed, some question the need for treating a luteal phase defect. Traditionally, treatment consists of progesterone vaginal suppositories 25 mg twice daily or intramuscular progesterone 12.5 milligrams beginning in the luteal phase and continuing through 10 weeks' gestation.

Clomiphene citrate has also been used with success in treatment of LPD. Unfortunately, no controlled trials have been performed. Paradoxically, clomiphene citrate has been shown to induce LPD. Thus, its utility is questionable.

### Polycystic Ovary Syndrome

Patients suffering from PCO may have an increased risk for miscarriage. The mechanism of pregnancy loss in women who have polycystic ovaries is uncertain; however, it has been proposed that hypersecretion of LH causes premature aging of the oocyte. Ovulation induction and prevention of LH hypersecretion are mainstays of treatment.

## INFECTIOUS CAUSES OF EARLY PREGNANCY LOSS

Numerous genital pathogens have been associated with sporadic pregnancy loss. These include *Listeria monocytogenes*, *Mycoplasma* species, *Ureaplasma* species, *Salmonella typhi*, *Brucella* species, *Chlamydia trachomatis*, and *Treponema pallidum*. Herpes and other viral infections have also been associated with pregnancy loss. Infections caused by mycoplasma, or ureaplasma and *L. monocytogenes* have been associated with recurrent pregnancy loss and deserve further attention.

### Genital Mycoplasmas

Genital tract colonization by *M. hominis* and *Ureaplasma urealyticum* has been associated with poor pregnancy outcome, including recurrent abortion. The evidence suggesting this association suffers from poor design and lack of power. In addition, treatment of the couple before pregnancy, or of the woman during pregnancy, has convincingly been shown to improve pregnancy outcome. Regardless, women who have recurrent pregnancy loss may have cultures performed to detect the growth of the mycoplasmas prior to pregnancy. Doxycycline 100 mg twice daily for 14 days is the treatment of choice. Persistent or recurrent infection is very common. During pregnancy, a macrolide, such as erythromycin, should be administered.

## LISTERIA MONOCYTOGENES

*Listeria* is an uncommon cause of recurrent abortion. The organism can arise from the fecal or vaginal flora and is usually acquired from contaminated dairy products. Maternal bacteremia with secondary fetal infection is the most common source of pregnancy wastage. Penicillin is the treatment of choice for infection caused by *L. monocytogenes*.

## AUTOIMMUNE CAUSES OF PREGNANCY LOSS

Autoimmune events are thought to account for 5 to 40% of recurrent pregnancy losses. The mechanism of action of this process is loss of self-tolerance. The vast majority of pregnancy losses are from antiphospholipid antibodies, including lupus anticoagulant and anticardiolipin antibody. Death occurs in the first or second trimester, frequently after *cardiac activity* has been detected. In women who have recurrent pregnancy loss, the incidence of anticardiolipin antibodies is 2 to 5%. The incidence of a positive lupus anticoagulant in recurrent pregnancy loss is 0.3 to 2%. There is a large amount of overlap, with both of these antibodies being positive in 60% of cases.

These antiphospholipid antibodies include those of the immunoglobulin G (IgG) and immunoglobulin M (IgM) classes, and these react against negatively charged phospholipids. Theories of how antiphospholipid antibodies cause pregnancy loss include inhibition of the thrombolytic system, thrombosis, infarction of the placenta, and abnormal prostacyclin metabolism.

Antiphospholipid syndrome is said to occur when an antiphospholipid antibody is associated with any of the following events: pregnancy loss, arterial or venous thrombosis, autoimmune thrombocytopenia, or autoimmune hemolytic anemia. Other rarer features that have been associated with antiphospholipid syndrome include livedo, chorea, pulmonary hypertension, and chronic leg ulcers. Thus, a thorough examination should be performed in patients suspected of having antiphospholipid syndrome.

Tests for anticardiolipin antibodies and lupus anticoagulant should be administered to women who have recurrent pregnancy losses. Routine testing for antinuclear antibodies (ANA) is not recommended. Numerous studies failed to find an association between an isolated positive ANA and pregnancy loss.

Treatment of antiphospholipid syndrome is noted in Table 3–6. Prednisone, low-dose aspirin (LDA) and heparin treatment have been studied most extensively in patients who have antiphospholipid antibodies and recurrent pregnancy loss. Prednisone suppresses production of antiphospholipid antibodies, whereas LDA inhibits platelet aggregation, increases the amount of prostacyclin, and decreases thromboxane production. Uniformly, pregnancy outcomes in treated patients were shown to be markedly improved over those in patients who received no treatment. Unfortunately, there are significant side effects associated with long-term prednisone therapy, including diabetes, hypertension, weight gain, and infection. Recently, subcutaneous heparin has gained popularity owing to its ability to prevent placental thrombosis. Heparin and LDA in combination appear to be the treatment of choice in antiphospholipid syndrome, with a live birth rate higher than 75 to 80% and significantly decreased pregnancy complications compared with treatment with prednisone. Complications of long-term heparin therapy include thrombocytopenia caused by the production of antiplatelet antibodies and osteoporosis complicated by fracture.

## UNEXPLAINED PREGNANCY LOSS

### Deficiency of Maternal Blocking Antibodies

The majority of pregnancy losses do not have a detectable underlying etiology. A proposed etiology is impaired maternal immunotolerance to the semiallogenic conceptor, resulting in a deficiency of maternal blocking antibodies. This theory makes the following assumptions:
1. There is an artificial maternal cell immune response in all pregnancies, which must be blocked.
2. Blocking antibodies develop in successful pregnancies.
3. In the absence of blocking antibodies, abortion of the fetus occurs.

**Table 3–6** Treatment of Antiphospholipid Syndrome During Pregnancy

---
Aspirin 80 mg daily
Heparin 10,000 to 15,000 U subcutaneously daily
Prednisone 60 mg to 80 mg orally daily
---

Unfortunately, none of the suppositions have been conclusively validated. In addition, many women who have successful pregnancies do not produce blocking antibodies.

### Human Leukocyte Antigen Sharing

Another theory of recurrent miscarriage is that human leukocyte antigen (HLA) similarity between maternal and paternal antigens results in the inability to produce maternal blocking antibodies. HLA antigens are the major determinants of histocompatibility in humans. These are derived from HLA genes on the short arm of chromosome 6 and are present on most nucleated cells in the body. Allogenic reactions are determined by the degree of incompatibility between cells. In theory, paternal HLA antigens induce a maternal allogenic reaction. If there is a high degree of HLA antigenic sharing, there is no maternal allogenic response and pregnancy loss occurs.

One problem with this theory is that research has not supported the concept that an intact maternal immune system is necessary for maintaining a normal pregnancy. In fact, genetically identical laboratory animals have been bred for generations without recurrent pregnancy loss.

Despite lack of substantiation, many treatments have been proposed for HLA compatibility to improve pregnancy outcome, and these treatments center around leukocyte immunization. The most popular method for alloimmune treatment is injecting the partner's leukocytes to improve maternal tolerance. Interpreting the results of leukocyte immunization has been difficult because of a lack of controlled trials. Many studies fail to control the fact that a woman who has recurrent pregnancy loss can have a 60 to 70% successful pregnancy rate without any treatment.

At present, the use of leukocyte immunization remains controversial at best. Controlled studies have not shown a statistically significant increase in births, although one study did show that there may be a slight increase in the live birth rate if adjustment is made for maternal age. Other immunization regimes, which have been shown to have no advantage over control groups, include third-party donor cells, trophoblast membrane infusion, and intravenous immunoglobulin.

## RECOMMENDATIONS FOR EVALUATION OF RECURRENT PREGNANCY LOSS

As stated previously, there is a debate over whether a workup for recurrent pregnancy loss should be performed after two or three losses. Many clinicians now begin a workup after two losses in women over 35 years of age or in women who are very anxious. We

**Table 3–7** Initial Workup for Recurrent Pregnancy Loss

HISTORY
Gestational age at time of loss
Establish whether cardiac activity was documented before previous losses
Obstetric and gynecologic history
Symptoms associated with antiphospholipid syndrome

PHYSICAL
Fibroid uterus or uterine anomalies
Signs of DES exposure

LABORATORY TEST
Lupus anticoagulant
Anticardiolipin antibody
Hysterosalpingogram
Endometrial biopsy
Parental karyotypes

DES = diethylstilbestrol.

recommend beginning a workup after two losses only if the previous pregnancies have included a documented viable pregnancy with *cardiac* activity present (Table 3–7).

## REFERENCES

Berry CW, Brambati B, Eskes TK, et al: The Euro-Team Early Pregnancy protocol for recurrent miscarriage. Hum Reprod 10:1516–1520, 1995.
Cook C, Pridham D: Recurrent pregnancy loss. Curr Opin Obstet Gynecol 7:357–366, 1995.
Daya S: Issues in the etiology of recurrent spontaneous abortion. Curr Opin Obstet Gynecol 6:253–259, 1994.
Fedele L, Bianchi S: Habitual abortion: Endocrinological aspects. Curr Opin Obstet Gynecol 7:351–356, 1995.
Geva E, Amit A, Lerner-Giva L, et al: Autoimmunity and reproduction. Fertil Steril 67:599–611, 1997.
Hill J: Sporadic and recurrent spontaneous abortion. Current problems in obstetrics. Gynecol Fertil 17:113–164, 1994.
Hutchins F: Uterine fibroids: Diagnosis and indication for treatment. Obstet Gynecol Clin North Am 22:459–465, 1995.
Katz V, Kuller J: Recurrent miscarriage. Am J Perinatol 11:386–397, 1994.
Leeuwen I, Branch D, Scott J: First trimester ultrasonography findings in women with a history of recurrent pregnancy loss. Am J Obstet Gynecol 168:111–114, 1993.
March C: Intrauterine adhesions. Obstet Gynecol Clin North Am 22:491–505, 1995.
Patton P: Anatomic uterine defects. Clin Obstet Gynecol 37:705–721, 1994.
Rai R, Clifford K, Regan L: The modern preventative treatment of recurrent miscarriage. Br J Obstet Gynaecol 103:106–110, 1996.
Rai R, Cohen H, Dave M, et al: Randomized controlled trial of aspirin and aspirin plus heparin in pregnant women with recurrent miscarriage associated with phospholipid antibodies. BMJ 314:253–257, 1997.
Scott J: Immunotherapy for recurrent miscarriage. The Cochrane Library 1:1–8, 1995.
Scott J: Recurrent miscarriage: Overview of recommendations. Clin Obstet Gynecol 37:765–773, 1994.
Silver R, Branch W: Recurrent miscarriage: Autoimmune considerations. Clin Obstet Gynecol 37:745–760, 1994.
Stern J, Coulam C: Current status of immunologic recurrent pregnancy loss. Curr Opin Obstet Gynecol 5:252–259, 1993.
Stirrat GM: Recurrent miscarriage. I: Definition and epidemiology. Lancet 336:673–675, 1990.

# 4

# Ectopic Pregnancy

THOMAS G. STOVALL

An ectopic pregnancy occurs when the blastocyst implants in any tissue other than the endometrium that lines the uterus. An ectopic pregnancy, which may be tubal, abdominal, ovarian, or uterine in its location (Table 4–1), occurs once in every 40 to 100 pregnancies.

## Epidemiology

The incidence of ectopic pregnancy has increased during the last two decades. The National Hospital Discharge Survey conducted by the National Center for Health Sciences obtains comprehensive data regarding ectopic pregnancies, and this information is compiled by the Centers for Disease Control. The incidence of ectopic pregnancy has tripled since 1970, increasing annually through 1994, but more recently the incidence has leveled off. This condition causes major maternal mortality, adversely affects future reproductive prospects, and contributes significantly to the economic burden of health care for women.

**Table 4–1** Sites of Occurrence

- Fallopian Tube, 97% of ectopic pregnancies occur in the tube (most commonly in the ampullary portion followed by the isthmic and interstitial portions)
- Abdominal Pregnancy, 1.0%
  Primary: A primary abdominal pregnancy occurs when fertilization and implantation take place in the peritoneal cavity
  Secondary: A secondary abdominal pregnancy is more common and occurs when implantation follows tubal abortion or rupture
- Uterine, 1.5%
  Cornual ectopic pregnancies are usually difficult to diagnose; bleeding may be profuse if rupture occurs
  Cervical implantation occurs in and around the internal cervical os; in this rare condition, patients present with profuse bleeding early in pregnancy
- Ovarian Pregnancy, rare, 0.5%
- Heterotrophic Pregnancy, 1 of every 30,000 ectopic pregnancies is a combined intrauterine and ectopic gestation

## Morbidity and Mortality

Despite the reduction in mortality for ectopic pregnancy, this condition remains a major cause of maternal mortality, causing 5 to 6% of all maternal deaths in the United States. However, the death rate decreased dramatically from 1970 to 1976, and continued to fall from 1977 to 1986. In 1984, 39 women died as a result of ectopic pregnancy; 33 died in 1985; and 36 died in 1986. The case fatality rates, for these 3 years ranked between 4.2 and 5.2 deaths out of a total of 10,000 ectopic pregnancies. A study of 86 deaths, which occurred among 102,100 cases of ectopic pregnancy in the United States during 1979 and 1980, revealed that 77% of these women sought medical care, 100% complained of pain, and 85% died as a result of acute hemorrhage. Error in diagnosis occurred in 49% of the cases, in which ectopic pregnancies were commonly confused with gastrointestinal disorders, intrauterine pregnancy, or pelvic inflammatory disease. More than half of these deaths might have been prevented if patients or providers had acted more expeditiously. Eclopic pregnancy is the leading cause of maternal mortality in the first trimester and the single leading cause of maternal deaths in black women. Although morbidity has been markedly reduced because of early diagnosis and better treatment methods, it is still substantial.

Overall, the pregnancy rate following an ectopic gestation is only 60%. The chance of a live birth following surgical treatment of an ectopic pregnancy is approximately 40%. The recurrent rate of ectopic pregnancy for patients who have had a previous tubal ectopic pregnancy is 15 to 20%. The recurrence rate is dependent on several variables, including treatment modality, status of the contralateral tube, and other associated infertility factors, as well as the underlying etiology of the ectopic pregnancy itself.

## Etiology

The reasons for increased numbers of ectopic pregnancies are not clearly understood, but they can be attributed in part to better reporting, improved diagnostic tools for the detection of this condition, and acquired risks for this disease in the reproductive population of women (Table 4–2). The most significant risk factor is scarring of the pelvic viscera caused by previous infection. Pelvic infection increases the chance of a woman's having an ectopic pregnancy and also greatly reduces her subsequent fertility. The incidence of pelvic infection has also been increasing. Reparative pelvic surgery, previous sterilization, gamete technology (intrafallopian or intrauterine placement of a gamete or zygote), congenital tubal anomalies, and diethylstilbestrol (DES) exposure in utero contribute to the occurrence of ectopic pregnancies. However, these factors are much less important than acquired pelvic disease (caused by previous infection or pelvic surgery). Finally, as a national trend, many women are deferring childbirth until late in their reproductive lives. The risk of ectopic gestation is greater in older women, and this sociologic shift has occurred with sufficient magnitude to become an important contributor to the incidence of ectopic pregnancy. Smoking also appears to be an independent risk factor for development of ectopic pregnancy.

## Diagnosis

Before to the last two decades, most women (85%) who had an ectopic pregnancy were diagnosed only after tubal leakage or rupture occurred. Quantitation of human chorionic gonadotropin (hCG) and serum progesterone combined with pelvic sonography can now diagnose a tubal pregnancy before it ruptures (Table 4–3). When symptoms are present, abdominal pain occurs in 85 to 100% of women who have an ectopic pregnancy. The pain is caused by peritoneal stretching of the expanding fallopian tube or blood in the peritoneal cavity as a result of tubal regurgitation or rupture. Unfortunately, abdominal pain is a common gynecologic complaint.

The second most common symptom associated with extrauterine pregnancy is abnormal vaginal bleeding that occurs as the result of insufficient hormonal support of the decidualized endometrium. The triad of pelvic pain, abnormal vaginal bleeding, and an adnexal mass represents the classic hallmark of an ectopic pregnancy. Unfortunately, the severity of the symptoms and their common association are dependent upon the duration of the gestation at the time when the patient seeks medical attention. This triad is present in only one third of ectopic gestations, and it usually occurs in advanced cases. In general, the adnexal mass of an ectopic pregnancy develops late, and its detection by vaginal examination is made difficult by the patient's discomfort.

The general procedure for establishing a diagnosis of ectopic pregnancy includes an abdominal-pelvic examination, an assessment of hemodynamic stability, ultrasonography, and laboratory testing (Table 4–4). A general abdominal palpation should identify tenderness, peritoneal irritation, guarding, and bowel sounds. The pelvic examination should estimate the position, size, and consistency of the uterus and describe any adnexal mass or tenderness. The cervix

**Table 4–2** Risk Factors for Ectopic Pregnancy

Previous pelvic inflammatory disease
Previous pelvic surgery
Tubal ligation
Previous ectopic pregnancy
Concomitant IUD use
Assistive reproductive technology
Advanced maternal age
DES exposure
Smoking

IUD = intrauterine device; DES = diethylstilbestrol.

**Table 4–3** Symptoms of Ectopic Pregnancy

| | |
|---|---|
| Pain, 100% | Nausea, 25% |
| Amenorrhea, 75% | Syncope, 10% |
| Bleeding, 65% | Tissue passage, 5% |

**Table 4–4** General Physical Examination and Basic Laboratory Testing

| | |
|---|---|
| Vital signs | CBC |
| Orthostatic changes (tilt) | Urine or serum pregnancy testing |
| Abdominal palpation | Blood type + Rh factor |
| Pelvic examination | |

CBC = complete blood count.

should be inspected to determine whether the product of conception is in the os (incomplete abortion) or if the os is dilated (inevitable abortion). Vital signs should be monitored, including pulse and blood pressure. The pulse and blood pressure testing can be repeated with the patient in the upright position to identify hemodynamic compromise (postural hypotension is characterized by a rise in pulse rate of 20 beats per minute, a drop in diastolic blood pressure of 15 mm Hg, or both).

Basic laboratory testing should include a blood count to assess hemoglobin or hematocrit levels. A urine or serum pregnancy test should be done, because, if negative, the likelihood of an ectopic pregnancy is very small. Importantly, the patient's blood type and Rh factor should be obtained to determine whether RhoGAM (anti-Du IgG) is indicated.

A slight elevation in temperature may be found (rarely above 101°F [38°C]), especially if there is a hemoperitoneum that is uncomplicated by concurrent infection. Blood pressure and pulse rate are usually normal, although a slight tachycardia associated with pain or anxiety is not uncommon. Tachycardia and hypotension are seen with ruptured ectopic pregnancy, although young healthy women have a considerable cardiovascular reserve; therefore, blood loss may be quite extensive before any noteworthy changes in heart rate and blood pressure are manifest.

When an ectopic pregnancy is ruptured, an acute abdomen and shock are often encountered. The patient complains of generalized crampy lower quadrant pain, often accompanied by referred pain in the shoulder, which is a result of diaphragmatic irritation caused by the presence of intraperitoneal blood. Other signs and symptoms may be obscured by pain and bowel sounds. This condition requires swift diagnostic confirmation, initial emergency measures, and immediate surgery. One should not, however, be misled by the patient who appears to be in no distress, because there is great variation in the presentation of patients who have significant intra-abdominal bleeding. When an unruptured ectopic pregnancy is present, the patient is usually a symptomatic or has only minor symptoms that could be attributed to an intrauterine pregnancy. In this situation, diagnosis is based upon a careful history, risk factor assessment, physical examination, pregnancy testing, serum progesterone screening, ultrasonography, dilatation and curettage, and laparoscopy.

Referred shoulder pain, if present, results from diaphragmatic irritation caused by a hemoperitoneum. The severity of such pain does not correlate with the amount of intra-abdominal bleeding. Listlessness, syncope, and fainting while straining at bowel movement are less commonly seen. Other subjective symptoms of pregnancy, such as breast tenderness, nausea, and urinary frequency are seen in 50 to 75% of patients.

## PELVIC EXAMINATION

With a ruptured ectopic pregnancy, the pelvic examination is typically characterized by a markedly tender abdomen, with pain on cervical motion or palpation of the uterus or adnexae. The cul-de-sac may be distended, the blood causing the septum to bulge into the posterior vaginal fornix.

The cervix may be normal in appearance, or it may be discolored (bluish) and soft. Some degree of cervical motion tenderness is common. The cervix may be dilated, with passage of blood and, occasionally, tissue, this latter manifestation is often confused with incomplete or threatened abortion. The decidual tissue is cast. It is passed, whole or in fragments, as the viability of the gestation wanes.

The uterus may be soft, tender, and enlarged, or it may seem normal. Deviation of the uterus to one side may indicate the presence of an adnexal mass, but this may represent a large corpus luteum as well as an ectopic gestation. A cornual pregnancy may palpably simulate an enlarged uterus.

A discrete adnexal mass or fullness is found in less than half of the patients who have ectopic pregnancies; therefore, the absence of an adnexal mass does not rule out an ectopic pregnancy. Conversely, a palpable mass may represent a corpus luteum of early pregnancy or an other ovarian neoplasm; therefore, the presence of a palpable adnexal mass does not equate with the existence of an ectopic pregnancy.

## PATHOLOGY

A fertilized ovum is implanted into the tubal mucosa. Rapid invasion of a trophoblast follows, with an extension from the tubal lumen into the connective tissue between the serosa and the endosalpinx. A hematoma in this space grows as the pregnancy advances, leading to bleeding from the distal aspect of the tube.

- Diagnosis is made of chorionic villi in the tube.
- Decidual reaction occurs in the uterine mucosa.
- An Arias-Stella reaction occurs, which is not

specific for ectopic pregnancy. This reaction is characterized by the presence of large epithelial cells with large nuclei and hypertrophic irregular nucleoli.

## LABORATORY TESTING AND DIAGNOSTIC PROCEDURS

Laboratory examination and diagnostic procedures are needed, because the history, physical examination, and assessment of risk factor are significant in fewer than 50% of cases. In an unruptured ectopic pregnancy, a correct diagnosis cannot be made without further testing. A complete blood count (CBC) is mandatory for determining the patient's hematologic status as a potential surgical candidate. Pregnancy testing is essential.

The levels of hCG secreted in normal gestations differ from those secreted in abnormal gestations; therefore, measurements of his hormone can be highly predictive of both gestational normalcy and early pregnancy abnormalities (Table 4–5). hCG doubles in a normal pregnancy at approximately 2 day intervals during the first 42 days of gestation. The amount of hCG produced varies with gestational age. The rate of hCG doubling is more rapid in early gestation (1.4 to 1.5 days to double) than in a pregnancy approaching 7 to 8 weeks (3.3 to 3.5 days to double). After approximately 7 to 8 weeks of gestation, the hCG titer peaks and then declines. As a consequence, hCG doubling is generally not helpful after 7 to 8 weeks of gestation. Clinically, after about 5 to 6 weeks of gestation, the measurement of hCG doubling is unimportant. Tubal pregnancies have a slower doubling time, and a 85% of them show less than a 66% increase in hCG concentration in a 48-hour interval. An abnormal doubling time, however, is not uniformly associated with an abnormal gestation. Fifteen percent of normal intrauterine pregnancies have slow hCG doubling. Additionally, hCG doubling times cannot discriminate between an ectopic pregnancy and an intrauterine abortion.

Current urinary pregnancy tests using monoclonal antibody technology are very sensitive (often to 50 mIU/ml β-hCG); if the test is positive, a pregnancy, but not its location, is established; if the test is negative, a pregnancy at any location is very unlikely. If the physician wishes to use quantitative β hCG titers in analyzing the pregnancy, a more sensitive serum pregnancy test should be done. Radioimmunoassay (RIA) for hCG using β-hCG antibodies (RIA for β-hCG) is very sensitive and capable of detecting gestation as early as 8 to 10 days postfertilization owing to a test sensitivity of 0.5 to 10 mIU/ml of serum. RIA for β-hCG is pregnancy-specific because the antibody is raised against the β-subunit of hCG, which is different from the β-subunit of the luteinizing hormone of (LH). With a negative β-hCG, an ectopic pregnancy can be effectively discounted. Each physician must learn which tests are available in his or her hospital, as well as the sensitivities and characteristics of each. hCG, produced by the syncytiotrophoblast, indicates a pregnancy but does not identify its location. Because hCG levels may be low in an ectopic pregnancy, the more sensitive the test, the higher the frequency of positive results. hCG concentrations, plotted individually or in a serially comparative manner against the duration of amenorrhea, have little diagnostic value because the actual times of ovulation and conception are not known for most patients. Also, 10% of women who have a normal gestation have a single hCG level lower than the 90% confidence limits set for a particular gestational age. A combined pregnancy, multiple ectopic pregnancies, or a viable ectopic pregnancy may not fit this pattern and may demonstrate relatively high hCG titers. Rarely, non–pregnancy-associated ectopic production of hCG caused by carcinoma of the bronchus, stomach, liver, pancreas, or breast, or by multiple myeloma or melanoma may confuse the clinical situation.

## SERUM PROGESTERONE

The progesterone concentration in an ectopic pregnancy is generally lower than the normal concentration found in an intrauterine pregnancy. In retrospective studies, Yeko and associates and Matthews and

**Table 4–5** Human Chorionic Gonadotropin (hCG)

- Detectable in maternal serum 8 days after the LH surge
- Rises exponentially to peak at about 8–10 wk of gestation (dated from LMP); thereafter falls to nadir from 16–24 wk
- At a serum concentration of >10,000 mIU/ml, the doubling time of hCG among different individuals is more varied
- In ectopic pregnancy, hCG generally increases more slowly than during normal pregnancy, with a 50–66% rise over 48 hr; interassay variability 10–15%
- Plateaued levels are the most predictive of ectopic pregnancy

Use in nonlaparoscopic algorithm:

- Persistent abnormal rise (<50% in 48 hr); undergo D&C if hCG at 62,000 mIU/ml
- Plateaued level (±15%), undergo D&C
- Used to time vaginal ultrasonogram at hCG levels of ≥2000 mIU/ml; Third International Preparation can visualize intrauterine sac in all normal IUPs
- Fall in hCG level following D&C
- A plateaued or rising level after D&C indicates persistent trophoblastic tissue
- Level ≤50,000 rarely (<0.1%) associated with ectopic pregnancy

LH = luteinizing hormone; LMP = last menstrual period; D&C = dilatation and curettage; IUP = intrauterine pregnancy.

associates demonstrated that all ectopic pregnancies were associated with a serum progesterone lower than 15 ng/ml, whereas all normal intrauterine pregnancies had progesterone levels equal to, or greater than, 15 ng/ml.

At the University of Tennessee, Memphis, our initial prospective study using serum progesterone revealed a considerable overlap in progesterone values for normal and abnormal pregnancies. Subsequent to this initial investigation, additional studies have been completed. At present, we have obtained serum progesterone samples in approximately 10,000 first-trimester pregnancies. The results of these trials confirm the role of serum progesterone in the diagnosis of ectopic pregnancy.

Serum progesterone may be used as a screening test for abnormal pregnancy. Only 1 to 2% of abnormal pregnancies (abortions or ectopic pregnancies) are associated with a progesterone level greater than, or equal to 25 ng/ml. Serum progesterone is also helpful in identifying a nonviable pregnancy. Although it is uncommon (1:10,000) to identify a viable pregnancy in association with a serum progesterone less than, or equal to, 5.0 ng/ml, two cases have been seen. Both patients had viable intrauterine pregnancies in association with a serum progesterone of 3.9 ng/ml.

## ULTRASONOGRAPHY

In the patient who is not acutely ill and who has a positive pregnancy test and findings suggestive of an ectopic pregnancy, ultrasonography is indicated. At defined hCG titers, ultrasonography is excellent for identifying an intrauterine pregnancy, because the gestational sac is clearly seen against the homogenous uterine shadow (Table 4–6). The prominent ring of echoes against the uniform density of the uterus of an intrauterine pregnancy is recognized by transabdominal ultrasound at 5 to 6 weeks of gestation measured from the first day of the last menstrual period, when the chorionic sac is 10 mm in diameter. Fetal heart activity is seen at 7 weeks of gestation. Transvaginal ultrasonography is able to identify an intrauterine pregnancy 1 to 2 weeks earlier. When an intrauterine pregnancy is demonstrated, an extrauterine pregnancy is effectively excluded (except for a rare combined pregnancy). Quantitative values for β-hCG may aid in evaluation of the sonographic images. It has been suggested that a range of 6000 to 6500 mIU/ml of β-hCG may be used as a "discriminatory hCG zone" for transabdominal ultrasound, and hCG levels for a transvaginal ultrasound scan are in the range of 1500 to 2000 mIU/ml hCG. The pregnancy may be assumed to be ectopic if it is not identified in the intrauterine position. Below these values, the sonographic diagnosis of intrauterine pregnancy may not be possible. In this case, serial evaluation or combination testing with other diagnostic modalities may be indicated.

Care must be taken not to confuse an early normal intrauterine pregnancy with a nonviable blighted ovum, characterized by an intrauterine echo with an irregular internal wall shadow, a volume of less than 2.5 ml, and the absence of a fetal pole. A blighted ovum, and to a lesser extent, an early intrauterine pregnancy, may in turn be confused with a decidual cast.

With all the sophistication of analysis and technique presently available, it is important to keep in mind the scope of disorders that may confuse an ultrasonographic evaluation of the pelvis for ectopic pregnancy. A differential list of the common ultrasonographic findings is presented in Table 4–1. Rarely, an ectopic pregnancy may be sonographically identified in the adnexa or other extrauterine positions, thus fulfilling Kobayashi's ultrasonographic criteria for ectopic pregnancy: diffuse, amorphous uterine echoes; uterine enlargement; absence of an intrauterine sac; an extrauterine irregular mass or a poorly defined extrauterine mass containing some echoes; and, at the same time, visualization of an extrauterine ectopic fetus.

When using transabdominal scanning, it is important to provide adequate bladder distention. The distended bladder pushes the bowel and other structures away from the top of the uterus so that their shadows do not confuse the ultrasonographic picture coming from within the uterus, and, in addition, the bladder provides an anatomic reference point for the many structures found in the pelvis. Such distention may be provided by giving the patient fluids (either orally or intravenously) or by placing a Foley catheter and distending the bladder with sterile saline solution. Care must be taken to neither overdistend nor underdistend the bladder. Overdistention is a common error that causes flattening and deformation of the uterus and any structures that may be contained therein. An exception is found in the case of the retroverted uterus, however, in which "overdistention" may help to achieve resolution of the intrauterine details by straightening the uterus. With transva-

**Table 4–6** Role of Transvaginal Ultrasound

- Identify gestational sac, which essentially excludes a diagnosis of ectopic pregnancy
- Identify ectopic pregnancy >3.5 cm in greatest dimension which is a contraindication to medical therapy
- Identify adnexal cardiac activity, which is a relative contraindication to medical therapy
- Color Doppler scanning allows differentiation of a complete abortion, an incomplete abortion, and an early intrauterine pregnancy before visualization of a gestational sac

ginal scanning, bladder distention is neither required nor desired.

## CULDOCENTESIS

Culdocentesis is a test that was popular before the development and widespread availability of rapid hCG measurements and sensitive sonography. Culdocentesis determines the presence of a hemoperitoneum. This test is 90% predictive of blood in the abdomen when the result is positive, and just as reliable when the result is negative. To be positive, the hematocrit of blood peritoneal fluid should be greater than 15%. However, culdocentesis is invasive and painful. If fluid is not seen in the cul-de-sac on vaginal sonography, culdocentesis is usually nondiagnostic. Therefore, in my practice, I generally perform culdocentesis only when clinically significant fluid is visualized, and if the information derived from the test will alter management of the case.

## DILATATION AND CURETTAGE

Examination of endometrial tissue is indicated in the presence of an abnormal pregnancy of uncertain location. Such tissue examination has not been useful in the diagnosis of ectopic pregnancy if the Arias-Stella reaction is found, because it is absent in about half to three fourths of patients, and, like the decidual reaction, it may be associated with other disorders. The absence of chorionic villi, however, is highly suggestive of either ectopic pregnancy or completed abortion, and further investigation involving repeat hCG testing is indicated. In some circumstances, intrauterine pregnancy may be possible in a patient whose clinical presentation suggests ectopic pregnancy.

## DIAGNOSTIC LAPAROSCOPY

Diagnostic laparoscopy is the gold standard for diagnosis and should be used when there is uncertainty of diagnosis. When the patient is hemodynamically stable and without a significant hemoperitoneum, diagnostic laparoscopy allows direct evaluation of the pelvis. This procedure permits an early diagnosis of an unruptured ectopic pregnancy. When an unruptured ectopic gestation is discovered, conservative treatments are more likely to be feasible. A contraindication to laparoscopy is an unstable patient. Abdominal hernia or repair is a relative contraindication to laparoscopy, as is the presence of an ileus.

## COMBINATION TESTING

Because no single noninvasive modality can diagnose an ectopic pregnancy in all situations, algorithms combining several of the previously mentioned diagnostic modalities are useful (see Table 4–6). A nonlaparoscopic algorithm is now available. The rationale is that a combination of diagnostic modalities may facilitate medical management of many ectopic pregnancies without laparoscopy. The following observations form the basis for this belief:

1. Transvaginal ultrasonography (TVU) can readily identify an intrauterine gestational sac with an hCG level greater than, or equal to, 2000 mIU/ml.
2. An hCG titer that is plateaued or that increases less than 50% over 45 hours is predictive of a nonviable pregnancy.
3. Chorionic villi can be recovered and identified by curettage; thus confirming a nonviable intrauterine pregnancy.
4. A rising hCG titer showing no villi following curettage suggests viable trophoblastic tissue.
5. TVU, a technique more sensitive than transabdominal ultrasonography, can be used to detect an ectopic pregnancy less than, or equal to, 3.5 cm in size, which is suitable for nonsurgical treatment.
6. Outpatient administration methotrexate is safe and effective for the treatment of ectopic pregnancy.

Employing these diagnostic tools, a prospective trial was conducted in which 34 patients were randomized into one of two groups:

1. Patients who had confirmatory diagnostic laparoscopy before methotrexate therapy
2. Patients who received immediate methotrexate therapy

All of the 17 patients who were presumptively diagnosed as having an ectopic pregnancy and who underwent laparoscopy did indeed have an ectopic pregnancy. In this series, laparoscopy did not add either to the safety or to the success of medical therapy. This randomized trial demonstrated the nonsurgical algorithm to be 100% accurate in the diagnosis of unruptured ectopic pregnancy.

# Surgical Management

Surgical management of an ectopic pregnancy is the mainstay of treatment and the standard to which other treatments are compared. All ectopic pregnancies can be managed surgically, but, under certain circumstances, surgical management is the only alternative. Obviously, if a patient comes to the emergency department in hypovolemic shock, the need for surgical intervention is not questioned. However, in the stable individual, indications for the use of surgery are outlined in Table 4–7. Other than the unstable

**Table 4–7** Indications for Surgical Treatment of Ectopic Pregnancy in Stable Patients

1. Patient refuses medical management
2. Ectopic implantation >3.5 cm in greatest dimension by ultrasonography
3. Evidence of rupture by ultrasonography
4. Unsure diagnosis
5. Previous tubal ligation
6. Contraindication to medical therapy

---

patient in hypovolemic shock, most women who have ectopic pregnancies are candidates for laparoscopic intervention. It is estimated that 4 to 5% of women who have ectopic pregnancies present in shock. Excluding another 5 to 10% who would require conversion for treatment from laparoscopy to laparotomy, over 80% of women could be treated via laparoscopy. In the hands of an experienced laparoscopist, the rate of conversion to laparotomy should remain low.

Both laparotomy and laparoscopy have been extensively used for the diagnosis and management of ectopic pregnancy. Laparoscopic treatment requires a greater degree of surgical skill but is thought to decrease cost and postoperative hospital stay. Laparoscopic management also avoids the risk of laparotomy. Laparotomy is generally indicated if:
1. The patient is hemodynamically unstable.
2. The skills of the surgeon favor laparotomy.
3. The patient has a contraindication to laparoscopy.
4. The ectopic pregnancy is cornual or abdominal.

Several published reports have compared laparoscopy with laparotomy for the treatment of ectopic pregnancy in women who are hemodynamically stable. Outcome factors, such as days of hospitalization, blood loss, operating time, cost, pain medication use, adhesion formation, and subsequent pregnancies have been studied.

Vermesh and associates randomizly assigned 60 women who had unruptured ectopic pregnancies smaller than 5 cm to either laparoscopy or laparotomy linear salpingostomy. Mean blood loss was statistically less for laparoscopy (79 ml) when compared with laparotomy (195 ml). However, two patients in the laparoscopy group required laparotomy to achieve hemostasis after the salpingostomy was performed. No differences were noted in incidence of postoperative fever or wound infection. One patient in each group required a second operation for rising hCG levels after surgery. Hospital stay was shorter per patient (1.4 vs. 3.3 days) for laparoscopy. This translated to a savings of $1500. Postoperative hysterosalpingogram showed patency in the involved tube in 16 of 20 (80%) laparoscopy patients and 17 of 19 (89%) laparotomy patients. Subsequent pregnancy rates were also not different.

Brumsted and associates compared laparoscopy and laparotomy for the treatment of ectopic pregnancy, randomizing 25 women to each group. The postoperative length of stay was significantly shorter in the laparoscopy group (1.34 vs. 3.42 days), as was return to normal activity (8.7 vs. 25.7 days). Postoperative pain, as measured by the number of doses of intramuscular or intravenous analgesia, was also significantly less in the laparoscopy group (0.84 vs. 4.64).

Murphy and associates prospectively assigned 26 women who had suspected ectopic pregnancies to treatment with laparoscopy and 37 women to laparotomy in a university-based residency training program. Operative and postoperative parameters were similar to those in previously reported studies. Patients treated by laparoscopy had reduced estimated blood loss (62 vs. 115 ml) and reduced need for analgesia (26 vs. 58 mg). The length of stay was also shorter (26 vs. 634 hours), as were the patient hospital charges ($5528 vs. $6793). Finally, patients who underwent laparoscopy had a shorter time to the return of normal activity (17 vs. 62 days).

Sultana and associates reviewed 126 cases of ectopic pregnancy at the Cleveland Clinic Foundation and compared rates of pregnancy and term deliveries among women who had had laparoscopic salpingostomy, laparotomy with salpingostomy, or laparotomy with salpingectomy. Crude pregnancy rates were no different among any of the three study groups. A history of previous infertility was a significant predictor of subsequent pregnancy rates. As noted earlier, Vermesh and associates noted no difference in subsequent outcomes in women who had salpingostomy by laparoscopy or laparotomy.

In summary, the laparoscopic approach is associated with equal or shorter operating times, shorter hospital stays and convalescence, lower analgesic needs, and potentially lower costs. However, other factors must be considered.

There is evidence to suggest that the conservative laparoscopic approach of salpingostomy has a higher incidence of persistent trophoblast than does laparotomy. Seifer and associates found that 15.5% (16 of 103) of women who underwent laparoscopic salpingostomy had persistent hCG levels compared with only 1.8% (1 of 54) of women who had salpingostomy via laparotomy. Murphy and associates found that three patients who had laparoscopic salpingostomy had a persistent hCG titer compared with none in those who underwent laparotomy. However, the study group of Vermesh and associates showed no differences in persistent hCG levels after laparoscopy or laparotomy, although the incidence of persistent trophoblast is lower after laparoscopic salpingostomy. Regardless of the method of treatment, hCG levels must be followed until they are negative so that persistence can be diagnosed and treated.

Lundorff and associates performed second-look laparoscopy on 73 women who had been treated by laparoscopy or laparotomy for ectopic pregnancy. Adhesions were statistically more common on both the involved and contralateral sides in women who underwent laparotomy.

When the ectopic pregnancy is managed surgically, several concepts must be considered, regardless of whether the ectopic pregnancy is managed by laparoscopy or laparotomy. Although the contralateral fallopian tube often appears normal on gross inspection, as many as half have significant microscopic abnormalities. Careful inspection of the tube is important (with discussion of findings in the operative note), but microsurgical intervention is not advisable at the initial surgery. Ablative surgery (salpingectomy, salpingo-oophorectomy, hysterectomy) may be necessary if irreparable damage has been done to the reproductive structures. When possible, however, conservative surgical procedures (salpingostomy, partial salpingectomy) should be performed, especially when the patient desires to maintain her maximal reproductive capability. In general, the initial surgery should be restricted to removal of the ectopic pregnancy and preservation of as much of the reproductive tract as possible. Reconstructive surgery should be done at a second operation after tissue edema and hyperemia have resolved and after a complete reproductive evaluation of the patient has been completed.

## SPECIFIC SURGICAL MANAGEMENT

The choice of surgical procedure depends on the specific implantation site of the ectopic pregnancy, the amount of anatomic damage done by the ectopic pregnancy (whether ruptured or unruptured), and the patient's desire for future fertility. In each case, the operating surgeon must weigh these factors to decide upon the appropriate surgical approach.

Ipsilateral salpingectomy is the most commonly performed procedure, primarily because it is rapid, simple, and effective. The procedure is indicated if the fallopian tube is damaged beyond repair or if the extra time needed for a nonablative procedure is not justified based on the patient's desire for future fertility. When a salpingectomy is performed, care must be taken to preserve the vascular supply of the ipsilateral ovary.

Oophorectomy is indicated only if the ovary is damaged beyond salvage or if the ovary shows a pathologic condition for which oophorectomy is indicated. Ipsilateral oophorectomy was formerly the commonly used management technique, because it was thought to reduce recurrence of ectopic pregnancy caused by ovum transmigration and the associated delay in ovum pickup. There is no evidence to support this concept. Thus, all viable ovarian tissue should be retained.

Hysterectomy may be indicated if there is extensive damage to the reproductive tract or if there is concomitant disease of the uterus, which, under other circumstances, would warrant hysterectomy. Hysterectomy as a routine procedure is not indicated, even if both fallopian tubes are damaged, because in vitro fertilization and other techniques are available for the couple who desire pregnancy.

Cornual resection has been advocated in the past to decrease the incidence of repeat ectopic pregnancy, especially the isthmic type. However, no data support its effectiveness, and it may actually lead to an increased incidence of interstitial ectopic pregnancy and uterine rupture. In addition, if an intrauterine pregnancy follows cornual resection, delivery may have to be performed by cesarean section because of the risk of uterine rupture at the site of the cornual resection.

Linear salpingostomy (with and without closure) is performed, if possible, on the antimesenteric border of the tube to minimize disruption of the blood supply to the fallopian tubes. The decision of whether to close the incision is controversial and is left to the surgeon. Segmental resection and subsequent reanastomosis are used in isthmic tubal pregnancy when linear salpingostomy is not feasible because of the extent of damage to the fallopian tube. Whether to proceed with anastomosis at the first operation is an individual surgical decision. Anastomosis does provide a nidus for infection. Rh immunoglobulin (RhoGAM) should be administered to all Rh-negative, unsensitized women within 72 hours of surgery for ectopic pregnancy.

# Nonsurgical Management

In an effort to eliminate the risk of surgery, a number of medical regimens and agents have been studied. At the present time, methotrexate (MTX) appears to be the agent of choice for medical management. MTX has been used extensively for the treatment of trophoblastic disease and for the treatment of placental tissue left in situ after exploration for an abdominal pregnancy. In 1982, Tanaka and associates treated an unruptured interstitial ectopic gestation with a 15-day course of intramuscular MTX. Following this, a few case reports described limited experience with use of MTX in unusual presentations of ectopic pregnancies. Miyazaki in 1983 and Ory in 1986 published the first clinical studies using MTX as the primary treatment for ectopic pregnancy.

To expand and validate these early reports, a prospective outpatient treatment protocol was begun at the University of Tennessee, Memphis. Our initial report detailed 36 patients who were treated with MTX and citrovorum factor (CF). Thirty-four (94.4%) of these patients had a successful outcome, with complete resolution of their ectopic pregnancy. Two patients experienced rupture after chemotherapy. In 1 patient, the ectopic pregnancy ruptured 23 days after treatment. There were no major chemotherapy-related side effects, and only 3 of 36 (8.3%) patients experienced a minor side effect. From this study, the following conclusions were drawn:

1. Individualized dosing of outpatient MTX-CF can be safely managed on an outpatient basis, even in an indigent population.
2. Ectopic pregnancy rupture can occur up to 23 days after chemotherapy initiation.
3. Fetal cardiac activity is a relative contraindication to medical therapy.

One hundred patients were treated with the multidose outpatient protocol, a 96% success rate. Cardiac activity in an ectopic pregnancy is not an absolute contraindication to medical therapy. The multidose protocol is shown in Table 4–8. When using this protocol, CF should be given on the day following the MTX dose, even if no further MTX is indicated. Patients are instructed to refrain from sexual intercourse until there is complete resolution of the ectopic pregnancy (hCG <15 mIU/ml), to avoid vitamins containing folic acid, and not to use alcohol while taking MTX. As an additional precaution, patients are asked to use oral contraceptives or double-barrier contraception for 1 to 2 months following treatment or until a hysterosalpingogram can be obtained (usually after the first or second menstrual period following treatment completion). Patients who have iron deficiency anemia are given iron sulfate, 325 mg, two or three times per day. RhoGAM is given if the patient is Rh negative. Absolute contraindications to MTX therapy include active liver or renal disease and tubal rupture. Using this protocol, our incidence of MTX-related side effects was approximately 3 to 4%. All side effects were mild, and the incidence of failure (nonresponders or tubal rupture) was approximately 5%.

Weekly intramuscular administration of MTX without CF (Table 4–9) has been reported for the treatment of nonmetastatic gestational trophoblastic disease. Single-dose MTX for ectopic pregnancy was first reported by Stovall and associates. The initial report detailed 31 patients who were treated with a single injection of MTX (50 mg/m$^2$) without CF rescue, using the same criteria as the multidose protocol. Twenty-nine of 30 (96.7%) patients were successfully treated. No patients experienced side effects. The number of patients was expanded to include 120 patients who were treated with this protocol. Patients had a mean hCG titer before treatment initiation of $3950 \pm 1193$ mIU/ml. TVU visualized cardiac activity in 14 (11.9%) patients, but an ectopic pregnancy was visualized in 113 (94.2%) patients. One hundred thirteen of 120 (94.2%) patients were successfully treated, with 4 (3.3%) of these patients requiring a second dose on day 7. The mean time to achieve pregnancy was $3.1 \pm 1.1$ months. To date, 315 patients have been reported with similar results in other studies.

Ransom reported that a serum progesterone level of less than 10 ng/ml was useful in predicting resolution of an ectopic pregnancy that was treated with MTX, whereas a serum progesterone higher than

**Table 4–8** Outpatient Multidose Protocol for Methotrexate Treatment

| Day | Time | Therapy |
|---|---|---|
| 1. | Variable | CBC, SGOT, MTX, β-hCG, Blood type+Rh, BUN, Creatinine |
| 2. | 8:00 AM | CF, β-hCG |
| 3. | 8:00 AM | MTX, β-hCG |
| 4. | 8:00 AM | CF, β-hCG |
| 5. | 8:00 AM | MTX, β-hCG |
| 6. | 8:00 AM | CG, β-hCG |
| 7. | 8:00 AM | MTX, β-hCG |
| 8. | 8:00 AM | CF, β-hCG |

CBC = complete blood count with differential and platelet count
SGOT = Serum glutamic oxalacetic, transaminase, U/L
MTX = Intramuscular methotrexate, 1.0 mg/kg
β-hCG = Quantitative beta-human chorionic gonatropin mIU/ml
CF = Intramuscular citrovorum, 0.1 mg/kg
BUN = Blood urea nitrogen

MTX is alternated with CF until there is a decrease in the hCG titer. If MTX has been given, it is always followed by CG.

**Table 4–9** Single-Dose Methotrexate Protocol

| Day | |
|---|---|
| 0 | hCG, D&C, CBC, SGOT, BUN, Creatinine, Blood Type+Rh |
| 1 | MTX, hCG |
| 4 | hCG |
| 7 | hCG |

- If <15% decline in hCG titer between days 4 and 7, give second dose of MTX 50 mg/m$^2$ on day 7
- If ≥15% decline in hCG titer between days 4 and 7, follow weekly until hCG <10 mIU/ml. If <15% decline, repeat 50 mg/m$^2$ dose on day 7
- In those patients not requiring D&C (hCG >2,000 mIU/ml before treatment initiation), days 0 and 1 were combined
- Endometrial curettage performed only on patients with an hCG titer <2,000 mIU/ml at the time of treatment initiation

hCG = human chorionic gonadotropin; D&C = dilatation and curettage; CBC = complete blood count; SGOT = serum glutamin oxalacetic transaminase; BUN = blood urea nitrogen; MTX = methotrexate.

10 ng/ml was associated with MTX treatment failure. The data of Stovall and of Lipscomb support this finding. Henry and Gentry reported 61 patients who had a gestational sac size smaller than 3.5 cm. Of the 61 patients, 16 required a second dose, and 52 (85%) were successfully treated. hCG was measured on days 1, 4, 7, and 10, and patients were given a second dose of MTX for any two rising hCG titers or for a plateauing hCG after day 7. Four of nine patients who had surgical intervention had an unruptured ectopic pregnancy. D&C was not performed before treatment in patients who had an hCG titer of less than 2000 mIU/ml.

Reproductive function following MTX-CF treatment was studied in a group of 57 patients who were successfully treated. Reproductive function was assessed by studying time to resolution, return of menses, tubal patency on hysterosalpingogram, time to pregnancy, and pregnancy outcome. In this study, MTX-CF treatment of unruptured ectopic pregnancy assisted in the restoration of tubal anatomy and did not impair the return of menses. Most importantly, the pregnancy rates following this form of therapy appeared to be better than those achieved by traditional surgical methods, and they were comparable to rates achieved by laparoscopic salpingostomy.

Pregnancy outcome following systemic therapy was reported by Stovall and associates in two separate reports. The first was in a group of 14 patients who attempted pregnancy after multidose intramuscular MTX. Of 44 patients available for follow-up (2 to 15 months), 14 desired and were attempting pregnancy. Eleven of 14 patients (78.6%) become pregnant, with 10 of 11 (90.9%) having an intrauterine pregnancy and with 1 (9.1%) having an extrauterine pregnancy. The mean time in this group from first attempt to achievement of pregnancy was 2.3 (range of 1 to 4 months) months. More recently, Stovall and associates reported a group of 49 patients who attempted pregnancy after completion of a single dose of intramuscular MTX. Of these 49 women, 39 (79.6%) became pregnant, with 34 pregnancies (87.2%) being intrauterine and 5 (12.8%) being ectopic pregnancies. The mean time from first attempt to achievement of pregnancy was 3.2 ± 1.1 months. Currently, the intrauterine pregnancy rate remains at 86%, with an ectopic pregnancy recurrence rate of 14%.

## INJECTION OF POTASSIUM CHLORIDE OR MTX BY ULTRASONOGRAPHIC LAPAROSCOPY

Injection of MTX into a tubal gestation by an ultrasonographically guided needle or at laparoscopy has been described with successful outcome. There have been numerous reports showing varying degrees of success. Potential advantages to this technique include a one-time injection, with the avoidance of potential systemic complications of MTX. The use of laparoscopy has the obvious disadvantage of requiring laparoscopy, and the results to date have not been as good as those achieved with intramuscular administration of MTX. Because the success rate for this method is not equivalent to that achieved with intramuscular administration of MTX, this form of treatment cannot be recommended until further studies are undertaken. Other agents used have included potassium chloride (KCl), prostaglandins, and hyperosmolar glucose.

## METHOTREXATE PROPHYLAXIS

Graczykowski and associates reported a group of 116 women who were randomized to receive either a single dose of MTX (50 mg/m$^2$) or to function as control group (n = 62). Persistence was defined as a rise in the serum hCG level or a decline of less than 20% between two consecutive measurements taken 3 days apart. One woman in the prophylactic group (1.9%) and 9 in the control group (14.5%) had persistence.

# Rare Types of Ectopic Pregnancy

**Combined Pregnancy.** Because the diagnosis of combined pregnancy is usually missed at the time of the first treatment, the morbidity is increased. How much it is increased over that of "simple" tubal ectopic pregnancy or "simple" spontaneous abortion is unknown because of the rarity of combined pregnancy. Once the correct diagnosis of combined pregnancy is made, a management appropriate for each pregnancy of the set must be formulated. The fetal salvage rate for the intrauterine component of the combined pregnancy is about 1:3, the most likely event being spontaneous abortion in the first trimester. The possibility of the need for diagnostic dilatation, suction, and curettage should be made known to the patient.

**Abdominal Pregnancy.** This condition occurs in 1:1136 to 1:7931 births. Maternal mortality is rare, although maternal morbidity is high because the diagnosis is made preoperatively in less than half of cases and there is extensive damage to the abdominopelvic organs associated with hemorrhage. A 10 to 20% overall fetal salvage rate is described for abdominal pregnancy. With a 10% chance of the infants being normal, the reported incidence of severe structural deformity ranges from 37 to 75%. Of surviving infants, a third to a half have some degree of deformity.

The diagnosis of primary abdominal pregnancy is uncommon and must meet the criteria established by Studdiford. These criteria include:
1. Presence of normal tubes and ovaries and no evidence of recent or past pregnancy
2. No evidence of uteroplacental fistula
3. Presence of a pregnancy related exclusively to the peritoneal surface and early enough to eliminate the possibility of secondary implantation following primary tubal nidation

Secondary abdominal pregnancy results from early tubal abortion or, most commonly, from tubal rupture. In addition to the classic triad of amenorrhea, pain, and abnormal uterine bleeding, signs and symptoms of abdominal pregnancy may include persistent nausea and emesis, unusually painful fetal movements, and severe abdominal cramping not characteristic of round ligament pain. Characteristic findings on physical examination include abnormal fetal presentation, palpation of the uterus separate from the fetal parts, or a cervix displaced from its expected position if the abdominal pregnancy is advanced.

After 16 weeks of gestation, fetal ossification allows direct visualization of the fetus, and fetal parts are often located posterior to the lumbar spine in a true lateral radiograph of the pelvis. Transabdominal ultrasonography and TVU are more commonly used and can also be diagnostic.

The management of abdominal pregnancy is to remove the fetus surgically. The placenta is also removed if possible in an en bloc dissection. Otherwise, it is left in situ to avoid the hemorrhage that will ensue if it is disturbed from its abnormal implantation site. Complications include secondary hemorrhage, intestinal obstruction, and infection.

**Ovarian Pregnancy.** This condition occurs in 11:40,000 deliveries. Incidence increases with use of an intrauterine device (IUD). The diagnostic criteria of Spiegelberg are used to confirm the presence of an ovarian pregnancy:
1. The tube, including the fimbria ovarica, must be intact.
2. The gestational sac definitely occupies the normal position of the ovary.
3. The sac is connected to the uterus by the ovarian ligament.
4. Ovarian tissue is demonstrable in the walls of the sac.

The history and physical examination are similar to those required for tubal ectopic pregnancy with two exceptions:
1. Continued menses, which may appear normal, seem to be relatively common in patients with ovarian pregnancy.
2. An adnexal mass is felt more often in patients who have an ovarian pregnancy (80 to 90% of cases) than in patients who have a tubal ectopic pregnancy.

Management includes surgical removal of the ectopic pregnancy as indicated, although preservation of as much ovarian tissue as possible is appropriate.

**Cervical Pregnancy.** The morbidity and potential for mortality is high in women have this condition because of the associated profuse hemorrhage and the surgical treatment often required, which is hysterectomy. Cervical pregnancy demonstrates amenorrhea, but the vaginal bleeding is painless rather than painful. Upon examination, the cervix is soft, thinwalled, round rather than conical, and disproportionally large. The examination is often confusing, with the cervical-uterine complex referred to as an hourglass-shaped uterus.

If the patient has a strong desire for pregnancy in the future, an attempt may be made at sharp curettage. Vaginal packing is sometimes helpful in controlling the profuse bleeding that may ensue. Cervical cerclage-type procedures that ligate the cervical branch of the uterine artery have been reported to help in the control of bleeding in this situation, and these may be tried. If the bleeding cannot be controlled, abdominal hysterectomy is required. When diagnosis is made early, usually by ultrasonography, treatment with MTX has been reported to be successful and is probably the treatment of choice.

# Future Directions

The future holds much promise for the treatment of this disease state. Earlier diagnosis is making more conservative treatment possible. Nonlaparoscopic medical management is proving to be feasible in many cases. The development of a single test, or set of tests, which will predict resolution without any form of intervention, will further reduce the morbidity associated with treatment and will raise the hope that future reproductive potential will be increased.

## REFERENCES

Bengtsson G, Bryman I, Thorburn J, et al: Low dose oral methotrexate as second line therapy for persistent trophoblast after conservative treatment of ectopic pregnancy. Obstet Gynecol 79:589–591, 1992.

Brandes MC, Youngs DD, Goldstein DP, et al: Treatment of cornual pregnancy with methotrexate: Case report. Am J Obstet Gynecol 1551:655, 1986.

Brumsted J, Kessler C, Gibson C, et al: A comparison of laparoscopy and laparotomy for the treatment of ectopic pregnancy. Obstet Gynecol 71:899–892, 1988.

Cacciatore B, Stenman UH, Ylostalo P: Comparison of abdominal and vaginal sonography in suspected ectopic pregnancy. Obstet Gynecol 73:770, 1989.

Chotiner JC: Nonsurgical management of ectopic pregnancy associated with severe hyperstimulation syndrome. Obstet Gynecol 66:740, 1985.

Clark LC, Raymond S, Stanger J, et al: Treatment of ectopic pregnancy with intraamniotic methotrexate: A case report. Aust N Z J Obstet Gynaecol 29:84,85, 1989.

Cowan BD, McGehee RP, Gates GH: Treatment of persistent ectopic pregnancy with methotrexate and leukovorum rescue: A case report. Obstet Gynecol 67:50S, 1986.

Cowen BD, Morrison JC: Management of ectopic pregnancy. In Plauché W, Morrison JC, O'Sullivan MJ (eds): Surgical Obstetrics. Philadelphia, WB Saunders, 1992.

Dorfman SF, Groimes DA, Cates W Jr, et al: Ectopic pregnancy mortality, United States 1979 to 1980. Clinical aspects. Obstet Gynecol 64:386, 1984.

Ectopic Pregnancy — United States, 1987. MMWR 39:401, 1980.

Egarter C, Fitz R, Spona J, et al: Treatment of tubal pregnancy with prostaglandins: A multicenter study. Geburstshilfe Fauenheilkd 49:808–812, 1989.

Egarter C, Husslein P: Treatment of tubal pregnancy by prostaglandins. Lancet, May 4, 1989.

Emerson DS, Cartier MS, Alter LA, et al: Diagnostic efficacy of endovaginal color Doppler through imaging in an ectopic pregnancy screening program. Radiology 183:413, 1992.

Farabow WS, Fulton JW, Fletcher V Jr, et al: Cervical pregnancy treated with methotrexate. N C Med J 44:910, 1983.

Feichtinger W, Kemeter P: Treatment of unruptured ectopic pregnancy by needling of sac and injection of methotrexate or PGE2 under transvaginal sonography control. Arch Gynecol Obstet 246:85–89, 1989.

Feichtinger W, Kemetre P: Conservative treatment of ectopic pregnancy by transvaginal aspiration under sonographic control and methotrexate injection. Lancet 1:381, 1987.

Fritz MA, Guo S: Doubling time of human chorionic gonadotropin (hCG) in early normal pregnancy: Relationship to hCG concentration and gestational age. Fertil Steril 47:584–589, 1987.

Graczykowski JW, Mishell DR: Methotrexate prophylaxis for persistent ectopic pregnancy after conservative treatment by salpingostomy. Obstet Gynecol 99:118–122, 1997.

Henry MA, Gentry WL: Single injection of methotrexate for treatment of ectopic pregnancies. Am J Obstet Gynecol 171:1584–1587, 1994.

Higgins KA, Schwartz MB: Treatment of persistent trophoblastic tissue after salpingostomy with methotrexate. Fertil Steril 45:427, 1986.

Hreshchyshyn MM, Naples JD Jr, Randle CL: Amethopterine in abdominal pregnancy. Am J Obstet Gynecol 93:286, 1965.

Kadar N, Caldwell BV, Romero R: A method of screening for ectopic pregnancy and its indications. Obstet Gynecol 58:162–166, 1981.

Kadar N, Freedman M, Zacher M: Further observation on the doubling time of human chorionic gonadotropin in early asymptomatic pregnancy. Fertil Steril 54:783–787, 1980.

Kjer JJ, Knudsen LB: Ectopic pregnancy subsequent to laparoscopic sterilization. Am J Obstet Gynecol 160:1202, 1989.

Ksauppila A, Rantakyla P, Huhtaniemi I, et al: Trophoblastic markers in the differential diagnosis of ectopic pregnancy. Obstet Gynecol 55:295, 1980.

Laatikainen T, Tuomiuaara L, Kaar K: Comparison of a local injection of hyperosmolar glucose solution with salpingostomy for the conservative treatment of tubal pregnancy. Fertil Steril 60:80–84, 1993.

Lang P, Weiss PAM, Mayer HO: Local application of hyperosmolar glucose solution in tubal pregnancy. Lancer 2:922–993, 1989.

Latrop JC, Bowles GE: Methotrexate in abdominal pregnancy. Report of a case. Obstet Gynecol 32:81, 1968.

Leach RE, Ory SJ: Modern management of ectopic pregnancy. J Reprod Med 34:324, 1989.

Leeton J, Davison G: Nonsurgical management of unruptured tubal pregnancy with intra-amniotic methotrexate: Preliminary report of two cases. Fertil Steril 50:167, 1988.

Lindblom B, Lakklfelt B, Hahlin M, et al: Local prostaglandin F2 injection for termination of ectopic pregnancy. Lancet 1:776, 1987.

Lipscomb GH, Bran D, McCord ML, et al: Analysis of three hundred fifteen ectopic pregnancies treated with single-dose methotrexate. Am J Obstet Gynecol 178:1354–1358, 1998.

Lundorff P, Hahlin M, Kalifelt B, et al: Adhesion formation after laparoscopic surgery in tubal pregnancy: A randomized trial versus laparotomy. Fertil Steril 55:911–995, 1991.

Matthews CP, Coulson PB, Wild RA: Serum progesterone levels as an aid in the diagnosis of ectopic pregnancy. Obstet Gynecol 68:390, 1986.

McCord ML, Muram D, Buster JE, et al: Single serum progesterone as a screen for ectopic pregnancy: Exchanging specificity and sensitivity to obtain optimal test performance. Fertil Steril 66:513–516, 1996.

Menard A, Cruquat J, Mandelbrot L, et al: Treatment of unruptured tubal pregnancy by local injection of methotrexate under transvaginal sonographic control. Fertil Steril 54:47–50, 1990.

Miyakaki Y: Nonsurgical therapy of ectopic pregnancy. Hokkaido Igaku Zasshi 58:132, 1983.

Mottla GL, Rulin MC, Guzick DS: Lack of resolution of ectopic pregnancy by intratubal injection of methotrexate. Fertil Steril 57:685–687, 1992.

Murphy AA, Nager CW, Wujek JJ, et al: Operative laparoscopy versus laparotomy for the management of ectopic pregnancy: A prospective trial. Fertil Steril 57:1180–1185, 1992.

Ooi DS, Perkins SL, Claman P, et al: Serum human chorionic gonadotrophin levels in early pregnancy. Clin Chim Acta 181:281, 1989.

Ory SJ, Villanueva AL, Sand PK, et al: Conservative treatment of ectopic pregnancy with methotrexate. Am J Obstet Gynecol 154:1299, 1986.

Pansky M, Bukovsky J, Olin A, et al: Reproductive outcome after laparoscopic local methotrexate injection for tubal pregnancy. Fertil Steril 60:85–87, 1993.

Paulson G, Kuint S, Labecker B, et al: Laparoscopic prostaglandin injection in ectopic pregnancy: Success rate according to endocrine activity. Fertil Steril 63:473–477, 1995.

Pittaway D, Wentz AC, Maxon W, et al: The efficacy of early pregnancy monitoring with serial chorionic gonadotropin determinations and relay-time sonography in an infertility population. Fertil Steril 44:190, 1985.

Pittaway D: Diagnosis of ectopic pregnancy. Obstet Gynecol 68:440, 1986.

Porreco RP: Percutaneous, ultrasound-directed ablation of ectopic pregnancy with methotrexate: A report of three cases. J Reprod Med 1992;37:36306

Ransom MX, Garcia AJ, Bohrer M, et al: serum progesterone as a predictor of methotrexate success in the treatment of ectopic pregnancy. Obstet Gynecol 83:1033–1037, 1994.

Ribic Paucel JM, Novak-Antolic Z, Urhovec I: Treatment of ectopic pregnancy with prostaglandin E$_2$. Clin Exp Obstet Gynecol 16:106–109 1989.

Robertson De, Moye MA, Hansen JH, et al: Reduction of ectopic pregnancy by injection under ultrasound control. Lancet 1:974–975, 1987.

Seifer DB, Gutmann JN, Grant MD, et al: Comparison of persistent ectopic pregnancy after laparoscopic salpingostomy versus salpingostomy at laparotomy for ectopic pregnancy. Obstet Gynecol 81:378–382, 1993.

Shalev E, Megory E, Romano S, Weiner E, et al: Interstitial pregnancy—Successful treatment with methotrexate. Isr J Med Sci 25:239,240, 1989.

St. Clair JT, Whealer DA: Methotrexate in abdominal pregnancy. JAMA 21:529, 1969.

Storring PL, Gaine-Des RE, Bangham DR: International reference preparation of human chorionic gonadotropin for immunoassay: Potency estimated in various bioassays and protein binding assay systems and international reference preparation of the alpha and beta subunits of human chorionic gonadotropin for immunoassay. J Endocrinol 84:295, 1980.

Stovall TG, Ling FW, Buster JE: Outpatient chemotherapy of unruptured ectopic pregnancy. Fertil Steril; 51:435, 1989.

Stovall TG, Ling FW, Cope BJ, et al: Preventing ruptured ectopic pregnancy with a single serum progesterone. Am J Obstet Gynecol 160:1425–1431, 1989.

Stovall TG, Ling FW, Buster JE: Reproductive performance after methotrexate treatment of ectopic pregnancy. Am J Obstet Gynecol 162:1620, 1990.

Stovall TG, Ling FW, Gray LA: Single dose methotrexate for ectopic pregnancy. Obstet Gynecol 77:754, 1991.

Stovall TG, Ling FW, Gray LA, et al: Methotrexate treatment of unruptured ectopic pregnancy: A report of 100 cases. Obstet Gynecol 77:749, 1991.

Stovall TG, Ling FW: Single dose methotrexate: An expanded clinical trial. Am J Obstet Gynecol 168:1759–1765, 1993.

Stovall TG, Ling FW: Ectopic pregnancy: Diagnostic and therapeutic algorithms minimizing surgical intervention. J Reprod Med 38:807–812, 1993.

Sultana CJ, Easley K, Collins RL: Outcome of laparoscopic versus traditional surgery for ectopic pregnancies. Fertil Steril 57:285–289, 1992.

Tanaka T, Hayaski H, Kutsuzawa T, et al: Treatment of interstitial ectopic pregnancy with methotrexate: Report of a successful case. Fertil Steril 37:851, 1982.

Timor-Tritsch IE, Montequdo A, Matera C, et al: Sonographic evolution of cornual pregnancies treated without surgery. Obstet Gynecol 79:1044–1049, 1992.

Tulandi T, Atri M, Bret P, et al: Transvaginal intratubal methotrexate treatment of ectopic pregnancy. Fertil Steril 58:98–100, 1992.

Tulandi T, Bret PM, Atri M, et al: Treatment of ectopic pregnancy by transvaginal intratubal methotrexate administration. Obstet Gynecol 77:627–630, 1991.

Vermesh M, Graczyhowski JW, Sauer MV: Reevaluation of the role of culdocentesis in the management of ectopic pregnancy. Am J Obstet Gynecol 162:411, 1990.

Vermesh M, Silva PD, Rosen GF, et al: Management of unruptured ectopic gestation by linear salpingostomy: A prospective, randomized clinical trial of laparoscopy versus laparotomy. Obstet Gynecol 73:400–404, 1989.

Vetorp M, Vejerslev LO, Ruge S. Local prostaglandin treatment of ectopic pregnancy. Hum Reprod 4:464–467, 1989.

Yeko TR, Gorrill JM, Hughes LH, et al: Timely diagnosis of ectopic pregnancy using a single blood progesterone measurement. Fertil Steril 48:1049, 1987.

Yeko TR, Mayer JC, Parsons AK, et al: A prospective series of unruptured ectopic pregnancies treated by tubal injection with hyperosmolar glucose. Obstet Gynecol 85:265–268, 1995.

Zilber U, Pansky M, Bukovsky I, et al: Laparoscopic salpingostomy versus laparoscopic local methotrexate injection in the management of unruptured ectopic gestation. Am J Obstet Gynecol 175:600–602 1996.

# 5

# Dysmenorrhea and Pelvic Pain

GARY H. LIPSCOMB

Complaints of dysmenorrhea and other types of pelvic pain or pelvic discomfort are commonly encountered by practitioners who provide care to women. While many such complaints are amenable to routine remedies, others are less easily resolved. Although persistent pain is rarely life threatening, it is frequently debilitating, and, by its very nature, often causes frustration for both physician and patient. By definition, pain that persists for longer than 6 months is considered chronic pain. This chapter attempts to present a logical and methodical approach to the workup and treatment of patients who have dysmenorrhea and other forms of pelvic pain, with particular attention to pain that persists despite routine therapeutic measures.

Traditionally, the gynecologic approach to pelvic pain has focused on the female reproductive tract organs as the sole source of pain. This excessively narrow approach, sometimes referred to as "gynevision," may fail to recognize other common contributors to pelvic pain (e.g., gastrointestinal tract, urinary tract, or psychological factors). This way of thinking tends to encourage a surgical approach, in which the organic pathology of the reproductive tract is a top priority. This overly simplistic view serves neither the patient nor the physician caring for her. A more comprehensive approach, which is centered around the idiosyncratic needs of the individual patient, offers a better methodology for dealing with pelvic pain.

This chapter focuses on various aspects of the comprehensive approach needed to establish a complete diagnosis and a comprehensive scheme for managing pelvic pain in general as well as some of the more difficult to treat subtypes. Regardless of whether individual physicians choose to treat all these subtypes themselves or whether they elect to refer part or all of such treatments to other health professionals, a basic knowledge of the etiology and treatment of these conditions is necessary. Curing all patients who have chronic pelvic pain is an idealistic and admirable goal, but it is also important to be able to recognize those patients who would be helped best by learning pain management, with goals of having a minimally disrupted lifestyle, performing normal daily activities, and maintaining a positive self-image. Strategies for management of these patients will also be presented.

## Dysmenorrhea and Predominantly Cyclic Pelvic Pain

It is estimated that 30 to 50% of women of childbearing age suffer from cyclic pelvic pain. In 10 to 15%

of these women, symptoms are severe enough to interfere with performance of normal activities. Although the cyclic nature of the pain implies a causal relationship to the female reproductive system, care must be taken to differentiate symptoms truly related to menstruation from symptoms aggravated by body changes occurring during the menstrual cycle. The practitioner must also differentiate cyclic pain unrelated to the menstrual cycle from the pain of true dysmenorrhea.

Dysmenorrhea is broadly divided into two categories: primary and secondary. Unlike many other diagnoses (e.g., infertility, amenorrhea), the terms "primary" and "secondary" do not imply a temporal meaning but instead relate to causality. In secondary dysmenorrhea, a readily identifiable cause (e.g., fibroids, endometriosis) is found, whereas in primary dysmenorrhea there is no such cause.

Primary dysmenorrhea has been experienced to some degree by most women at some time in their lives. The pain is characteristically sharp or cramping and generally occurs during the first 3 days of menstruation. The location of the pain is generally in the suprapubic area, but it may radiate to the back, inner thighs, or deep pelvis. Nausea, with or without vomiting, and diarrhea may also occur. Dyspareunia, even during menstruation, is uncommon and should suggest another pathology. The diagnosis of primary dysmenorrhea is one of exclusion, that is, no abnormalities are found on history or physical that might reasonably be the cause of the dysmenorrhea.

Patients who have secondary dysmenorrhea often have symptoms in addition to cyclic pain that may suggest the underlying etiology. Heavy menstrual flow with dysmenorrhea suggests a diagnosis of uterine leiomyomata, adenomyosis, or endometrial polyps. Likewise, cyclic pain in a patient who has primary amenorrhea suggests outflow obstruction. Gastrointestinal, urinary, or musculoskeletal complaints should alert the physician to the possibility of a nongynecologic process. Diagnosis and management of these entities are discussed at greater length in the section that follows.

# Predominantly Noncyclic Pelvic Pain

## Gastrointestinal Causes

It has been estimated that as many as 60% of referrals for chronic pelvic pain may be attributed to a gastrointestinal origin, particularly irritable bowel syndrome. Because of the visceral innervation of the bowel, it is often difficult to differentiate lower abdominal pain of gynecologic origin from that of gastrointestinal origin. Unfortunately, lower abdominal pain in women is not infrequently interpreted as pelvic pain by both the patient and the physician.

## Urinary Tract Causes of Pelvic Pain

Pain originating in the urinary tract may be difficult to differentiate from pain in gynecologic sources, because these organ systems have a common embryologic origin. Thus, the urinary tract should always be considered in the differential diagnosis of pelvic pain, particularly when the standard gynecologic evaluation is inconclusive.

## Musculoskeletal Causes of Chronic Pelvic Pain

The musculoskeletal system is perhaps the most common source of nongynecologic chronic pelvic pain. Unfortunately, the musculoskeletal evaluation is also the most frequently overlooked component of the comprehensive evaluation of the patient who has chronic pelvic pain.

# History and Physical Examination

A complete history is essential for proper evaluation of any patient who has chronic lower abdominal or pelvic pain. The patient should be questioned about the character of her pain, as well as its duration, frequency of occurrence, location, and any radiation patterns. Any exacerbating or alleviating factors should be determined. It should also be noted whether the severity of the pain is stable or whether it has improved or worsened with time. The relationship, if any, of the pain to the menstrual cycle, sexual activity, bladder and bowel function, and emotional state may prove critical.

Particular attention should be focused on past surgical procedures or presumptive episodes of pelvic inflammatory disease (PID). The patient's psychological response to her pain and its effect on her lifestyle, family, and friends should also be determined, if possible. The patient should be questioned about the effect of any previous treatment on the pain, regardless of whether such treatment was medically mandated or self-administered.

The classic gynecologic approach of dividing the pain into cyclic and noncyclic categories may help to determine whether the origin of the pain is related to the menstrual cycle. Table 5–1 lists the differential

**Table 5–1** Differential Diagnosis of Cyclic and Noncyclic Pelvic Pain

| PREDOMINANTLY CYCLIC PAIN |
|---|
| Mittelschmerz |
| Primary dysmenorrhea |
| Secondary dysmenorrhea |
|     Endometriosis |
|     Adenomyosis |
|     Endometritis |
|     Cervical stenosis |
|     Intrauterine device (IUD) |
|     Leiomyomata |
| Premenstrual syndrome |

| PREDOMINANTLY NONCYCLIC PAIN |
|---|
| Pelvic inflammatory disease |
| Pelvic adhesions |
| Displacement of the uterus |
| Symptomatic pelvic relaxation |
| Chronic pelvic pain without organic abnormalities |
| Musculoskeletal disorders |
| Urinary tract disorders |
| Gastrointestinal tract disorders |
| Psychogenic/psychological factors |

diagnosis of chronic pelvic pain and provides a generally accurate starting point for categorizing the causes of pelvic pain. The two lists are not mutually exclusive, because patients who have conditions that commonly produce cyclic pain may occasionally present with noncyclic pain and vice versa. The physician must also be wary of non–menstrual-related pain that may be exacerbated by the menstrual cycle; that is, dysmenorrhea must be differentiated from pelvic pain that is constant throughout the month but exacerbated at the time of the menstrual cycle.

If the pain does appear to be cyclic or related to menstruation, a detailed menstrual history should be obtained. This should include the time of menarche, the regularity and length of the cycle, the number of days of bleeding, and an approximate quantification of blood loss. It should be determined whether this pain has been present since menarche or whether it is a relatively new phenomenon.

Symptoms of urgency, frequency, and dysuria may indicate an acute or chronic urinary tract problem. Likewise, recurrent episodes of urinary tract infection that yield negative urine cultures should raise suspicion of the presence of a chronic inflammatory process of noninfectious etiology. A history of hesitancy of urination or incomplete emptying may indicate a disorder of the urethra or bladder neck. Postcoital voiding difficulties are strongly associated with urethral syndrome secondary to chronic urethritis. Likewise, dyspareunia is a common accompaniment of a urethral syndrome.

A careful history may reveal details that suggest a gastrointestinal etiology. Bowel habits are a particularly useful source of information. Abdominal pain associated with irritable bowel syndrome characteristically improves following a bowel movement and is often worse after eating. There may also be a sense of rectal fullness or incomplete rectal evacuation. Hard, pellet-like stools in the rectum are also suggestive of irritable bowel syndrome. Exacerbation of pain during times of stress is a common finding. Correlation of pain with food intake should be discussed. Patients who have infrequent bowel movements associated with pain during or preceding evacuation may have only chronic constipation; however, patients who have diarrhea should be evaluated for intrinsic bowel disease as a possible underlying etiology. Dyspareunia is frequently gynecologic in origin, but it is present in many women who have irritable bowel syndrome.

Some factors that may indicate a musculoskeletal source of pain include poor posture, scoliosis, unilateral standing habits, marked lumbar lordosis, discrepancy of leg length, abnormal gait, abdominal wall trigger points or tenderness, a history of low back trauma, and a previous normal laparoscopy.

Once the history is obtained, this information should be used in directing the physical examination. A complete physical examination is essential, and certain aspects of the examination warrant particular attention. The patient's posture and walk should be noted. Generally poor posture, slouching, or standing with the weight on one leg may suggest a possible musculoskeletal etiology. A gentle abdominal examination should be performed to search for masses and areas of tenderness. Special attention to superficial palpation is critical in identifying musculoskeletal pain. If a painful area is encountered, the patient should be questioned as to whether this pain reproduces the complaint for which she is being evaluated. If pain on palpation increases or remains constant during voluntary tightening of the abdominal musculature, the pain usually stems from the abdominal wall rather than the visceral area. This maneuver can be accomplished easily by asking the patient to elevate her head or both legs from the examination table while the examiner applies gentle pressure to the painful area. A brief neurologic examination of the lower extremity reflexes should be performed. Abnormal reflexes or pain on straight leg raises may indicate a possible herniated disk, and this should signal the need for a more extensive neurologic evaluation.

Before the bimanual examination is performed, gentle palpation of the introitus, possibly with a moistened cotton swab, can aid in identifying vestibulitis, a variant of pelvic pain that often presents as a new-onset of entrance dyspareunia. A monomanual (one-handed) pelvic examination should precede the traditional bimanual examination because it can aid in differentiating pain that is caused by the abdominal wall from an etiology within the pelvis. Gentle palpation of the relaxed levator muscles with a posteriorly directed index finger helps to diagnose levator spasm. The patient should be asked to contract the levator muscles during palpation with the index finger as a further aid in identifying muscular pain. The same finger is then rotated anteriorly to gently palpate the urethra and the bladder base. The physcian should include a complete monomanual internal evaluation of cervical motion tenderness and vaginal fornix pain before the bimanual examination is performed. The physician can thus avoid mislabeling the lower abdominal muscular pain elicited on bimanual examination as some other pelvic pathologic condition, such as adhesions caused by PID.

The examiner should pay particular attention to the size, mobility, and tenderness of the uterus and adnexa. A mildly enlarged, boggy, tender, symmetrical uterus suggests adenomyosis or perhaps fibroid tumors. A markedly enlarged or asymmetrically enlarged uterus is more consistent with the presence of fibroids. A uterus with poor mobility may indicate fibrosis caused by endometriosis. Any nodularity or induration of the uterosacral ligaments, which would also suggest endometriosis, should be further assessed by a rectal examination. Specific notation should be made as to whether the uterus itself is tender and whether it is actually the source of the complaints of pain. This is a pivotal concern if a hysterectomy is subsequently considered. Similar information should be obtained regarding both adnexa. A rectovaginal examination is necessary for obtaining an adequate evaluation of any induration or nodularity of the uterosacral ligaments caused by endometriosis. Tenderness localized over the sigmoid colon in the absence of inflammatory signs is frequently present in patients who have irritable bowel syndrome, whereas a tender mass in the left lower quadrant in a febrile patient suggests diverticulitis.

In many instances of suspected urinary dysfunction, a 24-hour voiding diary can be helpful in providing insight into the frequency of voiding, episodes of leakage, and amount of fluid intake. For example, frequency at night may relate to sensory problems of the bladder and urethra, whereas constant voiding throughout the day may suggest limited bladder capacity as a result of an intrinsic bladder condition.

A cursory neurologic examination of the lower extremities and the perineal area should be performed. The tone and sensation of the pelvic floor musculature should be ascertained during the pelvic examination. Excessive tone or tenderness of the levator ani musculature may indicate an underlying urethral or bladder disorder; for example, spasm of the levator ani has been suggested as one of the causes of pain in patients who have interstitial cystitis. In these patients, gentle palpation of the urethra, the bladder trigone, and the base frequently identifies a specific source of pain.

Nongynecologic causes of chronic pelvic pain should always be thoroughly evaluated and ruled out before any surgical therapy is attempted. Of particular concern should be possible contributions of the gastrointestinal tract (e.g., irritable bowel syndrome) or urogynecologic causes (e.g., chronic urethritis, interstitial cystitis, and musculoskeletal factors).

The typical bimanual pelvic examination may be a poor discriminator of the cause of pelvic pain because it simultaneously evaluates the abdominal wall, the vaginal wall, and the tissues in between. For example, in the bimanual evaluation of the anteverted uterus, the two examining hands palpate the abdominal wall (including skin, subcutaneous tissue, fascia, and muscle), uterus, bladder, and vaginal wall. The initial use of the monomanual pelvic technique, as previously described, helps to prevent mislabeling pain that is actually located in the abdominal wall and the levator muscle as uterine or adnexal pain. Careful palpation of the rectus muscles in both relaxed and tensed states can often elicit the patient's pain. The lateral borders of the abdominal rectus muscles, as well as their insertion site into the symphysis, are particularly common sites of tenderness.

Slocumb has suggested that hypersensitive areas of the abdominal wall (trigger points) are the most common cause of pelvic pain. These trigger points are hyperirritable areas that are tender when compressed, and they may also generate referred pain and tenderness. Trigger points typically manifest themselves after some type of muscle strain, and they can often be found within a taut band of skeletal muscle. Trigger points can respond dramatically to specific therapy. In his classic study, Slocumb used trigger-point injections of local anesthetic agents to treat 122 patients who had chronic pelvic pain. More than 50% of the patients in this study became pain-free. Only 13 patients had surgery, and all patients who received only injections in the abdominal wall were reported to have had a successful response. Those who had vaginal trigger points had an 84.6% response rate to the injections.

## Laboratory Evaluation

Laboratory studies are of limited use in evaluating patients who have dysmenorrhea. Blood counts are occasionally helpful for assessing blood loss in patients who have excessive bleeding, as are sedimentation rates in identifying a chronic inflammatory process.

Ultrasonography and other radiologic modalities rarely provide additional helpful information, except in cases in which the physical examination is either inadequate or suspicious but not conclusive for a particular condition. In fact, these imaging techniques may often further confuse the diagnosis by identifying a small physiologic ovarian cyst or other benign process. This misleading information may then result in additional unnecessary tests and, occasionally, even unnecessary surgery. Diagnostic laparoscopy is usually reserved for patients in whom additional pathology is suspected based on the history and physical examination, or for patients who respond poorly to nonsteroidal agents and oral contraceptive pills.

Although the history and physical examination are the most effective method of ruling out acute and most chronic conditions, the differential diagnosis of irritable bowel syndrome includes inflammatory bowel disease as well as malignancy. Thus, performing a thorough workup to exclude these conditions is appropriate. Laboratory tests may include taking a complete blood count and a stool sample to check for occult blood and white cells. A plain film of the abdomen may reveal radiologic evidence of acute or chronic disease. Likewise, ultrasonography may detect gallstones, ascites, or the presence of an intra-abdominal mass. In selected patients, flexible sigmoidoscopy, colonoscopy, or a barium enema may be helpful and appropriate.

Cystourethroscopy should be considered in all women who have chronic pelvic pain of suspected urologic origin. The urethra and the bladder mucosa can be inspected, and any evidence of chronic infection or structural deformities, such as diverticula or tumors, can be visualized. Although cystourethroscopy is usually performed in the office setting without anesthesia, for painful conditions, such as interstitial cystitis, cystourethroscopy may require general anesthesia. In these cases, the procedure should be performed in a hospital or outpatient surgical setting. Findings of erythema and exudate in patients who have pelvic pain and irritable urinary symptoms without other bladder pathology are consistent with urethral syndrome caused by chronic urethritis. In the patient who has no demonstrable findings but who has significant symptoms, urethral spasm should be considered. In patients who are suspected of having interstitial cystitis, the bladder is filled and allowed to remain distended for 1 minute. It is then emptied and refilled. Patients who have interstitial cystitis develop characteristic submucosal hemorrhages and petechiae after this double-fill cystoscopy.

## Treatment

The underlying pathophysiology in patients who have primary dysmenorrhea relates to prostaglandins; therefore, the mainstay of treatment is use of nonsteroidal anti-inflammatory drugs (NSAIDs). Generally, the similarities between NSAIDs are such that practitioners need only be familiar with one or two agents. Although the chemical structures of NSAIDs are so similar that marked clinical differences would not be expected in response to administration of different NSAIDs, patients who have poor or partial response to one NSAID may respond well to a different agent. Apparently subtle differences in the site or mechanism of action are responsible for this phenomenon.

Hormonal agents are frequently prescribed for dysmenorrhea. The most common of the hormonal agents is the oral contraceptive pill (OCP). OCPs are widely used for relief of primary dysmenorrhea in patients who do not desire pregnancy. No one pill has been shown to be superior to another in this regard; thus, physicians should use the OCP with which they are most familiar for this purpose. OCPs are generally prescribed on a 28-day cycle (21 days of hormone followed by 7 hormone-free days), but they can be used continuously (no hormone-free days) in an attempt to produce amenorrhea if patients still have dysmenorrhea during withdrawal bleeding. Unfortunately, breakthrough bleeding is common and often limits the use of this regimen. Medroxyprogesterone acetate (Depo-Provera) may also be used to induce hypomenorrhea or amenorrhea in these patients. However, only 50% of patients can be expected to become totally amenorrheic in the first year of use. Likewise gonadotropin-releasing hormone (Gn-RH) agonists have been used to obtain amenorrhea, but their use is limited by the high cost of therapy and association with bone loss when long-term use is contemplated. Their use for dysmenorrhea should probably be reserved for therapy of symptomatic endometriosis.

Although all the previously mentioned modalities for treatment of primary dysmenorrhea may also be used as treatment for secondary dysmenorrhea, results are frequently less than satisfactory. Only specific therapy for the cause of secondary dysmenorrhea can ultimately give satisfactory results.

There is no known detectable structural or biochemical abnormality associated with irritable bowel syndrome, but activation of hypersensitive receptors in the bowel wall caused by physiologic distention or contraction may be responsible for the pain. Studies also suggest that the conscious threshold for perception of visceral sensation in the form of pain is altered in patients who have irritable bowel syndrome. In addition, a large number of women who have this syndrome have proved to have a coexisting psychopathology, such as somatization disorder, anxiety disorder, or depression, as well as other psychological syndromes.

Current medical treatment for irritable bowel syndrome is generally unsatisfactory, and 30 to 70% of patients have continued symptoms even after long-term treatment. Treatment primarily consists of reassurance, education, stress reduction, bulk-forming agents, anxiolytics, and low-dose tricyclic antidepressants (Table 5–2). The single most effective therapy is use of bulk-forming agents. Anticholinergic agents are generally ineffective. In many instances, multidisciplinary pain management is appropriate for these patients, just as it is for any patient who has chronic pelvic pain.

No one specific therapy is uniformly successful for patients who have urethral syndrome. However, one treatment that can be initiated in all cases is modification of voiding habits. Patients are taught to tighten and relax their pelvic floor musculature to gain control of voluntary—or learned—spastic behavior of the urethral sphincter. Additionally, bladder retraining by use of regular voiding schedule drills aids the patient's ability to better control the urge and need to void.

In patients who have suspected chronic urethritis, the use of low-dose antibiotic therapy with trimethoprim-sulfamethoxazole or nitrofurantoin for bedtime suppression is appropriate. Normally, a 3- to 6-month trial is employed. Urethral dilatation is an often performed as therapy for urethral syndrome. The mechanism of action is unclear, but it may be attributable to the opening of the obstructed and inflamed periurethral glands. Summit, reporting on a group of patients who initially presented with complaints of pelvic pain and dyspareunia, showed that therapy with long-term suppressive antibiotics and serial urethral dilatation resulted in marked improvement or resolution in these patients, all of whom had reduced pain and who were subsequently able to resume sexual activity without discomfort.

Other treatments for urethral syndrome, which have been used with variable success, include anxiolytics, psychotherapy, periurethral steroid injections, and internal urethrotomy. Because these patients present with a confusing or changing clinical picture, consultation with a urologist or urogynecologist may be very helpful in diagnosing and treating this syndrome.

Treatment for interstitial cystitis is aimed at treating the inflammation or correcting the bladder wall permeability. Hydrodistention performed at the time of the diagnosis may itself be therapeutic. Similarly, behavior modification using increasing voiding intervals can produce similar results. Tricyclic antidepressants have been used to provide sedative effects as well as pain relief through peripheral neuroblockade and central stimulation. Use of dimethyl sulfoxide (DMSO) as an intravesical instillation is one of the more frequently used medical therapies. Surgical therapy has been used, but it should be considered a last resort.

In the patient who has demonstrable trigger points, injection with a local anesthetic may be a useful therapeutic and diagnostic aid. The use of 1- to 1.5-inch, 22-gauge needle is recommended for injection into the superficial musculature. Although smaller gauge needles cause less discomfort on skin penetration, they have the disadvantage of being less able to mechanically disrupt a trigger point, and they also reduce the clinician's sensitivity in detecting passage through the various tissue planes. Smaller needles may also be too flexible, sliding around taut muscle bands and masking the tactile clues that a clinician may use.

When a trigger point is injected, an aseptic technique should be used. The patient should also be forewarned that she may feel a muscle twitch or flash of referred pain during the insertion. The palpating finger should maintain tension on the skin as various

**Table 5–2** Treatment Options for Chronic Pelvic Pain

| GENERAL MEASURES |
| --- |
| Multidisciplinary management |
|   NSAIDs |
|   Psychological support |
|   Antipsychotic medications |
| Irritable bowel syndrome |
|   Bulk-forming agents |
| Musculoskeletal etiology |
|   Multidisciplinary management |
|   Physical therapy |
|   Trigger point injections |
|   NSAIDs |
| Urinary tract etiology |
|   Urethral syndrome |
|     Voiding schedule |
|     Suppressive antibiotics |
|     Urethral dilatation |
|     Anxiolytics |
|     Surgical therapy |
|   Interstitial cystitis |
|     Hydrodistention |
|     DMSO |
|     Voiding schedule |
|     Surgical therapy |
| Primary dysmenorrhea |
|   NSAIDs |
|   Oral contraceptive pill |
| Secondary dysmenorrhea |
|   NSAIDs |
|   Oral contraceptive pill |
|   Specific therapy for etiology |

| SURGICAL MEASURES |
| --- |
| Diagnostic laparoscopy |
| Adhesiolysis |
| Uterine suspension |
| Uterosacral nerve ablation |
| Presacral neurectomy |
| Hysterectomy |

NSAIDs = nonsteroidal anti-inflammatory drugs; DMSO = dimethyl sulfoxide.

injection tracts are made. If a trigger point is not identified directly, the injection may be less effective but still useful diagnostically. Successful injection results in a loss of tenderness and relaxation of the tight band of muscle, if that was originally present. The patient should also be able to note a symptomatic difference when palpating the area.

Although any of the local anesthetic agents may be used for trigger point injections, bupivacaine 0.25% is my agent of choice. Volumes of 1.0 ml or less are commonly adequate to produce a clear diagnostic test. Interestingly, the pain relief often extends for a far longer period of time than would be predicted by the normal duration of action of the drug. This time frame is frequently longer with subsequent injections and may reflect recovery of normal muscle and nerve function.

Relief of pain after trigger point injection helps the patient to understand that the source of the pain is at least partially musculoskeletal and not necessarily from gynecologic causes, such as an ovarian cyst, endometriosis, or infection. When used in this fashion, trigger point injections can clearly be diagnostic and, as shown by Slocumb, can also be therapeutic, either alone or in a series of injections. Relief of pain from one source may uncover pain from other causes; therefore, trigger point injections should be viewed as helpful adjuvants in an overall management plan.

Physical therapy, when included in a multidisciplinary approach, has been very successful in managing patients who have chronic pelvic pain derived from a musculoskeletal source. Referral to a physical therapist for further evaluation or more intensive physical therapy instruction than can be provided by the practitioner is frequently helpful in these patients. In cases in which such referral is unavailable or impractical, the use of NSAIDs, muscle relaxants, and heat application may be effective. Initial use of these agents on a scheduled rather than an as-needed basis for the first 1 to 2 weeks of treatment is recommended. These medications may also be used in conjunction with physical therapy.

## Psychiatric Factors in Pelvic Pain

All patients who have pelvic pain undergo adaptive responses to their pain. What might otherwise be perceived as an abnormal response to pain may, based on the duration of symptoms, be very normal. With passage of time, the patient goes through a normal series of significantly altered emotional states in response to chronic pain, starting at what is often an unknown baseline. Initially, the patient has high expectations, but, with the passage of time, frustration and despair predominate, and the patient gives up hope of improvement. "Doctor shopping," hostility, and, eventually, clinical depression occur as the patient passes through these stages. The physician needs to keep these emotional changes in perspective when interpreting the patient's words and actions.

For patients who have chronic pain, the exercise of trying to differentiate mental from physical pain is not useful, because mental factors, such as clinical depression, anxiety, and anger, are clearly part of the patient's perception of discomfort. In this regard, patients who have chronic pelvic pain are not different from patients who have other types of chronic pain. The patient's response to pain is affected by such varied factors as the cultural value placed on pain tolerance and display of emotion; the patient's perception of the risk involved with the pain; and work, social, financial, and idiosyncratic considerations.

As with any other disease process, psychiatric illness may be totally unrelated to the chronic pain, or it may be a contributory factor that must be dealt with to achieve improvement in the patient's pain. It is beyond the scope of this chapter to discuss diagnosis and management of major psychiatric illnesses, such as manic-depressive disorders or schizophrenia. Patients who have these disorders are often best managed in close collaboration with mental health professionals. However, because it is impossible to totally separate the relationship of mind and body in relation to chronic pelvic pain, we will attempt to discuss briefly some common psychiatric issues frequently encountered in the patient who has chronic pelvic pain.

One particular psychiatric disorder frequently encountered in patients who have chronic pelvic pain is somatization. In patients who have this disorder, emotional problems may be manifested as physical complaints. The emotional state of these patients may adversely affect their adaptation to a mild but persistent pain. There are multiple physical complaints for which there is no identifiable organic basis. In these cases, nonthreatening psychological and psychiatric intervention may be of therapeutic benefit. In general, these patients need ongoing supportive care; that is, no cure is anticipated. Principles of managing somatization are based on the patient's ongoing need for sanctioned caretaking and the tendency to express problems of the mind in the language of the body. These principles, which can also be modified for the treatment of the syndrome of chronic pain in general, are summarized as follows:

1. See the patient at regular intervals to preclude the need for the patient to use symptoms as a "ticket of admission" to the medical system.
2. Accept the patient's need to be considered ill. The patient should be told that even if symp-

toms improve, the illness will probably always be present. Promise understanding and support rather than complete relief, which can be a threat as much as a reward to some patients. Emphasizing management rather than cure can help the patient gain a more realistic view of her condition.
3. Do not make physician contacts contingent on physical complaints. If the patient knows that the patient-physician relationship will continue even when the patient feels well, the use of symptoms as a means of ensuring access to the physician will decrease.
4. Do not prolong contact with the patient in response to an increase of symptoms. A specific visit length discourages the patient from having more symptoms in order to see the physician more extensively.
5. Allow the patient to structure the content of the discussions. Open-ended questions, such as, "How are you feeling?," are usually sufficient to allow the patient this option.
6. Minimize secondary gain. If the patient is receiving monetary compensation for the illness, improvement is likely to be both financially and emotionally threatening. The family should be helped to avoid reorganizing their lives around the patient's illness, and they should be encouraged to gradually increase their demands that the patient function more effectively as a family member regardless of her level of well-being.
7. Teach the patient to express emotions in words. When the patient describes a situation in which a strong emotion, such as anger, should have been experienced, but pain or some other physical sensation was felt instead, ask, "Were you angry, too?" If the patient responds that anger did not cause the pain, point out that anger and pain are two different states that may or may not have anything to do with each other, but both are important to physicians who wish to treat the whole patient.
8. Control strong reactions to the patient. Patients who covertly refuse to cooperate often arouse strong feelings in their physicians, which can result in the physician's expressing hostility or an argumentative approach to the patient. Such responses by the physician tell the patient not to return unless symptoms become worse, or they may cause the patient to behave with excessive hostility or retreat into a state of isolation.
9. Remain alert for intercurrent medical illness. Changes in the patient's symptoms that cannot be explained by new stressors or unavailability of the physician may mean that the patient is expressing a new medical problem in characteristic ways, which make it appear to be an outgrowth of the original functional complaint.

## Sexual Abuse History

Many patients who have chronic pain have a history of abusive family relationships, which have impacted upon their childhood, adulthood, or both. Sexual victimization has been particularly linked to a later development of chronic pelvic pain. This complicates both the evaluation and the treatment of women who have chronic pelvic pain. For example, the use of antidepressant medications appears to be less efficacious in women who have a history of sexual victimization. These patients may also be less able to develop a close relationship with their physicians, a situation that may make long-term therapeutic attempts less effective. Because of the high risk of other psychiatric illness, such as anxiety and mood disorders, these patients may not easily fall within the purview of the typical physician who initially sees most victims of sexual abuse. The most important factor for the clinician and the patient is that the physician be made aware of the patient's sexual trauma. The initial evaluation of a patient who has chronic pelvic pain should include a gentle inquiry directed toward current or past sexual or physical abuse. For example, "Have you ever been touched against your will, either as a child or an adult?" is one possible entry statement. Recognition of this factor may help frame future discussions and therapeutic interventions, including supportive listening, use of community resources, referral to support groups, and treatment with antidepressants.

## Role of Antidepressants in Chronic Pelvic Pain

The use of antidepressant medication may prove beneficial in the patient who has difficulty coping with chronic pain or with the emotional demands that the illness may cause on the family unit. A clinical trial of these medications given at bedtime often results in the patient's experiencing an enhanced quality of sleep as well as an overall improvement in adjustment to her illness. Tricyclic antidepressants also may provide pain relief through peripheral neuroblockade and central stimulation in addition to their other actions. In a meta-analytic review of 39 controlled antidepressant trials, Onghena and Van Houdenhove found that on average, the chronic pain patient who was treated with an antidepressant had less pain than 74% of such patients who received a placebo.

Amitriptyline, an antidepressant with sedative effects, is a good choice when such agents are needed for the treatment of chronic pain. It should not be used in patients who are taking monoamine oxidase inhibitors or in those who have cardiovascular disorders, particularly arrhythmias. Common side effects are related to anticholinergic effects and include urinary retention, dry mouth, and constipation. Serious side effects include myocardial infarction, cardiac arrhythmias, and bone marrow depression. Dosages of amitriptyline start at 25 mg at bedtime and can be increased to 150 mg if needed. Other antidepressants, such as nortriptyline, imipramine, and fluoxetine, have also been used successfully. Nortriptyline may be started, using 25 mg at bedtime and increasing by 25 mg every 3 to 4 days thereafter as tolerated, with a maximum dosage of 100 mg per day. Fluoxetine may be given at a dosage of 20 mg per day. Sertraline may be given at a dosage of 50 mg per day.

## Role of Surgical Management in Chronic Pelvic Pain

Surgery is often a logical extension of a thorough diagnostic and therapeutic management scheme for patients who have chronic pelvic pain. In particular, diagnostic laparoscopy remains the best procedural choice when a diagnostic dilemma exists. For a clinician who is not trained in surgery, this requires referral to a specialist. For the nonsurgical clinician to make an appropriate referral, some knowledge of the required procedure is necessary. Therefore, we will attempt to briefly review surgical options that are frequently performed in treating chronic pelvic pain.

### Diagnostic Laparoscopy

Diagnostic laparoscopy has four roles in the management of the pelvic pain patient:
1. Patient reassurance
2. Documentation of adhesive disease
3. Elimination of diagnostic errors
4. Histologic documentation

Diagnostic laparoscopy can result in a therapeutic response in patients who may be anxious about neoplasia, infection, or any other pelvic etiology of their pain. Thus, physicians should not minimize the importance of reassuring these patients and making nonsurgical interventions in the management of their chronic pelvic pain. This reassurance is potentially aided by the use of a videocassette recording or photographs taken at the time of surgery.

Documentation of pelvic adhesions is necessary if therapeutic surgery is contemplated. Overall, the patient's history and physical examination have been shown to be very poor predictors of whether the patient actually has pelvic adhesions. However, a pelvic examination with two abnormal findings has been shown to predict the presence of pelvic adhesions in 74% of patients. These data show that all patients who present with chronic pelvic pain do not necessarily need diagnostic laparoscopy, regardless of historical or physical findings. Moreover, in the absence of such findings, patients who have chronic pelvic pain may sometimes be best served initially by nonsurgical therapy.

Diagnostic laparoscopy does eliminate presumptive treatment of suspected pathology by providing direct visualization of pelvic structures. The presence and extent of significant pathology, such as endometriosis, pelvic infection, or adhesions, can be documented both for baseline comparative purposes and for proper selection of therapy. However, approximately 30% of patients who have chronic pelvic pain can be expected to have normal findings. In these patients, as I have mentioned previously, reassurance can potentially be therapeutic.

In no group of patients is histologic documentation more important than in those who have suspected endometriosis. Recent evidence indicates that many endometrial implants may not fit the classic description of black or blue lesions. Many conditions can simulate endometriosis; therefore, numerous biopsies should be taken of classic lesions as well as of any areas of the peritoneum that appear abnormal. It is certainly not unusual at the time of laparoscopy to find that patients who have a history of PID actually have endometriosis as the cause of their pain.

### Adhesiolysis

Surgical lysis of adhesions, whether by laparoscopy or laparotomy, would, at first glance, appear to be the logical therapy for patients who have documented adhesive disease caused by PID. Unfortunately, there is no documented evidence that adhesions always cause such pelvic pain. As previously indicated, only a small percentage of patients who have chronic pelvic pain have documented adhesive disease. Other studies have shown a comparable incidence of adhesions in both chronic pelvic pain patients and control patients. Nevertheless, in a study of 100 patients who were followed for a minimum for 6 months, Chan found that adhesiolysis produced complete or partial pain relief in 65% of patients, whereas 20.9% said the pain was unchanged, and 11.6% had more severe pain. This type of information is useful when counseling patients who are considering adhesiolysis. These patients should receive the following information:
1. Adhesions are present but may not be the cause of pain.

2. Adhesiolysis may not provide relief, or the pain may become worse.
3. Adhesions may form again and result in further pain.

**Uterine Suspension**

Although uterine retrodisplacement is an unusual occurrence, it may be associated with pelvic pain. The mere presence of retrodisplacement is not an indication for a suspension procedure, because as many as one third of all women may have a retroverted uterus. Typically, symptoms associated with uterine retroversion include a pressure sensation in the pelvis, the low back, or both. In addition, deep thrust or "bump" dyspareunia is a common symptom. *No surgical therapy for symptomatic retrodisplacement should be undertaken without a successful trial of a pessary.* Such a trial would entail placement of a pessary (Smith's or Hodge's) to effect anteversion of the uterus. Uterine anteversion should relieve the pain if it is caused by retrodisplacement, and removal of the pessary should result in a return of pain.

In an older patient who does not desire future childbearing, vaginal hysterectomy is appropriate. In a younger patient, uterine suspension may be considered. The modified Gilliam suspension, in which the round ligaments are drawn through an opening near the internal inguinal ring and sutured to the fascia, is an excellent and classic choice for suspension. The laparoscopic procedure is a more modern approach, in which the round ligament is drawn up to the abdominal wall through two additional puncture sites and sutured to the rectus sheath.

**Uterosacral Nerve Ablation and Presacral Neurectomy**

Uterosacral nerve ablation appears to have only a limited role in the management of chronic pelvic pain. This procedure transects the afferent pain fibers within the uterosacral ligaments. Significant relief of dysmenorrhea has been reported in 60% of patients whose symptoms were refractory to oral contraceptives and NSAIDs with laparoscopic uterosacral nerve ablation (LUNA).

In my opinion, uterosacral nerve ablation offers a secondary line of therapy for dysmenorrhea only. It can be performed at the time of diagnostic laparoscopy in those patients who do not respond to medical therapy. Potential long-term complications, which have not been evaluated, include loss of cervical support and creation of large denuded areas posterior to the uterus. This denudation may heighten susceptibility to adhesion formation in the area of the tubes and ovaries. The proximity of the ureters is also of concern to the gynecologic surgeon. It should be noted that this procedure should be reserved only for patients who have dysmenorrhea and not chronic pelvic pain. Considering that adhesions from PID are most likely to occur in the adnexal area, the role of LUNA should be quite limited.

Presacral neurectomy has also been advocated by some authors for patients who have central pelvic pain. Current indications for presacral neurectomy are for relief of dysmenorrhea, deep thrust dyspareunia, sacral backache, and chronic recurrent pain in the center of the pelvis. In patients who have chronic pelvic pain, Lee and associates reported a group of 50 patients who underwent presacral neurectomy after failed medical therapy for chronic pelvic pain, including dysmenorrhea and selected cases of dyspareunia. They found a success rate of 73% in relieving dysmenorrhea, 77% in relieving dyspareunia, and 63% in relieving pelvic pain. Including the bilateral uterosacral ligaments in this procedure did not increase the success rate. There was an 18% lateral pain recurrence but no recurrence of dysmenorrhea. We recommend that presacral neurectomy be reserved only for cases that fail all other conservative measures.

**Hysterectomy**

Although hysterectomy is usually reserved for those patients who do not obtain pain relief from medical or conservative surgical therapy, chronic pain remains the third most common indication for hysterectomy. A study at the University of Tennessee, Memphis, evaluated the long-term outcome of 99 women who underwent hysterectomy for pelvic pain of at least 6 months' duration. All these patients had symptoms and findings on physical examination that were suggestive of disease confined to the uterus. Patients who had previously documented extrauterine disease or uterine weight in excess of 200 g were excluded from this review. Twenty-two patients had persistent pelvic pain, even after hysterectomy. Five patients described their pain as being worse than before surgery. Information such as this regarding the likelihood of postoperative pain relief should be shared with all patients who consider undergoing hysterectomy for pelvic pain of presumed uterine origin. Although a 75% cure rate may be appealing to some patients, others may prefer to explore other nonsurgical approaches when given these odds.

# Summary

The basic diagnostic and therapeutic approaches to the patient with pelvic pain have been described above (see Table 5–2). Using this rationale allows the practicing physician to evaluate and realistically manage, or appropriately refer, most patients who have pelvic pain. The key to the management of patients who have pelvic pain, especially those who have long-standing chronic pain, is to use any and all available diagnostic and therapeutic modalities to identify the source or sources of the pain and to direct therapy accordingly. By having at least a working knowledge of the various diagnostic and therapeutic modalities available to the patient, the individual clinician can help the patient to understand the nature of chronic pelvic pain generally and her own pelvic pain specifically.

## REFERENCES

Chan C, Wood C: Pelvic adhesiolysis: The assessment of symptom relief by 100 patients. Aust N Z J Obstet Gynecol 25:295, 1985.

Fernandes M, Seebode J: Urologic causes of pelvic pain in the female. *In* Weiss G (ed): Clinical Consultations in Obstetrics and Gynecology. Philadelphia: WB Saunders, 1991, pp 46–53.

Lee RB, Stone K, Magelssen D, et al: Presacral neurectomy for chronic pelvic pain. Obstet Gynecol 68:517–521, 1986.

Milburn A, Reiter RC, Rhomberg AT: Multidisciplinary approach to chronic pelvic pain. *In* Ling FW (ed): Contemporary Management of Chronic Pelvic Pain. Obstet Gynecol North Am 20:643, 1993.

Onghena P, Van Houdenhove BV: Antidepressant-induced analgesia in chronic non-malignant pain: A meta-analysis of 39 placebo controlled studies. Pain 49:205, 1992.

Powell EM, Wattenburg CA: Treatment of urethritis in the female: With a clinical and pathological study. J Urol 72:392, 1954.

Rubelowski J, Machiedo G: Gastrointestinal causes of pelvic pain. *In* Weiss G (ed): Clinical Consultations in Obstetrics and Gynecology. Philadelphia, WB Saunders, 1991, pp 41–45.

Slocumb J: Neurologic factors in chronic pelvic pain: Trigger points and the abdominal pelvic pain syndrome. Am J Obstet Gynecol 149:536, 1984.

Summitt R, Ling F: Urethral syndrome presenting as chronic pelvic pain. J Psychosom Obstet Gynecol 12:77, 1991.

Walling MK, Reiter RC, O'Hare MW, et al: Abuse history and chronic pain in women: I & II. Prevalences of sexual and physical abuse. Obstet Gyecol 84:193, 1994.

# 6

# Leiomyoma

LARA J. BURROWS
THOMAS E. ELKINS

Uterine leiomyomas (fibroids) are the most common neoplasms of the female pelvis. They occur in approximately 20 to 25% of women of reproductive age. Their distribution appears to be worldwide, and they are more common in black women. True estimates of their prevalence are unknown because the majority of leiomyomas are asymptomatic. These tumors are the most common indication for hysterectomy, accounting for approximately 30% of all procedures in two large collaborative trials from the United States. They account for approximately 67% of all hysterectomies performed among middle-aged women. Leiomyomas rarely occur before menarche and typically regress after menopause, implicating estrogen as a promotor of this growth.

## Pathology

By definition, a leiomyoma is a benign neoplasm composed of smooth muscle cells with variable amounts of fibrous stroma. Each of the cells comprising leiomyomas is of identical glucose-6-phosphate-dehydrogenase electrophoretic type, which suggests that leiomyomas are unicellular in origin. Although the exact stimulus to the development of leiomyomas is not known, it is generally accepted that they are influenced by estrogen and progesterone. Evidence for this as outlined by Silverberg and Kurman includes the following:

1. The rarity of leiomyomas before menarche and their usual regression after menopause
2. Occasional rapid growth and hemorrhagic degeneration of leiomyomas associated with pregnancy and clomiphene and progestin treatment
3. Regression of leiomyomas after treatment with gonadotropin-releasing hormone (Gn-RH) agonists.
4. Increased mitotic activity in leiomyomas during the secretory phase of the menstrual cycle.
5. Ultrastructural evidence of increased differentiation (myofilaments, dense bodies) in leiomyoma cells cultured with estrogen and progesterone
6. The presence of estrogen and progesterone receptors in leiomyoma cells, with variation in their concentration during the menstrual cycle

As described by Prayson and associates, features that are assessed by the pathologist when examining a leiomyoma, include its anatomic location, the presence of extrauterine extension, size, gross appearance, the degree of histologic cellularity, nuclear atypia and mitotic activity, as well as characterization of any necrosis that may be present. Atypical gross or microscopic features are worrisome. There are many subtypes of leiomyoma that must be distinguished from leiomyosarcoma both grossly and microscopically.

This chapter presents a classification system of smooth muscle tumors as outlined by Silverberg and Kurman.

# Leiomyoma

## GROSS FINDINGS

In approximately two thirds of women who have uterine leiomyoma, multiple myomas are present. Leiomyomas are usually found in the myometrium of the uterine corpus; however, they can also originate in the cervix and, occasionally, in the broad ligament (intraligamentous leiomyoma), thus creating uncertainty when the adnexa is evaluated on bimanual examination. Rarely, vaginal, urethral, or vulvar leiomyomas are detected or even intravenous leiomyomatosis may be encountered, and the presence of these unusual tumors confounds the findings on physical examination. Leiomyomas that occur in the uterine corpus are described with regard to their location: submucosal, intramural, or subserosal. Uncommonly, submucosal leiomyomas are pedunculated, which can produce cervical dilatation and prolapse through the external os. These "aborting fibroids" are prone to ulceration and secondary infection. They may also be mistaken for endocervical or endometrial polyps on pelvic examination. Even more uncommon is the pedunculated subserosal leiomyoma, which may become attached to an adjacent pelvic or abdominal structure from which it derives a new blood supply that enables it to subsequently detach from the uterus (parasitic leiomyoma).

In gross appearance, leiomyomas vary in size from small, incidental findings to huge tumors weighing more than 100 lb. Most leiomyomas are firm, spherical, well-circumscribed tumors within the myometrium. Their cut surface is typically white to tan with a whorled appearance. Variations in this appearance include hemorrhage; hyalinization; hydropic, myxoid, or mucinous degeneration; true necrosis; and calcification. These features are important because they may also be seen in leiomyosarcoma. Patients who are pregnant, postpartum, or who are using oral contraceptives or other progestational agents may have leiomyomas that undergo hemorrhagic infarction (also called red or carneous degeneration).

## MICROSCOPIC FINDINGS

Typical leioimyomas constitute almost all uterine smooth muscle tumors and are characterized by an admixture of bland, smooth muscle cells, fibroblasts, and collagen. The smooth muscle cells are generally arranged in anastomosing whorled fascicles of uniform fusiform cells. In contrast to leiomyosarcoma, the nuclei have a uniform appearance. Mitotic figures are infrequent, and there is never nuclear atypia.

The variants of uterine leiomyoma listed in the International Society of Gynecological Pathologists' Classification are cellular, epithelioid, and bizarre leiomyoma and lipoleiomyoma. A *cellular leiomyoma* is a benign tumor that is significantly more cellular than the surrounding myometrium. They are clinically and grossly indistinguishable from other leiomyomas but it is noteworthy because hypercellularity is also one of the characteristics of a leiomyosarcoma.

One form of cellular leiomyoma, as mentioned previously, is the *hemorrhagic cellular leiomyoma* (apoplectic leiomyoma). Venous thrombosis and congestion with interstitial hemorrhage are responsible for the color of such a leiomyoma, which is undergoing "red degeneration." This tumor is characterized by multifocal areas of hemorrhage noted on gross appearance in addition to increased mitotic activity confined to a narrow zone around the hemorrhage. The cellularity, hemorrhage, and mitotic activity can be misleading and may give rise to the erroneous diagnosis of a leiomyosarcoma. However, the clinical history, lack of atypia, and focal distribution of the mitotic activity point to the diagnosis of a hemorrhagic leiomyoma.

**Epithelioid Leiomyoma.** These are benign, smooth-muscle tumors that resemble epithelial cells. They are composed of round or polygonal cells as opposed to the spindled cells seen in typical leiomyomas. They tend to be solitary and softer than the typical leiomyoma and are often yellow or gray. This type of leiomyoma is divided into *leiomyoblastoma*, *clear all leiomyoma*, and *plexiform* leiomyoma, all of which are rare and clinically very similar to typical leiomyomas except that a plexiform leiomyoma is often an incidental microscopic finding, measuring only a few millimeters in diameter. Predicting the clinical behavior of these tumors can be challenging. Plexiform leiomyomas are considered completely benign and *most* leiomyoblastomas and clear cell leiomyomas are also clinically benign, but the exact criteria for distinguishing benign from malignant tumors in this group have not yet been clarified. Therefore, some feel it is safest to classify some tumors in this group as "smooth muscle tumors of uncertain malignant potential."

**Bizarre Leiomyoma.** This is a benign tumor characterized by pleomorphic and symplastic giant cells. These masses resemble typical leiomyoma in gross appearance; however, microscopically, they can be difficult to distinguish from leiomyosarcoma.

**Lipoleiomyoma.** These tumors resemble ordinary

leiomyoma, but they also contain benign adipocytes. They are rare and occur mostly in postmenopausal women.

## Leiomyosarcoma

Leiomyosarcoma by definition is a malignant tumor showing smooth muscle differentiation. This is a rare tumor, representing slightly more than 1% of all corporeal malignant tumors. It is generally found in postmenopausal women and is not associated with any known risk factors. Contrary to previous beliefs, a leiomyosarcoma can rarely be proven to arise in or from a benign leiomyoma and is thought to arise de novo. The signs and symptoms are similar to those produced by a benign leiomyoma; however, the presence of a rapid increase in the size of a uterine tumor after menopause ought to arouse suspicion. The diagnosis of leiomyosarcoma is most commonly made at the time of a hysterectomy.

On gross appearance, leiomyosarcomas usually appear very different from benign leiomyomas. They are generally solitary, large, and poorly-circumscribed, with a soft, fleshy consistency and a gray yellow to pink color, with foci of hemorrhage and necrosis. In advanced cases, they may show evidence of extension beyond the uterine corpus. Microscopically, most leiomyosarcomas show the triad of hypercellularity, atypia, and numerous mitotic figures. Two variant leiomyosarcomas, the epithelioid and myxoid types, are noteworthy because they can be difficult to distinguish from benign leiomyomas of similar type.

The natural history of these tumors is poorly understood. Generally, leiomyosarcomas have spread beyond the confines of the uterine corpus at the time of initial diagnosis. Lymph node metastases are uncommon, but distant metastases to the lung, liver, and bone do occur. Treatment is predominantly surgical, consisting of a total abdominal hysterectomy and bilateral salpingo-oophorectomy. Radiotherapy and single-agent chemotherapy have not been found to significantly alter the natural history of the disease. For stages I and II disease, 5-year survival rates are approximately 40 to 50%.

## Smooth Muscle Tumors of Uncertain Malignant Potential

Smooth muscle tumors of uncertain malignant potential are those that cannot be diagnosed definitively as benign or malignant by using the generally accepted criteria. If the diagnosis is made, the reason should be specific.

## Other Smooth Muscle Tumors

Metastasizing leiomyomas appear benign and after several years metastasize to extrauterine tissues. Most metastases are pulmonary, although some are attached to pelvic and extrapelvic soft tissues. These lesions usually occur several years after hysterectomy and are frequently compatible with many additional years of life.

Intravenous leiomyomas are rare, benign, smooth muscle proliferations involving the myometrial veins. On gross appearance, they are worm-like masses of firm to soft tissue seen within the veins of the uterus. It is not uncommon to find extensions into the inferior vena cava or the right side of the heart.

## Clinical Features

It is estimated that 10 to 40% of leiomyomas are symptomatic, thus, the majority are asymptomatic. Although any form of abnormal bleeding is possible, these patients most commonly have menorrhagia, the precise etiology of which is not completely understood. The theories that increased uterine bleeding is caused by ulcerated submucous tumors, and that the uterine cavity is expanded by submucous leiomyoma, are now controversial, although the correlation between severe menorrhagia and an associated submucous myoma is not uncommonly seen. Current theories imply that enhanced bleeding may be caused by increased vascularity or by alteration in the endometrial microvasculature, such as congestion and dilatation. A common result of all abnormal uterine bleeding is iron deficiency anemia, which may not be amenable to iron therapy in the presence of uterine leiomyomata.

Pain is not an uncommon consequence of leiomyoma. Some women have been noted to have a chronic dull backache when a leiomyoma of moderate size is present in a retroverted uterus; others may have dysmenorrhea or dyspareunia. Acute pain associated with low-grade fever and localized uterine tenderness occurs (especially in a postpartum or pregnant patient) with red degeneration of a leiomyoma or with torsion of a pedunculated subserous tumor. This pain can be excruciating and can produce a clinical picture consistent with an acute abdomen. Usually, these events are self-limited and can be managed conservatively after more serious illnesses have been ruled out. There are also reports of women who have leiomyoma and who develop severe abdominal pain while taking luteinizing hormone–releasing hormone (LH–RH) analogs for leiomyoma shrinkage.

Chronic pelvic pain is atypical, except when confused with increasing pelvic pressure.

Pelvic pressure, lower urinary tract symptoms, and impingement on adjacent viscera are common in many women who have leiomyomas that are large. Uterine size is usually estimated based on an equivalent gestational size in weeks. A uterus greater than a 12-week size is considered large and can be palpated on abdominal examination. Depending on the size and location of the leiomyoma, if these tumors are larger than a 10- to 12-week size, they may compress or displace the ureters, the bladder, or the rectum, producing chronic hydroureter or hydronephrosis, renal malfunction, urinary retention, abdominal enlargement, constipation, or rectal pressure symptoms. The enlarged uterus can compress the bladder, resulting in urinary frequency and stress incontinence. There have been rare instances of leiomyoma occurring in the female urethra or bladder itself, but the vast majority of these are asymptomatic.

Reproductive disorders, including infertility, recurrent spontaneous abortion, and preterm labor, have been attributed to uterine leiomyoma. There are no controlled studies to date that support a causal association between uterine leiomyoma and adverse reproductive outcomes, with the rare exception of bilateral tubal obstruction stemming from a cornual leiomyoma, which causes infertility. Performance of a hysterosalpingogram should be considered in patients who have palpable leiomyomas and infertility or recurrent abortions. Myomectomies have been helpful in such settings, although definitive, prospective, controlled studies have not shown a clear benefit in every situation. Leiomyomas occasionally complicate pregnancy by causing obstruction, uterine inversion, or rapid growth. Myomectomies are not recommended during pregnancy because of hemorrhagic complications and the risk of pregnancy loss. Red degeneration seems to be more common both postpartum and during pregnancy and should be suspected in a woman who has acute pain and tenderness and known leiomyomas but no other identifiable cause of her symptoms.

Other complications include ulceration and secondary infection of a prolapsing cervical leiomyoma, which can cause fever and a leukocytosis. Ascites has been reported, and polycythemia caused by autonomous production of erythropoietin by a leiomyoma has also been reported.

Leiomyosarcomas typically arise in the fifth or sixth decade of life, and the incidence increases with each succeeding decade. Clinically, these tumors are associated with abnormal bleeding and rapid uterine enlargement. There is a uniformly poor prognosis in the postmenopausal years, regardless of the clinical stage at the time of diagnosis. Stage I and II tumors (confined to the uterus) seem to have a more favorable prognosis in premenopausal women, and hysterectomy is usually curative.

# Diagnosis

The pelvic examination is the primary method of leiomyoma diagnosis. A leiomyoma may be suspected based on a bimanual examination that reveals an enlarged, firm, nontender, and irregularly shaped uterus. Although experienced clinicians can be highly accurate (the diagnosis of a uterine leiomyoma can be established with approximately 95% confidence on the basis of examination), it is often important to obtain objective confirmation before treatment. Pelvic ultrasonography has revolutionized how leiomyomas are diagnosed and treated and has proved to be the most useful imaging study available.

A proper ultrasound examination should provide answers regarding uterine volume, the number of leiomyoma, their location relative to the endometrial stripe, evaluation of the adnexa, and a cursory scan of the kidneys to rule out hydronephrosis. Ultrasonography can also document interval growth with serial studies. Although ultrasonography is an invaluable tool in assessing uterine leiomyomas, it is not recommended routinely for women who have obvious leiomyomas because it has not been shown to improve long-term clinical outcomes beyond those obtained with appropriate clinical assessment. Magnetic resonance imaging is also highly accurate in ways similar to ultrasonography; however, the expense of this test limits its usefulness.

The improved efficacy of pelvic ultrasound in differentiating leiomyomas from other pelvic pathologies has all but eliminated the indication for hysterectomy based on uterine size alone, especially since uteri beyond 16 to 20 weeks of gestational size are rarely asymptomatic. Because ultrasonographic assessment evaluates the adnexal structures accurately in the majority of cases, the diagnostic test for hysterectomy occasioned by leiomyomas that interfere with physical examination of the adnexa is now obsolete.

Other imaging studies include the hysterosalpingogram, which is not a primary indication for the evaluation of leiomyoma. This is usually performed as part of an evaluation before myomectomy to assess the chance of future fertility after surgery. The computed tomography (CT) scan has not proved to be useful in the diagnosis of leiomyoma.

Laboratory testing should include a Papanicolaou smear if routinely indicated, a hematocrit study if the patient has menorrhagia, and a urinalysis if she has urinary complaints. If the patient has a history of a bleeding disorder, a coagulation profile is indicated. In women who have abnormal bleeding or who are at risk for endometrial neoplasia, an endometrial biopsy is indicated.

# Management

The available treatment options for uterine leiomyoma include both nonsurgical and surgical modalities.

## EXPECTANT MANAGEMENT

Expectant management consists of serial histories and physical examinations at clinically indicated intervals. If the tumors are stable and slow growing, yearly follow-up with optimization of symptom control is a viable option. Whether or not the patient has leiomyomas, the treatment of menorrhagia should be the same, namely, a trial of at least two nonsteroidal anti-inflammatory drugs on a scheduled (as opposed to an as-needed) basis. Although antiprostaglandin therapy has been shown to reduce menstrual blood loss by 30 to 50% in women who have menorrhagia, patients who have leiomyoma-associated menorrhagia may respond less consistently to these agents. Low-dose oral contraceptives and progestins might be effective alternative treatments. Patients who have symptoms associated with leiomyoma should usually be offered a trial of conservative management before considering surgical therapy.

## MEDICAL MANAGEMENT

Gonadotropin-releasing hormone (GnRH) agonists are analogs of gonadotropin-releasing hormone. With continuous administration, they suppress the pituitary-ovarian axis with a subsequent hypoestrogenic state (sometimes referred to as pseudomenopause). It has been shown that there is a median reduction in uterine volume of 50%, and the greatest effect is seen 12 weeks after initiation of therapy, with no further reduction in uterine size observed between 12 and 24 weeks. Upon discontinuing the treatment, there is a rapid rate of regrowth of the leiomyoma. The preoperative reduction of tumor size before hysterectomy for either minimizing blood loss or facilitating a vaginal hysterectomy is controversial. A reduction in intraoperative blood loss has not consistently been reported, and there does not appear to be a reduction in the likelihood of blood transfusion.

The side effects of these medications, which are caused primarily by the hypoestrogenic state they induce, include hot flushes, mood changes, vaginal dryness, decreased libido, and loss of bone density, which may or may not be permanent. Therefore, the use of GnRH analogs are recommended only for the following cases:
- Treating a large submucous tumor to facilitate hysteroscopic resection
- Awaiting imminent onset of menopause (in the perimenopausal age group)
- Decreasing tumor size and symptoms before surgery

Newer treatment options regarding Gn-RH analogs include "add-back" therapy. When a patient is being treated for an indefinite period of time with Gn-RH analogs, after 12 weeks of therapy low doses of estrogen and progesterone are added. This type of therapy is still considered to be investigational, and further studies must be performed before this option can be accepted as an appropriate treatment for leiomyoma.

## ENDOSCOPIC RESECTION

Many studies have documented the effectiveness of hysteroscopic diagnosis and resection of submucous leiomyoma, but long-term follow-up has demonstrated that approximately 20% of patients require additional treatment within 5 to 10 years after initial resection. Some studies have demonstrated that laparoscopic myomectomy is a safe and reliable treatment option, but it is difficult to perform technically and not available universally. In the future, after further investigation, endometrial ablation by neodymium:yttrium-aluminum-garnet (Nd:YAG) laser may be a viable treatment alternative for smaller submucous leiomyomas.

## MYOMECTOMY

The principal reason for performing a myomectomy in a patient who has abnormal bleeding associated with leiomyoma is uterine conservation for the preservation of fertility. Over the long term, myomectomy seems to be a safe, effective and usually permanent treatment option. Preoperative criteria currently endorsed by the American College of Obstetricians and Gynecologists (ACOG) are as follows:
- Failure to conceive or recurrent pregnancy loss
- Presence of leiomyomas of sufficient size or specific location to be a probable factor
- No more likely explanation exists for the failure to conceive or recurrent pregnancy loss

## HYSTERECTOMY

Hysterectomy is considered to be the definitive treatment for uterine leiomyoma in symptomatic women

who have completed childbearing. ACOG criteria for hysterectomy for the indication of uterine leiomyoma are as follows:
- Presence of 1 to 3 asymptomatic leiomyomas of palpable size abdominally and are a concern to the patient
- Excessive uterine bleeding
  —Profuse bleeding with flooding or clots or repetitive periods lasting more than 8 days
  —Anemia due to acute or chronic blood loss
- Pelvic discomfort caused by myomas
  —Acute and severe pain
  —Chronic lower abdominal or low back pressure
  —Bladder pressure with urinary frequency not due to urinary tract infection

In the past, hysterectomy was recommended in asymptomatic women who had uteri larger than 12 weeks size who did not desire fertility. Recommending a hysterectomy based on uterine size alone is no longer a standard of care. Currently, unless there is an indication for a hysterectomy for other medical reasons, these patients can be managed expectantly (assuming the leiomyomas are slow-growing and asymptomatic). In patients who have large cervical leiomyomas, broad ligament myomas, or uterine size of 16 gestational weeks or larger, evaluations for ureteral obstruction and renal dysfunction should be done before the course of management is undertaken.

## UTERINE ARTERY EMBOLIZATION

Uterine artery embolization is a new and investigational technique for the treatment of uterine leiomyomas. Preliminary studies in women who had large, symptomatic leiomyomas have shown considerable improvement in their symptoms. While these results appear promising, the long-term efficacy and safety of this treatment modality require further investigation.

## ENDOSCOPIC CRYOTHERAPY

Laparoscopic insertion of a cryotherapy probe into the core of a myoma less than 6 cm in diameter has been reported to be helpful in some settings in avoiding more invasive surgery.

## REFERENCES

ACOG Technical Bulletin, No. 192, May 1994.

Bradley EA, Reidy JF, Forman RG, et al: Transcatheter uterine artery embolisation to treat large uterine fibroids. Br J Obstet Gynecol 105:235–240, 1998.

Buttram VC Jr, Reiter RC: Uterine leiomyomata: Etiology, symptomatology, and management. Fertil Steril 36:433–445, 1981.

Cornella JL, Larson TR, Lee RA, et al: Leiomyoma of the female urethra and bladder: Report of twenty-three patients and review of the literature. Am J Obstet Gynecol 176:1278–1285, 1997.

Davis KM, Schlaff WD: Medical management of uterine fibromyomata. Obstet Gynecol Clin North Am 22:727–738, 1995.

Derman SG, Rehnstrom J, Neuwirth RS: The long-term effectiveness of hysteroscopic treatment of menorrhagia and leiomyomas. Obstet Gynecol 77:591–594, 1991.

Dubusson JB, Chapron C: Uterine fibroids: Place and modalities of laparoscopic treatment. Eur J Obstet Gynecol Reprod Biol 65:91–94, 1996.

Farrer-Brown G, Beilby JOW, Tarbit MH: Venous changes in the endometrium of myomatous uteri. Obstet Gynecol 38:743–751, 1971.

Friedman AJ, Hoffman DI, Comite F, et al: Treatment of leiomyoma uteri with leupride acetate depot: A double-blind, placebo-controlled, multi-center study. Obstet Gynecol 77:720–725, 1991.

Gambone JC, Reiter RC, Lench JB, et al: The impact of a quality assurance process on the frequency and confirmation rate of hysterectomy. Am J Obstet Gynecol 163:545–550, 1990.

Garcia CR: Management of the symptomatic fibroid in women older than 40 years of age. Obstet Gynecol Clin North Am 22:337–348, 1993.

Garry R, Erian J, Grochmal SA: A multi-centre collaborative study into the treatment of menorrhagia by Nd:YAG laser ablation of the endometrium. Br J Obstet Gynecol 98:357–362, 1991.

Greenberg MD, Kazamel TIG: Medical and socioeconomic impact of uterine fibroids. Obstet Gynecol Clin North Am 22:625–636, 1995.

Hutchins FL: Uterine fibroids. Obstet Gynecol Clin North Am 22:659–665, 1995.

Kjerulff KH, Langenberg P, Seidman JD, et al: Racial differences in severity, symptoms and age at diagnosis. J Reprod Med 41:483–490, 1996.

LaMorte AI, Lalwani S, Diamond MP: Morbidity associated with abdominal myomectomy. Obstet Gynecol 82:897–900, 1993.

Pernoll ML: Current Obstetric & Gynecologic Diagnosis and Treatment. E. Norwalk, CT, Appleton & Lange, 1994, 731–736.

Prayson RA, Hart WR: Pathologic considerations of uterine smooth muscle tumors. Obstet Gynecol Clin North Am 22:637–656, 1995.

Silverberg SG, Kurman RJ: Tumors of the uterine corpus and gestational trophoblastic disease. *In* Atlas of Tumor Pathology, Series 3, Fascicle 3. Washington, DC, Armed Forces Institute of Pathology, 1991.

Vollenhoven BJ, Lawrence AS, Healy DL: Uterine fibroids: A clinical review. Br J Obstet Gynaecol 97:285–298, 1990.

# 7

# Lower Genital Tract Infection

S. GENE McNEELEY, JR.

Lower genital tract infections are among the most commonly treated gynecologic conditions. They include vulvovaginal and cervical infections. They are frequently associated with vaginal discharge and odor and vulvo vaginal pruritus. Genital tract ulcers or masses may be present.

Vaginal discharge is a common symptom of sexually transmitted diseases (STDs). More than 12 million sexually transmitted infections are reported annually in the United States. Many billions of healthcare dollars are expended annually for treatment of these infections and their sequelae. In particular, women experience complications of many STDs that are often undiagnosed and untreated. These disorders include chronic pelvic pain, infertility, and ectopic pregnancy.

## Vaginitis

Vaginitis is a clinical syndrome characterized by vaginal discharge with or without vulvovaginal itching. Vaginal odor is a common complaint.

### BACTERIAL VAGINOSIS

Bacterial vaginosis (BV) is a clinical syndrome characterized by a homogeneous vaginal discharge, malodor, and pruritus. BV is the most commonly occurring vaginal infection and is caused by replacement of the normal *Lactobacillus* species in the vagina with high concentrations of anaerobic pathogens. The most frequently identified of these are species of *Bacteroides*, *Peptostreptococcus*, *Mobiluncus*, *Prevotella*, and *Mycoplasma*, as well as *Gardnerella vaginalis*. BV is not considered a sexually transmitted disease. In the classic sense; however, it is associated with extensive sexual experience, that is, frequent intercourse and multiple sexual partners. Approximately half of the women who have BV are asymptomatic. This condition is associated with pelvic inflammatory disease, postabortion endometritis, and posthysterectomy soft tissue infections. In the pregnant patient, BV has been linked with poor pregnancy outcome, including preterm delivery, premature rupture of membranes, and delivery of low birth-weight infants.

### VULVOVAGINAL CANDIDIASIS

Most vaginal yeast infections are caused by *Candida albicans*, and they account for approximately 35 to 40% of all vaginal infections. Approximately 75% of women experience at least one episode of vulvovaginal candidiasis (VVC). Typical symptoms include pruritus and a cottage cheese–like discharge. Vulvovaginal burning, dysuria, and dyspareunia are also common symptoms. Over the past two decades, there appears to have been a trend toward a greater prevalence of non-*albicans* species, including *C. tropicalis*, *C. glabrata*, and *Saccharomyces cerevisiae*. The clinical significance of these non-*albicans* species is uncertain; however, they tend to be less susceptible to over-the-counter medications (miconazole and clotrimazole). VVC is uncommon in postmenopausal women, unless they are taking hormone replacement therapy or receiving tamoxifen for breast cancer.

## TRICHOMONAS VAGINITIS

*Trichomonas vaginalis* is responsible for approximately 10% of vaginal infections. Although the organism is not invasive, it causes an intense inflammatory response. Like many other sexually transmitted pathogens, approximately 50% of women who have trichomonas vaginitis are symptom-free. When symptoms are present, they frequently include a profuse vaginal discharge, dysuria, and dyspareunia. *Trichomonas vaginalis* is associated with a poor pregnancy outcome, including premature rupture of the membranes and premature delivery.

# Mucopurulent Cervicitis

Mucopurulent cervicitis (MPC) is characterized by a mucopurulent discharge arising from the glandular cells of the cervix. Approximately half of all cases of MPC are caused by *Chlamydia trachomatis* or *Neisseria gonorrhoeae*, which are sexually transmitted pathogens. Infected women are frequently asymptomatic, but vaginal discharge and postcoital vaginal bleeding are common symptoms. Cervicitis is the most common clinical manifestation of infection caused by *C. trachomatis* or *N. gonorrhoeae*. Untreated gonorrhea and chlamydia infections during pregnancy have been associated with poor pregnancy outcome and clinical infection of the newborn infant. Treatment during pregnancy has been shown to improve the pregnancy outcome and prevent vertical transmission to the newborn infant.

## CHLAMYDIA

Approximately four million infections occur annually, primarily in young women aged 14 to 24. Approximately 75% of women who have chlamydia cervicitis are asymptomatic, and half of the women who are infected develop pelvic inflammatory disease. Many women who have upper genital tract infections are also asymptomatic. Thus, screening for chlamydia may reduce the incidence of pelvic inflammatory disease by 60%. Symptoms of chlamydia infection include atypical abdominal pain, vaginal discharge, and irregular or postcoital bleeding. Approximately 50% of women who have gonococcal cervical infections test positive for chlamydia.

## GONORRHEA

There are approximately two million gonococcal infections in the United States annually. The majority of women who have these infections are asymptomatic. The incidence rate of gonorrhea has declined since 1974, with a decrease of 17% between 1995 and 1996. Approximately 30% of gonococcal isolates demonstrate resistance to penicillin, tetracycline, or both. In addition to infections of the cervix, *N. gonorrhoeae* also causes Bartholin's gland infection, sepsis, migratory polyarthritis, and endocarditis. When present, genital symptoms include vaginal discharge and abnormal bleeding. Approximately 15% of women who have gonococcal cervicitis develop pelvic inflammatory disease.

# Genital Ulcers

Genital ulcers are a common manifestation of sexually transmitted diseases. Genital herpes infections account for approximately 60 to 70% of genital ulcers. The remaining 30 to 40% of infectious genital ulcerations include syphilis, chancroid, and lymphogranuloma venereum. Some patients experience severe pain with genital ulcers. Many patients, however, are asymptomatic or have minimal symptoms, emphasizing the need for a thorough workup of genital ulceration. Approximately 75% of women who have genital ulcers will have a laboratory-confirmed diagnosis after completion of the evaluation. Genital ulceration is an important risk factor for human immunodeficiency virus (HIV) transmission. Chronic genital ulceration is a symptom of HIV infection.

## GENITAL HERPES

The herpes simplex virus (HSV) type 2 is the most common cause of genital herpes. It has been estimated that approximately 30 million persons in the United States have had genital herpes infections. Symptoms are most severe in *primary genital herpes* infections. In addition to multiple small painful ulcers, systemic symptoms are present. *First episode nonprimary herpes* is caused by HSV-2 in patients who have a history of HSV-1 infection. The first episode of nonprimary infection includes symptoms and signs whose severity and duration are midway between those of primary disease and symptoms and signs of recurrence. Systemic symptoms are uncommon in recurrent infections. Approximately half of the patients who have genital herpes experience a recurrence within 6 months of the initial clinical infection. *Recurrent genital herpes* outbreaks are usually characterized by milder symptoms, fewer ulcers, and shorter duration. *Asymptomatic shedding* in HSV is intermittent and occurs in the majority of women.

## SYPHILIS

Syphilis is caused by *Treponema pallidum*. Following an epidemic of syphilis in the late 1980s, there was a dramatic drop in the number of cases reported. A 77% decline in the rate of primary and secondary syphilis in women occurred between 1990 and 1996. There has been a similar decline in cases of congenital syphilis. Often, the primary or local infection is not detected. The primary chancre of *primary syphilis* occurs at the site where *T. pallidum* enters the body. Hematogenous dissemination of the spirochete lasts for 2 to 6 weeks, resulting in a rash and generalized adenopathy (*secondary syphilis*). The woman enters the latent phase of syphilis, which is asymptomatic. *Early latent* syphilis is defined as infection of less than 1 year's duration. Approximately a third of untreated patients develop *tertiary syphilis* 1 to 20 years after the primary infection. End-organ target sites include the heart, the aorta, the eye, the brain, and the musculoskeletal system.

## CHANCROID

Chancroid is an uncommon infection caused by *Haemophilus ducreyi*. It is predominantly endemic in the southwestern United States. Symptoms include pain at the site of ulceration and regional adenopathy. Approximately 10% of patients who have chancroid also have syphilis or genital herpes infections.

## LYMPHOGRANULOMA VENEREUM

Lymphogranuloma venereum (LGV) is also an uncommon infection and is frequently misdiagnosed. The infection is caused by L1, L2, and L3 *Chlamydia* serotypes, which are considered to be the more invasive than other *Chlamydia* serotypes. Clinical manifestations include genital ulceration, lymphadenopathy, and proctitis. Late manifestations include rectal stricture, anal fissures, genital fistulas, and genital elephantiasis.

# Human Papillomavirus Infection

Human papilloma virus (HPV) infection of the genital tract is common. Approximately 1% of Papanicolaou (Pap) smears show evidence of HPV infection, and genital warts have been reported to occur in more than 6% of women aged 20 to 34.

## CONDYLOMA ACUMINATA

These are benign epithelial tumors that affect the anogenital region. Genital warts are associated with infection by HPV types six and 11. The vulva is the most frequently affected site, but the cervix, the vagina, the urethra, and the anus are also commonly infected.

## DYSPLASIA

This condition is frequently associated with HPV types 16, 18, 31 33, and 35. Intraepithelial neoplasia usually involves the cervix, although other genital tract tissues can be affected. This is discussed more thoroughly in Chapter 42.

## SUBCLINICAL INFECTIONS

These are common and, by definition, asymptomatic. They are frequently diagnosed during the evaluation of an abnormal Pap smear. Methods are available to detect the HPV DNA and RNA types; however, the clinical utility of HPV typing has not been determined. Screening for subclinical genital HPV infections is not recommended.

# Risk Factors

## VAGINITIS

There is significant overlap of risk factors for vaginitis and other sexually transmitted infections of the lower genital tract. Risk factors for developing BV include frequency of sexual activity and multiple sexual partners. Use of an intrauterine device (IUD) is also a risk factor for bacterial vaginosis. Contraceptive methods play a role in vaginal yeast infections, which occur more frequently in women using IUDs and barrier methods of contraception. Low-dose oral contraceptives do not increase the risk of vaginal yeast infections. Other important risk factors for vaginal yeast infections include diabetes, recent antibiotic use, immunodeficiency states (including HIV) and tight-fitting underclothes and pantyhose. Risk factors for trichomonas vaginitis are similar to those for other STDs.

## SEXUALLY TRANSMITTED INFECTIONS

The most important risk factor for developing an STD is exposure. Important demographic characteristics include marital status, race (non-white), and a socially disadvantaged station. STDs occur more frequently in women who are younger than 24 years of age and in those who use either no protection or a nonbarrier method of contraception. The presence of another STD, as well as alcohol and drug abuse, are additional risk factors for acquiring an STD. Sexual behavior, particularly as it relates to the number of partners, the rate of acquiring partners, and sexual practices (e.g., anal intercourse) are significant risk factors for acquiring a sexually transmitted infection. As mentioned previously; the presence of an ulcerative STD significantly increases the risk of infection with HIV.

# Physical Findings

## INSPECTION

Before focusing attention on the pelvic examination, it is important for the physician not to overlook nongenital manifestations of STDs. For example, the extremities and trunk should be inspected for the characteristic rash of secondary syphilis. The primary chancre of syphilis is frequently extragenital. Likewise, examination of the extremities may reveal evidence of arthritis, or pustules may be present on the palmar surface of the hands; both these findings are suggestive of systemic gonococcal infections. Lymphadenopathy is present in women who have either primary or first episode nonprimary genital herpes infections, lymphogranuloma venereum, or chancroid. Indeed, inguinal adenitis is a characteristic feature of chancroid, occurring in 50% of patients. It is most often unilateral. The bubos subsequently become fluctuant and rupture through the skin.

## DETAILED GENITAL TRACT EXAMINATION

The external genitalia should be inspected thoroughly. Generalized erythema, with or without discharge, is characteristic of VVC or other dermatoses. The presence, size, and number of lesions should be noted. Specifically, if ulceration is present, multiple small painful ulcers are suggestive of genital herpes infection. The ulcer seen with chancroid is also tender but much larger and usually solitary. The primary chancre of syphilis is typically nontender and has smooth raised edges. Condyloma latum, seen in secondary syphilis, is raised and flat, whereas condyloma acuminatum appears as a fleshy exophytic growth. The primary lesion of LGV often appears as a vesicle or papule in the posterior forchette.

After introduction of the speculum into the vagina, the presence and characteristics of the vaginal discharge should be noted. A normal vaginal discharge appears clear or flocculent and comparisons between normal discharges and the abnormal discharges of VVC, BV, and trichomonas are listed in Table 7-1.

**Table 7-1** Characteristics of Normal and Abnormal Vaginal Secretions

| Condition | Patient Concern | Discharge | Vaginal pH | Amine Odor | Microscopic Appearance |
|---|---|---|---|---|---|
| Normal | None | White, flocculent | 3.8–4.2 | Absent | Lactobacilli |
| Candida vulvovaginitis | Itching<br>Burning<br>Discharge | White, cottage cheese-like<br><br>May be increased | <4.5 | Absent | Mycelia<br>Budding yeast<br>Pseudohyphae with preparation |
| Bacterial vaginosis | Discharge<br>Bad odor, may be worse after intercourse | Thin homogeneous<br>Whitish gray<br>Adherent<br>Often increased | >4.5 | Present, fishy | Clue cells<br>Coccoid bacteria<br>No WBCs |
| Trichomonas vaginitis | Itching<br>Frothy discharge<br>Bad odor<br>Dysuria | Yellow, green, frothy<br><br>Adherent<br>Increased | <4.5 | Present<br><br>Fishy (not always) | Trichomonads<br>WBCs >10/hpf |

KOH = potassium hydroxide; WBCs = white blood cells; hpf = high-power field.

Table 7–2  Diagnostic Criteria for Bacterial Vaginosis

| Excellent Predictors | Predictive Value % + | Predictive Value % − | Poor Predictors | Predictive Value % + | Predictive Value % − |
|---|---|---|---|---|---|
| Odor on alkalinization | 94 | 93 | Homogeneous discharge | 42 | 88 |
| Clue cells on saline suspension | 90 | 99 | pH >4.5 | 52 | 94 |
| *Mobiluncus* sp on saline suspension | 99 | 57 | Background bacteria | 61 | 97 |
| Clue cells and odor | 99 | 92 | | | |

Adapted from Thomason JL: Statistical evaluation of diagnostic criteria for bacterial vaginosis. Am J Obstet Gynecol 162:155–160, 1990.

Erythema of the vagina is characteristic of VVC and trichomonas. Small punctate lesions of the vagina and cervix can be seen in trichomonas infections.

In a patient who has MPC, the cervix appears erythematous and friable; for example, bleeding can be induced by placing the vaginal speculum or touching the cervix with a swab or spatula. The MPC discharge appears yellow to green when placed on a cotton-tipped applicator.

After the speculum is removed, a gentle bimanual examination should be performed. Specifically, an attempt should be made to elicit signs of upper genital tract infection (pelvic inflammatory disease) as evidenced by adnexal or uterine tenderness or pain on cervical motion.

## Laboratory Evaluation

The laboratory evaluation of vaginitis is straightforward. The pH can be determined by means of pH paper. A pH of more than 4.5 is typical of BV and infection with trichomonas. Vaginal secretions can be suspended in a normal saline solution, and the wet preparation of the vaginal discharge can be examined. A 10% potassium hydroxide (KOH) solution is added to a second slide. The presence of an amine odor (whiff test) is suggestive of BV. The diagnostic criteria for BV are listed in Table 7–2. Trichomonal organisms and clue cells can be identified by a microscopic examination of the saline suspension. The characteristic pseudohyphae of *C. albicans* infection are usually detected by a microscopic examination of the KOH slide. A fungal culture can be very helpful in diagnosing non-*albicans* infections as well as recurrent VVC. Culture of vaginal secretions for *Gardnerella vaginalis* is not recommended.

After excess mucus is removed from the cervix, a culture or DNA probe test for infection with gonorrhea and chlamydia should be obtained. MPC is diagnosed by the presence of more than 10 polymorphonuclear cells in a Gram's stain specimen.

The presence of a genital ulcer requires a complete laboratory evaluation. Coinfection with other sexually transmitted pathogens is common. Culture for HSV is preferable to an antigen test. A culture for *H. ducreyi* should also be performed. If the primary chancre of syphilis is present, a darkfield examination is the most sensitive method for diagnosis. Otherwise, serologic testing including confirmation with a direct immunofluoresence test for *T. pallidum* should be performed. HIV testing should be performed on all women who have genital ulcers caused by *T. pallidum* or *H. ducreyi* and is recommended for women who have ulcers due to HSV.

## Treatment

### BACTERIAL VAGINOSIS

A variety of topical and systemic medications are effective for treating bacterial vaginosis. All patients who have symptomatic BV require treatment. Evidence suggests that women undergoing elective suction abortion should be screened and treated for BV. Treatment options for this infection are listed in Table 7–3. Recurrence of BV is common, occurring in 20 to 40% of women. Treatment with a 14-day course of 0.75% metronidazole gel followed by weekly applications has been modestly effective. Treatment of sexual partners has not been shown to improve treatment outcome.

Table 7–3  Treatment for Bacterial Vaginosis

| | |
|---|---|
| Metronidazole | 500 mg PO bid for 7 d |
| Clindamycin cream, 2% | One full applicator (5 g) intravaginally qhs for 7 d |
| Metronidazole gel, 0.75% | One full applicator (5 g) intravaginally qd for 5 d |

PO = orally.

## VULVOVAGINAL CANDIDIASIS

For patients who have infections with mild-to-moderate symptoms occurring on a sporadic basis, treatment with a 1-, 3- or 7-day course of any of the antifungal agents listed in Table 7–4, is indicated. Women who have severe symptoms or an infection occurring in an abnormal host (immunosuppressed) may require treatment for 10 to 14 days. *C. glabrata* and *Torulopsis glabrata* are less susceptible to the topical azoles. Therefore, treatment with terconazole is indicated. Both ketoconazole and fluconazole have been shown to be effective in the suppression of recurrent VVC. Fluconazole is recommended because of a reduced potential for hepatotoxicity (Table 7–4).

## TRICHOMONAS

The recommended treatment for trichomonal vaginitis is a single dose of metronidazole, 2 g orally. Metronidazole 500 mg twice daily for 7 days is an alternative regimen with lower compliance.

## CHLAMYDIA

Recommendations for treating uncomplicated chlamydial infections of the cervix are listed in Table 7–5.

**Table 7–4** Treatment of Vulvovaginal Candidiasis

| *Recommended Regimens* |
|---|
| INTRAVAGINAL AGENTS |
| Butoconazole, 2% cream, 5 g intravaginally for 3 d*† |
| Clotrimazole, 1% cream, 5 g intravaginally for 7–14 d*† |
| Clotrimazole, 100-mg vaginal tablet for 7 d* |
| Clotrimazole, 100-mg vaginal tablet, 2 tablets for 3 d* |
| Clotrimazole, 500-mg vaginal tablet, one tablet in a single application* |
| Miconazole, 2% cream, 5 g intravaginally for 7 d*† |
| Miconazole, 200-mg vaginal suppository, one suppository for 3 d*† |
| Miconazole, 100-mg vaginal suppository, one suppository for 7 d*† |
| Nystatin, 100,000-unit vaginal tablet, one tablet for 14 d |
| Tioconazole, 6.5% ointment, 5 g intravaginally in a single application*† |
| Terconazole, 0.4% cream, 5 g intravaginally for 7 d* |
| Terconazole, 0.8% cream, 5 g intravaginally for 3 d* |
| Terconazole, 80-mg vaginal suppository, one suppository for 3 d* |
| ORAL AGENT |
| Fluconazole 150-mg tablet PO, one tablet in a single dose |

PO = orally.
*These creams and suppositories are oil based and may weaken latex condoms and diaphragms. Refer to the condom product labeling for additional information.
†Over-the-counter (OTC) preparations.

**Table 7–5** Treatment for Infections with *Chlamydia*

| RECOMMENDED REGIMENS FOR NONPREGNANT WOMEN | |
|---|---|
| Azithromycin | 1 g PO in a single dose |
| Doxycycline | 100 mg PO bid for 10 d |
| **ALTERNATIVE REGIMENS** | |
| Erythromycin base | 500 mg PO qid for 7 d |
| Erythromycin ethylsuccinate | 800 mg PO orally qid for 7 d |
| Ofloxacin | 300 mg PO bid for 7 d |
| **RECOMMENDED REGIMENS FOR PREGNANT WOMEN** | |
| Erythromycin base | 500 mg PO qid for 7 d |
| Amoxicillin | 500 mg PO tid for 7 d |
| **ALTERNATIVE REGIMENS FOR PREGNANT WOMEN** | |
| Erythromycin base | 250 mg PO qid for 14 d |
| Erythromycin ethylsuccinate | 800 mg PO qid for 7 d |
| Erythromycin ethylsuccinate | 400 mg PO qid for 14 d |
| Azithromycin | 1 g PO in a single dose |

PO = orally.

A test of cure is not recommended for nonpregnant patients. Women who have lymphogranuloma venereum should receive doxycycline, 100 mg orally (PO) twice a day for 21 days. For patients who are allergic to doxycycline, erythromycin, 500 mg orally, four times a day for 21 days should be prescribed.

## GONORRHEA

Uncomplicated gonococcal infections of the cervix can be treated with single-dose therapy. PO regimens include cefixime, 400 mg; ciprofloxacin, 500 mg; and ofloxacin, 400 mg. Ceftriaxone, 125 mg intramuscularly (IM), is also effective. All patients who have gonorrhea should receive empiric treatment for chlamydia.

## GENITAL HERPES

Three antiviral agents have been shown to be effective in treating primary and recurrent genital herpes infections and in the suppressing of multiple frequent recurrences. Although all three agents demonstrate comparable effectiveness, famciclovir and valaciclovir offer the advantage of once or twice a day dosing (Table 7–6). After 1 year of continuous suppression, antiviral therapy should be discontinued and the frequency of recurrent infections should be assessed.

## SYPHILIS

Treatment recommendations for syphilis are listed in Table 7–7. Therapy should be monitored with serial

## Table 7–6  Treatment of Genital Herpes

| RECOMMENDED REGIMENS | |
|---|---|
| Acyclovir | 400 mg PO tid for 7–10 d |
| Acyclovir | 200 mg PO q4hr for 7–10 d |
| Famciclovir | 250 mg PO tid for 7–10 d |
| Valaciclovir | 1 g PO bid for 7–10 d |

| RECOMMENDED REGIMENS FOR EPISODIC RECURRENT INFECTION | |
|---|---|
| Acyclovir | 400 mg PO tid for 5 d |
| Acyclovir | 200 mg PO q4hr for 5 d |
| Acyclovir | 800 mg PO bid for 5 d |
| Famciclovir | 125 mg PO bid for 5 d |
| Valaciclovir | 500 mg PO bid for 5 d |

| RECOMMENDED REGIMENS FOR DAILY SUPPRESSIVE THERAPY | |
|---|---|
| Acyclovir | 400 mg PO bid |
| Famciclovir | 250 mg PO bid |
| Valaciclovir | 250 mg PO bid |
| Valaciclovir | 500 mg PO d |

PO = orally.

Venereal Disease Research Laboratory (VDRL) titers. A four-fold decline in the titer should occur over a 3-month period. Treatment failures should be retreated.

## CHANCROID

Chancroid also responds to single-dose antibiotic therapy. Recommended regimens include azithromycin, 1g PO in a single dose or ceftriaxone, 250 mg IM. Multidose regimens include ciprofloxacin, 500 mg PO, twice daily for three days or erythromycin 500 mg PO four times a day for 7 days.

## GENITAL WARTS

Treatment of genital warts is determined by the site and extent of wart growth and patient preference (Table 7–8). Patient-applied methods are recommended for the initial treatment of external genital warts (EGW) that have a total volume smaller than 10 cm³. Topical treatments include podophyllin, tri-

## Table 7–7  Treatment of Syphilis

| PRIMARY, SECONDARY, AND EARLY LATENT SYPHILIS | |
|---|---|
| Benzathine penicillin G | 2.4 million U IM in a single dose |

| LATE LATENT SYPHILIS OR LATENT SYPHILIS OF UNKNOWN DURATION | |
|---|---|
| Benzathine penicillin G | 7.2 million U total, administered as 3 doses of 2.4 million U IM each, at 1-wk intervals |

IM = intramuscularly.

## Table 7–8  Treatment for Genital Warts

| External Genital Warts, Recommended Treatments | |
|---|---|
| PATIENT—APPLIED: | |
| Podofilox, 0.5% solution or gel | Apply to visible genital warts bid for 3 d, followed by 4 d of no therapy; may be repeated as necessary for a total of four cycles. |
| Imiquimod, 5% | Apply imiquimod cream with a finger hs three times a wk for as long as 16 wk. Treatment area should be washed with mild soap and water 6–10 hr after the application. |
| PROVIDER—ADMINISTERED: | |
| Cryotherapy | Every 1 to 2 wk |
| Podophyllin resin, 10–25% | Applied to each wart and allowed to air dry. The preparation should be thoroughly washed off 1–4 hr after application to reduce local irritation. Repeat weekly if necessary. |
| TCA or BCA, 80–90% | Apply a small amount only to warts and allow to dry. Repeat weekly if necessary. |
| Surgical removal | By excision, curettage, or electrosurgery |

| Alternative Treatments | |
|---|---|
| Intralesional interferon | Laser surgery |

| Cervical Warts | |
|---|---|
| Cryotherapy | |

| Vaginal Warts | |
|---|---|
| Cryotherapy | |

| Urethral Meatus Warts | |
|---|---|
| Cryotherapy | Podophyllin, 10–25% |

| Anal Warts | |
|---|---|
| Cryotherapy | Surgical removal |
| TCA or BCA, 80–90% | |

TCA = Trichloro acetic acid; BCA = Bichloro acetic acid.

chloroacetic acid, bichloroacetic acid, and imiquimod 5% cream, which has now been approved for treatment of EGW. Treatment efficacy for topical therapy varies from 30 to 90%. For extensive EGW and warts that fail to respond to topical therapy, biopsy should be performed before treatment is initiated with alternative regimens.

Warts can be removed in the outpatient setting by means of cryotherapy, electrodessication, laser, and electrocautery. Since HPV infections are multifocal, all clinically apparent disease should be treated. A Pap smear should be obtained from all women who have EGW, and colposcopy with biopsy performed as indicated. Any suspicious lesion should be excised.

## Counseling and Follow-up

STD prevention strategies should be reviewed with the patient during treatment. These include the use of barrier methods of contraception and the concomitant use of spermicides. Patients' drug and alcohol use should be addressed and referral for treatment should be indicated. All sexual partners should be treated or referred for treatment. A test of cure is recommended for women who have gonorrhea, and VDRL titers should be followed as described previously. Women who have ulcerative STDs should be tested for HIV. A Pap smear should be obtained from all women who have EGW because HPV infection is frequently multifocal.

### REFERENCES

1998 guidelines for treatment of sexually transmitted diseases. Centers for Disease Control and Prevention. MMWR 47:1–111, 1998.

Brunham R, Iwin B, Stamm WE, et al: Epidemiological and clinical correlates of *C. trachomatis* and *N. gonorrhoeae* infection among women attending an STD clinic. Clin Res 29:47A, 1981.

Corey L, Spear PG: Infections with herpes simplex viruses (1). N Engl J Med 314:686, 1986.

Corey L, Spear PG: Infections with herpes simplex viruses (2). N Engl J Med 314:749, 1986.

Corey L: Genital herpes. *In* Holmes K. ed: Sexually Transmitted Diseases. New York, McGraw-Hill, 1990, p 515.

Eschenbach DA: Epidemiology and diagnosis of acute pelvic inflammatory disease. Obstet Gynecol 55:142, 1980.

Eschenbach DA, Hillier SL, Critchlow C, et al: Diagnosis and clinical manifestations of bacterial vaginosis. Am J Obstet Gynecol 158:819, 1988.

Hillier SL, Nugent RP, Eschenbach DA, et al: Association between bacterial vaginosis and preterm delivery of a low-birth-weight infant. N Engl J Med 333:1737, 1995.

Kent HL: Epidemiology of vaginitis. Am J Obstet Gynecol 165:1168–1176, 1991.

Larsson PG, Platz-Cristensen JJ, Thejis H, et al: Incidence of pelvic inflammatory disease after first trimester legal abortion in women with bacterial vaginosis after treatment with metronidazole: A double-blind, randomized study. Am J Obstet Gynecol 166:100, 1992.

McGregor JA, French JI, Richter R, et al: Antenatal microbiologic and maternal risk factors associated with prematurity. Am J Obstet Gynecol 163:1465, 1990.

Paavonen J, Kiviat N, Brunham RC, et al: Prevalence and manifestations of endometritis among women with cervicitis. Am J Obstet Gynecol 152:280, 1985.

Pearlman MD, McNeeley SG: A review of the microbiology, immunology and clinical implications of *Chlamydia trachomatis* infections. Obstet Gynecol Surv 47:448, 1992.

Sobel JD: Vulvovaginal candidiasis. *In* Holmes K (ed): Sexually Transmitted Diseases. New York, McGraw-Hill, 1990, p 515.

Sobel JD: Fluconazole maintenance therapy in recurrent vulvovaginal candidiasis. Int J Gynecol Obstet 37:17, 1997.

Soper DE, Bump RC, Hurt WG: Bacterial vaginosis and trichomoniasis vaginitis are risk factors for cuff cellulitis after abdominal hysterectomy. Am J Obstet Gynecol 163: 1016, 1990.

Thomason JL: Statistical evaluation of diagnosic criteria for bacterial vaginosis. Am J Obstet Gynecol 162:155–1990.

# 8

# Pelvic Inflammatory Disease

DAVID E. SOPER

More than 1 million women are treated for pelvic inflammatory disease (PID) in the United States each year. An excess of 250,000 women are hospitalized with this diagnosis annually, and as many as 150,000 women undergo surgical procedures, many involving hysterectomy. In addition, the outpatient management of PID involves between 2 and 3 million physician visits annually. Direct costs (those associated with spending for health services) and indirect costs (output lost due to disease or premature death) are projected to approach 10 billion dollars annually by the year 2000, with an increasing proportion covered by public payment sources.

Although there has been a decreased incidence of hospitalization for acute PID since 1983, the average annual number of women visiting private physicians for this disorder has increased, suggesting a higher proportion of women who have clinically mild disease associated with *Chlamydia trachomatis*. Although rates of *Neisseria gonorrhoeae* infection have been decreasing since the 1970s, *C. trachomatis* remains the most common sexually transmitted bacterial disease in the United States. There is increasing emphasis on the recognition and diagnosis of atypical PID, which suggests that symptomatic disease is only the tip of the iceberg with respect to the overall morbidity associated with this insidious infection.

## Definitions

The majority of PID in the United States is caused by an ascending infection. This ascending infection is manifested by a continuum of genital tract inflammation from the cervix (mucopurulent endocervicitis) to the fallopian tube (salpingitis). Recognition of this inflammatory continuum can be helpful in establishing a diagnosis of PID. *Leukorrhea* is noted in more than 90% of women who have laparoscopic salpingitis. Simply put, leukorrhea is present when microscopy of the vaginal secretions reveals a predominance of polymorphonuclear leukocytes. This inflammatory cell predominance reflects endocervical as well as endometrial inflammation. *Bacterial vaginosis (BV)* is commonly associated with PID, and the diagnostic criteria of homogeneous discharge, abnormal vaginal pH (>4.5), presence of clue cells, and a positive whiff test should be assessed. *Mucopurulent endocervicitis* is noted when there is a yellow or green endocervical exudate associated with a plethora of leukocytes in the endocervical secretions. Friability of the endocervical mucosa is common and bleeding is easily induced. In addition, erythema and edema of the zone of ectopy are commonly present. Histologic evidence of *endometritis* (≥5 neutrophils per ×400 field in endometrial surface epithelium together with one or more plasma cells per ×120 field in endometrial stroma) is highly predictive of upper genital tract infection and visual salpingitis. However, the gold standard for the diagnosis of PID remains laparoscopic visualization of the fallopian tubes. The minimal criteria for the visual confirmation of *acute salpingitis* include pronounced hyperemia of the tubal surface, edema of the tubal wall, and a sticky exudate on the tubal surface of the fimbriated ends when they are patent. *Mild salpingitis* is associated with the above minimal visual criteria. In addition, the tubes are freely mobile and the ostia appear patent. The tubes may be covered with a sticky exudate. *Moderate salpingitis* is associated with more pronounced inflammation. There are patchy fibrin deposits on the serosal surfaces and the tubes are not freely movable. Adhesions are loose and moist and a paraphimotic appearance may be present. The fimbria may appear adherent. *Severe salpingitis* reveals intensely congested peritoneal surfaces. Pelvic organs adhere to each other and pyosalpinx or *tubo-ovarian complex* formation may be present.

## Common Causes of PID

### MICROBIOLOGY

The microbiology of pelvic inflammatory disease has been defined by the use of lower genital tract cultures for the sexually transmitted organisms *N. gonorrhoeae* and *C. trachomatis* in patients who have a clinical diagnosis of PID. In an attempt to further describe the microbiology of the upper genital tract, telescoping endometrial sampling devices and culdocentesis have been used to culture the endometrium and extract purulent material from the cul de sac of patients who have PID. Both of these techniques are associated with some contamination of the specimen by either resident vaginal or cervical flora, or both. Use of the laparoscope allows investigators to sample the sites of infection without the possibility of contamination by microorganisms in the vagina or cervix (see Table 8–2).

Both *C. trachomatis* and *N. gonorrhoeae* have been cultured from the cervix, endometrium, and fallopian tubes of patients who have laparoscopically confirmed salpingitis. *Haemophilus influenzae* appears to be increasingly associated with acute salpingitis. This microorganism has been isolated from the cervix and fallopian tubes of patients who have laparoscopically proven salpingitis. In most cases, these patients are severely affected, with pyosalpinx formation being the rule. This microorganism is highly virulent and is capable of monoetiologic disease similar to that seen with *N. gonorrhoeae*. It appears to originate in the endocervix and ascends into the upper genital tract.

Other microorganisms that are not thought to be sexually transmitted have also been implicated in the pathogenesis of salpingitis. Originally, culdocentesis studies suggested that as many as 80% of cases were associated with mixed infections of both aerobic and anaerobic microorganisms. However, a certain amount of contamination by resident vaginal flora occurred with this procedure. North American laparoscopic studies confirm a polymicrobial etiology of acute salpingitis in 30 to 40% of cases. These organisms are particularly found in cases associated with tubo-ovarian abscesses. These "BV microorganisms" ascend from the vagina, the cervix, or both. In many cases, it appears that this polymicrobial infection is the result of bacterial superinfection following the initiation of the inflammatory process by *N. gonorrhoeae*. Microorganisms of particular importance include *Escherichia coli* and gram-negative anaerobic rods, such as *Prevotella* species. The *Prevotella* group of microorganisms is particularly important, because many of these isolates produce penicillinase, making them resistant to penicillins and first-generation cephalosporins. In unusual cases, appendicitis or Crohn's disease can lead to a polymicrobial salpingitis by contiguous spread of microorganisms from the bowel.

## Diagnostic Strategies

**Risk Factors.** Determining a woman's risk for PID is essential for timely, reliable diagnosis (Table 8–1). Factors associated with the development of disease may be assessed in relation to the following risks (and risk factors may be viewed as either increasing risk or as exerting a protective effect):
- Exposure to the infectious agent
- Acquisition of the infection upon exposure
- Progression to upper genital tract infection (UGTI)

Risk factors for the development of PID primarily involve the patient's exposure to the sexually transmitted pathogens, *N. gonorrhoeae* and *C. trachomatis* (see Table 8–1). Sexually active young women who have multiple sexual partners are at the highest risk. In addition, biological characteristics associated with young age may contribute to the evolution of lower genital tract infections (LGTI) into PID. These characteristics include a low prevalence of protective antibodies, a large zone of cervical ectopy, and greater penetrability of the cervical mucus. Reports suggest that bacterial vaginosis may also be related to the

**Table 8-1** Risk Factors for Pelvic Inflammatory Disease

Age <25 years
    Correlated with sexual behavior
    Lower prevalence of protective antibodies
    Larger zone of cervical ectopy
    Greater penetrability of cervical mucus
Microbiologic
    LGTI
        *Neisseria gonorrhoeae*
        *Chlamydia trachomatis*
        Bacterial vaginosis
    Behavioral risks that increase chance of LGTI
        Multiple sexual partners
        Sexual intercourse with high-risk men
            Lower socioeconomic class
            Ethnicity
Facilitate transport to the upper genital tract
    Iatrogenic procedures
        Dilatation and curettage
        IUD insertion
        Hysterosalpingogram
    Patient practices
        Douching

LGTI = lower genital tract infection; IUD = intrauterine device.

development of PID. This complex alteration of vaginal flora leads to an increase in the concentration of potentially pathogenic bacteria, particularly gram-negative anaerobic rods (BV microorganisms) in the endocervix, the vagina, or both.

Race and socioeconomic status have traditionally been assumed to be markers for sexual behavior. These two markers appear to correlate with risky sexual behavior and increased risk for sexually transmitted diseases (STDs) in black men of low socioeconomic status, This, in turn, results in an increased risk for LGTI and, subsequently, PID, in their female sexual partners.

Risk factors that promote the progression of LGTI to PID facilitate the movement of bacteria through the cervical mucus barrier and into the endometrium and fallopian tubes. These include iatrogenic factors, such as intrauterine device (IUD) insertion; dilatation and curettage; and hysterosalpingography, which may directly transport microorganisms to the upper genital tract. Moreover, patients themselves can increase their risk for the development of PID by douching. Douche fluid may enter the uterine cavity, depending on the anatomy of the cervical canal, the viscosity of the cervical mucus, and the douching technique used.

Contraceptive practices also play a role in the development of PID. The risk of PID associated with IUD use is primarily confined to the time of insertion. For women who do not have risk factors for PID, IUD use poses little risk of tubal infection. Barrier methods of contraception (condoms or diaphragm in conjunction with vaginal spermicides) decrease the risk of acquiring STDs and, therefore, protect against the development of PID. Oral contraceptives have a dichotomous role in the prevention of PID. Use of oral contraceptives increases the risk for acquiring LGTI infection caused by *Chlamydia*, probably because these contraceptives create a large zone of cervical ectopy. Data have also revealed that women who have unrecognized endometritis are more likely to use oral contraceptives than women who have recognized PID. However, using oral contraceptives decreases the risk of symptomatic PID and the severity of salpingitis in patients who develop the disease. This decreased risk may be related to enhancement of cervical mucus, which acts as a barrier to UGTI. Moreover, use of oral contraceptives decreases menstrual blood loss and, therefore, decreases the inoculum caused by retrograde menstruation. An important caveat that remains is the fact that the risk of tubal infertility is unchanged in patients who use oral contraceptives, suggesting that "silent" PID may play a role in these patients.

**Symptoms** (Table 8–2). Lower abdominal pain is the most frequent symptom noted in patients who have PID. This reflects UGTI involving the endometrium, fallopian tubes, and the peritoneum, either alone or in combination with the endometrium and the fallopian tubes. The pain is generally bilateral and is not necessarily severe. Associated symptoms generally reflect infection of other anatomical structures with *N. gonorrhoeae* or *C. trachomatis*. For example, endocervicitis may be manifested by the complaint of an abnormal vaginal discharge. Symptoms of urethritis, such as dysuria, urgency, and frequency, may be due to concomitant infection of the urethra. Breakthrough bleeding in patients who are taking the birth control pill or persistent vaginal spotting following elective termination of pregnancy are other signs that may herald the onset of PID. These complaints are common sequelae of endometritis, which, if left untreated, may progress to salpingitis. Systemic symptoms, such as fever and associated nausea, with or without vomiting, reflect peritoneal inflammation and severe clinical disease.

**Physical Examination and Laboratory Tests** (Table 8–3). Physical findings consistent with a diagnosis of PID include the presence of leukorrhea, cervical mucopus, or both. A saline preparation of the vaginal secretions should be examined microscopically for the presence of white blood cells. Leukorrhea can be

**Table 8–2** Diagnosis of Pelvic Inflammatory Disease: Symptoms

| | |
|---|---|
| Lower abdominal pain | Metrorrhagia |
| Vaginal discharge | Fever |
| Urethritis | Nausea and/or vomiting |
| Proctitis | |

**Table 8–3** Diagnosis of Pelvic Inflammatory Disease: Signs

| Signs of LGTI | Cervical motion tenderness |
| --- | --- |
| Leukorrhea* | Bilateral adnexal tenderness |
| Mucopurulent endocervicitis† | Palpable adnexal swelling |
| Lower abdominal tenderness | Temperature >38°C |

LGTI = lower genital tract infection.
*>1 White blood cell (WBC) per epithelial cell with microscopy of vaginal secretions.
†Green or yellow endocervical secretions on a Q-Tip inserted into the endocervical canal or ≥30 WBCs of cervical mucus.

defined as more than one polymorphonuclear leukocyte per vaginal epithelial cell. After the ectocervix is cleansed with a large cotton swab, the endocervical canal should be swabbed with a Q-Tip. The Q-Tip should then be inspected for a green or yellow color. In addition, after this material is streaked on a slide, it should be examined microscopically for the presence of white blood cells. More than 30 polymorphonuclear leukocytes per oil immersion field indicates the presence of mucopurulent cervicitis and chlamydial or gonococcal infection. In a patient who presents with lower abdominal pain, the presence of bilateral adnexal tenderness, together with signs of an LGTI (e.g., mucopus, leukorrhea, or both), is associated with the laparoscopically confirmed diagnosis of acute salpingitis in 65% of cases.

Additional clinical findings supportive of infection and inflammation improve the specificity of the clinical diagnosis of PID. Elevated temperature, palpation of an adnexal complex, leukocytosis, elevated erythrocyte sedimentation rate or C-reactive protein, and purulent material obtained by culdocentesis are considered adjunctive criteria for the diagnosis of PID. A positive test for LGTI caused by *N. gonorrhoeae* or *C. trachomatis*, evaluated either alone or in conjunction with the aforementioned criteria, also confirms the same diagnosis. The specificity of the clinical diagnosis of PID increases to more than 90% when two or more of these criteria are associated with the findings of pain, adnexal tenderness, and leukorrhea (Table 8–4).

Endometrial biopsy is another technique used to document UGTI. When compared with laparoscopically confirmed salpingitis, endometritis detected by biopsy had a sensitivity of 89%, a specificity of 67%, a positive predictive value of 84%, and a false-negative rate of 22% in the diagnosis of PID. The procedure, which uses a Pipelle endometrial suction curette, can be performed easily in the physician's office or in the emergency room as part of the evaluation of a patient suspected of having acute salpingitis. In addition, biopsy is indispensable in evaluating the endometrium of patients who are undergoing diagnostic laparoscopy. Patients who fail to meet criteria for the visual diagnosis of acute salpingitis may have an acute or chronic endometritis as the sole source of their symptoms.

Use of the laparoscope has greatly enhanced understanding of the pathophysiology of PID; however, routine use of the laparoscope for obtaining a diagnosis of PID is not useful. The majority of patients who have a clinical diagnosis of PID respond promptly to antimicrobial therapy. Moreover, patients who do not have visually confirmed salpingitis still require antimicrobial therapy, because the majority of these patients have endometritis. Diagnostic laparoscopy should be considered for patients in whom the diagnosis is in question, especially if there is a possibility of an ectopic pregnancy. Also, patients who fail an initial outpatient course of antibiotics rarely have visually confirmed salpingitis; therefore, laparoscopy should be considered for diagnosis. Many of these patients have an alternative, treatable diagnosis, such as endometriosis.

## Atypical or "Silent Salpingitis"

More than half of women who have tubal infertility have no history of PID. Antibodies to *C. trachomatis* are often present in asymptomatic women who have either an ectopic pregnancy or a distal tubal occlusion. In addition, morphologic changes of the fallopian tube mucosa and physiologic alterations of the ciliated epithelium are similar in patients who have tubal factor infertility with or without clinically overt salpingitis. Moreover, it is not uncommon to find endometrial infection with *C. trachomatis* in asymp-

**Table 8–4** Clinical Diagnosis of Pelvic Inflammatory Disease: Criteria*

| Criteria | Specificity (%) |
| --- | --- |
| **MAJOR** | |
| Lower abdominal pain | |
| Signs of LGTI | |
| Bilateral adnexal tenderness | 61 |
| **MINOR** | |
| Fever | |
| Palpable adnexal swelling | |
| Leukocytosis | |
| Elevated C-reactive protein | |
| Positive test for gonorrhea or *Chlamydia* | |
| Major + one Minor | 78 |
| Major + two Minor | 90 |
| Major + three Minor | 96 |

LGTI = lower genital tract infection.
*From Westrom L, Mardh PA: Salpingitis. In Holmes KK, Mardh PA, Sparling PF, et al (eds): Sexually Transmitted Diseases. New York, McGraw-Hill, 1984. With permission of The McGraw-Hill Companies.

tomatic women who have serum anti-*Chlamydia* antibodies. Women who have bacterial vaginosis may also have associated endometritis. These data suggest the probability that patients may develop a tubal infection without typical clinical signs of pelvic infection, the so-called silent salpingitis. In some patients who have absence of pelvic pain, symptoms such as metrorrhagia, abnormal vaginal discharge, or urinary tract symptoms may represent the clinical manifestations of PID. To address this issue and improve the treatment capture rate for these patients, the concept of "think PID" should be adopted. In much the same way as the "think ectopic" concept promoted recognition of ectopic pregnancy before the use of serum pregnancy tests, this concept increases awareness of subtle and often subclinical signs of UGTI, prompting evaluation and treatment.

Diagnostic criteria for silent salpingitis must not, therefore, be excessively stringent and that should reflect the subacute or relatively asymptomatic nature of this entity (Table 8–5). Patients who have risk factors with bilateral adnexal tenderness and signs of LGTI or bacterial vaginosis, even in the absence of a complaint of pelvic pain, should be treated as if they have acute salpingitis until more information is available. Obviously, the diagnosis of silent salpingitis is less specific than that of overt PID, but this is acceptable, considering how much there is to be gained from the prompt treatment of patients who have UGTI.

## Treatment

Current guidelines for the treatment of PID reflect the concern that a significant number of cases are associated with polymicrobial infection. Recommended regimens provide empiric, broad-spectrum coverage of likely etiologic pathogens while maintaining an emphasis on coverage of both *N. gonorrhoeae* and *C. trachomatis*. Institutional availability, cost-control efforts, patient acceptance, and regional differences in antimicrobial susceptibility must all be considered when a treatment regimen is considered. Antibiotic regimens are listed in Table 8–6.

Ambulatory management of PID includes administration of a single injection of a β-lactam antibiotic followed by a 14-day course of doxycycline and met-

**Table 8–5** Diagnostic Criteria: Silent Salpingitis

Signs of LGTI
Bilateral adnexal tenderness

LGTI = lower genital tract infection.

**Table 8–6** 1998 Centers for Disease Control Treatment Guidelines for Pelvic Inflammatory Disease

**Inpatient Treatment**

Regimen A
  *Cefotetan*, 2 g IV q12h, or *cefoxitin*\* IV 2 g q6hr
  PLUS
  *Doxycycline*, 100 mg q12hr PO or IV
Regimen B
  *Clindamycin*, 900 mg IV q8hr
  PLUS
  *Gentamicin*, loading dose IV or IM (2 mg/kg), followed by a maintenance dose (1.5 mg/kg) q8hr
One of the above regimens is given for at least 24 hr after the patient clinically improves.
Continue therapy with
  *Doxycycline*, 100 mg PO bid to total 14 d (Clindamycin, 450 mg PO qid for 14 d may be considered as an alternative.)

**Outpatient Treatment**

Regimen A
  *Ofloxacin*, 400 mg PO bid for 14 d
  PLUS
  *Metronidazole*, 500 mg PO bid for 14 d
Regimen B‡
  *Ceftriaxone*, 250 mg IM or equivalent cephalosporin or *cefoxitin*, 2 g IM plus probenicid 1 g PO in a single dose concurrently once
  PLUS
  *Doxycycline*, 100 mg PO bid for 14 d

IV = intravenously; PO = orally; IM = intramuscularly.
\*Other cephalosporins, such as ceftizoxime, cefotaxime, and ceftriaxone, which provide adequate coverage for gonococcal and other facultative gram-negative aerobic and anaerobic infections, may be given in appropriate doses.
‡Theoretical limitations in regimen B's coverage of anaerobes may require the addition of metronidazole, which also treats bacterial vaginosis, frequently associated with PID.

ronidazole. Parenteral administration of the β-lactam antibiotic ensures compliance. Ceftriaxone and doxycycline maximize coverage against the gonococcus and *Chlamydia*. Metronidazole provides treatment for bacterial vaginosis, which is commonly associated with PID, and coverage for a possible anaerobic UGTI. All patients who are treated in an ambulatory setting should return for repeat evaluation within 72 hours if they notice no improvement in their symptoms.

Some patients may benefit from parenteral therapy or hospitalization (Table 8–7). Generally, patients who have severe clinical disease, those who are unable to tolerate oral administration of antibiotics, or those who meet both of these criteria should be hospitalized. As mentioned before, patients who have a questionable diagnosis should be admitted, and diagnostic laparoscopy should be considered. This is especially true in cases of early pregnancy complicated by PID, because ectopic pregnancy must be ruled out. Women who have tubo-ovarian abscesses should receive parenteral therapy and the decision for hospitalization should be based on the severity of their clinical disease.

**Table 8–7** Indications for Parenteral Therapy and/or Hospitalization for Pelvic Inflammatory Disease

---

Uncertain diagnosis
    Pregnancy and PID = R/O ectopic
    Failure to respond to outpatient therapy
Severe clinical disease
    Temperature >39°C
    Upper peritoneal signs
Suspected pelvic or tubo-ovarian abscess
Questionable compliance with outpatient regimen
Nausea/vomiting precludes oral therapy

---

PID = pelvic inflammatory disease; R/O = rule out.

Both inpatient antibiotic regimens (see Table 8–6) cover *N. gonorrhoeae* and *C. trachomatis* as well as anaerobes and facultative bacteria. The combination of doxycycline with cefotetan or cefoxitin is recommended when sexually transmitted organisms are thought to play a role in the etiology of PID. The combination of clindamycin and an aminoglycoside provides excellent coverage for mixed anaerobic and aerobic infections. Both regimens have been extensively studied and are associated with clinical cure rates in the 90% range.

Parenteral antibiotics should be continued until a therapeutic response is reached. This response should include total lysis of fever, normalization of the white blood cell count, total disappearance of abdominal rebound tenderness, and marked amelioration of pelvic organ tenderness. Most patients respond within 5 to 6 days; however, patients who have tubo-ovarian abscess formation may have an even longer recovery cycle. Patients should continue to receive an oral antibiotic, usually doxycycline, until they complete a 14-day course of therapy. Patients who have *Chlamydia*-associated PID may have a clinical response to antibiotics that is not directed at this organism. Such patients may continue to have positive cultures despite becoming asymptomatic. The reason for this may be that the microorganism has been inhibited but not killed. This raises the possibility of an ongoing subclinical infection that could cause continued tubal damage. Therefore, treatment of *Chlamydia*-associated PID should not only depend upon a clinical response but also upon eradication of the microorganism as documented by a negative follow-up culture. In experimental chlamydial infections, as well as in trachoma, host immune response is enhanced by subsequent infections, thus precipitating more local tissue damage.

Anaerobic microorganisms may also persist in the endometrium of women who have a clinical response to therapy with an antibiotic, such as ciprofloxacin, which is not active against these microorganisms. Concern about the tendency of these microorganisms to cause continued UGTI has prompted the addition of metronidazole to the regimen A outpatient treatment recommendation (see Table 8–6).

Treatment of PID involves more than just antibiotic therapy (Table 8–8). Sexual partners of patients treated for PID should be evaluated for STDs. This is true even for partners who fail to test positive for *N. gonorrhoeae* or *C. trachomatis*. Approximately one third of male sexual contacts of patients who have gonococcal PID test positive for gonococcus, and many are asymptomatic. Moreover, even sexual contacts of patients with nongonococcal PID have a 15% incidence of culture-proven *N. gonorrhoeae*. Chlamydia infection also occurs commonly in sexual contacts of women who have PID and is present in 35% of male sexual partners. Epidemiologic treatment for uncomplicated LGTI in sexual contacts of patients who have PID is in order. These individuals should receive a β-lactam antibiotic, such as ceftriaxone, plus 7 days of oral doxycycline or, single dose azithromycin. In addition, screening these individuals for sexually transmitted diseases may shed new light on the pathogenesis of PID in the index patient as well as eliminate a reservoir of reinfection. Indeed, in many cases, it is not the patient's exposure to multiple sexual partners that puts her at risk but rather one sexual partner who has had contact with many different sexual partners and who is infected and asymptomatic.

## Tubo-Ovarian Abscess

Tubo-ovarian abscess (TOA) formation, the most severe consequence of PID, complicates approximately 15% of cases. The pathophysiology is identical to that of uncomplicated salpingitis, except that, presumably through an ovulation site, microorganisms gain entry to the ovarian stroma. This leads to destruction of the ovary and formation of an abscess cavity. Alternatively, loculations of pus can occur between pelvic structures, such as the tube, ovary, and uterus. In many cases, the bowel is also involved. These loculations act as abscess cavities and lead to persistent inflammation and destruction of the adjacent organs. Moreover, intraluminal pus from pyosalpinx formation is also involved.

**Table 8–8** Therapeutic Approach to the Patient with Pelvic Inflammatory Disease

---

Antibiotics
Follow-up
Treatment of sexual partners
Education regarding STDs

---

STD = sexually transmitted disease.

The clinical diagnosis of TOA is based upon the previously noted criteria for the diagnosis of PID in conjunction with a palpable adnexal complex. This adnexal complex can be further characterized by ultrasonography or computed tomography (CT). The complex may actually appear to be a "bag of pus," or it may only represent side-to-side agglutination of pelvic structures in association with tissue induration.

Initially, treatment of a TOA should consist of parenteral administration of broad-spectrum antibiotics. Hospitalization should be considered for women who have severe clinical symptoms. Within 72 hours, the patient should begin showing a therapeutic response, with subjective improvement of symptoms, decreasing white blood cell count, and lysis of fever. If there is a suspicion of abscess rupture, or if the patient fails to respond to antibiotic therapy within 72 to 96 hours, surgical exploration should be considered. The conservative approach of unilateral adnexectomy and drainage is appropriate if future fertility or hormone production is desired. Total abdominal hysterectomy with bilateral salpingo-oophorectomy should be reserved for patients who are not desirous of future fertility, or in cases in which overwhelming sepsis has developed. Drainage of TOAs performed under guidance of a laparoscope or CT scan is being performed with increasing frequency and is successful in selected cases.

## Sequelae

Major sequelae resulting from PID include tubal factor infertility, ectopic pregnancy, chronic abdominal pain, and recurrent infection (Table 8–9). Infertility resulting from salpingitis is directly proportional to the severity of the inflammatory reactions of the tubes. In addition, the number of episodes of salpingitis increases the risk of the patient for tubal factor infertility. The infertility rate after a single episode of severe salpingitis appears to be close to 27%; this falls to a low of 6% in patients who have only mild disease. Patients who are taking oral contraceptives at the time of their diagnosis appear to have an improved prognosis. Not only are they less likely to develop salpingitis in the first place, but they generally have a less severe grade of salpingitis if they do develop

**Table 8–9** Sequelae Associated with Pelvic Inflammatory Disease

Tubal factor infertility
Ectopic pregnancy
Chronic lower abdominal pain
Recurrent pelvic infection

upper tract disease. Rates of tubal factor infertility also increase with subsequent episodes of PID. The patient who has had three or more episodes of salpingitis runs a 50 to 60% risk of tubal factor infertility. Fertility prognosis does not appear to be related to the microbial etiology of acute salpingitis.

There has been a fourfold increase in the number of ectopic pregnancies occurring in the United States since 1970. This increase appears to be related to the concomitant increase in the number of cases of PID over the same period of time. Patients who have a history of PID have a four- to eightfold increased risk for ectopic pregnancy. In addition, patients who have an antibody to *C. trachomatis* also have an increased risk for the development of ectopic pregnancy.

Chronic lower abdominal pain occurs at a rate of up to 20% in patients who have a history of PID. This pain is attributed to pelvic adhesive disease, with more than two thirds of these patients being infertile. Compounding this problem is the presence of dyspareunia in more than half of these cases.

Finally, recurrence of PID is common, with a rate as high as 25%. Distorted tubal architecture may increase the risk of subsequent infection because the host immune factors are impaired. Patients who have PID have increased likelihood of becoming reinfected with the same sexually transmitted pathogens that caused their upper tract inflammation in the first place.

**Fitz-Hugh-Curtis Syndrome.** This disorder is characterized by violin string adhesions between the liver and the anterior abdominal wall in women who have gross pathologic evidence of previous tubal infection. It consists of a continuum of acute perihepatitis associated with acute salpingitis and followed by the formation of perihepatic adhesions. Both *N. gonorrhoeae* and *C. trachomatis* have been isolated from the liver capsule of patients who have Fitz-Hugh-Curtis syndrome. The severity of perihepatic adhesions is associated with the severity of pelvic adhesions, suggesting that the process is progressive, as is the case with pelvic adhesions. Occasionally, chronic right upper quadrant pain occurs, which necessitates laparoscopic lysis of adhesions.

## Prevention

The most cost-effective approach in managing PID and its associated sequelae is prevention (Table 8–10). Because the majority of PID is caused by sexually transmitted pathogens, specifically *N. gonorrhoeae* and *C. trachomatis*, aggressive diagnosis and treatment of LGTI must be undertaken. This includes not only liberal therapy for mucopurulent endocervicitis but

**Table 8–10** Prevention of Pelvic Inflammatory Disease

Control of LGTIs
    Liberal therapy for MPC
    Increased public awareness
    Screen and treat for *Chlamydia*
    Stricter attitudes concerning sexual relationships
    AIDS awareness
    Minimize iatrogenic risk

LGTI = lower genital tract infection; MPC = mucopurulent cervicitis; AIDS = acquired immunodeficiency syndrome.

also an increased public awareness of the dangers of lower tract infection with these pathogens. In addition, educating women about the earliest signs of abnormality, such as an abnormal vaginal discharge, will prompt them to seek health care, and, finally, educating physician providers to "think PID" will go far to decrease the morbidity associated with overt or "silent" salpingitis. Physicians can also minimize iatrogenic risks by providing appropriate screening and prophylaxis for patients who are undergoing upper genital instrumentation, such as hysterosalpingogram.

## REFERENCES

Burkman RT: Intrauterine devices and pelvic inflammatory disease: Evolving perspectives on the data. Obstet Gynecol Surv 51 (suppl):S35–S41, 1996.

Burnham RC, Binns B, Guijon F, et al: Etiology and outcome of acute pelvic inflammatory disease. J Infect Dis 158:510–517, 1988.

Cates W, Rolfs RT, Aral SO: Sexually transmitted diseases, pelvic inflammatory disease, and infertility: An epidemiologic update. Epidemiol Rev 12:199–220, 1990.

CDC: 1998 Guidelines for treatment of sexually transmitted diseases. MMWR Morb Mortal Wkly Rep 47:79–85, 1998.

Chow AW, Malkasian KL, Marshall JR, et al: Acute pelvic inflammatory disease and clinical response to parenteral doxycycline. Antimicrob Agents Chemother 7:133–137, 1975.

Cleary RE, Jones RB: Recovery of *Chlamydia trachomatis* from the endometrium in infertile women with serum antichlamydial antibodies. Fertil Steril 44:233–235, 1985.

Cramer DW, Schiff I, Schoenbaum SC, et al: Tubal infertility and the intrauterine device. N Engl J Med 312:941–947, 1985.

Crombleholme WR, Schachter J, Ohm-Smith M, et al: Efficacy of single-agent therapy for the treatment of acute pelvic inflammatory disease with ciprofloxacin. Am J Med 87:142S–147S, 1989.

Cunningham FG, Hauth JC, Gilstrap LC, et al: The bacterial pathogenesis of acute pelvic inflammatory disease. Obstet Gynecol 52:161–164, 1978.

Eschenbach DA, Hillier S, Critchlow C, et al: Diagnosis and clinical manifestations of bacterial vaginosis. Am J Obstet Gynecol 158:819–828, 1988.

Eschenbach DA, Buchanan TM, Pollock HM, et al: Polymicrobial etiology of acute pelvic inflammatory disease. N Engl J Med 293:166–171, 1975.

Fish ANJ, Fairweather DVI, Oriel JD, et al: Isolation of *Chlamydia trachomatis* from endometriums of women with and without symptoms. Genitourin Med 1988;64:75–77, 1988.

Gilstrap LC, Herbert WNP, Cunningham FG, et al: Gonorrhea screening in male consorts of women with pelvic infection. JAMA 238:965–966, 1977.

Hillier SL, Kiviat NB, Hawes SE, et al: Role of bacterial vaginosis-associated microorganisms in endometritis. Am J Obstet Gynecol 175:435–441, 1996.

Holmes KK: Lower genital tract infections in women: Cystitis, urethritis, vulvovaginitis, and cervicitis. *In* Holmes KK, Mardh PA, Sparling PF, et al (eds): Sexually Transmitted Diseases, 2nd ed. New York, McGraw-Hill, 1990.

Jacobson L, Westrom L: Objectivized diagnosis of acute pelvic inflammatory disease: Diagnostic and prognostic value of routine laparoscopy. Am J Obstet Gynecol 1969;105:1088–1098, 1969.

Kiviat NB, Wolner-Hanssen P, Eschenbach DA, et al: Endometrial histopathology in patients with culture-proved upper genital tract infection and laparoscopically diagnosed acute salpingitis. Am J Surg Pathol 14:167–175, 1990.

Korn AP, Hessol N, Padian N, et al: Commonly used diagnostic criteria for pelvic inflammatory disease have poor sensitivity for plasma cell endometritis. Sex Transm Dis 22:335–341, 1995.

Landers DV, Sweet RL: Current trends in the diagnosis and treatment of tuboovarian abscess. Am J Obstet Gynecol 151:1098–1110, 1985.

Monif GRG: Significance of polymicrobial bacterial superinfection in the therapy of gonococcal endometritis-salpingitis-peritonitis. Obstet Gynecol 55:154S–161S, 1980.

Moore DE, Cates WJ Jr: Sexually transmitted diseases and infertility. *In* Holmes KK, Mardh P-A, Sparling PF, et al (eds): Sexually Transmitted Diseases, 2nd ed. New York, McGraw-Hill, 1990.

Moss TR, Hawkswell J: Evidence of infection with *Chlamydia trachomatis* in patients with pelvic inflammatory disease: Value of partner investigation. Fertil Steril 1986;45:429–30, 1986.

Ness RB, Keder LM, Soper DE, et al: Oral contraception and the recognition of endometritis. Am J Obstet Gynecol 176:580–585, 1997.

Paavonen J, Aine R, Teisala K, et al: Comparison of endometrial biopsy and peritoneal fluid cytologic testing with laparoscopy in the diagnosis of acute pelvic inflammatory disease. Am J Obstet Gynecol 1985;151:645–650, 1985.

Patton DL, Moore DE, Spadoni LR, et al: A comparison of the fallopian tube's response to overt and silent salpingitis. Obstet Gynecol 1989;73:622–630, 1989.

Peipert JF, Boardman L, Hogan JW, et al: Laboratory evaluation of acute upper genital tract infection. Obstet Gynecol 87:730–736, 1996.

Peterson HB, Walker CK, Kahn JG, et al: Pelvic inflammatory disease: Key treatment and issues and options. JAMA 266:2605–2611, 1991.

Reichert JA, Valle RF: Fitz-Hugh-Curtis syndrome, a laparoscopic approach. JAMA 236:266–268, 1976.

Rolfs RT, Galaid EI, Zaidi AA: Pelvic inflammatory disease: Trends in hospitalizations and office visits, 1979 through 1988. Am J Obstet Gynecol 166:983–990, 1992.

Scholes D, Stergachis A, Heidrich FE, et al: Prevention of pelvic inflammatory disease by screening for cervical chlamydia infection. N Engl J Med 334:1362–1366, 1996.

Soper DE, Peipert J, Ness R, et al: The utility of readily available clinical tests in predicting pelvic inflammatory disease in women presenting with pelvic pain. Las Croabas, Puerto Rico, Infectious Disease Society for Ob/Gyn August 6–9, 1997.

Soper DE, Brockwell NJ, Dalton HP, et al: Observations concerning the microbial etiology of acute salpingitis. Am J Obstet Gynecol 170:1014–1017, 1994.

Soper DE, Brockwell NJ, Dalton HP: False positive cultures of the cul-de-sac associated with culdocentesis in patients undergoing elective laparoscopy. Obstet Gynecol 164:134–138, 1991.

Svensson L, Mardh PA, Westrom L: Infertility after acute salpingitis with special reference to *Chlamydia trachomatis*. Fertil Steril 40:322–327, 1983.

Sweet RL, Draper DL, Schacter J, et al: Microbiology and pathogenesis of acute salpingitis as determined by laparoscopy: What is the appropriate site to sample? Am J Obstet Gynecol 138:985–989, 1980.

Sweet RL, Draper DL, Hadley WK: Etiology of acute salpingitis: Influence of episode number and duration of symptoms. Obstet Gynecol 58:62–68, 1981.

Sweet RL, Schachter J, Robbie MO: Failure of β-lactam antibiotics to eradicate *Chlamydia trachomatis* in the endometrium despite apparent clinical cure of acute salpingitis. JAMA 250:2641–2645, 1983.

Washington AE, Aral SO, Grimes DA, et al: Assessing risk for pelvic inflammatory disease and its sequelae. JAMA 266:2581–2586, 1991.

Wasserheit JN, Bell TA, Kiviat NB, et al: Microbial causes of proven pelvic inflammatory disease and efficacy of clindamycin and tobramycin. Ann Intern Med 104:187–193, 1986.

Westrom L, Mardh PA: Salpingitis. *In* Holmes KK, Mardh PA, Sparling PF, et al (eds): Sexually Transmitted Diseases. New York, McGraw-Hill, 1984.

Westrom L: Incidence, prevalence, and trends of acute pelvic inflammatory disease and its consequences in industrialized countries. Am J Obstet Gynecol 138:880–892, 1980.

Westrom L: Effect of acute pelvic inflammatory disease on fertility. Am J Obstet Gynecol 121:707–713, 1975.

Wolner-Hanssen, Eschenbach DA, Paavonen J, et al: Association between vaginal douching and acute pelvic inflammatory disease. JAMA 263:1936–1941, 1990.

Wolner-Hanssen P, Eschenbach DA, Paavonen J, et al: Decreased risk of symptomatic chlamydial pelvic inflammatory disease associated with oral contraceptive use. JAMA 263:54–59, 1990.

# 9

# Pelvic Mass

LARA J. BURROWS
THOMAS E. ELKINS

Pelvic masses are commonly encountered in clinical practice and can be difficult to evaluate. They may range from a simple ovarian cyst to an advanced malignancy. Many conditions present as a pelvic mass, and when this condition is evaluated multiple organ systems have to be considered. The differential diagnosis of a pelvic mass and the evaluation of its significance vary in accordance with different stages of the patient's reproductive life. This chapter discusses the differential diagnosis at each stage and outlines basic guidelines for proper evaluation and treatment.

## Ovarian Cysts in Newborns

Generally, functional cysts (those related to the physiologic functioning of the ovary) are uncommon before puberty, with the exception of those found in neonates. The etiology of a pelvic mass in a newborn is most likely a functional cyst on the fetal ovary resulting from maternal hormone stimulation in utero. This type of cyst may be diagnosed in utero by ultrasonography or it may be recognized as an asymptomatic abdominal mass secondary to displacement of the cyst upward into the abdomen from the narrow fetal pelvis. The evaluation and treatment of the neonate who has a large follicular cyst involves a thorough physical examination followed by an assessment of its characteristics via abdominal ultrasonography. Usually, the ultrasonogram reveals a simple ovarian follicular cyst that regresses after the first few months of life. Observation is an appropriate means of treatment, but symptoms of ovarian torsion should be explained to the caregivers. If the cyst does not regress, ultrasonographically guided drainage may be performed.

## Ovarian Cysts in Children

The appearance of a pelvic mass is rare in childhood (Table 9–1) until puberty, and its presence suggests a neoplastic process. Abdominopelvic masses in chil-

Table 9–1  The Differential Diagnosis of Pelvic Mass in Newborns and Children

| Newborns | |
|---|---|
| Functional ovarian cyst | |
| **Children** | |
| Ovarian | Lymphoma |
| Teratoma | Burkitt's tumor |
| Dysgerminoma | Gastrointestinal |
| Wilms' tumor | Musculoskeletal |
| Neuroblastoma | |

dren are usually nongynecologic in origin and are related to the presence of Wilms' tumor or a neuroblastoma. Ovarian neoplasms are the most commonly occurring genital neoplasm in children and these tumors account for only 1% of tumors in this age group. The majority of ovarian neoplasms are benign, but a 35% malignancy rate requires referral to a specialist. Most ovarian neoplasms in this age group are of germ cell origin. Should they produce estrogen or testosterone, it may present clinically as precocious puberty or masculinization.

The symptoms of ovarian neoplasms in children may be nonspecific and include nausea, vomiting, chronic abdominal pain, fullness, and urinary complaints related to the size of the tumor. Adnexal masses in childhood may manifest as acute and severe pain related to torsion or infarction, mimicking acute appendicitis. Intermittent severe abdominal pain may represent intermittent adnexal torsion, which may progress to a pelvic mass with congestion followed by subsequent infarction. The child's caregiver or physician may note an increase in abdominal girth because the adnexa in a child is located in the abdomen. Evaluation should include an abdominal and a rectal examination.

In patients who have a stable adnexal mass, it is appropriate to perform pelvic ultrasonography for further assessment. A timely referral to a specialist is required, and he or she may wish to perform alternative imaging studies. The use of tumor markers in this age group does not affect preoperative management, and it is usually reserved for postoperative follow-up.

## Adnexal Masses in Adolescents

Young women between menarche and 20 years of age constitute an age group in which pelvic masses become increasingly common and complex. The differential diagnosis of the pelvic mass (Table 9–2) is broader for reasons pertaining to the menstrual cycle and the functioning ovary, the onset of sexual activity, and the possibility of pregnancy. The majority of adnexal masses in this age group appear as functional cysts. Benign and malignant neoplasms, even though uncommon, must be considered in the differential diagnosis.

With the onset of menarche, abnormalities of müllerian development may become apparent. These rare anomalies can produce obstruction in the reproductive outflow tract, resulting in a buildup of menstrual blood in the vagina (hematocolpos) or the uterus (hematometra), which may then lead to palpable pelvic masses. A dilated uterine horn may also present as a mass.

**Table 9–2** Differential Diagnosis of Pelvic Mass in Adolescent Girls

| **Obstructive genital lesion** | |
| --- | --- |
| Imperforate hymen | Blind uterine horn |
| **Ovarian** | |
| Functional  Germ cell tumor | Other ovarian neoplasm |
| **Tubal** | |
| Paratubal cyst  Ectopic gestation | Tubo-ovarian abscess  Pyosalpinx |
| **Uterine** | |
| Cornual ectopic gestation  Leiomyoma | Pregnancy, including molar gestation |
| **Gastrointestinal** | |
| Appendiceal abscess | |

With the onset of ovulation, the functional ovary begins to produce physiologic ovarian cysts, which may become symptomatic throughout the reproductive years. Physiologic follicular cysts can arise from normal ovarian function, failure of a mature follicle to rupture at ovulation, or bleeding into a follicle after ovulation. Additionally, the functional ovary allows fertility and a potential for pregnancy. Pregnancy in either a uterine or an extrauterine location is a major cause of pelvic mass in this age group and must always be considered.

With the onset of sexual activity, pelvic infections and salpingitis not uncommonly may progress to pyosalpinx or tubo-ovarian abscess. When an infectious pelvic mass is evaluated, an appendiceal abscess must be considered as well. Adolescents often present with symptomatic pelvic masses, because they are usually otherwise healthy and do not seek care on a regular basis.

The evaluation of patients in this age group consists of a complete history and physical examination. This should include a detailed menstrual history, including the presence of dysmenorrhea, as well as a sexual history, including contraceptive use. Congenital obstructive lesions often occur in association with absent menstrual cycles but with cyclic lower abdominal pain. The physical examination enables the clinician to identify hematocolpos secondary to an imperforate hymen. A blind uterine horn presents with cyclic menstrual bleeding as well as severe cyclic pelvic pain and a pelvic mass on examination. Approximately one third of patients who have congenital reproductive tract abnormalities also have urinary tract abnormalities, including pelvic kidney, renal agenesis, horseshoe kidney, or an abnormality in the collecting ducts. An intravenous pyelogram is recommended for further assessment of the urinary tract.

Although the majority of adolescent pelvic masses are physiologic cysts, adnexal masses in this age group are occasionally neoplastic in origin. The majority of these neoplasms are benign cystic teratomas (dermoid cyst). These cysts are generally between 5 and 10 cm in diameter and have a 15% chance of bilaterality. They are slow growing and usually do not cause symptoms. Dysgerminomas and malignant tumors, usually of germ cell origin, are also encountered in this age group. All patients who have adnexal masses require a complete evaluation, including a gynecologic examination, pregnancy testing, and a complete blood count as indicated by the clinical condition. An abdominal radiograph may also be helpful in the diagnosis of a teratoma, which often has calcifications and a fat pad. Color Doppler velocimetry of adnexal tumors is capable of detecting flow-velocity waveforms. These waveforms reflect low peripheral resistances that are likely to be the result of the process of neovascularization of tumors. Velocimetry techniques are evolving, and this may prove to be a reliable method in characterizing ovarian neoplasms.

Functional ovarian cysts may be followed and treated symptomatically with nonsteroidal anti-inflammatory drugs if the size of the cyst is smaller than 5 cm and the patient has no evidence of an acute abdomen. Adding oral contraceptives does not affect the resolution of a current ovarian cyst; however, it allows suppression of future ovulation. Thus, a particular cyst can be followed over time, and future symptomatic ovarian cysts can be prevented from occurring. In this group, ultrasonography is not required as long as a follow-up examination is performed within 4 to 6 weeks. Patients who have cysts larger than 5 cm, or a cyst that does not resolve in 4 to 6 weeks, should have a pelvic ultrasonogram performed. The use of vaginal and abdominal ultrasonography can often help to characterize the adnexal mass.

Patients who have severe pain and those who have cysts larger than 10 cm require operative intervention (Table 9–3). In the past, surgical managment of adnexal cystic masses consisted of laparotomy. Some clinicians believe that ultrasonographically guided percutaneous aspiration of these cysts may be helpful, particularly in the pediatric population. Others have reservations about this treatment, because it may impair future fertility or lead to spillage of malignant cells into the abdomen. Moreover, the cysts have a high rate of recurrence. Others believe that under certain cirumstances, the enucleation of an adnexal mass at operative laparoscopy is sometimes superior to aspiration. This approach is not commonly used, and its success is highly dependent upon the skill of the endoscopist.

Other common causes of pelvic masses in adolescents relate to pregnancy and infection. Adolescents often deny and avoid treatment for pregnancy. A pregnancy test should be performed on any adolescent who is questionably pregnant. Ectopic pregnancy should be suspected in those who have abdominal pain, a normal-sized uterus, a positive pregnancy test, and who have had a pelvic ultrasonogram performed. The management of ectopic pregnancy is reviewed extensively in Chapter 4.

Patients who have pyosalpinx or tubo-ovarian abscess should be admitted to the hospital for parenteral antibiotic therapy. The diagnosis and management of pelvic inflammatory disease are reviewed in Chapter 8. Laparoscopy is recommended for women in whom the diagnosis is uncertain or who show slow or inadequate clinical improvement. Ultrasonographically guided aspiration in conjunction with antibiotic instillation for the treatment of a tubo-ovarian abscess is an easy and safe alternative therapy for patients in whom treatment with systemic antibiotics has failed. Appendectomy can be performed via laparoscopy or laparotomy.

## Pelvic Masses in Women of Reproductive Age (20 to 45 Years of Age)

This age group has an expanded differential diagnosis for possible etiologies of a pelvic mass. There are many nongynecologic causes in this age group (Table 9–4). In women of reproductive age, however, a pelvic mass usually arises from the genital tract (Table 9–5). As previously discussed in relation to the adolescent patient, the clinician must always consider pregnancy as a potential cause of a pelvic mass, because an ectopic pregnancy can be life threatening. An ectopic gestation must be considered in pregnant patients who have adnexal fullness or a mass, and it must be ruled out by an appropriate evaluation, as mentioned previously.

The adnexa is most commonly involved in conditions that appear as a pelvic mass. The mass may arise

**Table 9–3** Surgical Emergency

Ruptured ectopic gestation
   Tubal
   Cornual
   Abdominal
Torsion of the adnexa
Ruptured tubo-ovarian abscess
Ruptured hemorrhagic ovarian cyst (hemodynamically compromised)

**Table 9–4** Nongynecologic Causes of Pelvic Mass

**Gastrointestinal**

| | |
|---|---|
| Cecal carcinoma | Appendiceal abscess |
| Crohn's disease at terminal ileum | Rectosigmoid carcinoma |
| Sigmoid colon diverticulitis | |

**Urinary Tract**

| | |
|---|---|
| Urologic neoplasm | Pelvic kidney |

**Retroperitoneal tumors**

| | |
|---|---|
| Lymphoma | Soft tissue neuromas |
| Anterior meningocele | Retroperitoneal cyst |
| Neurogenic tumors | |
| Neurofibromas | |

**Vascular**

| | |
|---|---|
| Iliac aneurysm | Arteriovenous fistula |

**Peritoneum**

| |
|---|
| Peritoneal cysts |

**Metastatic**

| | |
|---|---|
| Gastrointestinal primary tumor | Breast tumor |

from the uterus, the fallopian tube, or the ovary. In reproductive-aged women, the most common adnexal mass is a physiologic ovarian cyst, and the most common neoplasm is a benign cystic teratoma.

Several conditions involving the fallopian tube may result in a pelvic mass as well. Most commonly, this is related to a paratubal cyst or the sequelae of a previous salpingitis, with occlusion of the fallopian tube resulting in pyosalpinx, hydrosalpinx, or a tubo-ovarian abscess.

The evaluation and treatment of an intrauterine pregnancy, an ectopic pregnancy, or a functional ovarian cyst in women of reproductive age are the same as those for the adolescent group. If expectant management does not result in resolution of the mass, if symptoms exceed 6 weeks, or if symptoms become severe, the woman should be referred to a gynecologist for a consultation. Patients who have worsening symptoms or who have multiple or complex cysts should be referred immediately for further evaluation.

A paratubal cyst usually presents asymptomatically as a unilocular cyst found on ultrasonography. The cyst may or become symptomatic if it undergoes torsion. Tubo-ovarian abscesses have been reported to occur in as many as one third of women hospitalized with salpingitis. A tubo-ovarian abscess is one of the most common causes of pelvic mass in reproductive-aged women, and it is the most common intra-abdominal abscess in premenopausal women. As mentioned earlier, the patient who has this diagnosis typically presents with abdominal or pelvic pain associated with elevated temperature and an elevated white blood cell count. Physical examination reveals lower abdominal or pelvic tenderness and cervical motion tenderness. These patients often have peritoneal signs, and it is frequently difficult to palpate a mass on bimanual examination. Thus, a pelvic ultrasonogram should be obtained for all patients who have a suspected tubo-ovarian abscess.

Laboratory tests that are helpful include a complete blood count with differential, screening for sexually transmitted diseases (including human immunodeficiency virus), blood cultures, and a sedimentation rate. Antibiotic therapy is successful in most women. Even with excellent cure rates in the acute phase, however, the clinician must keep in mind that many of these patients will subsequently require surgical intervention.

Other adnexal masses in the reproductive years may involve any known ovarian tumor, including metastatic disease. The most common neoplastic ovarian mass is the benign cystic teratoma. Even though the presence of an adnexal malignancy is rare before the age of 40, ovarian cancer must be considered in patients who have suspicious findings (such as a positive family history) on physical examination or imaging studies.

Endometriosis, involving implants of benign endometrial tissue outside the endometrium, may manifest as a pelvic mass in this age group. This condition is most commonly seen in nulliparous white women between the ages of 35 and 45. Implants may be present on one or both ovaries, forming large cysts called endometriomas (chocolate cysts). They are usually symptomatic, and the patient complains of cyclic pelvic pain, pressure, and dyspareunia. Definitive diagnosis requires a diagnostic laparoscopy.

Polycystic ovarian syndrome, a common cause of infertility among reproductive-aged women is seen uncommonly in association with a pelvic mass. Often,

**Table 9–5** Differential Diagnosis of Pelvic Mass in Reproductive-Aged Women

**Uterine**

| | |
|---|---|
| Leiomyoma | Pregnancy, including molar gestation |
| Cornual ectopic | |

**Cervical**

| |
|---|
| Neoplasm |

**Tubal**

| | |
|---|---|
| Paratubal cyst | Pyosalpinx |
| Ectopic gestation | Hydrosalpinx |
| Tubo-ovarian abscess | |

**Ovarian**

| | |
|---|---|
| Functional | Endometrioma |
| Neoplastic | |

these patients are hirsute and obese. They have bilaterally enlarged ovaries and a history of menstrual irregularities.

A pelvic mass related to the uterus or cervix is not uncommon in reproductive-aged women. The examination of the uterus and cervix is an essential component in the evaluation of a pelvic mass in this age group. In the United States, leiomyomas are found in 10% of white women and 30 to 40% of African-American women who are past the age of 35. In any of the varied locations of myomas, degeneration, infarction, and infection can occur. These symptoms can be associated with a pelvic mass, significant lower abdominal and pelvic pain, and abnormal bleeding. Uterine leiomyomas are usually asymptomatic, but when symptoms occur, the most common is menorrhagia. Asymptomatic enlargement of the uterus does not require surgical therapy. Leiomyomas are discussed further in Chapter 6.

## Pelvic Masses in Perimenopausal and Postmenopausal Women (Past 45 Years of Age)

In this age group, the presence of a pelvic mass must be considered very carefully because neoplasms from both genital and other organ systems occur more frequently (Table 9–6). Ovarian cancer affects 1 in 70 women in their lifetimes. Two thirds of these cancers are an advanced stage (III or IV) at diagnosis, and ovarian cancer causes more deaths than any other genital tract malignancy. In 80% of these cases, women are past the age of 50. Thus, the clinician should be concerned whenever a pelvic mass is discovered in a postmenopausal woman. In addition, every patient in the perimenopausal and postmenopausal age group who has a pelvic mass must be considered for gastrointestinal diverticula and cancers. Primary tumors from the musculoskeletal system and genitourinary and lymphatic tracts are also more common in this age group. Metastatic tumors to the ovaries include gastrointestinal and breast cancers. *BRCA1*, the breast cancer susceptibility gene, accounts for approximately 5 to 10% of breast cancers. Mutations in *BRCA1* and *BRCA2* also indicate a greatly increased risk of ovarian cancer, approaching 40% incidence. The medical actions that should follow a negative or positive test result have not been completely elucidated.

The benign genital conditions, such as uterine leiomyomas and endometriosis, that occur in the reproductive-aged group are seen less commonly in this age group, and they do not require surgical therapy as often. In the postmenopausal age group, the incidence of uterine leiomyomas is 30% in white women and 40 to 50% in African-American women. These neoplasms are hormone-dependent; therefore, they usually regress following menopause.

Uterine myomas and endometriosis can be considered in the differential diagnosis of pelvic masses in this age group, but malignant tumors, including adenocarcinomas, sarcomas, and mixed mesodermal tumors, are most commonly present in this age group. Additionally, uterine tumors must be considered in the postmenopausal patient who has an enlarging uterine mass. Sarcomatous elements within the uterus may manifest as a rapidly growing mass, sometimes associated with pain and tenderness. Likewise, adnexal masses occurring in the postmenopausal female can be benign, but the likelihood of malignancy increases with age.

The evaluation and treatment of the perimenopausal and postmenopausal woman must include a thorough evaluation of other organ systems. The clinician must inquire about gastrointestinal complaints and history of a breast mass or lesions. If the history or physical examination indicates that another organ system is involved, appropriate screening tests must be performed, including a mammogram, a barium enema, and either a flexible sigmoidoscopy or a colonoscopy.

The evaluation of a pelvic mass of gynecologic origin must be complete, and a malignancy from the vagina, cervix, uterus, fallopian tubes, or ovaries must be ruled out. A history of any previous gynecologic surgery or tumors must be reviewed, and previous operative and pathology records must be obtained. The date of the patient's last gynecologic examination allows the physician to determine whether the mass is growing rapidly. Any visible abnormality of the

**Table 9–6** Differential Diagnosis of Pelvic Mass in Perimenopausal and Postmenopausal Women

| **Uterine** | |
|---|---|
| Leiomyoma | Neoplasm |
| **Cervical** | |
| Neoplasm | |
| **Fallopian Tube** | |
| Paratubal cyst | Neoplasm |
| **Ovarian** | |
| Neoplasm Benign Malignant | |

vulva, vagina, or cervix should be biopsied and sent for pathologic study. A cytologic smear may be obtained from the cervix or vaginal cuff if this has not recently been performed. A pelvic mass associated with postmenopausal bleeding or menstrual irregularities should be evaluated with an endometrial biopsy. Referral should not be delayed, however, if an endometrial biopsy performed for an enlarged uterus is negative for hyperplasia or cancer. The presence of leiomyoma in the postmenopausal woman is not in itself an indication for surgery, but an enlarging postmenopausal myoma is suspicious for a leiomyosarcoma and the patient should be referred for further evaluation and possible surgical removal.

A pelvic mass detected on pelvic examination in a patient who has a normal cervix and uterus suggests the fallopian tubes or ovaries as a possible source of the adnexal mass. The fallopian tube is an uncommon source of a pelvic mass in postmenopausal women, because infectious etiologies are extremely rare and pregnancy does not occur in this age group. Fallopian tube carcinoma is rare, accounting for less than 1% of all genital cancers. The classic presentation is a watery cervical discharge, pain, and menorrhagia with a pelvic mass. Management of fallopian tube carcinoma is similar to that of ovarian cancer.

The primary concern caused by an adnexal mass in the postmenopausal women is ovarian cancer. A proper history should include questions regarding abdominal discomfort, increased abdominal girth, and previous surgical therapy, along with other general questions about such topics as weight loss, changes in appetite, and fevers. The physical examination, like all gynecologic examinations of a pelvic mass, should include a rectovaginal examination and testing for occult blood. The ovaries in postmenopausal women should not be palpable and their tangible presence should arouse suspicion.

In the past, the primary means of diagnosing a pelvic mass was by physical examination and history. The use of ultrasonography has been shown to be more precise in detecting ovarian tumors than the pelvic examination. Ultrasonography has proved to be invaluable in evaluating pelvic masses and, as mentioned earlier, color-flow Doppler imaging seems promising, but its exact role has yet to be determined. With the routine use of ultrasonography, simple, unilateral, unilocular cysts measuring less than 5 cm, without septations or ascites, are unlikely to be malignant and often the progression of these cysts can be followed conservatively without risk to the patient. The patient should be seen initially at 6-week intervals. If there is any progression of the cyst on ultrasonography or if there is an elevation in serum CA 125 levels, surgical exploration is mandatory. Factors that increase the likelihood of an ovarian malignancy include size larger than 10 cm, ascites, and bilaterality. A CA 125 tumor marker test should be ordered in the postmenopausal patient who has a pelvic mass, however, its utility as a screening test is not clear.

## REFERENCES

American College of Obstetricians and Gynecologists: ACOG Technical Bulletin. Number 192–May 1994.

Ansbacher R, Mills EM, Thrush JC, et al: Ectopic pregnancy and maternal mortality in Michigan. Am J Gynecol Health III 4:118, 1989.

Asadourian LA, Taylor HB: Dysgerminomas: An analysis of 105 cases. Obstet Gynecol 33:370, 1969.

Boring CC, Squires TS, Tong T: Cancer statistics, 1991. CA Cancer J Clin 41:19, 1991.

Bradley EA, Reidy JF, Forman RG, et al: Transcatheter uterine artery embolisation to treat large uterine fibroids. Br J Obstet Gynaecol 105:235, 1998.

Caruso A, Caforio L, Testa AC. et al: Transvaginal color Doppler ultrasonography in the presurgical characterization of adnexal masses. Gynecol Oncol 63:184, 1996.

Caruso PA, Marsh MR, Minkowitz S, et al: An intense clinical pathologic study of 305 teratomas of the ovary. Cancer 27:343, 1971.

Caspi B, Zalel Y, Lurie S, et al: Ultrasound-guided aspiration for relief of pain generated by simple ovarian cysts. Gynecol Obstet Invest 35:121, 1993.

Caspi B, Zalel Y, Or Y, et al: Sonographically guided aspiration: An alternative therapy for tubo-ovarian abscess. Ultrasound Obstet Gynecol 7:439, 1996.

Cosun ME, Kennedy RJL: Ovarian tumors in infants and children. Am J Dis Child 76:127, 1948.

Culter SJ, Young JL (eds): Third National Cancer Survey: Incidence Data. Washington, DC, National Cancer Institute. *In* Monograph 41, U.S. Department of Health, Education, and Welfare publication, National Institutes of Health, 1975, pp 75–77.

Dennerstein G: Ultrasound guided aspiration of ovarian cysts (letter). Aust N Z J Obstet Gynaecol 36:223, 1996.

DePriest PD, Gallio HH, Pavlik EJ, et al: Transvaginal sonography as a screening method for the detection of early ovarian cancer. Gynecol Oncol 65:408, 1997.

DiSaia PJ, Creasman WT: The adnexal mass and early ovarian cancer. *In* DiSaia PJ, Creasman WT (eds): Clinical Gynecologic Oncology. St. Louis, Mosby–Year Book, 1993, pp 302–332, 484.

Gerber B, Muller H, Kulz T, et al: Simple ovarian cysts in premenopausal patients. Int J Gynecol Obstet 57:49, 1997.

Goldstein SR: Postmenopausal adnexal cysts: How clinical management has evolved. Am J Obstet Gynecol 175:1498, 1996.

Goldstein SR, Snyder JR, Schwartz LB: Clinical management of simple postmenopausal adnexal cystic masses detected on ultrasonography. Female Patient 22:15, 1997.

Kedar N, Caldwell BV, Romereo R: A method of screening for ectopic pregnancy and its indications. Obstet Gynecol 58:162, 1981.

Keith SC, London SN, Weitzman GA, et al: Serial transvaginal ultrasound scans and beta-human chorionic gonadotropin levels in early singleton and multiple pregnancies. Fertil Steril 59:1007, 1993.

Landers DV, Wolner-Hanssen P, Paavonen J, et al: Combination antimicrobial therapy in the treatment of acute pelvic inflammatory disease. Am J Obstet Gynecol 164:849, 1991.

Marana R, Caruana P, Muzii L, et al: Operative laparoscopy for ovarian cysts: Excision vs. aspiration. J Reprod Med 41:435, 1996.

Mueller CW, Thompkins P, Lapp WA: Dysgerminomas of the ovary: An analysis of 427 cases. Am J Obstet Gynecol 60:153, 1950.

Peterson WF, Prevost EC, Edmunds FT, et al: Benign cystic teratoma of the ovary: A clinico-statistical study of 1007 cases with a review of the literature. Am J Obstet Gynecol 70:568, 1955.

Petterson F (ed): Annual Report on the Results of Treatment in Gynecologic Cancer, International Federation of Gynecology and Obstetrics, Stockholm, 1990, p 20.

Ross DW: BRCA1: Genetic testing and hereditary breast and ovarian cancer. Arch Pathol Lab Med 121:754, 1997.

Rulin MC, Presin AL: Adnexal masses in postmenopausal women. Obstet Gynecol 70:578, 1987.

Russell DJ: The female pelvic mass: Diagnosis and management. Med Clin North Am 79:6, 1995.

Soper DE, Despres B: A comparison of two antibiotic regimens for treatment of pelvic inflammatory disease. Obstet Gynecol 72:7, 1988.

Stenchever MA: Differential diagnosis of major gynecologic problems by age groups. In Mishell DR, Stenchever MA, Droegemueller W, et al (eds): Comprehensive Gynecology. St. Louis, CV Mosby, 1997, p 161.

Sweet RI, Gibbs RS: Pelvic infection and abscess. In Sweet RL, Gibbs RS (eds): Infectious Diseases of the Female Genital Tract. Baltimore, Williams & Wilkins, 1990, p 90.

Sweet RL, Schachter J, Landers DV, et al: Treatment of hospitalized patients with acute pelvic inflammatory disease: Comparison of cefotetan plus doxycycline and cefoxitin plus doxycyline. Am J Obstet Gynecol 158:736, 1988.

Walters MD, Gibbs RS: A randomized comparison of gentamycin-clindamycin and cefoxitin-doxycycline in the treatment of acute pelvic inflammatory disease. Obstet Gynecol 75:867, 1990.

Wiesenfeld HC, Sweet RL: Progress in the management of tuboovarian abscess. Clin Obstet Gynecol 36:433, 1993.

# 10

# Pediatric and Adolescent Gynecology*

## DAVID MURAM

The reproductive tract of a female child differs in structure and function from that of the adult female, and the physician who cares for young patients should be familiar with these differences. Moreover, these anatomic differences require the use of specially designed instruments (e.g., vaginoscope, virginal vaginal speculum) if the examination is to be performed without causing undue discomfort and subsequent anxiety for the patient about future examinations.

This chapter reviews some of the common gynecologic disorders that the primary care provider may encounter in the pediatric and adolescent age groups. For a more extensive review, the reader should consult other resources.

## Anatomic and Physiologic Considerations

Immediately following birth and during the first few weeks of life, the female newborn responds to maternal estrogens. The effects of such stimulation may be seen for 6 weeks and sometimes even longer. The most obvious sign, breast budding, occurs in nearly all children born at term. Sometimes the breast enlargement is marked and may be accompanied by a discharge from the nipples. This breast enlargement requires no treatment, and repeated examinations may lead to bruising or infection of the breast tissue. At birth, the vagina is about 4 cm long. The uterus is enlarged, measuring 4 cm in length. It has no axial flexion and the ratio of the cervix to the corpus is 3:1. The external genitalia are affected by maternal estrogens as well. The labia majora are bulbous and the labia minora are thick and protruding. The clitoris in the newborn appears relatively large. Vaginal discharge is frequently present (Fig. 10–1). The ovaries, which arise from the $T_{10}$ level, are abdominal organs in early childhood and are not palpable on pelvic or rectal examination.

During early childhood, the genital tract receives very little estrogen stimulation. The labia majora are flat and the labia minora and hymen are extremely thin (Fig. 10–2). The clitoris is relatively small. The vagina measures 5 cm in length and the mucosa is thin and atrophic. The vagina is colonized with mixed bacterial flora, and the pH is neutral or slightly alkaline. The uterus is very small, and the cervix is flush with the vaginal vault.

When a girl is between 8 and 10 years of age, the external genitalia begin to show signs of estrogen stimulation. The mons pubis thickens, the labia majora fill out, the labia minora become rounded, and the hymen thickens. The vagina grows to 8 cm in

---

*David Muram retains copyright for original figures contributed to this chapter.

PEDIATRIC AND ADOLESCENT GYNECOLOGY 83

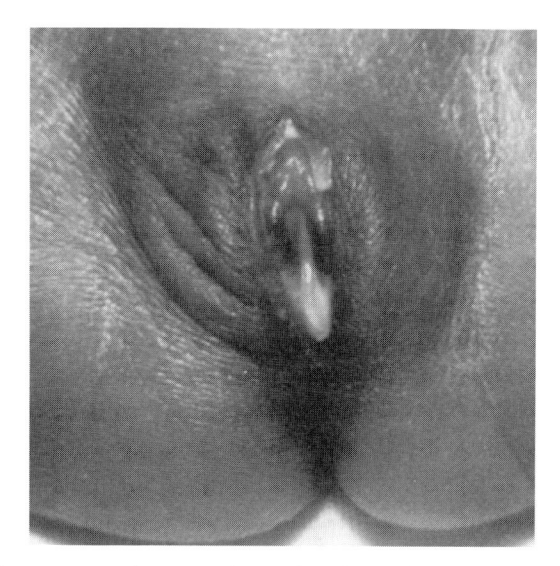

**Figure 10–1** The external genitalia of a newborn female. Note the hypertrophy and turgor of the vulvar tissue and the large amount of vaginal secretions. (From Ransom SB, McNeeley SG [eds]: Gynecology for the Primary Care Provider. Philadelphia, WB Saunders, 1997, p. 248.)

descend into the true pelvis. Secondary sexual characteristics develop rapidly during the late childhood period. Accelerated somatic growth (adolescent growth spurt) occurs, followed by breast development and sexual hair growth. The body habitus becomes rounded, especially in the shoulders and hips.

## Examination Strategies

### EXAMINATION OF THE PREPUBERTAL PATIENT

Young children are very sensitive to the physician's attitude. They react positively to someone who is kind, warm, and patient. These young patients must be assured that the examination, although perhaps uncomfortable, embarrassing, or both, is not painful. The girl's mother often accompanies her to the examination room. The mother's presence during the examination may provides comfort and a sense of security to the child. A young child (≤5 years of age) may be held on the mother's lap, with the mother supporting the child's legs (Fig. 10–3). An older child can lie on the examination table, but the use of stirrups is generally not necessary. The patient should place her hands on the dorsal aspects of her lower thighs, flexing her knees and abducting her legs.

After the general examination is completed, the

length. The mucosa becomes thicker, and the maturation index shows intermediate cells and, occasionally, superficial cells. The uterine corpus grows, and the ratio of cervix to corpus is 1:1.

During puberty (ages 10 to 13 years), the external genitalia acquire an adult appearance. The vagina reaches its adult length (10 to 12 cm) and the mucosa becomes thick and moist. The vaginal secretions are acidic and contain lactobacilli. The uterine corpus becomes twice as large as the cervix, and the ovaries

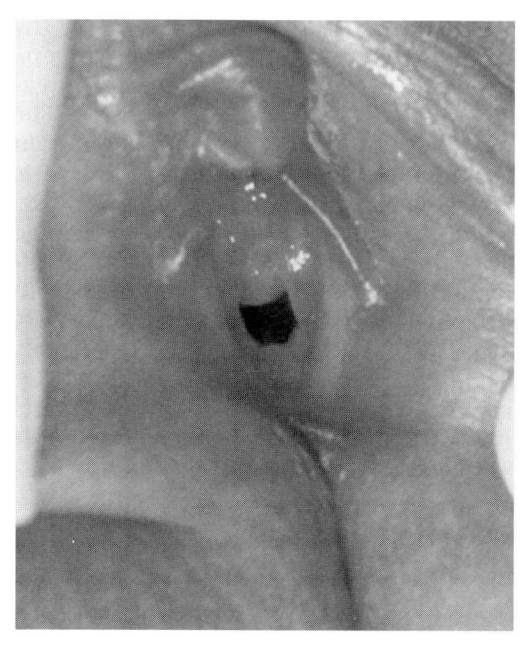

**Figure 10–2** The external genitalia of a child 3 years of age. (From Ransom SB, McNeeley SG [eds]: Gynecology for the Primary Care Provider. Philadelphia, WB Saunders, 1997, p. 248.)

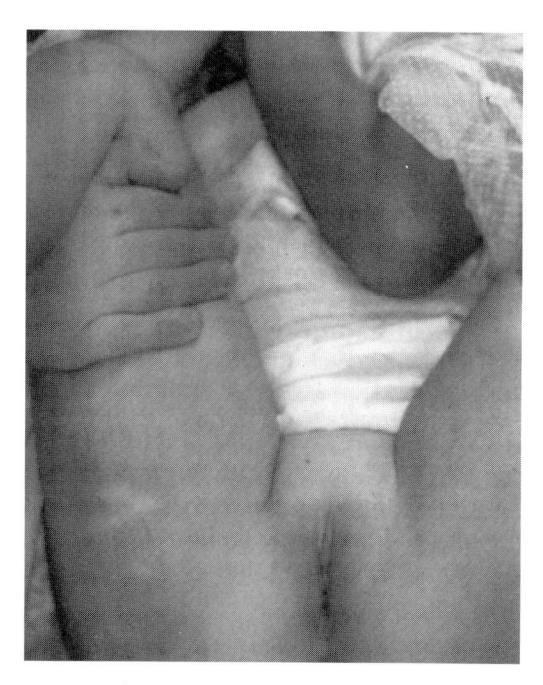

**Figure 10–3** The examination of a young girl who is seated on her mother's lap. The mother supports the child's legs, thereby providing an excellent view of the genital area. (From Ransom SB, McNeeley SG [eds]: Gynecology for the Primary Care Provider. Philadelphia, WB Saunders, 1997, p. 249.)

child's breasts should be inspected and palpated. At the onset of breast growth, the examiner may feel a small, firm, flat "button" beneath the nipple. Prominence of the nipple and breast development in a child younger than 8 years of age may be the first signs of sexual precocity. The ovaries of a premenarcheal child are situated high in the pelvis, and ovarian neoplasms grow toward the midabdomen; therefore, light palpation of the abdomen elicits the needed information.

The examiner exposes the vulva and vestibule by exerting light lateral downward pressure on both sides of the perineum. Signs of hormonal stimulation in early childhood, or their absence when they should be evident, may indicate abnormal pubertal development. Enlargement of the clitoris may indicate increased androgenic stimulation and virilization. The examiner should look for skin lesions, vaginal discharge, perineal excoriations, ulcers, and tumors. In addition, the patency of the hymenal orifice should be confirmed.

It is impossible to perform a digital vaginal examination in a child if the size of the hymenal opening is normal for age; for example, the average hymeneal orifice in a 6-year-old girl is 4 to 6 mm. In all prepubertal children, the hymenal orifice is smaller than 10 mm. However, a gentle rectal digital examination can be easily accomplished and should not cause pain. Nonetheless, accurate intrapelvic evaluation is often difficult because of the relatively small size of the uterus, the size and location of the ovaries, and the firmness of the abdominal wall. If the presence of a pelvic tumor is strongly suspected, other diagnostic procedures, such as ultrasonography, magnetic resonance imaging (MRI), or computed tomography (CT), should be performed, regardless of the findings of the rectoabdominal examination.

If the child refuses an intrapelvic examination or if the examination is occasioned by an acute injury, it is advisable to use sedation or, preferably, general anesthesia. Forcible examination is not justified. Not only is it psychologically traumatic to the patient, but she may be injured by the instruments if she struggles to free herself.

Use of vaginal instrumentation is not a routine part of the gynecologic examination of young patients, but it may be required for evaluation of the upper vagina, observation and removal of foreign bodies, or assessment of vaginal trauma after a penetrating injury. Many types of instruments have been used to separate the vaginal walls (e.g., nasal speculum, otoscope, vaginoscope, flexible urethroscope). If the examination is performed in an office setting, the patient must be relaxed and cooperative. Xylocaine jelly is placed at the vaginal introitus and on the instrument. The physician should show the instrument to the girl before inserting it. She should be allowed to touch the lubricated instrument and to become familiar with its slippery, cool surface. The instrument should then be placed against her inner thigh and she should be reminded of the cool, slippery, and unusual feeling. Only then should the instrument be inserted through the hymenal orifice.

If the examination is performed under general anesthesia, I prefer to use a water cystoscope. The labia minora are pressed together to retain the water in the vagina. This maintains distention and facilitates visualization of the vaginal walls. The water irrigates any secretions, blood, or debris and provides an unobstructed view (Fig. 10–4).

## EXAMINATION OF THE ADOLESCENT PATIENT

An adolescent's first trip to the gynecologist is often fraught with fear and apprehension. Friends may have told her harrowing stories they have heard about vaginal examinations. The patient may be concerned that the physician will discuss with her parents the particulars of her visit or the findings of the examination. Therefore, the physician must spend time putting the patient at ease and winning her confidence. The adolescent must understand that she, not her mother, is the patient. The girl herself is asked to provide pertinent medical information required for the medical record. Questions about sexual behavior and venereal diseases require a delicate approach and, obviously, such questions should not be asked with the girl's mother present. After the history has been obtained, the girl should be given a brief description of what the examination entails. She and her mother may need to be assured that her hymen will not be injured and that the examination will not be painful, although she may feel uncomfortable or embarrassed.

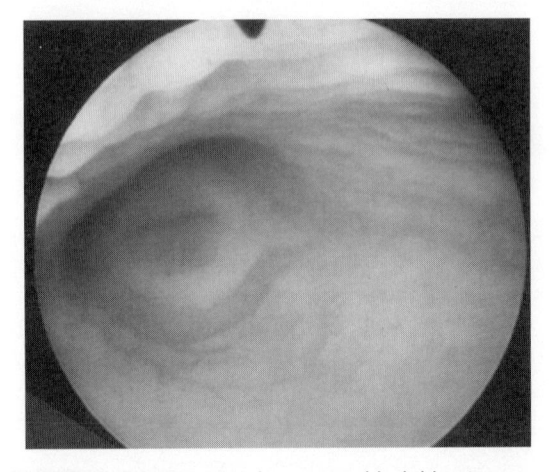

**Figure 10–4** Vaginoscopy of a 2-year-old child using a water cystoscope. The vagina is distended and the examiner has a clear panoramic view of the entire vagina and cervix. (From Ransom SB, McNeeley SG [eds]: Gynecology for the Primary Care Provider. Philadelphia, WB Saunders, 1997, p. 250.)

The examination is performed in the presence of a female assistant whose role is to give constant reassurance to the young patient. After the mother has left the room is the time to ask the patient sensitive questions about sexual activity, contraception, and exposure to sexually transmitted diseases (STDs). Examination of the breasts is an integral part of the physical examination of every female patient. In addition, the physician should provide the adolescent with instruction on breast self-examination.

During the genital examination, the physician should provide an explanation of what is being done. The patient may even be shown a direct view of her own genitalia, using a mirror or a videocolposcope. After the external genitalia have been inspected, a speculum is inserted into the vagina. The hymenal orifice of most virginal adolescents is about 1.0 cm in diameter. A narrow speculum can be inserted without difficulty. The Huffman-Graves long-bladed speculum, which is specifically designed to reach the cervix, is preferable to the short-bladed pediatric speculum. Patients who are sexually active, or those who have a large hymenal opening, can undergo a bimanual examination, but the physician may elect to insert only one finger into the vagina. Patients who have a hymenal orifice that is too small for digital examination should undergo a rectoabdominal examination.

After the examination is performed, the girl should have an opportunity to talk privately with the examiner. The examination and findings are discussed with the parent, or parents, only after the physician and patient have completed their discussion and agreed on what should be held in confidence. Under no circumstances should the physician violate the patient's request for privacy. If the physician believes the parents should be aware of certain details, the patient must be advised and persuaded that for her own benefit this information should be released to her parents.

## Common Disorders in Premenarcheal Girls

### VULVOVAGINITIS

Vulvovaginitis is the most common gynecologic disorder in children; perineal hygiene is often inadequate and contamination by stool and other debris is common. Because of the lack of estrogen, the vaginal mucosa is thin and atrophic and has low resistance to infectious organisms.

Vulvovaginitis can be divided into three major etiologic groups:

1. Nonspecific vulvovaginitis denotes a polymicrobial infection associated with disturbed local homeostasis caused by contamination (e.g., poor perineal hygiene, foreign body).
2. Secondary inoculation denotes an infection with a specific organism that causes a primary infection elsewhere (e.g., pharyngitis, septic sore throat). Infection of the vagina occurs after bacteremia or inoculation by the patient's hands.
3. Specific infection denotes a specific primary vaginal infection, most commonly sexually transmitted (e.g., gonorrhea).

The symptoms of vulvovaginitis vary from minor vulvar discomfort or relatively intense perineal pruritus to a sensation of burning and are accompanied by a foul-smelling vaginal discharge that may range in quantity from minimal to copious. This irritating discharge inflames the vulva and may cause the child to scratch the area to the point of bleeding. Acute vulvovaginitis may denude the thin vulvar or vaginal mucosa, but bleeding is usually minimal, merely staining the vaginal secretions. Inspection of the genitalia usually reveals a sore, reddened area, which may be either confined to the vestibule or extended laterally to the thighs and posteriorly to the anus (Fig. 10–5).

The clinical appearance alone is often sufficient to establish the diagnosis of vulvovaginitis. A laboratory evaluation of the secretions may suggest the specific etiology for the inflammatory process and may include the following:

1. Wet mount preparation for
   a. White and red blood cells
   b. Vaginal epithelial cells (determine estrogenic effect)
   c. Mycotic organisms (potassium hydroxide [KOH] preparation)
   d. *Trichomonas* spp.
   e. Parasitic ova

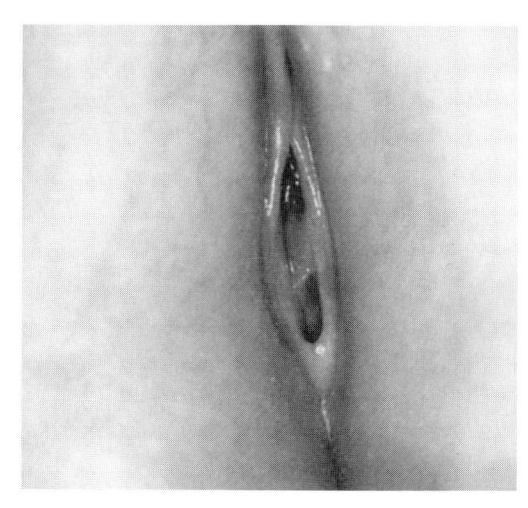

**Figure 10–5** The genitalia of a five-year-old girl who has vulvovaginitis. The inflammation extends laterally from the vestibule to the thighs and posteriorly to the anus. (From Ransom SB, McNeeley SG [eds]: Gynecology for the Primary Care Provider. Philadelphia, WB Saunders, 1997, p. 251.)

Table 10-1  Selected Anogenital Infections in Children

| Disease | Clinical Features | Diagnostic Workup | Treatment |
|---|---|---|---|
| ENTEROBIASIS<br>Infestation with small (1-cm) white worms. Child ingests eggs, which hatch in the stomach; the larvae migrate to the cecum. The worms migrate by night to the perianal region to deposit eggs. | Symptomatic individuals complain of nocturnal perianal pruritus and sleeplessness. | Identification of eggs or worms. In the morning, press adhesive tape against the perianal skin, and look for the eggs. | Single oral dose of mebendazol (100 mg). Piperazine salt or pyrvinium pamoate may also be used. All bedding must be changed and washed. Treat all individuals living in the house. |
| GONORRHEA<br>Usually caused by sexual contact. Commonly infected sites include vagina, rectum, pharynx, and conjunctiva. | Some individuals may have asymptomatic colonization, but most develop vulvovaginitis accompanied by erythema, purulent vaginal discharge, pruritus, and dysuria. Upper genital tract infections are rare in children. | DNA probes may be useful. Use selective cultures. It is recommended that isolates obtained from children be stored at −70°C for additional confirmatory testing. | For uncomplicated infections, a single dose of ceftriaxone, 125 mg intramuscularly, or spectinomycin, 40 mg/kg. Use a longer course of therapy for complicated infections. |
| CHLAMYDIA TRACHOMATIS<br>Primary modes of transmission are direct contact with infected secretions at birth and sexual contact. Perinatal exposure may result in colonization of the vagina and rectum. | Asymptomatic colonization of the genital tract may occur, but children often have symptoms of vaginitis, urethritis, and, occasionally, rectal pain. | Cell culture, using a monolayer of susceptible cells (e.g., McCoy cells) is regarded as the optimal method. DNA probes may prove useful. Antigen detection testing is not recommended in children. | Erythromycin (30–50 mg/kg/d) is the treatment of choice for children ≥8 years of age. Doxycycline (200 mg/d) is recommended for children older than 8 years of age. |
| SYPHILIS<br>After the neonatal period, syphilis is often acquired through sexual contact. Other modes of transmission are rare. | Primary syphilis: A painless chancre appears at an average of 21 days after exposure, with regional lymphadenopathy. The chancre heals within 4–6 weeks. Secondary stage shows symmetric mucocutaneous lesions and lymphadenopathy. Mucous patches appear on mucosal surfaces and condylomata lata occur in intertriginous areas. | Dark-field examination identifies the *Treponema pallidum*. Nontreponemal antibody tests are the RPR and the VDRL. These are used for initial screening or determining the activity of the disease. Specific serologic tests are the FTA-ABS and the MHA-TP. | Children who have primary, secondary, and early latent syphilis should be treated with benzathine penicillin, 50,000 U/kg. Do not exceed 2.4 million units. Congenital and neurosyphilis: Administer penicillin G, 200,000–300,000 U/kg/d for 10–14 d. |
| GENITAL HERPES<br>The virus enters the mucosal surfaces through an epithelial break. Sexual contact is the most common source of childhood genital herpes. | Painful vesicular lesions after 2–20 days, with inguinal adenopathy, fever, malaise, nausea, and headaches. The lesions later ulcerate and may become infected. Urinary retention may develop. Recurrences are less severe. | Isolation of the virus from suspicious lesions. False-negative cultures if cultured from lesions with decreased viral shedding. False-positive cultures in children who have herpes zoster. Antigen detection testing is not recommended. | Some clinicians treat children with acyclovir. Others use only symptomatic treatment: sitz baths, topical anesthetics, and drying agents. |
| CONDYLOMA ACUMINATA<br>Infection with HPV, which infects the germinal layer of the epithelium. The majority of perinatally acquired cases of HPV have been reported in children aged 2 years and younger. In older children who have genital HPV, sexual transmission is most common. | Prepubertal children are more likely to have periurethral and perianal condylomata. Upper genital tract infection is rare, but the anal canal is often infected. The lesions appear as flesh-colored verrucous growths and are often asymptomatic. The friable nature of condyloma may result in vaginal or rectal bleeding, dysuria, vaginal discharge, or painful defecation. | The diagnosis is often established by careful clinical inspection. Application of 3–5% acetic acid on a compress for 10–15 minutes may elicit the classic acetowhite appearance. Biopsy may be indicated in some cases. | Spontaneous regression has been described in some children. The use of topical agents is limited by the discomfort. CO₂ laser allows control over depth of tissue destruction and avoids much of the scarring. Recurrence rates are almost 30%. Interferon has been used only sporadically in children. |

FTA-ABS = fluorescent treponemal antibody absorption test; HPV = human papilloma virus; MHA-TP = microhemagglutination assay–*Treponema pallidum*; RPR = rapid plasma reagin; VDRL = Venereal Disease Research Laboratory

2. Smears for Gram's stain
3. Bacterial cultures, and, in selected patients, cultures for mycotic organisms

If a child has a documented first-time infection, vaginoscopy can be delayed. However, vaginoscopy is indicated in children who have recurrent vaginal infections that are refractory to treatment, or if there is a foul-smelling bloody discharge. In these patients, vaginoscopy also serves to exclude the presence of foreign bodies or neoplasms.

Regardless of the etiology of the infection, the physician should stress the importance of good perineal hygiene. The girl should be instructed to wipe the genitalia and anus from front to back. Sitz baths and mild soap remove debris and secretions from the vulva. Lukewarm soapy water also provides symptomatic relief by soothing the skin and reducing swelling. In children who have severe vulvovaginitis, the vaginal mucosa may be denuded. For these patients, a short course of topical estrogen promotes healing of vulvar and vaginal tissues. A small quantity of Premarin vaginal cream should be applied twice daily for 5 to 7 days. Steroid creams may be necessary for alleviating itching in patients who suffer from intense pruritus. The physician may prescribe triamcinolone, 0.025%, or hydrocortisone cream, 1%, to be applied to the affected area twice daily for 5 to 7 days.

These measures are sufficient for treating most children who have nonspecific vaginitis. In rare instances, allergic reactions to creams or chemical agents (e.g., detergents, bubble bath foam) have been documented. In these cases, discontinuation of contact with the allergens alleviates the symptoms and prevents recurrence. Antibiotic therapy is usually not required for children who have nonspecific vaginitis unless they develop superimposed infections.

Antibiotic therapy is required to treat children who have sexually transmitted diseases. Before initiating antibiotic therapy, the physician should determine the exact etiology of the disease. If a specific organism is isolated, the patient should be treated with an appropriate antibiotic agent. Occasionally, when the patient suffers from an intense inflammatory reaction, the physician may choose to initiate antibiotic therapy before the culture results are available. In these cases, a broad-spectrum antibiotic agent can be used (e.g., ampicillin, 50 to 100 mg/kg per day) until the results of the bacteriologic studies are available. A change in the antibiotic regimen may be required if the isolated organism is resistant to ampicillin. Table 10–1 lists some of the anogenital infections that occur in children and strategies for managing such infections.

## FOREIGN BODIES

The presence of a foreign body in the vagina induces an intense inflammatory reaction, resulting in a bloody, foul-smelling discharge. In most instances, the foreign body is lodged accidentally in the vagina, and the child does not recall the incident. Even if the girl has intentionally inserted the foreign object into the vagina, she will rarely admit to having done so.

The most commonly found objects are small pieces of toilet paper. These appear as amorphous conglomerates on grayish material in which white and red blood cells are embedded (Fig. 10–6). They are often seen on the posterior wall of the lower third of the vagina. They can be seen easily when the labia are separated and the perineum is pushed downward. Radiographs are of little value in the diagnosis, because most foreign bodies are not radiopaque. Many of these objects can be irrigated and removed with warm saline. Vaginoscopy is indicated for the removal of large foreign bodies or to confirm that no other foreign objects are present in the upper vagina.

Occasionally, when a solid foreign body is left in the vagina for a prolonged period of time, it may become embedded in the vaginal mucosa and may even penetrate the rectovaginal or vesicovaginal septum to the rectum or bladder, respectively, creating fistulous tracts.

## LICHEN SCLEROSUS

Vulvar pruritus may be caused by any of several vulvar or perineal dermatologic disorders. These conditions are often not limited to the vulva but affect other body areas as well. Lichen sclerosus of the vulva is a hypotrophic dystrophy. Although it mainly affects women in the postmenopausal age group, it is occasionally seen in young children. Symptoms consist of vulvar irritation, dysuria, and pruritus. Examination of the vulva shows flat, ivory–colored papules, which may coalesce into plaques and may have pronounced

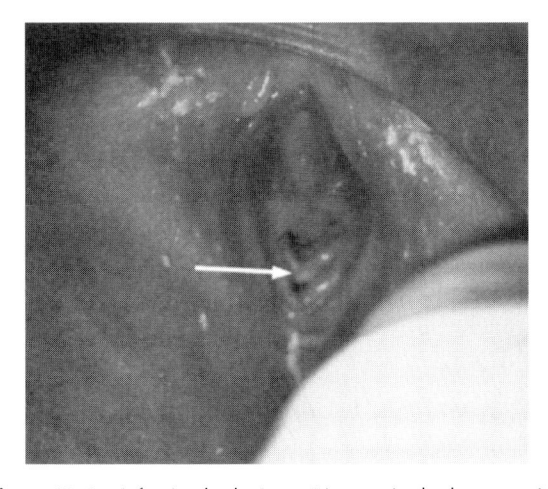

**Figure 10–6** A foreign body *(arrow)* is seen in the lower vagina. (From Ransom SB, McNeeley SG [eds]: Gynecology for the Primary Care Provider. Philadelphia, WB Saunders, 1997, p. 256.)

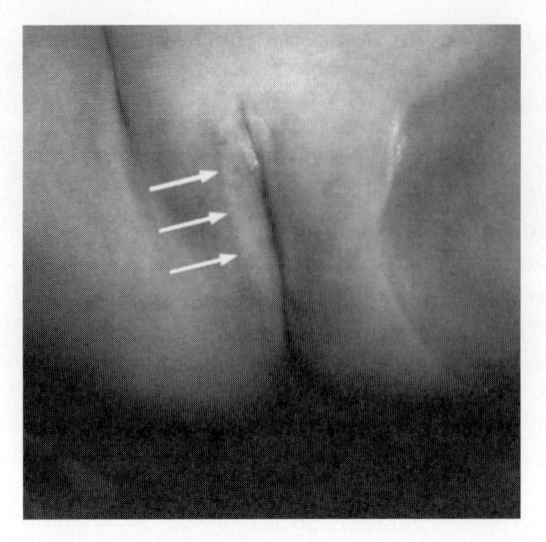

**Figure 10–7** Lichen sclerosus of the vulva in a 6-year-old child. The margins of the lesion are clearly defined (arrows). (From Ransom SB, McNeeley SG [eds]: Gynecology for the Primary Care Provider. Philadelphia, WB Saunders, 1997, p. 257.)

vascular markings. In extreme cases, the lesion may involve the entire vulvar surface (Fig. 10–7). The lesion does not extend laterally beyond the middle of the labia majora nor does it encroach into the vagina. Nonetheless, the clitoris, the posterior fourchette, and the anorectal area are frequently affected. The lesions tend to bruise easily, forming bloody blisters that are susceptible to secondary infections. The affected skin may bleed after minor trauma (e.g., friction from tight-fitting jeans or riding a bike). Some of these patients manifest genital bleeding without a history of trauma and are mistakenly thought to be victims of sexual abuse.

The experienced physician is generally able to establish the diagnosis of lichen sclerosus based upon the clinical features and the typical appearance of the affected skin. When the lesion is atypical or the diagnosis is in doubt, a skin biopsy is required. The histologic features are quite typical. The biopsy specimen shows flattening of the rete pegs, hyalinization of the subdermal tissues, and keratinization.

Lichen sclerosus in children has no malignant potential. Treatment consists of improved local hygiene, reduction of trauma, and short-term use of hydrocortisone cream for alleviating the intense pruritus. Treatment may be repeated if exacerbations occur. The long-term use of estrogen or testosterone is not recommended in children because feminization or virilization may result depending upon the medication used.

Patients often experience marked improvement in symptoms and appearance of the skin lesions after going through puberty. Review of the literature suggests that up to 50% of these cases improve significantly or recover during puberty, 30 to 45% experience no change in symptoms, and 5 to 10% experience worsening of the disease.

## LABIAL ADHESIONS

Labial adhesions in prepubertal children are believed to be relatively common. Huffman considers that girls aged 2 to 6 years are most likely to be affected; however, others have found the highest frequency occurs in children who are younger than 2 years of age. Many physicians believe that the incidence of labial adhesions is significantly more widespread than records indicate, because many girls with this condition are asymptomatic, and the findings are often not recorded in the medical chart.

The etiology of labial adhesions is not known, but it is probably related to low levels of estrogens in the prepubertal child. It is suggested that the thin skin covering the labia may be denuded as a result of local irritation and scratching. The labia then adhere in the midline, and, as re-epithelialization occurs on both sides, the labia remain fused in the midline (Fig. 10–8). Some authorities have reported that labial adhesions are more prevalent in prepubertal girls who have been sexually abused. It is possible that abusive activities cause denudation of the vulvar tissues, with subsequent labial agglutination.

The diagnosis of labial adhesions is made by visual inspection of the vulva. The examiner can see a thin avascular line of fusion in the midline. As mentioned,

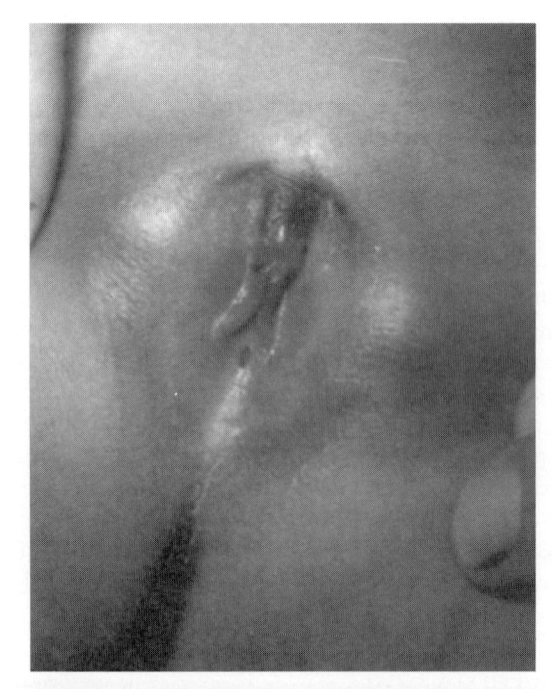

**Figure 10–8** Labial adhesions in a young girl. Note the translucent vertical line in the center, where the labia are fused together. (From Ransom SB, McNeeley SG [eds]: Gynecology for the Primary Care Provider. Philadelphia, WB Saunders, 1997, p. 257.)

most children who have minor degrees of labial adhesion are asymptomatic. When symptoms do occur, they usually relate to interference with urination or to the accumulation of urine behind the fused labia. Dysuria and recurrent vulvar or vaginal infections are the apparent symptoms. On rare occasions, when complete occlusion is present, urinary retention may occur.

If the patient is asymptomatic, no treatment is required for a minimal to moderate degree of labial fusion. When the degree of fusion is significant or the child is symptomatic, a short course of treatment with Premarin vaginal cream, applied twice daily for 7 to 10 days, may separate the labia. At times, the fused labia respond only partially to treatment with estrogen. In such cases, when the patient is cooperative, the physician can separate the labia in the office. A few minutes after application of a generous amount of 5% lidocaine (Xylocaine) ointment, a small probe is inserted through the opening between the labia and gently passed along the line of fusion, teasing the labia apart. If medical treatment fails or if severe urinary symptoms exist, surgical division of the fused labia is indicated.

Recurrence of labial adhesions is common because the estrogen-deficient state persists until puberty. Meticulous perineal hygiene and removal of irritants from the vulva may prevent recurrence. The condition usually resolves spontaneously after puberty.

## URETHRAL PROLAPSE

The urethral mucosa of patients who suffer from urethral prolapse protrudes through the meatus and forms a hemorrhagic, tender vulvar mass that bleeds easily (Fig. 10–9). The etiology of this condition is unknown. Capraro suggested that there is redundancy of the urethral mucosa associated with laxity in the support of the urethra. This predisposition is further aggravated by the increased intra-abdominal pressure caused by coughing, sneezing, or straining. Although the lack of estrogenic effect has been considered to be a contributing factor, hormonal studies have failed to show differences between affected and nonaffected girls.

The typical appearance and location of the mass, which is separate from the vagina, enable the physician to establish the diagnosis. The urethral orifice can often be seen in the center of the mass. When the lesion is small and urination is unimpaired, a short course of topical estrogens is beneficial. Resection of the prolapsed tissue should be considered if urinary retention is present, if the lesion is large and necrotic, or if the child is examined under anesthesia.

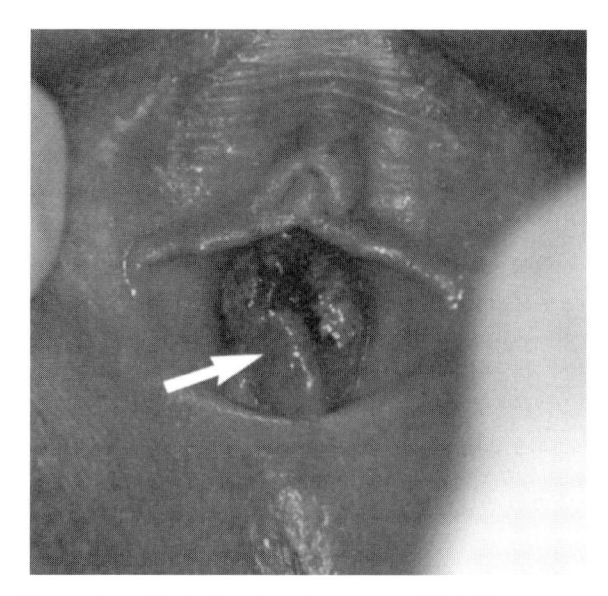

**Figure 10–9** Urethral prolapse in a 6-year-old child. (From Ransom SB, McNeeley SG [eds]: Gynecology for the Primary Care Provider. Philadelphia, WB Saunders, 1997, p. 259.)

## GENITAL TUMORS

Although uncommon, genital tumors must be considered whenever a girl is found to have a chronic genital ulcer, a nontraumatic swelling of the external genitalia, tissue protruding from the vagina, a foul-smelling bloody discharge, abdominal pain, genital enlargement, virilization, or premature sexual maturation. Despite the rarity of these tumors, virtually every type of genital neoplasm reported in adults has also been found in girls younger than 14 years of age, and about half of these are found to be malignant.

Most benign tumors of the vagina that occur in children are unilocular cystic remnants of the mesonephric duct. Other benign neoplasms include teratomas, hemangiomas, simple cysts of the hymen, retention cysts of the paraurethral ducts, benign granulomas of the perineum, and condylomata acuminata.

Small cysts of the mesonephric duct (Gartner's cyst) do not require surgery if the patient is asymptomatic. However, large cysts may interfere with urination or vaginal drainage, thereby requiring surgical treatment. The cyst is opened, most of the accessible cyst wall is removed, and the edges undergo marsupialization to prevent future reaccumulation of fluid. Obstruction of a paraurethral duct may form a relatively large cyst, distorting the urethral orifice. Simple excision or marsupialization is, again, the recommended treatment. Teratomas usually appear as cystic masses arising from the midline of the perineum. Although teratomas in this area are often benign, they may recur locally; therefore, a generous margin of healthy tissue should be excised around the periphery. Capillary hemangiomas usually disappear as the child grows older and thus they require no therapy. In contrast, cavernous hemangiomas are composed of vessels of considerable size, and injury to them may cause serious hemorrhage. For this reason, surgery is the optimal treatment for patients who have cavernous hemangiomas.

Embryonal carcinoma of the vagina (botryoid sarcoma) appears most commonly in the very young age group (<3 years old). In a very young child, the tumor is often situated in the lower vagina, whereas in an older child (>10 years old), the tumor more often affects the upper vagina or the cervix. The tumor arises from the lamina propria (from the undifferentiated mesenchyme), spreads rapidly beneath the vaginal epithelium, and infiltrates the vaginal wall, forcing it to bulge into a series of polypoid growths that contain abundant edematous stroma and dilated blood vessels. The loose myxomatous nature of the matrix gives it the characteristic soft and grape-like, or botyroid, appearance (Fig. 10–10). The growths may be hemorrhagic or ulcerated. The neoplasm may also infiltrate nearby pelvic structures (e.g., bladder, rectum, pelvic cavity).

The diagnosis is confirmed by histologic examination of a biopsy specimen. Mircroscopically, these masses contain poorly differentiated round or spindle-shaped cells, the rhabdomyoblasts. The cambium layer, described as a dense zone of primitive cells located just beneath the overlying basement membrane of the epithelium, is another histologic feature.

The management and prognosis of childhood pelvic rhabdomyosarcoma have improved markedly over the last three decades, evolving from a position of primary radical excision with no adjuvant treatment to a combined treatment modality of chemotherapy with subsequent limited surgery or radiotherapy. Survival has not been compromised in the process. Initial treatment of embryonal carcinoma consists of combination chemotherapy, usually vincristine, actinomycin-D, and cyclophosphamide. Further surgical excision or radiation therapy may be necessary after the course of chemotherapy is complete.

## GENITAL TRAUMA

Prepubertal girls often sustain genital injuries. Accidental injuries usually occur as a result of a fall, and the child presents with hematomas, lacerations, or a penetrating injury. Such injuries often affect the external genitalia and the perineum. The perineum and the vulva are extremely vascular, and the subcutaneous tissues are loosely arranged; therefore, blood accumulates under the skin and forms a hematoma, which appears as a rounded, tense, tender swelling. The size of the hematoma depends on the amount of bleeding (Fig. 10–11). A small vulvar hematoma can be controlled by exerting pressure with an ice pack. A large hematoma, or one that continues to increase in size, should be incised, with removal of clotted blood and ligation of bleeding vessels. If the source of the bleeding cannot be found, the cavity should be packed with gauze and a pressure dressing applied. The pack is removed in 24 hours. The prophylactic use of broad-spectrum antibiotics is advisable. The vulva should be kept clean and dry. If the urethra is obstructed by the hematoma, it is necessary to insert a suprapubic catheter. A pelvic radiogram may be

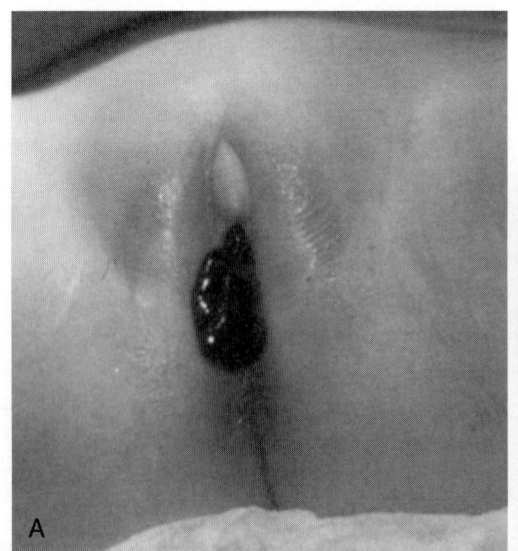

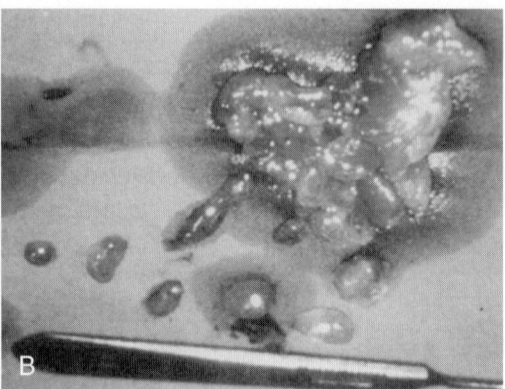

**Figure 10–10** *A*, Botryoid sarcoma that appears as a hemorrhagic growth extruding from the vagina. *B*, Note the appearance of the lesion. The cystic structures are loosely connected and have the appearance of grapes. This is the origin for the name sarcoma botryoides. (From Ransom SB, McNeeley SG [eds]: Gynecology for the Primary Care Provider. Philadelphia, WB Saunders, 1997, p. 260.)

PEDIATRIC AND ADOLESCENT GYNECOLOGY  91

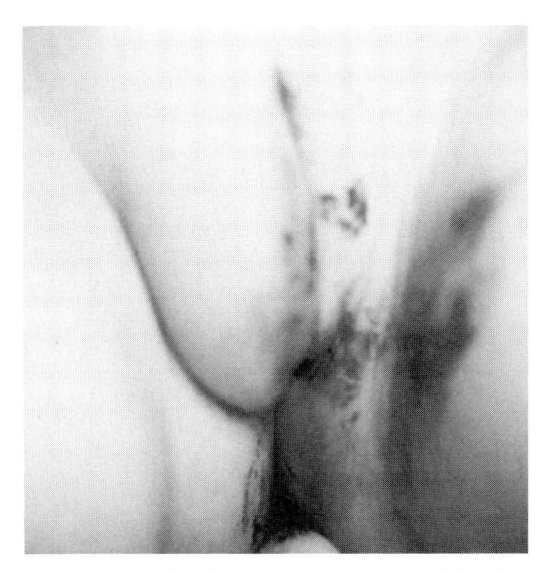

**Figure 10–11** A vulvar hematoma in a 12-year-old girl, caused by a straddle injury. (From Ransom SB, McNeeley SG [eds]: Gynecology for the Primary Care Provider. Philadelphia, WB Saunders, 1997, p. 261.)

indicated in selected patients to rule out a fracture of the pelvis.

Most vaginal injuries occur when an object penetrates the vagina through the hymenal opening. Such penetration causes a laceration of the hymenal ring. Tearing of the hymen occurs as the vagina is entered by a blunt object (e.g., digital or penile penetration). As the unestrogenized hymen has only limited elasticity, the shearing force causes the hymen to tear. The tear may then extend to either the vaginal wall or the perineum (Fig. 10–12). Bleeding is often minimal, and the patient has no acute symptoms. However, penetration in the very young patient is often associated with a significant vaginal injury. The thin vaginal mucosa, which has limited distensibility, is lacerated along with the hymen. When penile pressure on the introitus is directed toward the posterior vaginal wall, the hymen tears from its posterior aspect and the laceration secondarily enlarges to involve the posterior vaginal wall. With further penetration, the rectovaginal septum is torn, and the tear extends into the rectum. All patients who have experienced acute hymenal injuries should have a detailed examination to exclude injuries to the upper vagina.

Injuries of the vagina or rectum may present surgical difficulties because of the small caliber of the organs involved. Small instruments are required, as well as proper exposure and assistance. Vaginal lacerations should be repaired in a single layer. Care must be taken to begin the repair from the apex of the tear. A continuous locking suture (Vicryl 3-0) is often satisfactory for approximating the tissues and controlling bleeding. The perineal tear and the anal sphincter are approximated only upon completion of the vaginal repair. This delay affords the surgeon better access into the narrow vagina. If the laceration extends to the vaginal vault, surgical exploration of the pelvic cavity is needed to rule out extension into the broad ligament or peritoneal cavity, because this could cause injuries to intra-abdominal organs. The examiner must confirm the integrity of the bladder and bowel by inspection, catheterization, and rectal palpation.

## CONGENITAL MALFORMATIONS

Anomalies of the genitalia may be divided into two major categories: those that suggest sexual ambiguity (intersex problems), and those that do not. In this section, some of the common abnormalities affecting the external and internal genitalia are discussed. For a more detailed discussion of the various anomalies

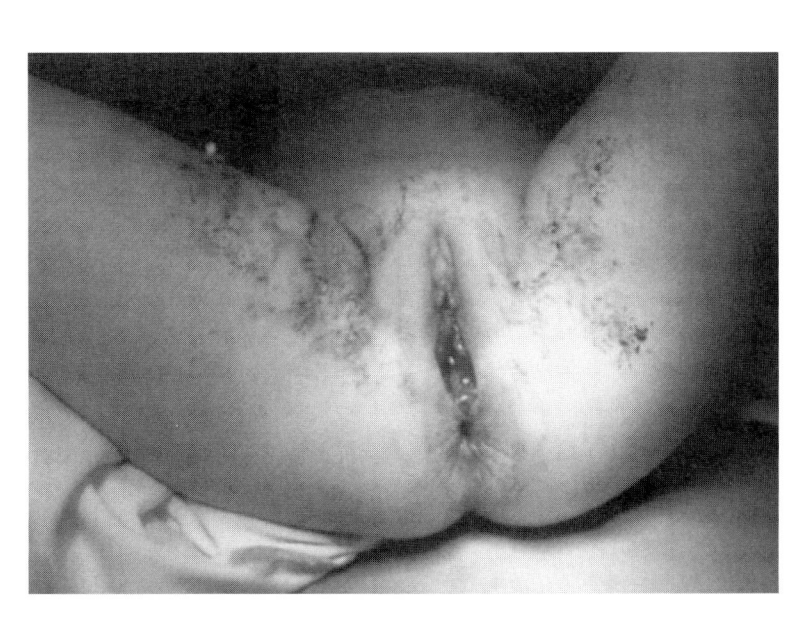

**Figure 10–12** Vaginal laceration following sexual assault of a 2-year-old girl. (From Ransom SB, McNeeley SG [eds]: Gynecology for the Primary Care Provider. Philadelphia, WB Saunders, 1997, p. 261.)

## Ambiguous Genitalia

Ambiguous genitalia denote a partial or incomplete virilization of the external genitalia (Fig. 10–13). Ambiguous genitalia occur in genetic females who were virilized in utero, in undervirilized males, or in true hermaphrodites. In general, exposure to androgens after 12 weeks of gestation leads to only clitoral hypertrophy. Examination of the genitalia reveals an enlarged clitoris with a normal vestibule, urethra, and vagina. The labia majora are altered by redundancy, wrinkling, and skin pigmentation. Exposure to androgens at early stages of embryologic development leads to clitoral hypertrophy, but, in addition, it causes retention of the urogenital sinus and fusion of the labioscrotal folds. In severely virilized individuals, the labia are fused in the midline to form a median raphe. The area of fusion may be partial, or it may extend the entire distance from the perineum to the phallus. When fusion is extensive, the fused labia form a wrinkled, pouch-like structure that resembles the scrotum in a male who has cryptorchidism. The vaginal opening is absent. Instead, a single opening is present, which extends to a common passage connecting the urethra and the vagina. The müllerian and gonadal development remain unaffected because neither is androgen-dependent. The medical management and surgical correction of genital ambiguity are beyond the scope of the primary care provider. A multidisciplinary team approach is best suited for comprehensive management of these patients.

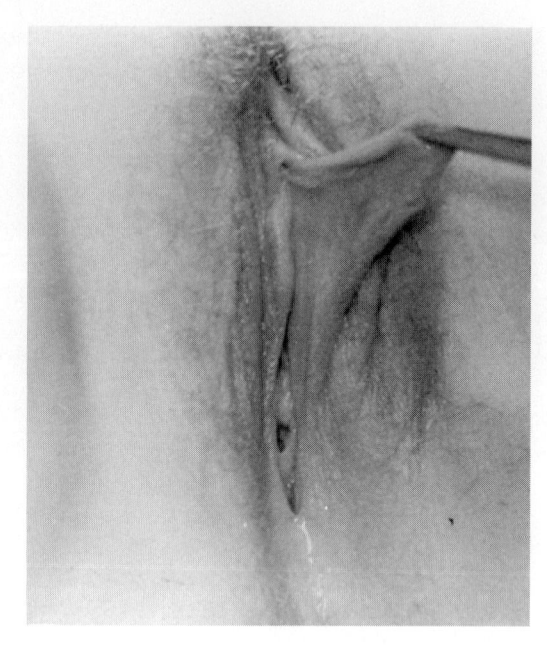

**Figure 10–14** Hypertrophy of the labia minora in a 10-year-old girl. (From Ransom SB, McNeeley SG [eds]: Gynecology for the Primary Care Provider. Philadelphia, WB Saunders, 1997, p. 264.)

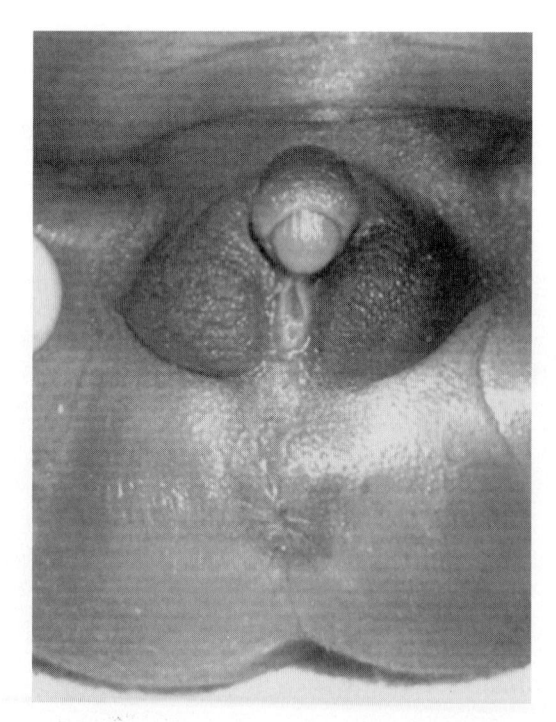

**Figure 10–13** Ambiguous genitalia of a female child, caused by congenital adrenocortical hyperplasia. (From Ransom SB, McNeeley SG [eds]: Gynecology for the Primary Care Provider. Philadelphia, WB Saunders, 1997, p. 262.)

## Anomalies of the Vulva and Labia

As in any other part of the body, minor differences in the contour or size of vulvar structures are not unusual. Often, there is considerable variation in the distance between the posterior fourchette and the anus, or between the urethra and the clitoris, giving the vulva an individual appearance. There is also considerable variation in the size and shape of the labia minora. One labium may be considerably larger than the other, or both labia may be unusually large (Fig. 10–14). Labial enlargement and asymmetry have been wrongly assumed to be the result of masturbation. The physician should reassure the patient that these individual characteristics are simply minor variations that require no treatment. If the asymmetry is significant, or if the labia would be pulled into the vagina during intercourse, the hypertrophied labia may be trimmed surgically.

## Anomalies of the Clitoris, Epispadias, and Bladder Exstrophy

Clitoral enlargement in an infant almost invariably suggests exposure to elevated levels of androgens.

Enlargement of the clitoris may be caused by a benign neoplasm (e.g., neurofibromatosis, lymphangioma, fibroma). In these cases, the physician should excise the neoplasm, thereby reducing the clitoris to normal size.

Splitting or duplication of the clitoris is caused by the failure of the corpora to fuse in the midline. A bifid clitoris usually occurs in conjunction with bladder exstrophy, epispadias, and absence or cleavage of the symphysis pubis. The labia majora are widely separated and the labia minora are separated anteriorly. They can, however, be traced posteriorly around the vaginal orifice. The vaginal orifice is narrow and the vagina is shortened and rotated anteriorly. The pelvic floor is incomplete, and uterine prolapse is often observed in these patients (Fig. 10–15). Other congenital anomalies may be present (e.g., spina bifida). At puberty, pubic hair growth is absent over the midline. Major urologic reconstruction is required immediately, but the gynecologic defects can be repaired during the adolescent years.

## Anomalies of the Hymen

Variations in the appearance of the hymen are extremely common. The orifice may vary in diameter from very small to very large. There may be one or

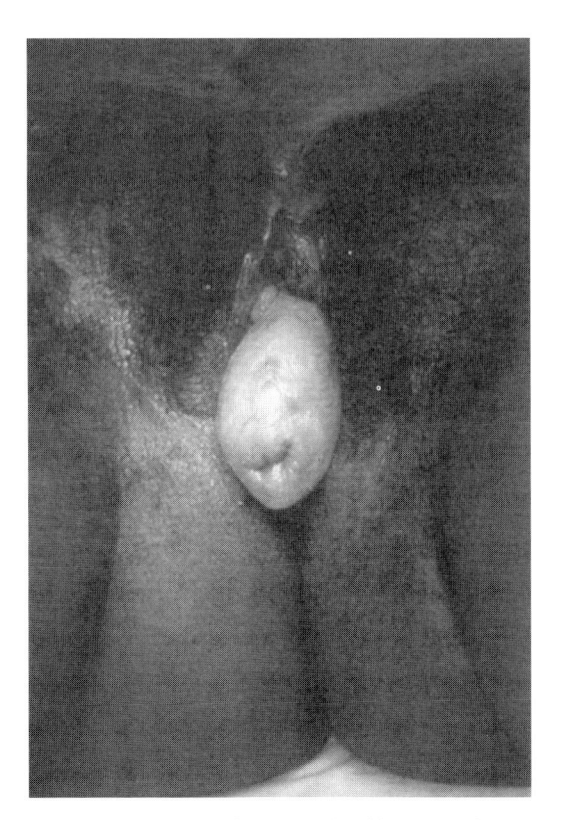

**Figure 10–15** Uterine prolapse with bladder exstrophy in a 15-year-old girl. (From Ransom SB, McNeeley SG [eds]: Gynecology for the Primary Care Provider. Philadelphia, WB Saunders, 1997, p. 264.)

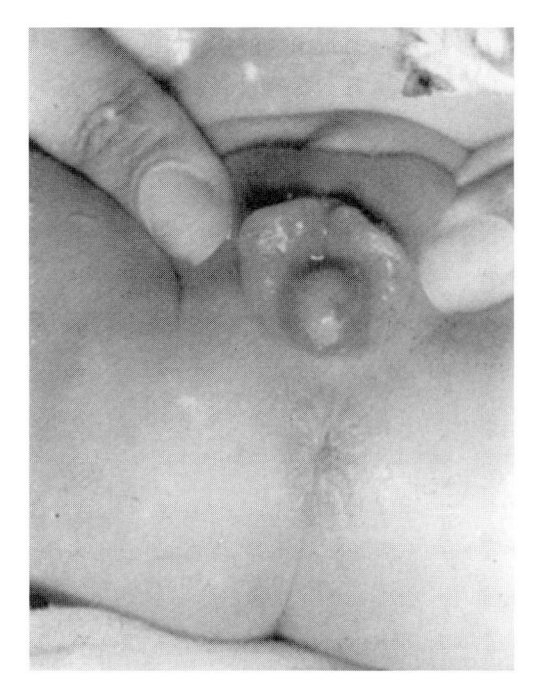

**Figure 10–16** Mucocolpos secondary to an imperforate hymen. (From Ransom SB, McNeeley SG [eds]: Gynecology for the Primary Care Provider. Philadelphia, WB Saunders, 1997, p. 264.)

more small orifices. A thick medial ridge separating two lateral hymenal orifices may suggest a septate vagina. The hymenal diaphragm may be a thin membrane, or a thickened and fibrous one, forming a firm partition. Occasionally, what initially appears to be an imperforate hymen is found to have one or more tiny openings, and this is called a microperforate hymen.

Although most of these variants are of no clinical significance, hymenal anomalies require surgical correction if they block the escape of vaginal secretions or menstrual fluid, interfere with intercourse, or prevent an indicated vaginoscopy or treatment of a vaginal disorder. An imperforate hymen occurs when the hymen forms a solid membrane without an aperture (Fig. 10–16). It is assumed that an imperforate hymen represents a persistent portion of the urogenital membrane. It occurs when the mesoderm of the primitive streak abnormally invades the urogenital portion of the cloacal membrane. When the vagina is obstructed, accumulation of vaginal secretions may distend the vagina, forming a mucocolpos or hydrocolpos. When this occurs, the thin hymenal membrane is stretched out, forming a bulging, shiny, thin protuberance. Unless a mucocolpos is diagnosed and the fluid drained, the distended vagina will form a large mass that may interfere with urination, and, at times, the mass may be mistaken for an abdominal tumor.

## Anomalies of the Vagina

### Failure of Vertical Fusion

Transverse vaginal septa are the result of faulty canalization of the embryonic vagina. These septa may have no opening (complete or obstructive) or may have a small central aperture (incomplete or nonobstructive). They are usually found in the midvagina but may occur at any level. If the septum is located in the upper vagina, it is likely to be patent (incomplete), whereas a septum located in the lower part of the vagina is frequently complete.

An incomplete septum is usually asymptomatic. The central aperture allows egression of vaginal secretions and menstrual flow from the vagina. However, a complete septum results in signs and symptoms similar to those of an imperforate hymen. Unfortunately, the diagnosis of a transverse vaginal septum is often delayed until after menarche. At this time, menstrual blood is trapped behind an obstructing membrane. If the diagnosis of complete septum is established before menarche, an incision should be made to create an aperture for outflow of discharges. Incision of a complete septum should be done only when the upper vagina is distended and the membrane is bulging. The distention confirms the presence of an upper vaginal segment, which facilitates the procedure and reduces the risk of injury to adjacent structures.

## Failure of Longitudinal Fusion

When the distal ends of the müllerian ducts fail to fuse properly, the mesenchymal tissue between the ducts forms a longitudinal septum that divides the vagina lengthwise. If the patient is asymptomatic, the longitudinal septum requires no treatment. Division of the septum is indicated if dyspareunia is present, if obstruction of drainage from one half of the vagina is noted, or if the physician suspects that a septum would interfere with the vaginal delivery of an infant.

## Vaginal Agenesis

Individuals who have Rokitansky's syndrome are genetically female. They develop normally in adolescence and have all the usual feminine attributes, but the müllerian ducts fail to grow and, therefore, the uterus and vagina do not form. However, the external genitalia are normal. A ruffled ridge of tissue represents the hymen; inside, there is an indentation marking the spot where the introitus would normally be found.

Other developmental defects are often present. These may affect the urinary tract (45–50%), the spine (10%), and, less frequently, the middle ear and other mesodermal structures. Therefore, at some time during their childhood, individuals who have vaginal agenesis should undergo an evaluation of the urinary tract and the spine as well as an assessment of their hearing. In addition, a chromosomal analysis should be performed for all patients who have vaginal agenesis to rule out the rare instances in which this condition represents the effects of testicular activity. An exploratory laparotomy is not indicated in these patients, and the absence of a uterus can be confirmed by a pelvic sonogram.

Creation of a functional vagina is the objective in correcting vaginal agenesis, and this should be deferred until the patient is considering an active sexual life. Several techniques have been used. Frank, and later Ingram, described the nonoperative creation of a vagina using graduated vaginal dilators. The method is risk-free, but it requires motivation and the cooperation of the patient. She is given a series of dilators of graduated sizes and lengths and is taught how to place them against the vaginal dimple while applying constant pressure. This maneuver is repeated daily for 20 to 30 minutes, using progressively wider and longer dilators. The procedure takes a few months to complete and requires persistence and patience.

If vaginal dilatation fails, the vaginal space between the urethra and the bladder anteriorly, and the perineal body and the rectum posteriorly, can be developed surgically. This cavity is then lined by a split-thickness skin graft that overlies a plastic or soft silicone mold (McIndoe's procedure). An alternative

**Table 10–2** Sexual Development in Girls

| | **Breast Development** |
|---|---|
| STAGE 1 | Preadolescent. Elevation of papilla only. |
| STAGE 2 | Breast bud stage. Elevation of breast and papilla as small mound. Enlargement of areolar diameter. |
| STAGE 3 | Further enlargement and elevation of breast and areola with no separation of their contours. |
| STAGE 4 | Projection of areola and papilla to form a secondary mound above the level of the breast. |
| STAGE 5 | Mature stage. Projection of papilla only caused by recession of the areola to the general contour of the breast. |

| | **Pubic Hair** |
|---|---|
| STAGE 1 | In preadolescent, the vellus over the pubes is developed only up to the adominal wall, i.e., there is no pubic hair. |
| STAGE 2 | Sparse growth of long, slightly pigmented downy hair, straight or curled, chiefly along the labia. |
| STAGE 3 | The hair is considerably darker, coarser, and more curled. The hair spreads sparsely over the junction of the pubes. |
| STAGE 4 | The hair is now adult in type, but the area covered is still considerably smaller than it is in the adult. There is no spread to the medial surface of the thighs. |
| STAGE 5 | The hair is adult in quantity and type with distribution of the horizontal (or classically "feminine") pattern. The hair has spread to the medial surface of the thighs but not up the linea alba or elsewhere above the base of the inverse triangle. (The spread up the linea alba occurs late and is rated stage 6). |

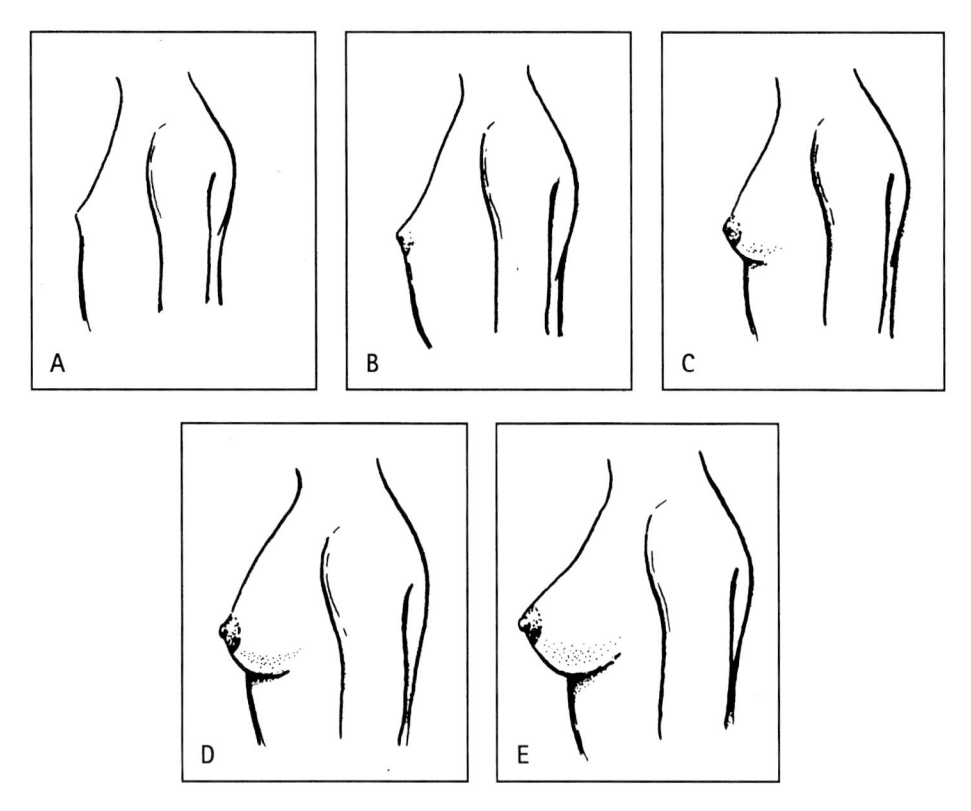

**Figure 10–17** Tanner staging of breast development. These arbitrary intervals of continuous pubertal breast development are useful for the documentation of the extent and progression of puberty. (From Goldfarb AF [ed]: Atlas of Clinical Gynecology. Philadelphia, Current Medicine, 1998.)

procedure is the Williams vulvovaginoplasty, which uses the labia majora to construct a coital pouch. A loop of bowel can also be used to create a functional vagina.

## Puberty

During puberty, secondary sexual development occurs, maturation of sex organs takes place, and reproductive capability is attained. Puberty begins with the first sign of secondary sexual development and continues until ovulation commences. These changes occur largely as a result of maturation of the hypothalamic-pituitary-ovarian (HPO) axis. At the onset of puberty, there is an increase in the amplitude and frequency of pulsatile gonadotropin-releasing hormone (GnRH) secretion. This sets off the cascade of hormonal and physical changes that constitute pubertal development. The mechanism that initiates this increase in GnRH production is unknown, although the timing of puberty correlates better with skeletal maturity than with chronologic age. GnRH stimulates the pituitary gland, which then produces follicle-stimulating hormone (FSH) and luteinizing hormone (LH), both of which stimulate the ovary to produce sex steroids. The pubertal growth spurt is related to the increased secretion of sex steroids, growth hormone (GH), and somatomedin insulin-like growth factor 1 [IGF-1].

The visible physical changes of puberty generally proceed in the following manner: breast development (thelarche), growth acceleration, appearance of pubic and axillary hair (pubarche or adrenarche), and onset of menstruation (menarche). The onset of thelarche and pubarche in North American girls is variable, with a mean of 10.9 and 11.2 years, respectively. Peak growth velocity occurs almost 2.5 years later and precedes the onset of menses (mean age 12.7 years). Regular ovulation, which occurs approximately 20 months later, marks the completion of the pubertal cycle. The interval between the onset of thelarche and menarche is 2.3 ± 1.0 years and is independent of the age at which thelarche occurs. Marshall and Tanner recorded the progression of pubertal development of English girls. Their classification (Table 10–2) is useful in following pubertal growth in adolescents (Figs. 10–17 and 10–18).

The chronologic span of puberty is wide but not infinite. The normal range for thelarche is 8.0 to 13 years. Sexual precocity is defined as the onset of sexual maturation at any age that is 2.5 standard deviations of total scores (SDs) earlier than the norm. At present, the appearance of any of the secondary

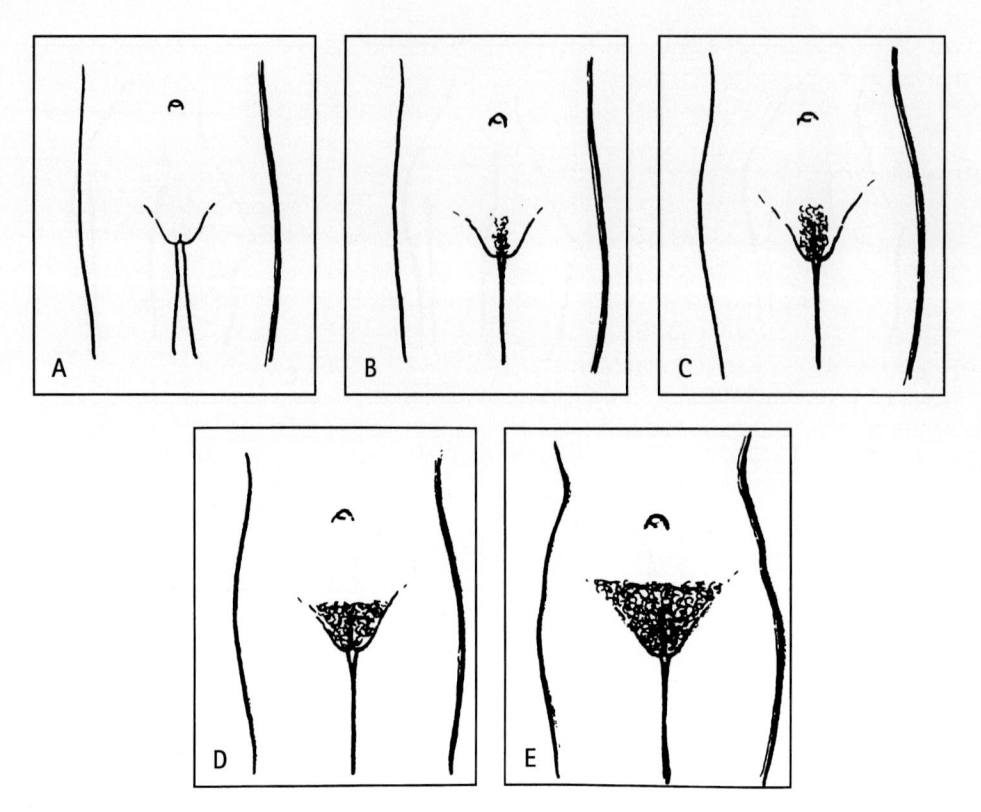

**Figure 10–18** Tanner staging of pubic hair development. Like the Tanner stages of breast development, these are markers in a continuous developmental process. (From Goldfarb AF [ed]: Atlas of Clinical Gynecology. Philadelphia, Current Medicine, 1998.)

sexual characteristics before a girl is 8 years of age, or onset of menarche before she is 10 years of age, is considered precocious. Similarly, puberty is thought to be delayed if no signs of sexual development have begun by age 13 or if there is absence of menarche by age 15.

## DELAYED PUBERTY

Delayed sexual development is defined as the absence of normal pubertal events at an age more than 2.5 SDs from the mean. However, the physician need not always delay evaluation until these criteria are met. The concerns of the patient, her family, or the referring physician are compelling enough reasons for initiating an evaluation. Because some degree of sexual maturation occurs in more than 30% of patients who have gonadal dysgenesis, an investigation is necessary if a girl experiences a delay in progression of pubertal development.

Patients who have an abnormal puberty may be classified according to gonadal function. Thus, patients are divided into three major clinical groups according to secondary sexual development.
1. Delayed menarche with adequate secondary sexual development (i.e., primary amenorrhea). The disorders that cause this delay have been collectively referred to as eugonadism.
2. Delayed puberty with inadequate or absent secondary sexual development. These types of disorders have been collectively referred to as hypogonadism. If FSH levels are high, the patient is said to have hypergonadotropic hypogonadism, and if they are low, the patient is said to have hypogonadotropic hypogonadism.
3. Delayed puberty and heterosexual secondary sexual development (i.e., virilization).

The various disorders are listed in Table 10–3.

### Adequate Secondary Sexual Development

Patients who have functioning ovaries but delayed sexual maturation in their mid-teens usually consult a physician for treatment of primary amenorrhea. They have a well-formed female configuration with appropriately developed breasts. Most of these patients (~80%) suffer from inappropriate LH feedback, anovulatory cycles, unopposed estrogens, and, sometimes, an excess of androgen production. Primary amenorrhea may persist until the patient is challenged with a progestin. After the patient experiences withdrawal bleeding, she should be monitored for continued menstrual function, because anovulation can persist. Patients who have continued amenorrhea are treated with cyclic progestins, which are administered monthly, or every other month, to ensure endometrial shedding and prevent potentially heavy menstrual bleeding. Obviously, if the patient is sexually active, birth control pills are preferable to cyclic progestins. Anovulation and the resulting endocrine disturbance (i.e., distortion of the estrogen-to-androgen ratio) is also encountered in adolescents who have postnatal adrenogenital syndrome or polycystic ovarian disease. The signs and symptoms are similar in these conditions, and when hyperandrogenism is present, the physician should evaluate adrenal function.

The possibility that an adolescent may become pregnant before she menstruates is highly unlikely, but it must be excluded in patients with delayed menarche.

Congenital anomalies of the paramesonephric (müllerian) structures account for ~20% of cases of primary amenorrhea. The most frequent defect is congenital absence of the uterus and the vagina. Other anatomic causes of amenorrhea include imperforate hymen, transverse vaginal septa, agenesis of the cervix, and partial or complete agenesis of the vagina. These anomalies have been described elsewhere in this chapter. Gynecologic examination supplemented by sonography establishes the diagnosis of these congenital anomalies.

Adolescents who have complete androgen insensitivity may also have primary amenorrhea. This condition is reltatively rare and accounts for only 1% of patients who have primary amenorrhea. These patients are genetic males who have testes that develop normally and produce adequate amounts of androgens. End-organ tissues (e.g., sexual hair, genitalia) are not responsive to androgens. The fetus develops along female lines, but the müllerian ducts regress under the influence of the müllerian inhibiting substance. The newborn infant appears to be a normal female because the external genitalia appear normal. During puberty, adequate breast development is often seen secondary to small amounts of unopposed estrogen produced by the testes. Pubic and axillary hair are scant and often missing (Fig. 10–19). Only a short or blind vaginal pouch is present, and the testes are often palpable in the inguinal canals. After pubertal development is complete, the patient should undergo extirpation of the gonads and vaginal reconstruction.

## Inadequate Secondary Sexual Development

Constitutional delay of puberty is a normal variant in which pubertal development and biochemical markers are as expected for a younger child. Patients who have this condition have been labeled "late bloomers." The absence of pubertal signs (including the pubertal growth spurt) often concerns the patient when her adolescent friends have secondary sexual features and characteristic increases in height. Excluding other causes of delayed sexual maturation helps to establish the diagnosis of constitutional delay. However, it is often difficult to distinguish between constitutional delay and hypogonadotropic hypogonadism. When the diagnosis of constitutional delay is considered, the patient must be kept under observation until she begins to have normal menstrual cycles. Occasionally, an adolescent requires hormonal replacement therapy because of the emotional distress caused by the delay and the associated immature appearance.

Isolated deficiency of gonadotropin-releasing factor, often associated with intracranial anomalies and anosmia (Kallmann's syndrome [*KAL*]), is uncommon. The cause for this disorder is the lack of production of adhesion molecules coded by the *KAL* gene located on the X chromosome. These patients fail to develop secondary sexual features and blood levels of gonadotropins are very low. A rise in gonadotropin levels is normally expected following a GnRH challenge test. Estrogen therapy is used to initiate and later sustain sexual development. Ovulation should be induced with menotropins (Pergonal) or GnRH should be given when fertility is desired.

A pituitary or parasellar tumor, particularly craniopharyngioma, pituitary adenoma, or prolactinoma, must be considered in the evaluation of a patient who has delayed sexual maturation. Weight loss caused by severe dieting, marked protein deficiency, and fat loss

**Table 10–3** Delayed Sexual Maturation

**Delayed Menarche With Adequate Secondary Sexual Development**

Inappropriate HPO axis feedback mechanism
Anatomic defect
   Obstructed outflow tract
   Vaginal agenesis
Complete androgen insensitivity syndrome

**Delayed Puberty (No Signs of Secondary Sexual Development)**

Gonadal failure (hypergonadotropic hypogonadism)
Constitutional delay
   Chronic illness
   Weight loss
   Gymnasts
Hypothalamic pituitary failure

**Delayed Puberty With Virilization**

XY female
Virilizing tumors
Congenital adrenal hyperplasia

HPO = hypothalamic-pituitary-ovarian axis.

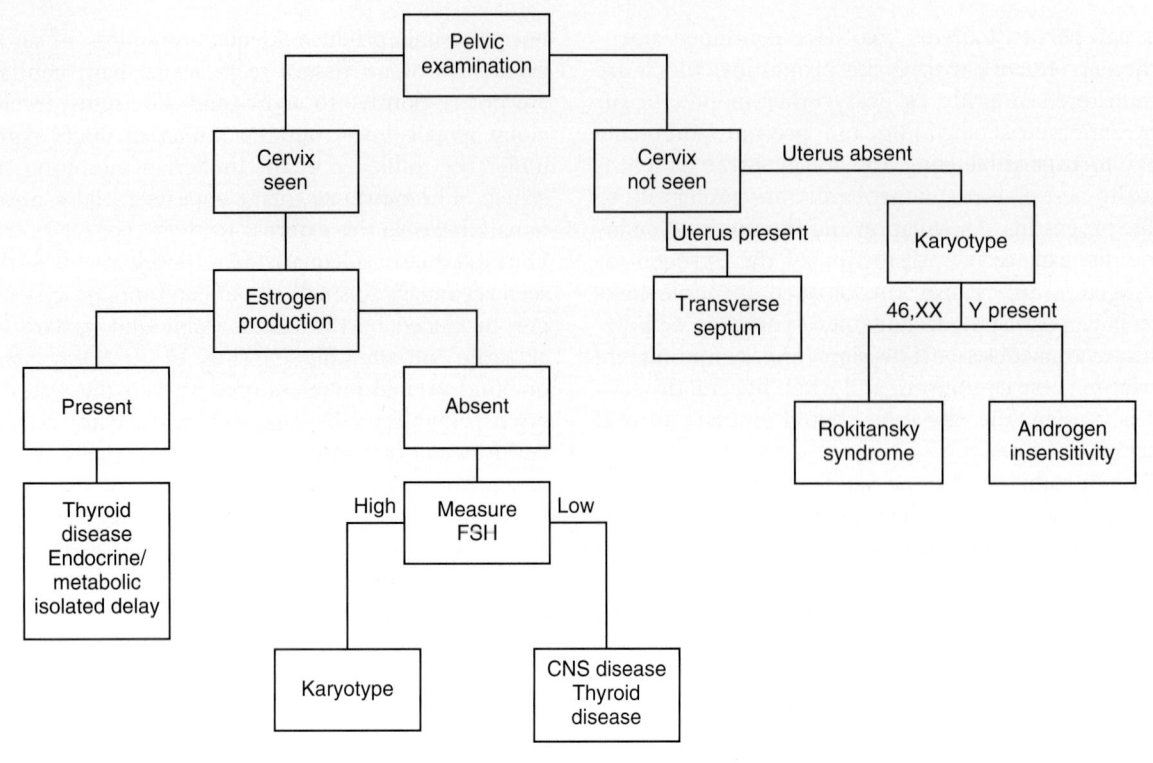

**Figure 10–19** The diagnostic workup of patients who have delayed sexual maturation.

without notable loss of muscle (often seen in athletes) may also delay or suppress hypothalamic pituitary maturation.

Many patients who have delayed sexual development suffer from gonadal failure, which is associated with a marked elevation of serum FSH levels. Most of these patients suffer from a loss of X-chromosome material and important ovarian determinant genes. Mosaicism with two or more cell lines, one containing an abnormal X chromosome, is probably more common than nonmosaic abnormalities. Certain somatic abnormalities are often seen in patients who have gonadal dysgenesis (e.g., short stature, webbing of the neck, shield chest, coarctation of the aorta). Replacement hormonal therapy given in a cyclic manner is the treatment of choice. When a Y chromosome complement or derivative is discovered, gonadectomy is indicated because of the possibility of neoplastic changes in the retained gonad.

Some patients who have ovarian failure may have normal sex chromosomes (46,XX). In these patients, ovarian failure may be secondary to etiologies other than privation of X-chromosome material. An autosomal recessive form of ovarian failure has been determined in some families. Other etiologies of follicular depletion include chemotherapy, irradiation, infections (e.g., mumps), infiltrative disease processes of the ovary, autoimmune diseases, and other known environmental agents. However, it is also possible that submicroscopic X-chromosome deletions in the ovarian determinant region resulted in ovarian failure.

The resistant ovary syndrome is characterized by delayed menarche or primary amenorrhea, a 46,XX karyotype, high FSH levels, and ovaries that do not respond to endogenous gonadotropins despite apparently normal follicle apparatus. It is assumed that absence of follicular receptors for gonadotropins is responsible for ovarian failure in these patients. These individuals have high FSH levels and a normal chromosomal constitution. Estrogen replacement therapy should be initiated to prevent long-term complications (e.g., vaginal dryness, osteoporosis).

## Delayed Puberty and Heterosexual Secondary Sexual Development

Virilization at puberty is caused by elevated androgens from adrenal or gonadal sources. These may be the result of an enzyme deficiency (e.g., late onset congenital adrenal hyperplasia) or a neoplasm (e.g., Leydig's cell tumor). A small group of patients who have this condition are male pseudohermaphrodites; that is, adolescents who are being reared as girls, have female external genitalia, intra-abdominal or ectopic malfunctioning testes, and a normal 46,XY chromosomal constitution.

## Evaluation of Patients Who Have Delayed Sexual Development

Determination of gonadal function for categorization into eugonadal, hypogonadal, or virilized patient groups can be accomplished by obtaining a medical history and performing a physical examination. Staging of pubertal development by the Tanner classification is important in determination of gonadal function. The presence of breast development signifies previous gonadal function. A vaginal smear can determine whether the gonad is continuing to produce estrogen. Examination of the pelvis and rectum can identify patients who have an obstructed outflow tract, as well as those who have congenital absence of the vagina and uterus. Further confirmation of patients with Rokitansky's sequence is dependent on a karyotype to identify normal 46,XX complement and a pelvic sonogram to confirm uterine absence and ovarian presence (Fig. 10–19).

Absence of pubic hair is suggestive of the androgen insensitivity syndrome (Fig. 10–20). Karyotype analysis can identify 46,XY individuals who have testicular feminization syndrome. Patients who have complete pubertal development, evidence of continued estrogen production, and normal müllerian systems probably have inappropriate positive feedback and, hence, chronic anovulation. Progesterone challenge in such patients is helpful; a withdrawal bleed signifies a normal müllerian system and continued estrogen production.

If breast development is minimal, the usual diagnosis is hypogonadism. Serum gonadotropin assays are performed for further elucidation; elevated FSH levels suggest gonadal failure. Other endocrine profiles should be obtained if hypothyroidism, congenital adrenal hyperplasia, or Cushing's syndrome is suspected. Karyotyping is necessary in patients who have gonadal failure. Gonadal extirpation is required when Y-chromosome material is identified.

Low FSH levels suggest interference with hypothalamic pituitary maturation and gonadotropin release. Skull films and prolactin assays must be obtained for all patients to rule out the more serious irreversible causes, such as pituitary tumors. Appropriate endocrine evaluation can identify the occasional patient who has hypothyroidism or congenital adrenal hyperplasia and the rare patient who has Cushing's syndrome. Diagnosis of KAL syndrome is suspected in hypogonadotropic patients who have associated anosmia but is confirmed only after GnRH challenge tests are performed. The presumed diagnosis of physiologic delay is made by exclusion of all other causes and by the FSH and LH release patterns that occur following GnRH challenge.

## EARLY PUBERTAL DEVELOPMENT

Isosexual precocious puberty is defined as the onset of secondary sexual development in a child younger than 8 years of age or menarche in a child younger than 10 years of age. Sexual precocity may result from premature activation of the HPO axis and is referred to as true precocious puberty, or GnRH-dependent precocious puberty. Alternatively, the signs of puberty may result from endogenous sex steroids produced by the ovaries or adrenal glands, or they may appear after a child has been exposed to estrogens from exogenous sources. In these cases, the HPO axis remains inactive and these disorders are labeled as pseudoprecocious puberty or GnRH-independent precocious puberty. Occasionally, for reasons that remain unclear, only one sign of pubertal development is present, such as breast development, pubic hair, or menstruation (Table 10–4).

True precocious puberty affects both sexes but is up to eight times more common in girls. The peak incidence of true precocious puberty occurs between the ages of 4 and 5 years. These patients have no abnormality except for the very early development of pubertal changes, which progress faster than normal but in an orderly sequence (Fig. 10–21). Gonadotro-

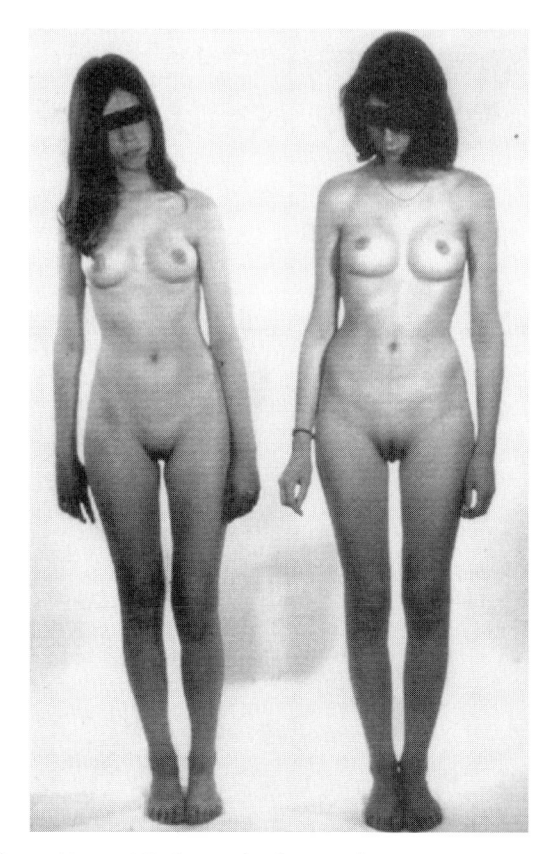

**Figure 10–20** XY sisters who have androgen insensitivity syndrome. (Courtesy of Professor Sir John Dewhurst. From Ransom SB, McNeeley SG [eds]: Gynecology for the Primary Care Provider. Philadelphia, WB Saunders, 1997, p. 268.)

### Table 10–4  Early Sexual Maturation

**Complete Forms**

Mature HPO axis (GnRH-dependent precocious puberty)
    Constitutional precocious puberty
    Central nervous system lesions
        Congenital defects, tumors, cysts
            after irradiation: Trauma, inflammation
        Hypothalamic hamartoma
Immature HPO axis (GnRH-independent precocious puberty)
    Exposure to estrogens
        In the food chain
        Medications
    Endogenous estrogen production
        Functional ovarian cysts
        Ovarian neoplasms
        Other hormone-producing neoplasms
McCune-Albright syndrome

**Incomplete Forms**

Premature thelarche
Premature adrenarche
Premature menarche

GnRH = gonadotropin-releasing hormone.

---

pins, estrogens, and LH response to GnRH stimulation are within the normal pubertal range. Follicular development occurs and pregnancies have been reported. Girls who have idiopathic precocious puberty have some loss of adult height as a result of accelerated bone maturation. However, in other respects, prognosis is favorable and future menstrual pattern and fertility in this group of patients are expected to be normal.

### Central Nervous System Lesions

Central nervous system (CNS) lesions (e.g., tumors, hydrocephalus, severe head injuries, irradiation therapy, meningitis, encephalitis) may cause early sexual development. Usually pubertal development in these patients is slower than normal and may progress gradually over several years. Clinical findings (apart from the early pubertal development) are related to the nature of the primary CNS lesion. When such lesions are large, concurrent neurologic deficit may be present. Treatment of such patients is directed toward the primary disorder, and patients who are precociously pubescent are treated symptomatically. Prognosis is determined by the nature of the primary CNS lesion. For example, primary pituitary tumors that secrete gonadotropins are unusual and rare causes of precocious puberty.

In some of these patients, a computed tomographic scan of the brain occasionally demonstrates the presence of small hypothalamic hamartomas. Such hamartomas of the tuber cinereum are not true neoplasms but rather congenital malformations of ectopic GnRH neurosecretory cells. These neoplasms do not increase in size and, therefore, there is no indication for surgical removal. Precocious pubertal development can be controlled by the use of GnRH agonists.

### GnRH-Independent Precocious Puberty

In these disorders, the production of sex steroids is independent of hypothalamic GnRH production. In other words, these disorders are not an expression of early maturation of the HPO axis. Accidental ingestion of estrogens (e.g., estrogen-containing food) or prolonged use of creams containing estrogens are possible (yet uncommon) causes of early feminization. If such exposure is documented, prompt discontinuation is the proper treatment.

The prepubertal ovary may give rise to large follicular cysts that are capable of estrogen production. In addition, other benign tumors of the ovary (e.g., teratoma, cystadenoma) are capable of either producing estrogens or of inducing the surrounding ovarian tissue to produce sex steroids. Finally, granulosa cell tumors capable of estrogen production are a rare

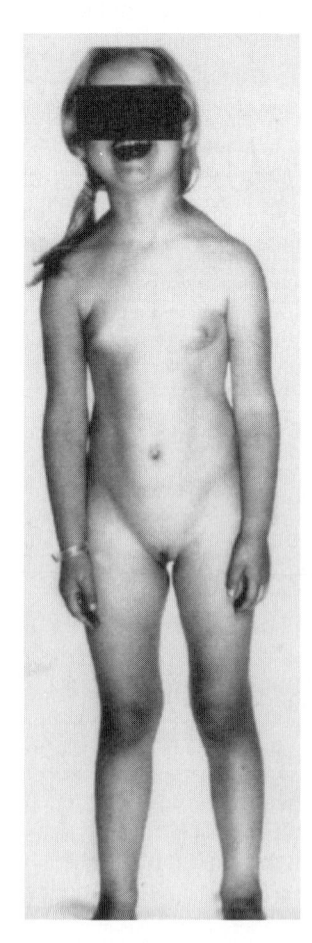

**Figure 10–21** Precocious puberty in a 4-year-old child. (From Ransom SB, McNeeley SG [eds]: Gynecology for the Primary Care Provider. Philadelphia, WB Saunders, 1997, p. 272.)

cause of feminization in a prepubertal child. Other tumors of extragonadal origin may produce estrogens, and these include hepatomas and adrenal adenomas; however, these neoplasms are extremely rare.

### McCune-Albright Syndrome

The diagnosis of McCune-Albright syndrome is established by the presence of the typical clinical triad of polyostotic fibrous dysplasia, irregular cutaneous pigmentation, and precocious puberty. Other endocrinopathies may be present. The McCune-Albright syndrome has been attributed to defects in the LH receptor that interfere with the synthesis of cyclic adenosine monophosphate (cAMP), which is the intracellular messenger required for estrogen production. This results in an autonomous hyperfunction of the ovaries. Estrogen secretion is episodic, although it corresponds to ovarian follicular development and regression. Children who have this syndrome usually manifest symptoms at a younger age than do those who have idiopathic precocious puberty. Vaginal bleeding occurs early, and is generally the first sign of puberty. The diagnosis is made on the basis of the skin pigmentation (Fig. 10–22) and the presence of typical bone lesions or pathologic fractures.

The prognosis is unfavorable. Adult height is significantly reduced, not only because of early epiphyseal closure but also because of skeletal abnormalities and associated pathologic fractures of the long bones. In addition, most women who have this disorder suffer from severe menstrual abnormalities and infertility.

### Incomplete Forms of Pubertal Development

Occasionally, for reasons that remain unclear, only one sign of pubertal development is present (e.g., breast development, pubic hair, or menstruation). This developmental abnormality is possibly caused by transient elevations in levels of circulating steroid hormones produced by small follicular ovarian cysts, or, alternatively, it may be caused by the extreme sensitivity of the end organ to the very low prepubertal levels of sex hormones. However, such isolated development may also be the first sign of true precocious puberty, and re-evaluation at regular intervals is indicated.

### Premature Thelarche

Premature thelarche is defined as the isolated development of breast tissue in girls younger than 8 years of age. This disorder is most common in children between 1 and 3 years of age, but it may occur earlier, and it may affect one or both breasts. On examination, the somatic growth pattern is not accelerated, bone age is not advanced, and estrogen levels are within the normal-low, prepubertal range. The diagnosis is made by exclusion of other disorders, such as hypothyroidism. Surgical biopsy of the breast is contraindicated, because the biopsy procedure may inadvertently excise a relatively large portion of breast tissue, causing permanent damage. Follow-up is necessary to identify patients in whom such breast development heralds the onset of true precocious puberty. The prognosis is favorable: 32% of patients have spontaneous regression, 54% experience no change, and breast size increases in only 11%. Pubertal development is unaffected and menstrual pattern and fertility are reported to be normal.

### Premature Pubarche

Premature pubarche is the isolated development of pubic or axillary hair in a child younger than 8 years of age, without other signs of precocious puberty. Such hair growth may be idiopathic and of no clinical significance. In some series, these individuals tend to be slightly taller than average, with marginally ad-

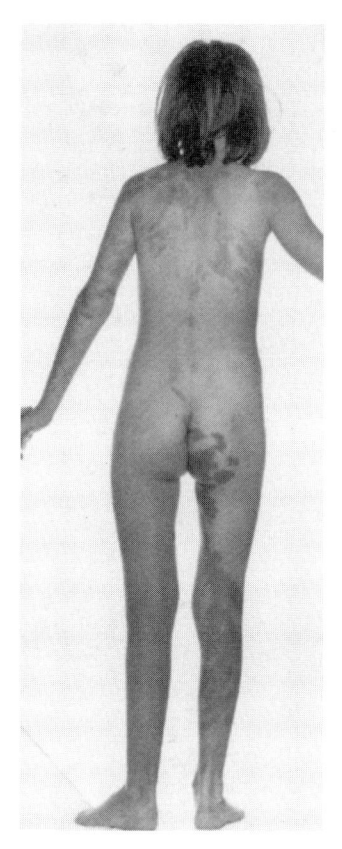

**Figure 10–22** Café-au-lait lesions in a child who has McCune-Albright syndrome. (From Ransom SB, McNeeley SG [eds]: Gynecology for the Primary Care Provider. Philadelphia, WB Saunders, 1997, p. 273.)

vanced bone age and slightly elevated dehydroepiandrosterone sulfate (DHEAS) levels in the blood.

However, early pubarche may also be a sign of excess androgen production caused by an enzyme deficiency (e.g., congenital adrenal hyperplasia) or a tumor (e.g., Leydig's cell tumor). A thorough evaluation of adrenal and gonadal function, as well as assessment of androgen production, is necessary to exclude such abnormalities. Thus, the diagnosis of idiopathic premature pubarche is made only after such an evaluation fails to detect a developmental abnormality.

Premature Menarche

Premature menarche denotes the appearance of cyclic vaginal bleeding in the absence of other signs of secondary sexual development in girls who are younger than 10 years of age. Growth and development are appropriate for age, and bone age is not advanced. The genitalia do not show signs of estrogenic stimulation. The response of the pituitary gland to GnRH challenge is the same as that of prepubertal children.

The diagnosis is formulated by exclusion of all other causes of vaginal bleeding. The diagnosis is confirmed when the cyclic nature of the bleeding becomes apparent. Prognosis for these girls is excellent; adult height is not reduced, their future menstrual pattern is normal, and fertility potential remains unimpaired.

**EVALUATION OF THE PATIENT WHO HAS ACCELERATED SEXUAL DEVELOPMENT**

The evaluation of a child who manifests early sexual maturation requires a detailed history, with particular consideration given to the onset and progression of growth and secondary sexual features, use of medications, history of head injury or CNS lesions, and family history of early sexual maturation. A complete physical examination should include an evaluation of height, weight, Tanner staging of breast and pubic hair development, as well as a search for pigmented nevi or neurofibromata. Growth should be plotted on standard growth charts and on growth velocity charts. Careful rectoabdominal palpation may identify patients who have large ovarian lesions.

Initial laboratory testing of patients who are suspected of undergoing true precocious puberty consists of an evaluation of plasma estrogen levels (or an evaluation of estrogen effect of a vaginal smear), determination of bone age by a left hand and wrist radiograph, a pelvic sonogram, and CT or magnetic resonance imaging (MRI) of the skull. LH and FSH responses to GnRH challenge may confirm the diagnosis.

If only breast development is present, the laboratory evaluation consists of an evaluation of plasma estrogen levels and serum prolactin levels, as well as thyroid function tests when clinically indicated. A radiograph of the left hand and wrist is performed to determine bone age. If these tests are normal, the diagnosis of premature thelarche is highly likely. Absence of further development confirms the diagnosis.

Initial laboratory evaluation of patients who have isolated pubic hair development requires analysis of plasma androgen levels, 17α-hydroxyprogesterone, and ACTH stimulation and suppression tests when clinically indicated. A radiograph of the left hand and wrist is performed to determine bone age. If all these tests are normal, the diagnosis of premature adrenarche is highly likely. Absence of further development confirms the diagnosis.

## Therapy

Treatment of patients who manifest early sexual development is dependent upon the exact etiology. Patients who have incomplete puberty (e.g., premature thelarche, premature adrenarche) require only observation and periodic follow-up visits. Gonadal or adrenal neoplasms should be surgically excised. Patients who have congenital adrenal hyperplasia require corticosteroid replacement therapy. Patients who have neoplasms may require surgery or irradiation, depending upon histologic features and the location of the lesion.

Treatment of patients who have true precocious puberty is aimed at the suppression of gonadotropin secretion. The most common treatment at present is the administration of GnRH agonists. These drugs lower the pituitary gland's production rate and secretion of gonadotropins. Within the first 6 months of therapy, girls who receive this treatment experience reduction in breast size and amount of pubic hair as well as cessation of menstrual periods. The ovaries and uterus decrease in size. GnRH agonist therapy also increases their final adult height.

# Common Gynecologic Disorders in Adolescents

### ABNORMAL UTERINE BLEEDING

Excessive or irregular bleeding from the vagina is a common disorder of menstrual function. Although few adolescents have an organic lesion that causes such bleeding, most of these patients suffer from dysfunctional uterine bleeding (DUB), a condition defined as abnormal bleeding from the uterine endometrium, which is unrelated to anatomic lesions of the genital tract. Almost all cases in the adolescent age group stem from anovulation that results in a total lack of progesterone production. DUB is only a symptom; before therapy can be instituted, the more serious causes of genital bleeding in the adolescent age group should be ruled out (Table 10–5).

Anovulatory uterine bleeding tends to follow one of several patterns, and the specific pattern depends on the duration and intensity of estrogen stimulation of the endometrium. In the presence of continuous high levels of estrogen, uninterrupted endometrial proliferation occurs. When estrogen levels become insufficient to support further endometrial growth or maintain endometrial integrity, desquamation and bleeding occur. The menstrual cycle of these patients is usually longer than the average span of the ovulatory cycle, and bleeding is often heavy. In the presence of continuous low circulating levels of estrogen, endometrial growth extends for a longer period, with a greater interval of amenorrhea between successive menstrual periods. The bleeding may be heavy and prolonged. In the presence of fluctuating levels of estrogens, there is an increase in the frequency of bleeding episodes. The patient often has more than one bleeding episode each month. With each decline in circulating estrogen levels, endometrial integrity is compromised and bleeding ensues.

The diagnosis of DUB is based on the patient's history, general physical examination, pelvic examination, and (rarely) selected laboratory tests. It requires the exclusion of all organic causes of abnormal vaginal bleeding. In the case of a typical teenager who has DUB, the history reveals irregular periods from the time of menarche, with a heavy flow that lasts several days or even weeks. Generally, the physical examination is normal. A Papanicolaou smear is obtained at the time of the pelvic examination. It is often useful to obtain a simple vaginal smear for a cytologic evaluation (maturation index). Although there is no typical anovulatory pattern, a progesterone-dominated maturation index is consistent with the presence of an ovulatory cycle and might, therefore, suggest a diagnosis other than dysfunctional bleeding (e.g., pregnancy). To complete the evaluation of a patient who has presumed dysfunctional uterine bleeding, the following tests should be included: pregnancy test; urinalysis; complete blood count; serum prolactin level; and, in selected cases, thyroid function tests. Although an endometrial biopsy is often performed in adult patients, it is seldom necessary in a teenager.

The possibility of an underlying coagulation disorder needs to be considered in the adolescent patient who has perimenarcheal menorrhagia. Idiopathic thrombocytopenic purpura and von Willebrand's disease are the most common occurrences. The physician should inquire about episodes of easy bruising, epistaxis, and gingival bleeding. A thorough physical examination, blood smear, and coagulation screen should be performed routinely for any patient who has severe menorrhagia or prolonged episodes of dysfunctional bleeding. The coagulation screen should include prothrombin time (PT), partial thromboplastin time (PTT), phase platelet count, and bleeding time. This relatively simple screen effectively rules out all but rare hematologic disorders. These tests should be performed before transfusion and administration of hormones are initiated.

A simple classification based on hemoglobin con-

**Table 10–5** Differential Diagnosis of Dysfunctional Uterine Bleeding

**Pregnancy Complications**

Abortion
Ectopic pregnancy
Trophoblastic disease

**Benign and Malignant Neoplasms of the Genital Tract**

Endometrial polyp
Cervical polyp
Vaginal adenosis
Vaginal carcinoma
Cervical carcinoma
Granulosa-theca cell tumor
Endometriosis
Leiomyoma

**Genital Tract Infection**

Vaginitis
Cervicitis
Vaginal foreign body
IUCD
Salpingo-oophoritis

**Endocrinopathies**

Polycystic ovarian disease
Hyperprolactinemia
Hypothyroidism
Hyperthyroidism

**Administration of Drugs or Hormones**

**Trauma**

**Coagulation Disorders**

Idiopathic thrombocytopenia purpura (ITP)
von Willebrand's disease

**Chronic Systemic Illness**

Liver cirrhosis
Renal failure

ITP = idiopathic thrombocytopenic purpura; IUCD = intrauterine contraceptive device.

centration is required for effective clinical management (Table 10–6). Patients who have hemoglobin levels greater than 12 g/dl are considered to have a mild disturbance (group I); those who have hemoglobin levels between 10 and 12 g/dl are thought to have a moderate abnormality (group II); and those who have a hemoglobin level of less than 10 g/dl are believed to have a severe problem (group III). For group I patients, reassurance and explanation are necessary, along with a periodic review of the patient's progress. The patient is given a menstrual calendar and encouraged to take a daily dietary iron supplement. The majority of these patients spontaneously convert to normal menstrual cycles within 1 or 2 years. For group II patients, the bleeding is severe enough to warrant intervention. Oral contraceptive pills (OCPs) may be prescribed for a short period of time. The pill reverses the effects of estrogens and prevents further endometrial proliferation. The use of OCPs should be considered in all sexually active girls. Girls who are not sexually active may choose to use intermittent progestin therapy, which interrupts long periods of amenorrhea. The physician can prescribe medroxyprogesterone acetate (Provera), 10 mg daily, for 5 to 7 days every 35 to 40 days. This is an excellent cycle regulator because it allows spontaneous menses to occur between treatment cycles.

Some group III patients need emergency hospital management. Patients who are bleeding heavily or who become hypotensive require transfusions and fluid replacement. Associated pathology, specifically involving complications of pregnancy and coagulopathy, must be excluded. In one series, 20% of all adolescent patients who required hospitalization for DUB were found to suffer from a coagulation disorder. Regardless of the cause, the bleeding may be controlled in most patients by administration of estrogens or, sometimes, progestins. In a few rare instances, when primary medical management has failed, dilatation and curettage may be required. Initial hormonal hemostasis may be achieved by the administration of conjugated estrogens (Premarin), 20 to 25 mg, intravenously every 4 hours for a maximum of six doses. It is usually unnecessary to continue parenteral estrogen therapy beyond 24 hours. Continued bleeding beyond this time is an indication for diagnostic dilatation and curettage. Concurrently, a progestational agent (e.g., norgestrel; ethinyl estradiol [Ovral]) is given. An initial loading dose of two tablets is followed by one tablet four times daily, and the dose is tapered gradually over the succeeding month. Despite the dosage, this regimen is well tolerated and antiemetics are seldom required.

After a period of intense hormonal therapy, 6 months of cyclic therapy with conventional combined OCPs is undertaken. It is expected that the withdrawal flow will be within normal bounds and regular, and that each successive cycle will be accompanied by a progressive reduction in endometrial height. After 6 months, the patient is reassessed. If she is sexually active, continued treatment with an OCP is required. Otherwise, the patient may be allowed to menstruate without medication. Careful follow-up is undertaken to assess the timing and duration of menses with the aid of a menstrual calendar and to treat any relapses that may occur. If the anovulatory pattern recurs, medroxyprogesterone acetate (Provera) is used as described for group II patients. By adhering to this medical protocol of initial hormonal hemostasis followed by cyclic regulation of menses and continuous long-term observation, unnecessary dilatation and curettage can be avoided. Thus, surgical management may be reserved for the small percentage of patients who fail to respond to conservative measures.

In general, adolescent menstrual problems are viewed with optimism and 50% of adolescents who have DUB return to a regular menstrual pattern within 4 years following menarche. However, if anovulation persists longer than 4 years, the chance of recovery is low. The risks of exposure to continued

**Table 10–6** Management of Dysfunctional Uterine Bleeding

| |
|---|
| **Hgb >12 g/dl** |
| Reassurance |
| Menstrual calendar |
| Iron supplement |
| Periodic re-evaluation |
| **Hgb 10–12 g/dl** |
| Reassurance and explanation |
| Menstrual calendar |
| Iron supplement |
| Cyclic progestin therapy or OCP |
| Re-evaluation in 6 months |
| **Hgb <10 g/dl** |
| *No Active Bleeding* |
| Explanation |
| Transfusion or iron supplement |
| OCP |
| Re-evaluation in 6–12 months |
| *Acute Hemorrhage* |
| Transfusion |
| Fluid replacement therapy |
| Hormonal hemostasis (IV Premarin) |
| Intensive progestin therapy |
| Dilatation and curettage when hormonal hemostasis fails |
| OCP for 6–12 months |

OCP = oral contraceptive pill.

unopposed estrogen stimulation must then be considered.

## DYSMENORRHEA

Dysmenorrhea affects almost half of all female adolescents today and is probably the most frequently encountered gynecologic disorder. The term *dysmenorrhea* is derived from the Greek language, and although it means difficult monthly flow, it is commonly used to refer to painful menstruation. Dysmenorrhea is classified as primary or secondary. Primary dysmenorrhea has no detectable pelvic pathology, whereas in secondary dysmenorrhea, the pain is the result of an existing pelvic disease.

Adolescent dysmenorrhea often begins shortly after menarche (within 6 to 12 months) and coincides with the onset of ovulatory cyles. The patient complains of colicky pain that begins several hours before or just at the onset of menstrual flow. The pain is described as crampy and usually begins in the midpelvis, radiating to the back and sometimes to the legs. The pain is most severe during the first day of menstruation but may last for 2 or 3 days. In more than half of patients, the pain is accompanied by other systemic signs, including nausea and vomiting, fatigue, diarrhea, headaches, and irritability. In rare instances, syncopal attacks have been reported. Patients who have primary dysmenorrhea have reported diminishing symptoms with increasing age. In some, the pain may disappear after the birth of their first child.

The clinical features of primary dysmenorrhea are quite typical. These include onset of pain at or shortly after menarche. The pain begins shortly before or immediately after menstruation and disappears completely within 2 or 3 days. The pelvic examination is normal.

It is now well accepted that in many adolescents who have primary dysmenorrhea, the production and release of endometrial prostaglandin give rise to abnormal uterine activity. The patient perceives this abnormal activity as cramps or pain. It has been shown that the intensity of abnormal uterine activity is related to the amount of prostaglandin released into the menstrual flow from the degenerating decidua. Prostaglandin levels are highest during the first 48 hours of menstruation. In addition to uterine hyperactivity, prostaglandin may give rise to pain by directly affecting nerve endings.

Both oral contraceptive pills (OCPs) and prostaglandin inhibitors were found to be highly effective in the treatment of dysmenorrhea. The use of OCPs was found to be effective in at least 90% of women who have primary dysmenorrhea. OCPs suppress endometrial proliferation, resulting in an endocrine environment similar to that of the early proliferative phase of the menstrual cycle, when prostaglandin levels are lowest. An OC is the drug of choice for sexually active teens who need contraception as well.

Prostaglandin inhibitors are used mainly in young patients who do not wish to use contraception. The treatment is given only during the first 2 or 3 days of the menstrual cycle. It inhibits cyclic endoperoxide synthesis or acts through the cyclic endoperoxide cleavage enzyme system. As a result, endometrial prostaglandin synthesis is suppressed, uterine activity is normal, and menstrual cramps are alleviated.

## SECONDARY DYSMENORRHEA

In secondary dysmenorrhea, the pain is caused by an existing pelvic pathology. Cases of endometriosis have been reported in adolescents who have obstructive genital malformations. At times, there is a history of a previous pelvic inflammatory disease. Although pain in adolescents is often presumed to represent primary dysmenorrhea, it is now well accepted that in some patients endometriosis may occur soon after the onset of menarche. If the patient fails to respond to medical therapy, she should be evaluated further to exclude pelvic pathology. Diagnostic laparoscopy is indicated to establish the diagnosis of endometriosis. The treatment for secondary dysmenorrhea is directed toward the underlying pelvic disorder.

## REFERENCES

Ben-Ami T, Boichis H, Hertz M: Fused labia. Clinical and radiological findings. Pediatr Radiol 7:33, 1978.

Berkowitz CD, Elvik SL, Logan MK: Labial fusion in prepubescent girls: A marker for sexual abuse? Am J Obstet Gynecol 156:16, 1987.

Capraro VJ, Bayonet-Rivera NP, Magosas I: Vulvar tumor in children due to prolapse of urethral mucosa. Am J Obstet Gynecol 108:572, 1970.

Carpenter SEK, Rock JA: Pediatric and Adolescent Gynecology. New York, Raven Press, 1992.

Centers for Disease Control: Sexually transmitted diseases treatment guidelines. MMWR 42:1, 1993.

Chatman DL, Ward AB: Endometriosis in adolescents. J Reprod Med 27:156, 1982.

Claessens EA, Cowell CA: Acute adolescent menorrhagia. Am J Obstet Gynecol 139:277, 1981.

Crist WM, Garnsey L, Beltangady MS, et al: Prognosis in children with rhabdomyosarcoma: A report of the intergroup rhabdomyosarcoma studies I and II. Intergroup Rhabdomyosarcoma Committee. J Clin Oncol 8:443, 1990.

DeVore GR, Owens O, Kase N: Use of intravenous Premarin in the treatment of dysfunctional bleeding—A double-blind randomized control study. Obstet Gynecol 59:285, 1982.

Dewhurst SJ: Female Puberty and Its Abnormalities. Edinburgh, UK, Churchill Livingstone, 1984.

Dewhurst J: Congenital malformations of the lower urinary tract. Clin Obstet Gynaecol 5:51, 1978.

Dewhurst J: Lichen sclerosus of the vulva in childhood. Pediatr Adolesc Gynecol 1:149, 1983.

Emans SJ, Laufer MR, Goldstein DP: Pediatric and Adolescent Gynecology, 4th ed. Philadelphia, Lippincott-Raven, 1998.

Frank R: Formation of artificial vagina without operation. Am J Obstet Gynecol 35:1053, 1938.

Goldfarb AF (ed): Atlas of Clinical Gynecology. Philadelphia, Current Medicine, 1998.

Goldstein DP, deCholnoky C, Emans SJ: Adolescent endometriosis. J Adolesc Health Care, 1:37, 1980.

Griffin JE, Edwards C, Madden JD, et al: Congenital absence of the vagina. The Mayer-Rokitansky-Kuster-Hauser syndrome. Ann Intern Med 85:224, 1976.

Grunberger W, Fisch LF: Pediatric gynecological outpatient department. A report on 600 patients. Wien Klin Wochenschr 94:614, 1982.

Hammerschlag MR, et al., Microbiology of the vagina in children: Normal and potentially pathogenic organisms. Pediatrics 62:57, 1978.

Hammerschlag M: Pitfalls in the diagnosis of sexually transmitted diseases in children. In The Advisor, American Professional Society on the Abuse of Children (APSAC), 1989, pp 4–5.

Heger A, Emans JE (eds): Evaluation of the Sexually Abused Child. New York, Oxford University Press, 1992.

Ingram JM: The bicycle seat stool in the treatment of vaginal agenesis and stenosis: A preliminary report. Am J Obstet Gynecol 140:867, 1981.

Jenny C, Kirby CP, Fuquay D: Genital lichen sclerosus mistaken for child sexual abuse. Pediatrics 83:597, 1989.

Jones HW Jr, Rock JA: Reparative and Constructive Surgery of the Female Genital Tract. Baltimore: Williams and Wilkins, 1983.

Kaneti J, Lieberman E, Moshe P, et al.: A case of ambiguous genitalia owing to neurofibromatosis: Review of the literature. J Urol 140:584, 1988.

Kaplowitz PB, Cockrell JL, Young RB: Premature adrenarche. Clinical and diagnostic features. Clin Pediatr 25:28, 1986.

Marshall WA, Tanner JM: Variations in the pattern of pubertal changes in girls. Arch Dis Child 44:291, 1969.

McIndoe AH, Banister JB: An operation for the cure of congenital absence of the vagina. J Obstet Gynaecol Br Emp 45:490, 1938.

Mercer LJ, Mueller CM, Hajj SN: Medical treatment of urethral prolapse. Adolesc Pediatr Gynecol 1:182, 1988.

Mills JL, Stolley PD, Davies J, et al., Premature thelarche: Natural history and etiologic investigation. Am J Dis Child 135:743, 1981.

Muram D: Genital tract injuries in the prepubertal child. Pediatr Ann 15:616, 1986.

Muram D: Labial adhesions: A possible marker of sexual abuse. JAMA 259:352, 1988.

Muram D: Vaginal bleeding in children and adolescents. Obstet Gynecol. Clin North Am 17:389, 1990.

Muram D: Congenital malformations. In Copeland LJ (ed): Textbook of Gynecology. Philadelphia, WB Saunders, 1993, pp 121–141.

Muram D: Vaginoscopy. In Stovall T, Ling F (eds): Atlas of Benign Gynecologic Surgery. 1994.

Muram D, Dewhurst SJ, Grant DB: Premature menarche: A follow-up study. Arch Dis Child 58:142, 1983.

Muram D, Elias S: The treatment of labial adhesions in prepubertal girls. Surg Forum 34:464, 1988.

Muram D, Grant DB, Dewhurst SJ: Precocious puberty: A follow-up study. Arch Dis Child 59:77, 1984.

Muram D Jones CE: The use of video-colposcopy in the gynecologic examination of children and adolescents. Adolesc Pediatr Gynecol 6:154, 1993.

Neinstein LS, Goldenring J, Carpenter S: Nonsexual transmission of sexually transmitted diseases: An infrequent occurrence. Pediatrics 74:67, 1984.

Newton AWJ, Soule EH, Hamoudi AB: Histopathology of childhood sarcomas, intergroup rhabdomyosarcoma studies I and II: Clinicopathologic correlation. J Clin Oncol 6:67, 1988.

Pokorny SF: Configuration of the prepubertal hymen. Am J Obstet Gynecol 157:950, 1987.

Redmond CA, Cowell CA, Krafchik BR: Genital lichen sclerosus in prepubertal girls. Adolesc Pediatr Gynecol 1:177, 1988.

Rock JA: Surgery for anomalies of the Müllerian ducts. In Thompson J, Rock J (eds): Te Linde's Operative Gynecology. Philadelphia, JB Lippincott 1992, pp 603–646.

Rock JA, Azziz R: Genital anomalies in childhood. Clin Obstet Gynecol 30:682, 1987.

Sanfilippo J, Muram D, Lee P, et al (eds): Pediatric and Adolescent Gynecology. Philadelphia, WB Saunders, 1994.

Shenker A, Weinstein LS, Moran A et al: Severe endocrine and nonendodocrine manifestations of the McCune-Albright syndrome associated with activating mutations of stimulatory G protein GS. J Pediatr 123:509, 1993.

Shulman LP, Elias S: Developmental abnormalities of the female reproductive tract: Pathogenesis and nosology. Adolesc Pediatr Gynecol 1:230, 1988.

Simpson JL: Disorders of Sexual Differentiation: Etiology and Clinical Delineation. New York, Academic Press, 1976.

Smith RP: Primary dysmenorrhea and the adolescent patient. Adolesc Pediatr Gynecol 1:23, 1988.

Southam AL, Richart RM: The prognosis for adolescents with menstrual abnormality. Am J Obstet Gynecol 94: 637, 1966.

Stovall TG, Muram D: Urinary retention secondary to labial adhesions. Adolesc Pediatr Gynecol 1:203, 1988.

Styne DM: New aspects in the diagnosis and treatment of pubertal disorders. Pediatr Clin North Am 44:505, 1997.

Sweet RL, Gibbs RS (eds): Infectious Diseases of the Female Genital Tract. Baltimore, William & Wilkins, 1990.

Velcek FT, Kugaczewski JT, Klotz DH, et al: Surgical therapy for urethral prolapse in young girls. Adolesc Pediatr Gynecol 2:230, 1989.

Williams EA: Congenital absence of the vagina. A simple operation for its relief. J Obstet Gynecol Br Commonw 71:511, 1964.

Yen SSC, Jaffe RB: Reproductive Endocrinology, 2nd ed. Philadelphia, WB Saunders, 1986.

# 11

# Hysterectomy

ROBERT A. HAMMER
MELVIN V. GERBIE

Since 1845, when Atlee introduced a surgical technique for removal of the uterus, hysterectomy has become the most commonly performed nonobstetric surgical procedure in the United States, with one woman out of every three undergoing the procedure by the age of 65. In the first half of the twentieth century hysterectomy became the preferred surgical modality for resolving functional and anatomic gynecologic disturbances. The reasons for the increased popularity of this procedure were the following:
1. Barrier contraceptive methods were only moderately effective.
2. Modern medical techniques of evaluating and controlling uterine bleeding were lacking.
3. Anesthetic and surgical safety were undergoing continual improvement.

Although the annual rate of hysterectomies has decreased by over 100,000 since 1978, there are still more than 500,000 hysterectomies performed in the United States each year, with significant national economic impact. Yet, despite the extent to which it is performed, the indications for hysterectomy remain controversial.

The American College of Obstetrics and Gynecology (ACOG) published guidelines in 1989 and again in 1994, describing preoperative criteria that had to be met before abdominal or vaginal hysterectomy could be performed. The Criteria Sets, updated yet again in 1997, list specific requirements for confirming indications documenting actions to be taken before performance of hysterectomy, and contraindications to the procedure. In an attempt to assess the extent to which suitable guidelines for hysterectomy were maintained, Bernstein and associates devised a scoring system to evaluate appropriate performance of hysterectomy. They used a random sample of managed care medical records of patients who had undergone hysterectomy. Overall, 58% of these patients had hysterectomies performed for appropriate reasons. In 25% of cases, the rationale for surgery was unclear, and in 16%, hysterectomy was judged to be clinically inappropriate. The authors believed these findings justified a rationale for decreasing the rate of unnecessary hysterectomies. However, even though appropriateness criteria may be useful in comparing procedures among populations, this method should not be used for managing care of individual patients.

There were large inter-regional variations in the rates of hysterectomies performed, particularly for discretionary indications. These variations suggest the need for more definitive practice guidelines. In this chapter, indications, alternatives, surgical techniques, prophylactic oophorectomy, prophylactic antibiotics, the use of preoperative gonadotropin-releasing hormone (GnRH) agonists, surgical complications, and long-term sequelae of hysterectomy are reviewed.

# Major Indications for Hysterectomy

## UTERINE FIBROID TUMORS

Leiomyomata, also known as leiomyomas or fibroid tumors, are the most common neoplasms of the female genital tract. They are found in 20 to 50% of women, depending on age and method of assessment, and appear with increasing frequency in women who are in their 30s and 40s. Most leiomyomas change slowly or not at all, but they may produce symptoms if they increase in size, undergo degenerative changes, or impact on the endometrial cavity. Leiomyomas currently account for approximately 30% of all hysterectomies performed in the United States. Most frequently, the symptoms include excessive bleeding, pelvic pain, or pelvic pressure. Although leiomyomas occur in fewer than 3% of pregnancies and usually have no effect on pregnancy outcome, they can contribute to recurrent abortion, placental abruption, premature labor, malpresentation, dystocia, postpartum hemorrhage, and puerperal infection.

### Asymptomatic Fibroid Tumors

The percentage of hysterectomies performed on asymptomatic women is unknown, but it is likely that a substantial proportion of large uteri are removed only because of their size. In a review by Reiter and associates 16 of 40 (40%) of women who had uteri larger than 12 weeks' gestational size removed by hysterectomy were asymptomatic. Although no objective grounds for this criterion have been provided, several theoretical arguments have been advanced to justify hysterectomy for an asymptomatic patient with a uterus larger than 12-week gestational size: increased risk for development of symptoms; interference with clinical evaluation of the adnexa, which could delay detection of ovarian cancer; early detection of uterine leiomyosarcoma; and prevention of increased operative morbidity. Reiter provides evidence for questioning the rationale of these hypothetical concerns.

Because no clinical guidelines exist to predict the likelihood of future symptoms in patients who have asymptomatic myomas, surgery should be deferred until symptoms develop, avoiding unnecessary expense and operative risks in patients who may remain free of symptoms. However, clinical experience suggests that as myomas enlarge beyond 12 weeks' gestational size, symptoms of abdominal enlargement and pressure are frequent and surgery may become necessary.

The contention that large uterine leiomyomas could delay diagnosis of ovarian cancer by interfering with clinical evaluation of the adnexa is valid only to the extent that pelvic examination can be shown to detect ovarian cancer at an early, curable stage. However, 75% of ovarian carcinomas are diagnosed only after the disease has spread beyond the confines of the ovary. In addition, transvaginal ultrasonography is an excellent means of adnexal evaluation, even in the presence of large uterine leiomyomas. Finally, surgery has not been recommended routinely in other settings in which adnexal evaluation is compromised, such as in obese women or in those who do not receive routine gynecologic care. Therefore, there appears to be no rationale for recommending hysterectomy for large uteri on the basis of ovarian cancer prophylaxis.

Another common argument for routine removal of large myomatous uteri is concern about the possible presence of leiomyosarcoma. The mortality rate reported for hysterectomy performed for benign indications in premenopausal women (1.0 to 1.6 per 1000) is greater than the incidence of leiomyosarcoma discovered incidentally in uteri that were removed because of presumed leiomyomas (one per 2000). Furthermore, the prognosis for leiomyosarcoma diagnosed in premenopausal women appears to be generally favorable, even when it has been discovered incidentally. With the possible exception of a rapidly growing, isolated uterine tumor, there is little evidence to support routine hysterectomy on the basis of risk for leiomyosarcoma in asymptomatic women who have large uteri.

There is also no scientific basis for the concern that expectant management of asymptomatic fibroid tumors would increase the risk of perioperative complications if hysterectomy became indicated after the uterus enlarged further. In 1992, Reiter demonstrated that women who had a uterine size larger than 12 weeks' gestation were no more likely to suffer perioperative complications than those who had smaller uteri. No significant increase in estimated blood loss or need for blood transfusions in women with larger uteri was noted.

Thus, hysterectomy for completely asymptomatic leiomyomas is indicated only in rare circumstances. Silent ureteral obstruction caused by uterine compression warrants operation; however, this condition occurs infrequently and is generally limited to women who have uteri larger than 12 weeks' gestational size or those who have intraligamentous tumors. In postmenopausal women, uterine growth raises concern about the presence of leiomyosarcoma, and hysterectomy may be necessary for definitive diagnosis. In premenopausal women, this malignancy is a very rare cause of rapid enlargement. As imaging techniques improve, they are likely to have a greater role in the noninvasive evaluation of enlarging leiomyomas in premenopausal women.

## Preoperative Evaluation

If the preoperative diagnosis is unclear, pelvic ultrasonography by combined transvaginal and abdominal approaches is the initial (and, in most instances, the only) technique needed to image the female pelvis. The advantages of ultrasonography are relatively low risk to the patient, its widespread availability, its good level of patient acceptance, and its reasonable cost. Identification of submucous tumors or small intramural tumors may be aided by hysteroscopy, hysterosalpingography, or sonohysterography (Fig. 11–1).

## Management Alternatives

Patients who have menometrorrhagia and leiomyomas should be evaluated for other causes of uterine bleeding. Endometrial adenocarcinoma should be ruled out in women who have risk factors. Patients who have chronic anovulation may, after appropriate treatment, experience resolution of their symptoms without surgery. Hysteroscopy can play a diagnostic and therapeutic role. Studies on the use of hysteroscopic myomectomy have shown short-term efficacy rates of 75 to 90%, with a need for repeat hysteroscopy of hysterectomy in 20% of cases. Thus, it is worthwhile to consider a conservative approach for managing pedunculated or submucous leiomyomas.

In patients who have dysmenorrhea or pelvic pain, etiologies other than fibroid tumors should be excluded before surgical intervention is entertained.

## Pharmacologic Therapy

The factors involved in the initiation and growth of leiomyomata uteri remain poorly understood. Traditionally, estrogen has been considered the major promoter of myoma growth. Therapeutic trials using danazol and progestins have shown that although

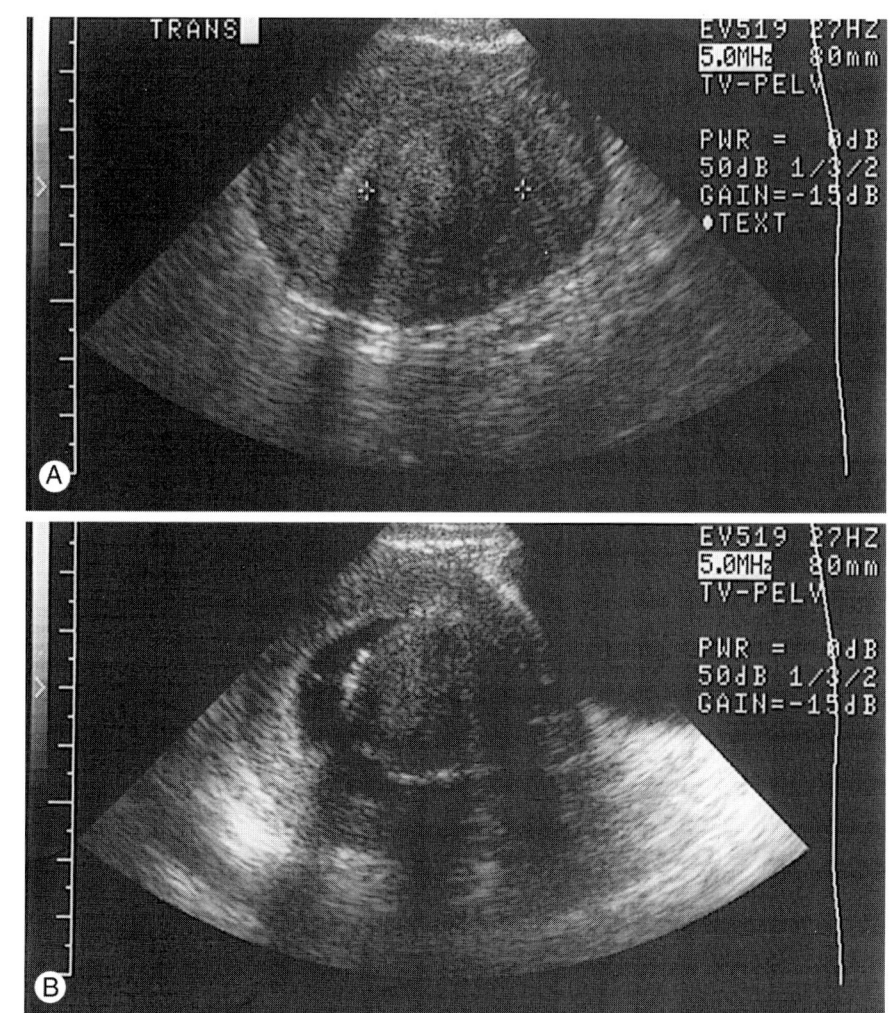

**Figure 11–1** *A, B,* Identification of submucous or small intramural tumors by sonohysterography.

these agents can successfully induce amenorrhea, they have never been demonstrated to produce uterine and leiomyoma shrinkage, moreover; they have a high rate of side effects. Current observations by Rein and associates provide biochemical, histologic, and clinical evidence supporting an important role for progesterone in the growth of uterine leiomyomas.

Increasingly, pharmacologic treatment of leiomyomata uteri has focused on GnRH agonists. Efficacy of GnRH agonists in decreasing uterine size has been demonstrated, with mean reduction in uterine volume of 40 to 50% in approximately 80% of patients. Maximum reduction in uterine volume occurs within 3 months. An increase in numbers of leiomyomas and uterine size and a return to pretreatment menstrual patterns occurs 3 to 12 months after cessation of therapy.

Studies evaluating bone density changes in women treated with GnRH agonists for up to 6 months have reported no significant decrease. Yet, because of concerns regarding bone resorption and the transient nature of uterine size reduction with GnRH agonist therapy, no long-term medical regimen currently exists for managing patients who have uterine fibroids. GnRH agonist therapy with add-back estrogen is currently under investigation. Pending study outcomes, this combination approach may be especially appropriate in patients who are close to menopause.

The predominant usefulness of GnRH agonists in the management of uterine fibroids is in their preoperative role. GnRH agonists reduce symptoms, but the increase in preoperative hemoglobin concentration, coupled with decreased intraoperative blood loss, may also decrease the potential for blood transfusion. Decreases in uterine and myoma volumes may allow conversion from an abdominal to a vaginal hysterectomy or to an abdominal approach via a more cosmetic incision. Fibroid shrinkage combined with an atrophic endometrium may facilitate endoscopic resection of subserosal or submucosal tumors, potentially averting hysterectomy.

## Dysfunctional Uterine Bleeding

Dysfunctional uterine bleeding accounts for 20% of hysterectomy cases in the United States. Once systemic and organic etiologies of abnormal uterine bleeding have been excluded, symptoms can be controlled by hormonal therapy in the majority of patients, obviating the need for hysterectomy. When the condition persists despite therapy and interferes with the patient's lifestyle, hysterectomy may be indicated. Consideration should be given to endometrial ablation for this condition.

## Chronic Pelvic Pain

Chronic pelvic pain is a common and often frustrating problem in clinical gynecology and is the indication for 10% of hysterectomies. Management of this condition by removal of the uterus remains controversial. Organic etiologies for chronic pelvic pain include fibroid tumors, endometriosis, and adhesions. Evaluation of the gastrointestinal and urinary tracts, and the musculoskeletal system should be performed if symptoms are unexplained. Because psychosomatic processes can have an impact on pelvic symptoms, these disorders must also be excluded. Notably, 40 to 60% of patients who have unexplained chronic pelvic pain have a history of childhood sexual abuse. Medical therapy, including nonsteroidal anti-inflammatory drugs (NSAIDs) and oral contraceptives, should be tried for at least 6 months before resorting to extirpative surgery. Presacral neurectomy or bilateral segmental resection of uterosacral ligaments has been reported to benefit up to 70% of patients who have pain of uterine origin, although neither treatment has been shown to offer lasting relief. In reviewing the current evidence for the efficacy of hysterectomy for chronic pain, two factors must be considered:
1. Current data are based on observational and retrospective studies
2. Success rates of hysterectomy for chronic pelvic pain may be overestimated, because patients who have persistent pain after hysterectomy may focus on other organ systems and seek treatment from other specialists.

In 1990, Stovall and Ling published long-term follow-up data (mean 21.6 months) on 99 of 104 eligible premenopausal women who had chronic pelvic pain that was attributed to uterine disease. Patients were excluded if a previous laparoscopy or finding of a hysterectomy suggested nonuterine pelvic disease. Histologic examination of specimens revealed no pathology in 65.7%. Leiomyomas were found in 12.1%, adenomyosis in 20.2%, and both in 2.2%. Seventy-eight percent of patients had no significant pain at the time of follow-up. Although these results are encouraging, unless patient selection criteria are strict, surgical outcomes are certain to be less impressive.

## Endometriosis

Endometriosis affects 5 to 15% of premenopausal women. If initial medical management of symptoms fails, laparoscopy is warranted to establish the diagnosis. The choice of treatment must then be individualized for the patient to achieve therapeutic goals, which should be based on established efficacy rates. Medical therapies and conservative surgical treatment are appropriate as initial modalities for symptomatic patients. If such therapy fails to relieve associated symptoms and childbearing is completed, definitive surgical therapy may be indicated.

Intractable pain caused by endometriosis accounts for 20% of hysterectomies. Although most studies indicate that the incidence of recurrence is low after hysterectomy with oophorectomy, the question remains as to whether bilateral oophorectomy is required to achieve a permanent cure. Retrospective studies comparing hysterectomy with bilateral oophorectomy to hysterectomy alone have revealed widely discordant results. In 1995, Namnoun and associates published a retrospective cohort study of symptom recurrence and reoperation after hysterectomy, with and without ovarian conservation. With a mean length of 58 months of follow-up, 62% of women whose ovaries were spared had recurrent symptoms, and 31% required further surgery, compared with 10.1% and 3.7%, respectively, when ovaries were removed.

## Premalignant and Malignant Disease

Five percent of hysterectomies are performed in patients who have endometrial hyperplasia. Surgery is not indicated for hyperplasia without atypia because medical therapy is effective and the risk of progression to carcinoma is low (Table 11–1). In contrast, because of the high rate of progression to malignancy in patients who have atypical hyperplasia, hysterectomy is the treatment of choice. Medical management should be reserved *only* for patients who are poor surgical candidates, those who wish to preserve fertility, or those in whom the cytologic atypia is focal. Medically managed patients who have atypical hyperplasia need long-term follow-up with endometrial sampling. Patients whose symptoms are refractory or intolerant to medical management should also undergo hysterectomy.

Ten percent of all hysterectomies are categorized as therapy or surgical staging in patients who have cancers of the cervix, endometrium, uterus, ovary, or fallopian tube, and, occasionally, in patients who have gestational trophoblastic disease. Although the vast majority of patients who have cervical dysplasia can be treated conservatively, a role remains for hysterectomy in those who are nondesirous of pregnancy and who have high-grade cervical dysplasia that persists or recurs after conservative treatment. Adenocarcinoma in situ lesions of the cervix are becoming more frequently diagnosed. Long-term progression rate of patients who have these lesions are poorly documented, and conization procedures are frequently performed; nonetheless, hysterectomy is an acceptable choice of treatment of this condition. Hysterectomy remains the treatment of choice for microinvasive squamous cell lesions of the cervix except in selected patients.

## Genital Prolapse

Approximately 15% of hysterectomies are performed to correct genital prolapse. In asymptomatic patients who have mild-to-moderate pelvic prolapse, clinical observation or pessary use are the mainstays of management. Symptoms of pelvic pressure, dyspareunia, urinary incontinence, incomplete defecation, rectal discomfort, external lesions, and ulceration of the externalized mucosa necessiate intervention. Nonsurgical therapy generally consists of the use of a pessary combined with estrogen cream and pelvic floor strengthening via Kegel's exercises, vaginal cones, or transvaginal electric nerve stimulation. Hysterectomy remains the standard of care for treatment of patients who have symptomatic pelvic organ prolapse. With the increasing desire of patients for uterine conservation, most reconstructive techniques can be modified to retain the uterus.

Although these patients commonly have multiple defects, including uterine descensus, which require correction, patients who have a well-supported uterus and who undergo colporrhaphy for cystocele, rectocele, or both may not require hysterectomy. There is no evidence that removal of the uterus improves the success rates for these operative procedures or that a later reoperation will be necessary.

The benefit for patients who have concomitant hysterectomy and surgery for urinary stress incontinence remains controversial. In 1975, Green found a 97% cure rate in patients who underwent hysterectomy and a Marshall-Marchetti-Krantz (MMK) operation, compared with an 81% cure rate after an MMK

Table 11–1 Endometrial Hyperplasia: Risk of Progression to Carcinoma

| Type of Hyperplasia | Progression to Cancer (%) |
| --- | --- |
| WITHOUT ATYPIA | |
| Simple (cystic without atypia) | 1 |
| Complex (adenomatous without atypia) | 3 |
| WITH ATYPIA | |
| Simple (cystic with atypia) | 8 |
| Complex (adenomatous with atypia) | 29 |

operation only. For a time, it was common policy to perform hysterectomy and surgical correction of incontinence together. However, other researchers have found no improvement in the cure rate for incontinence with this combined procedure. In 1988, Langer prospectively randomized to MMK, either with or without hysterectomy, 45 patients who required surgery for correction of genuine stress urinary incontinence, unaccompanied by uterine disease or pelvic floor defects. There were no differences in outcome success in either group. Similar results have been found by others.

## Tubo-ovarian Abscess

Tubo-ovarian abscess (TOA), a known sequela of pelvic infection, has been reported to occur in 3 to 16% of patients who have been hospitalized because of salpingitis. It is generally accepted that rupture of a TOA is an indication for immediate surgical intervention. However, there is still considerable controversy about the management of the unruptured TOA. There is a general trend toward a more conservative approach in both the timing and extent of surgical intervention for an unruptured TOA, especially in nulliparous patients.

Overall, studies indicate that antibiotic therapy is successful in 33 to 74% of patients. Although the rate of subsequent intrauterine pregnancy is low (9.5% to 13.8%), future reproductive capability is a significant concern to most patients who have TOAs and plays a major role in efforts for a more conservative therapeutic approach.

Although a definitive cure can be achieved in most patients treated by hysterectomy and bilateral salpingo-oophorectomy (BSO), unilateral salpingo-oophorectomy may be adequate therapy in the surgical management of unilateral TOA. Rivlin and Hunt reported their results with the use of conservative surgery and peritoneal lavage in 113 patients who had ruptured TOAs. Overall, hysterectomy was required in only 3% of the cases. In a study by Landers and Sweet, total hysterectomy and contralateral salpingo-oophorectomy were subsequently required in only 10.5% of patients who initially underwent unilateral salpingo-oophorectomy. Of the patients who were treated with antibiotics alone, 10% required subsequent laparotomy for pelvic pain or persistence of the mass, although long-term follow-up data were available for only 58 of the 175 patients.

In summary, an initially conservative approach using antimicrobials in the management of an unruptured TOA is appropriate. The antibiotic regimen should include clindamycin because of its activity against the gram-negative anaerobic rods commonly associated with abscess formation and because of its ability to penetrate the human neutrophil. However, if the patient does not begin to show a response within a reasonable amount of time (48 to 72 hours), or if there is suspicion of rupture of the TOA, surgical intervention should be undertaken, and a conservative approach (i.e., unilateral salpingo-oophorectomy) should be considered if preservation of reproductive potential is desired.

## Familial Cancer Syndromes

In women whose family history makes them prone to ovarian cancer, the risk of ovarian neoplasm may be as high as 50%, and they may elect to have prophylactic oophorectomy after they have completed their childbearing. Hysterectomy, however, is not warranted unless the patient has a clear-cut indication for surgery. For a woman who has Lynch II syndrome (familial preponderance of breast, endometrial, ovarian, and nonpolyposis colon cancer), prophylactic oophorectomy and hysterectomy are appropriate after completion of childbearing.

## Obstetric Indications

Hysterectomy in the obstetric patient is performed for life-saving indications, the most common of which is uncontrollable postpartum hemorrhage casued by uterine atony, placenta accreta, or uterine rupture. Further discussion on the indications and technique of cesarean hysterectomy is beyond the scope of this chapter.

## Supracervical Hysterectomy

Before the 1960s, supracervical amputation of the uterus was the standard hysterectomy technique for excision of benign pelvic lesions. Removal of the cervix was associated with considerable morbidity from infection and intraoperative bleeding. Improvements in anesthesia, surgical technique, and postoperative care reduced this morbidity, and prevention of cervical cancer justified removal of the cervix in most cases. However, as a result of the purported detrimental effects of total hysterectomy (discussed later in this chapter), the interest in performing supracervical hysterectomy has recently increased.

In specific instances, supracervical hysterectomy is extremely practical. During an emergency operation, if excessive bleeding has occurred and the patient has become unstable, or if disseminated intravascular coagulation is present, supracervical hysterectomy is preferred. During a cesarean hysterectomy, the inferior and lateral margins of the cervix can be difficult to palpate, and there is increased risk of injury to the ureters and bladder, in such a case, supracervical hysterectomy should be considered. Finally, for cases in which the pouch of Douglas is obliterated by endometriosis or adhesions, it may be prudent to perform a supracervical procedure if it is not otherwise contraindicated.

# Alternatives to Hysterectomy

## MYOMECTOMY

Myomectomy is 80% effective in reducing menorrhagia caused by submucosal leiomyomas. However, the procedure has an incidence of morbidity similar to that of hysterectomy, and, within 20 years of myomectomy, one of four women who has undergone this surgery subsequently requires a definitive procedure for recurrent symptoms. Generally, myomectomy should be reserved for women of reproductive age who desire future fertility. As in hysterectomy, GnRH agonist treatment may play a preoperative role in the management of women scheduled for myomectomy. In a double-blind, placebo-controlled trial, Friedman and associates reported that treatment with leuprolide acetate depot, 3.75 mg every 4 weeks for 12 weeks before myomectomy, reduced intraoperative blood loss in women who had uterine leiomyomas that were at least 600 ml in volume (189 ml versus 390 ml, $P<0.01$).

## UTERINE ARTERY EMBOLIZATION

Uterine artery embolization (UAE) has been successfully employed in the treatment of women who have hypervascular pelvic masses, including abdominal pregnancy, arteriovenous malformation, and bleeding caused by cervical cancer. In addition, its use has been advocated as first-line therapy for patients who have postpartum and postoperative bleeding that is refractory to local measures.

Recent preliminary experience with UAE as therapy for women who have symptomatic uterine fibroid tumors has shown promise. Goodwin and associates noted a significant (40%) reduction in mean uterine volume at 2 months, and impressive short-term results (mean follow-up 5.8 months) with respect to menorrhagia (6 of 7 improved) and pelvic pain (8 of 9 improved). UAE gives the gynecologist another alternative in managing patients who have fibroid tumors. It may be especially appropriate for patients who have troublesome bleeding but who are poor surgical candidates, for those who wish to maintain their uterus for psychosocial reasons, or for those who otherwise decline surgical therapy. As with ligation of any or all of the hypogastric, uterine, or ovarian arteries, an effect on fertility is not anticipated, but data are currently limited.

## ENDOMETRIAL ABLATION

Elimination of menorrhagia by hysteroscopically directed endometrial ablation (EA) is reported in 70 to 90% of cases, although recurrences occur in 15 to 25% of patients. EA, using rollerball or electroexcision, offers the advantages of shorter operating and recovery times, decreased perioperative complications, and high satisfaction rates (90%), although success may decrease over time. The subsequent surgery rate within 3 years of EA is approximately 20%. Thermal balloon techniques recently became available and may increase the use of ablation procedures. Long-term outcomes and the question of whether endometrial ablation may affect the early detection of endometrial carcinoma require further investigation.

# Determining the Route of Hysterectomy

In the United States, total abdominal hysterectomy (TAH) is currently performed more commonly than total vaginal hysterectomy (TVH) for treatment of patients who have benign diseases by a ratio of 3:1. Several factors have been implicated:
1. There is less emphasis on vaginal surgery in resident training programs.
2. Clear guidelines are lacking for selecting appropriate candidates for TVH.
3. The adnexa must be evaluated or removed or both evaluated and removed.
4. The majority of physicians habitually use TAH in their practice style.

The ACOG (1990) stated that the choice of route of hysterectomy "depends on the patient's anatomy and the surgeon's experience," and that vaginal hysterectomy is usually performed in women with mobile uteri no larger than 12 weeks' gestational size (280 g), especially if there is uterine descent. However, much larger uteri may be removed vaginally if the surgeon is experienced in reducing techniques, such as morcellation, bivalving, and coring, as discussed later.

The practice style and personal preference of the

surgeon play a significant role in operation selection. In a report on 502 women who had elective inpatient hysterectomies performed by 16 experienced gynecologists, Dorsey noted that, although no nulliparous patients and no patients who had an estimated uterine size greater than 12 weeks of gestation underwent total vaginal hysterectomy, 16.6% and 30.6% of patients who had laparoscopically assisted vaginal hysterectomy (LAVH) had these characteristics, respectively. This fact also suggests strongly that the surgeons who would have used TAH for these patients used LAVH instead.

There is overwhelming evidence that vaginal hysterectomy has a substantial cost advantage over either of the other two procedures. The mean operating time is consistently less for the vaginal hysterectomy group compared with groups who undergo either of the other two approaches, with the LAVH group requiring the longest operating time. However, the higher costs associated with longer operating room times for LAVH compared with TAH may be offset by the costs associated with shorter length of stay.

Van Den Eeden reported that patients who underwent abdominal hysterectomy were significantly slower to return to normal activity than patients who had either TVH or LAVH. TVH clearly results in lower costs and utilization. In addition, they had more favorable functioning, less pain, more energy and vitality, and higher activity profiles than patients who underwent either TAH or LAVH.

Currently, TAHs are performed more often for removal of leiomyomas and known or suspected gynecologic malignancy, whereas TVHs are performed more often for prolapse or bleeding, and LAVHs are performed more often in the presence of endometriosis. Overall, LAVH has increased the use of the vaginal route for uterine removal and has quite possibly spurred a renewed vigor in the use of vaginal hysterectomy without laparoscopic assistance.

## GUIDELINES FOR VAGINAL HYSTERECTOMY

Despite the guidelines for vaginal hysterectomy outlined by the ACOG and many textbooks, uterine size may be less important than access and mobility. Other considerations include the need for concurrent procedures. In general, there are five factors that may create difficulty in executing an exclusively vaginal hysterectomy: a vagina narrower than the width of two finger breadths, a subpubic arch of less than 90 degrees, a bituberous diameter of less than 9 cm, obesity with protuberant buttocks or massive thighs, and congenital abnormalities of the vagina or cervix. Exposure, however, may be facilitated by performing an episiotomy or Schuchardt's incision, using appropriate retractors, and having experienced surgical assistants. Uterine descensus is best assessed with the patient under anesthesia, in cases in which cervical traction may yield unexpected mobility in uteri previously thought to be inaccessible. If the enlarged uterus is immobile, a laparoscopic survey may be warranted, especially when the patient's history is compatible with intra-abdominal adhesions.

## GUIDELINES FOR LAPAROSCOPICALLY ASSISTED VAGINAL HYSTERECTOMY

It has been suggested that LAVH can extend the option of vaginal hysterectomy to many patients who were not previously considered candidates. However, it is not clear in which patients preliminary laparoscopy should be performed or how much of the operation should be done with the laparoscope. A previous cesarean section or another previous pelvic operation is not in itself an indication for LAVH.

In light of its high costs in many centers, specific guidelines incorporating uterine size, risk factors, and uterine and adnexal mobility and accessibility would be useful in selecting the appropriate candidates for LAVH. In fact, laparoscopy may have its greatest value in this regard; it can be used primarily to *determine* the route of hysterectomy. Kovac has proposed a scoring system used at a preliminary laparoscopy in patients who are rescheduled for hysterectomy. Using this system, the need for laparoscopic techniques to permit a vaginal operation may be considerably less than some investigators have proposed. Further randomized trials are needed.

## GUIDELINES FOR ABDOMINAL HYSTERECTOMY

Patients who are not candidates for TVH or LAVH should undergo TAH. Although it is not an absolute contraindication to TVH or LAVH hysterectomy for suspected or known malignancy is usually performed via the abdominal approach. When uterine size or configuration impairs access to uterine vessels, the abdominal route for hysterectomy may be prudent.

## GUIDELINES FOR PROPHYLACTIC OOPHORECTOMY

The abdominal route is occasionally chosen in order to guarantee removal of the ovaries. In 1996, Kovac and Cruikshank attempted to establish objective guidelines for choosing the route of oophorectomy. The degree of ovarian descent was graded by means of a modified system that was previously used to classify pelvic organ prolapse (Table 11-2).

Kovac postulated that "any ovary that was grade I or higher should be visible and accessible for transvaginal removal by most gynecologic surgeons." Of 875 patients, 99.9% had ovaries that were, or could have been, removed based on this postulate. The ovaries were grade II in 813 patients (92.9%) and grade III in 40 patients (4.6%). Before selecting other approaches (LAVH or TAH) that may have greater morbidity, surgeons should document the inability to remove the ovaries transvaginally.

## GUIDELINES FOR CONCURRENT OOPHORECTOMY AND HYSTERECTOMY

Prophylactic oophorectomy performed concurrently with hysterectomy for benign disease remains controversial. Advantages include the prevention of ovarian neoplasms, alleviation of symptoms attributable to continued ovarian function, and elimination of the risk of reoperation for adnexal pathology. Because methods for early detection of ovarian malignancy are not available, prevention of the disease is the primary indication for prophylaxis. The reported incidence of ovarian cancer in women who have undergone a previous hysterectomy is unclear, stemming largely from inconsistent duration and extent of follow-up. Inversely, of all women who have ovarian cancer, the reported incidence of previous hysterectomy with ovarian conservation varies from less than 1% to 14%.

The impact of prophylactic oophorectomy on the incidence of ovarian cancer is also a subject of debate. It has been estimated that 700 prophylactic oophorectomies would be required to prevent one case of ovarian cancer. Additionally, this procedure may not offer total protection in women from families prone to ovarian cancer. In one study involving 28 women from 16 such families, 3 subjects who had previously undergone prophylactic oophorectomy developed intra-abdominal carcinomatosis that was histologically indistinguishable from ovarian cancer. It is thought that in these patients the entire coelomic epithelium may be at risk for malignancy.

Disadvantages of surgical castration include the need for subsequent hormonal replacement therapy and the potential for diminished self-image and adverse effects on libido. According to the National Center for Health Statistics, the frequency with which bilateral oophorectomy accompanies hysterectomy has increased 36% (between 1965 and 1984) to 50% (between 1988 and 1990). Thirty-seven percent of women who are younger than the age of 45 and who undergo hysterectomy now have bilateral oophorectomy, compared with 68% of women who are older than 45 years of age. For all groups, bilateral oophorectomy is significantly more likely to be performed during abdominal rather than vaginal surgery. The indications for ovarian removal should be similar regardless of whether abdominal, laparoscopic, or vaginal hysterectomy is being performed. Current guidelines for women who are not members of high-risk families suggest that prophylactic oophorectomy should be recommended in women who are undergoing hysterectomy and who are older than 45 years of age.

## Postoperative Vaginal Papanicolaou Screening

There are conflicting recommendations regarding whether Papanicolaou smears should be performed in women who have undergone hysterectomy for benign disease. The only analytic study that controlled successfully for previous premalignant or malignant disease suggested that hysterectomy for benign disease is not associated with an increased risk for vaginal cancer. Currently, there is insufficient evidence to recommend routine vaginal smear screening in women who have undergone total hysterectomy for benign disease and who have no history of premalignant or malignant genital disease and no history of maternal diethylstilbestrol (DES) exposure. Critical examination of other purported risk factors may help clarify whether there are subpopulations of women who are at sufficiently increased risk of vaginal cancer to warrant screening.

## Technique

It is not within the purview of this chapter to describe detailed hysterectomy technique. Many surgical

**Table 11-2** Grading System for Ovarian Descent During Vaginal Hysterectomy

| | |
|---|---|
| GRADE 0 | No descent |
| GRADE I | Traction on ovaries brings descent into the long-axis plane of the vagina halfway between the ischial spines and the midvagina |
| GRADE II | With traction on the ovary between the midvagina and the hymenal ring |
| GRADE III | Ovaries can be brought past the hymenal ring with traction |

Adapted from Kovac SR, Cruikshank SH: Guidelines to determine the route of oophorectomy with hysterectomy. Am J Obstet Gynecol 175:1483, 1996.

atlases and texts are available, as are an increasing number of videotapes and other multimedia. All emphasize preoperative evaluation for indications and medical complications, systematic technique, adequate assistance, preparation for unexpected events or findings, avoidance of blind and mass clamping, and recognition and correction of complications during the procedure or in the early postoperative period.

Adequate exposure is vital in reducing operative injury to any abdominal organ or blood vessel. In abdominal surgery, care should be taken in choosing an incision to optimize visualization and mobilization of the pelvic structures, the bowel, and the urinary tract. When exposure of the pelvis is suboptimal, the vertical incision can be extended, and a Pfannenstiel incision can be converted to a Maylard incision.

One important point needs emphasis: To reduce the risk of injury, the path of the ureter must be identified throughout its entire pelvic course for every abdominal and laparoscopic hysterectomy, especially in the presence of adnexal or intraligamentous pathology, which may significantly distort its course. At vaginal hysterectomy, the surgeon should have a comprehensive understanding of the anatomic relationships between the ureter and the uterosacral-cardinal ligament complex and between the ureter and the infundibulopelvic ligament.

Many techniques for the effective vaginal removal of enlarged uteri were developed in the late 1800s, when laparotomy was complicated by poor anesthetic techniques and high mortality rates. Today, there is a renewed interest in alternatives to lapartomy, attributable in part to laparoscopic advances and economic demands for shorter hospitalizations and quicker return to work. These demands require the modern surgeon to become familiar with reliable surgical methods for extirpating large uteri.

Uteri up to 14 weeks of gestation in size can be removed by the vaginal approach with simple morcellation. The limiting factors in larger uteri are access to the uterine arteries and the shape of the lower uterine segment. Large uterine size alone is not a major impediment to safe TVH or LAVH. A large cervical myoma obliterating the vaginal fornices may make anterior and posterior colpotomies difficult to execute. Direct infiltration with vasoconstrictors with subsequent enucleation may avoid the need for laparotomy. The most challenging uterine shape is a smoothly diffuse uterine enlargement associated with a short cervix and limited space lateral to the isthmus, preventing division of the uterosacral-cardinal ligament complex and uterine arteries. If an intraligamentous leiomyoma is suspected, a preliminary intravenous pyelogram to determine the course of the ureters may be warranted.

Before any morcellation technique is attempted during TVH, anterior and posterior colpotomies must be performed, uterosacral-cardinal attachments must be divided, and the uterine arteries must be secured.

# Complications

The mortality rate of hysterectomy for benign nonobstetric indications ranges from 6 to 11 fatalities per 10,000 cases. In obstetric cases, the mortality rate is 29 to 38 per 10,000, and 70 to 200 per 10,000 cases when performed for oncologic reasons. Morbidity rates generally range from 24% vaginal procedures to 43% for abdominal procedures. Complication rates for LAVH vary, depending on the skill of the surgeon and the extent of the disease, and may be lower than rates for TAH and TVH, especially for laparoscopic supracervical hysterectomies.

The effect of any type of hysterectomy on other functions should be considered. It has been estimated that bladder abnormalities may develop in 20 to 30% of patients. Sexual dysfunction reportedly occurs in 20% of patients. A sense of loss accompanied by depression may also occur in patients who have preoperative psychiatric disorders.

## URETERAL INJURY

Approximately 30% of all ureteral injuries are attributed to gynecologic procedures. However, the incidence of such injuries during major gynecologic surgery ranges from 0.3 to 7%. Although the greatest absolute number of injuries occur during TAH (two thirds), there is some debate as to which approach puts the ureter at highest risk. Nichols has suggested that the risk of ureteral injury during a TVH is greater, because the ureters may be pulled down to the uterus by the uterine artery. However, Hofmeister and Kamina have suggested that there is a margin of ureteral safety during each step of a TVH. Cruikshank provides objective evidence that the transection and retraction of the uterosacral-cardinal ligament complex serves to pull the ureter out of the operative field during TVH.

Although the ureters are *statistically* located well away from the uterosacral ligaments in patients who have a prolapsed uterus, this is not invariably so, and, therefore, special care must always be taken. Care must also be taken to avoid ureteral kinking during repairs of large cystocele. As the use of operative laparoscopy has increased, the rates of transection, thermal injury, and stapling damage of the ureters have also increased and appear to be directly related to the surgeon's skill. Cystoscopy with indigo carmine to confirm ureteral patency should be considered in high-risk cases.

The sites of ureteral injury that occur during hysterectomy are diagrammed in Figure 11–2. Although the risk of ureteral injury cannot be completely eliminated, it can be dramatically reduced with identification and meticulous technique (Table 11–3).

## POSTOPERATIVE INFECTION AND PROPHYLACTIC ANTIBIOTICS

The most common complication associated with TVH is a postoperative pelvic infection. Such an infection usually takes the form of a cellulitis affecting the vaginal cuff or the entire pelvic floor. Occasionally, a vaginal cuff abscess or an intraperitoneal abscess may develop as a consequence of surgery. The incidence of operative-site infection after TVH has been reported to be as high as 70%, with an average occurence of 30 to 40%. Within the last two decades, a significant amount of basic and clinical research has been devoted to elucidating the pathophysiology of postoperative infections and evaluating a variety of measures for preventing or reducing the frequency of such infections.

The development of postoperative infection is dependent upon four factors: the size of the inoculum introduced into the surgical wound, the pathogenicity of the micro-organisms, the presence of tissue fluids favorable for growth of bacteria, and the host's inherent resistance to infection.

It has been well established that the vagina harbors a variety of pathogenic bacteria, gram-positive and gram-negative, aerobic and anaerobic. It is impossible to eliminate micro-organisms completely from the operative field, despite a thorough preoperative preparation with antibacterial agents. Incised tissue, incorporated into pedicles, rapidly becomes devitalized and necrotic, thus favoring the growth of pathogenic anaerobic bacteria. Within 48 hours after hysterectomy, an average of 4 ml of serosanguineous fluid, shown to support the growth of a variety of pathogenic bacteria, collects in the retroperitoneal space.

The goal of systemic antibiotic prophylaxis for surgical procedures is to reduce the size of the bacterial inoculum and change the characteristics of the culture medium at the operative site during the brief period of time when tissue defenses are impaired by the trauma of surgery. To be most effective in suppressing infection, antibiotics need to be administered before the bacteria are introduced into the tissue. When antibiotic administration is delayed longer than 3 hours from the time of bacterial inoculation, there is no beneficial effect of antibiotic prophylaxis.

With regard to duration of prophylaxis, several studies clearly demonstrate that prophylactic antibiotics, when indicated, do not need to be administered for extended periods to provide effective prophylaxis (1 to 3 doses).

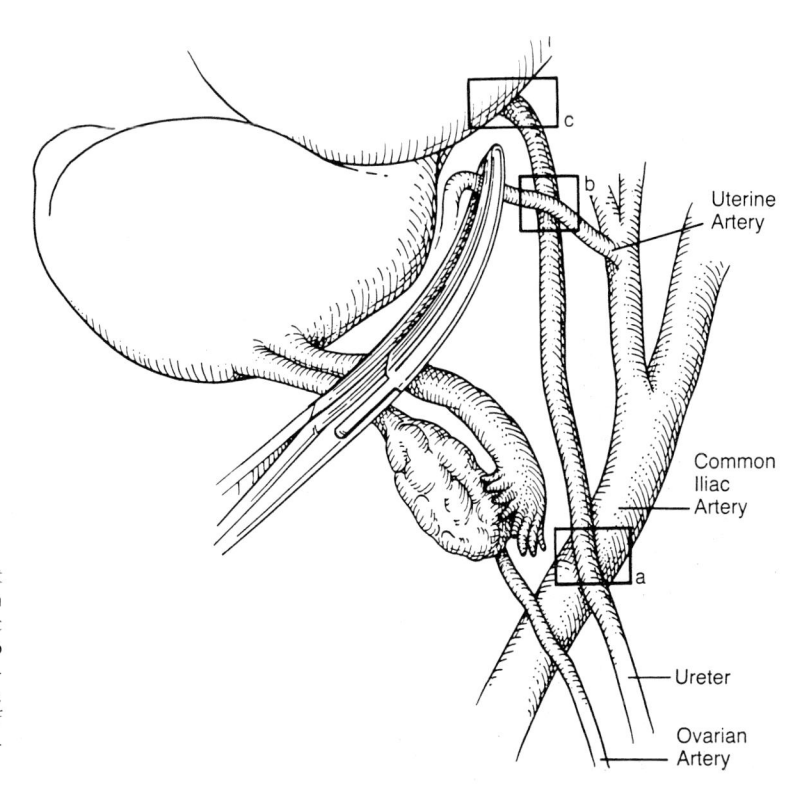

**Figure 11–2** Sites of possible injury to the right ureter. *A,* Where the ureter crosses the common iliac artery and is close to the infundibulopelvic ligament. *B,* Where the ureter passes medial to the uterine artery. *C,* Where the ureter turns medially, close to the cervix, to enter the bladder. (From Newton M, Newton ER: Complications of Gynecologic and Obstetric Management. Philadelphia, WB Saunders, 1988, p 50.)

**Table 11–3** Avoidance of Bladder and Ureteral Injuries in Abdominal Gynecologic Surgery

- Initial sharp dissection of bladder flap.
- Bladder instillation with methylene blue or sterile milk or intentional cystotomy for difficult cases.
- Observation for pericystic fatty tissue (a prebladder wall marker).
- Normalization of anatomy before the placement of clamps. Elevation of adherent pelvic organs completely away from the ovarian fossae prior to the placement of clamps and excision of tissue.
- At mimimum, limited retroperitoneal dissection in all major pelvic operations to visualize the ureter, especially when faced with uterine artery bleeding, retroperitoneal fibrosis, or adnexal masses.
- Palpation of the ureter after opening the retroperitoneal space along the pelvic sidewall at abdominal hysterectomy. The ureter's cord-like structure and the snapping sound made when it is plucked are distinctive. Division of the peritoneum anterior to the palpated ureter before clamping infundibulopelvic and/or utero-ovarian vessels usually ensures ureteral safety. If any questions about ureteral location exists after this maneuver, retroperitoneal dissection and direct ureteral visualization are prudent.
- Skeletonization of the uterine vessels and incision of the posterior peritoneum above the level of the uterosacral ligaments drops the ureters away from where the uterine vessels enter the uterus and cervix.
- Use of vein retractors, Penrose drains, or long malleable ribbon retractors to displace the ureter medially during hypogastric artery ligation, pelvic lymphadenectomy, or both.
- Careful, sharp dissection directly on the ureter anteriorly to perform ureterolysis when necessary.
- A "second bladder flap dissection" at the base of the cervix to ensure clear mobilization of the bladder away from the vaginal cuff after removal of the uterus and cervix during hysterectomy.
- A peritoneum-releasing incision between the uterosacral ligaments and the ureters when performing any culdoplasty procedure that involves uterosacral ligament plication.
- Intrafascial hysterectomy technique should be used whenever possible when dealing with benign disease. This is usually done with a V-shaped incision through the pubovesicocervical fascia, followed by placement of clamps medial to these incisions.
- When pelvic fibrosis prevents palpation or visualization of ureters, begin the retroperitoneal dissection above the bifurcation of the common iliac vessel, above the pelvic brim.
- At the time of cesarean hysterectomy, identification of the cervicovaginal junction may be very difficult, especially in the presence of complete cervical dilatation. In an emergency setting, supracervical hysterectomy reduces the risk of ureteral injury. When excising the cervix, extend the uterine incision downward anteriorly, identify the swollen cervical rim, and apply a Babcock or Allis clamp to the cervical edges. Cervical excision may then be undertaken without fear of excising excessive vaginal tissue and encroaching upon the ureters as they come near the vaginal cuff to enter the bladder trigone.
- Postoperative cystoscopy to identify bladder injury and confirm ureteral patency.

## ANTIBIOTICS IN VAGINAL HYSTERECTOMY

There have been a number of well-designed studies evaluating the use of antibiotic prophylaxis in TVH. Virtually every study has shown that antibiotic administration results in a striking decrease in the incidence of operative site infections and hence in a decrease in febrile morbidity. With the use of antibiotic prophylaxis, the incidence of pelvic infections has been reduced consistently to an average range of 5 to 20%, with an even more significant reduction in the incidence of the more serious types of postoperative infections and abscesses. The efficacy of prophylactic antibiotics applies to all patients undergoing vaginal hysterectomy, regardless of age, menopausal status, or phase of the menstrual cycle.

## SELECTION OF ANTIBIOTIC

In 1975, Ledger established basic guidelines for antibiotic prophylaxis. A prophylactic agent must fulfill the following criteria:

1. Have a spectrum of activity effective against those bacteria most likely to cause or initiate infection
2. Be present in tissue at the operative site in concentrations that will be effective against the most frequent infecting organisms
3. Have demonstrated clinical efficacy
4. Not be an antibiotic that is considered a first-line therapeutic agent
5. Not be responsible for toxicity to the patient
6. Not cause the emergence of resistant bacteria
7. Not cause superinfection
8. Be the least expensive but the most efficacious agent available.

Several studies have shown that the cephamycins, cephalosporins, and semisynthetic penicillins all achieve tissue levels well above the minimal inhibitory concentrations (MIC 90) of gram-positive and gram-negative aerobic and anaerobic bacteria. These antibiotics are capable of reducing the inoculum but not presenting opportunities for any one particular bacterium to dominate. Cefazolin (Kefzol, Ancef) and cephalexin (Keflex), first-generation cephalosporins, have proved as effective as second- and third-generation agents, including cefoxitin.

## ANTIBIOTICS IN ABDOMINAL HYSTERECTOMY

Patients undergoing TAH are at less risk for postoperative pelvic infection, presumably because the pelvic cavity is less likely to be contaminated by bacteria from the lower genital tract. Contamination occurs at the end of the TAH procedure, with incision into the vagina. The period of exposure to bacteria is brief and is followed almost immediately by an infusion of irrigation solution, a step not routinely performed after TVH.

To evaluate the efficacy of antibiotic prophylaxis in abdominal hysterectomy, a meta-analysis by Mittendorf and associates compiled the data from 30 individual studies of 3752 patients. Compared with efficacy rates of vaginal hysterectomy, results are more contradictory. The average reduction of febrile morbidity, pelvic infections, and wound infections was limited to 12, 5, and 5% respectively. Although comparison of the overall rates of operative-site infection among women given antibiotic (9.7%) and among those given placebo (20.4%) is statistically significant ($P<0.001$), because of the limited statistical power of most studies, perioperative antimicrobial treatment was found to be superior to placebo in only 6 of 19 trials. Discrepant findings among different centers emphasize the importance of institutional decisions about the necessity for—and benefits to be expected from—prophylaxis after TAH.

Preoperative vaginal colonization or cervical infection appears to have an important impact on postoperative infection. Two recent reports implicated bacterial vaginosis and trichomonal vaginitis as risk factors for postoperative pelvic infection. None of the women studied were given prophylaxis, and postoperative infection rates for the two groups were 36% and 35%, respectively. The rates of infection among women without evidence of these risk factors was 11% and 4%, respectively. Studies are needed to determine the impact of prophylaxis on outcome in such cases.

In summary, clear benefits or prophylactic antibiotics in vaginal hysterectomy are to be expected. Overall, the data are currently not convincing that the majority of patients undergoing TAH can benefit from antibiotic prophylaxis. Therefore, institutional policy must be established for prophylaxis with TAH and LAVH. Patients should be evaluated for risk factors, such as obesity, peripheral vascular disease, diabetes, collagen disease, and previous history of postsurgical infection. If used, the recommended prophylaxis is 1 or 2 g of cefazolin as described for TVH. The surgeon still has the most important role in preventing infection, and antibiotic prophylaxis serves only as an adjunct to the surgeon's abilities. Tissue handling must be meticulous, good hemostasis must be achieved, and tissue pedicles should be small.

### POSTOPERATIVE VAGINAL VAULT PROLAPSE OR ENTEROCELE

Vaginal eversion after hysterectomy has traditionally been thought of as a problem caused by an enterocele that was not repaired at the time of TVH performed for correction of prolapse. However, half of the patients who have posthysterectomy vaginal eversion, the condition develops after TAH performed for reasons other than prolapse. In addition, this theory does not explain why some patients have an enterocele with a well-supported vaginal apex after hysterectomy, whereas others have both an enterocele and vaginal eversion. Via cadaveric dissection, DeLancey studied the role of individual structures involved in vaginal support. He provided a straightforward description of vaginal support and factors leading to pelvic floor defects in the posthysterectomy patient. The upper third of the vagina (level I) is suspended from the pelvic walls by vertical fibers of the paracolpium, which is a continuation of the cardinal ligament. In the middle third of the vagina (level II), the paracolpium attaches the vagina laterally to the arcus tendineus and fascia of the levator ani muscles. The vagina's lower third fuses with the perineal membrane, the levator ani muscles, and the perineal body (level III). The paracolpium in level I forms the critical factor that differentiates apical vaginal eversion from posthysterectomy cystocele-rectocele or enterocele (level II defects).

Preoperative and intraoperative recognition of anterior, posterior, and apical vaginal support defects are crucial. These defects should be corrected at the time of hysterectomy. Uterosacral ligament shortening, attachment of the cardinal ligaments to the vaginal cuff cul-de-sac obliteration, and intrafascial hysterectomy technique are surgical methods that can reduce posthysterectomy vaginal prolapse and enterocele.

## Long-Term Sequelae

### SEXUAL FUNCTIONING

Sexual function and dysfunction are endpoints that are extermely difficult to measure objectively. The overwhelming evidence suggests that total hysterectomy has little if any effect on sexual functioning, including the ability to achieve orgasm. Yet, planned supracervical hysterectomy is being performed increasingly for the ostensible patient benefit of improved sexual function. Short-term studies suggest this advantage, although the data are of a preliminary nature. Because of effective cervical cancer screening, supracervical hysterectomy is a viable alternative in selected patients without a history of cervical disease.

### PSYCHOLOGICAL SEQUELAE AND CLIMACTERIC COMPLAINTS

Current medical opinion that hormonal changes do not occur after simple hysterectomy may be incorrect.

A survey based on 6622 women ranging from 39 to 60 years of age showed that women in all age groups who have had a hysterectomy with one or both ovaries preserved report more severe climacteric symptoms (flushes or sweating and vaginal dryness) than women who have not had a hysterectomy. In a study by Oldenhave, women who have had hysterectomies, especially those aged 39 to 41 years, reported significantly more vasomotor complaints, vaginal dryness, and atypical complaints mimicking nonpsychotic psychiatric disturbances (anxiety and depression) than did women of the same age who had experienced a normal climacteric. The literature indicates that women who have undergone hysterectomy with ovarian conservation are over-represented with regard to cardiovascular disease, osteoporosis and osteoarthritis, depression, and sexual problems (i.e., vaginal dryness, dyspareunia, and decreased libido). A mean acceleration of 4 years in postmenopausal follicle-stimulating hormone and luteinizing-hormone levels has been observed in women who have had hysterectomy without oophorectomy.

# Conclusion

With adherence to the changing guidelines for hysterectomy, along with the increasing availability of less invasive and less morbid alternatives, gynecologists can perform this operation with more confidence, knowing that it is the optimal procedure. Individualization is extremely important in choosing specific treatment, and both patient and surgeon must realize that all management decisions require ongoing evaluation and potential for change. It is essential that gynecologists remain knowledgeable regarding published surgical success rates in addition to their individual outcomes.

## REFERENCES

ACOG Technical Bulletin #111: Prophylactic Oophorectomy. Washington, DC, American College of Obstetricians and Gynecologists, December 1987.

Allahabadia GN, Nalawady V, Patkar VD, et al: The Sion test. Aust N Z J Obstet Gynecol 32:67, 1992.

American College of Obstetrics and Gynecology Task Force on Quality Assurance: Quality Assurance: Quality Assurance in Obstetrics and Gynecology. Washington, DC, American College of Obstetrics and Gynecology, 1989.

American College of Obstetrics and Gynecology Task Force on Quality Assurance: Quality Assurance and Improvement in Obstetrics and Gynecology. Washington, DC, American College of Obstetrics and Gynecology, 1994.

Atlee WL: Case of a successful extirpation of a fibrous tumor of the peritoneal surface of the uterus by the large peritoneal section. Am J Med Sci 9:309, 1845.

Bardequez AD: Uterine Leiomyomas in pregnancy. Clin Consult Obstet Gynecol 2:53–57, 1990.

Bernstein SJ, McGlynn EA, Siu AL, et al: The appropriateness of hysterectomy: A comparison of care in seven health plans. JAMA 269:2398, 1993.

Bolling DR, Plunkett GD: Prophylactic antibiotics for vaginal hysterectomies. Obstet Gynecol 41:689,1972.

Buttram VC, Reiter RC: Uterine leiomyomata—etiology, symptomatology and management. Fertil Steril 36:433, 1981.

Campbell S, Royston P, Bhan V, et al: Novel screening strategies for early ovarian cancer by transabdominal ultrasonography. Br J Obstet Gynaecol 97:304, 1990.

Carlson KJ, Nichols DH, Schiff I: Indications for hysterectomy. N Engl J Med 328:856, 1993.

Crosignani PG, Aimi G, Vercellini P, et al: Hysterectomy for benign gynecologic disorders: When and why? Postgrad Med 100:133, 1996.

Cruikshank SH, Kovac SR: Role of the uterosacral-cardinal ligament complex in protecting the ureter during vaginal hysterectomy. Int J Gynecol Obstet 40:141, 1993.

DeLancey JO: Anatomic aspects of vaginal eversion after hysterectomy. Am J Obstet Gynecol 166:1717, 1992.

Dicker RC, Greenspan JR: Complications of abdominal and vaginal hysterctomy among women of reproductive age in the United States. Am J Obstet Gynecol 144:841, 1982.

Dicker RC, Greenspan JR, Strauss LT, et al: Hysterectomy among women of reproductive age: Trends in the United States, 1970–1978. JAMA 248:323, 1982.

Dorsey JH, Steinberg EP, Holtz PM: Clinical indications for hysterectomy route: Patient characteristics or physician preference? Am J Obstet Gynecol 173:1452, 1995.

Elkins T: Syllabus: The simple vesicovaginal fistula. 7th Annual Urogynecology and Disorders of the Female Pelvic Floor Conference. Mayo Clinic, Scottsdale, 1998.

Ferenczy A, Gelfand M: The biologic significance of cytologic atypia in progesterone-treated endometrial hyperplasia. Am J Obstet Gynecol 160:126, 1989.

Fetters MD, Fischer G, Reed BD: Effectiveness of vaginal Papanicolaou smear screening after total hysterectomy for benign disease. JAMA 275:940, 1996.

Franssen AMHW, Willemsen WNP, Corbey RS, et al: Subcutaneous injection or infusion of gonadotropin-releasing agonist buserelin in the treatment of enlarged uteri harboring leiomyomata. Eur J Obstet Gynecol Reprod Biol 40:221, 1991.

Freidman AJ, Hoffman DI, Comite F, et al: Treatment of leiomyomata uteri with leuprolide acetate depo: A double-blind placebo-controlled multicenter study, the Leuprolide Study Group. Obstet Gynecol 77:720, 1991.

Freidman AJ, Sobel S, Rein MS, et al: Efficacy and safety considerations in women with uterine leiomyomas treated with GnRH-releasing hormone agonists: The estrogen threshold hypothesis. Am J Obstet Gynecol 163:1114, 1990.

Gath D, Cooper P, Day A: Hysterectomy and psychiatric disorder. I: Levels of psychiatric morbidity before and after hysterectomy. Br J Psychiatr 140:335, 1982.

Goodwin SC, Vedantham S, McLucas B, et al: Preliminary experience with uterine artery embolization for uterine fibroids. J Vasc Interv Radiol 8:517, 1997.

Graves EJ: Detailed diagnoses and procedures. In: National Hospital Discharge Survey: United States, 1990. Vital Health Stat 13:118, 1991.

Green TH: Urinary stress incontinence: Differential diagnosis, pathophysiology, and management. Am J Obstet Gynecol 122:368, 1975.

Hannigan EV, Gomez LG: Uterine leiomyosarcoma: A review of prognostic clinical and pathological features. Am J Obstet Gynecol 134:557, 1979.

Hasson HM: Cervical removal at hysterectomy for benign disease: Risks and benefits. J Reprod Med 38:781, 1993.

Hasson HM: Incidence of endometriosis in diagnostic laparoscopy. J Reprod Med 16:135–138, 1976.

Herman JM, Homesley HD, Dignan MB: Is hysterectomy a risk factor for vaginal cancer. JAMA 256:601, 1986.

Hofmeister FJ, Wolfgran RC: Methods of demonstrating measurement relationships between vaginal hysterectomy ligatures and the ureters. Am J Obstet Gynecol 83:938, 1962.

Jequier AM: Urinary symptoms and total hysterectomy. Br J Urol 48:437, 1976.

Kamina P: De l'anatomie a la technique de l'hysterectomie vaginale. Rev Fr Gynecol Obstet 85:435, 1990.

Klempner MS, Styrt B: Clindamycin uptake by human neutrophils. J Infect Dis 144:472, 1981.

Kovac SR, Cruikshank SH, Retto HF: Laparoscopy-assisted vaginal hysterectomy. J Gynecol Surg 6:185, 1990.

Kovac SR: Guidelines to determine the route of hysterectomy. Obstet Gynecol 85:18, 1995.

Kovac SR, Cruikshank SH: Guidelines to determine the route of oophorectomy with hysterectomy. Am J Obstet Gynecol 175:1483, 1996.

Kurman RJ, Kaminski PF, Norris HJ: The behavior of endometrial hyperplasia. A long-term study of "untreated" hyperplasia in 170 patients. CA Cancer J Clin 56:403, 1985.

Landers DV, Sweet RL, Tubo-ovarian abscess: Contemporary approach to management. Rev Infect Dis 5:876, 1983.

Langer R, Ron-E1 R, Neuman M, et al: The value of simultaneous hysterectomy during Burch colposuspension for urinary stress incontinence. Obstet Gynecol 72:866, 1988.

Loffer FD: Removal of large symptomatic intrauterine growths by the hysteroscopic resectoscope. Obstet Gynecol 76:836, 1990.

Lu PY, Ory SJ: Endometriosis: Current management. Mayo Clin Proc 70:453, 1995.

Lumsden MA, West CP, Thomas E, et al: Treatment with the gonadotrophin releasing hormone-agonist goserelin before hysterectomy for uterine fibroids. Br J Obstet Gynaecol 101:438, 1994.

Lynch HT, Conway T, Lynch J: Hereditary ovarian cancer. *In* Sharp F, Mason WP, Leake RE (eds): Ovarian Cancer: Biologic and Therapeutic Challenges. Cambridge, Chapman and Hall Medical, 1990, p 719.

Lyons TL: Laparoscopic supracervical hysterectomies: A comparison of morbidity and mortality results with laparoscopic assisted vaginal hysterectomies. J Reprod Med 38:763, 1993.

Mann WJ, Koonings PP: Ureteral injuries in gynecologic surgery. Int Urogynecol J 4:361, 1993.

Mattingly RF, Thompson JD: Operative Gynecology, 6th ed. Philadelphia, JB Lippincott, 1985, p 218.

McGowan L: Ovarian cancer after hysterectomy. Obstet Gynecol 69:1024, 1979.

Mittendorf R, Aronson MP, Berry RE, et al: Avoiding serious infections associated with abdominal hysterectomy: A meta-analysis of antibiotic prophylaxis. Am J Obstet Gynecol 169:1119–1124, 1993.

Morley GW: Indications for hysterectomy. *In*: TeLind's Operative Gynecology Updates. Philadelphia, JB Lippincott Co, 1993.

Namnoum AB, Gehlbach DL, Hickman TN, et al: Incidence of symptom recurrence after hysterectomy for endometriosis. Fertil Steril 64:898, 1995.

Newton M, Newton E (eds). Complications of Gynecologic and Obstetric Management. Philadelphia, WB Saunders Company, 1988, p 50.

Nezhat CH, Nezhat F, Roemisch M, et al: Laparoscopic trachelectomy for persistent pelvic pain and endometriosis after supracervical hysterectomy. Fertil Steril 66:925, 1996.

Nichols DH: Vaginal hysterectomy. *In* Nichols DH, Randalp CL (eds): Vaginal Surgery, 3rd ed. Baltimore, Williams and Wilkins, 1989.

Nielsen K: Carcinoma of the cervix following supracervical hysterectomy. Acta Radiol 37:335, 1952.

O'Connor H, Broadbent JA, Magos AL, et al: Medical Research Council randomized trial of endometrial resection versus hysterectomy in management of menorrhagia. Lancet 349:897, 1997.

Oldenhave A, Jaszmann LJB, Everaerd W, et al: Hysterectomized women with ovarian conservation report more severe climacteric complaints than do normal climacteric women of similar age. Am J Obstet Gynecol 168:765, 1993.

Parys BT, Haylen BT, Hutton JL, et al: The effects of simple hysterectomy on vesicourethral function. Br J Urol 64:594, 1989.

Pelosi MA, Kadar N: Laparoscopically assisted hysterectomy for uteri weighing 500 g or more. J Am Assoc Gynecol Laparosc 1:405, 1994.

Pokras R, Hunagel V: Hysterectomy in the United States, 1965–1984. Am J Public Health 78:852, 1988.

Precis IV: An update in obstetrics and gynecology. Washington, DC, American College of Obstetricians and Gynecologists, 1990, p 197.

Randall CL, Hall DW, Armenia CS: Pathology in the preserved ovary after unilateral oophorectomy. Am J Obstet Gynecol 84:1233, 1962.

Ransom SB, McNeeley SG, White C, et al: A cost analysis of endometrial ablation, vaginal hysterectomy, abdominal hysterectomy, and LAVH in the treatment of primary menorrhagia. J Am Assoc Gynecol Laparosc 4:29, 1996.

Rein MS, Freidman AJ, Stuart JM, et al: Fibroid and myometrial steroid receptors in women treated with gonadotropin-releasing hormone agonist leuprolide acetate. Fertil Steril 53:1018, 1990.

Rein MS, Barbieri RL, Friedman AJ: Progesterone: A critical role in the pathogenesis of uterine myomas. Am J Obstet Gynecol 172:14, 1995.

Reiter RC, Wagner PL, Gambone JC: Routine hysterectomy for large asymptomatic uterine leiomyomata: A reappraisal. Obstet Gynecol 79:481, 1992.

Richardson GS, Scully RE, Nikrui N: Common epithelial cancer of the ovary. N Engl J Med 312:415, 1985.

Rivlin ME, Hunt JA: Ruptured tuboovarian abscess. Is hysterectomy necessary? Obstet Gynecol 50:519, 1977.

Serra GB, Panetta V, Colosimo M, et al: Efficacy of leuprorelin acetate depo in symptomatic fibromyomatous uteri: The Italian Multicentre Trial. Clin Ther 14(suppl):57, 1992.

Shekelle PG, Kahan JP, Bernstein SJ, et al: The reproducibility of a method to identify the overuse and underuse of medical procedures. N Engl J Med 338:1888, 1998.

Stovall TG, Ling FW, Crawford DA: Hysterectomy for chronic pelvic pain of presumed uterine etiology. Obstet Gynecol 75:676, 1990.

Tobacman JK, Greene MH, Tucker MA, et al: Intraabdominal carcinomatosis after prophylactic oophorectomy in ovarian-cancer-prone families. Lancet 2:795, 1982.

Van Den Eeden SK, Glasser M, Mathias SD, et al: Quality of life, health care utilization, and costs among women undergoing hysterectomy in a managed-care setting. Am J Obstet Gynecol 178:91, 1998.

Verkauf BS: Changing trends in treatment of leiomyomata uteri. Curr Opin Obstet Gynecol 5:301, 1993.

Vilos GA, Vilos EC, Pendley L: Endometrial ablation with a thermal balloon for the treatment of menorrhagia. J Am Assoc Gynecol Laparosc 3:383, 1996.

Vollenhoven BJ, Lawrence AS, Healy DL: Uterine fibroids: A clinical review. Br J Obstet Gynaecol 97:285, 1990.

Walker E, Katon W, Harrop-Griffiths J, et al: Relationship of chronic pelvic pain to psychiatric diagnoses and childhood sexual abuse. Am J Psychiatr 145:75, 1988.

Wilcox LS, Koonin LM, Pokras R, et al: Hysterectomy in the United States, 1988–1990. Obstet Gynecol 83:549, 1994.

Wingo PA, Huezo CM, Rubin GL, et al: The mortality risk associated with hysterectomy. Am J Obstet Gynecol 152:803, 1985.

# 12

# Laparoscopy

STEVEN J. ORY

Laparoscopy is currently the most commonly performed gynecologic surgical procedure. Applications for laparoscopic surgery have dramatically expanded over the past 15 years as a consequence of numerous technical advances. Many surgical procedures that previously could only be accomplished via laparotomy can now be performed endoscopically, with many advantages accruing to the patient. These include decreased cost associated with surgery performed in an ambulatory setting, more rapid recuperation and return to normal activities, less postoperative pain and fewer requirements for analgesia, and more acceptable cosmetic results. Although laparoscopic procedures have not been shown to be more effective than comparable procedures performed via laparotomy, most series have demonstrated comparable efficacy.

Technical improvements include the introduction of new laparoscope designs; better light sources, such as xenon, for use in laser-powered lamps; video chip cameras; rapid insufflation devices that permit a continuous pneumoperitoneum to be maintained; and a broader selection of operative instruments, including special devices for laparoscopic suturing.

## Equipment

Several different options are available for the laparoscope itself. A straight laparoscope provides the clearest view of pelvic structures. If the laparoscope is outfitted with an operative channel, the head of the laparoscope is either offset 45 degrees from the longitudinal axis of the laparoscope or placed parallel to the main body of the laparoscope, with a right-angle optic attachment permitting direct introduction of an operative instrument and functional use of the laparoscope. The operative laparoscope offers an additional operative port but it has the disadvantages of significantly decreased maneuverability and visibility, particularly with low light settings.

Several choices are available for the optics of the laparoscope. The ocular lens may be offset 0 to 30 degrees. The zero-degree lens has generally been most popular and provides a straight-ahead view. The 30-degree optic, or foreoblique, lens has the advantage of providing an oblique view of the structure at the end of the laparoscope and may be preferred if a beam splitter is used. This has greater applicability in confined spaces and is a preferable optic for a hysteroscope. Laparoscopes are available with varying diameters, from 2 to 10 mm.

Xenon light sources provide the most intense cold light for endoscopy and have largely replaced previous halogen light sources. They are particularly well adapted to the video chip camera and photodocumentation. The fiberoptic light cables that provide the light source for the laparoscope are critical for optimal illumination. The efficiency of light transmission increases with the cord diameter, and most cables provide a cord diameter comparable with the laparoscope. The fibers can be easily fractured, which diminishes light transmission.

The chip video camera has undergone many technical refinements. The current generation of lightweight cameras mount securely on the laparoscope; they provide superb image quality and can be easily focused and controlled from the handset. They provide a highly accurate and reliable image for one or more television monitors and can also be used for video recording and still photography. Beam-splitter video cameras, which permit direct viewing through the laparoscope with simultaneous video camera imaging on the monitors are still available, but most laparoscopic procedures are now performed without direct viewing through the laparoscope. Although initially requiring more training and skill, operating from video monitors permits assistants to have the same view of the operative field as the surgeon. This approach also allows the operator to assume a more technically effective and comfortable posture while performing laparoscopic operations.

Most laparoscopic procedures are now performed with high-flow insufflators that permit a pneumoperitoneum to be maintained with a preset intra-abdominal pressure. High-flow insufflators are essential for preserving adequate abdominal distention and clearing smoke from the operative field when extensive operative procedures employing the laser or electrocautery are used. All such insufflators have a regulator to control the pressure and flow rate of the insufflation. They also have a pressure gauge that reflects the actual intra-abdominal pressure, and a flow ball or other indicator to confirm patency of the system. If intra-abdominal pressure is excessive, venous return to the heart is impeded and increased ventilatory pressure is required to sustain the patient.

Additional instruments unique to laparoscopy include several variations of the Veres needle for insufflation. Also, several permanent and disposable trocars and sleeves are available in varying diameters for introduction of the laparoscope and operative instruments. A variety of suction irrigation systems are available, permitting rapid evacuation of fluid and gas from the abdomen. Irrigation fluids can be forcibly directed to the operative site. Suction devices can be connected to wall suction and filtering systems to prevent recirculation within the operating room. Some suction-irrigation probes also include a cautery, which allows the surgeon to aspirate, irrigate, and achieve hemostasis with the same instrument.

Equipment for ensuring hemostasis should be available in the operating room before the onset of the procedure. Both bipolar and unipolar cautery can be safely used for this. Various electrocautery power sources are available, activated either by foot pedal or by controls mounted on the device. The current generation of electrosurgical units employ high-frequency, low-voltage generators and are much improved over the previously available spark-gap units. Incision of tissues, a basic surgical technique, can be accomplished through the laparoscope with laparoscopic scissors of various designs, a laparoscopic scalpel inserted through a 5-mm sheath, an electrocautery, or a laser.

## ELECTROCAUTERY AND LASER

Electrocautery and laser both break down tissue by using high-power density energy systems to produce tissue heating and destruction. In the case of electrocautery, energy is produced in the form of electrons, whereas photons are coherently produced with the laser. Upon impact with tissue, electrons and photons generate energy. This in turn is absorbed by intracellular components that produce thermal damage. The degree of peripheral heating is influenced by the vascularity and density of the tissue; heat is dissipated through the vascular and lymphatic systems. Both laser and electrocautery seal the vessels and lymphatics but also produce ischemia and adjacent tissue necrosis. This field effect can be minimized with electrocautery and laser systems that pulse the energy, allowing intermittent dissipation of heat through the vascular and lymphatic channels. The power density and watts per $cm^2$ reflect the energy delivered to the tissue, and the area of thermal damage is inversely related to the power density. The power density can be calculated by the equation

$$Pd = W \times 100/sa^2.$$

Pd represents the power density, W is the power in watts, and sa is the surface area in millimeters of the laser beam or electrocautery tip. In order to minimize the field effect or zone of thermal damage, a Pd of greater than 2500 $W/cm^2$ should be maintained for the carbon dioxide laser using pulsed waveforms; and a Pd greater than 5000 $W/cm^2$ should be used for continuous waveform energy sources, including electrocautery. When endometriotic tissue is being vaporized with continuous waveform energy power, densities of 1000 to 4000 $W/cm^2$ are acceptable. The field effect rapidly increases, and additional undesired tissue damage occurs if the Pd decreases below these limits. This may be desirable when working in highly vascular tissues to maintain the hemostatic properties of the energy, but it is undesirable when it is important to minimize subsequent adhesion formation.

The carbon dioxide laser has been the most extensively used laser in laparoscopic surgery. It offers the advantages of greater safety and lower cost than those of other lasers. The argon laser, the neodymium: yttrium-aluminum-garnet (Nd:YAG) laser, and the potassium-titanyl-phosphate (KTP-532) laser have also been successfully used through the laparoscope, but their additional cost has limited their availability. All have unique properties, with differences in color absorption of the beam, wavelengths, beam-scattering effects, and depth of penetration.

### SUTURING INSTRUMENTS

Several techniques have been developed for the placement of sutures by the laparoscope. Laparoscopic suturing requires substantial technical proficiency and practice. Modified surgical needles can be introduced through the laparoscope and ligatures placed with special laparoscopic needle holders. Once placed, knots can be secured either intra-abdominally or by extracorporeal techniques in which the knot is placed outside the abdomen and passed down through a laparoscopic sleeve. Several techniques have been developed to secure these knots, including a modified fisherman's knot and the Roeder and Duncan knots. Pretied loops in a variety of suture materials are available. These loops can be placed over tissue and secured by cinching the knots into place. There are also a variety of stapling devices and clip applicators, the former capable of simultaneously dividing and ligating tissues with a row of staples. Titanium clips can be applied to vessels for hemostasis.

### TISSUE REMOVAL

Several techniques can be employed to remove tissue through the laparoscope. Often the tissue to be removed is larger than the 5- or 10-mm diameter of the accessory sleeves. The tissue may be divided in the abdomen by laparoscopic morcellators or scissors and forceps and removed from the abdomen piecemeal. Often, it is desirable to use a 5-mm sheath instead of a 10-mm one. There are several plastic and Silastic pouches available, which can be introduced into the abdomen through a 10-mm sleeve. These pouches are large enough to contain most gynecologic specimens (e.g., cysts, ovaries, fallopian tubes, ectopic pregnancies). Once the tissue is placed within the pouch, a pursestring can be drawn, securing the specimen within the pouch. If the specimen cannot be easily removed through a 10-mm sleeve, the sleeve can be withdrawn, and the incision can be extended slightly to permit removal of the intact specimen inside the pouch.

## Technique

### ANESTHESIA

General anesthesia is preferred by most surgeons for performing laparoscopy. In order to ensure adequate ventilation with increased intra-abdominal pressure in the Trendelenburg position, endotracheal intubation is essential. Violent contractions of the diaphragm and abdominal musculature can be avoided, and maximal visibility can be achieved only when the patient is fully relaxed. This state of relaxation can be achieved by administration of a succinylcholine drip.

Local anesthesia offers greater respiratory safety than is obtained with general anesthesia, and it may be used for short diagnostic procedures in selected patients. Modern analgesics, including midazolam and alfentanil, permit greater patient comfort; however, these drugs result in depressed respiration, and, therefore, supplemental oxygen provided by nasal cannula is recommended. If this technique is employed, surgery must be smooth and deliberate, and abrupt motion must be avoided to maintain patient comfort. The insufflating gas can be either carbon dioxide or nitrous oxide. Nitrous oxide is associated with less peritoneal irritation than carbon dioxide, which produces carbonic acid, but it may be associated with more intestinal distention. Nitrous oxide does support combustion, but it has been safely used for electrocoagulation. It is absorbed from the bloodstream approximately 60% as rapidly as carbon dioxide.

## Pneumoperitoneum

Most surgeons prefer to establish a pneumoperitoneum before introducing the laparoscopic trocar and sleeve. However, successful techniques for safe introduction of a 10-mm trocar without previous creation of a pneumoperitoneum have been described. The use of a Veres needle may reduce the risk of injury to the bowel but not to the large vessels. After introducing the Veres needle, correct intra-abdominal placement can be confirmed by several tests, including injection of saline into the abdomen. Also, if the insufflator registers negative pressure, the Veres needle may be attached to the insufflation tubing before initiating insufflation to confirm the intra-abdominal position. If the abdominal skin is grasped and elevated lateral to the umbilicus, a negative intra-abdominal pressure registers on the pressure gauge. This is a highly reliable test for confirming intra-abdominal placement. After correct placement is confirmed, the initial flow rate should be 1 L/min or less until a pneumoperitoneum is established. Obese patients may require additional abdominal distention and intra-abdominal pressure as high as 20 to 25 mm Hg before trocar insertion. After the laparoscope has been correctly positioned, maintenance pressures for the insufflator should not exceed 16 to 20 mm Hg.

## TROCAR AND SLEEVE INSERTION

Insertion of the 10-mm laparoscopic trocar and sleeve should be performed with the operative table in a horizontal position. Insertion performed with the patient in the Trendelenburg position has been associated with major vascular injuries. Several techniques have been described, including elevation of the abdominal wall and direct insertion using only intra-abdominal pressure for resistance. The trocar should be sharp before it is introduced into the patient. Newer disposable trocars with protective sheaths that ensure sharpness and offer some protection are available; however, vascular and bowel injuries have been reported with the sheathed trocars as well. Special care should be taken with patients who have had multiple previous abdominal procedures and those otherwise suspected of having significant intra-abdominal adhesions. Some surgeons prefer to pass a spinal needle connected with a syringe filled with saline before introducing the trocar. This permits delineation of a free space below the umbilicus. Alternatively, performing an open laparoscopy technique, such as that described by Hasson, may help minimize the risk of vessel and bowel injury.

Most operative laparoscopic procedures require placement of one to three ancillary trocars in sleeves. These are usually 5 mm in diameter. For most diagnostic procedures, a single midline suprapubic trocar may be placed. If two ports are required, they should be placed at least 4 cm above the pubic symphysis and generally lateral to the edge of the rectus muscles to avoid the inferior epigastric vessels. Transilluminating the abdominal wall with the laparoscope may help identify vessels.

## Procedures

### INDICATIONS

Most gynecologic operations performed via laparotomy have been attempted through the laparoscope. The list of successful laparoscopic procedures continues to expand (Table 12–1). Laparoscopic procedures are generally performed for evaluation and treatment of pelvic pain, infertility, ectopic pregnancy, and pelvic masses. Tubal ligation performed at laparoscopy is the most commonly performed sterilization procedure. Laparoscopy may also play a role in the evaluation and delineation of müllerian anomalies in patients who have ambiguous genitalia, allowing identification of internal genitalia. Laparoscopy is still used in assisted reproductive technologies, although to a lesser extent now that most oocyte retrievals are performed with transvaginal ultrasonography. Laparoscopy is still used for gamete intrafallopian transfer (GIFT) and zygote intrafallopian transfer (ZIFT).

**Table 12–1** Laparoscopic Gynecologic Procedures

1. Adhesiolysis
2. Appendectomy
3. Laparoscopic-assisted vaginal hysterectomy (LAVH)
4. Myomectomy
5. Neosalpingostomy
6. Oophorectomy
7. Ovarian cystectomy
8. Ovarian wedge resection and ovarian drilling procedures
9. Salpingectomy (complete or partial for ectopic pregnancy)
10. Salpingo-oophorectomy
11. Salpingostomy or salpingotomy for ectopic pregnancy
12. Sterilization
13. Transection of uterosacral ligaments (laparoscopic uterine nerve ablation [LUNA] procedure)
14. Uterine suspension
15. Vaporization and excision of endometriosis
16. Suspension of bladder neck (Burch or Marshall-Marchetti-Krantz procedure)

LUNA = laparoscopic uterine nerve ablation.

For patients who have chronic pelvic pain, laparoscopy is frequently part of the evaluation. Laparoscopy is indicated after a physical examination has been performed, and after appropriate studies, including ultrasonography and laboratory evaluations, have either been inconclusive or if they further support the need to perform this procedure. Acute and chronic pelvic infections, endometriosis, ectopic pregnancy, adnexal torsion, hemorrhagic ovarian cysts, and non-gynecologic problems, including appendicitis, are routinely diagnosed by laparoscopy. Less commonly, pelvic foreign bodies, including displaced intrauterine devices and complications of hysteroscopy, can be evaluated and treated by laparoscopy.

Laparoscopy is an essential part of a comprehensive infertility evaluation. Not all infertile patients require laparoscopy, but patients who have signs and symptoms of endometriosis and tubal disease should undergo laparoscopy early in their evaluation. However, with improvements in the assisted reproductive technologies, the relative benefit of laparoscopy in patients who have tubal disease and endometriosis is less clear than it was previously. Patients who have extensive disease, including endometrioma formation, may benefit from surgery, particularly if in vitro fertilization is to be considered in the future. Patients who have distal tubal occlusion and large hydrosalpinx formation may improve their chances of success with in vitro fertilization by undergoing salpingectomy before proceeding with in vitro fertilization. Patients who have less extensive disease may benefit from confirmation of disease, repair of minor abnormalities, and lysis of pelvic adhesions.

Patients who have unexplained infertility should

also consider undergoing laparoscopy, because as many as 50% of these individuals have abnormalities found by laparoscopy. This is particularly true when empiric treatments, such as superovulation therapy with or without intrauterine insemination, have been unsuccessful. Laparoscopy performed for infertility should include the careful inspection of all pelvic organs, including the undersurface of both ovaries and tubes and an assessment of tubal patency; this examination is usually accomplished by means of transcervical injection of dye.

Ectopic pregnancy can often be diagnosed without resorting to laparoscopy, and such patients may be candidates for nonoperative medical therapy. However, a substantial proportion of patients who have ectopic pregnancy require laparoscopy because they defy current medical diagnostic algorithms. They present with pain or hypovolemia, or they elect surgical treatment. If laparoscopy is required for diagnosis, treatment should be accomplished at the time of surgery, because there is no apparent advantage in using subsequent medical treatment in this instance. Requirements for laparoscopic treatment include hemodynamic stability and an accessible pelvis.

Laparoscopy is well suited for the diagnostic evaluation of pelvic masses, and often treatment can be instituted at the same time. A variety of benign neoplasms, including ovarian endometrioma, pedunculated myomas, and peritubal cysts, can be safely and effectively removed through the laparoscope. Rupture of dermoid cysts at the time of laparoscopic resection has been reported to produce chemical peritonitis. There have been 42 cases of laparoscopic excision of ovarian neoplasms subsequently determined to be malignant. In questionable cases, it is preferable to perform a minilaparotomy or laparotomy to avoid an intra-abdominal spill. The preoperative assessment of adnexal masses is essential in the selection of appropriate candidates for laparotomy.

## CONTRAINDICATIONS

Absolute contraindications to laparoscopy include uncontrolled intra-abdominal bleeding with hypovolemia, diaphragmatic hernia, bowel obstruction, severe ileus, and cardiopulmonary compromise in the presence of large undiagnosed masses. Relative contraindications to laparoscopy include known or suspected extensive abdominal or pelvic adhesions, intrauterine pregnancy, ascites, and morbid obesity.

# Operations

## PELVIC ADHESIONS

The laparoscope has a number of theoretical surgical advantages that make it well suited for the treatment of pelvic adhesions, including the opportunity to use magnification, fine atraumatic instruments, and copious irrigation. Lysis of adhesions by laparoscopic scissors, electrocautery, and laser has produced results comparable with those achieved by laparotomy if pelvic pain and infertility have been the outcomes measured. Treatment is generally intended to restore the normal anatomic position and range of motion of the pelvic structures. Fimbrioplasty or neosalpingostomy can be performed with the same instruments that are used to treat distal tubal occlusion. Pregnancy rates following tubal surgery are correlated with the degree of damage, but overall they are disappointing, with only about 30% of patients who have distal tubal occlusion achieving successful intrauterine pregnancy after surgery.

## ENDOMETRIOSIS

Laparoscopy and laparotomy provide the only methods of definitively confirming the diagnosis of endometriosis. Moreover, these two procedures offer the opportunity of staging the disease. Endometriosis can usually be treated at the time of laparoscopy. The intent of the procedure is to excise or destroy all visible endometriotic lesions and lyse all adhesions that restrict normal mobility to the tubes and ovaries. This is undertaken to treat associated pain or infertility. Endometriotic implants may assume a variety of appearances, and it may be difficult to identify all lesions in the patient who has extensive disease.

Ovarian endometriomas represent a unique therapeutic challenge. They can often be detected before laparoscopy by ultrasonography. Recurrence is common and treatment should be directed toward removal of the entire cyst. This is usually performed by opening and draining the endometrioma. Then the cyst wall is grasped and carefully removed with gentle traction from the attached ovarian tissue. Simple aspiration of the cyst and hormonal suppression are almost invariably associated with recurrence.

## ECTOPIC PREGNANCY

Studies comparing laparoscopic treatment of ectopic pregnancy with treatment performed via laparotomy have documented shorter hospitalization, more rapid convalescence, lower cost, and comparable future fertility. Operative time is generally reduced when experienced surgeons perform the procedure, and the requirements for postoperative analgesia are fewer with laparoscopy as well. Before proceeding to surgery, the surgeon should have a full understanding of the patient's reproductive plans. Salpingectomy should be performed in patients who do not desire subsequent pregnancy or in cases of irreparable tubal damage. Salpingectomy may also be indicated if hemostasis cannot be achieved with a conservative procedure or if the patient has had prior ectopic pregnancies in the same tube.

Linear salpingostomy is the treatment of choice for patients who have ampullary ectopic pregnancies. This procedure can be accomplished by making an incision with electrocautery, laser, or scissors over the site of maximal extension of the ectopic pregnancy. The ectopic gestation is then gently removed from the tube, and hemostasis is achieved by use of bipolar or microtip unipolar cautery. All tissue should be gently removed from the tubal lumen with forceps or irrigation.

Patients who have isthmic ectopic pregnancy generally have extensive distortion of the tubal lumen, making linear salpingostomy impractical. If significant tubal distortion occurs, segmental resection of the affected portion of the tube may be necessary. These patients may undergo tubal anastomosis at a later date. They are at risk for future ectopic pregnancy in the distal segment of the tube if this is left detached from the uterus, although this is an uncommon event.

## LAPAROSCOPIC-ASSISTED VAGINAL HYSTERECTOMY

Laparoscopic-assisted vaginal hysterectomy (LAVH) was initially described in 1989, and since then it has evolved substantially. The principal advantage of LAVH is in allowing patients who would otherwise require abdominal hysterectomy to receive some of the advantages of vaginal hysterectomy, including shorter hospitalization, more rapid recuperation and resumption of normal activities, and decreased need for postoperative analgesia. LAVH also permits the surgeon to perform an oophorectomy in patients whose ovaries might be difficult to remove vaginally. LAVH is associated with a longer operative time than vaginal hysterectomy, increased cost in most series, and a potentially greater complication rate, including bladder and ureter injury, operative hemorrhage, and postoperative infections. There is considerable controversy regarding the definition and indications for LAVH. LAVH may refer to vaginal hysterectomy performed following laparoscopic oophorectomy, or it may involve performing virtually the complete hysterectomy through the laparoscope. Procedures that are performed in association with LAVH include lysis of adhesions, treatment of endometriosis, and division of the infundibular pelvic ligaments for removal of the ovaries.

Generally, laparoscopy is performed first to assess the feasibility of LAVH and to free the uterus of any adhesions. If oophorectomy is then elected, the infundibular pelvic ligament is divided. If the ovaries are to be spared, the utero-ovarian ligament is divided. The round and broad ligaments can also be divided through the laparoscope, and the resection of the vesicouterine reflection may be initiated. Vascular pedicles can be secured with automatic stapling and cutting devices, laparoscopic sutures, or cautery clips. The uterine arteries and cardinal ligaments are generally secured during the vaginal portion of the operation after the anterior and posterior cul-de-sacs have been entered. Both of the uterine arteries may be ligated laparoscopically as well.

The choice of surgical approach is determined by the indication, the patient's condition, and the surgeon's expertise and training. As more data become available, the specific role of this procedure should be more clearly defined.

## OOPHORECTOMY AND CYSTECTOMY

Laparoscopic oophorectomy and cystectomy can be performed easily with a variety of techniques. Simple cysts can be aspirated with a needle or suction irrigator. Alternatively, cysts can be excised from the ovary using cautery, laser, or scissors for incising the ovarian cortex and dissecting the cyst free of the adjacent parenchyma. Irrigation can be used to facilitate the dissection. Most cystectomies do not require sutures to close the ovarian cortex, but if the resulting defect is large, a few interrupted, fine, absorbable sutures may be placed to reapproximate the edges.

A variety of techniques have been used to perform oophorectomy. If the location of the ureter is uncertain, it may be desirable to open the broad ligament and identify the ureter, but this is usually not necessary. Division of the infundibular pelvic ligament can be accomplished with an automatic cutting and stapling device, bipolar cautery and scissors, or suture and scissors.

## OTHER OPERATIONS

Laparoscopic myomectomy is a controversial procedure. Pedunculated myomas may be easily removed with laser, electrocautery, or bipolar cautery and scissors. Laparoscopic removal of intramural myomas is technically more difficult, and this procedure was previously associated with uterine dehiscence and hemorrhage.

Several laparoscopic bladder neck suspension procedures have been performed. Success rates compare favorably with those performed using a traditional abdominal approach. However, available data are limited to date.

## Complications

Laparoscopy is overall a very safe procedure. The true incidence of complications is unknown, because most laparoscopic complications are unreported. The mortality rate associated with laparoscopy is 2.5 to 8.0 per 100,000 cases. Death generally occurs as a result of cardiac arrest, gas embolism, hemorrhage, or bowel perforation. Pelvic abscesses and wound infections are rare. Direct trauma to the uterus, bladder, gallbladder, spleen, and liver have all been described. Perforation of the stomach, aspiration of gas contents, and insufflation of the small and large bowel have also been described. The most common vascular injury is damage to the inferior epigastric vessels during insertion of the ancillary trocars. Perforation of the aorta, the vena cava, or the iliac vessels by the Veres needle or the trocar are rare but life threatening. Immediate laparotomy and vascular surgery consultation are necessary to manage these complications.

Bowel injuries may result from sharp, direct trauma caused by the Veres needle or the trocar, or thermal injury may be caused by the electrocautery or the laser. Small, clean, discrete injuries caused by the Veres needle may not require further management. Burns and larger trocar injuries require immediate intervention. The decision to proceed with primary closure versus diverting colostomy is determined by the size and duration of the injury and the degree of contamination. Burns require resection of the viable tissue around the injury to ensure that any occult damage is removed.

Injury of the bladder is the most common urinary tract complication of laparoscopy. It can usually be avoided by drainage of the bladder before the procedure and insertion of ancillary trocars at least 4 cm above the pubic symphysis. Veres needle injuries may not require additional treatment, but a larger trocar injury necessitates surgical closure. Ureteral injury also requires immediate repair and stent placement.

Bowel herniation into the laparoscopic incision has been reported to be associated with the use of larger caliber laparoscopic instruments. Taking care to avoid retracting the bowel with the laparoscopic instruments at the time of their removal and appropriate fascial closure may avoid this complication.

## Future of Laparoscopy

As emphasis on cost containment increases, operative laparoscopic procedures will continue to undergo critical evaluation of their efficacy and cost effectiveness. However, laparoscopy is certain to have a secure role in the future. The development of a 2-mm minilaparoscope, which will allow diagnostic and limited operative procedures to be performed in an outpatient or office setting, will likely have an expanded role in this context. Microendoscopes have also been developed for evaluation of the fallopian tubes. Their role and value have yet to be defined.

### REFERENCES

Bahary CM, Gorodeski IG: The diagnostic value of laparoscopy in women with chronic pelvic pain. Ann Surg 11:672, 1977.

Boike GM, Miller CE, Spirtos NM, et al: Incisional bowel herniations after operative laparoscopy: A series of 19 cases and review of the literature. Am J Obstet Gynecol 172:1726, 1995.

Bruhat MA, Mage G, Manhes H, et al: Laparoscopy procedures to promote fertility: Ovariolysis and adhesiolysis: Results of 93 selected cases. Acta Eur Fertil 14:113, 1983.

Dmowski WP: Pitfalls in clinical, laparoscopic and histologic diagnosis of endometriosis. Acta Obstet Gynecol Scand (suppl)123:29, 1984.

Donnez J: $CO_2$ laser laparoscopy in infertile women with endometriosis and women with adnexal adhesions. Fertil Steril 48:390, 1987.

Drake TS, Grunert GM: The unsuspected pelvic factor in infertility investigation. Fertil Steril 34:27, 1980.

Fayez JA, Vogel MF: Comparison of different treatment methods of endometriomas by laparoscopy. Obstet Gynecol 78:660, 1991.

Fried AM, Rhodes RA, Morehouse IR: Endometrioma: Analysis and sonographic classification of 51 documented cases. South Med J 86:297, 1993.

Grimes DA: Frontiers of operative laparoscopy: A review and critique of the evidence. Am J Obstet Gynecol 166:1062, 1992.

Hasson HM: A modified instrument and method for laparoscopy. Am J Obstet Gynecol 110:886, 1971.

Hopkins H: Optical principles of the endoscope. In Berci G (ed): Endoscopy. New York, Appleton-Century-Crofts, 1976.

Hunt RB, Cohen SM: Discussions of salpingostomy. In Current Problems in Obstetrics, Gynecology, and Fertility. Vol. 9. Chicago, Year Book, 1986.

Jarrett JC: Laparoscopy: Direct trocar insertion without pneumoperitoneum. Obstet Gynecol 75:725, 1990.

Johns DA, Carrera B, Jones J, et al: The medical and economic impact of laparoscopically assisted vaginal hysterectomy in a large, metropolitan, not-for-profit hospital. Am J Obstet Gynecol 172:1709, 1995.

Keckstein J, Ulrich U, Sasse V, et al: Reduction of postoperative adhesion formation after laparoscopic ovarian cystectomy. Hum Reprod 11:579, 1996.

Krebs HB: Intestinal injury in gynecologic surgery: A ten-year experience. Am J Obstet Gynecol 155:509, 1986.

Luciano AA, Whitman G, Maier DB, et al: A comparison of thermal injury, healing patterns, and postoperative adhesion formation following a $CO_2$ laser and electromicrosurgery. Fertil Steril 48:1025, 1987.

Maiman M, Seltzer V, Boyce J: Laparoscopic excision of ovarian neoplasm subsequently found to be malignant. Obstet Gynecol 77:563, 191.

Martin DC (ed): Intra-abdominal Laser Surgery. Memphis, Resurge, 1986.

Mettler L, Giesel H, Semm K: Treatment of female infertility due to tubal obstruction by operative laparoscopy. Fertil Steril 32:384, 1979.

Reich H, Maher PJ, Wood C: Laparoscopic hysterectomy. Baillieres Clin Obstet Gynaecol 8:799, 1994.

Summitt RL Jr, Stovall TG, Lipscomb GH, et al: Randomized comparison of laparoscopy-assisted vaginal hysterectomy with standard vaginal hysterectomy in an outpatient setting. Obstet Gynecol 80:895, 1992.

# 13

# Office Hysteroscopy and Suction Curettage in the Evaluation of Abnormal Uterine Bleeding

MILTON GOLDRATH

Dilatation and curettage (D&C) has long been considered the method of choice for investigating abnormal uterine bleeding and obtaining samples of endometrium for histologic examination. In 1975, approximately 977,000 patients underwent diagnostic D&C in short-stay, nonfederal hospitals (Grimes, 1982). Although this number had dropped by 65% in 1991, according to data from the National Health Survey, 1997, D&C is probably still one of the most commonly performed operations in the United States today. Because of the current emphasis on containing cost of health care, there has been increasing motivation to find less expensive outpatient procedures to substitute for diagnostic D&C performed in the hospital. In addition to being expensive, a hospital procedure is inconvenient and time-consuming. Initially, there was a move to outpatient procedures instead of the usual 2-day hospital admission. This trend reduced costs; however, the increasing costs of hospital operation necessitated raising the charges even for outpatient surgery—to very high levels.

Many authors have shown that in an office setting, aspiration curettage without cervical dilatation is a reliable and acceptable method of endometrial sampling (Grimes 1982; MacKenzie and Bibby, 1978; Creasman and Weed, 1976; Hale et al, 1976; Hofmeister, 1976; and Lutz et al, 1977). As menopause approaches, women experience increased incidence of atypical hyperplasias and endometrial cancer. It is, of course, the gynecologist's prime responsibility to rule out endometrial carcinoma and to detect lesions that precede cancer in patients who have abnormal bleeding. The various studies mentioned earlier show that aspiration curettage equals and perhaps surpasses conventional D&C in its ability to detect endometrial carcinoma. It is noted in these studies that on rare occasions, endometrial carcinoma may be missed by all methods previously described.

It is recognized by gynecologists that the incidence of carcinoma, especially in younger women, is very low. The primary reason for performing diagnostic curettage in these patients is to find the etiology of menstrual abnormalities that can be remedied, such as endometrial polyps, and submucosal leiomyomas. A large number of these symptomatic lesions may be missed by endometrial biopsy and aspiration curettage. It has long been the gynecologist's view that conventional D&C is more likely to result in discovery of submucosal leiomyomas because the operator can feel them with the curet, whereas a similar level of tangibility cannot be experienced with the commonly used suction cannula. In addition, during conventional D&C, exploration with a polyp forceps often results in the removal of endometrial polyps that were missed by curettage.

In reality, experience has shown that many submucosal leiomyomas have been missed despite repeated curettage, and that many leiomyomas that were "found" by curettage were not actually present at the time of hysterectomy, and that many endometrial polyps that were not discovered by D&C were specimens removed when hysterectomy was eventually performed to relieve patients' symptoms. MacKenzie and Bibby (1978) conducted a retrospective study of more than 1000 patients who had undergone diagnostic curettage. They noted that unsuspected pelvic or endometrial lesions were found in 34 of 160 patients who had had hysterectomy after initial curettage.

Although most gynecologists still maintain that D&C is by far the most reliable technique for diagnosing endometrial abnormalities, the sensitivity and specificity of D&C are difficult to assess, because without removal of the uterus, the true incidence of intrauterine lesions is unknown. Stock and Kanbour (1975) evaluated the completeness of curettage performed immediately before hysterectomy. They found that in 60% of patients, less than half of the uterine cavity was curetted, and in 16% of specimens less than one fourth of the cavity had been curetted. Therefore, it is not surprising that endometrial polyps, submucosal myomas, or small endometrial carcinomas are missed at routine curettage. Word and associates (1958) demonstrated that 49 of 512 patients who had undergone hysterectomy after curettage had residual endometrial polyps. Clearly, the curet left many polyps undetected.

Hysteroscopy is indicated in any situation in which intrauterine visualization can enhance diagnostic accuracy and define therapy (Valle, 1978). The most common indication for hysteroscopy is abnormal uterine bleeding.

## Surgical Technique

Hysteroscopy is performed with a 4-mm hysteroscope in a 5-mm sheath, using carbon dioxide ($CO_2$) as a distending medium. Rarely, a low-viscosity medium (saline) is used in patients who are bleeding. A small flexible hysteroscope is used by some surgeons. Paracervical block with 5 ml of 1% mepivacaine injected into the base of each cardinal ligament decreases the patient's discomfort. *After injection, at least 2 minutes should elapse before hysteroscopy is performed.* I have encountered no untoward effects resulting from paracervical block, but attention must be given to the amount of drug used and the syringe must be carefully aspirated before each injection. The concomitant use of epinephrine in this area tends to produce transient tachycardia and hypertension and does not seem necessary when 1% mepivacaine is used.

The patient is placed in the usual lithotomy position on a regular examination table. The position of the uterus is determined by bimanual examination. A Graves speculum, a Sims double-ended, or other open-sided speculum is used to visualize the cervix. The cervix is grasped with a single-tooth tenaculum, and the vagina and cervix are wiped with an antiseptic solution.

It is helpful and much more comfortable for the operator if the patient's buttocks are elevated. Most gynecologic examination tables allow this. $CO_2$ is delivered through the hysteroscope sheath, using one of various types of purpose-designed hysteroscopic delivery systems. *It is important that a laparoscopy insufflator not be used, for this may deliver large amounts of $CO_2$ under pressure and may prove disastrous.* A 150-watt bulb delivers light through the fiberoptic cable. This is not adequate for photographic purposes. With a flow rate of 30 to 35 ml of $CO_2$ per minute, and a maximum pressure of 50 to 100 mm Hg, the hysteroscope is advanced through the endocervical canal. The canal in front of the scope is inspected, and the endometrial cavity is entered under direct vision. The entire cavity is surveyed, including the cornual regions, the fundus, and the anterior and posterior walls down to the isthmus. With moderate experience, this procedure may take only 30 to 40 seconds. Usually, the scope is then removed, and a 6-mm flexible suction cannula attached to a 50-ml syringe is inserted. The uterine cavity is aspirated thoroughly by suction while the cannula is slowly scraped and rotated over the entire surface of the uterus. It has been found that small polyps can often be removed with this size cannula. All patients who have abnormal uterine bleeding undergo endometrial sampling by suction curettage immediately after the hysteroscopy is performed.

If a small, discrete lesion is to be biopsied, the hysteroscope can be used with an operating sheath through which a small biopsy forceps may be introduced. This is rarely used in clinical practice.

The patient experiences minimal discomfort, and this is further decreased by paracervical block. Only rare patients have severe discomfort. In general, patients have more discomfort from suction curettage than from hysteroscopy. Patients are discharged immediately after completion of the procedure. A few patients have shoulder pain caused by passage of $CO_2$

through the fallopian tubes and ascent to the diaphragm. Although gynecologists are aware of this phenomenon, patients should be warned, because it is often frightening.

Goldrath and Sherman (1985) reported on 423 procedures. Some patients underwent the procedure twice and one patient three times. Patient ages ranged from 24 to 94 years. This age distribution was similar to that of patients who had D&C performed in the hospital. Indications for hysteroscopy and suction curettage were standards for diagnostic D&C, which had been used by gynecologists for many years. It should be noted that 149 (37%) of their patients were initially seen for treatment of menorrhagia. This reflected the large number of patients who were referred for laser ablation of the endometrium (Goldrath et al, 1981). Eighty-four patients had postmenopausal bleeding or spotting. Ten of these postmenopausal patients had an endometrial carcinoma. One had an adenocarcinoma high in the endocervix. Two additional patients who had intermenstrual spotting also had adenocarcinoma of the endometrium.

Corson and Brooks (1983) reported significant findings in 64% of patients with abnormal or menopausal bleeding, or both, whom they examined hysteroscopically. Goldrath and Sherman (1985) reported hysteroscopic or pathologic diagnoses, or both, related to patients' initial symptoms. In addition to miscellaneous findings unrelated to patients' symptoms (e.g., synechiae, diethylstilbestrol [DES] uterus, septate uterus, hemiuterus), significant hysteroscopic diagnoses were made in 181 of the 406 procedures (45%). This is an extremely high yield compared with other published reports for diagnostic D&C (MacKenzie and Bibby, 1978). Minute polyps, which are often seen hysteroscopically, were also considered a normal variant and not significant. Similarly, endometrium with secretory appearance, which is often polypoid, was not considered abnormal. The most common abnormality seen hysteroscopically in this series was submucosal leiomyoma (N = 87). It should be noted that in 28 of these cases there were no palpable myomas on bimanual examination.

In 4 cases, the hysteroscopic examination was considered unsatisfactory because the patients had large amounts of secretory endometrium. Toward the end of a normal menstrual cycle, the thick, succulent, secretory endometrium prevents proper examination. These 4 patients returned after their menstrual period, and in all 4 a satisfactory examination was accomplished. Hysteroscopic examinations in the proliferative phase of the cycle are strongly advised. The procedure is much more satisfactory in the presence of flattened endometrium, and when performed in the follicular phase of the cycle, it does not interfere with the luteal phase of pregnancy.

Of interest was the fact that in 5 patients, hysteroscopic examination failed to show the submucosal myomas previously diagnosed by D&C. MacKenzie and Bibby (1978) similarly reported seven *disappearing leiomyomas* in their large series of diagnostic curettages.

The incidence of adenocarcinoma of the endometrium (3%) was consistent with the incidence of endometrial carcinoma found by D&C in other series. A similar incidence of endometrial hyperplasia was found. It should be noted that in each of these carcinoma cases the isthmus and cervix were examined. One showed involvement by carcinoma and was confirmed histologically at hysterectomy. Usually patients with postmenopausal bleeding have their endocervix curetted separately before undergoing D&C. However, with the current technique, fractional curettage can probably be carried out after the hysteroscopic portion of the procedure without risking contamination by endometrial fragments. This should confirm the hysteroscopic impression of whether there is cervical involvement, which is considered important in staging endometrial carcinoma.

To answer the question, "Can we eliminate the hospital diagnostic D&C?" we must address the following points: safety, adequacy of specimen and diagnostic accuracy, convenience, discomfort, benefits of examination under anesthesia; and evaluation of therapeutic effects. These parameters were discussed thoroughly by Grimes (1982) in his excellent reappraisal of diagnostic D&C. In comparing safety of the procedure and adequacy of specimens, Vabra aspiration compared very favorably with D&C. It is only logical to expect that combining $CO_2$ hysteroscopy with suction curettage will improve results.

Lindemann (1979) reported no infections in 1500 consecutive patients who underwent $CO_2$ hysteroscopies. Taylor and Hamou (1983) reported no infections in their last 3000 patients who had $CO_2$ hysteroscopies. Perforations of the uterus are very rare in all series. It seems that risk of perforation is greater when *operative* procedures are being performed through the hysteroscope. The technique of passing the hysteroscope through the cervix into the endometrial cavity under direct vision seems to reduce the risk of perforation greatly. Perforation during performance of hysteroscopy seems to occur less frequently than during D&C.

Grimes (1982) compared the diagnostic accuracy of Vabra aspiration to that of D&C and noted that Vabra aspiration appeared to be sensitive in diagnosing adenocarcinoma but less sensitive in detecting polyps. The decreased sensitivity of aspiration curettage in detecting polyps can certainly be remedied by use of $CO_2$ hysteroscopy before performance of suction aspiration. In addition, use of a 6-mm suction curet often results in removal of polyps and negates the necessity of doing a therapeutic curettage. In many cases, the cervix can be dilated and a forceps inserted for removal of visualized endometrial polyps. There is no doubt that hysteroscopy reveals many more submucosal leiomyomas than suction curettage or D&C. In addition, hysteroscopy should avoid the "finding" of submucosal leiomyomas that are not present.

Hale and associates (1976) compared the adequacy of specimens for histopathologic examination by routine D&C, using a flexible suction cannula. They found the suction cannula to be far superior to the rigid curet for obtaining adequate sample specimens. They also observed that the technique minimizes damage to the basal endometrium and perhaps decreases occurrence of synechiae.

Though administration of general anesthesia for D&C is a very safe procedure, there are certainly complications associated with it. No complications were associated with use of paracervical block in Goldrath and Sherman's (1985) series.

If the cost of office hysteroscopy combined with suction curettage is compared with outpatient D&C, there is no contest. As previously stated, the hospital charge for this procedure, including preoperative care, operating room, and postanesthetic recovery room, is very high. To these are added the professional fees of the anesthetist, the gynecologist, and the pathologist. Suction D&C with hysteroscopy in an office setting incurs only a surgical fee and a fee for pathologic examination of tissue removed. Compared with the cost of hospital procedures, the savings realized from performance of the office-based procedure would be enormous.

In discussing convenience, of course, there is no comparing an office visit with a trip to the hospital, even for outpatient surgery. The office procedure is done during a routine visit and it adds only about 5 to 10 minutes to the total time of the visit. A trip to the hospital entails at least 1 day out of a person's usual routine. If a general anesthetic is used, the patient is often groggy the next day as well. In addition, the patient needs someone to accompany her to the hospital and to take her home from the hospital. After office hysteroscopy and suction curettage, patients leave and drive themselves home or to work with no aftereffects from the procedure.

Although examination under anesthesia occasionally yields findings that are beneficial to the patient, I do not believe they are germane to this discussion. Usually these findings have nothing to do with the reason for the D&C. In current gynecologic practice, there are certainly ample methods for diagnosing hidden pathology other than examination under anesthesia (e.g., ultrasonography, computed tomography [CT]).

In discussing therapeutic effects of diagnostic D&C, any direct effect is inconceivable unless some pathology is discovered and removed. Grimes (1982) is of the same opinion. It is more likely that the improvement of menstrual disturbances, which occasionally occurs following diagnostic curettage, is more coincidental than causal. Haynes and associates (1977) measured blood loss in women who had had D&C for menorrhagia and found that after the first month there was no lessening in the amount of blood lost. This has also been our impression. The combined use of $CO_2$ hysteroscopy and suction curettage yields many more cases of patients who have endometrial polyps and submucosal myomas amenable to proper treatment by therapeutic curettage, by myomectomy, or by other appropriate means.

Although hysteroscopy is a new procedure for most gynecologists, its use is proliferating. It is a procedure that is learned readily. It should be taught to residents during their training. Graduate courses in hysteroscopy are available, and gynecologists who plan to use this procedure are highly recommended to take such a course. The clarity of view with $CO_2$ hysteroscopy is quite astounding. Most gynecologists are familiar with the appearance of the uterine cavity and its possible contents; therefore, they rapidly become confident about making hysteroscopic observations. As with most new diagnostic procedures, errors may be made at first; however, ample safeguards are provided by performing follow-up suction curettage after hysteroscopy in all of these cases.

In conclusion, performance of $CO_2$ hysteroscopy in combination with suction curettage, using a flexible 6-mm cannula is a superior alternative to performance of routine D&C, and, at greatly diminished cost, it provides greater accuracy, more convenience, enhanced safety, and a higher degree of comfort. Currently $CO_2$ hysteroscopy with suction curettage is used as the primary diagnostic procedure in all patients for whom a diagnostic D&C has previously been indicated. In rare instances in which hysteroscopy with suction curettage cannot be completed as an office procedure, the same operation should be performed in a hospital operating room.

## REFERENCES

Corson SL, Brooks PG: Experience with the Hamou colpomicrohysteroscope. J Reprod Med 28:654–658, 1983.

Creasman WT, Weed JC: Screening techniques in endometrial cancer. Cancer 38:436–440, 1976.

Goldrath MH, Fuller TA, Segal S: Laser photovaporization of endometrium for the treatment of menorrhagia. Am J Obstet Gynecol 140:14–19, 1981.

Goldrath MH, Sherman AI: Office hysteroscopy and suction curettage: Can we eliminate the hospital diagnostic dilatation and curettage? Am J Obstet Gynecol 155:220–229, 1985.

Grimes DA: Diagnostic dilatation and curettage: A reappraisal. Am J Obstet Gynecol 142:1–6, 1982.

Hale RW, Reich IA, Joiner JM, et al: Histopathologic evaluation of uteri curetted by flexible suction cannula. Am J Obstet Gynecol 125:805–808, 1976.

Haynes PJ, Hodgson H, Anderson AB, et al: Measurement of

menstrual blood loss in patients complaining of menorrhagia. Br J Obstet Gynaecol 84:763–768, 1977.

Hofmeister FJ: Endometrial biopsy: Another look. Am J Obstet Gynecol 118:773–777, 1974.

Lindemann HJ: $CO_2$ hysteroscopies today. Endoscopy 11:94–100, 1979.

Lutz MH, Underwood PB Jr, Kreutner A, Mitchell KS: Vacuum aspiration: An efficient out-patient screening technique for endometrial disease. Southern Medical Journal 70:393–395, 1977.

MacKenzie IZ, Bibby JG: Critical assessment of dilatation and curettage in 1029 women. Lancet 2:566–568, 1978.

Stock RJ, Kanbour A: Pre-hysterectomy curettage. Obstet Gynecol 45:537–541, 1975.

Taylor PJ, Hamou JE: Hysteroscopy. J Reprod Med 28:359–389, 1983.

Valle RF: Hysteroscopy. Obstet Gynecol Annu 7:245–283, 1978.

Word B, Gravlee LC, Wideman GL: The fallacy of simple uterine curettage. Obstet Gynecol 12:642–648, 1958.

# 14

# Genital Tract Prolapse

DEE ELLEN FENNER

Genital tract prolapse or pelvic organ prolapse (POP) is bulging or protrusion of the pelvic organs into or out of the vaginal canal. It is a condition most commonly seen in adult multiparous women. Genital tract prolapse results from damage to the normal neuromuscular and fascial supports of the pelvic organs. Genital tract prolapse should be thought of as a hernia. As with other hernias, there is a tear in the fascia, allowing protrusion or prolapse of the underlying viscera. In general, there is no pathology associated with the organ (i.e., bladder, uterus, bowel) that is prolapsing.

## Pelvic Support

The primary support of the pelvic organs is the levator ani muscle complex. With the urethral and anal sphincter muscles and the overlying endopelvic fascia, the levator ani muscles comprise the pelvic floor (Fig. 14–1). The levator ani muscles are attached to the bony pelvis anteroposteriorly and laterally to the arcus tendineus levator ani and ischial spine. The anterior separation, called the levator hiatus, allows the passage of the urethra, vagina, and rectum. Inferiorly, the levator hiatus is covered by the urogenital diaphragm. The posterior midline fusion of the levator muscles by the anococcygeal ligament forms the levator plate. The resulting sling of muscle acts as primary support for the pelvic viscera, which is suspended by the endopelvic fascia (Fig. 14–2). In the female who is standing, the pelvic floor is in the horizontal position, providing a flap valve system on which the pelvic organs are pinned, preventing downward vertical prolapse of the organs through the hiatus.

Physiologically, these muscles are different from most skeletal muscles in that they exhibit constant activity except during voiding and defecation. This constant basal tone keeps the urogenital hiatus closed. If this resting tone is decreased or lost by neuromuscular damage, the hiatus widens and dilates and the pelvic organs descend. If the endopelvic or ligamentous supports are also weakened or torn, prolapse occurs. Besides providing normal tonic contraction and support, the pelvic floor must respond to rises in intra-abdominal pressure, such as coughing or straining. The puborectalis muscles contain type I (slow-twitch) muscle fibers that maintain long-term steady tone, and type II (fast-twitch) muscle fibers that provide rapid increase in muscle strength in response to increased abdominal pressure.

The levator ani muscles have dual innervation. The pelvic surface is innervated by direct branches from the second, third, and fourth sacral nerves, and the perineal surface receives innervation through the pudendal nerve. The pudendal nerve also arises from S2, S3, and S4, passes through Alcock's canal, and divides into three branches to innervate the levator ani, perineum, and clitoris. Because of its location

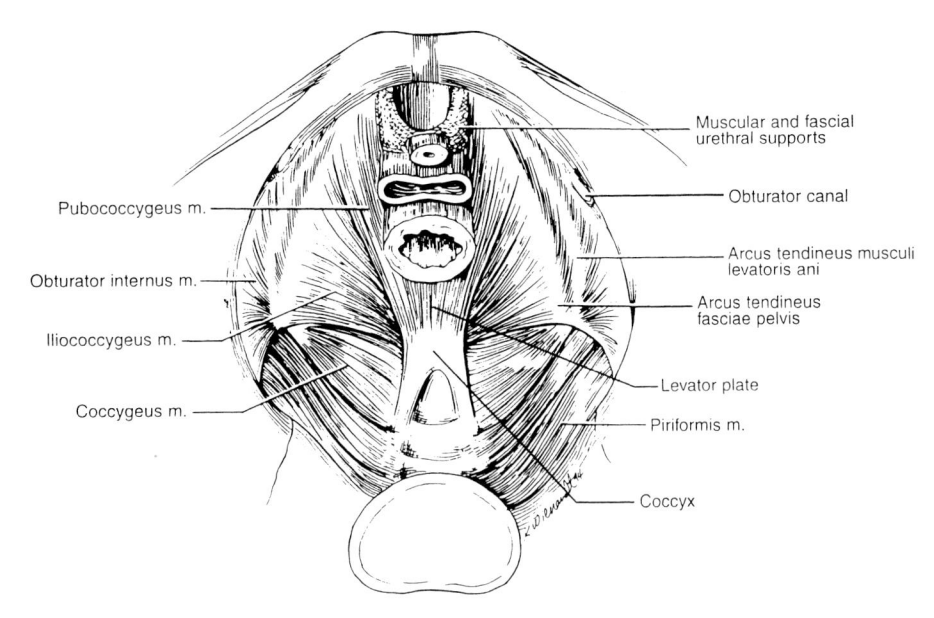

**Figure 14–1** A view of the pelvic floor from above with the bladder, vagina, and rectum removed. (From Brubaker LT, Saclarides TJ [eds]: The Female Pelvic Floor: Disorders of Function and Support. Philadelphia, FA Davis, 1996, p 11.)

and course, it is at risk for stretch and pressure injuries during vaginal delivery.

The endopelvic fascia is a visceral fascia composed of collagen fibers, elastin, smooth muscle, and neurovascular elements. Unlike other fascial or ligamentous supports, the endopelvic fascia not only serves to suspend the pelvic organs but also permits flexibility and distention.

The endopelvic fascia extends from the level of the uterine artery to the fusion of the vagina and the levator ani. The endopelvic fascia envelops the bladder, urethra, vagina, cervix, rectum, and anal canal (Fig. 14–3). This capsule, or envelope, connects the pelvic organs to the parietal fascia and bone. Special names and importance have been given to parts of the endopelvic fascia, depending on their location and function. The superior, or apical, portions of the endopelvic fascia are known as the uterosacral ligaments. They suspend the vagina to the pelvic side wall and presacral fascia. Damage to these supports

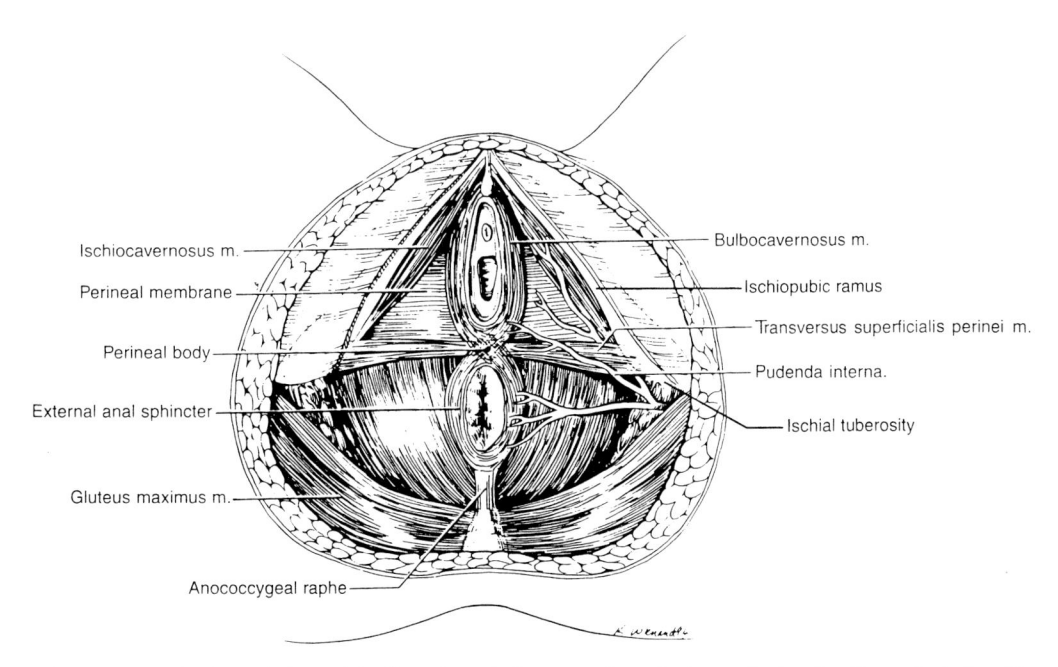

**Figure 14–2** A view of the pelvic floor from below, cut through the anal triangle. (From Brubaker LT, Saclarides TJ [eds]: The Female Pelvic Floor: Disorders of Function and Support. Philadelphia, FA Davis, 1996, p 13.)

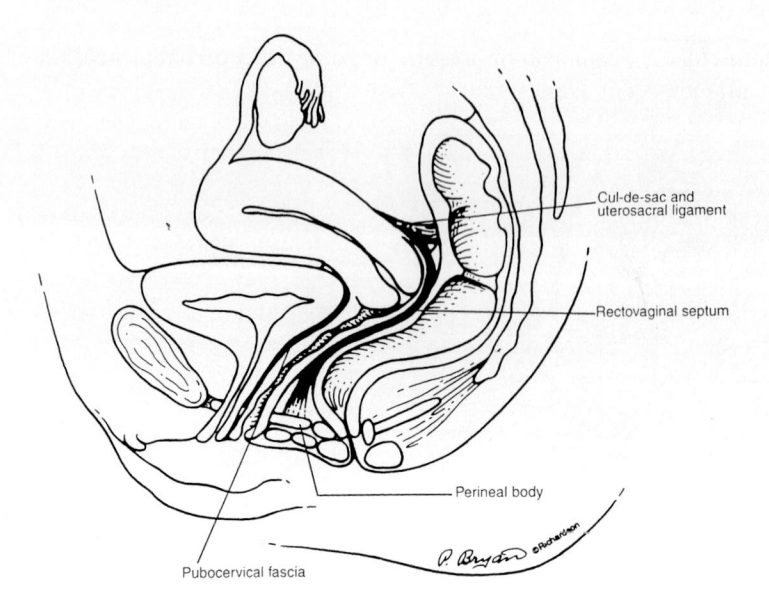

**Figure 14–3** The endopelvic fascia envelops the pelvic organs from the uterosacral ligaments to the perineal body. (From Brubaker LT, Saclarides TJ (eds): The Female Pelvic Floor: Disorders of Function and Support. Philadelphia, FA Davis, 1996, p 18.)

results in prolapse of the uterus or vaginal apex. The endopelvic fascia attached to the uterus is called the parametrium and is composed of the cardinal ligaments laterally and the uterosacral ligaments superiorly. The endopelvic fascia that supports the vagina is called the paracolpium and is divided into the pubocervical fascia anteriorly and the rectovaginal fascia posteriorly. The paracolpium is attached laterally to the arcus tendineus fascia pelvis. Detachment of the pubocervical fascia from the arcus tendineus fascia pelvis may cause cystoceles. The rectovaginal fascia fuses with the perineal body to anchor the endopelvic fascia, thus providing a continuous capsule of fascia suspended from the uterosacral ligaments to the perineal body.

How the neuromuscular and endopelvic fascial supports work together to prevent genital tract prolapse, while at the same time allowing urination, defecation, sexual function, and childbirth, is a complex anatomic and physiologic relationship that is difficult to visualize and understand. Nevertheless, understanding this relationship is vital in order to prevent, treat, and surgically correct genital tract prolapse. An excellent analogy is the concept of a boat tied to a dock. The boat represents the pelvic organs, the water supporting the boat represents the levator ani muscles, and the ropes, or moorings, tying the boat to the dock represent the endopelvic fascia. As long as the water (levator ani muscles) functions normally, the boat (pelvic organs) sits high in the water. The moorings, which are not stretched or placed on tension, help stabilize the boat's position. As the water is drained (strength of the levator muscles weakens or relaxes), the boat begins to sink. More tension and weight is placed upon the moorings (endopelvic fascia). As the water (muscular support) decreases, eventually the moorings (fascial supports) are broken and the boat (pelvic organs) prolapses.

# Etiology

During the course of evolution, as women attained an erect, bipedal posture, increasing pressure and strain were placed on the pelvic floor muscles, nerves, and fascial supports. With chronic increases in intra-abdominal pressures and acute episodes of damage from childbirth, heavy lifting, or constipation, the pelvic floor support is weakened and overcome by intra-abdominal pressures, resulting in genital tract prolapse.

Genital tract prolapse is rarely seen in a neurologically intact nulliparous woman. Pregnancy, labor, and vaginal delivery are thought to be the primary factors contributing to the development of genital tract prolapse. Vaginal delivery places a tremendous amount of stretch and pressure on the pelvic floor musculature and nerve supply. Stretching and pressure on the sacral plexus and pudendal nerves that supply the levator ani muscles lead to denervation of the pelvic floor muscles. Levator denervation has been found in 50% of women who have symptomatic genital tract prolapse. Women who have vaginal deliveries have been found to have prolonged pudendal nerve motor latencies, a measure of nerve conductance. Subsequent reinervation of the levator ani muscles occurs in most women in the first 6 months after vaginal delivery, but some women have long-term neuromuscular damage to the pelvic floor. In parous women who have genital tract prolapse, histologic and electromyographic evidence of levator denervation is apparent. Current investigations are aimed at discovering women who are at risk for permanent damage and determining how the obstetrician can help. Episiotomy does not appear to be protective in preventing genital tract prolapse, but length of the second stage and the use of forceps may play a role in neuromuscular damage. Besides the neuromuscular damage, vaginal childbirth stretches and tears the endopelvic fascial supports of the pelvic viscera. These tears, or hernias, in combination with loss of muscle support, lead to the downward displacement of the pelvic organs.

Other chronic and repetitive increases in intra-abdominal pressure also increase the risk of genital tract prolapse. Heavy lifting, chronic constipation, obstructive pulmonary disease, chronic cough secondary to cigarette smoking, ascites, pelvic tumors, or obesity can predispose a woman to prolapse.

Women who have intrinsically abnormal collagen are also at risk for genital tract prolapse. A collagen abnormality or neuromuscular disease should be suspected in a nulliparous patient who develops genital tract prolapse. These disease processes include spina bifida occulta, joint hypermobility, and Ehlers-Danlos and Marfan syndromes. Connective tissue undergoes dynamic turnover and remodeling with age. Collagen cross-links occur with age and stabilize the molecule, but may prevent remodeling and flexibility. There are also racial differences in collagen. Zacharin attempted to measure anatomic differences between Asians and whites in trying to explain differences in the prevalence of stress incontinence and genital tract prolapse between the two groups. He reported that the fascia of the pelvic structures of the cadavers of Chinese women was dense and thick compared with that of the cadavers of white women.

How estrogen affects the support of the pelvic floor is probably multifactorial. Estrogen receptors have been found in the bladder, urethra, and vagina, as well as in the connective tissue and muscular supports of the pelvic floor. Estrogen affects collagen content by either inhibiting its breakdown or increasing its rate of synthesis. Progesterone acts as a smooth muscle relaxer and increases joint hypermobility. Increased collagen synthesis may be responsible for the therapeutic effect of estrogen replacement therapy. Loss of estrogen also causes decreased vascularity of the pelvic organs. Estrogen therapy at the time of menopause helps preserve the integrity of the vaginal supports and prevents vaginal atrophy. Although estrogen therapy is generally accepted as adjunctive treatment for genital tract prolapse, further investigation is needed to establish its effect on the natural history of POP and its therapeutic role.

## Signs and Symptoms of Genital Tract Prolapse

The signs and symptoms of genital tract prolapse are quite varied and not always consistent with the amount of organ prolapse. Although some women complain of pressure or pain with a partial protrusion of the anterior or posterior vaginal wall, others may be totally unbothered by a complete vault eversion. It is essential that the physician listen to the patient and that her care be matched to her symptoms.

Common symptoms associated with genital tract prolapse are listed in Table 14–1. Because these defects are pelvic floor hernias, symptoms often arise after the patient has been standing for prolonged periods or after increases in intra-abdominal pressure. Many times, the symptoms subside after the patient lies down.

Patients who are incontinent should have some urodynamic evaluation before undergoing surgery. Occult urinary incontinence may be present in as many as 40% of women who have genital tract prolapse and who do not complain of urinary incontinence. The patient should be carefully evaluated before reconstructive surgery is performed, and the prolapse should be reduced so that potential incontinence problems after surgery can be addressed.

Many patients also complain of constipation, straining, or difficult defecation. It is important to obtain a thorough history of the patient's gastrointestinal complaints, so that chronic constipation can be separated from obstructed defecation or the need to support the perineal body or rectum in order to defecate. The latter problem is associated with the presence of a rectocele and may be corrected by surgical repair. However, chronic constipation and straining may actually be the cause of the patient's genital tract prolapse rather than the result. Medical therapy, including stool softeners, dietary modification, and fluid intake, should be tried rather than surgery for management of symptoms.

## Evaluation

Clinical evaluation of genital tract prolapse should begin with assessment of the neuromuscular function of the pelvis. Sacral reflexes can be checked by gently touching the labia majora or periclitoral skin with a cotton swab. Spontaneous contraction of the levator

**Table 14–1** Signs and Symptoms of Pelvic Organ Prolapse

| |
|---|
| Vaginal bulge |
| Pelvic pressure |
| Pulling sensation in the vagina |
| Lower back pain |
| Urinary incontinence, urgency, or retention |
| Difficult defecation |
| Vaginal spotting from ulceration |
| Dyspareunia |

muscles or the external anal sphincter indicates that the reflex is intact. This reflex is present in only 90% of women. Strength and function of the pelvic floor can be assessed by placing the index finger of the examining hand on the posterior fourchette and asking the patient to squeeze her pelvis as if she is trying to stop urinating or by asking her to perform a Kegel contraction.

The vagina should also be assessed for atrophy and hypoestrogenic effects. The vagina is pale, thin, and without rugae if there is not enough estrogen stimulation.

Genital tract prolapse is best examined by Valsalva's maneuver with the patient in the standing position to maximize the prolapse. The patient should be asked if her prolapse is at its worst to ensure maximum assessment. Because of the difficulty observing and determining specific defects when the patient is in the standing position, she should also be examined in the lithotomy position. With use of the posterior blade of a Graves' speculum, the anterior wall, apex, and posterior wall can inspected. Lateral defects of the anterior wall can be evaluated by placing a ring forceps in the lateral sulcus of the vagina. If the anterior wall prolapse disappears, the patient has a paravaginal defect. Measurements are taken again with maximum strain, using the hymen as the zero reference point (Fig. 14–4). Although many grading and classification systems have been published, a system for quantifying and staging pelvic organ prolapse has been approved by the International Continence Society, the American Urogynecologic Society, and the Society of Pelvic Surgeons. This grading system, known as the Pelvic Organ Prolapse Quantification Profile, or POP-Q, has been shown to be reproducible by separate examiners. The system allows a series of examinations for site-specific defects in the same patient so that the progression of her prolapse can be followed. In addition, patients who have similar conditions can be grouped for study and surgical outcomes, which helps to expand knowledge of this problem. A ruler, a uterine sound, index finger, or any calibrated instrument can be used to obtain the measurements. Although the system appears complicated at first, it is easily learned and examinations may be performed quickly.

Physical examination alone may not always be accurate in delineating all pelvic floor defects. This is especially true in patients who have had previous reconstructive surgeries. Patients who have only a posterior or anterior compartment defect may have an enterocele behind the rectocele or a cystocele that is not palpable by pelvic examination. Before initiating surgical treatment, some clinicians advocate obtaining a defecating proctogram to assess the presence of an enterocele.

## Classification of Genital Tract Prolapse

Traditionally, POP has been classified by the organ located behind the bulge (i.e., cystocele or rectocele). Since POP is actually different sites of herniation through which more than one viscous protrusion can be seen, the hernias should be classified as occurring in the anterior compartment, apex, or posterior compartment of the endopelvic fascia.

**Anterior Compartment.** Breaks in the endopelvic fascia can occur along any site in the anterior vaginal wall. With downward pressure, the bladder or urethra descends. The most commonly occurring tears or detachments are paravaginal tears along the lateral sulci of the vagina, transverse tears of the pubocervical fascia. Midline tears under the urethra occur with least frequency. Paravaginal tears can be unilateral or bilateral. Transverse tears may result in a midline cystocele or anterior enterocele.

**Apex.** The loss of apical support leads to uterine descent or prolapse if the uterus is in situ or vaginal vault prolapse if the patient has undergone hysterectomy. An enterocele, or peritoneal sac containing small bowel, may descend behind the prolapsing uterus between the posterior wall and the rectum. After a hysterectomy, an enterocele may occur anterior to the apex, through the apex, or posterior to the apex, depending on the location of the fascial break.

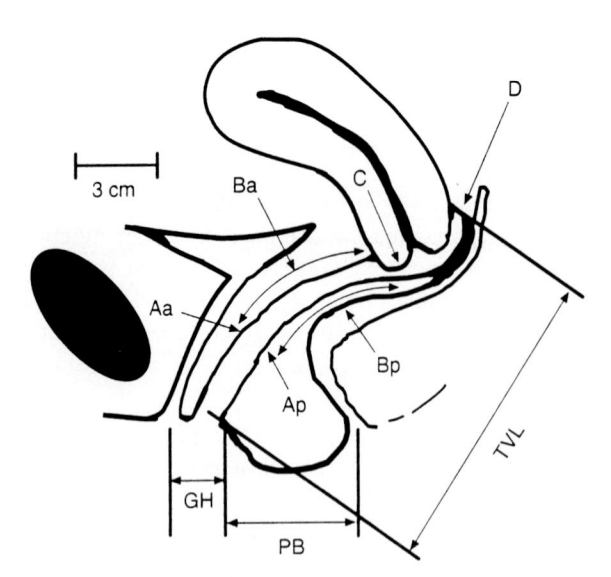

**Figure 14–4** Six sites (points Aa, Ba, C, D, Bp, and AP), genital hiatus (GH), perineal body (PB), and total vaginal length (TVL) used for pelvic organ support quantitation. (From Bump RC, Mattiasson A, Bo K, et al: The standardization of terminology of female pelvic organ prolapse and pelvic floor dysfunction. Am J Obstet Gynecol 175:10–17, 1996.)

**Posterior Compartment.** A bulge in the posterior wall of the vagina can be a rectocele, an enterocele, or even a sigmoidocele, depending on the organ that "reaches" the hernia first. The herniation is the result of a defect or attenuation in the rectovaginal fascia known as Denonvilliers' fascia. A rectocele can also be the result of detachment of the rectovaginal septum from the perineal body. A deficient perineal body is caused by a poorly reconstructed or healed obstetric tear or episiotomy.

## Treatment

Ironically, the best treatment for POP is prevention. Currently, childbirth is the leading cause associated with damage to the neuromuscular and fascial supports of the pelvic organs. Risk factors include forceps deliveries, prolonged pushing in the second stage of labor, third-degree lacerations, macrosomia, and multiparity. Although not all of these factors can be modified, careful attention to the pelvic floor at the time of delivery and at repair of the episiotomy may be preventive.

Certain health and lifestyle changes may also help prevent or deter POP. Managing obesity, constipation, heavy lifting, straining, chronic cough, or smoking cessation can lessen strain on the pelvic floor. Estrogen replacement therapy can improve vascular flow to the vagina, leading to healthier tissues.

Pelvic floor exercises or Kegel's maneuver can help strengthen the levator ani muscles to add support to the pelvic organs. Proper instruction may be needed to ensure that the patient is capable of performing the exercise.

Regardless of surgical indication, prophylaxis at the time of hysterectomy, by reattaching apical supports, can prevent vaginal vault prolapse.

Pessaries can provide excellent treatment for many women. Various sizes and shapes are available, including some with urethral support. Preferably, the women should also be given estrogen replacement therapy, orally or transvaginally, to thicken the vaginal epithelium and deter erosion. Pessaries must be removed and cleaned periodically, either by the patient or by her health-care provider, to prevent a pressure ulcer. Although it is not a cure, a pessary can give excellent symptomatic relief.

### SURGERY

Surgeries for pelvic organ prolapse should be planned to correct the anatomic defects or hernias in the endopelvic fascia. Not all patients have the same defects and, therefore, not every patient should receive an identical surgical procedure. After careful examination and evaluation, considering the specific defects and concomitant diagnosis, such as stress incontinence, the surgeon should decide with the patient the appropriate surgical procedure.

**Anterior Compartment.** Surgeries to correct defects in the anterior compartment should be directed at the site of fascial tear. A paravaginal defect is repaired by reattaching the vaginal sulcus to the arcus tendinius. This surgery may be performed abdominally by entering the space of Retzius or transvaginally by dissecting laterally, perforating the endopelvic fascia, and then reattaching the vaginal sulcus to the arcus. Permanent sutures should be used. A transverse defect is best repaired with an anterior colporrhaphy. Transvaginally the mucosa is incised in the midline and dissected off the bladder. The endopelvic fascia is then dissected sharply off the vaginal mucosa. The fascia is then plicated in the midline in one or more layers. Careful attention should be given to the highest stitches, or apical plication, as this is the most common site of recurrence. Trimming the vaginal mucosa should be done with caution so as not to narrow or shorten the vagina.

**Apex.** Uterine prolapse is generally treated by vaginal hysterectomy and resuspension of the vaginal cuff to shortened uterosacral ligaments, or, if they are overly attenuated, to the sacrospinous ligament. If an abdominal approach is preferred for performing anti-incontinence surgery or for other abdominal pathology, an abdominal hysterectomy with uterosacral plication or sacrocolpopexy can be performed. Whether performed abdominally or vaginally, after a hysterectomy the cul-de-sac should be closed to help prevent enterocele formation.

A McCall's culdoplasty, which shortens and reattaches the apex to the uterosacral ligaments, can be performed at the time of vaginal hysterectomy or surgical repair of vaginal vault prolapse. Two or three sutures are passed through the vaginal cuff, high on the left uterosacral ligament. They are then pulled in a purse-string fashion across the cul-de-sac, through the right uterosacral ligament, and back through the cuff. This procedure provides suspension and posterior traction of the apex as well as obliterating the enterocele sac. Excellent long-term results have been obtained.

Sacrospinous ligament suspension offers an excellent alternative to weakened natural supports. The ligament is accessed through the opened vaginal apex or through a posterior vaginal wall incision. Under direct visualization, two or more stitches are placed through the ligament and then attached to the vaginal apex to be tied snugly. The enterocele sac is closed separately by purse-string sutures. The abdominal sacrocolpopexy attaches the vagina via graft to the longitudinal ligament overlying the sacrum. Two stitches are placed through the ligament after careful dissection of the presacral space. The graft is then attached to the vaginal apex, extending down the posterior and anterior walls after dissection of the peritoneum, rectum, and bladder. Generally, three or more pairs of permanent sutures are used to attach the graft. The enterocele is closed with a Halban or Moschowitz procedure. Again, good long-term results have been reported.

A colpocleisis, complete or partial, is a very good procedure for repair of uterine prolapse or vaginal vault prolapse for a woman who does not wish to retain sexual function. By removing only the vaginal mucosa, and then suturing the anterior and posterior vaginal walls together, the vaginal space is obliterated, blocking the prolapse. The procedure is quick, has minimal risk, and develops few complications.

**Posterior Compartment.** A posterior compartment defect repair is dependent on the location and the prolapsed organ. A posthysterectomy enterocele should have a high intraperitoneal ligation with repair of the overlying fascial defect. The traditional technique for repairing a fascial defect in the posterior wall is to make a diamond-shaped incision in the skin overlying the perineal body, extend the incision in the midline to the vaginal apex, dissect the endopelvic fascia from the vaginal mucosa, plicate in the midline, excise excess mucosa, and close. Many have advocated plication of the levator ani muscles in the midline to add support. This practice is not anatomically correct and may cause dyspareunia.

In a fashion similar to repair of anterior wall defects, attempts have been made to repair posterior wall defects anatomically. With careful dissection, transverse and horseshoe-shaped breaks can be identified in the fascia and repaired. Long-term studies evaluating this modified repair for improved anatomic and functional outcome are ongoing. A detached rectovaginal septum that causes a distal rectocele can be repaired by transversely suturing the rectovaginal septum to the perineal body. This is in contrast to the traditional side-to-side rectocele plication. If a deficient perineal body is present, it should be repaired first to provide an anchor for attaching the septum.

To correct the deficient perineal body, a triangle-shaped incision is made and careful dissection is performed in an attempt to identify the retracted bulbocavernosus and transverse perinei muscles. Side-to-side sutures are placed to reapproximate the muscles in the midline.

# Conclusion

Pelvic organ prolapse is a problem that can seriously affect the quality of life for a woman. New diagnostic and surgical procedures are providing better understanding of the causes and aiding in the development of successful treatments. With a better understanding of the etiology and pathophysiology of POP, we will be able to help prevent many women from developing POP, and, for those who do, we will be able to provide better care.

### REFERENCES

Bonney V: The principles that should underlie all operations for prolapse. J Obstet Gynaecol Br Empire 41:669–683, 1943.

Brubaker L, Resky S, Smith C, et al: Pelvic floor evaluation with dynamic fluoroscopy. Obstet Gynecol 82:1–6, 1993.

Bump RC, Mattiasson A, Bo K, et al: The standardization of terminology of female pelvic organ prolapse and pelvic floor dysfunction. Am J Obstet Gynecol 175:10–17, 1996.

DeLancey JO: Anatomic aspects of vaginal eversion after hysterectomy. Am J Obstet Gynecol 166:1717–1724, 1992.

DeLancey JO: Anatomy and biomechanics of genital prolapse. Clin Obstet Gynecol 36:897–909, 1993.

Morley GW, DeLancey JO: Sacrospinous ligament fixation for eversion of the vagina. Am J Obstet Gynecol 168:1669–1677, 1993.

Norton PA: Pelvic floor disorders: The role of fascia and ligaments. Clin Obstet Gynecol 36:926–938, 1993.

Richardson ACR, Edmonds PB, Williams NL: Treatment of stress urinary incontinence due to paravaginal fascial defect. Obstet Gynecol 57:357, 1981.

Richardson DA, Bent AE, Ostergard DR: The effect of uterovaginal prolapse on uerthrovesical pressure dynamics. Am J Obstet Gynecol 146:901–905, 1983.

Sleep J, Grant A: West Berkshire perineal management trial: Three year follow up. Br Med J 295:749, 1987.

Smith ARB, Hosker GL, Warrell DW: The role of partial denervation of the pelvic floor in the aetiology of genitourinary prolapse and genuine stress incontinence. A neurophysiological study. Br J Obstet Gynaecol 96:24–28, 1989.

Smith P, Heimer G, Norgren A, et al: Steroid hormone receptors in the pelvic muscles and ligaments in women. Gynecol Obstet Invest 30:27–30, 1990.

Snooks SJ, Swash M, Mathers SE, et al: Effect of vaginal delivery on the pelvic floor: A 5-year follow-up. Br J Surg 77:1358–1360, 1990.

Snooks SJ, Swash M, Setchell M, et al: Injury to innervation of pelvic floor sphincter musculature. Lancet ii:546–550, 1984.

Timmons MC, Addison WA, Addison SB: Abdominal sacral colpopexy in 163 women with posthysterectomy vaginal vault prolapse and enterocele. Evolution of operative techniques. J Reprod Med 37:323–327, 1992.

Webb MJ, Aronson MP, Ferguson LK, et al: Posthysterectomy vaginal vault prolapse: Primary repair in 693 patients. Obstet Gynecol 92:281–285, 1998.

White GR: Cystocele: A radical cure by suturing lateral sulci of the vagina to the white line of pelvic fascia. JAMA 21:1707–1710, 1909.

Zacharin RF: A Chinese anatomy—the pelvic supporting tissues of the Chinese and Occidental female compared and contrasted. Aust N Z J Obstet Gynecol 17:1–11, 1977.

# 15

# Sexuality

SALLY A. KOPE

Women, sexuality, and the medical profession have had an intricate relationship dating back to the beginning of rudimentary medical practice. For example, until modern times (approximately the mid-20th century), a girl's hymen was considered to be co-owned by her and her future husband. Hymenal integrity was often overseen by the medical profession, even though for a century physicians have agreed that the presence or absence of a hymen proves nothing about a woman's sexual experience. Menstruation was poorly understood until the 1920s, when the relationship between estrogen and the menstrual cycle was determined. In the Victorian era, medical practitioners pondered whether a woman's brain and her ovaries could work simultaneously and whether strenuous physical and mental work would overtax her health. What a confounding environment—for the physician and for the patient—as far as understanding women's sexuality. Social change, awareness of women's rights and needs regarding their sexual health, medical advances, reliable birth control, and changing mores have contributed to enhanced understanding of female sexuality.

As health practitioners enter the next millennium, they draw on the work of pioneers in the field of human sexuality. Masters and Johnson studied human sexuality in the 1960s. They analyzed the human sexual response cycle and developed treatment interventions to help couples who were having problems in achieving arousal and orgasm. In the 1970s, Helen Singer Kaplan addressed the sexual response from a multifactorial approach, which included looking at sexual response medically, psychologically, and in the context of a woman's relationships. She introduced the concept of sexual desire and its complexities as the hub of sexual response. Kinsey, and later Gagnon, brought public attention to people's private sexual behavior.

Because all aspects of sexuality became legitimate topics of study, it was inevitable that sexual dysfunction would become a subject for investigation in its own right. Sexual problems are organized into two categories: paraphilic behavior and sexual dysfunction.

**Paraphilic Behavior.** This is defined as an inappropriate sexual response to a person, a situation, or an object (e.g., pedophilia, a paraphilic condition in which children are regarded as objects of sexual desire by an adult or an older teen). Paraphilic behavior may derive from psychological or character disorders and requires specialized evaluation and treatment.

**Sexual Dysfunction.** This disorder is caused by or can be a medical or psychological problem or is induced by trauma (e.g., dyspareunia, pain with sex, may cause low sexual desire because the pain becomes something to avoid; therefore, sexual activity becomes something to avoid). It is important to note here that the health-care practitioner from whom a woman receives her gynecologic care is the professional she is most likely to approach with questions about sexuality.

Therapy for problems of sexuality has evolved into a "biopsychosocial" model. The patient's biologic or physiologic state is assessed, her psychological resilience is measured, and the social context in which the sexual problem occurs is examined. For example, a patient who is undergoing treatment for infertility may complain of plummeting sexual interest. Biologically, she may be affected by the hormone treatment she is receiving. Psychologically, she may be reacting to the chronicity of stress and repeated monthly reminders of her infertility. Socially, she may be confronted with reminders of her infertility when coworkers and family members announce pregnancies. All of these factors are given equal consideration when an evaluation of this patient's sexual problem is made.

A chapter cannot be written about women's sexuality without acknowledging the impact of the media and commercialization on this aspect of women's lives. In 1 week, adolescent girls are exposed to more glossy, unrealistic representations of female perfection and exaggerated depictions of sexual behavior than their grandmothers encountered throughout their entire adolescence. All too frequently, this exposure causes young women to feel chronic dissatisfaction with their bodily image, and this may send them on an unhealthy quest for a model's perfection. The hyper–self-consciousness that women feel about their body image frequently manifests itself as inhibited sexual desire or avoidance.

## The Person of the Patient and Her Relationships

Each patient has her own values, cultural influences, ethnicity, personality structure, developmental stage, sex education, socioeconomic status, and the unique roles she plays in her world. The patient is in a dilemma when these factors compete with one another. For example, a 33-year-old woman comes to an appointment with her gynecologist for an annual examination. She has several children and describes her marriage as strong, but she has recently lost sexual interest to the point where she avoids sexual relations. When she is asked about birth control, she becomes tearful and confides that she lacks confidence in the method of family planning that she and her husband have used throughout their marriage, which is in accordance with their religious values. She feels guilty about avoiding sex, but she is even more worried about becoming pregnant. Her moral dilemma, then, is deciding which value should have the most weight. Sometimes, just bringing a dilemma to the surface of awareness (i.e., in this case, recognizing the connection between her avoiding sex and her fear of pregnancy) can illuminate the solution.

Most complaints about sexual difficulty come from women who are involved in a relationship. The quality of the relationship is a significant determinant of the outcome of treatment. For example, if a woman complains that her partner shows no sexual interest whatsoever in her but demonstrates frequent sexual interest in others, the relationship, rather than lack of sexual desire, is likely to be the problem. Education, encouragement, and the expectation that the patient will assume responsibility for her own well-being are ongoing conjunctive aspects of all medical treatment. Certainly, the treatment of sexual dysfunction is highly dependent on the patient's willingness to assume responsibility for actively seeking solutions.

A healthy sexual relationship exerts a positive effect on a marriage. Conversely, a sexually dysfunctional or nonsexual relationship has a profoundly negative effect on the marriage and drains the relationship of power and vitality. Long-standing sexual problems discourage both the patient and the clinician who is treating her. Sometimes, a sexual dysfunction is resolved only to recur at a later time, causing even more discouragement by its relapse than by its original presentation. Factors that contribute to the chronicity of a sexual dysfunction include duration; lack of motivation to resolve the issue; cessation of affectionate or sensual contact; and ambivalence about trying again, having an affair, or obtaining divorce.

When women seek help for a low level of sexual desire, the persistence and scope of the problem may offer some indication about the type of therapy needed. The concern may be handled effectively with patient education, or a referral for individual sexual therapy or couple therapy may be more appropriate. Deep-seated anger toward the partner, entrenchment of the sexual problem, resistance to any suggestion of personal responsibility for change, and sexual aversion are indicators that a more systematic and therapeutic approach to the problem is indicated.

## Sexual Response Cycle

The description of the sexual response cycle remains a useful guideline for health-care practitioners in determining appropriate treatment interventions when problems occur. Although the science is relatively new, practitioners continue to draw from a constantly evolving body of medical and psychological knowledge about how women function and respond sexually.

The sexual response cycle is referred to as a triphasic model: desire, arousal, and orgasm. The *desire* phase refers to a woman's energy for and interest in sexual activity, alone or with a partner, and the motivation to follow through on that interest. Desire is also referred to in academic literature as libido, drive, and sexual motivation. The *arousal* phase refers to the physiologic signs of arousal, such as lubrication, and the psychological response refers to stimulation. Sex therapists do not refer to the physical signs of the arousal phase as the readiness to engage in sexual intercourse. This is because sexual intercourse is not an endpoint of sexual arousal. The range of sexual activity potentiated by the signs of sexual arousal includes masturbation, oral-genital contact, mutual masturbation, and a range of sensual and sexual activities that may or may not include vaginal penetration. The *orgasm* phase refers to the release of accumulated sexual tension. This is a physiologic response with an intense psychological component.

## DESIRE PHASE OF SEXUAL RESPONSE

Sexual desire, or libido, is a normal drive. Women regularly act on opportunities for sexual expression, including sex with a partner or masturbation, unless there are influences that thwart this normal drive. In no phase of the sexual response cycle is the impact of psychological and relational issues more prominent. Sexual desire is also regulated by biologic factors. Of course, responding behaviorally to sexual desire cues also means that the circumstances are reasonably conducive to accommodating sexual behavior. For example, a woman may look forward all week to her partner's return from a business trip, and she may imagine a romantic reunion. On the night of his scheduled return, if she is beginning to have symptoms of a severe head cold, the sexual feelings she may have been entertaining in anticipation will be dampened considerably.

Patients need to understand that desire and drive do not define the quality of the sexual experience. Women are often passive participants, too frequently expecting their partners to be responsible for their sexual responsiveness. Sex therapists play down the role of *spontaneity* in sexual desire. Often sexual activity, just like other daily life activities, requires planning to be successful.

## SEX HORMONES IN SEXUAL DESIRE

The brain organizes and interprets sexual stimuli so that they are experienced as sexual feelings. Hormones, specifically estrogen and androgens, are integral to female sexuality. Sexual behavior is not *predictable* according to hormone levels in women. Sexual desire and receptivity are known to be cyclic in females of all species except women. Although androgens and estrogen influence women's sexual responsiveness and sensitivity, hormones are only one variable in a complex system that determines women's responsiveness.

**Estrogen.** The term *estrogen* is derived from the words *estrus* (meaning excitement) and *generate*. Estrogen certainly affects the physical climate of a woman's body in a positive way by maintaining the elasticity and density of the tissues of the vulva and the vagina and by contributing to lubrication. Studies attempting to establish the link between estrogen and women's sexual desire have been conducted primarily with women who have had a dramatic decline in estrogen brought about by menopause or oophorectomy. These studies indicate that women report a positive relationship between estrogen and sexual desire, and this goes beyond the issues of physical comfort and well-being.

**Androgens.** Androgens have been associated with sexual desire in both men and women. These hormones, which are produced by the gonads and adrenal glands—specifically, testosterone—are present at a rate up to 20 times higher in men than in women. This does not mean that men have a 20 times greater sex drive as women. It does mean that a woman's sexual response is initiated at a lower level of testosterone than a man's. The effect of testosterone is regulated by the central nervous system. In studies conducted to determine the impact of supplemental testosterone in women who complain of a low level of sexual desire, it appears that supplemental androgens may influence women's *reported* interest, but they seem to have little influence on increasing actual sexual *activity* with their partners. This supports the concept that sexual desire in a woman is multifactorial, including developmental changes, body image, experience with intimacy, and expectations of her partner.

## AROUSAL PHASE OF SEXUAL RESPONSE

The arousal phase of sexual response is defined by the physical and psychological presence of signs of excitement. Psychologically, a woman's focus of concentration narrows toward rising sexual tension, and physically her body reflects the state of heightened arousal. The subjective experience of the intensity of sexual arousal is connected to the context in which the arousal occurs—masturbation or partner sex—and the feelings and emotions attached to the context.

### Vasocongestion and Lubrication

During the period of heightened sexual arousal, which may last moments or much longer, a woman's blood pressure rises and her pulse rate increases. Erectile tissue of the vulva, breasts, and nipples engorges with blood that is temporarily prevented from outflow. In many women, the clitoris becomes erect. The labia majora become engorged and retract, and the labia minora become engorged with blood.

The presence of lubrication is considered to be the feature of female sexual arousal that is analogous to a male's erection. Lubrication occurs within the walls of the vagina through transudation. When the walls of the vagina have become engorged, they push minute beads of lubrication through glands located in the walls of the vagina.

### Internal Organ Response to Sexual Arousal

With the exception of wetness from lubrication, a woman is not generally aware of internal signs of sexual arousal. The external genitals are engorged and highly sensitive, increasing their receptivity to sexual stimulation. The internal organs do not have as many nerve endings, so physical sensation is not as accentuated internally.

The uterus expands and is elevated during sexual arousal. The position of the cervix is also altered by sexual arousal. The upper portion of the vagina balloons, and the portion nearest the vaginal introitus swells, so that it surrounds or seems to clasp a finger or penis.

### Orgasm Phase

The orgasm phase—the briefest phase of the sexual response cycle, lasting only seconds—refers to the release of accumulated sexual tension, optimally through orgasm. This is not necessarily a *spontaneously occurring event*: Orgasm in women may be more a learned than a spontaneous response. Studies tracking pubertal development in boys and girls show a direct connection between puberty and ejaculation for boys. For girls, social factors seem to be much stronger in determining orgasm than the onset of puberty connected with hormonal changes. Orgasm is a subjective experience of sensation. Although technology exists to measure the number and intensity of pelvic contractions during orgasm, a woman's report of her feelings of pleasure may not correlate with the mechanical findings. In fact, orgasm is frequently most intensely experienced through masturbation but most satisfactorily experienced through partner sex.

### Physiologic Aspects of Orgasm

Striated muscles of the pelvic floor and the genital and anal areas contract involuntarily and rhythmically during orgasm. The contractions may be strong and intense or weaker and more rippling. The uterus contracts during orgasm as well. The uterine contractions may not be felt at all. Low, or widely fluctuating, estrogen levels may make the uterine contractions painful. These contractions can be an associated side effect of childbirth or a symptom of menopause or perimenopause. The clitoris triggers orgasm, although its pleasurable pulsations are most frequently experienced in the pelvis and the entire genital region. Many women do not experience orgasm through sexual intercourse. They require other stimulation, often in the form of direct clitoral stimulation. There are no reliable statistics for determining *how many* women require this type of stimulation, but what needs to be stressed is that this need is *normal and not a sexual dysfunction*. A woman does not have a refractory period. She is capable of multiple orgasms, although this capacity has been highly sensationalized: Multiple orgasms are not always desirable to a woman. Further stimulation can be uncomfortable rather than pleasurable for a woman who is physically quite sensitive after orgasm.

## ILLNESS, TREATMENT, AND SEXUAL RESPONSE

Patients often leave acute care settings when concerns about recovery, disease course, treatment, and pain management are still very serious preoccupations. For example, a 37-year-old patient is released from the hospital 30 hours after a hysterectomy and oophorectomy. Before the patient is discharged, wound care, follow-up appointments, and general health needs must be discussed; therefore, it would probably be inappropriate to discuss changes in sexual desire, arousal, and orgasm at this time. This is, however, the right time to build a bridge for addressing future problems. "Other women's experiences tell me that you may have some questions about the effect of your surgery on your sexual functioning. I want you to know that we will discuss these questions whenever you are ready to talk about them." The point is not to address sexual concerns in a context that doesn't make sense, but rather to set the stage for returning to this important topic at a more appropriate time.

Chronic illness and medical treatment can have a devastating impact on all functional aspects of the sexual response cycle. It is also common to have sexual problems secondary to the original medical condition or treatment.

Pain and restriction of movement frequently blunt sexual interest or response. Both pain and lack of flexibility—and one is often linked to the other—can be invisible to other people. When either becomes chronic, the coping abilities of both the patient and her partner can become overtaxed. At a time when many of their other resources are also likely to be depleted, they find that resuming sexual activity will also require adaptations and changes for which they may have no preparation or experience. Avoidance of sexual activity after chemotherapy—one of many possible scenarios—is common. The partner may hesitate to initiate intimate contact out of fear of causing pain or distress. The patient may feel undesirable or fearful. Both parties may be uncertain of what to do, so the avoidance continues. This issue can be anticipated by the medical practitioner, and counseling can become a normal part of the follow-up appointment. Ask questions, even if the woman is not obviously in a partnership or if she is much older than you, the interviewer. Some direct inquiries are the following: "Have you resumed sexual activity?" "Is sex working satisfactorily for you?" "Do you have any pain or apprehension about having sexual relations?" "Are you avoiding sexual activity?" "Is your partner having any problems with your sexual relationship?" Another approach is the indirect technique: "Most patients at this point in their recovery/treatment/course of illness have questions about sex. One common concern is whether resuming sexual activity could cause another heart attack/relapse/increase of pain," and so on.

Occasionally, a medical intervention actually causes a psychogenic sexual dysfunction. Such iatrogenic problems mimic symptoms of post-traumatic stress disorder (PTSD) and the patient can be treated in much the same way as is a victim of sexual assault.

> Hilda, a 61-year-old woman, began to have flashbacks when her husband touched her vulva gently several months after she had had radiation implant surgery for cervical cancer. She felt a wave of panic. Her jaw clenched and she felt tears beginning. She remembered the fear and isolation she had felt when other people were physically segregated or heavily shielded from her during the treatments. After Hilda experienced this strong reaction, she and her husband mutually decided that they would speak with a counselor about her negative reactions to her husband's sexual approach. They were both relieved, although still concerned, to learn from the counselor that emotional memories—memories of trauma—may be stored in a way that makes recall of those memories seem as if they were happening again. In addition, the couple learned that even in a situation where there was no present danger, such as Hilda's being touched gently by her husband of many years, painful memories could be evoked. As the husband touched his wife, her triggered recall was that of her vulva's being touched by someone other than herself or her trusted husband, and touched in a way that was painful and frightening. Her emotional responses were involuntary. Gradually, as they talked about her response, and practiced careful re-entry into the world of intimate touch—with Hilda in control at all times—the powerful negative emotional response was replaced by the positive rebuilding of their intimate life together.

This is not to imply that treatment should not occur when PTSD or other psychological problems are a real concern. Disease treatment *cannot* be neglected or delayed because of psychosexual concerns. The sensitive clinician, however, can make a dramatic difference in the outcome. Preparing the patient and her partner as much as possible for the procedures she will be undergoing is an essential factor. This takes time and may require repetition, but such preparation can positively influence the long-term outcome. Frequently, physicians and medical practitioners are concerned that if invasive or unpleasant aspects of medical intervention are outlined, the very process of informing a patient in detail could cause the disordered response. In my experience, patients can manage distressing or painful treatments much more readily if they know what to anticipate at each step.

Frequently used medications can cause sexual problems that range from blunting sexual desire to influencing the physical signs of arousal to changing orgasm patterns. The choice should not be to abandon an appropriate medication. The dilemma comes from the fact that patients sometimes quit their medications with little guidance if they experience a negative sexual side effect. A collaborative, candid, and ongoing dialogue with the patient can help minimize the *flight into noncompliance* that often occurs when a patient panics because of a medication side effect.

Patients can learn to compensate for the negative effects of medication on desire or orgasm. A specific example is a woman who is taking a selective serotonin reuptake inhibitor (SSRI). The medication works well for the control of the patient's depression. She is reluctant to keep taking the medication, however, because she is having difficulty achieving orgasm. Encouraging the patient to experiment with a change in the intensity and duration of stimulation amounting to almost *relearning* the orgasmic response has been a successful technique for many patients. In fact, the patient's benefit has often been an orgasm of increased intensity because of the prolonged phase of peak sexual arousal before orgasm is achieved. Of course, encouraging a patient to experiment with her sexual response is variably successful and highly dependent upon the patient's motivation or resistance in assuming responsibility for her own sexual response.

## Pain Disorders

The Diagnostic and Statistical Manual of Mental Disorders lists two types of sexual pain disorders: dyspareunia and vaginismus. The subtypes of these disorders include both psychological and physical (secondary to a medical condition) causes of the pain disorder. The diagnostic manual describes dyspareunia as pain that accompanies intercourse (Table 15–1), and vaginismus as pain that interferes with intercourse. In describing the disorders as they relate to sexual intercourse, diagnostic categories are too narrow to encompass all the ways in which pain disorders can impact sexual functioning. Interference with penetration is only one of a range of negative consequences women may experience with pain disorders. Some women may experience pain during any sexual activity. The categories do not take into consideration women whose sexual relationships do not include penetration, either by choice or by circumstance. I use the term *dyspareunia* to refer to deep-thrust pain experienced during intercourse or attempts at intercourse, pain that accompanies vasocongestion (sexual arousal), or pain caused by stimulation of the vaginal introitus or vulva. The prime consideration is whether pain interferes with sexual pleasure or inhibits sexual activity. Common symptoms connected with dyspareunia are burning, rawness, itching, stinging, and irritation.

Dealing with chronic pain connected with sexual activity is daunting for the patient, the patient's partner, and the treating clinician. Pain disorders have often been dismissed or attributed to psychological reasons; but, in fact, the origins may be medical or undetermined. Psychological sequelae are common and expected if a patient experiences chronic pain connected with sexual activity. Pain may be continual or intermittent or limited to sexually stimulating activity.

## VULVAR DISORDERS AND VAGINISMUS

Vulvar disorders that cause pain are generally classified into subsets of *vulvodynia*, although—like *fever*—this is not a diagnostic category. The term refers to chronic vulvar pain, characterized by symptoms such as itching, rawness, burning, stinging, stretching, swelling, or throbbing. Some patients complain of associated problems, such as sleep difficulties and temporomandibular joint (TMJ) disorder caused by chronically clenching their teeth against the pain symptom. Many subsets of disease are included in the category called vulvodynia. These may include some dermatologic problems, such as lichen planus and lichen sclerosis. Some sexually transmitted diseases have been found to cause chronic vulvar discomfort: genital herpes infection, human papillomavirus, and *Trichomonas*. Hypersensitivity reactions to soap, topical medications, hygiene products, and surgery are common causes of vulvar pain.

There are two major categories of vulvodynia: organic, in which the etiology of the problem is known; and essential, in which the cause is not identified. There is no relationship between vulvodynia and the subsequent development of vulvar cancer.

Vulvar vestibulitis is a subset of vulvodynia. With this disorder, there is diffuse or point tenderness in the vulvar vestibule. Many women who have vulvar vestibulitis have symptoms of pain and point tenderness for months or years and can trace the beginning of their pain to having given birth or to having chronic vulvovaginal infections or other illnesses. However, no specific etiology of vulvar vestibulitis has been found. In some cases, chronic yeast infections are identified as the basis of the problem.

Vaginismus is characterized by an involuntary spasm that occurs in the musculature of the pelvic floor near the vaginal introitus, making penetration painful or impossible. The *Diagnostic and Statistical Manual of Mental Disorders* lists this as a psychological disorder, and it certainly can be linked with fear of penetration, but the origin and tenacity of this symptom are not completely understood. We know that women who have vaginismus frequently have sexual desire, and the ability to achieve orgasm remains intact. They can experience the physiologic signs of arousal, such as lubrication, but, despite motivation and desire, they still cannot achieve enough pelvic floor relaxation to permit vaginal penetration.

Many women who have chronic vulvar discomfort develop an associated pelvic floor musculature tension or vaginismic response. Sometimes, the symptoms of one disorder are difficult to differentiate from another. For example, secondary vaginismus related to vulvar pain may not remit when the original vulvar disease is eliminated. The patient still experiences and reports pain when attempts at sexual penetration are made. Often, the same terms are used to describe the pain, such as "burning."

## EFFECTIVE TREATMENT FOR VULVAR PAIN AND VAGINISMUS

**Medical Evaluation.** A thorough medical and psychosocial evaluation should be performed for patients

**Table 15–1** Conditions Associated With Dyspareunia

| Introital Dyspareunia | Deep-Thrust Dyspareunia |
|---|---|
| Anatomic abnormalities | Cystitis |
| Bartholin's gland/cyst/abscess | Endometriosis |
| Dermatitis | Fibroid uterus |
| External genital infections | Genital prolapse |
| Human papillomavirus | Interstitial cystitis |
| Lichen sclerosus | Ovarian cyst |
| Urethritis | Pelvic inflammatory disease |
| Vaginal atrophy | Vaginismus |
| Vaginismus | |
| Vulvar intraepithelial neoplasia | |
| Vulvar vestibulitis | |
| Vulvodynia | |

who have chronic vulvar pain or vaginismus. Establishing a working alliance with the patient and her partner is imperative. For many patients, the validation of their pain is the first step in this process. These patients may have suffered for months or years with painful sexual experiences. In a case where the origin of the pain is unknown, the patient's physician and other medical practitioners have often been stymied. Sometimes, both patient and practitioner conclude that the cause must be psychological. There appears to be no correlation between vulvodynia and physical or sexual abuse or an unpleasant first sexual experience. This is worth noting, because some practitioners have speculated that patients who have vulvar pain symptoms may be more likely to be abuse victims.

Although there is almost always a psychological component to suffering pain in conjunction with sexual activity, it is still very likely that the patient is experiencing pain from an organic cause that has not been identified. A referral to a specialty clinic for vulvar disease or a consultation with an expert in this field is indicated for patients whose condition has become chronic. It is frequently helpful for the sex therapist to work in conjunction with the patient's gynecologist or other health-care practitioner in addressing physical aspects of the patient's sexuality.

**Addressing Issues of Sexuality and Pain.** Pain-based sexual dysfunction, even if it is obviously secondary to a disease process, has a psychological impact on the patient and her partner. The patient's pain affects her partner directly, and normally neither she nor her partner has found a strategy that is effective against the pain. The partner does not want to contribute to the pain. Simply reassuring the patient or couple that frustration and avoidance in dealing with pain are normal responses can be helpful in reducing the feeling of isolation.

It can be effective to facilitate a couple's expansion of their sexual repertoire to include sexual and sensual activities that do not depend on sexual intercourse or penetration. For some patients who have chronic pain, even physiologic sexual arousal causes distress as the agitated tissues become engorged with blood. This represents a challenge to the patient, her partner, and the treating clinician. Psychoeducation can be helpful, even if it doesn't, in itself, result in pain relief. Sensual, nonsexual exercises can help with psychological connection. Patients may benefit from the connection with other patients, either in a group or through the Internet.

**Relief Measures.** Certainly, anything that gives the patient substantial relief from symptoms of pain will decrease her anxiety about pain related to sexual activity and will thus have a positive effect on her sexual functioning. These measures must be determined on a case-by-case basis and may be as simple as recommending the use of all-cotton underwear or prescribing a topical anesthetic for relief of pain during intercourse.

**Dilator Treatment and Physical Therapy.** Education of the patient about her body, her internal organs and their placement, her pelvic floor muscles, her pelvic skeletal structures, and her vulva is imperative. Some patients who have long-standing pain have literally "divorced" their genitals. For them to be in touch with their bodies is an important step in regaining control. Physical therapy is an excellent adjunctive treatment for patients who have vulvar pain or vaginismus. Physical therapists who are trained in the rehabilitation of pelvic floor muscles work with women in a process of biofeedback. An internal sensor is placed in the anus or vagina and the pelvic floor muscles are stimulated. The patient is trained to control muscle tension by tensing and relaxing pelvic muscles. She can observe her progress on a monitor. If she is averse to touching her own genitals or having anyone else touch them, the therapist can guide the process very gently, with the patient in control at all times. Biofeedback therapy is equally effective for vaginismus and vulvar pain.

Dilator therapy can be helpful in desensitizing the pelvic floor muscles in patients who have vaginismus or vulvar pain. Vaginal dilators are smooth, plastic, non pliable cylinders, shaped much like tampons. They are made in graduated sizes from extra small to the approximate size of an erect penis and are available through medical supply companies. They were originally designed for use by women who had undergone vulvar or vaginal reconstructive surgery or treatment. Pliable dilators are highly preferable but difficult to locate. The pliable dilator is more "user friendly." Some creative patients have discovered that catalogs featuring sexual toys have small, pliable, dilator-like items that are effective. Instructions about dilator therapy are important and need to be specific. The patient should come for follow-up appointments no more than 2 weeks apart. Assessing the patient's motivation in performing dilator therapy is essential. Many patients are reticent or averse to practicing dilator therapy, but they are also reluctant to speak about their concerns. This puts the treating clinician in the untenable position of unwittingly directing the patient to experience penetration she does not want. It is imperative to establish clearly that dilator therapy is within the patient's control and cannot be effective unless she is motivated for reasons of her own.

Pain caused by deep thrusting should, of course, be medically evaluated and treated on a case-by-case basis. Patients may learn to position themselves for sexual activity in such a way as to avoid pain. Some patients are very adaptable and have no difficulty experimenting to find comfortable positions for themselves. Other couples may avoid sexual contact for years because they have neither addressed the issue of pain with sexual activity, nor found ways to compensate for such a complication. One couple avoided lovemaking for years after the woman had hip replacement surgery and found that flexing her legs was difficult and painful. The couple had not considered that she could keep her legs closed while her husband flexed his legs around her. Although penetration was shallow with intercourse in this position, they were able to achieve satisfactory and stimulating sexual contact.

## Trauma and Sexual Dysfunction

A traumatic event that happened in a woman's past, such as sexual or physical assault (at any age), can, and often does, impact on her current sexual functioning. Memories involving strong emotions are consolidated and stored differently from declarative memories. They are retained as visceral sensations, such as anxiety or panic, or visual images, such as flashbacks or nightmares. This is a normative way of recording trauma. These emotional memories can come back with powerful force. For some people, they may fade over time, but for others, the memories, when recalled, can be as vivid as the original experience. The memories may be accompanied by adrenal responses as well, including hyper-responsiveness to stimuli, such as an exaggerated startle or other fear response, avoidance or numbing (i.e., the fight or flight or freeze response to stimuli).

Unfortunately, responses can occur even when present-day circumstances are desirable. An odor, a gesture, a touch, or a word can trigger an emotional response from a threatening situation in one's history. For example, a husband who is caressing his wife's neck lovingly may cause her to react suddenly with terror. She may begin to breathe shallowly and then struggle to push his hand away. By the time he has collected himself and turned on the light in the room, she is unaccountably in tears. Because they have experienced her flashback responses in the past, they both put the facts together and discover that the husband's loving gesture triggered in his wife memory of a rape that had happened years before, when the wife had awakened to find a stranger who had one hand over her mouth and the other at her throat. Her response to her husband's gesture was extreme, but, nevertheless, it occurred with all of its emotional impact. Although she is aware that she is in no current danger, her emotional cues provided an entirely different signal.

Bessel van der Kolk's work in the Trauma Clinic at Harvard Medical School was directed toward the complexities of neurobiologic treatment strategies for individuals who are paralyzed in the throes of their trauma experience. Psychopharmacology is increasingly playing a role in the management of intrusive symptoms. Reliving the traumatic event experience to achieve catharsis is currently considered to be an outmoded psychological approach for helping patients to master their experience. Current treatment strategies acknowledge the patient's trauma and the ramifications of the experience but the focus is instead on symptom control. Cognitive behavioral strategies, such as keeping journals or a diary of symptoms, assist patients to find their own positive methods of symptom management. Self-help programs are also useful because they provide a type of "natural support system."

Guided-touch exercises are encouraged for patients and their partners. The process of integrating new responses into painful past experiences is complex and requires determined effort and commitment, but many women accomplish this successfully.

## Sex Therapy

Before the age of self-help books and the information highway, sex therapy was often a primary avenue for educating patients about sexuality and sexual functioning. Now, although information is not always reliable, it is most certainly plentiful, so individuals and couples often manage their own symptoms and achieve their own self-help cures. Nevertheless, sex therapy remains a legitimate, integral discipline, which is in demand in the field of psychotherapy. Moreover, sex therapy is frequently effective as adjunctive intervention in medical treatment. It is not a case of couples no longer seeking sex therapy—it is just that patients appear more often with more complicated sexual problems than they did in the past. Those who are dealing with entrenched sexual problems may have depleted their ability to cope with and manage such problems. As stated earlier, this can have a significantly negative effect on an individual or a couple's overall sense of well-being. As Dr. William Masters says, "Sex is a quality-of-life issue."

When and how does a physician or other medical practitioner refer a patient to a sex therapist? The American Association of Sex Educators, Counselors, and Therapists (P.O. Box 238, Mount Vernon, IA 52314-0238 USA) maintains a comprehensive and up-to-date list of all certified sex therapists, educators, counselors, and supervisors. Sex therapists are clinicians who are trained in psychotherapy and treatment of couples. They are aware of the social and psychological aspects of sexuality and issues of intimacy. Many times, what appears to be a straightforward sexual problem—such as discrepant sexual desire (a situation in which one partner wants sexual activity much more frequently than the other) turns out to be much more of a problem related to the couple, such as how they manage power dynamics in their relationship.

It would be ideal if sex therapists could publish a comprehensive set of techniques to employ for various sexual problems, running through the list of dysfunctions that occur with each phase of the sexual response cycle and matching a treatment technique to the specific problem. It is no more realistic to think this could happen than it would be to diagnose a patient's persistent vaginal bleeding without being able to check her vital signs, conduct an examination, and ask questions. Sex therapy, like all disciplines, is contextual. Good sex therapy works closely with medical treatment and uses solid therapy techniques ranging from those oriented toward insight to cognitive behavior or theories of family systems.

## REFERENCES

American Psychiatric Association: The Diagnostic and Statistical Manual of Mental Disorders: Washington, D.C., 1994.

American Psychiatric Association: Diagnostic Criteria from DSM-IV. Washington, D.C., 1994, pp 237–240.

American Psychiatric Association: Sexual and Gender Identity Disorders. *In* American Psychiatric Association: Quick Reference to the Diagnostic and Statistical Manual of Mental Disorders: DSM IV. Washington, D.C., 1994, pp 233–249.

Brumberg JA: The Body Project. New York, Random House, 1997, p 150.

Burleson M, Gregory WL, Trevathan WR: Heterosexual activity: Relationship with ovarian function. Psychoneuroendocrinology 20:405–421, 1995.

Crenshaw TL, Crenshaw JP: Sexual Pharmacology: Drugs That Affect Sexual Function. New York, Norton, 1996, p 64, xv, 95.

Crenshaw TL, Crenshaw JP: Sexual Pharmacology: Drugs That Affect Sexual Function. New York, Norton, p xv.

Crenshaw TL, Goldberg JP: Sexual Pharmacology: Drugs That Affect Sexual Function. New York, Norton, p 95.

Edwards L, Mason M, Phillips M, et al: Childhood sexual and physical abuse: Incidence in patients with vulvodynia. J Reprod Med 42:135–139, 1997.

Foley SM: Contemporary sex therapy. *In* Lectenberg R, Ohl DA (eds): Sexual Dysfunction: Neurologic, Urologic and Gynecologic Aspects. Philadelphia, Lea & Febiger, 1994.

Foley SM: Psychogenic sexual dysfunction. *In* Lectenberg R, Ohl D (eds): Sexual Dysfunction: Neurologic, Urologic and Gynecologic Aspects. Philadelphia, Lea & Febiger, 1994, pp 189–193.

Frederickson HL, Wilkins-Haug L: Ob/Gyn Secrets, Philadelphia, Hanley and Belfus, 1997, p 63.

Haseltine FP, Redmond GP, Wentz AC, et al: Androgens and women's health. Am J Med 98:1A–111S, 1995.

Hutchinson KA: Androgens and sexuality. Am J Med 98(suppl):111S–115S, 1995.

Interview with physical therapists Stephanie Ruseckas and Andrea Sanfield, Beaumont Hospital Royal Oak Michigan, on site, February 26, 1997.

Kaplan HS: The New Sex Therapy: Active Treatment of Sexual Dysfunction. New York, Brunner/Mazel, 1981, p 33.

Kitzinger S: Woman's Experience of Sex: The Facts and Feelings at Every Stage of Life. New York, Penguin, 1983, p 203.

Lectenberg R, Ohl D (eds): Sexual Dysfunction: Neurologic, Urologic and Gynecologic Aspects. Philadelphia, Lea & Febiger, 1994, p 35.

Masters WH, Johnson VE, Kolodny RC: Masters and Johnson on Sex and Human Loving. Boston, Little, Brown, 1986, pp 57–60.

McCarthy BW: Chronic sexual dysfunction: Assessment, intervention and realistic expectations. J Sex Educ Ther 22:51–56, 1998.

van der Kolk B: The body keeps the score: Memory and the evolving psychobiology of posttraumatic stress. Harv Rev Psychiatry 1:253–255, 1994.

# 16

# Urinary Incontinence: Strategies for Evaluation and Nonsurgical Management

CAROL GRAHAM
VERONICA T. MALLETT

Urinary incontinence can be both a physically and mentally devastating disorder. The social stigma, debilitation, and embarrassment associated with incontinence may lead to social isolation and depression. It is estimated that 10 million American adults suffer with urinary incontinence. Health-care costs for management of urinary incontinence alone have been estimated to be more than $10 billion annually. Although urinary incontinence is not a life-threatening illness, the impact on one's quality of life may be profound. The societal cost of urinary incontinence is very difficult to measure but may equal or even exceed the economic costs of managing incontinence.

Although both men and women suffer from incontinence, women are four times more likely to be affected, according to the UPRNet Study by Lagace. It is well established that the prevalence of incontinence increases with advancing age. Similarly, susceptibility to the disease processes and functional impairments that contribute to urinary incontinence also increases with age. In two studies conducted among women of reproductive age, Samuelsson and Turan independently found the prevalence of incontinence to be between 25 and 28%, whereas the prevalence among women aged 65 and older is slightly higher and has been reported to be between 30 and 50%. Among institutionalized women the prevalence of urinary incontinence has been reported to be as high as 80%. By the year 2050, it has been estimated that 21% of the population will be 65 and older. Therefore, the potential growth of the incontinent patient population presents a formidable challenge to the health-care community.

Reports of incontinent patients who do not seek evaluation and treatment are also of concern. Samuelsson and Turan determined that between 85 and 91% of women of reproductive age who have symptoms of incontinence have never sought treatment. These findings are consistent with those of other studies. Factors that may prevent patients from seeking help include embarrassment, fear of surgery, or the perception that physicians lack interest in their problem. More commonly, however, patients may believe that incontinence is a normal and inevitable part of aging.

As the population ages, urinary incontinence will continue to escalate, as will the costs of its management. It is important that health-care providers become familiar with the symptoms, evaluation, and management of urinary incontinence. Providers must become proficient in identifying those who suffer from incontinence. Once identified, patient education, evaluation, and treatment can then be implemented. This chapter provides strategies for the evaluation and nonsurgical management of the incontinent patient.

## Incontinence Symptoms

Different pathophysiologic mechanisms can contribute to the development of urinary incontinence. Incontinence symptoms may help define the pathophysiology underlying the development of incontinence. Stress incontinence may be experienced by women who have urethral diverticula or urethral sphincter dysfunction, as well as by those who have experienced anatomic relocation of the continence unit after increase of intra-abdominal pressure. Detrusor instability may be secondary to inflammation, neuropathic changes, obstruction, or other alterations, the etiologies of which are unknown. Therefore, the approach to the incontinent patient begins with an understanding of the types of incontinence symptoms she may experience. Because of the underlying complexity of the continence mechanism, symptoms of incontinence may not be predictive of the patient's actual diagnosis.

**Stress Incontinence.** Urine loss occurs with increased intra-abdominal pressure caused by coughing, sneezing, laughing, or exercising. It is important to point out that loss of urine with stress is a nondiagnostic symptom. More than 50% of patients who have other incontinence types complain of stress incontinence.

**Urge Incontinence.** The loss of urine is associated with the strong feeling of needing to void. This incontinence symptom may be present in patients who have detrusor instability and genuine stress incontinence. Only 25% of patients who have this complaint actually have urodynamically confirmed detrusor instability.

**Mixed Incontinence.** Urine leakage occurs when both urge and stress incontinence symptoms are present. Mixed incontinence may be caused by a different pathophysiologic entity from the one that triggers the isolated symptoms of urge or stress incontinence. Thus, patients who have mixed incontinence may initially require referral for urodynamic testing.

**Overflow Incontinence.** Uncontrollable urine loss occurs secondary to an overdistended bladder. Patients may experience either urge or stress incontinence, or both, because of excessive bladder volume. Bladder distention initiates a detrusor contraction that in turn causes urine loss. However, in most cases, the contraction is too weak for the bladder contents to empty completely. High residual urine volumes accumulate. During increases in abdominal pressure or movement, the overfilled bladder pressure exceeds the urethral pressure and urine loss occurs.

**Continuous Incontinence.** Leakage of urine occurs all the time. This symptom is unusual and may be associated with the presence of a fistula or a congenital defect. Most congenital defects are identified by pediatricians and thus represent an unlikely cause of incontinence in the older patient population. While obstetric fistulas are rare in industrialized countries, patients who have had previous gynecologic or urologic surgery may be at increased risk for urogenital fistulas. Scarring from previous surgery or radiation can also contribute to a fibrosed, open urethra, which can then produce continuous incontinence.

**Unknown Incontinence.** The loss of urine occurs without preceding symptoms or warning signs. Women may identify the loss of urine only when wet undergarments are noted during toileting or clothing changes. This symptom may indicate a neurologic or psychiatric disorder.

**Incontinence During Intercourse.** Uncontrollable urine loss happens during sexual intercourse. Different pathophysiologic mechanisms of incontinence can produce this symptom. This complaint, however, may be the primary reason a patient seeks help. It is important to explore this issue thoroughly.

## History

To evaluate the incontinent patient adequately, a thorough history must be developed. In addition to defining symptoms related to the type of incontinence, it is important to determine the following:
- Duration of symptoms
- Changes in either the severity or character, or both, of the symptoms
- Use of incontinence products and quantity used per time period
- Activities that produce or exacerbate symptoms
- Effect on patients' daily living routine or social life

### Table 16-1  Urinary Symptoms

| Symptom | Description |
| --- | --- |
| Urgency | Strong desire to void |
| Frequency | Passage of urine at least every 2 hours or more than seven times per d |
| Nocturia | Being awakened from sleep by the urge to void; passage of urine more than two times per night |
| Enuresis | Involuntary passage of urine while sleeping |
| Hematuria | Passage of blood in the urine, either gross or microscopic |
| Dysuria | Painful passage of urine usually not associated with incontinence |
| Pneumaturia | Gas passage in the urine; may occur after intercourse or genitourinary tract instrumentation; may also be a symptom of a fistulous tract between the gastrointestinal and urinary tracts |

- Previous treatment for this condition and outcome of treatment
- Previous surgery for this problem or other related conditions

Other urologic symptoms that should be identified in the history are listed in Table 16–1. Symptoms of urgency and frequency may be indicative of an unstable bladder but may also be symptomatic of interstitial cystitis. Pain syndromes, including dysuria and suprapubic pain, are usually not associated with incontinence. Once a urinary tract infection is ruled out as a pain source, patients who have pain syndromes should be referred for further investigation. Alterations in voiding habits should be explored (Table 16–2).

**Gynecologic-Obstetric History.** The gynecologic history may identify associated pathology. For example, prolapse disorders are common in patients who have various types of incontinence. Frequently, patients who have prolapse complain of pelvic pressure, vaginal bulging, lower abdominal pain, or all of these. Endometriosis and leiomyomas can also directly involve the urinary tract. In addition, uterine enlargement secondary to leiomyomas can also impact bladder function. A history of chronic pelvic pain, dyspareunia, and dysmenorrhea may alter incontinence therapy. Radical pelvic surgery can significantly affect urinary tract physiology and produce dysfunction.

A detailed obstetric history should be included, with information about any complicated or operative vaginal deliveries. Any history of extensive lacerations or episiotomies should be documented. Transient incontinence problems that occurred after deliveries should be noted.

**Medical History.** The general medical history is equally important in making an evaluation of incontinence. Patients who have pulmonary disorders, such as asthma, chronic obstructive pulmonary disease, and chronic bronchitis, may experience excessive coughing. Chronic coughing may weaken the continence support system as well as increase the severity of the condition. Medications used to treat various cardiac diseases, including congestive heart failure, can affect the continence mechanism. Gastrointestinal problems are important to identify because irritable bowel syndrome has been associated with detrusor instability. Patients who have urinary incontinence may also frequently experience fecal and gas incontinence. The presence of fecal and gas incontinence may signify a primary bowel disorder or neurologic abnormality. Trauma, previous surgeries, or obstetric complications may contribute to the development of urinary, fecal, and gas incontinence. A history of chronic constipation may indicate prolonged stress on the continence support system.

Endocrine disorders, such as diabetes mellitus and thyroid dysfunction, can also significantly affect urinary function. Although the pathogenesis of diabetic lower urinary tract dysfunction is not known, it is thought to be similar to diabetic neuropathy in other systems. Classic diabetic cystopathy involves impaired bladder sensation followed by a progressive decrease in detrusor contractility, which ultimately results in urinary retention and possible infection. Patients who have thyroid disease have an increased risk of developing detrusor instability; however, the etiology is unclear.

**Neurologic.** An intact neurologic system is essential for normal functioning of the urinary system. A lesion located at any level of the nervous system can adversely affect urologic function. The incidence of bladder neuropathies is high, even in the more common neurologic disorders (e.g., diabetic neuropathy, multiple sclerosis, stroke, lumbar disk disease, and parkinsonism). Patients who have lower urinary tract complaints are more likely to have a neurologic abnormality. It is important to elicit any history of

### Table 16-2  Voiding Abnormalities

| Symptom | Explanation |
| --- | --- |
| Hesitancy | Difficulty initiating urine stream |
| Intermittent stream | Urinary flow repetitively interrupted |
| Poor stream | Urine stream with reduced flow force |
| Straining to void | Abdominal straining to effect urination |
| Incomplete emptying | Sensation of bladder fullness after voiding |
| Postmicturition dribble | Urine loss experienced after normal urination |
| Acute urinary retention | Sudden onset of voiding inability that may lead to painful overdistention of the bladder; this usually requires emergency catheterization |

neurologic dysfunction as well as any history of back trauma or back surgery.

**Psychiatric.** Psychiatric disorders can also affect the urinary tract. In a 1997 survey, Bonney and associates found that incontinence was more prevalent in schizophrenic patients than in a similar group of patients who had mood disorders. Many of the anticholinergic medications used to treat psychiatric disorders can cause urinary retention and, therefore, contribute to overflow incontinence. The impact of incontinence and loss of bodily control on psychiatric health must also be considered.

**Medication.** The medication history is of primary importance to explore. Many prescription medications, as well as over-the-counter preparations, may detrimentally affect the urinary tract (Table 16–3). Slightly altering the medication prescribed or the dosing regimen may be critical in decreasing urinary symptoms.

**Social.** Social habits should also be reviewed with the patient. The type of fluid intake and the volume of consumption should be considered in the evaluation. It is important to determine the amount of alcoholic and caffeinated beverages the patient consumes, because alcohol and caffeine can alter urinary tract function. This information can be recorded prospectively by the patient in an intake/output diary. Abuse of alcohol and other substances may directly affect the urinary system but can also lead to long-term neuropathic changes. Tobacco abuse may contribute to chronic pulmonary problems and thereby impact the continence support system.

In assessing the history of the elderly incontinent patient, it is important to recognize that there may be transient contributing factors to urinary dysfunction. Transient causes of incontinence affect 30% of community-dwelling elderly patients and 50% of those who are acutely hospitalized. These transient causes must be ruled out as contributing factors to the elderly patient's incontinence problem. Resnick has adeptly formulated a mnemonic that facilitates recall of these transient factors:

- D  Delirium (confusional state)
- I  Infection—urinary (only symptomatic)
- A  Atrophic urethritis, vaginitis
- P  Pharmaceuticals
- P  Psychological, especially severe depression
- E  Excessive urine output (e.g., congestive heart failure [CHF], hyperglycemia)
- R  Restricted mobility
- S  Stool impaction

Compiling a comprehensive history is an important first step in evaluating the incontinent patient. Moreover, the history should provide insight for defining the final diagnosis. Based on the history and the physical examination, the physician can individualize the necessary extent and type of further evaluation. However, caution is needed in evaluating the diagnostic accuracy of the patient's history. Symptoms are important to explore, but the history alone may not be reliable in predicting a final diagnosis. In an analysis of 535 women, Cundiff found that pure symptoms identified fewer than 50% of patients who had diagnoses of stress incontinence, detrusor instability, or mixed incontinence. Jensen and associates evaluated 19 articles that addressed the clinical evaluation of urinary incontinence. The results of this analysis sug-

Table 16–3  Over-the-Counter and Common Prescription Medications Affecting the Continence Mechanism

| Agent | Effects |
| --- | --- |
| Caffeine | Lower urethral pressure can result from excessive caffeine intake |
| Calcium channel blockers | May decrease smooth muscle contractility and contribute to urinary retention with overflow incontinence |
| Loop diuretics | Produces significant diuresis; rapid increase in urine production may overstress continence mechanism, especially in immobile patients |
| Anticholinergic agents: Antidepressants Antihistamines Antipsychotics Antispasmodics Opiates Donnatal Antiparkinsonian agents Benztropine mesylate | Impaired detrusor contractility leading to urinary retention with secondary overflow incontinence; agents are common in over-the-counter cold medications; in addition to anticholinergic effects, antipsychotics can produce sedation and movement disorders |
| Sympatholytics (prazosin, phenoxybenzamine) | α-adrenergic antagonists decrease urethral sphincter tone |
| Sympathomimetics (decongestants) | α-adrenergic agonists increase urethral sphincter tone and lead to urinary retention; common in over-the-counter cold preparations |
| Alcohol | Diuresis with impaired sensorium and mobility may stress a compromised continence mechanism |

Data from Urinary Incontinence Guideline Panel: Urinary incontinence in adults: Clinical practice guideline. Rockville, MD, Agency for Health Care Policy and Research. Public Health Service, US Department of Health and Human Services 1992, Agency for Health Care Policy and Research (AHCPR) publication no. 92-0038.

gest that the patient's history is an inaccurate predictor of the final urodynamic diagnosis. Therefore, additional information is required to assess the incontinent patient properly.

## Physical Examination

**Pelvic Examination.** A general physical examination is performed. When the general physical examination is completed, the pelvic examination is performed. The pelvic examination should assess the neurologic function, estrogen status, pelvic pathology, and presence of pelvic relaxation. Ideally, the patient should have a comfortably full bladder at the time of the examination. This assists in evaluating pelvic relaxation disorders and in performing the stress test.

**Neurologic.** In addition to a brief general neurologic examination, a more focused examination can assess the integrity of the lumbosacral and pelvic areas. The lumbosacral spine should be palpated to identify possible abnormalities. Muscle strength and deep tendon reflexes should be evaluated. In addition, the patient should be asked to abduct her toes to evaluate the integrity of the lower sacral segments. The examination of perineal sensation can be performed with the patient in the dorsal lithotomy position. Presence of the anal reflex can be determined by lightly stroking the perianal region and observing the resulting anal contraction (anal "wink"). Similarly, the bulbocavernosus reflex is elicited by lightly touching the clitoris and observing an anal contraction. The "cough reflex" is a pelvic floor contraction stimulated by a cough. The absence of all three reflexes may indicate a lesion of S2–S4 in the presence of other neurologic findings. Since these reflexes may be difficult to elicit in some women, the absence of one reflex is not indicative of neurologic abnormality.

**Estrogen Status and Prolapse Assessment.** The genitalia should be evaluated for signs of estrogen deprivation. Atrophic vaginitis and urethritis, decrease in vaginal rugae, and presence of a urethral caruncle or urethral prolapse can be signs of hypoestrogenism. The urethra and surrounding Skene's glands should be palpated for evidence of inflammation and the presence of purulent drainage. Palpation of the urethra may also reveal the presence of a diverticulum, which can produce incontinence symptoms. The anatomic positioning of the urethral meatus should be evaluated, because abnormal displacement may be a sign of urethral hypermobility.

Pelvic relaxation can be assessed by using the posterior blade of a metal Graves or Pederson speculum. Placing the speculum in such a way as to retract either the posterior or the anterior vaginal wall allows observation of prolapse defects of the opposite vaginal wall. When the speculum is retracted posteriorly, the patient is encouraged to cough and then perform the Valsalva maneuver. Excursion of the anterior vaginal wall is noted with each maneuver. This examination is performed similarly for the posterior wall assessment. The bivalve speculum can be used to evaluate uterine prolapse or posthysterectomy vaginal vault prolapse. The speculum can be placed to support the anterior and posterior walls in such a way that uterine descensus and vault prolapse can be observed when the patient coughs and executes the Valsalva maneuver. Assessment of prolapse should also include an examination with the patient in the standing position. A rectovaginal examination using this position can help distinguish an enterocele from a rectocele. Anal tone can also be assessed at this time.

**Stress Test.** As mentioned previously, the incontinent patient should be examined with a comfortably full bladder. Examination of the patient with a full bladder facilitates performance of the stress test as well as assessment of pelvic relaxation. The stress test is performed in an attempt to reproduce any symptoms of stress incontinence or cough-induced urge incontinence. While in the supine position, the patient is encouraged to cough or bear down. Movement of the urethra and the bladder neck accompanied by loss of urine with the cough strongly suggests that the patient has stress incontinence. Detrusor instability is suspected if there is delayed urine loss or a large-volume loss. The patient must confirm that the examination is reflective of her symptoms. If the stress test is negative in the supine position, the test must be repeated in the standing position.

Patients who have significant prolapse may remain continent secondary to kinking of the urethra. To unmask incontinence in this group, the stress test should be performed with either a pessary in place or with the support of a speculum. Once the prolapse is reduced (with care taken to avoid urethral obstruction), the stress test can be performed as detailed above.

**Postvoid Residual and Urethral Mobility Assessment.** After the stress evaluation is completed, the patient may empty her bladder. A residual volume can then be measured. The remainder of the pelvic examination can also be completed, because an empty bladder is preferable for performance of the bimanual examination and assessment of pelvic floor muscle strength. With the patient in the supine position, a sterile catheter is used to obtain the residual volume that is recorded. A residual volume of more than 50 ml may reflect voiding dysfunction and requires further testing. The specimen may also be used for urinalysis and assessment of urinary infection. A 14-French (F) plastic catheter can be used to obtain the specimen and left in place to evaluate bladder neck mobility in place of the Q-Tip.

The Q-Tip test is a method of evaluating bladder neck mobility (Fig. 16–1). The presence of bladder neck mobility, however, is not diagnostic of stress incontinence. Documenting mobility of the bladder neck is important because many anti-incontinence procedures are performed to stabilize the urethrovesical junction. Patients who undergo concomitant surgeries for stress incontinence and lack bladder neck mobility have a higher surgical failure rate. To perform the test, either the plastic catheter or a sterile, lubricated Q-Tip (more commonly used) is inserted just beyond the bladder neck. The resting angle is measured in relation to the horizontal axis. These measurements can most easily be taken using an orthopedic goniometer. The excursions of the Q-Tip or catheter are measured as the patient contracts her pelvic floor, coughs, and performs the Valsalva maneuver. A resting angle or a Q-Tip excursion of more than 30 degrees can be suggestive of urethral and bladder neck mobility.

Other methods of assessing urethrovesical junction mobility include inspection and palpation, bead-chain cystourethrography, and ultrasonography. Inspection and palpation of the bladder neck have proven reliable in the assessment of bladder neck mobility; however, the evaluation may be inaccurate in certain patients. Urethrovesical descent may be difficult to distinguish in patients who have redundant periurethral tissue. Alternatively, descent of the bladder neck during stress may be missed in a young nulliparous woman. Bead-chain cystourethrography is now an outmoded method of urethral assessment. This was a popular procedure in the 1960s and 1970s. It was discovered, however, that static radiographic measurements taken of the urethrovesical angles were not reflective of mobility or predictive of incontinence.

Ultrasonography has proved to be a promising method of urethral mobility assessment. Caputo and Benson compared the Q-Tip assessment to ultrasonographic measurements of urethrovesical mobility. Using ultrasonography as the standard, the Q-Tip test was found to be less accurate for mobility measurement. Other authors recommend use of the vaginal transducer to measure urethrovesical mobility in relation to the symphysis pubis. This method has been shown to be reproducible, reliable, and productive of minimal artifact. The limiting factors to widespread usage of ultrasonographic assessment are cost and accessibility. In most general office practices, use of the Q-Tip is sufficient for documenting urethral mobility.

**Bimanual Examination and Pelvic Floor Assessment.** Pelvic pathology is assessed by performance of the bimanual examination. Any possible pelvic abnormalities that might contribute to the urologic symptoms should be examined and evaluated when they are discovered. When the bimanual examination is performed, the physician can easily evaluate the pelvic floor musculature and muscle strength by palpating the posterior vaginal wall with two gloved digits. The patient is instructed to perform a pelvic floor contraction (e.g., "Stop your urine stream," "Hold back gas," or "Squeeze my fingers"), holding it as

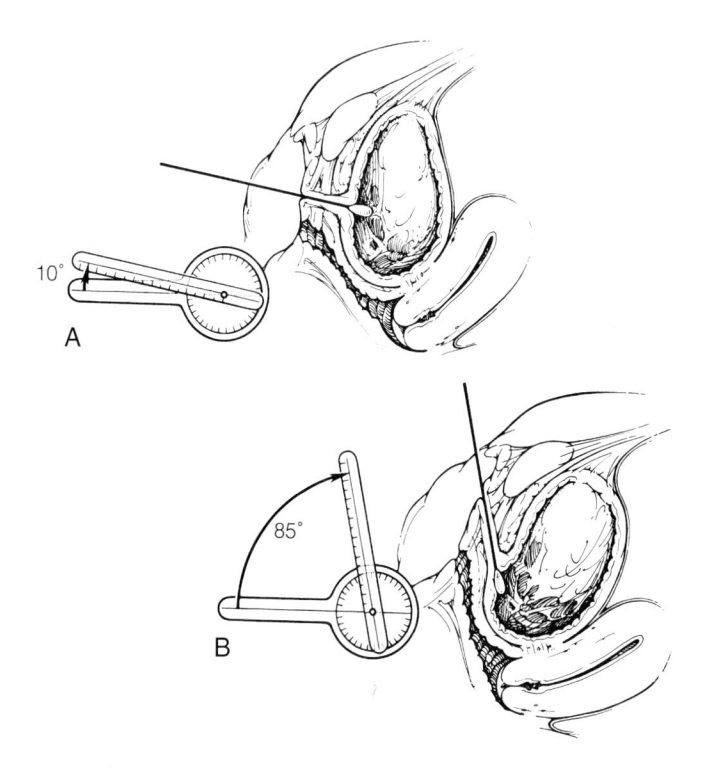

Figure 16–1 Urethral mobility assessment using Q-Tip test. A, Using an orthopedic goniometer, the resting angle is measured in relation to the horizontal axis. B, During Valsalva's maneuver, straining angle is measured. (From Mallett VT, Richardson DA: Gynecologic urology. In Nichols DG, Sweeney PJ [eds]: Ambulatory Gynecology. Philadelphia, JB Lippincott, 1995, pp 314–341.)

**Table 16–4** Assessing Pelvic Floor Muscle Contractions

| Score | Assessment |
|---|---|
| 0/5 | No contraction |
| 1/5 | Contraction <1 sec |
| 2/5 *weak* | Contraction for 1–3 sec. Hold and/or fingers not elevated |
| 3/5 *moderate* | Contraction for 4–6 sec. Hold and fingers elevated; repeat 3× |
| 4/5 *strong* | Contraction 7–9 sec. Hold and fingers elevated; repeat 3× |
| 5/5 *unmistakably strong* | Rapid contraction with elevation for >9 sec; repeat 4× |

long as possible. Using three repetitions, the contractions are then scored on the basis of strength and duration (Table 16–4). The score provides a baseline measurement for assessing future change or assessing progress of physical therapy, if prescribed. This examination should also include an assessment of muscle symmetry and the presence of tenderness. As the patient contracts the pelvic floor, any asymmetry of muscle movement or muscle elevation should be noted.

## Laboratory Testing

Currently, the laboratory testing recommended for urinary incontinence assessment is limited. It is most important to test for urinary infection (urinalysis, micro ± urine culture) because a lower urinary tract infection may cause incontinence symptoms. Asymptomatic bacteriuria and urinary tract infections are common in all age groups, but the incidence increases as a woman ages, as does incontinence. Ideally, urinary infection should be ruled out before instrumentation occurs. Chemical dipsticks may be helpful in screening before catheterization is performed. Persistent pyuria or hematuria with a negative urine culture mandates further evaluation. Glucosuria or proteinuria may reveal underlying medical problems that may contribute to incontinence. Patients at risk of urinary tract obstruction (e.g., severe prolapse disorders, overflow incontinence) should have blood urea nitrogen and serum creatinine tests performed to rule out renal impairment. Patients who have an unstable bladder should be screened for thyroid abnormalities. Hypercalcemia can contribute to incontinence in the elderly; therefore, a serum calcium level should be obtained in the appropriate clinical setting.

## Urinary Diaries

Patients should complete 24-hour and 7-day urinary diaries (Figs. 16–2 and 16–3). The diaries provide prospective and semiobjective information, which can be compared with the history. In addition, the severity and nature of incontinence can be objectively determined. The 24-hour diary requires measurement of voided volumes and assessment of episodes of incontinence. Symptoms, such as urge and pain, can be noted along with the amount of fluid volume consumed. The 24-hour diary identifies high-output and infrequent voiders. Other information obtained from the 24-hour diary includes the following:

1. Diurnal variation
2. Total voided volume in 24 hours
3. Largest single voided volume
4. Mean voided volume
5. Voiding frequency.

The International Continence Society has defined a patient's functional bladder capacity as the patient's largest voided volume recorded in the 24-hour diary.

The 7-day diary requires recording of voiding as well as stress and urge incontinence events. Numeric totals are recorded for events occurring between midnight and 6 AM. Since no measurements are required, this diary is more convenient for patients to complete. The 7-day diary is an excellent tool to use before and after therapy in the assessment of treatment efficacy.

## Pad Tests

Pad tests can be performed either to document incontinent episodes or to quantify the amount of urine loss. There are several different pad tests, none of which has been universally recommended. Short-term tests are usually performed in the office or laboratory during a 1- to 2-hour period, whereas long-term tests

**Table 16–5** International Continence Society Pad Test (Modified) Sample Schedule—Short-Term Test

Patient begins test without voiding
Preweighed pad is positioned and 1-hr test begins
Patient drinks 500 ml of sodium-free beverage
Over the next 30 min, patient walks and climbs up and down equivalent of one flight of stairs
Following activities are performed in remainder of hour:
    a. Standing from sitting 10 times
    b. Coughing vigorously 10 times
    c. Running in place for 1 min
    d. Bending to pick up small object from floor 5 times
    e. Washing hands in running water for 1 min
After completion of 1-hr test, pad is removed and weighed
If patient believes test is representative, patient voids and amount is recorded
If test is not reflective of patient's symptoms, test is repeated without voiding

# URINARY INCONTINENCE: EVALUATION AND NONSURGICAL MANAGEMENT

Name          Date        Time You Awoke / Time You Went to Bed

| Enter Time of Void or Leak | Amount of Urine Voided (cc (or ml) | Amount Leaked 1 2 3 (See key on bottom page) | Did You Have Urge With Leak | Activity When Leakage Occurred | Fluid Intake (cc or oz) |
|---|---|---|---|---|---|
| | | | | | |

**Key: Mark Each Episode of Leaking With:**
1. Damp pad or a few drops
2. Wet pad or underwear
3. Soaked pad or emptied bladder

**Figure 16-2** Twenty-four hour voiding diary.

are performed at home over a 24- to 48-hour period. If the stress test fails to demonstrate incontinence or if quantification of incontinence is desired, a pad test can be performed. To prepare for the short-term test, a patient may take phenazopyridine hydrochloride (200 mg 1 to 2 hours before the scheduled test) and have a comfortably full bladder (pyridium pad test). Alternatively, the patient's bladder can be filled in a retrograde manner with methylene blue-tinted sterile saline. The patient is then instructed to perform various physical maneuvers, which may be individualized if patients have physical limitations. The pad should be weighed before and after testing. Both the presence and quantity of leakage can be documented. In 1983, the International Continence Society proposed a standardized 1-hour pad-weighing test, which has been used in most studies of pad tests. An updated outline of the test schedule is detailed in Table 16–5. Some authors (Lose and associates and Versi and associates) recommend that short-term tests be used with caution given the low negative predictive value and the low level of reproducibility of the tests.

Long-term pad tests may have advantages in the assessment of incontinence. In recent studies, long-term tests were found to have a higher level of reproducibility. For the long-term pad-weighing tests, patients are provided with absorbent pads, a letter balance for pad weighing before and after use, in-

**Figure 16–3** Seven-day voiding diary.

|  | 6 AM | 7 AM | 8 AM | 9 AM | 10 AM | 11 AM | 12 PM | 1 PM | 2 PM | 3 PM | 4 PM | 5 PM | 6 PM | 7 PM | 8 PM | 9 PM | 10 PM | 11 PM | 12 AM | No. of voids from midnight to 6 AM | No. of leaks from midnight to 6 AM | No. of pads used each day |
|---|---|---|---|---|---|---|---|---|---|---|---|---|---|---|---|---|---|---|---|---|---|---|
| Sample | E |  | S E | | E | S | | E S | | S | | E | S | | E | | E | | | 2 | NONE | 3 |
| Day 1 | | | | | | | | | | | | | | | | | | | | | | |
| Day 2 | | | | | | | | | | | | | | | | | | | | | | |
| Day 3 | | | | | | | | | | | | | | | | | | | | | | |
| Day 4 | | | | | | | | | | | | | | | | | | | | | | |
| Day 5 | | | | | | | | | | | | | | | | | | | | | | |
| Day 6 | | | | | | | | | | | | | | | | | | | | | | |
| Day 7 | | | | | | | | | | | | | | | | | | | | | | |

Mark each void or leak with:
   E  When you empty your bladder
   S  When you leak with cough, sneeze, exercise, etc.
   U  When you leak with a strong urge

Type of pad used:
   \_\_\_\_\_ Mini
   \_\_\_\_\_ Regular
   \_\_\_\_\_ Maxi

Patient name:                                                              Date:

Signature of study coordinator or physician after review of the diary:

structions, and a test protocol. Patients are encouraged to perform their daily activities and not avoid situations in which leakage might occur. Pads are weighed before and after use and the measurements recorded. Practical advantages of the long-term test include no requirement of supervision by staff and the comfort of testing in the home environment. Given the less stressful testing situation, patients may feel more comfortable about demonstrating incontinence. This testing is easy for most patients to perform regardless of medical problems or disability.

## Simple Cystometry

The previously described incontinence evaluation, as outlined in Table 16–6, should be completed before nonsurgical therapy is initiated. The recommended evaluation strategy is straightforward and simple to perform in the office. Moreover, it does not require a significant investment in equipment. If, however, the testing remains inconclusive, questionable, or surgical therapy is indicated, additional testing must be performed. It is important to confirm and define the incontinence type before surgery is undertaken.

The simple cystometrogram can easily be incorporated into the office examination if necessary (Fig. 16–4). The test is usually begun after the patient has emptied her bladder. With the patient in the dorsal lithotomy position, the urethral meatus is prepared with iodine and a 12- to 14-F red rubber catheter is inserted. The residual volume is measured and recorded and urine sent for evaluation, if necessary. With the catheter in place, cystometry is performed to determine the presence of bladder instability. The catheter is attached to a 60-ml catheter-tip syringe. The bladder is filled in 60-ml increments with warmed sterile saline. Volumes are noted (eyeballed) as the patient is questioned regarding the following points:

1. First desire to void
2. Sensation of fullness
3. Maximum holding capacity

This last volume represents the cystometric capacity. Normal first desire to void usually occurs between 150 and 250 ml. A first sensation at less than 100 ml is abnormal. Strong desire to void usually occurs at volumes greater than 250 ml, and cystometric capacity is normally between 400 and 600 ml.

The syringe is also monitored closely during the filling phase. If the saline level is noted to rise 15 ml or more without evidence of increased abdominal pressure, bladder instability is strongly suspected. If the stress test has not already been performed, it can be done at this time. Before the catheter is removed, some of the fluid should be drained to achieve a comfortable fullness. The stress test with the patient in the supine and standing positions can now be performed as previously detailed. Wall and associates demonstrated that when compared with multichannel subtracted cystometry, simple cystometry with a stress test had positive and negative predictive values of 83.3 and 70.2%, respectively, for the diagnosis of detrusor instability. Similarly, they found that positive and negative predictive values for the demonstration of stress incontinence were 82 and 84.4%, respectively. They concluded that simple bladder filling is a reliable method of diagnosing urinary incontinence in uncomplicated patients.

**Table 16–6** Strategy for Evaluation of Urinary Incontinence (Minimum Assessment for Medical Management)

### HISTORY
Incontinence and urinary symptoms
Impact on daily activity
Surgical/medical/social problems affecting urinary tract
Medications

### GENERAL PHYSICAL EXAMINATION

### PELVIC EXAMINATION

| Full Bladder | Full or empty bladder | Empty bladder |
|---|---|---|
| Prolapse | Estrogen assessment | Pelvic mass |
| Stress test | Neurologic | Postvoid residual |
|  | Pelvic floor muscle strength | Urethral hypermobility |
|  |  | Empty supine stress test |

### LABORATORY TESTING
Urinalysis
Culture and sensitivity
TSH, serum creatinine/BUN, calcium (if indicated)

### URINARY DIARIES
24 hour
7 day

### PAD TEST
Document incontinent episodes, quantity of urine loss, or both

BUN = blood urea nitrogen; TSH = thyroid-stimulating hormone.

## Complex Urodynamic Testing

Most patients who have uncomplicated incontinence problems can be initially evaluated using the previously described strategy. However, certain patients require complex testing before surgical therapy can be performed. Patients who may benefit from multi-

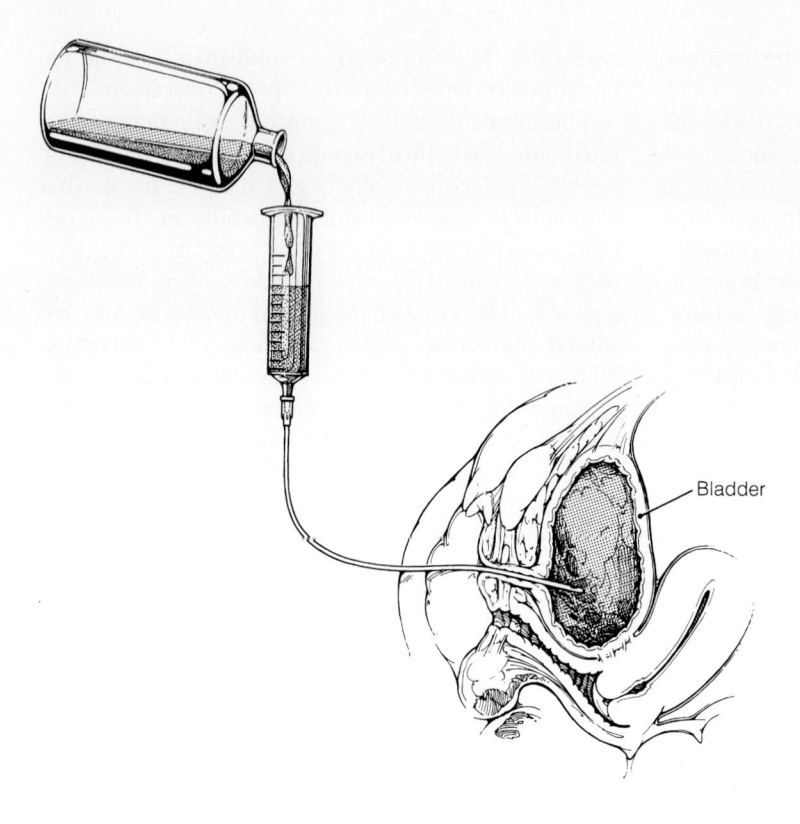

**Figure 16–4** Basic setup for simple cystometrogram. The supine position is illustrated. (From Mallett VT, Richardson DA: Gynecologic urology. *In* Nichols DG, Sweeney PJ (eds): Ambulatory Gynecology. Philadelphia, JB Lippincott, 1995, pp 314–341.)

channel subtracted urodynamic testing include the following:

- Older than 50 years of age (greater risk of detrusor instability or mixed incontinence)
- History of incontinence or prolapse surgery
- History of radical pelvic surgery, pelvic irradiation, or both
- No urethral hypermobility; no evidence of anterior vaginal relaxation
- Severe pelvic organ prolapse (greater than grade 2)
- Continuous incontinence
- Possible urethral diverticulum
- Hematuria with negative urine culture
- Inconclusive or confusing office evaluation

A complete urodynamic examination is usually performed in a laboratory setting and includes complex cystometry, urethral pressure profilometry, and uroflowmetry. Fluoroscopic assessment can be added to any one of these tests.

## Multichannel Subtracted Cystometry

Complex cystometry measures bladder volume and pressure, abdominal pressure, subtracted detrusor pressure, and filling rate simultaneously during bladder filling. Patients are usually placed in the sitting position at a 45-degree angle for urodynamic testing. Alternatively, testing may be performed while the patient stands or ambulates. Using catheters with special transducers (e.g., microtip transducers), the patient's bladder is filled with sterile saline at 75 to 100 ml/min (slower rates may be used if instability is a problem). As the bladder is filled, the patient is instructed to note when she senses a first urge to void, a full bladder, and maximum holding capacity. Bladder and true detrusor pressures are measured during filling and detrusor activity is recorded. True detrusor pressure is calculated by subtracting abdominal pressure (the pressure transducer is placed vaginally or rectally) from bladder or vesical pressure. An increase in true detrusor pressure associated with leaking and urgency confirms detrusor instability. Bladder atony or noncompliance can also be documented by assessment of detrusor pressure changes with filling.

Provocative testing is usually performed if bladder instability has not yet been demonstrated. Once a full bladder capacity is achieved or 300 ml has been infused, filling is stopped and the patient is asked to cough and then perform Valsalva's maneuver. If these fail to stimulate a detrusor contraction, further provocative testing with running water can be performed. If stress incontinence or detrusor instability has not been documented at this point, the patient should be challenged in the standing position. With a full bladder, the standing patient is asked to cough, bear down, heel bounce, and listen to running water. Bladder stability is then confirmed if no detrusor contractions are documented in the sitting or standing position.

Ambulatory cystourethrovaginometry is an alternative to stationary cystometry. Ambulatory testing was developed to enhance detection of patients who have incontinence and who are unable to demonstrate their leakage in the urodynamics lab. The ambulatory setup and catheter placement are similar to those used for stationary cystometry. The catheters, however, must either be taped or sutured in place. Leakage can be recorded using pads with special sensors or conductance rings on the catheter (distal to the urethral pressure transducer). Kulseng-Hanssen recently reported that the sensitivity of ambulatory cystourethrovaginometry is higher than stationary urodynamic recording in detecting bladder instability. Porru and Usai, in a study of 46 patients, found that extramural ambulatory urodynamics detected motor urgency and urge incontinence twice as frequently as did stationary urodynamic evaluation. Advantages of ambulatory cystometry also include antegrade bladder filling, which is more natural. Patients may also feel more relaxed about demonstrating incontinence episodes if the stress of performing is removed. From Kulseng-Hanssen's literature study on cystometry reproducibility, it was also found that an extracorporally fixed urethral pressure catheter produces an unreliable recording. As the technology improves, ambulatory testing may be a more successful method of urodynamic assessment.

## Pressure Profilometry

Urethral pressure profilometry measures urethral pressure changes over urethral length. Bladder filling is discontinued while the pressure profile is generated. An empty bladder urethral profile can be recorded before bladder filling is initiated. A urethral profile at maximum bladder capacity can be performed after cystometrogram testing is completed. This profile can either be generated manually or by use of sophisticated equipment. By slow, steady, manual withdrawal of the urethral catheter from the bladder to the urethral meatus, a pressure profile is created. Alternatively, automated equipment generates the pressure profile curve by coordinating the chart speed and the speed of the catheter puller. The functional urethral length is that portion of the curve where the urethral pressure exceeds the bladder pressure, when both pressures are measured simultaneously. Total urethral length is the functional length plus the remaining urethral length extending to the meatus.

Urethral closure pressure is calculated by subtracting bladder pressure from urethral pressure. The maximum closure pressure represents the greatest pressure difference between the detrusor and the urethra. A maximum closure pressure less than or equal to 20 cm $H_2O$ suggests a low-pressure urethra and intrinsic sphincter deficiency. Patients who have low urethral pressures may experience a higher failure rate after surgical treatment with retropubic procedures.

During the urethral pressure assessment, a cough profile is obtained. The patient is asked to cough forcefully at several points during the urethral profile test. Ideally, the patient should cough during the ascent, peak, and descent of the urethral profile curve. The deflection of the curve as the patient coughs represents the pressure transmission ratio (PTR). The ratio can be calculated by dividing the change in urethral closure pressure by the change in bladder pressure and multiplying by 100. Genuine stress incontinence is associated with a PTR of less than 90%. In a study of 145 women, Richardson found the cough profile to have low sensitivity (41%) but high specificity (92%). However, many of the subjects who had stress incontinence in this study population had a normal cough profile. The authors cautioned against use of the cough profile as the only diagnostic information in making clinical decisions. Although the cough profile can provide important additional information, the stress test is still considered the gold standard.

## Uroflowmetry

Uroflowmetry, performed to assess voiding dysfunction, uses a special commode containing a calibrated electronic flowmeter that generates a flow tracing. During simple flowmetry, peak flow, mean flow rate, flow time, voiding time, time to peak flow, and volume voided are usually measured. A normal peak flow rate is 15 to 20 ml/sec. Rates of less than 15 ml/sec suggest an obstructed outflow tract; however, a patient must void at least 150 to 200 ml for the study to be meaningful.

Pressure-flow voiding studies add bladder, urethral, and abdominal pressure changes to the simple flowmetry measures. Pressure-flow studies provide assessment of voiding mechanisms and provide differentiation among detrusor contraction, pelvic relaxation, and abdominal straining. Patterns of obstructive voiding can also be determined using pressure-flow studies. Obstruction is considered if a patient's flow rate is less than 15 ml/sec with a detrusor contraction pressure higher than 50 cm $H_2O$.

In addition to the measurements listed above, flow curves are important to evaluate when interpreting voiding function. Typically, a normal flow pattern is represented by a bell-shaped curve that is indicative of a normal detrusor contraction with pelvic relaxation to effect micturition. Patients who use abdominal assistance to void demonstrate a flow curve with superimposed spikes. Flow patterns with interrupted sharp peaks or with a low, plateau-like curve usually are indicative of significant voiding dysfunction.

## Urethrocystoscopy

Endoscopic evaluation of the urethra and bladder can detect urethral inflammation, urethral diverticula, interstitial cystitis, and various bladder lesions. This procedure can be performed easily in the office setting if appropriate training for the examiner has been completed. With application of intraurethral anesthetic jelly, patients usually tolerate the procedure without great discomfort. Endoscopy can be an important adjunct to the urodynamic evaluation. If a urethral diverticulum is suspected or a postoperative patient presents with postoperative symptoms that cause concern, cystoscopy should be performed. Urethrocystoscopy, however, has limited use in the diagnosis of genuine stress incontinence. Versi and associates challenged the diagnostic value of cystoscopy in the detection of an open bladder neck. In their study, they found an open bladder neck in 50% of asymptomatic menopausal women. When comparing urethrocystoscopy with standard urodynamics, Scotti and associates found cystoscopy to be an insensitive predictor of stress urinary incontinence.

## Treatment

Once the evaluation is complete and a diagnosis defined, a management plan can be developed. Patient treatment preference is an important consideration when an individualized therapy program is being created. Behavioral modification, pelvic floor muscle physical therapy with biofeedback or electrical stimulation, pharmacotherapy, and continence devices are all nonsurgical treatment modalities that may be effective incontinence therapies. Most of these therapies can be used for both detrusor instability and stress incontinence. Karram and associates recently demonstrated the success of nonsurgical therapy. Of 202 incontinent women studied, 59% (119) were subjectively cured or improved with nonsurgical therapy. The researchers concluded that all incontinent women should be initially offered nonsurgical therapy. Nonsurgical conservative therapies for genuine stress incontinence and detrusor instability are outlined in subsequent sections.

## Pharmacotherapy

**Estrogens.** For many years, estrogens have been used for the treatment of incontinence and other female lower urinary tract disorders. Estrogen has been used to treat both detrusor instability and stress incontinence. Symptoms of frequency, urgency, and urge incontinence may diminish after estrogen therapy. For the treatment of stress incontinence, estrogen combined with an α-adrenergic agonist has been shown to be more effective than either agent alone. The therapeutic efficacy of estrogen, however, remains controversial because few randomized, placebo-controlled prospective studies have been conducted to evaluate estrogen's efficacy in incontinence therapy. In a recent randomized, placebo-controlled study, Fantl and associates evaluated the effects of estrogen supplementation on incontinence symptoms. They found no significant improvement in clinical measures or quality of life. However, their study was limited by the short-term use of oral estrogen without vaginal estrogen therapy.

In planning an estrogen regimen, it is important to note that local delivery of systemic estrogen may be decreased if significant urogenital atrophy is present. To enhance submucosal vascularity, vaginal estrogen administration is recommended initially with or without systemic therapy. Therapy consists of one-half or one full applicator of any vaginal estrogen cream (Premarin, Estrace, or Ogen) placed daily for 2 to 4 weeks. Estring (estradiol delivered via silicone ring) can also be inserted vaginally for 3 months. As the atrophy improves, local maintenance therapy can be continued with one-half applicator once or twice weekly or discontinued if systemic therapy is ongoing. See Table 16–7, which summarizes the pharmacotherapy for treatment of stress urinary incontinence, detrusor instability, or both.

### STRESS URINARY INCONTINENCE

**Sympathomimetic Agents.** Enhancement of urethral sphincter tone is the goal of stress incontinence pharmacotherapy. Smooth muscle contraction is stimulated by α-receptor agonists, which increase bladder outlet resistance. These medications may cure up to 14% of patients, with marked improvement demonstrated in 30 to 60%. Ephedrine and phenylpropanolamine are the α-agonists most commonly prescribed for the treatment of stress incontinence. Ephedrine, a noncatecholamine sympathomimetic, directly stimulates both α- and β-adrenergic receptors and also acts peripherally to release norepinephrine. The recommended dosage for incontinence therapy is 25 to 50 mg three or four times a day. A stereoisomer

**Table 16–7** Pharmacotherapy of Urinary Incontinence

| Medication | Treatment for: Stress Incontinence | Treatment for: Detrusor Instability | Recommended Dosage |
|---|---|---|---|
| **ESTROGEN** | | | |
| Local or creams | + | + | Initial: 1/2–1 applicator q hs × 2–4 wk<br>Maintenance: 1/2 applicator 2 ×/wk |
| Systemic | + | + | Depends on estrogen type and mode of delivery |
| **SYMPATHOMIMETIC AGENTS** | | | |
| Ephedrine | + | – | 25 mg tid–50 mg qid |
| Pseudoephedrine | + | – | 15 mg bid–60 mg qid |
| Phenylpropanolamine | + | – | Available in over-the-counter appetite suppressants and decongestants |
| Tablets | | | 25 mg bid–50 mg qid |
| Sustained release | | | 75 mg bid |
| **TRICYCLIC ANTIDEPRESSANTS** | | | |
| Imipramine (Tofranil) | + | + | 10 mg bid–75 mg bid |
| Doxepin (Sinequan) | + | + | 50 mg qhs ± 25 mg q AM |
| **ANTICHOLINERGIC AGENTS** | | | |
| Propantheline bromide (Pro-Banthine) | – | + | 15–30 mg q 4–6 hr (administer 30 min before meals) |
| Hyoscyamine (Cystospaz) | – | + | .15–.30 mg qid |
| Hyoscyamine sulfate (Levsin/SL) | – | + | .125–.250 mg qid sublingual/PO |
| Hyoscyamine sulfate (Cystopaz-M) | – | + | .375 mg bid |
| Tolterodine (Detrol) | – | + | 1–2 mg bid |
| **ANTISPASMODIC AGENTS** | | | |
| Oxybutynin (Ditropan) | – | + | 2.5 mg bid–5.0 mg tid |
| Dicyclomine (Bentyl) | – | + | 10–20 mg tid |
| **CALCIUM ANTAGONIST** | | | |
| Nifedipine (Procardia) | – | + | 10–20 mg bid |

bid = two times daily; tid = three times daily; qid = four times daily; qd = every day.

of ephedrine, pseudoephedrine, is available over the counter (Actifed, Sudafed). Pseudoephedrine dosage recommendations range from 15 mg twice a day to 60 mg four times a day. The pharmacologic mechanism of phenylpropanolamine hydrochloride is similar to that of ephedrine, but phenylpropanolamine has less central nervous system activity. Many appetite suppressants and sinus decongestants contain phenylpropanolamine and can be obtained without a prescription. Therapeutic dosages for incontinence range from 25 mg twice a day to 50 mg four times a day. Sustained-release formulations with phenylpropanolamine are available but are combined with other possibly undesirable medications. Ornade Spansules contain chlorpheniramine and Entex LA contains guaifenesin. The recommended dosage for the sustained-release medications is 75 mg twice a day.

Sympathomimetic agents should be prescribed cautiously in patients who have cardiovascular disease, hypertension, or hyperthyroidism. Because of central nervous system stimulation, insomnia and anxiety can result from treatment. Other side effects that may cause concern include headache, tremor, palpitations, cardiac arrhythmias, and elevated blood pressure.

**Tricyclic Antidepressants.** Pharmacologic mechanisms of these agents include central and peripheral anticholinergic activity, reuptake inhibition of norepinephrine and serotonin, sedative activity (probably through central antihistaminic properties), and relaxation of bladder smooth muscle. Tricyclic antidepressants can be used to treat stress incontinence, detrusor instability, and mixed incontinence, given their range of pharmacologic activity. Reuptake inhibition of norepinephrine stimulates α-receptors with subsequent increase in bladder outlet resistance. Imipramine (Tofranil) is most commonly used. Because of sedation, the recommended starting dose is 25 mg at bedtime. The dosage is then titrated for the desired effect up to a maximum of 150 mg/day. The usual maintenance dose is 25 mg twice a day or four times a day. Elderly patients may require an initial dose of 10 mg. At the higher doses, patients may predominantly experience the anticholinergic side effects. These effects include weakness, fatigue, tremor, psychiatric changes, or parkinsonian responses to these medications, as well as postural hypotension or cardiac arrhythmias. Patients who have a cardiac history or a hypertensive disorder must be evaluated thoroughly before this medication is prescribed. In addition, use of imipramine in patients on monoamine oxidase inhibitors is contraindicated. Central nervous system toxicity can result and may lead to seizures, hyperpyrexia, and coma.

## DETRUSOR INSTABILITY

Anticholinergic agents, antispasmodic medications, tricyclic antidepressants, and calcium-channel blockers are the major pharmacologic classes of medications for treatment of detrusor instability. Medical therapy for detrusor instability can reduce incontinent episodes by 10 to 80% and cure 5 to 30% of these patients.

**Anticholinergic Agents.** Inadequate storage of urine may be related to bladder dysfunction, urethral abnormalities, or both. Postganglionic parasympathetic release of acetylcholine stimulates detrusor contractions by interaction with bladder smooth muscle cholinergic receptors. Atropine and other anticholinergic agents antagonize these smooth muscle receptors and depress normal contractile function of the bladder.

For treatment of detrusor instability, propantheline bromide (Pro-Banthīne) is the most commonly prescribed anticholinergic. It is a quaternary ammonium compound that is poorly absorbed after oral administration. The recommended adult oral dose is 15 to 30 mg every 4 to 6 hours; however, higher doses may be required because of poor absorption. The recommended schedule of administration of this medication is 30 minutes before meals for increased bioavailability. Hyoscyamine (Cystospaz) and hyoscyamine sulfate (Cystospaz-M, Levsin, Levsinex) are belladonna alkaloids with side effects and anticholinergic properties similar to those of atropine. A sublingual formulation of hyoscyamine sulfate is available, but randomized, controlled studies need to be completed to demonstrate its efficacy.

Side effects are a common problem with antimuscarinic agents because of the lack of selectivity for bladder muscle. Symptoms may include dry mouth, tachycardia, drowsiness, constipation, and blurred vision. These medications are contraindicated in patients who have narrow-angle glaucoma, myasthenia gravis, or impaired gastrointestinal motility. Conservative use of antimuscarinic medications is recommended in patients who have bladder outlet obstruction or cardiac disease.

Currently, tolterodine tartrate (Detrol) is the newest pharmacologic agent available for the treatment of detrusor instability. It is a potent, competitive, muscarinic receptor antagonist that has improved selectivity for bladder smooth muscle. Tolterodine tartrate is comparable to oxybutynin in efficacy, but the severity and incidence of dry mouth are much lower for tolterodine. The recommended initial dose of tolterodine tartrate is 2 mg twice a day. Based on side effects and response, the dose of tolterodine tartrate can be decreased to 1 mg twice a day.

**Antispasmodic Agents.** Medications in this group have direct smooth muscle relaxant activity. These antispasmodic agents reportedly interact with receptors that are metabolically distant from the cholinergic receptor and the other contractile receptor mechanism. In vitro, these agents relax smooth muscle by papaverine-like mechanisms. It is uncertain whether the atropine-like activity or the papaverine-like activity is primarily responsible for these agents' clinical effects. In addition, all medications possess varying degrees of anticholinergic and local anesthetic properties. The most effective medication for treatment of detrusor instability is oxybutynin chloride (Ditropan), a quaternary amine. The usual adult dose is 2.5 to 5.0 mg orally twice a day or three times a day. For patients who cannot tolerate the anticholinergic side effects of oxybutynin, dicyclomine (Bentyl) may be prescribed, because dicyclomine has less anticholinergic activity. The recommended dose is 10 to 20 mg three times a day. Side effects of and contraindications for these medications are similar to those for the anticholinergic agents discussed previously.

**Tricyclic Antidepressants.** Although tricyclics have systemic anticholinergic activity, selectivity for bladder smooth muscle is poor. Tricyclic medications act directly on bladder smooth muscle to inhibit contractility. This mechanism explains the efficacy of tricyclics for the treatment of detrusor instability. These agents are usually not the primary pharmacologic treatment for detrusor instability but may be preferred for patients who have mixed incontinence. Doxepin (Sinequan), another tricyclic antidepressant, has been shown to significantly decrease nighttime frequency and nighttime incontinence episodes. The dosage used in this study was 50 mg at bedtime with or without an additional 25 mg in the morning.

**Calcium Antagonists.** Calcium plays an integral role in excitation-contraction coupling in cardiac, striated, and smooth muscle. Calcium antagonists block the extracellular influx and intracellular release of calcium, which ultimately alters the excitation-contraction mechanism. This is a potentially effective mechanism in producing relaxation of bladder smooth muscle. However, the potent cardiovascular effects of these medications have limited their use to the very rare patient who has otherwise intractable detrusor instability. For patients who have intractable instability, the recommended dose of nifedipine for incontinence therapy is 10 to 20 mg twice a day.

# Nonpharmacologic Incontinence Therapy

A variety of therapeutic modalities are available for treatment of both detrusor instability and stress incontinence. The following section reviews treatment strategies that can be applied to both types of incontinence.

## PELVIC FLOOR EXERCISES

Pelvic floor muscle exercises, described by Kegel in 1948, have been used to treat both genuine stress urinary incontinence and detrusor instability. Repetitive voluntary contractions of the levator ani muscles stabilize and raise the urethrovesical junction into an intra-abdominal position. If these muscles can be effectively tightened during periods of increased abdominal pressure, improved pressure transmission results. In addition, contraction of the pelvic floor with onset of urgency symptoms may assist in controlling urgency and preventing urge incontinence. An effective pelvic floor training program includes the following:

1. Proper patient identification of muscles
2. Appropriate exercise program for strengthening muscles
3. Instruction of exercise application during periods of stress

Baseline assessment of pelvic floor strength should be noted so that intermittent evaluation of therapy can be performed. To help the patient identify the appropriate muscles, she can be instructed to "Stop your urine stream," "Hold back gas," or "Squeeze/tighten your muscles." However, this may not be effective guidance for some patients. Using the instructions, "Contract the muscles you would use if you were trying to stop your urine stream," Bump and associates demonstrated that only 60% of patients produced effective muscle contractions and that 25% performed Valsalva's maneuver. Patients who are unable to produce effective pelvic floor contractions after in-office guidance should be referred to a physical therapist.

An exercise program tailored to the patient's needs depends on the initial strength evaluation, the type and severity of incontinence, and the patient's physical abilities. To enhance muscle strength, it is important to perform exercises using both rapid and sustained contractions. This allows for recruitment of fast-twitch (rapid contractions) and slow-twitch muscle fibers (sustained contractions). Development of muscle strength requires hypertrophy of both muscle fiber types (fast-twitch and slow-twitch). Thus, an effective physical therapy program must incorporate exercises that enhance the development of both fiber types.

There is no universally accepted physical therapy program at present. An initial program may begin with holding exercises. The patient contracts her pelvic floor muscles and holds for 2 to 10 seconds, then releases for 10 seconds. As the patient becomes proficient, she increases the number of exercises performed and the length of time the contraction is held. Rapid contractions and resistance exercises should also be incorporated into the therapy program. Follow-up at regular intervals is recommended to ensure continued progress. Two months of regular exercise are usually necessary before improvement is apparent.

The effectiveness of pelvic floor exercises has been debated. Cure rates have been reported to range from 30 to 75%. In a recent study by Morkved and Bo, postpartum patients who participated in a specially designed pelvic floor exercise course were found to have significantly less urinary incontinence and a greater improvement in muscle strength when compared with control patients. Further studies are required to evaluate physical therapy programs adequately.

## VAGINAL CONES

Strengthening programs may be augmented by use of vaginal cones. Dacomed Corporation (Minneapolis, MN) produces specially designed graduated cones to assist in pelvic floor exercising. A set contains five cones of similar size but different weights (20 to 70 g). The cone is placed vaginally and the pelvic floor muscles are contracted to prevent the cone from falling out. Maintaining cone placement provides feedback to the patient regarding appropriate muscle use. The patient begins with the heaviest cone that can be retained vaginally. While walking and standing, the cone is held in place for 15-minute intervals twice daily. Once the cone is retained for two sessions or when the patient feels comfortable, she may graduate to the next cone weight. The long-term effectiveness of this treatment is unknown. Peattie and associates demonstrated a 68 to 79% improvement in patients who used vaginal cones for 4 weeks.

# Behavior Modification

Alteration of some behaviors may significantly improve the patient's incontinence or enhance the response to other therapies. Behavioral changes may be integrated in therapy programs for both stress incontinence and detrusor instability.

## STRESS INCONTINENCE

The urinary diary identifies patients who void infrequently or who overdrink. Instructing the infrequent voider to urinate at decreased intervals may minimize the incontinent episodes. For the overdrinker, altering fluid intake may be all that is needed to cure the problem. Activities that trigger incontinence episodes can be reviewed with the patient. Avoidance of these activities may be recommended and alternate activities suggested.

**Biofeedback.** Biofeedback is a form of behavioral modification that incorporates visual and auditory cues to alter unconscious physiologic processes. For stress incontinence, biofeedback may facilitate proper exercise technique and promote compliance. Burgio studied the efficacy of augmenting a pelvic floor muscle training program with biofeedback. In comparing verbal feedback with biofeedback, she demonstrated a 50% reduction of leakage after biofeedback. Stein and associates evaluated the use of biofeedback for stress incontinence therapy. They compared quantifiable patient symptoms and patients' subjective improvement scores before and after therapy and demonstrated a 36% success rate with biofeedback therapy. They concluded that biofeedback is only moderately effective.

## DETRUSOR INSTABILITY

For the treatment of bladder instability, behavioral modification is based on the theory that cortical control over the sacral micturition reflex has been lost or altered. Therapy is designed to help patients regain control of the involuntary detrusor contractions. The "bladder drill" is the most common technique of behavioral modification for detrusor instability. Using the bladder drill, patients should increase their voiding intervals, increase the capacity of the bladder, and decrease urgency and leakage.

The patient's initial voiding frequency is determined by the severity of urgency and leakage as indicated in the patient's voiding diaries. The patient must void regularly at a predetermined interval whether the urge to urinate is present or not. If the urge occurs at other times, the patient is taught to wait. Once the drill is mastered, she is then instructed to increase the voiding interval by 15- to 30-minute increments. Success is achieved when the voiding interval has been increased to between 2 and 3 hours, continence is regained, and urgency symptoms have resolved. Bladder drills have been shown to be effective in 50 to 90% of patients, with a relapse rate of 10 to 15%. Wyman and associates evaluated the efficacy of bladder training in improving quality of life for older women. In a randomized, controlled 6-week trial, their group demonstrated a significant and sustained quality of life improvement after bladder training.

Timed voiding is another behavioral technique used to treat some patients who have bladder instability. This technique may be effective in those patients who void infrequently and experience uninhibited detrusor contractions at bladder volumes of 400 ml and greater. For these patients, a regular voiding schedule with 2-hour intervals can be effective in controlling bladder instability.

**Biofeedback.** As in stress incontinence therapy, biofeedback can be used to augment pelvic floor rehabilitation in patients who have detrusor instability. Biofeedback can also be applied during cystometry. As the bladder is filled, bladder pressure is recorded. As bladder pressure increases, an auditory signal sounds with an intensity that varies according to the level of bladder pressure. Using these cues, the patient learns to control uninhibited contractions and bladder pressure. Burgio demonstrated a 33% cure rate for patients who were treated with biofeedback.

# Functional Electrical Stimulation

Functional electrical stimulation (FES) has been used in some areas of medicine for many years. In rehabilitation medicine, electrical stimulation has been applied to functional electrical prostheses for gait improvement. At the present time, pelvic floor electrical stimulation has become popular for the treatment of stress incontinence and detrusor instability.

## GENUINE STRESS INCONTINENCE

Electrical stimulation has been shown to be effective in the treatment of stress incontinence. Mechanisms of action affect several pathways:
 1. Direct stimulation of the efferent pudendal nerve activates urethral closure and stimulates

hypogastric fibers (which affect smooth periurethral fibers).
2. Stimulation of the pelvic nerve efferents produces increases in urethral intraluminal pressure.
3. Pelvic floor stimulation produces a reflex contraction of the periurethral striated and intrinsic striated sphincter; for FES to be effective, total or partial pelvic floor innervation is necessary.

Modes of treatment for stress incontinence include acute maximal (high-intensity, short-term) and chronic intermittent (low-intensity, long-term) stimulation. Chronic therapy involves many hours of treatment daily for 3 to 12 months. Weak electrical pulses that are used do not reach the sensory threshold. Poor patient acceptance of this protocol led to the development of acute maximal therapy. With acute maximal therapy, the current intensity is set just below the patient's pain threshold. Stimulation sessions are scheduled once or twice daily for 15 to 20 minutes. Stimulation frequencies of 20 to 50 Hz with a pulse duration of 1 to 5 milliseconds are optimal settings for producing pelvic floor contractions.

In a multicenter, placebo-controlled, randomized trial, Sand and associates compared an active pelvic floor stimulator with a sham device for the treatment of genuine stress incontinence. Patients randomized to the active device group expeienced a significant improvement in vaginal muscle strength and a significant decrease in weekly incontinence episodes compared with experiences of controls. Sixty-two percent of the experimental group demonstrated a 50% improvement in stress incontinence during pad testing, compared with improvement in 19% of the control group. Sand and associates concluded that pelvic floor electrical stimulation is effective treatment for stress incontinence.

**DETRUSOR INSTABILITY**

Electrical stimulation has also been shown to be effective in treating detrusor instability. In a multicenter, prospective, randomized trial, Brubaker and associates evaluated the efficacy of transvaginal electrical stimulation for urinary incontinence therapy. In patients who had detrusor instability, 49% of the active device group became stable on provocative cystometry, but no significant change in the sham group was noted. In the stress incontinent patients, no statistically significant differences between the active or sham device groups were found either before or after treatment.

Pudendal nerve stimulation produces detrusor relaxation through activation of the sympathetic nerves and inhibition of the parasympathetic nerves. It has been demonstrated that electrical stimulation also decreases cholinergic activity and increases detrusor β-receptor activity in experimental models. Both chronic intermittent (low-level, long-term) and acute maximal (high-level, short-term) therapies have been used to treat detrusor instability. As for stress incontinence, the acute maximal technique is preferred by patients. Frequency settings of 10 to 20 Hz with a pulse duration of 2 milliseconds are used to achieve bladder inhibition.

# Continence Devices

Pessaries have been used primarily to treat pelvic organ prolapse disorders, but pessary use can also improve incontinence. Pessary placement elevates the urethrovesical junction and thereby reapproximates the normal urethral position. As a result, urethral pressure transmission is improved. A variety of continence devices are now available and include vaginal and urethral (internal and external) devices. The Incontinence Ring (Milex Products, Inc.) is a modified ring pessary with a silicone ball, which is placed under the urethrovesical junction. The Incontinence Dish, the Gehrung pessary with ball, and the Hodge pessary with ball are also available (Milex Products, Inc.). Introl (UroMed) is a ring-shaped silicone vaginal device with two prongs on one end. When properly placed, it simulates the effects of a retropubic urethropexy without creating outflow obstruction. All of the vaginal continence devices must be properly fitted to optimize incontinence control and decrease side effects.

FemAssist (INSIGHT Medical) is a cylindric device made of silicone rubber and available in two sizes (3.5 cm and 2.6 cm). The device is compressed to create suction and then placed directly over the urethral meatus. The mild vacuum creates occlusion of the meatus. In clinical trials, 76.7% of the women subjects maintained dryness for more than 50% of the time with the use of the FemAssist device. Adverse events included discomfort (35%), urinary tract infection (10%), urethral irritation (6%), bleeding (5%), and discharge (3%). As with the vaginal devices, the FemAssist must be carefully sized.

Other barrier devices include Impress and CapSure (Bard). Impress is an external urethral occlusive device that covers the meatus using a gentle adhesive. CapSure is a silicone device similar to the FemAssist, but the contour of the CapSure device is different. The nipple-shaped shield works by creating a mild vacuum when the device is compressed. In the multicenter clinical study, CapSure was found to be very effective for controlling incontinence episodes. The percentages of completely dry study patients who had severe, moderate, or mild incontinence were

79, 87, and 88%, respectively. No study patients developed a symptomatic urinary tract infection and only 3.5% of patients developed asymptomatic bacteriuria.

# Conclusion

The management of urinary incontinence is a major health-care issue, which will become an increasing challenge in the new millennium. Health-care personnel must develop knowledge and effective skills for identifying, evaluating, and treating patients who have urinary incontinence. An essential component of successful incontinence management is patient education. Patients need to understand that urinary incontinence is never normal and that effective treatment is available for their condition. This chapter provides an overview of the diagnosis and medical management of urinary incontinence. A strategy for evaluation of the patient with incontinence is presented. This strategy can facilitate incontinence therapy so that future health-care challenges can be managed easily.

## REFERENCES

Abrams P, Blaivas JG, Stanton SL, et al: The standardization of terminology of lower urinary tract function. Scand J Urol Nephrol (suppl) 144:5–19, 1988.

Ahkstrom K, Sandahl B, Sjoberg B, et al: Effect of combined treatment with phenylpropanolamine and estriol, compared with estriol treatment alone, in postmenopausal women with stress urinary incontinence. Clin Obstet Gynecol 38:175–188, 1995.

Andersson KE, Persson K: The L-arginine/nitric oxide pathway and nonadrenergic, noncholinergic relaxation of the lower urinary tract. Gen Pharm 24:833–839, 1993.

Bergman A, Ballard CA, Platt LD: Ultrasonic evaluation of urethrovesical junction in women with stress urinary incontinence. J Clin Ultrasound 16:295–300, 1988.

Bonney WW, Gupta S, Hunter DR, et al: Bladder dysfunction in schizophrenia. Schizophrenia Res 25:243–249, 1997.

Bors E, Turner RD: History and physical examination in neurological urology. J Urol 83:759–767, 1960.

Bourcier AP, Juras JC: Nonsurgical therapy for stress incontinence. Urol Clin North Am 22:613–627, 1995.

Brubaker L, Benson JT, Bent A, et al: Transvaginal electrical stimulation for female urinary incontinence. Am J Obstet Gynecol 177:536–540, 1997.

Burgio KL: Urinary incontinence in the elderly: Bladder sphincter biofeedback and toilet skills training. Ann Intern Med 103:507–515, 1985.

Burgio KL: Behavioral training for stress and urge incontinence in the community. Gerontology 36(suppl 2):27–34, 1990.

Caputo RM, Benson JT: The Q-Tip test and urethrovesical junction mobility. Obstet Gynecol 82:892–896, 1993.

Chiarelli P: Incontinence: The pelvic floor function. Aust Fam Phys 18:949, 953, 954, 956, 957, 1989.

Consensus Conference: Urinary incontinence in adults. JAMA 261:2685–2690, 1989.

Cornella JL, Larson TR, Lee RA, et al: Leiomyoma of the female urethra and bladder: Report of twenty-three patients and review of the literature. Am J Obstet Gynecol 176:1278–1285, 1997.

Cundiff GW, Harris RL, Coates KW, et al: Clinical predictors of urinary incontinence in women. Am J Obstet Gynecol 177:262–267, 1997.

DuBeau CE: Interpreting the effect of common medical conditions on voiding dysfunction in the elderly. Urol Clin North Am 23:11–18, 1996.

Elbadawi A: Pathology and pathophysiology of detrusor in incontinence. Urol Clin North Am 22:499–512, 1995.

Elia G, Bergman A: Pelvic muscle exercises: When do they work? Obstet Gynecol 81:283–286, 1993.

Eriksen BC: Electrical stimulation. In Benson JT (ed): Female Pelvic Floor Disorders. New York, Norton Medical Books, 1992, pp 219–231.

Fall M, Erlandson BE, Carlsson CA, et al: The effect of intravaginal stimulation of the feline urethra and urinary bladder: Neuronal mechanisms. Scand J Urol Nephrol (suppl)44:19–30, 1977.

Fantl JA, Bump RC, Robinson D, et al: Efficacy of estrogen supplementation in the treatment of urinary incontinence. Obstet Gynecol 88:745–749, 1996.

Frimodt-Moller C: Diabetic cystopathy: Epidemiology and related disorders. Ann Intern Med 92:318–321, 1980.

Galloway NTM: Classification and diagnosis of neurogenic bladder dysfunction. Probl Urol 3:1–39, 1989.

Hadley ED: Bladder training and related therapies for urinary incontinence in older people. JAMA 256:372–379, 1986.

Herzog AR, Fultz NH: Prevalence and incidence of urinary incontinence in community-dwelling populations. J Am Geriatr Soc 38:273–281, 1990.

Jensen J, Nielsen FR, Ostergard DR: The role of patient history in the diagnosis of urinary incontinence. Obstet Gynecol 83:904–910, 1994.

Karram MM: Lower urinary tract infection. In Walters MD, Karram MM (eds): Clinical Urogynecology. St. Louis, Mosby–Year Book, 1993, pp 310–329.

Karram MM, Partoll L, Rahe J: Efficacy of nonsurgical therapy for urinary incontinence. J Reprod Med 41:215–219, 1996.

Kegel A: Progressive resistance exercise in the functional restoration of the perineal muscles. Am J Gynecol 56:238–249, 1948.

Klutke JJ, Bergman A: Hormonal influence on the urinary tract. Urol Clin North Am 22:629–639, 1995.

Kujansuu E: Patient history in the diagnosis of urinary incontinence and determining the quality of life. Acta Obstet Gynecol Scand (suppl)166:15–18, 1997.

Kulseng-Hanssen S: Reliability and validity of stationary cystometry, stationary cysto-urethrometry and ambulatory cysto-urethro-vaginometry. Acta Obstet Gynecol Scand (suppl) 166:33–38, 1997.

Lagace EA, Hansen W, Hickner JM: Prevalence and severity of urinary incontinence in ambulatory adults: An UPRNet Study. J Fam Pract 36:610–614, 1993.

Larsson G, Victor A: The frequency/volume chart in genuine stress incontinent women. Neurourol Urodyn 11:23–32, 1992.

Lose G: Uroflowmetry and pressure/flow study of voiding in women. Acta Obstet Gynecol Scand (suppl)166:43–47, 1997.

Lose G, Jorgensen L, Thunedborg P: 24-hour home pad weighing test versus 1-hour ward test in the assessment of mild stress incontinence. Acta Obstet Gynecol Scand 68:211–215, 1989.

Lose G, Jorgensen L, Thunedborg P: Doxepin in the treatment of female detrusor overactivity: A randomized double-blind crossover study. J Urol 142:1024–1026, 1989.

Lobel RW, Sand PK: The empty supine stress test as a predictor of intrinsic urethral sphincter dysfunction. Obstet Gynecol 88:128–32, 1996.

Mallett VT, Richardson DA: Gynecologic urology. In Nichols DG, Sweeney PJ (eds): Ambulatory Gynecology. Philadelphia, JB Lippincott, 1995, pp 314–341.

Morkved S, Bo K: The effect of postpartum pelvic floor muscle exercise in the prevention and treatment of urinary incontinence. Int Urogynecol J 8:217–222, 1997.

National Institutes of Health Consensus Development Conference Statement: Urinary incontinence in adults. Natl Inst Health Consensus Dev Conf Consensus Statement 7:1–11, 1988.

Ory MG, Wyman JF, Yu L: Psychosocial factors in urinary incontinence. Clin Geriatr Med 2:657–671, 1986.

Peattie AB, Plevnik S, Stanton SL: Vaginal cones: A conservative method of treating genuine stress incontinence. Br J Obstet Gynaecol 95:1049–1053, 1988.

Porru D, Usai E: Standard and extramural ambulatory urodynamic investigation for the diagnosis of detrusor instability-correlated incontinence and micturition disorders. Neurourol Urodyn 13:237–242, 1994.

Resnick NM: Voiding dysfunction in the elderly. *In* Yalla SV, McGuire EJ, Elbadawi A, et al: (eds): Neurourology and Urodynamics: Principles and Practice. New York, MacMillan, 1988, pp 303–330.

Resnick NM: Geriatric incontinence. Urol Clin North Am 23:55–74, 1996.

Richardson DA: Value of cough pressure profile in the valuation of patients with stress incontinence. Am J Obstet Gynecol 155:808–811, 1986.

Romanzi LJ, Heritz DM, Blaivas JG: Preliminary assessment of the incontinent woman. Urol Clin North Am 22:513–520, 1995.

Rozenzweig BA, Bhatia NN, Nelson AL: Dynamic urethral pressure profilometry pressure transmission ratio: What do the numbers really mean? Obstet Gynecol 77:586–590, 1991.

Samuelsson E, Victor A, Tibblin G: A population study of urinary incontinence and nocturia among women aged 20–59 years. Acta Obstet Gynecol Scand 76:74–80, 1997.

Sand PK, Richardson DA, Staskin DR, et al: Pelvic floor electrical stimulation in the treatment of genuine stress incontinence: A multicenter, placebo-controlled trial. Am J Obstet Gynecol 173:72–79, 1995.

Sand PK, Bowen LW, Panganiban R, et al: The low pressure urethra as a factor in failed retropubic urethropexy. Obstet Gynecol 69:399–402, 1987.

Scotti R, Ostergard D, Guillaume A, et al: Predictive value of urethroscopy as compared to urodynamics in the diagnosis of genuine stress incontinence. J Reprod Med 35:772–776, 1990.

Siltberg H, Victor A, Larsson G: Pad weighing tests: The best way to quantify urine loss in patients with incontinence. Acta Obstet Gynecol Scand (suppl 166) 76:28–32, 1997.

Smith JJ: Intravaginal stimulation randomized trial. J Urol 155:127–130, 1996.

Stanton SL, Ozsoy C, Hilton P: Voiding difficulties in the female: Prevalence, clinical and urodynamic review. Obstet Gynecol 90:919–933, 1983.

Stein M, Discippio W, Davia M, et al: Biofeedback for the treatment of stress and urge incontinence. J Urol 153:641–643, 1995.

Turan C, Zorlu CG, Ekin M, et al: Urinary incontinence in women of reproductive age. Gynecol Obstet Invest 41:132–134, 1996.

Ulmsten U: Some reflections and hypotheses on the pathophysiology of female urinary incontinence. Acta Obstet Gynecol Scand (suppl) 166:3–8, 1997.

Urinary Incontinence Guideline Panel: Urinary incontinence in adults: Clinical practice guideline. Rockville, MD, Agency for Health Care Policy and Research, Public Health Service, US Department of Health and Human Services 1992. AHCPR publication no. 92-0038.

US Bureau of the Census: Sixty-Five Plus in America. Current Population Reports, Special Studies. Washington, DC, US Government Printing Office. 23–178, 1992.

Van Kerrebroeck PE, Amarenco G, Thuroff JW, et al: Dose-ranging study of tolterodine in patients with detrusor hyperreflexia. Neurourol Urodyn 17:499–512, 1998.

Versi E, Cardozo LD, Studd JW: Internal urinary sphincter in maintenance of female continence. Br Med J Clin Res Ed 292:166, 167, 1986.

Versi E, Orrego G, Hardy E, et al: Evaluation of the home pad test in the investigation of female urinary incontinence. Br J Obstet Gynaecol 103:162–167, 1996.

Victor A: Pad weighing test—A simple method to quantitate urinary incontinence. Ann Med 22:443–447, 1990.

Victor A, Larsson G, Asbrink A-S: A simple patient-administered test for objective quantification of the symptom of urinary incontinence. Scand J Urol Nephrol 21:277–279, 1987.

Wall LL, Norton PA, DeLancey JOL: Evaluating symptoms. *In* Wall LL, Norton PA, DeLancey JOL (eds): Practical Urogynecology. Baltimore, Williams & Wilkins, 1993, pp 41–82.

Wall LL, Wiskind AK, Taylor PA: Simple bladder filling with a cough stress test compared with subtracted cystometry for the diagnosis of urinary incontinence. Am J Obstet Gynecol 171:1472–1479, 1994.

Walter S, Olesen KP: Urinary incontinence and genital prolapse in the female: Clinical, urodynamic and radiological examinations. Br J Obstet Gynaecol 89:393–401, 1982.

Walters MD, Diaz D: Q-Tip test: A study of continent and incontinent women. Obstet Gynecol 70:208–211, 1987.

Walters MD, Shields LE: The diagnostic value of history, physical examination, and the Q-Tip cotton swab test in women with urinary incontinence. Am J Obstet Gynecol 159:145–149, 1988.

Wein AJ: Pharmacologic treatment of incontinence. J Am Geriatr Soc 38:317–325, 1990.

Wein AJ: Neuromuscular dysfunction of the lower urinary tract. *In* Walsh PC, Retik AB, Stamey TA, et al (eds): Campbell's Urology, 6th ed. Philadelphia, WB Saunders, 1992, pp 573–642.

Wein AJ: Pharmacology of incontinence. Urol Clin North Am 22:557–577, 1995.

Weinberger MW: Conservative treatment of urinary incontinence. Clin Obstet Gynecol 38:175–188, 1995.

Wells TJ: Pelvic (floor) muscle exercise. J Am Geriatr Soc 38:333–337, 1990.

Wyman JF, Fantl JA, McClish DK, et al: Quality of life following bladder training in older women with urinary incontinence. Int Urogynecol J 8:223–229, 1997.

Wyman JF, Harkins SW, Fantl JA: Psychosocial impact of urinary incontinence in the community dwelling population. J Am Geriatr Soc 38:282–288, 1990.

Young SB, Pingeton DM: A practical approach to perimenopausal and postmenopausal urinary incontinence. Obstet Gynecol Clin North Am 21:357–379, 1994.

# 17

# Diseases of the Breast

CAROLYN JOHNSTON

This chapter presents a review of the breast examination, a practical approach to the evaluation of a palpable mass, and a discussion of several common breast disorders. Readers are referred elsewhere for a discussion of breast carcinoma and details of surgical technique.

## Breast Examination

A thorough breast examination is recommended as part of the annual gynecologic examination, regardless of whether a woman has any complaints. This can also provide an opportunity to review the techniques of breast self-examination (SBE), which women who are 20 years of age and older should be encouraged to perform on a regular monthly basis. If a woman is premenstrual, SBE is best accomplished during the week after her menstrual period when the breasts are least nodular, full, and tender. Instruction in SBE technique leads over time to increased sensitivity at the expense of decreased specificity. Those involved in health care make this recommendation for SBE, although substantial data supporting a reduction in mortality from breast cancer are lacking. Approximately 50% of all breast cancers are discovered by the patient. In women who are eligible for mammograms, the breast examination is complementary. SBE and mammogram should not be used as substitutes for each other, because approximately 16% of breast cancers are detected by examination only and 45% are detected by mammogram.

### INSPECTION

Look for congruence. Normal breasts may vary by as much as 10% in size, but larger discrepancies should be noted and explained.

Check for nipple retraction, inversion, erosions or lesions, and discharge. Assessment of nipple discharge is generally done during the palpation portion of the examination. Accessory nipples (polythelia) occur in approximately 1 to 2% of the population and are located along the midclavicular (milk) line that extends from the clavicle to the groin. Their appearance may be confused with that of nevi. They also may enlarge as well as become more deeply pigmented during pregnancy. Nipple inversion increases with age, may be unilateral or bilateral, and can be a normal finding, particularly if of long duration. Non-bloody nipple discharge can be elicited in most women by gently squeezing the nipple. Both spontaneous and elicited discharges are abnormal if they are bloody or serous and thus require additional evaluation to rule out carcinoma. Greenish discharge, associated with fibrocystic changes, can often be elicited from multiple ducts. Nipple discharge should be evaluated in light of drug, trauma, and pregnancy history.

Areas of skin retraction, erythema, thickening, or actual lesions should be noted and considered abnormal until proved otherwise. Retraction may be attributable to an underlying malignancy or to a previous biopsy scar. Skin retraction that is not immediately apparent may be elicited by the maneuvers of pectoral contraction, having the patient raise the arms above the head while the examiner gently molds the breast tissue around the site.

## PALPATION

Numerous examination techniques have been described, with the common denominator being the establishment of a systematic pattern that evaluates the nodal areas as well as the entire breast and minimizes the number of times the patient has to change position from sitting to supine.

Examination includes inspection of the nodes in the supraclavicular anterior cervical chain and axillary areas. Having the patient shrug her shoulders slightly facilitates palpation of the supraclavicular area, as does support of the patient's arm by the examiner during the axillary portion of the examination. This latter maneuver allows relaxation of the muscles and thus increases the ease of palpation. Small (<1 cm), rubbery, mobile lymph nodes that result from skin breaks or infection in the hands can often be palpated in the axillae. These lymph nodes are generally considered normal. Fixed, matted, firm, or large (> than 1 cm) lymph nodes are considered pathologic until proved otherwise.

Feel for dominant masses discrete from the surrounding breast tissue. Note any areas of tenderness and attempt to correlate them with examination findings. Include the axillary tail in the examination. In addition, some women have prominent—and sometimes separate or accessory—breast tissue in the axilla, which requires examination as well. The breast of an elderly woman should have scant glandular tissue unless she is taking hormone replacement therapy; therefore, asymmetry requires further evaluation and possibly biopsy. Thickening under a scar may represent normal postoperative healing, but this finding should be correlated with radiologic studies, data from previous examinations, and the histologic findings of the biopsy. Breast implants are usually placed behind the pectoralis muscle, pushing the breast tissue forward and compressing it. Small masses and thickening are best appreciated by bimanual examination. The patient should be upright, which serves to drop the breast tissue forward. Irregularities may signify scarring or rupture of the implant, which can then be confirmed by mammography, ultrasonography, or magnetic resonance imaging.

## CONCLUSION

Explain the findings to the patient and allow her to ask questions.

# Palpable Mass

A palpable breast mass must be interpreted in light of the patient's personal and family medical history, breast examination, and age. The risk of cancer within a palpable mass increases with age, such that in a woman younger than 25 years it is minimal, whereas it approaches 75% in a woman older than 70 years. Physical examination alone is often not sufficient, as noted earlier, and should be complemented by radiologic or cytologic evaluation, especially in women older than 25 years.

The cystic or solid nature of the mass should be determined. This is performed most efficiently by fine needle aspiration (FNA). Special attention should be paid to whether the cyst fluid is bloody and whether it resolves after aspiration. Nonbloody cyst fluid can be discarded because it is rarely associated with a malignancy. Residual palpable masses, recurrent cysts (after two or three aspirations), and bloody fluid require histologic evaluation because of a heightened chance of malignancy. Fewer than 20% of simple cysts refill and only 9% do so after two or three aspirations. Simple cysts with no associated mass or mammographic abnormalities can therefore be managed with repeat aspiration and a follow-up visit to confirm resolution 6 to 8 weeks after aspiration. Cysts in postmenopausal women should be analyzed with more suspicion. Breast cancer may appear as a predominantly cystic mass representing cystic degeneration of a high-grade tumor or intracystic papillary carcinoma. Ultrasonography can also be used to determine whether a mass is cystic or solid. Asymptomatic simple cysts that are stable over time do not require aspiration because their malignant potential is low. Patients who have otherwise nonsuspicious cysts may be sufficiently anxious to request aspiration. If a mammogram is indicated, it should be performed before the aspiration so as not to confuse an aspiration-induced alteration with a true mammographic abnormality.

Solid masses are managed according to size, age, cytologic results, and associated mammographic findings. For example, a confirmed fibroadenoma in a woman younger than 35 years can be safely followed and should be removed only because of patient distress or an increase in size or symptoms. However, solid masses in older women and those associated with mammographic abnormalities should be excised to rule out malignancy. Abnormal or nondiagnostic cytologic studies should also lead to biopsy. Similarly, if the size of a solid mass has increased over time, biopsy is mandatory. FNA of a palpable breast mass has a reported specificity of 98 to 100% and a sensitivity of 65 to 99%. False-negative and positive rates are 1 to 35% and 0.8 to 18%, respectively. The false-negative rate can be minimized by using more stringent criteria to define an unsatisfactory aspirate and by increasing the adequacy of sampling with several passes through the tissue. The positive predictive value is nearly 100% and the negative predictive value is 89%. Helvie and associates reported a similar sensitivity and specificity for FNA in the diagnosis of mammographically detected, nonpalpable breast lesions (97 and 94%, respectively). This versatile easy-to learn technique has been reviewed well by Wilkinson and associates. There is clearly a learning curve, so it is important to work closely with a cytopathologist to reduce the rate of unsatisfactory aspirates. Core needle biopsy can be used when the FNA material is nondiagnostic, insufficient, or suspected of being cancerous. Core needle biopsy can also be used to provide additional tissue for analytic studies. A cytopathologist can provide immediate interpretation of the FNA material, and if a diagnosis cannot be rendered, a core biopsy can be performed. A cost benefit has been demonstrated for needle sampling of lesions that are highly suspicious of malignancy or those that are clinically benign, with an estimated savings of $1100 per patient by avoidance of biopsy. Diagnostic accuracy is enhanced by using information from three sources: clinical examination, mammogram, and FNA. If all three are negative for malignancy, the incidence of a cancer is 0 to 0.7%. If, however, all three are positive, the incidence is 97 to 99%.

Persistent masses that cannot be clinically characterized as benign will certainly require biopsy, especially in women older than 35 years. Masses that are being followed conservatively should be re-evaluated by examination every 3 to 6 months for assessment of stability. Any change, with the exception of shrinkage, should lead to surgical intervention. See Figure 17–1 for a suggested algorithm.

Fat necrosis is a benign condition often caused by the trauma of accident, surgery (biopsy or mammoplasty), radiation therapy, infection, duct ectasia, injection of foreign substances, and autologous fat and reconstruction after mastectomy. Fat necrosis usually appears as a firm, superficial, painless, discrete or irregular mass, which at times is associated with thickening of the overlying skin. Mammographic findings include dystrophic calcifications and lipid cysts, although characteristics most often associated with malignancy may also be seen, such as speculated densities, skin thickening and retraction, and angular calcification. Diagnosis is established by biopsy; however, a well-documented history of trauma is suggestive of the correct answer.

Another post-traumatic breast mass is the hematoma. It can occur after accidental injury or after surgical injury, including FNA and biopsy (core needle biopsy, stereotactic wire localized biopsy, excisional biopsy). The incidence after excisional biopsy is 0.8 to 4%. A hematoma often drains spontaneously through the skin incision and requires no further therapy. An immediately enlarging hematoma or a secondarily infected hematoma requires surgical repair, including incision and drainage. A hematoma can make subsequent physical and mammographic examinations difficult by obscuring or mimicking a carcinoma.

Palpable masses in pregnant or lactating women should undergo similar evaluation. Surgery more extensive than FNA or excisional biopsy may require tocolysis. Interpretation of FNA results can be more difficult because of pregnancy-related hyperplastic changes with atypia, which may result in a false-positive diagnosis of cancer. If the FNA is nondiagnostic, core needle biopsy is noninvasive and could be performed; however, this procedure is seldom selected, primarily because of the possibility of milk fistula formation. Both pregnant and nonpregnant women have the same range of histologic abnormalities. Furthermore, there does not appear to be an increased incidence of malignant diagnoses in pregnancy.

# Infectious or Inflammatory Conditions

Both puerperal and nonpuerperal conditions of the breast are most often caused by bacterial infections with *Staphylococcus aureus* or streptococci after disruption of the epithelium at the nipple-areola complex. The infection may manifest as a variety of conditions, ranging from painful cellulitis to unifocal or multifocal abscesses. If untreated, cellulitis generally progresses to an abscess, especially in the puerperal state. A streptococcal infection is more likely to persist as a diffuse cellulitis, whereas staphylococcal infection appears early with suppuration and abscess formation.

The reported incidence of sporadic puerperal mastitis ranges from 1.4 to 8.9%, with abscess formation in 4.8 to 11% of cases. The causes are presumed to be nipple fissures and milk stasis, which encourage retrograde bacterial infection. Although it has been suggested that the determination of milk leukocyte and bacterial counts is diagnostically important, the treatment of puerperal mastitis is best dictated by clinical presentation and the early use of antibiotics and breast drainage as reported by Bland. A broad-

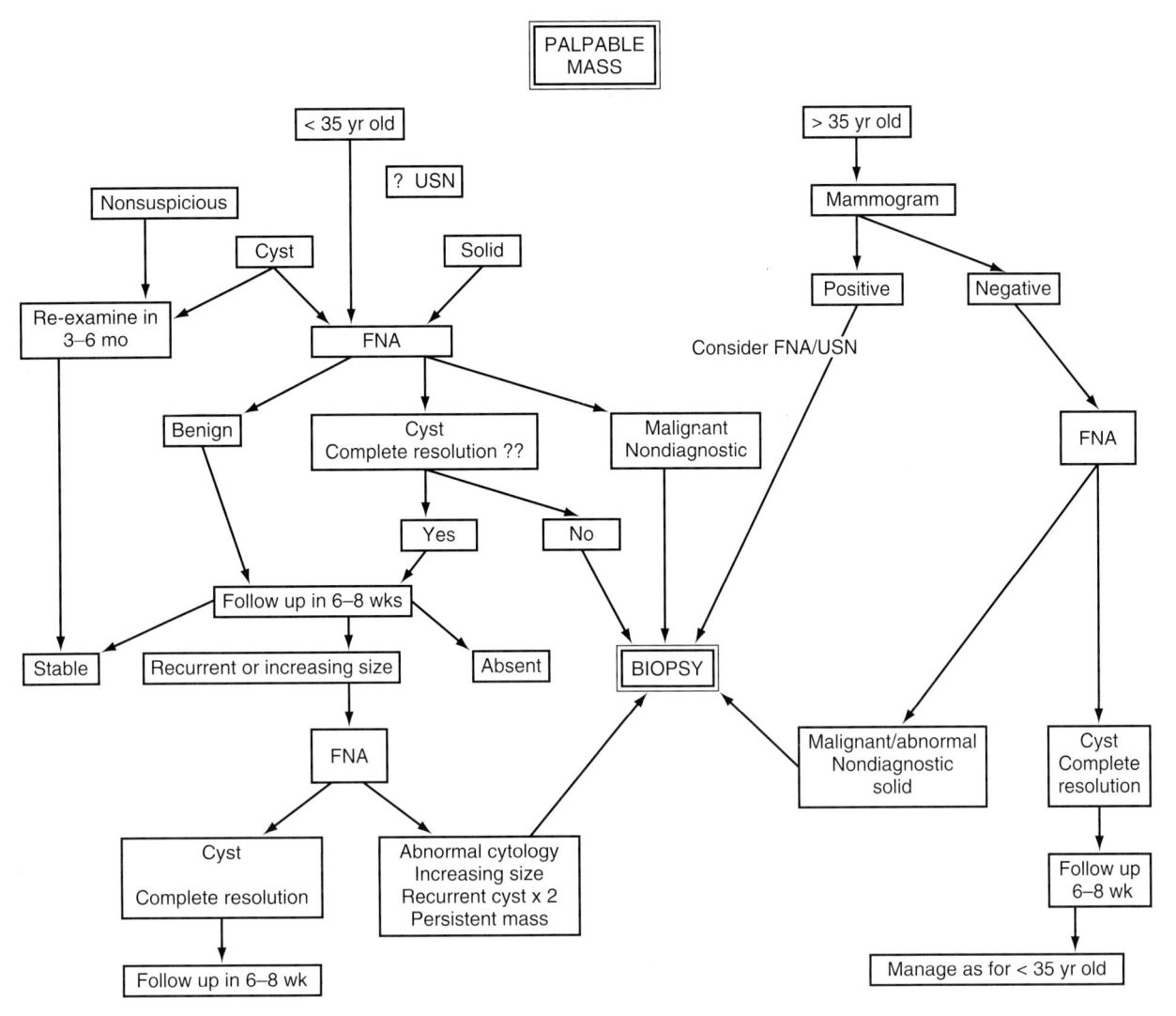

Figure 17–1. Evaluation of a palpable mass. FNA = fine needle aspiration; USN = ultrasound. (From Johnston C: Breast disorders. *In* Ransom SB, McNeeley SG (eds): Gynecology for the Primary Care Provider. Philadelphia, WB Saunders, 1997, p 32.)

spectrum antibiotic with good coverage of skin flora—the likely source of infection— is recommended. However, the ultimate choice of antibiotic can be guided by the results of Gram stains and cultures as well as sensitivities of the infecting organisms.

Cellulitis should be treated early and aggressively with local wound care and oral antibiotics. The application of local heat may also be appropriate. A penicillinase-resistant penicillin is the drug of choice for non–penicillin-allergic patients. Alternatively, a first-generation cephalosporin such as cefazolin can be used. Erythromycin can be used in penicillin-sensitive patients. All of these agents can be safely used in lactating or pregnant women. Lactating women should continue to breast-feed, use a breast pump, or both because either of these modalities has been shown to shorten the duration of symptoms and improve the outcome, with a reduction in the recurrence of infectious mastitis. In the treatment of puerperal mastitis, a combination of antibiotics and breast drainage ensures a good outcome up to 96% of the time, whereas no treatment or breast drainage alone leads to successful outcomes 15 and 50% of the time, respectively. Furthermore, the bacteria in the milk do not appear to be pathogenic to the breast-feeding infant. The choice of antibiotics for a lactating mother is dictated not only by the suspected causal organism but also by the tolerance of both mother and infant. Failure of the cellulitis to improve in 48 to 72 hours after the institution of broad-spectrum antibiotic coverage suggests the presence of an abscess or resistant organism.

An abscess requires incision and drainage—often under general anesthesia—thereby permitting adequate disruption of loculations and debridement of all infected tissue. Incisions are generally placed in a circumareolar location or in the direction of Langer's lines farther out on the breast. The decision to leave the wound open to heal by secondary intention or to close it primarily with a drain is left to the discretion of the surgeon. Chronic infections generally require healing by secondary intention after surgical debridement.

Nonpuerperal mastitis or other inflammatory conditions of the breast requires a thorough breast examination and mammogram. Infections not associated with an abscess or underlying mass or mammographic abnormality may be treated initially with antibiotics. Any residual mass, mammographic abnormality, or failure to respond to antibiotics should lead to a biopsy. Similarly, an abscess should be treated with incision and drainage, with representative tissue being sent for pathologic analysis. Several authors have documented superior response and decreased recurrence rates with excisional versus incisional techniques. The key to successful treatment of periareolar infections is adequate debridement and excision of any sinus tracts from the overlying nipple or areola. Readers are referred to reports by Maier and associates and Hartley and associates for suggested technical approaches to the treatment of periareolar abscesses. The potential sequelae of this approach include loss of nipple sensation and sloughing of the nipple and areolar skin, as well as recurrent abscesses and deformation; however, these sequelae should not deter surgical management. Biopsy of any inflammatory sites should include a sample of the overlying inflamed skin for assessment of dermal infiltration by carcinoma.

The differential diagnosis of nonpuerperal breast inflammation includes malignancy; duct ectasia; chronic or acute periareolar and subareolar infections; inflamed cysts; sarcoidosis; viral, fungal, tubercular, or parasitic infections; thrombophlebitis (see later section on Mondor's disease); and necrosis resulting from radiation or anticoagulation. Nonpuerperal breast abscesses tend to be more centrally located than those of the puerperium and are often indolent and chronic in nature. These are often thought to be related to duct ectasia. As with puerperal states, infections are often caused by *Staphylococcus aureus* or streptococci; however, anaerobic bacteria may also play a role, including *Bacteroides* species, enteroccocci, and anaerobic streptococci. Persistence of the infection despite surgical debridement and antibiotics should prompt a search for microabscesses, sinus tracts, resistant organisms, or slow-growing organisms, such as *Mycobacterium* species. The presence of foreign bodies in the nipple as a consequence of increasingly popular body piercing has been associated with a recalcitrant *M. chelonae* infection with sinus tract formation, presumably acquired through contamination of piercing equipment by tap water.

Duct ectasia involves the large and intermediate ductules of the breast. Histologically, the ducts are dilated and filled with inspissated secretions and keratin plugs. Periductal mastitis describes the associated inflammatory changes. Duct ectasia and periductal mastitis are most common in women aged 40 to 49 years, with periductal mastitis occurring at a slightly younger age. Its main clinical significance is its similarity to invasive carcinoma, from which it must be distinguished by biopsy. Mammographic features include nipple retraction, retroareolar duct dilation, and macrocalcification. Duct ectasia with periductal mastitis accounts for 1 to 2% of symptomatic breast disease. It is not associated with an increased risk for carcinoma, nor does there seem to be any relationship to parity or breastfeeding history, although patients who have periductal mastitis are more likely to use tobacco. Younger patients are more likely to have breast pain or a mass, whereas older patients more often have nipple retraction. This corresponds to the prominence of periductal inflammation and ductal dilatation on histologic examination in younger and older patients, respectively. Patients who have periductal mastitis are more likely to have had a previous episode than patients who have duct ectasia. Furthermore, the lesions of duct ectasia are not sterile, supporting a possible infectious etiology. It is unclear whether duct ectasia and periductal mastitis are two different entities or whether they are part of a continuum. Duct ectasia is in the differential diagnosis of bloody nipple discharge, nipple retraction, mammary fistula, palpable breast mass, and nonpuerperal breast abscess.

## Nipple Discharge

Elicited nipple discharge is often a normal finding. It can be elicited by gentle squeezing of the nipple-areolar complex or with a hand-held breast pump. Approximately 48% of all women and 70% of white women produce nipple secretions on manipulation. The amount and presence of nipple discharge depend on race, age, menopausal status, breast disease, and the amount of discharge produced. It may also be associated with drug ingestion, particularly with those drugs that alter serum prolactin levels. It does not appear to vary consistently with the phases of the menstrual cycle or with oral contraceptive or postmenopausal estrogen use. The color is variable, ranging from green or black to yellow or whitish, and the color may reflect chemical composition, such as cholesterol content. Cytologic examination of nipple aspiration fluid does not have a role in screening for breast cancer because of the limitations of fluid availability and specimen adequacy. Sensitivity for the detection of carcinoma is low (55%) but specificity is high (100%). However, cytologic studies can be useful adjunctive tools because some breast cancers are detected only by cytology.

Spontaneous nipple discharge is rare, comprising only 3 to 5% of breast complaints. Four types of discharge have been found to be associated with breast cancer in increasing frequency: serous, serosanguineous, sanguineous, and watery. These require further evaluation to rule out an underlying malignancy. In a cytologic study of 5305 nipple discharges from 3687 women, bloody discharge was present in 70% of cancer cases. In contrast, two different analyses found cancer to be present in only 4.8 and 5.9% of patients with spontaneous, symptomatic nipple discharge. Seltzer and associates evaluated the significance of age and nipple discharge and found that 4.4% of patients younger than 50 years of age and 32% older than 60 years of age who had a bloody nipple discharge had carcinoma. Cancer appears as an isolated abnormal discharge less than 1% of the time. Benign lesions, such as duct ectasia, products of fibrocystic changes, and intraductal papillomas, are the lesions most often associated with a spontaneous, heme-postive discharge. The presence of both an abnormal discharge and a mass should heighten the suspicion of malignancy. Cytologic examination of bloody or serous discharge can be useful in the absence of an associated mass.

The three most important parts of the clinical history are whether the discharge comes from one or multiple ducts, whether it is spontaneous, and whether it is associated with a mass. Discharge from a single duct is associated with a 4.07% relative risk (95% confidence interval [CI] = 2.7–6) of cancer, whereas that from multiple ducts carries the same risk as occurs in the general population.

Galactorrhea, or milky discharge, usually comes from multiple ducts bilaterally and is generally associated with lactation, elevated serum prolactin, or drug intake (especially phenothiazines and oral contraceptives). However, the most common causes of galactorrhea are idiopathic. Thus, a menstrual and drug history should be taken as part of the clinical examination. Other less common systemic disease etiologies include hypothyroidism, renal failure, and chest trauma, all of which cause an increase in serum prolactin levels. Cytologic analysis of nipple discharge during pregnancy and lactation can be difficult because blood may be found in the absence of an underlying lesion; hence, it is not indicated. A serum prolactin reading should be obtained at a time other than that of the breast examination, because breast stimulation can elevate serum levels and lead to a false concern over the presence of a prolactinoma. An estimated 2% of patients who have nipple discharge have prolactinomas. Serum prolactin levels greater than 20 ng/ml need further evaluation. Once an abnormality is ruled out, the patient can be reassured.

The treatment of choice for an abnormal nipple discharge is duct excision and removal of any concurrent mass. At times, palpation of a point around the nipple clearly elicits the discharge, and this area should be excised as well. Mammography should be performed in women who are older than 35 years of age and who are to undergo surgery for a nipple discharge, especially in those who do not have a palpable mass. Galactography has been demonstrated to identify ductal lesions, but because a histologic diagnosis is needed it may be an unnecessary expense. Proponents of the procedure suggest that because of the complexity of the duct system, galactography allows identification of abnormalities.

## Intraductal Papilloma

Intraductal papilloma is the most common benign papillary lesion. It arises from a larger duct, usually in the subareolar region. Intraductal papilloma is associated with unilateral, spontaneous serous (48%) or bloody (52%) discharge that represents the apparent symptom in 76% of patients and the only complaint in 43%. Twenty-four percent of patients have a palpable—usually subareolar—mass, and 33% have both a mass and a discharge. Mammograms are normal in approximately one third of patients. Ultrasonography is diagnostically useful, especially if it demonstrates a well-defined, smooth-walled, solid hypoechoic nodule or a lobulated, smooth-walled cystic lesion with solid areas. Dilated ducts are commonly seen. The differential diagnosis includes fibroadenoma, cystosarcoma phyllodes, and carcinoma. The mean age of occurrence (47.9 years) is older than that for other benign breast diseases, with the exception of duct ectasia. There may be an increased risk of carcinoma, especially for papillomas arising in the periphery of the breast. Ciatto and associates reported a 3.3 relative risk (RR) (95% CI = 1.60–6.13) of developing an ipsilateral breast cancer. Multiple peripheral papillomas are less common and are less often associated with nipple discharge but more likely to be larger and bilateral. In addition, multiple papillomas are more likely to be associated with subsequent development of carcinoma, possibly caused by the coexistent atypical hyperplasia. Overall, patients who have atypical ductal hyperplasia within papillomas appear to have a greater chance of subsequent disease—either recurrent papillomas or cancer.

The treatment is surgical duct excision, including the associated mass, with consistent long-term follow-up.

## Fibroadenoma

Fibroadenoma is the third most common neoplasm of the breast, ranking after gross cystic changes and carcinoma; it occurs most commonly in premenopausal women at a mean age of 33.9 years. Two-and-one-half percent occur in postmenopausal women, although they may constitute as many as 12% of all breast masses in this age group. They tend to occur and recur more frequently and at an earlier age in black women. Thirteen to sixteen percent of women have multiple or recurrent fibroadenomas. There appears to be an inverse association between oral contraceptive use and occurrence of fibroadenomas; the age-adjusted odds ratio for women younger than 45 years of age is 0.57 (94% CI = 0.42–0.79). The risk of an associated carcinoma is rare, with approximately 100 cases having been reported by 1985. Sixty-five to seventy-one percent of cancers within a fibroadenoma are lobular carcinoma in situ. Twenty-nine percent of patients were found to have a contralateral breast carcinoma. This fact is not surprising given the known risk associated with lobular carcinoma in situ. The prognosis is determined by the type and extent of malignancy and not by the origin within a fibroadenoma.

Fibroadenoma usually presents as an asymptomatic or slightly tender mass, which, if observed, grows slowly, taking 6 to 12 months to double in size. Most growth stops after the fibroadenoma reaches 2 to 3 cm. Occasionally, very large fibroadenomas develop, particularly in adolescents; hence their designation as juvenile fibroadenomas. These may grow rapidly but are almost always benign. Similarly, fibroadenomas may increase rapidly in size during pregnancy and be associated with pain and inflammatory changes that mimic a carcinoma.

Pathologically, fibroadenomas are characterized by a proliferating connective tissue stroma surrounding multiplication of ducts and acini. Either component may predominate; thus, appearances vary. Grossly, they are well delineated from the surrounding breast tissue and, despite appearances, are not truly encapsulated. Infarction, although infrequent (1:202), may make the differential diagnosis from carcinoma more difficult and may cause pain for the patient. Cytogenetic studies reveal some common chromosome aberrations in breast carcinomas and fibroadenomas, implying that specific fibroadenomas may have different pathologic significance. The histologic differential includes adenomas, phyllodes tumors, and fibromatosis.

Management may be surgical excision or expectant treatment, depending on patient age, tumor size, histologic confirmation, mammographic characteristics, and patient desires. Juvenile fibroadenomas are usually excised to avoid breast asymmetry and to preserve the maximum amount of normal tissue. Fibroadenomas can be followed safely in women who are younger than 25 years of age, and, some suggest, in those who are younger than 40 years of age. Of 92.1% of subjects who chose this option in a 2-year longitudinal study of 202 women, all were younger than 40 years of age. During the 2-year period, 8% of cytologically confirmed fibroadenomas enlarged and 26% resolved. Other authors have observed that 32% of these tumors increase in size. When followed conservatively in another study, the actuarial probability of disappearance was 46 and 69% at 5 and 9 years, respectively. Size (larger or smaller than 2 cm) or number (multiple vs. single) did not affect individual rate of resolution, although resolution was more frequent in women younger than 20 years of age. Therefore, age and time course should be discussed when patients are counseled regarding management. FNA was found to be associated with a sensitivity of 84 to 87% and a specificity of 76%. Any associated mammographic finding warrants a biopsy despite the FNA interpretation. Similarly, if cytologic testing reveals any suggestion of atypia, biopsy is necessary. Thus, conservative treatment based on a triple assessment of clinical examination, cytology, and sonogram or mammogram (if indicated) appears to be an appropriate management approach to fibroadenomas in women who are younger than 25—and possibly 40—years of age. If surgery is indicated, it can usually be performed on an outpatient basis under local anesthesia. Surgical excision is almost always indicated to exclude carcinoma for women who are older than 35 (possibly 40) years of age, although improved experience with core biopsy sampling techniques may obviate this recommendation.

## Phyllodes Tumor

The phyllodes tumor, also known as cystosarcoma phyllodes, is an uncommon fibroepithelial neoplasm that accounts for fewer than 1% of breast tumors in women. The phyllodes tumor is usually a palpable mass in premenopausal women. It differs from the fibroadenoma by its increased stromal cellularity, occurrence at a later age (median 45 to 50 years), increased tendency toward local recurrence after complete resection, more rapid growth, and higher rate of associated malignancy. An estimated 25% of these tumors are malignant. The most significant difficulty with phyllodes tumors is the inconsistency between histology and clinical behavior and the criteria for malignancy. Diagnosis with FNA is difficult because both stromal and epithelial elements must be present. Diagnostic failure of FNA in 22 to 86% of cases has been reported. The treatment of choice is surgical excision with margins of 2 to 3 cm and close follow-up, because local recurrences are frequent (20%). Treatment of any associated cancer is determined by its type and extent. Mammographic findings are not unique and may be confused with those of fibroadenomas.

## Mastodynia

Mastodynia, or mastalgia, refers to pain in the breast parenchyma without any specific underlying pathology. The incidence of mastodynia as a breast complaint is 45 to 84%. Typically, it is described as cyclic (40.1%) but may also be noncyclic (26.7%), or it may have other causes (33.2%). Some other causes, which when classified may help direct therapy, include trigger zone pain, Tietze's disease, duct ectasia, psychological depression, and Mondor's disease. The association of mastodynia with an underlying breast cancer is reported to be low, but it may be as high 24%. Attempts to correlate mastalgia with hormone and gonadotropin levels have been unsuccessful, despite the prominence of cyclicity.

Treatment consists of a history, breast examination, and radiologic studies, if indicated. An underlying malignancy should be excluded. Any palpable mass should be evaluated and possibly aspirated as indicated by age and consistency. After significant pathology and specific etiologies have been excluded, patients should be reassured of the normality of the situation.

Most women tolerate the cyclic breast swelling and tenderness associated with menstrual cycles. For those who do not, for whom lifestyle is altered, or for whom the pain becomes constant, no consistently adequate medical therapy currently exists. Symptomatic improvement has been reported with the use of drugs that induce a relative hypoestrogenic state, including danocrine, progestational agents, bromocriptine, tamoxifen, and oral contraceptives, but these agents are associated with side effects that may negate their benefit, such as physiologic stigmata of excessive androgens, altered liver function tests, adverse effects on lipid profiles, symptoms of menopause, nausea, vomiting, orthostasis, and thromboembolic complications. There are also a number of absolute contraindications to their use. Several nonendocrine treatments have also been used with variable results, including vitamin E, evening primrose oil (EPO), and abstinence from caffeine. The most consistently beneficial in reducing pain and nodularity are progesterone, danocrine, bromocriptine, tamoxifen, and evening primrose oil. In a prospective evaluation of patients who had refractory cyclic mastodynia, danocrine was more effective than EPO and bromocriptine. However, given the 50% clinical response rate, the ready availability, and the relatively few side effects, 3 g of EPO per day is a good first-line agent for treatment of patients who have cyclic mastalgia. In general, the symptomatic relief provided by any of these agents is unpredictable and often inadequate or short-lived, leaving the woman and her clinician frustrated. It is of interest that most women who have severe mastodynia have a rapid improvement in those symptoms at menopause.

A report of the successful use of a gonadotropin-releasing hormone (GnRH) analog for short-term treatment of women who have severe, painful fibrocystic breast disease demonstrated response rates of 81%. The mechanism of action is not completely understood. GnRH analogs have been used safely for as long as 6 months with no disruption of serum lipid profiles or induction of irreversible osteoporosis and with the addition of low-dose estrogen they may be used even longer. This may be a viable alternative to the previously mentioned therapies in women who have severe refractory cyclic mastalgia.

## Benign Breast Disease

Diffuse nodular irregularities throughout the breasts are referred to as fibrocystic disease (FCD), benign breast disease (BBD), or fibrocystic changes (FCC). The difficulty with the nomenclature results from the lack of a precise clinicopathologic correlation. This problem exists despite the attempt in 1945 of Foote and associates to define components of FCD: cysts, sclerosing adenosis, fibrosis, papillomatosis, and apocrine change. Nodular breasts presumably develop because of cyclic proliferative activity with incomplete resolution, caused either by excess hormonal stimulation or an exaggerated proliferative response by hypersensitive breast tissue. These fibrocystic changes are correlated with age and menstrual status and increase in the 10 to 15 years before menopause. Patients typically have complaints of a mass, lumpiness, or pain, which may or may not be cyclic.

The risk of developing a breast cancer given a history of FCC is uncertain. Most of the potential for an increased risk comes from the difficulty in examination resulting from multiple nonspecific nodules. Dupont and Page attempted to clarify the issue by re-evaluating 10,366 breast biopsies done for BBD. They were able to identify 70% of women who were not at high risk for breast cancer and 4% who had atypical proliferating lesions and who were at high risk. Thus, it appears that for the majority of women who have BBD, an increased risk of malignancy is not a valid concern.

Treatment for FCC requires a history and breast

examination. A mammogram should be obtained if the patient is older than 35 years of age and if the palpable changes are new since the last mammogram, even if it was performed within the preceding year. The primary goal of the evaluation should be to rule out malignancy. Multifocality and bilaterality suggest a diffuse process that is usually benign. An FNA or biopsy may be necessary for establishing a diagnosis. This should be performed after radiologic studies are completed. Conservative management is discussed in this chapter under Palpable Mass. If cyclicity is prominent and oral contraceptives are not contraindicated, they may be useful. If mastalgia predominates, several medical options and nonhormonal remedies exist. See the section on Mastodynia. Often, reassurance is the most effective therapy.

## High-Risk Lesions

High-risk lesions of the breast confer an increased risk of breast cancer that is further modified by familial and personal histories. The high-risk lesions identified by Dupont and Page are characterized by degrees of epithelial proliferation and atypia arising within either the ductal or lobular elements of the breast. For example, mild and moderate hyperplasia have three and five or more non–atypical cell layers above the basement membrane. Atypical hyperplasia is characterized by severaly abnormal cells that do not quite qualify for a diagnosis of carcinoma in situ within the ductal or lobular unit. Although these lesions are all associated with an increased risk of subsequent breast cancer, ductal (DCIS) and lobular (LCIS) carcinoma in situ are associated with the highest risk. Whether it is more likely to occur ipsilaterally or in both breasts depends on the ductal or lobular designation, respectively (Table 17–1).

Patients who have DCIS have an invasive malignancy discovered 2 to 3% of the time during performance of a mastectomy. Larger lesions are more likely to be associated with invasive disease. DCIS accounts for 5 to 8% of breast cancers and for more than 20% of mammographically detected cancers. It may also present as bloody nipple discharge or a palpable mass.

In contrast, LCIS is not usually clinically apparent and is an incidental finding on biopsy. It is associated with an 18 to 35% risk of subsequent breast cancer in either breast during long-term observation (15 to 24 years), in contradistinction to the approximate 10% increased risk of ipsilateral cancer seen with DCIS. LCIS accounts for 3% of invasive cancers.

The major difficulty with radial scars and sclerosing lesions is caused by their clinical and mammographic similarity to malignancies. Jenson and associates, however, found sclerosing adenosis to be an independent risk factor for breast cancer with an RR of 2.1; this decreased to 1.7 and increased to 6.7 when lesions with atypical hyperplasia were excluded and included, respectively.

Treatment of women who have many of these preinvasive lesions is completed in the process of diagnostic biopsy if the margins are free of disease. FNAs of proliferative lesions show cytologic features that are common to many malignancies; therefore, biopsy is recommended. Patients should be counseled regarding any increased risk of cancer. Estrogen replacement therapy appears not to be associated with a higher risk of cancer in patients who have atypical hyperplasia and LCIS as extrapolated from retrospective studies, but this has not been studied in a prospective fashion. Because LCIS is more common in premenopausal women, an estrogen relationship is frequently assumed, although it has not been substantiated. Dupont and associates found a lower RR of breast cancer in patients who had atypical ductal hyperplasia and who took estrogens than in those who

**Table 17–1** Preinvasive Breast Lesions: Associated Risk of Breast Cancer*

| Lesion | RR (−)FH | RR (+)FH |
|---|---|---|
| **NO SIGNIFICANT INCREASED RISK** | | |
| Radial scar | | |
| Duct ectasia | | |
| Fibroadenoma | | |
| Fibrocystic changes | | |
| **SLIGHT INCREASED RISK** | | |
| Sclerosing adenosis† | | |
| Intraductal papilloma (peripheral/atypical)‡ | 2.1 × | 2.1 × |
| Proliferative disease without atypia* | 1.5 × | 2.1 × |
| **HIGH RISK** | | |
| Atypical hyperplasia* | 3.5–4.0 × | 8.9 × |
| Atypical hyperplasia with calcifications* | 6.5 × | |
| **VERY HIGH RISK** | | |
| Ductal carcinoma in situ (DCIS)§ | 11 × | |
| Lobular carcinoma in situ (LCIS)¶ | 9–12 × | |

*Presented with consideration of family history (FH); first-degree relative with (+) or without (−) breast cancer. (Data from Dupont WD, Page DL: Risk factors for breast cancer in women with proliferative breast disease. N Engl J Med 312:146, 1985.)
†Jensen RA, Page DL, Dupont WD, et al: Invasive breast cancer (IBC) risk in women with sclerosing adenosis (SA). Cancer 64:1977, 1989.
‡Regardless of FH. (Adapted from Page DL, Salhany KE, Jenson RA, et al: Subsequent breast carcinoma risk after biopsy with atypia in a breast papilloma. Cancer 78:258, 1996.
§Regardless of FH. (Adapted from Page DL, Dupont WD, Rogers LW, et al: Intraductal carcinoma of the breast: Higher risk for subsequent invasive cancer predicted by more extensive disease. Cancer 49:751,1996.)
¶Regardless of FH. (Adapted from McDivitt RW, Hutter RVP, et al: In situ lobular carcinoma: A prospective follow-up study indicating cumulative patient risks. JAMA 201:96–100, 1982.)
(From Johnston C: Breast disorders. In Ransom SB, McNeeley SG (eds): Gynecology for the Primary Care Provider. Philadelphia, WB Saunders, 1997, p 37.)

did not; the ratio was 3.0:4.5. Estrogen should be used cautiously in these patients after extensive counseling regarding the relative personal risks and benefits, because newer information suggests that estrogen replacement therapy may increase the overall risk of breast cancer for all women regardless of previous pathology. In follow-up of atypical and in situ lesions, mammograms and physical examinations are initially conducted on a 6-month basis. DCIS is treated either with lumpectomy and radiation therapy or simple mastectomy. The latter procedure is associated with a 1% risk of recurrence, whereas the former procedure is associated with a 10% risk of recurrence in the ipsilateral breast. The addition of radiation therapy to surgical excision significantly reduces the recurrence risk of cancer or DCIS approximately sixfold. The role of postoperative irradiation is less clear for LCIS, which is treated with surgical excision and close observation or ipsilateral mastectomy. Gump surveyed medical oncologists to ascertain their treatment preferences for LCIS and found a slight majority in favor of close observation. Bilateral simple mastectomy may be considered in some instances because of the bilaterally increased risk of malignancy, especially for patients who have strong familial or personal risk factors, inability to undergo close observation, and a high level of anxiety. However, this decision must be made with input from patient, medical oncologist, surgeon, and plastic surgeon. The decision is not to be taken lightly because it has profound physical and psychological impact on the patient. Prophylactic mastectomy does not completely eradicate the risk of breast cancer because total removal of breast tissue is unlikely. Practically, this means that fewer than 1% of patients develop invasive cancer after subcutaneous mastectomy. Certainly, women who have had prophylactic mastectomy, which spares the nipple-areolar complex, need mammographic follow-up because they have significant residual breast tissue. Patients who have LCIS are also candidates for the ongoing National Surgical Adjuvant Breast and Bowel Project (NSABP) prevention trial using tamoxifen vs. placebo.

Bilateral prophylactic mastectomy may also be an option for women who have genetic markers for breast cancer, such as breast cancer (BRCA)-1 and BRCA-2, a strong family history of breast cancer, or high-risk lesions (as mentioned earlier) in conjunction with a positive family history.

## Mondor's Disease

Mondor's disease, or thrombophlebitis of the superficial veins of the breast (including the lateral thoracic, thoracoepigastric and, less commonly, the superficial epigastric veins), is an uncommon entity that is often thought to be associated with antecedent trauma, either surgical or nonsurgical, including biopsies, aesthetic or reconstructive procedures, the use of a body girdle, and intravenous drug use. Although not generally associated with a malignancy, a coexistent carcinoma has been reported in as many as 12.7% of cases, prompting Catania and associates to recommend a mammogram for any woman who has the diagnosis. Furthermore, the presence of a mass may necessitate a surgical biopsy to rule out an underlying carcinoma. Four stages of evolution occurring over 2 to 24 weeks have been described, consisting of thrombus formation with an associated inflammatory infiltrate (stage 1) with subsequent appearance of fibrous cords (stage 2) and multiple sites of recanalization (stage 3) until the entire vein is recanalized with a thick vessel wall and resolution of the perivascular inflammation (stage 4).

The diagnosis of Mondor's disease is easily made by history and examination. Typically, patients have pain and then an appearance of a palpable tender cord in the lateral aspect of one breast. Physical examination should be performed to rule out an associated mass that would require biopsy. Treatment consists of administration of nonsteroidal anti-inflammatory drugs and local heat application. Anticoagulants and antibiotics are not generally required. The time course from initial presentation to complete resolution ranges from 2 to 24 weeks.

## Paget's Disease

Paget's disease is a skin disorder occurring both on the nipple and in extramammary sites, with the latter being less common. Mammary Paget's disease is thought to arise from gland cells of the lactiferous ducts and thus represents an ascending carcinoma. Histologically, large pale-staining cells are seen above the basement membrane in the epidermis. Various immunohistochemical staining panels have been recommended to differentiate Paget's disease from other entities, including PAS, CAM 5.2, 21N, S-100, anti-EMA and anti-c-erbB-2.

Paget's disease generally manifests as an eczematoid, nonhealing lesion with crusting, scaling, and erythema; it is sometimes accompanied by a bloody discharge. Highly pigmented lesions have been reported and may be confused with malignant melanoma. Other differential diagnoses include Bowen's disease, eczema, nipple papillomatosis, and nipple adenoma. All nonhealing lesions of the nipple should be biopsied. This is easily performed with a punch biopsy after infiltration of the site with a local anesthetic. Cytologic scraping has been used in a limited number of patients with excellent diagnostic correlation and may represent a viable alternative to punch biopsy. When scrape cytology is negative or nondiagnostic, it should be followed by a confirmatory biopsy.

Many patients have an underlying carcinoma or ductal carcinoma in situ, although in as many as 40% of patients this may not be clinically detectable. The carcinoma is often multifocal (73%). Similarly, 10% of cases of Paget's disease may be diagnosed microscopically in retrospect after removal of a palpable malignancy. Mammography should be performed before biopsy is attempted, with the realization that as many as 64% of patients may not have a mammographically apparent underlying carcinoma.

Treatment depends on the existence and extent of the underlying carcinoma, but traditionally it has most often involved a mastectomy. Excision of the nipple-areolar complex alone is associated with an unacceptably high recurrence rate of 40 to 60% vs. a 5% rate with mastectomy of the whole breast, including the nipple-areolar complex. Experience with breast conservation therapy, including removal of the nipple-areolar complex and subsequent radiation therapy, is increasing and yielding acceptable rates of disease-free survival and local recurrence. Thus, this may represent a viable alternative to mastectomy for selected patients who have Paget's disease.

## Hormone Use and Breast Cancer

Whether or not to use hormone replacement therapy (HRT) in the postmenopausal years is a decision that is becoming increasingly difficult to make. Often, concern over a possibly modest (21%) increased risk of breast cancer outweighs the benefit of reduction in fatal coronary heart disease (49%) and in deaths from hip fractures (49%). The development of endometrial cancer is avoided by the addition of adequate progesterone. Ultimately, the choice to use HRT should include a discussion of these RRs in light of the patient's family and personal medical history.

Two studies of combined estrogen and progesterone replacement therapy in postmenopausal women failed to find an increased risk of breast cancer; in fact, a significantly reduced risk was found in this cohort. However, Colditz and associates in an update of the Nurses Health Study found an increased risk for users of combination therapy, as did Schairer and associates. In contrast, three studies, including one meta-analysis, showed an increased RR (1.1–1.7) of breast cancer in estrogen users. Steinberg and associates and Bergkvist and associates suggested that duration of use was important; they reported findings after more than 60 and 109 months, respectively.

Colditz and associates noted that current but not past users were at increased risk for breast cancer. Schairer and associates confirmed the increased RR and were able to attribute it to an increase in the incidence of in situ cancer.

It also remains unclear whether there is any relevance in the woman's being premenopausal or postmenopausal at the time of exposure to estrogen, or whether the type of exposure—estradiol vs. conjugated estrogen—is relevant. Although Bergkvist and associates reported a 1.8 RR of breast cancer in estradiol users and no increased risk in users of conjugated estrogens, their data were not significant. It is unclear why there should be a difference in RR, because both of these forms of hormone replacement create similar blood concentrations of estrone and estradiol.

The interpretation of the effect of oral contraceptives (OCP) on the development of breast cancer is difficult, especially because of changing formulations. However, a recent analysis showed a significant 1.3 RR (95% CI = 1.1–1.5) of breast cancer in OCP users. This risk was most prominent in the group who developed breast cancer before the age of 35 years, as well as for those who used it early and for more than 10 years. A meta-analysis of 90% of the published epidemiologic studies by the Collaborative Group on Hormonal Factors in Breast Cancer confirmed the findings of Brinton and associates that there is a slight increased risk of breast cancer in current users of OCP. Others have not noted an increased risk. Once again, the decision about whether to use OCP needs to include a consideration of this potential risk as well as the multiple well-documented benefits that would seem to outweigh the risks in a young woman who does not have a strong family history of breast cancer.

Ongoing drug development has created selective estrogen receptor modulators, such as tamoxifen and raloxifene, which both produce beneficial estrogen-like effects on bone and lipid metabolism. Tamoxifen, a triphenylethylene, produces both agonist and antagonist effects on uterine tissue and antagonist effects on mammary tissue. Tamoxifen has a well-established role in the treatment of primary and recurrent breast cancer and an emerging role in the prevention of breast cancer. Patients who cannot tolerate estrogen thus derive protective benefit against osteoporosis and cardiovascular disease but may somewhat increase their risk of endometrial cancer. Raloxifene, a benzothiophene, is purely an estrogen antagonist in uterine and mammary tissue. It appears to be potentially useful for women who can benefit from its lipid, cardiovascular, and bone-protective effects and for whom avoidance of endometrial—and possibly breast—effects is important. Unfortunately, vasomotor symptoms, such as hot flashes, are not controlled by raloxifene.

## Radiologic Studies and Associated Diagnostic Techniques

Mammography as a screening test in asymptomatic women who are 40 years of age or older reduces the mortality from breast cancer by 20 to 30%. Mammograms should be used according to the guidelines of the American Cancer Society. Exceptions include additional studies needed in the evaluation of a new palpable mass in women older than 20 years of age and a previous diagnosis of malignancy or a high-risk lesion, as well as a strong family history, particularly of premenopausal breast cancer. Despite the mammogram's contribution to a known reduction in mortality, many health insurance plans do not provide coverage for annual screening mammograms in women who are 50 years of age and older but do provide annual coverage for diagnostic mammograms, the definition of which can be variable. Therefore, it is important to be familiar with current indications for "diagnostic" mammograms and to note specifically the indication on the requisition (Table 17–2). Mammography should be used cautiously in pregnant women. The fetus should be shielded appropriately and the period of organogenesis should be avoided. Mammography alone has a specificity and sensitivity greater than 90%. It is less sensitive and specific in dense breasts. A hormonal or menstrual history should be provided with the mammogram request because of the recognized changes in density patterns secondary to HRT use. The location of any existing palpable mass should be documented and provided. The optimal threshold for intervention based on mammographic findings varies, depending on the patient population, perceived expense, and radiologist's experience. The typical percentage of malignancy in wire localization biopsies is 20 to 30%.

**Table 17–2** Accepted Indications for Diagnostic Mammography

Distinct signs and symptoms for which a mammogram is indicated
Personal history of breast, ovarian, endometrial, or colon cancer
Fibrocystic changes
Breast changes that persist, such as a lump, thickening, swelling, or dimpling
Skin irritation or discoloration of the breast
Nipple retraction
Nodularity within the breast
Persistent breast pain
Follow-up of an abnormal mammogram
History of a previous breast biopsy

Some acceptable indications for diagnostic mammography are included in this list. These indications are subject to change with time and may vary with insurance carrier. (Data from the Medicare B Bulletin for Michigan, September 1995.)

With the advent of higher resolution machines, ultrasonography has become a more versatile tool, although it still remains primarily an adjunct to mammography. Its fundamental roles are as follows: to distinguish a cystic mass from a solid mass, especially in a patient who refuses FNA or in whom the mass is nonpalpable and seen only on mammogram; and to facilitate FNA or core biopsy. Ultrasonography does not detect small lesions and calcifications well when compared with mammography. However, when a mass lesion is also present, ultrasonography can have a high sensitivity—95%—and specificity—87.8%—for the detection of microcalcifications.

At this time, computed tomography and magnetic resonance imaging (MRI) have no well-defined role in the routine evaluation of the breast. MRI appears best suited as a supplement to conventional breast imaging. Women for whom MRI might be most useful are those who have dense breasts, silicone augmentation, or postoperative scarring. MRI is also useful in monitoring responses to chemotherapy and in identifying foci of cancer in women who present with metastatic adenocarcinoma in the axilla and clinically negative mammographic lesions.

Positron emission tomography (PET) is an emerging technology. When used with $^{18}$F-fluorodeoxy-glucose (FDG), it appears to be most useful in characterization of malignant lesions and in their follow-up rather than in screening for malignancies.

Scintimammography is another less common method of nuclear medicine used to evaluate the breast. It employs $^{99}$Tcm-MIBI, which is taken up by breast tissue. Scintimammography appears to have a sensitivity similar to that of mammography and MRI for palpable masses but has greater specificity. It may be most useful in women who have dense breasts or in those who have had previous surgery and for whom other diagnostic modalities are inconclusive.

For a comprehensive review of newer methods of breast cancer imaging, consult the textbook by Adler and Wahl.

The use of stereotactic core needle biopsy is increasingly common. Typically, it is performed by radiologists using a 14-gauge needle, an automated gun with which to fire it, and stereotactic apparatus. After 5 to 15 passes are made through the abnormality, the specimens are sent for histologic review. Diagnostic concordance with surgical biopsy is high in experienced hands, and the sensitivity is 90 to 95% for the detection of breast cancer. Absolute indications for its use are still being modified. When the core specimen shows atypical ductal hyperplasia, surgical biopsy is indicated to rule out cancer because of the high chance of an associated malignancy. Other indications for surgical biopsy include frankly invasive malignancy, carcinoma in situ, nondiagnostic results, or insufficient tissue for analysis. Although wire-localized biopsy is the standard method of evaluating suspicious microcalcifications of the breast, experience with core biopsy for this indication is increasing, particularly for clustered microcalicifications. Core biopsy may also be useful in patients who have multifocal suspected mammographic abnormalities. It may eliminate the need for several wire-localized biopsies yet still give the information required to make a decision about the need for mastectomy. Core biopsy is more cost-effective than open surgical biopsy, especially for the analysis of indeterminate masses. As with many new techniques, credentialing requirements, criteria for core biopsy, and follow-up recommendations after core biopsy are variable.

## Chemoprevention

Chemoprevention refers to the use of drugs or non-pharmacologic substances for the purpose of preventing breast cancer.

Prevention trials for women at high risk for developing breast cancer are ongoing, especially with tamoxifen. The rationale for the use of tamoxifen in a preventive fashion emerged from trials that showed a significant reduction in repeat development of primary cancers in breast cancer patients who received tamoxifen.

Retinoids as a group suppress and prevent tumor growth. They are being evaluated in the prevention of breast cancer. A favorable interaction has been noted between 4-hydroxyphenylretinamide (4-HPR) and tamoxifen in breast cancer cell lines.

These compounds are not without harmful side effects. Therefore, until firm data become available, patients should not be encouraged to use them outside of a monitored trial situation. For example, tamoxifen is associated with gynecologic abnormalities, including an elevated risk of endometrial cancer, retinal damage, hepatic toxicity, and vasomotor symptoms, whereas retinoids are associated with changes in skin and mucous membranes, central nervous system side effects, ophthalmic and hepatic toxicity, and teratogenicity.

### REFERENCES

Adler DD, Wahl RL: New methods for breast cancer imaging. In Harris JR, Lippman ME, Morrow M, et al (eds): Diseases of the Breast. Philadelphia, Lippincott-Raven, 1996.

Al-jurf A, Hawk WA, Crile G: Cystosarcoma phyllodes. Surg Gynecol Obstet 146:358, 1978.

Andersen JA: Lobular carcinoma in situ of the breast: An approach to rational treatment. Cancer 39:2597, 1977.

Anonymous: Hormonal contraception. ACOG Technical Bulletin. No. 198—October 1994 (replaces No. 106, July 1987). American College of Obstetricians and Gynecologists. Int J Gynecol Obstet 48:115, 1995.

Arnold GJ, Neiheisel MB: A comprehensive approach to evaluating nipple discharge. Nurse Pract 22:96, 1997.

Azzopardi JG: Problems in Breast Pathology. Philadelphia, WB Saunders, 1979, pp 59–71.

Bassett L, Gold R, Cove H: Mammographic spectrum of traumatic fat necrosis: The fallibility of "pathognomonic" signs of carcinoma. Am J Roentgenol 130:119, 1978.

Bennett IC, Khan A, DeFreitas R, et al: Phyllodes tumors: A clinicopathological review of 30 cases. Aust N Z J Surg 62:628, 1992.

Benson EA: Management of breast abscesses. World J Surg 13:753, 1989.

Bergkvist L, Adami HO, Persson I, et al: The risk of breast cancer after estrogen and estrogen-progestin replacement. N Engl J Med 321:293, 1989.

Bernstein L, Deapen D, Ross RK: The descriptive epidemiology of malignant cystosarcoma phyllodes tumors of the breast. Cancer 71:3020, 1993.

Bland KI: Inflammatory, infectious and metabolic disorders of the mamma. In Bland KI, Copeland EM (eds): The Breast: Comprehensive Management of Benign and Malignant Diseases. Philadelphia WB Saunders; 1991, pp 87–109.

Brenner RJ, Rothman BJ: Detection of primary breast cancer in women with known adenocarcinoma metastatic to the axilla: Use of MRI after negative clinical and mammographic examination. J Magn Reson Imaging 7:1153, 1997.

Brinton LA, Daling JR, Liff JM, et al: Oral contraceptives and breast cancer risk among younger women. J Natl Cancer Inst 87:827, 1995.

Bryant HU, Dere WH: Selective estrogen receptor modulators: An alternative to hormone replacement therapy. Proc Soc Exp Biol Med 217:45, 1998.

Bundred NJ, Dixon JM, Chetty U: Mammillary fistula. Br J Surg 74:466, 1987.

Buscombe JR, Cwikla JB, Thakrar DS, et al: Scintigraphic imaging of breast cancer: A review. Nucl Med Commun 18:698, 1997.

Butler JA, Vargfas HI, Worthen N, et al: Accuracy of combined clinical mammographic cytologic diagnosis of dominant breast mass. Arch Surg 125:893, 1990.

Byrd BF, Bayer DS, Robertson JC, et al: Treatment of breast tumors associated with pregnancy and lactation. Ann Surg 155:940, 1962.

Camiel MR: Mondor's disease in the breast. Am J Obstet Gynecol 152:879, 1985.

Canny PF, Berkowitz GS, Kelsey JL, et al: Fibroadenoma and the use of exogenous hormones. A case-control study. Am J Epidemiol 127:454, 1988.

Cant PJ, Madden MV, Coleman MG, et al: Non-operative management of breast masses diagnosed as fibroadenoma. Br J Surg 82:792, 1995.

Cardenosa G, Eklund GW: Benign papillary neoplasms of the breast: Mammographic findings. Radiology 181:751, 1991.

Carter D: Intraductal papillary tumors of the breast: A study of 78 cases. Cancer 39:1689, 1977.

Carty NJ, Carter C, Rubin C, et al: Management of fibroadenoma of the breast. Ann R Coll Surg Engl 77:127, 1995.

Catania S, Zurrida S, Veronesi P, et al: Mondor's disease and breast cancer. Cancer 69:2267, 1992.

Chaudary MA, Millis RR, Davies GC, et al: The diagnostic value of testing for occult blood. Ann Surg 196:651, 1982.

Chiedozi LC: Mondor's disease. Relationship to use of body girdle. Trop Geogr Med 42:162, 1990.

Chua CL, Thomas A: Cystosarcoma phyllodes tumors. Surg Gynecol Obstet 166:302, 1988.

Ciatto S, Cariaggi P, Bulgaresi P: The value of routine cytologic examination of breast cyst fluids. Acta Cytol 31:301, 1987.

Ciatto S, Andreoli C, Cirillo A, et al: The risk of breast cancer subsequent to histologic diagnosis of benign intraductal papilloma follow-up study of 339 cases. Tumori 77:41, 1991.

Ciatto S, Bravetti P, Cariaggi P: Significance of nipple discharge clinical patterns in the selection of cases for cytologic examination. Acta Cytol 30:17, 1986.

Cohn-Cedarmark G, Rutqvist LE, Rosendahl I, et al: Prognostic factors in cystosarcoma phyllodes. A clinicopathologic study of 77 patients. Cancer 68:2017, 1991.

Colditz GA, Stampfer MJ, Willett WC, et al: Prospective study

of estrogen replacement therapy and risk of breast cancer in postmenopausal women. JAMA 264:2648, 1990.
Colditz GA, Hankinson SE, Hunter DJ, et al: The use of estrogens and progestins and the risk of breast cancer in postmenopausal women. N Engl J Med 332:1589, 1995.
Collins JC, Liao S, Wile AG: Surgical management of breast masses in pregnant women. J Reprod Med 40:785, 1995.
Cooper RA. Mondor's disease secondary to intravenous drug abuse. Arch Surg 125:807, 1990.
Coradini D, Biffi A, Pellizzaro C, et al: Combined effect of tamoxifen or interferon-beta and 4-hydroxyphenylretinamide on the growth of breast cancer cell lines. Tumour Biol 18:22, 1997.
Cosmacini P, Zurrida S, Veronesi P, et al: Phyllodes tumor of the breast: Mammographic experience in 99 cases. Eur J Radiol 15:11, 1992.
Dabski K, Stoll HL: Paget's disease of the breast presenting as a cutaneous horn. J Surg Oncol 29:237, 1985.
Delmas PD, Bjarnason NH, Mitlak BH, et al: Effects of raloxifene on bone mineral density, serum cholesterol concentrations, and uterine endometrium in postmenopausal women. N Engl J Med 337:1641, 1997.
Dennerstein L, Spencer-Gardner C, Gotts G, et al: Progesterone and the premenstrual syndrome: A double blind crossover trial. Br Med J (Clin Res Ed) 290:1617, 1985.
Dent DM, Cant PJ: Fibroadenoma. World J Surg 13:706, 1989.
DePalo G. Formelli F: Risks and benefits of retinoids in the chemoprevention of cancer. Drug Safety 13:245, 1995.
Devereux WP: Acute puerperal mastitis: Evaluation of its management. Am J Obstet Gynecol 108:78, 1970.
Dixon AR, Galea MH, Ellis IO, et al: Paget's disease of the nipple. Br J Surg 78:722, 1991.
Dixon JM: Periductal mastitis/duct ectasia. World J Surg 13:715, 1989.
Dixon JM, Anderson TJ, Lumsden AB, et al: Mammary duct ectasia. Br J Surg 70:601, 1983.
Dixon JM, Dobie V, Lamb J et al: Assessment of the acceptability of conservative management of fibroadenoma of the breast. Br J Surg 83:264, 1996.
Dixon JM, Ravisekar O, Chetty U, et al: Periductal mastitis and duct ectasia: Different conditions with different aetiologies. Br J Surg 83:820, 1996.
Donegan WL: Evaluation of a palpable breast mass. N Engl J Med 327:937, 1992.
Duncan JT, Walker J: Staphylococcus aureus in the milk of nursing mothers and the alimentary canal of their infants: Report to the Medical Research Council. J Hyg 43:474, 1942.
Dunn JM, Lucarotti ME, Wood SJ, et al: Exfoliative cytology in the diagnosis of breast disease. Br J Surg 82:789, 1995.
Dupont WD, Page DL: Risk factors for breast cancer in women with proliferative breast disease. N Engl J Med 312:146, 1985.
Dupont WD, Page DL, Rogers LW, et al: Influence of exogenous estrogens, proliferative breast disease, and other variables on breast cancer risk. Cancer 63:948, 1989.
Ernster VL, Goodson WH III, Hunt TK, et al: Vitamin E and benign breast "disease": A double-blind, randomized clinical trial. Surgery 97:490, 1985.
Fentiman IS, Caleffi M, Brame K, et al: Double blind, controlled trial of tamoxifen therapy for mastalgia. Lancet 1:287, 1986.
Fisher B: Early Breast Cancer Trialist Collaborative Group: Systemic treatment of early breast cancer hormonal, cytotoxic, or immune therapy. Lancet 339:1, 1992.
Fisher B, Constantino J, Redmond C, et al: A randomized clinical trial evaluating tamoxifen in the treatment of patients with node negative breast cancer who have estrogen receptor positive tumors. N Engl J Med 320:479, 1989.
Fisher B, Costantino JP, Redmond CK, et al: Endometrial cancer in tamoxifen treated breast cancer patients: Findings from the NSABP B-14. J Natl Cancer Inst 86:527, 1994.
Fisher ER, Leeming R, Anderson S, et al: Conservative management of intraductal carcinoma (DCIS) of the breast. J Surg Oncol 47:139, 1991.
Fletcher SW, Black W, Harris R, et al: Report of the International Workshop on Screening for Breast Cancer. J Natl Cancer Inst 85:1644, 1993.
Florentine BD, Cobb CJ, Frankel K, et al: Core needle biopsy. A useful adjunct to fine-needle aspiration in select patients with palpable breast lesions. Cancer 81:33, 1997.

Fondo EY, Rosen PP, Fracchia AA, et al: The problem of carcinoma developing in a fibroadenoma: Recent experience at Memorial Hospital. Cancer 43:563, 1979.
Foote FW, Stewart FW: Comparative studies of cancerous versus noncancerous breasts. I. Basic morphologic characteristics. II. Role of so-called chronic cystic mastitis in mammary carcinogenesis: Influence of certain hormones on human breast structure. Ann Surg 121:6, 1945.
Frantz VK, Pickren JW, Melcher GW, et al: Incidence of chronic cystic disease in so-called "normal breasts." A study based on 225 postmortem examinations. Cancer 4:762, 1951.
Funderburk WW, Syphax B: Evaluation of nipple discharge in benign and malignant diseases. Cancer 24:1290, 1969.
Gambrell RD, Maier RC, Sanders BI: Decreased incidence of breast cancer in postmenopausal estrogen-progestogen users. Obstet Gynecol 62:435, 1983.
Gateley CA, Maddox PR, Mansel RE: Mastalgia refractory to drug treatment. Br J Surg 77:1110, 1990.
Gateley CA, Miers M, Mansel RE, et al: Drug treatments for mastalgia: 17 years experience in the Cardiff Mastalgia Clinic. J R Soc Med 85:12, 1992.
Gibbard GF: Sporadic and epidemic puerperal breast infections. Am J Obstet Gynecol 65:1038, 1953.
Gilles R, Guinebretiere JM, Toussaint C, et al: Locally advanced breast cancer: Contrast enhanced subtraction MR imaging of response to preoperative chemotherapy. Radiology 187:493, 1993.
Goodnight JE Jr, Quagliana JM, Morton DL: Failure of subcutaneous mastectomy to prevent the development of breast cancer. J Surg Oncol 26:98, 1984.
Gorsky RD, Koplan JP, Peterson HB, et al: Relative risks and benefits of long-term estrogen replacement therapy: A decision analysis. Obstet Gynecol 83:161, 1994.
Green RA, Dowden RV: Mondor's disease in plastic surgery patients. Ann Plast Surg 20:231, 1988.
Griffith CD, Dowle CW, Hinton CP: The breast pain clinic: A rational approach to classification and treatment of breast pain. Postgrad Med J 63:547, 1987.
Gump FE: Lobular carcinoma in situ. Pathology and treatment. Surg Clin North Am 70:873, 1990.
Gump FE, Jicha DL, Ozella L: Ductal carcinoma in situ (DCIS): A revised concept. Surg 102:790, 1987.
Gupta RK, Simpson J, Dowle C: The role of cytology in the diagnosis of Paget's disease of the nipple. Pathology 28:248, 1996.
Haagensen CD: Adenofibroma. In Haagensen CD, Bodian C, Haagensen DE Jr (eds): Diseases of the Breast, 3rd ed. Philadelphia, WB Saunders, 1986, pp 267–283.
Haagensen CD: Anatomy of the mammary glands. In Haagensen CD, Bodian C, Haagensen DE Jr (eds): Diseases of the Breast, 3rd ed. Philadelphia, WB Saunders, 1986, pp 2–7.
Haagensen CD: Multiple intraductal papilloma. In Haagensen CD, Bodian C, Haagensen DE Jr (eds): Diseases of the Breast, 3rd ed. Philadelphia, WB Saunders, 1986, pp 176–191.
Haagensen CD: Physician's role in the detection and diagnosis of breast disease. In Haagensen CD, Bodian C, Haagensen DE Jr (eds): Diseases of the Breast, 3rd ed. Philadelphia, WB Saunders, 1986, pp 528–543.
Haagensen CD: Solitary intraductal papilloma. In Haagensen CD, Bodian C, Haagensen DE Jr (eds): Diseases of the Breast, 3rd ed. Philadelphia, WB Saunders, 1986, pp 138–162.
Haagensen CD, Bodian C, Haagensen DE: Lobular neoplasia (lobular carcinoma in situ). In Haagensen CD, Bodian C, Haagensen DE Jr (eds): Breast carcinoma: Risk and Detection. Philadelphia, WB Saunders, 1981, p 238.
Hadfield J: Excision of the major duct system for benign disease of the breast. Br J Surg 47:472, 1960.
Hajdu S, Espinosa MH, Robbins GF: Recurrent cystosarcoma phyllodes. A clinicopathologic study of 32 cases. Cancer 38:1402, 1976.
Hamed H, Caleffi M, Chaudary MA, et al: LHRH analogue for treatment of recurrent and refractory mastalgia. Ann R Coll Surg Engl 72:221, 1990.
Hammond S, Keyhani-Rofagha S, O'Toole RV: Statistical analysis of fine needle aspiration cytology of the breast. Acta Cytol 31:276, 1987.
Harms SE, Flamig DP, Hesley KL et al: Fat suppressed 3-D MR imaging of the breast. Radiographics 13:247, 1993.

Hartley MN, Stewart J, Benson EA: Subareolar dissection for duct ectasia and periareolar sepsis. Br J Surg 78:1187, 1991.

Hartrampf CR Jr, Bennett GK: Autogenous tissue reconstruction in the mastectomy patient: A critical review of 300 patients. Am Surg 205:508, 1987.

Helvie MA, Baker DE, Adler DD, et al: Radiographically guided fine needle aspiration of nonpalpable breast lesions. Radiol 174:657, 1990.

Hirst C, Davis N: Core biopsy for microcalcifications in the breast. Aust N Z J Surg 67:320, 1997.

Hitchcock A, Topham S, Bell J, et al: Routine diagnosis of mammary Paget's disease. A modern approach. Am J Surg Pathol 16:58, 1992.

Hoh CK, Schiepers C, Seltzer MA, et al: PET in oncology: Will it replace the other modalities? Semin Nucl Med 27:94, 1997.

Horl HW, Feller AM, Steinau HU, et al: Autologous injection of fatty tissue following liposuction—not a method for breast augmentation. Handchir Mikrochir Plast Chir 21:59, 1989.

Hughes LE, Mansel RE, Webster DJT: Breast pain and nodularity. In Benign Disorders and Diseases of the Breast. Concepts and clinical management. London, Balliere Tindall, 1989, pp 75–92.

Hunter TB, Roberts CC, Hunt KR, et al: Occurrence of fibroadenomas in postmenopausal women referred for breast biopsy. J Am Geriatr Soc 44:61, 1996.

Hutter RVP: Goodbye to fibrocystic disease (editorial). N Engl J Med 312:179, 1985.

Jensen RA, Page DL, Dupont WD, et al: Invasive breast cancer (IBC) risk in women with sclerosing adenosis (SA). Cancer 64:1977, 1989.

Johanson A, Sager EM: Contrast mammography in spontaneous bloody secretion from the nipple. Tidsskr Nor Laegeforen 110:3750, 1990.

Johnson WC, Wallrich R, Helurg EB: Superficial thrombophlebitis of the chest wall. JAMA 180:103, 1962.

Kaelin CM, Smith TJ, Homer MJ, et al: Safety, accuracy and diagnostic yield of needle localization biopsy of the breast performed using local anesthesia. J Am Coll Surg 179:267, 1994.

Kanitakis J, Thivolet J, Claudy A: p53 protein expression in mammary and extramammary Paget's disease. Anticancer Res 13:2429, 1993.

Kario K, Maeda S, Mizuno Y, et al: Phyllodes tumor of the breast: A clinicopathologic study of 34 cases. J Surg Oncol 45:46, 1990.

Kessinger A, Foley JF, Lemon HM, et al: Metastatic cystosarcoma phyllodes: A case report and review of the literature. J Surg Oncol 4:131, 1972.

King EB, Goodson WH: Discharges and secretions of the nipple. In Bland KI, Copeland EM (eds): The Breast: Comprehensive Management of Benign and Malignant Diseases. Philadelphia, WB Saunders, 1991, pp 61–62.

Kline TS, Lash SR: Nipple secretion in pregnancy; a cytologic and histologic study. Am J Clin Pathol 37:626, 1962.

Kline TS, Lash SR: The bleeding nipple of pregnancy and postpartum period; a cytologic and histologic study. Acta Cytol 8:336, 1964.

Lafaye C, Aubert B: The effect of local progesterone on benign breast diseases. 500 case studies. J Gynecol Obstet Biol Reprod 7:1123, 1978.

Lagios M: Duct carcinoma in situ. Pathology and treatment. Surg Clin North Am 70:853, 1990.

Lagios MD, Margolin FR, Westdahl PR, et al: Mammographically detected duct carcinoma in situ: Frequency of local recurrence following tylectomy and prognostic effect of nuclear grade on local recurrence. Cancer 63:618, 1989.

Layfield LJ, Glasgow BJ, Cramer H: Fine needle aspiration in the management of breast masses. Pathol Annu 24:23, 1989.

Layfield LJ, Mooney EE, Glasgow B, et al: What constitutes an adequate smear in fine-needle aspiration cytology of the breast? Cancer 81:16, 1997.

Leary WG Jr: Acute puerperal mastitis—A view. Calif Med 68:147, 1948.

Lee CH, Egglin TK, Philpotts L, et al: Cost-effectiveness of stereotactic core needle biopsy: Analysis by means of mammographic findings. Radiology 202:849, 1997.

Leis HP Jr: Gross breast cysts: Significance and management. Contemp Surg 39:13, 1991.

Liberman L, Cohen MA, Dershaw DD, et al: Atypical ductal hyperplasia diagnosed at stereotaxic core biopsy of breast lesions: An indication for surgical biopsy. AJR 164:1111, 1995.

Ligon RE, Stevenson DR, Diner W, et al: Breast masses in young women. Am J Surg 140:779, 1980.

Lucarotti ME, Dunn JM, Webb AJ: Scrape cytology in the diagnosis of Paget's disease of the breast (meeting abstract). Cytopathology 5:9, 1994.

Maier WP, Berger A, Derrick BM: Periareolar abscess in the nonlactating breast. Am J Surg 144:359, 1982.

Majmudar B, Rosales-Quintanta S: Infarction of breast fibroadenomas during pregnancy. JAMA 231:963, 1975.

March DE, Raslavicus A, Coughlin BF, et al: Use of breast core biopsy in the United States: Results of a national survey. AJR 169:697, 1997.

Marin-Bertolin S, Gonzalez-Martinez R, Velasco-Pastor M, et al: Mondor's disease and aesthetic breast surgery: Report of case secondary to mastopexy with augmentation. Aesthetic Plast Surg 19:251, 1995.

Marshall BT, Hepper JK, Zirbel CC: Sporadic puerperal mastitis: An infection that need not interrupt lactation. JAMA 233:1377, 1975.

McDivitt RW, Hutter RVP, Foote FW, et al: In situ lobular carcinoma: A prospective follow-up study indicating cumulative patient risks. JAMA 201:96, 1967.

Mendelson EB: Evaluation of the postoperative breast. Radiol Clin North Am 30:107, 1992.

Midulla C, Cenci M, De Iorio P, et al: The value of fine needle aspiration cytology in the diagnosis of breast proliferative lesions. Anticancer Res 15:2619, 1995.

Mitre BK, Kanbour AI, Mauser N: Fine needle aspiration biopsy of breast carcinoma in pregnancy and lactation. Acta Cytol 41:1121, 1997.

Moore MP, Kinne DW: Diagnosis and treatment of in situ breast cancer. Contemp Oncol 46–51, 1992.

Moskowitz M: The predictive value of certain mammographic signs in screening for breast cancer. Cancer 51:1007, 1983.

Murad TM, Contesso G, Mouriesse H: Nipple discharge from the breast. Ann Surg 195:259, 1982.

Nadji M, Morales AR, Girtanner RE, et al: Paget's disease of the skin. A unifying concept of histogenesis. Cancer 50:2203, 1982.

Newton M, Newton NR: Breast abscess: Result of lactation failure. Surg Gynecol Obstet 91:651, 1950.

Niebyl JR, Spence MR, Pharmley TH: Sporadic (nonepidemic) puerperal mastitis. J Reprod Med 20:97, 1978.

Norris HJ, Taylor HB: Relationship of the histologic appearance to behavior of cystosarcoma phyllodes: Analysis of ninety-four cases. Cancer 20:2090, 1967.

Ohuchi N, Abe R, Kasai M: Possible cancerous change of intraductal papillomas of the breast. A 3-D reconstruction study of 25 cases. Cancer 54:605, 1984.

O'Malley MS, Fletcher SW: US Preventive Services Task Force. Screening for breast cancer with breast self-examination. A critical review. JAMA 257:2196, 1987.

Orel SG: High-resolution MR imaging of the breast. Semin Ultrasound CT MR 17:476, 1996.

Organ CH Jr, Organ BC: Fibroadenoma of the female breast: A critical clinical assessment. J Natl Med Assoc 75:701, 1983.

O'Shaughnessy JA: Chemoprevention of breast cancer. JAMA 275:1349, 1996.

Ostrow LB, DuBois JJ, Hofer RA Jr, et al: Needle-localized biopsy of occult breast lesions. South Med J 80:29, 1987.

Ozzello L, Gump FE: The management of patients with carcinomas in fibroadenomatous tumors of the breast. Surg Gynecol Obstet 160:99, 1985.

Page DL, Dupont WD, Rogers LW, et al: Intraductal carcinoma of the breast. Cancer 49:751, 1982.

Page DL, Kidd TE Jr, Dupont WD, et al: Lobular neoplasia of the breast: Higher risk for subsequent invasive cancer predicted by more extensive disease. Hum Pathol 22:1232, 1991.

Page DL, Salhany KE, Jensen RA, et al: Subsequent breast carcinoma risk after biopsy with atypia in a breast papilloma. Cancer 78:258, 1996.

Page DL, Simpson JF: Benign, high-risk, and premalignant lesions of the mamma. In Bland KI, Copeland EM (eds): The Breast: Comprehensive Management of Benign and Malignant Diseases.

Philadelphia, WB Saunders, 1991, pp 113–116, 117–124, 126–128.

Parazzini F, LaVecchia C, Rlundi R, et al: Methylxanthine, alcohol-free diet and fibrocystic breast disease. A factorial clinical trial. Surgery 99:576, 1986.

Parker S, Burbank F, Tabar L, et al: Percutaneous large core breast biopsy: A multi-institutional experience. Radiology 1993:359, 1994.

Parker SH, Lovin JD, Jobe WE, et al: Nonpalpable breast lesions: Stereotactic automated large core biopsies. Radiology 180:403, 1991.

Pashby NL, Mansel RE, Hughes LE, et al: A clinical trial of evening primrose oil in mastalgia. Br J Surg 68:801, 1981.

Patey DH, Thackeray AC: Pathology and treatment of mammary-duct fistula. Lancet 2:871, 1958.

Paulus D: Benign diseases of the breast. Radiol Clin North Am 21:38, 1983.

Pearlman MD: *Mycobacterium chelonai* breast abscess associated with nipple piercing. Infect Dis Obstet Gynecol 3:116, 1995.

Peison B, Benisch B: Paget's disease of the nipple simulating malignant melanoma in a black woman. Am J Dermatopathol (suppl) 7:165, 1985.

Pennisi VR, Capozzi A: Subcutaneous mastectomy: An interim report on 1244 patients. Ann Plast Surg 12:340, 1984.

Petersson C, Pandis N, Rlzou H, et al: Karyotypic abnormalities in fibroadenomas of the breast. Int J Cancer 70:282,1997.

Petrakis NL, Lee RE, Miike R, et al: Coloration of breast fluid related to concentration of cholesterol, cholesterol epoxides, estrogen and lipid peroxides. Am J Clin Pathol 89:117, 1988.

Petrakis NL, Mason L, Lee R, et al: Association of race, age, menopausal status, and cerumen type with breast fluid secretion in nonlactating women, as determined by nipple aspiration. J Natl Cancer Inst 54:829, 1975.

Pick PW, Iossifides IA: Occurrence of breast carcinoma within a fibroadenoma. A review. Arch Pathol Lab Med 108:590, 1984.

Pierce LJ, Haffty BG, Solin LJ, et al: The conservative management of Paget's disease of the breast with radiotherapy. Cancer 80:1065, 1997.

Pike AM, Oberman HA: Juvenile (cellular) adenofibromas. A clinicopathologic study. Am J Surg Pathol 9:730, 1985.

Plu-Bureau G, Le MG: Oral contraception and the risk of breast cancer. Contraception Fertil Sex 25:301, 1997.

Preece PE, Mansel RE, Bolton PM, et al: Clinical syndromes of mastalgia. Lancet 2:670, 1976.

Pye JK, Mansel RE, Hughes LE: Clinical experience of drug treatments for mastalgia. Lancet 2:373, 1985.

Raju U, Vertes D: Breast papillomas with atypical ductal hyperplasia: A clinicopathologic study. Hum Pathol 27:1231, 1996.

Ravichandran D, Carty NJ, al-Talib RK, et al: Cystic carcinoma of the breast: A trap for the unwary. Ann R Coll Surg Engl 77:123, 1995.

Reed W, Oppedal BR, Eeg Larsen T: Immunohistology is valuable in distinguishing between Paget's disease, Bowen's disease, and superficial spreading malignant melanoma. Histopathology 16:583, 1990.

Rees BI, Gravelle IH, Hughes LE: Nipple retraction in duct ectasia. Br J Surg 64:577, 1977.

Ricciardi I, Ianniruberto A: Tamoxifen-induced regression of benign breast lesions. Obstet Gynecol 54:80, 1979.

Rickard MT: Ultrasound of malignant breast microcalcifications: Role in evaluation and guided procedures. Australas Radiol 40:26, 1996.

River L, Silverstein J, Grout J, et al. Carcinoma of the breast: The diagnostic significance of pain. Am J Surg 82:733, 1951.

Rongione AJ, Evans BD, Kling KM, et al: Ductography is a useful technique in evaluation of abnormal nipple discharge. Am Surg 62:785, 1996.

Rosen PP, Lieberman PH, Braun DW Jr, et al: Lobular carcinoma in situ of the breast. Am J Surg Pathol 2:225, 1978.

Rosen PP, Senie RT, Farr GH, et al: Epidemiology of breast carcinoma: Age, menstrual status, and exogenous hormone usage in patients with lobular carcinoma in situ. Surgery 85:219, 1979.

Rosenblatt R, Fineberg SA, Sparano JA, et al: Stereotactic core needle biopsy of multiple sites in the breast: Efficacy and effect on patient care. Radiology 201:67, 1996.

Rubin M. Horiuchi K, Joy N, et al: Use of fine needle aspiration for solid breast lesions is accurate and cost-effective. Am J Surg 174:694, 1997.

Salvadori B, Cusumano F, Del Bo R, et al: Surgical treatment of phyllodes tumors of the breast. Cancer 63:2532, 1989.

Samarasinghe D, Frost F, Sterrett G, et al: Cytological diagnosis of Paget's disease of the nipple by scrape smears: A report of five cases. Diagn Cytopathol 9:291, 1993.

Sartorius OW, Smith HS, Morris P, et al: Cytologic evaluation of breast fluid in the detection of breast disease. J Natl Cancer Inst 59:1073, 1977.

Sattin RW, Rubin GL, Wingo PA, et al: Oral contraceptive use and the risk of breast cancer. The Cancer and Steroid Hormone Study of the Centers for Disease Control and the National Institute of Child Health and Human Development. N Engl J Med 315:405, 1986.

Schairer C, Byrne C, Keyl PM, et al: Menopausal estrogen and estrogen-progestin replacement therapy and risk of breast cancer (United States). Cancer Causes Control 5:491, 1994.

Schmidt RA: Stereotactic breast biopsy. CA Cancer J Clin 44:172, 1994.

Seltzer MH Perloff LJ, Kelley RI, et al: The significance of age in patients with a nipple discharge. Surg Gynecol Obstet 131:522, 1970.

Semb C: Pathologico-anatomical and clinical investigations of fibroadenomatosis cystica mammae and its relation to other pathological conditions in the mamma, especially cancer. Acta Chir Scandinav (suppl) 64:1, 1928.

Shehi LJ, Pierson KK: Benign and malignant epithelial neoplasms and dermatological disorders. *In* Bland KI, Copeland EM (eds): The Breast: Comprehensive Management of Benign and Malignant Diseases, Philadelphia, WB Saunders, 1991, pp 227–228.

Sickles EA: Sonographic detectability of breast calcifications. Soc Photogr Instrom Eng J 419:51, 1983.

Sickles EA, Filly RA, Callen RW: Breast cancer detection with sonography and mammography: Comparison using state of the art equipment. Am J Roentgenol 140:843, 1983.

Sitakalin C, Ackerman AB: Mammary and extramammary Paget's disease. Am J Dermatopathol 7:335, 1985.

Snead DR, Vryenhoef P, Pinder SE, et al: Routine audit of breast fine needle aspiration (FNA) cytology specimens and aspirator inadequate rates. Cytopathology 8:236, 1997.

Souba WW: Evaluation and treatment of benign breast disorders. *In* Bland KI, Copeland EM (eds): The Breast: Comprehensive Management of Benign and Malignant Diseases. Philadelphia, WB Saunders, 1991, 723–724.

Stanford JL, Weiss NS, Voigt LF, et al: Combined estrogen and progestin hormone replacement therapy in relation to risk of breast cancer in middle aged women. JAMA 274:137, 1995.

Stanley MW, Tani EM, Rutqvist LE, et al: Cystosarcoma phyllodes of the breast: A cytologic and clinicopathologic study of 23 cases. Diagn Cytopathol 5:29, 1989.

Steinberg K, Thacker SB, Smith J, et al: A meta-analysis of the effect of estrogen replacement therapy on the risk of breast cancer. JAMA 265:1985, 1991.

Stomper PC, Bradley J, Voorhis V, et al: Mammographic changes associated with postmenopausal hormone replacement therapy: A longitudinal study. Radiology 174:487, 1990.

Sumkin JH, Perrone AM, Harris KM, et al: Lactating adenoma: US features and literature review. Radiology 206:271, 1998.

Swain SM: Ductal carcinoma in situ—incidence, presentation and guidelines to treatment. Oncology 3:25, 1989.

Swain SM: Ductal carcinoma in situ. Cancer Invest 10:443, 1992.

Sweeney DJ, Wylie EJ: Mammographic appearances of mammary duct ectasia that mimic carcinoma in a screening programme. Australas Radiol 39:18, 1995.

Thompson AC, Espersen T, Maigaard S: Course and treatment of milk stasis, noninfectious inflammation of the breast, and infectious mastitis in nursing women. Am J Obstet Gynecol 149:492, 1984.

Tobiassen T, Rasmussen T, Doberl A, et al: Danazol treatment of severely symptomatic fibrocystic breast disease and long-term follow-up—the Hjorring project. Acta Obstet Gynecol Scand (suppl) 123:159, 1984.

Tsuji T: Mammary and extramammary Paget's disease: Expression of Ca 15-3, Ka-93, Ca 19-9, and CD44 in Paget cells and adjacent normal skin. Br J Dermatol 132:7, 1995.

Urban JA: Excision of the major duct system of the breast. Cancer 16:516, 1963.

Veronesi U, DePalo G, Costa A, et al: Chemoprevention of breast cancer with fenretinide. IARC Scientific Publications 136:87, 1996.

Vielh P, Validire P, Kheirallah S, et al: Paget's disease of the nipple without clinically and radiologically detectable breast tumor. Histochemical and immunohistochemical study of 44 cases. Pathol Res Pract 189:150, 1993.

Vogel VG: High risk populations as targets for breast cancer prevention trials. 1991; 20:86, Prev Med.

Walt AJ, Simon M, Swanson GM: The continuing dilemma of lobular carcinoma in situ. Arch Surg 127:904, 1992.

Wang DY, Fentiman IS: Epidemiology and endocrinology of benign breast disease. Breast Cancer Res Treat 6:5, 1985.

Wapnir IL, Rabinowitz B, Greco RS: A reappraisal of prophylactic mastectomy. Surg Gynecol Obstet 171:171, 1990.

Wargotz ES, Norris HJ, Austin RM, et al Fibromatosis of the breast. A clinical and pathological study of 28 cases. Am J Surg Pathol 11:38, 1987.

Whitehead MI, Campbell S: Endometrial histology, uterine bleeding and oestrogen levels in women receiving oestrogen therapy and oestrogen/progesterone therapy. In Taylor R, Brush M, King R (eds): Endometrial Cancer. London, Balliere Tindall, 1978, pp 65–80.

Wilkinson EJ, Franzini DA, Masood S: Cytological needle sampling of the breast: Techniques and end results. In Bland KI, Copeland EM (eds): The Breast: Comprehensive Management of Benign and Malignant Diseases. Philadelphia, WB Saunders, 1991, pp 478–480.

Wilkinson S, Anderson TJ, Rifkind E, et al: Fibroadenoma of the breast: A follow-up of conservative management. Br J Surg 76:390, 1989.

Willis SL, Ramzy I: Analysis of false results in a series of 835 fine needle aspirates of breast lesions. Acta Cytol 39:858, 1995.

Wolber RA, Dupuis BA, Wick MR: Expression of c-erbB-2 oncoprotein in mammary and extramammary Paget's disease. Am J Clin Pathol 96:243, 1991.

Wynder EL, Lahti H, Laakso K, et al: Nipple aspirates of breast fluid and the epidemiology of breast disease. Cancer 56:1473, 1985.

Yang WT, Suen M, Metreweli C: Sonographic features of benign papillary neoplasms of the breast: Review of 22 patients. J Ultrasound Med 16:161, 1997.

Yim JH, Wick MR, Philpott GW, et al: Underlying pathology in mammary Paget's disease. Ann Surg Oncol 4:287, 1997.

# 18

# Prevention and Treatment of Postoperative Infections

DAVID L. HEMSELL

Because most gynecologic surgical procedures are elective, the gynecologist has the opportunity to optimize infection prevention. Infection occurring after surgical procedures is the most frequently observed morbid condition.

## Risk Categories

In the 1960s, virtually all patients who underwent any type of surgical procedure were given antibiotic starting with hospital admission and continued until discharge. It was quickly recognized that justification for this treatment was necessary to prevent unwarranted administration of antibiotic, because there were cases of significant sequelae after antibiotic administration to uninfected patients. The four defined classes of surgical procedure are presented in Table 18–1.

There is obviously overlap. Dilatation and curettage and cervical conization are *clean contaminated procedures*, yet the infection rate after either is so low that prophylaxis is not warranted. If a patient is immunocompromised or debilitated, then a dose of prophylaxis is warranted before conization, but there are no prospective data to confirm the need for such prophylaxis. There have been no prospective clinical trials evaluating prophylaxis with infertility surgery, and yet prophylaxis is universally administered for these *clean* procedures because of the drastic consequences of pelvic infection in an infertility patient. The infection rate observed after pregnancy termination is that of a clean procedure, but clinical trials have shown a decrease in infection associated with antibiotic administration, so prophylaxis is warranted.

It is much more difficult to ascertain true infection rates in gynecologic surgical procedures conducted in day surgeries or in surgicenters. Follow-up requires direct patient contact by a surveillance team. The overall infection rate in one study of 1241 women was 0.9% and was highest with tubal lavage, a procedure that has been shown to introduce bacteria into the peritoneal cavity. Prophylaxis should be given to women undergoing that procedure.

## Postoperative Infection Classification

In 1988, the Centers for Disease Control and Prevention (CDC) introduced definitions for nosocomial

**Table 18-1** Classes of Surgical Procedures, Infection Rates, and Antibiotic Use

| Class | Infection Rate (%) | Typical Procedure(s) | Antibiotic Administration |
|---|---|---|---|
| Clean | 1–5 | Laparoscopic procedures<br>Adnexal surgery | None |
| Clean contaminated | 5–15 | Hysterectomy<br>Laparoscopy with hydrotubation | Prophylactic |
| Contaminated | 15–25 | Laparotomy/laparoscopy for acute PID | Therapeutic |
| Dirty | >25 | Ruptured tubo-ovarian abscess | Therapeutic |

PID = pelvic inflammatory disease.

infection, Horan and associates modified the definitions and refer to them as surgical site infections (SSI). They are classified as either superficial or deep incisional (abdominal wall infections), or as organ or space infections. A schematic appears in Figure 18–1. SSI definitions are precise and are used primarily by surveillance infection control teams in reviewing records. All infections must occur within 30 days of the operative procedure unless an implant is left in place during the procedure, in which case the interval is extended to 1 year. The definitions require that the diagnosis be made by the surgeon or physician.

## SUPERFICIAL INCISIONAL INFECTION

This infection involves skin or subcutaneous tissue (or both) surrounding the abdominal incision, and requires at least one of the following variables:
1. Purulent drainage
2. Aseptically obtained fluid or tissue culture material from which organisms are isolated
3. At least one of the following signs or symptoms of infection:
   a. Pain or tenderness
   b. Localized swelling, redness, or heat
   c. An incision deliberately opened by the surgeon (unless the culture is negative)

Stitch abscesses are not included. A superficial seroma or hematoma can result in superficial dehiscence, which results in the same prolongation of hospital stay that is observed with infection. The treatment of patients is essentially the same as for patients who have infection. It is important to collect fluid aseptically for culture from the incision in question, even if it is believed to be just a seroma or hematoma. The bacteria isolated from such an infection are predominantly those of a pelvic operative site infection rather than gram-positive aerobic bacteria, which are usually isolated from skin infections.

## DEEP INCISIONAL INFECTION

When infection involves the deep soft tissues, as depicted in Figure 18–1, it is classified as a deep incisional infection. At least one of the following symptoms must be present:
1. Purulent drainage from a deep incision
2. Spontaneous dehiscence or deliberate opening of a deep incision by a surgeon because of at least one of the following:
   a. Temperature higher than 38°C
   b. Localized pain or tenderness (unless the culture is negative)
   c. An abscess or other infection of the deep tissues is identified by direct examination, during reoperation, or by radiologic or histopathologic examination.

Abdominal incision infections are much less common than those in the pelvis following hysterectomy or other gynecologic procedures. Deep infections oc-

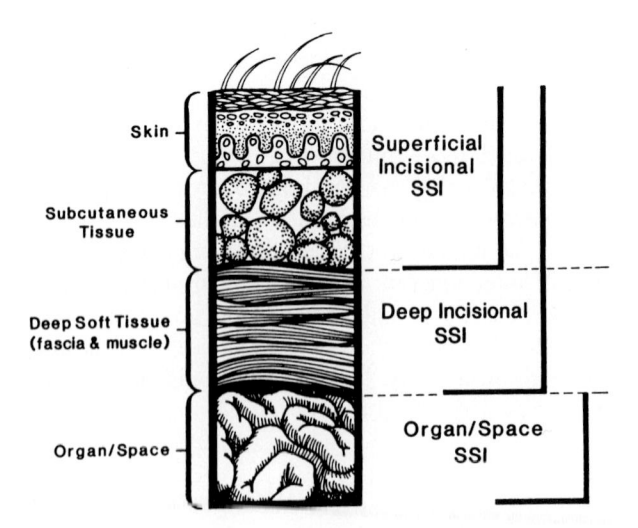

**Figure 18-1** Surgical site infection (SSI) classification. (From Horan TC, Gaynes RP, Martone WJ, et al: CDC definitions of nosocomial surgical site infections, 1992: A modification of CDC definitions of surgical wound infections. Am J Infect Control 20:271–274, 1992.)

cur infrequently enough that they could be classified as rare.

Since incisional infections normally develop on the fourth or fifth day after hysterectomy or other procedures, the patient is normally at home. For that reason, it is very important that patients be aware of the symptoms and signs of incisional or pelvic infections before they undergo surgery, and before discharge from the hospital, so that if infection develops, they will contact the surgeon promptly so that a diagnosis will be made and therapy will be initiated as early as possible.

## ORGAN OR SPACE INFECTIONS

This type of infection usually develops after hysterectomy and involves tissues deep in the incision, which were opened or manipulated during the surgical procedure. The majority of infections that develop after elective gynecologic surgery fall into this category. Qualifiers for this type of infection include at least one of the following:

1. Purulent drainage from a drain placed into the deep operative site
2. Organisms recovered from aseptic culture of fluid or tissue obtained from the infected site
3. Abscess or other infection diagnosed by direct examination, during reoperation, or by either radiologic or histopathologic means

# Posthysterectomy Infection

A CDC report of August 1997 indicates that hysterectomy is the second most frequently performed major surgical procedure among reproductive-aged women. It is estimated that approximately 40% of nosocomial infections that develop are the direct result of elective surgical procedures. Operative site infection significantly prolongs hospital stay and increases the cost of health care. That is especially true now that most elective cases are performed as same-day surgeries with postoperative observation that may extend in some centers from several hours after vaginal hysterectomy to several days after abdominal hysterectomy.

## RISK FACTORS

After the surgical procedure classification was developed, investigations were designed to identify demographic, diagnostic, or surgical variables associated with an increased risk for postoperative infection. The purpose of these investigations was to diminish the unnecessary administration of prophylactic antibiotic to all patients undergoing gynecologic surgery. Variables for infection after hysterectomy were not as uniform as those following cesarean section. Data compiled from multiple prospective randomized and blinded clinical trials indicated that all patients were at risk for infection after hysterectomy, and that single-dose antimicrobial prophylaxis was as effective as multidose therapy. The Infectious Disease Society of America, in developing quality standards for infectious diseases, found that vaginal and abdominal hysterectomy were procedures for which there were superior data that supported treating patients with antibiotic prophylaxis.

## VAGINAL SURGICAL MARGIN (CUFF) CELLULITIS (Fig. 18–2)

Vaginal surgical margin (cuff) cellulitis, a posthysterectomy infection, should theoretically be classified as a *superficial incisional infection*, but it is not. When the vagina is examined during the first several days following hysterectomy, criteria for infection are present. There are purulent secretions and a bimanual examination reveals that the vaginal surgical margin is tender, erythematous, and edematous. This is true regardless of patient symptoms, physical findings, temperature reading, and (or) leukocyte count. In reality, every woman develops vaginal cuff cellulitis after undergoing hysterectomy. If patients do not have symptoms and have a normal examination of the lower abdomen over the pelvic structures, neither a pelvic examination nor antibiotic therapy is necessary. A pelvic examination is always necessary before a patient is treated for a pelvic infection, however, and a diagnosis should be made.

If a patient develops a temperature elevation or has a subjective fever; symptoms of pelvic, lower abdominal, back, or upper thigh pain; lower abdominal discomfort in response to gentle, deep palpation; and there is tenderness of the vaginal surgical margin during bimanual examination, cuff cellulitis is present and requires antimicrobial therapy. This mild infection commonly develops in our indigent patient population after the patient is discharged from the hospital, and oral outpatient antimicrobial therapy is successful in curing it.

## PELVIC CELLULITIS (Fig. 18–3)

If the inflammatory response is not confined to the vaginal cuff, it extends laterally into the parametrial areas with resultant development of pain in the locations described previously. There is tenderness that was not present, and there is usually temperature elevation and leukocytosis. Symptoms and physical

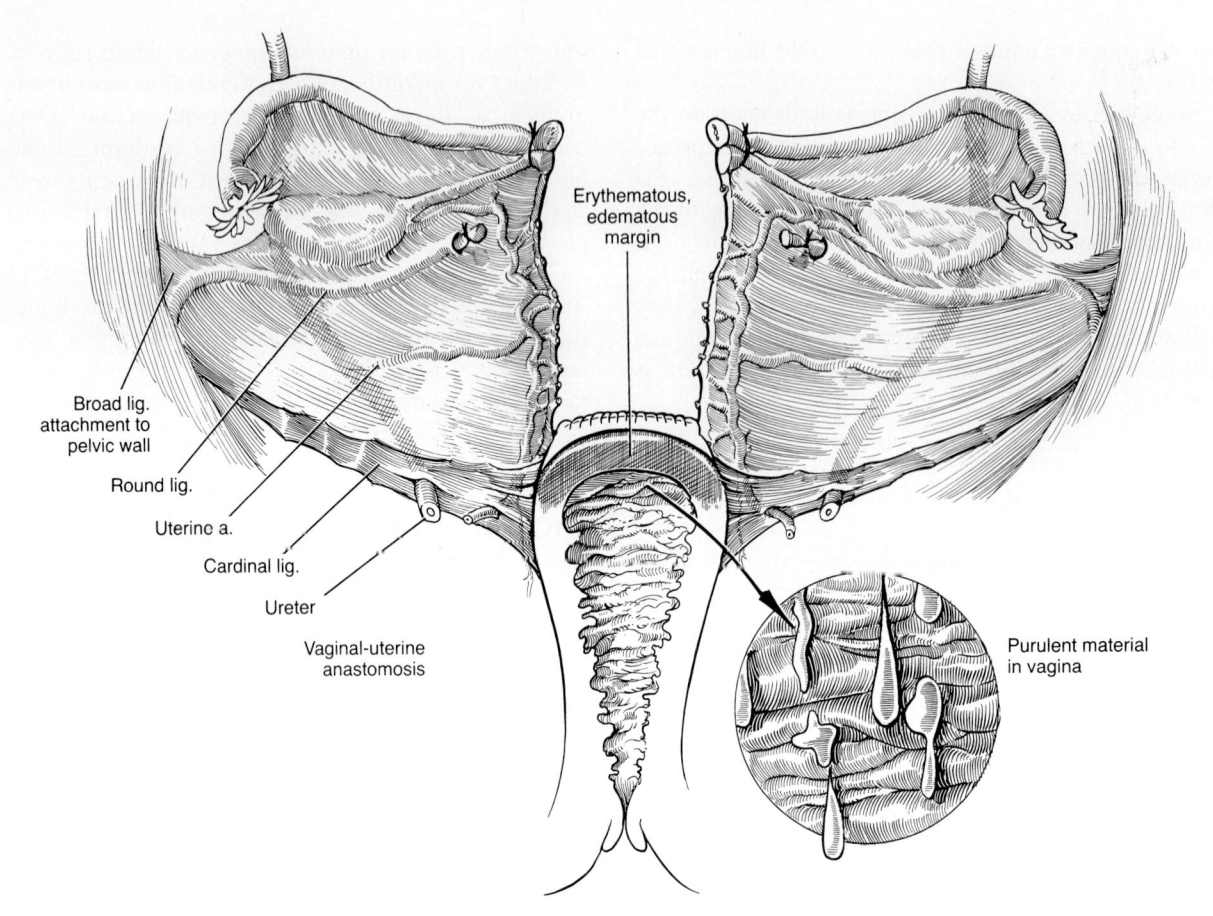

**Figure 18–2** Female pelvis during the first several days following hysterectomy. (From Copeland LJ: Textbook of Gynecology. Philadelphia, WB Saunders, 1993, p 564.)

findings are more pronounced on one side than on the other. Pelvic cellulitis frequently develops on the second or third postoperative day and is treated with parenteral antimicrobial therapy. Occasionally, patients develop this infection after hospital discharge and require readmission for therapy.

## ADNEXAL INFECTION (Fig. 18–4)

As depicted in Figure 18–4, infection may develop in retained adnexal structures. The characteristics of this infection are almost identical to those of pelvic cellulitis, with one exception: Bimanual examination reveals that the tenderness is not *in* but rather cephalad or posterior to the parametrial area or areas. This infection is usually unilateral. Infection in this location is uncommon except after hysterectomy, but it can occur after adnexal surgery. Parenteral antimicrobial therapy is indicated.

## CUFF OR PELVIC ABSCESS (Fig. 18–5)

After hysterectomy, between 20 and 200 ml of serum, blood, and lymph may collect between the vaginal surgical margin and the pelvic peritoneum if the cuff is closed. Before the universal practice of giving patients antibiotic prophylaxis for hysterectomy, surgeons did not appose the vaginal surgical margins but decreased infection by placing a running, locking suture around the circumference, leaving the cuff open for drainage. With prophylaxis, closing the vagina does not increase the postoperative infection rate.

This fluid collection is a superb growth medium for bacteria inoculated during the surgical procedure. Host defense mechanisms and antimicrobial prophylaxis usually prevent development of an abscess in this area, although rarely it does develop despite these measures. The appearance of the abscess is similar to that of pelvic cellulitis or adnexal infection, but symptoms do not develop until 1 or 2 days later and are more central. Bimanual examination reveals a tender mass that can be palpated immediately above the vaginal apex. Parenteral antimicrobial therapy is necessary, and mechanical drainage in a treatment room allows access to material for culture, decreases morbidity, and shortens therapy time.

## PELVIC HEMATOMA

A hematoma may also commonly develop in the space depicted in Figure 18–5, but it is undetected in the

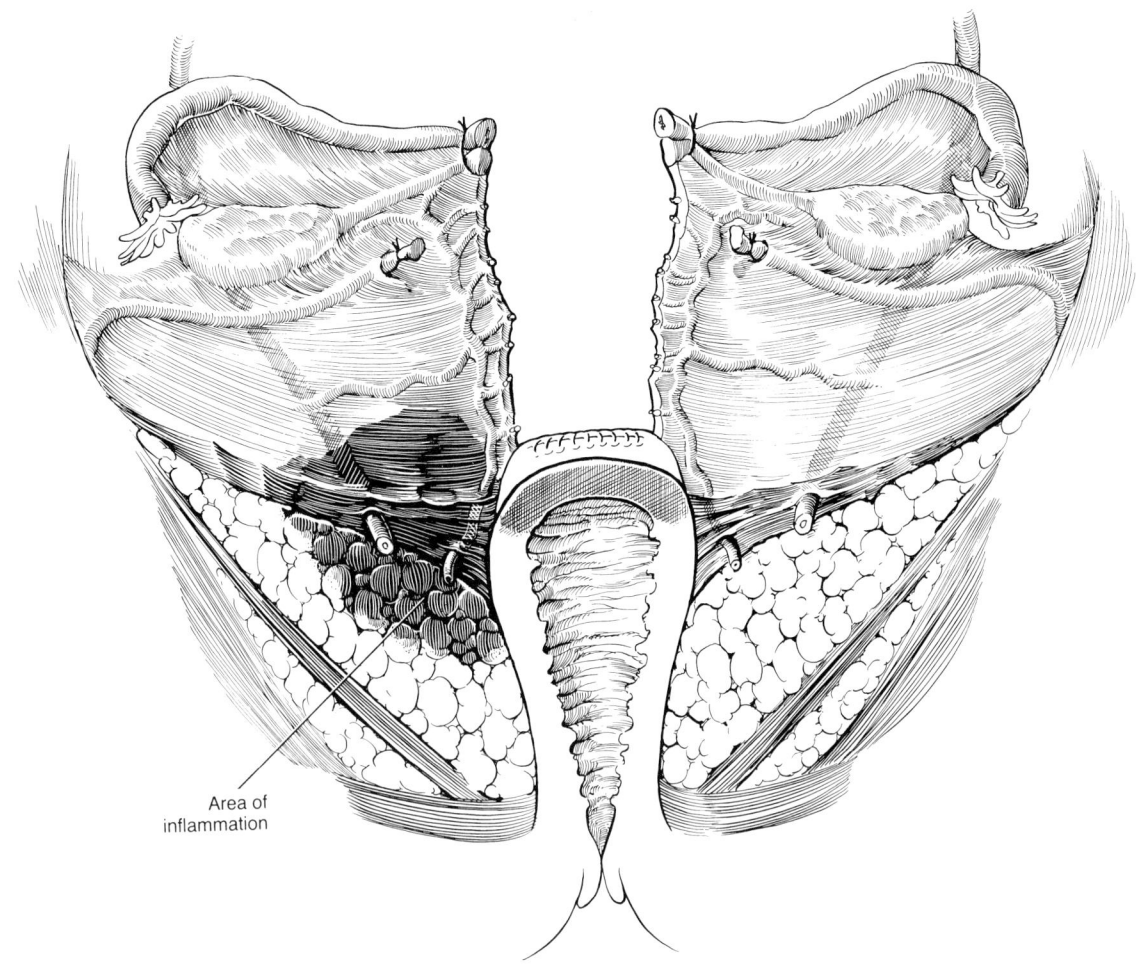

**Figure 18–3** Pelvic cellulitis. Female pelvis after hysterectomy with infection in the right parametrial area. (From Copeland LJ: Textbook of Gynecology. Philadelphia, WB Saunders, 1993, p 565.)

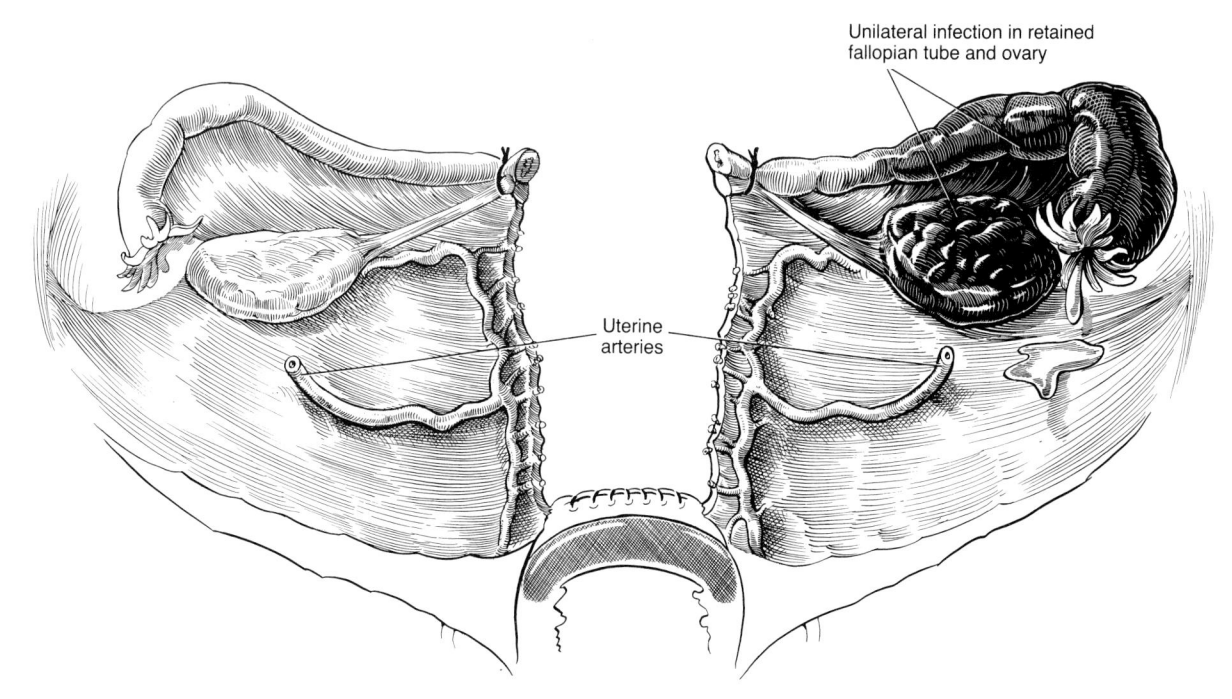

**Figure 18–4** Adnexal infection. Female pelvis following hysterectomy with cellulitis involving the right fallopian tube and ovary. (From Copeland LJ: Textbook of Gynecology. Philadelphia, WB Saunders, 1993, p 566.)

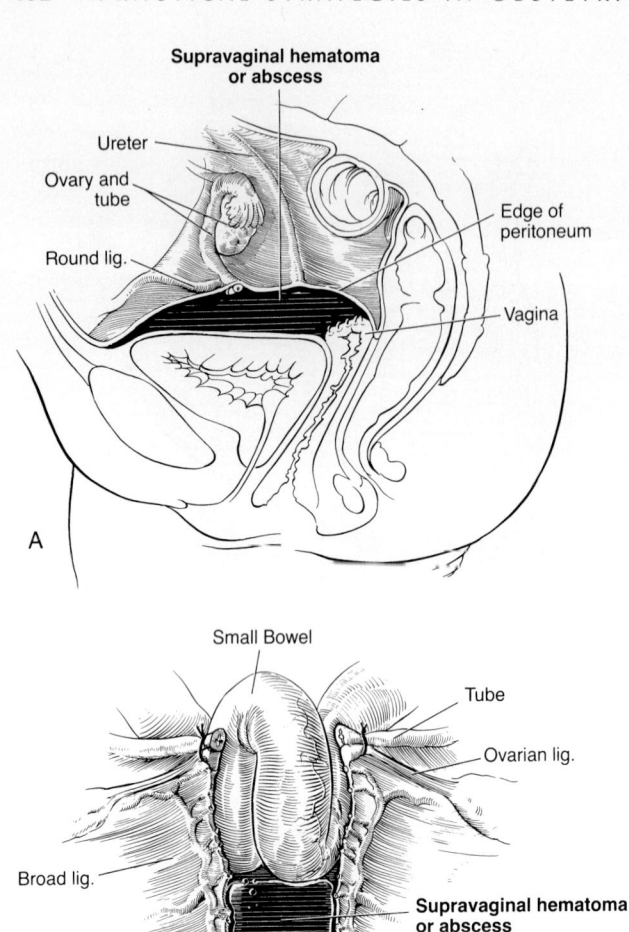

**Figure 18–5** Sagittal view of the female pelvis following hysterectomy with an abscess or hematoma in the extraperitoneal supravaginal space. (From Copeland LJ: Textbook of Gynecology. Philadelphia, WB Saunders, 1993, p 567.)

asymptomatic patient. Infection in such a hematoma is, however, uncommon. Early in the course, patients who have an infected hematoma manifest only a recurring temperature elevation. They have no symptoms and examination of the abdomen and pelvis are normal. The only suggestion of its presence is an unexplained postoperative drop in hemoglobin.

Vaginal probe sonography can identify a hematoma in this space before the structure is able to be palpated. Parenteral antimicrobial therapy should be initiated as soon as it is suspected or confirmed that a patient has an infected hematoma (i.e., before the onset of symptoms but after the development of temperature elevation.) This is one of the few occasions in which an asymptomatic woman with a normal examination should be treated for temperature elevation. If therapy is withheld, symptoms and signs of infection will develop and the therapy will be prolonged.

## FEBRILE MORBIDITY

In early gynecologic literature, febrile morbidity is frequently equated with infection requiring antimicrobial therapy. There are more than 30 different definitions for this nonspecific entity. It is more appropriately defined as recurring temperature elevation in women who have neither symptoms nor signs of infection and whose temperature elevation disappears without antimicrobial therapy. Women who have pelvic infection requiring antimicrobial therapy do have recurring temperature elevation, but it is associated with the development of symptoms and physical findings as described earlier. An elevated temperature is an indication for evaluating the patient. This evaluation should be general in scope and designed to identify an infectious process not only in the operative site but in any other site, or sites. History and physical examination are required, but laboratory testing other than culture is rarely beneficial.

## MICROBIOLOGY

Presented in Table 18–2 are bacteria recovered from a pelvic SSI performed on 192 women who had un-

Table 18–2  Bacteria Recovered From 192 Women With Pelvic Infections After Hysterectomy

| Bacterial Species | Number |
|---|---|
| GRAM-POSITIVE [654] | |
| **Aerobic Bacteria (369)** | |
| *Enterococcus faecalis* | 154 |
| *Staphylococcus epidermidis* | 119 |
| *Streptococcus* spp. | 56 |
| *Staphylococcus aureus* | 28 |
| *Streptococcus agalactiae* | 12 |
| **Anaerobic Bacteria (285)** | |
| *Peptostreptococcus* spp. | 258 |
| *Clostridium* spp. | 27 |
| GRAM-NEGATIVE [601] | |
| **Aerobic Bacteria (233)** | |
| *Escherichia coli* | 130 |
| *Klebsiella* spp. | 32 |
| *Proteus* spp. | 25 |
| *Enterobacter* spp. | 22 |
| *Citrobacter* spp. | 12 |
| Other *Enterobacteriaceae* | 12 |
| **Anaerobic Bacteria (368)** | |
| *Prevotella bivia* | 115 |
| *Bacteroides fragilis* group | 110 |
| *Prevotella* spp. | 60 |
| Other gram-negative rods | 39 |
| *Bacteroides* spp. | 20 |
| *Prevotella disiens* | 16 |
| *Fusobacterium* spp. | 10 |

dergone hysterectomy at Parkland Health and Hospital System. It can be seen that more gram-positive than gram-negative bacteria, and more anaerobic than aerobic bacteria were recovered from these infection sites. A mean of 6.5 species was recovered from these patients. It is impossible to ascertain which of these recovered species are truly pathogens and which are not. For that reason, therapy for patients with these polymicrobial infections is empiric and should provide a broad spectrum of coverage that includes many of the species presented in Table 18–2.

## Infection Treatment Regimens

In Table 18–3, are presented single-agent parenteral therapeutic regimens with documented efficacy in the treatment of women who have postoperative pelvic infections.

### CEPHALOSPORINS

This family of antibiotics is bactericidal and has a broad spectrum of in vitro activity that includes not only aerobic but also many anaerobic bacteria recovered from pelvic infection sites. Cefoxitin and cefotetan have the greatest anaerobic activity, but efficacy of these regimens has not been statistically superior to that observed with third-generation cephalosporins. First-generation cephalosporins are used for prophylaxis and not for treatment of postoperative infection in the United States.

### PENICILLINS

Penicillins are also bactericidal and have as their principal target gram-positive aerobic pathogens. The ureidopenicillins have an expanded spectrum of antibacterial activity with enhanced activity against gram-negative aerobic and anaerobic bacteria. Further spectrum expansion has resulted from the addition of a β-lactamase enzyme inhibitor to several penicillins. Inhibitors block the most frequently observed form of bacterial resistance in isolates recovered from pelvic infection sites (i.e., production of β-lactamase enzyme). The oral agent that has been used most extensively in the treatment of mild to moderate SSI is amoxicillin with sodium clavulanate (Augmentin) at a dose of 500 to 875 mg twice daily, depending on the clinical severity of the infection.

### CARBAPENEMS

This family of bactericidal β-lactam antibiotics has a very broad antibacterial spectrum and provides effi-

Table 18–3  Empiric Intravenous Single-Agent Regimens for Postoperative Pelvic SSI

| Regimen Family and Generic Name | Trade Name | Dose/Interval |
|---|---|---|
| **CEPHALOSPORINS** | | |
| Cefoxitin | Mefoxin | 2 g q6h |
| Cefotetan | Cefotan | 2 g q12h |
| Cefotaxime | Claforan | 1–2 g q8h |
| Cefoperazone | Cefobid | 2 g q12h |
| **UREIDOPENICILLIN** | | |
| Piperacillin | Pipracil | 4 g q6h |
| **CARBAPENEMS** | | |
| Imipenem/cilastatin | Primaxin | 500 mg q6–8h |
| Meropenem | Merrem | 1 g q8h |
| **PENICILLIN PLUS β-LACTAMASE INHIBITOR** | | |
| Ampicillin/sulbactam | Unasyn | 3 g q6h |
| Piperacillin/tazobactam | Zosyn | 3.375 g q6h |
| **QUINOLONE** | | |
| Trovafloxacin | Trovan | 300 mg IV then 200 mg PO q24h |

cacy at low concentrations. These antibiotics are usually reserved for initial regimen failure or for immunocompromised hosts, as is true for the expanded spectrum penicillin/β-lactamase inhibitor combination.

## QUINOLONES

Quinolone antibiotics are bactericidal and were originally used to treat patients who had urinary tract infection because of their activity against enterobacteriaceae. The Food and Drug Administration (FDA) has approved the quinolone trovafloxacin, which has a very broad spectrum and a prolonged half-life (11 hours) that allows once-daily dosing. With experience, it may be possible to initiate treatment of the patient with antimicrobial therapy and convert to oral therapy for home completion. Serum and tissue concentrations are comparable after intravenous (IV) and oral (PO) administration. The oral product is much less expensive.

# Combination Regimens

## CLINDAMYCIN/GENTAMICIN

Clindamycin (Cleocin) is a lincosamide antibiotic with activity against gram-positive aerobic and gram-positive and gram-negative anaerobic species. The standard dose is 900 mg administered IV every 8 hours. PO or IV administration result in comparable tissue and serum concentration. Although increasing clindamycin resistance among anaerobes has been reported for years, possible clinical evidence of that phenomenon in our patients has not become evident until the last several years. Substituting metronidazole for clindamycin results in resolution of the pelvic infection.

Gentamicin (Garamycin) is an aminoglycoside that is also bactericidal. Newer tested regimens include doses of 5 to 7 mg/kg given once daily by IV infusion over 1 hour. There have been no reports in postoperative gynecologic surgery patients who have operative site infection, but there are data in patients treated for acute pelvic inflammatory disease and postpartum metritis, either of which may be more serious for the patient and more difficult to cure than infection after gynecologic surgery.

## METRONIDAZOLE/GENTAMICIN/ AMPICILLIN

Metronidazole (Flagyl) is an antiprotozoal, antianaerobic, bactericidal antibiotic. Serum and tissue concentrations are equivalent after PO or IV administration. Although it is commonly given at an IV dose of 500 mg every 6 hours, the recommended loading dose is 15 mg/kg followed by 7.5 mg/kg every 6 hours for maintenance dosing. It is necessary to add ampicillin, 2 g every 6 hours, to metronidazole/gentamicin to provide gram-positive aerobic bacteria coverage.

# Special Antibiotics

## MONOBACTAM

Aztreonam (Azactam) is a bactericidal antibiotic that is active against most enterobacteriaceae, including *Pseudomonas aeruginosa*. Nephro- and ototoxicity, which are observed with aminoglycosides, are not seen with aztreonam. The standard dose of aztreonam is 1 g IV every 8 hours.

## VANCOMYCIN (VANCOCIN)

This bactericidal antibiotic is the agent of choice for patients who are truly penicillin-allergic and have infections caused by gram-positive aerobic bacteria. Overuse may result in development of vancomycin-resistant enterococci; *Enterococcus faecalis*, one of the most frequent isolates recovered from pelvic infection sites, is being seen in increasing numbers as cephalosporin prophylaxis use increases. A standard dose for vancomycin is 1 g every 12 hours.

## REFERENCES

Ad Hoc Committee of the Committee on Trauma Division, Division of Medical Sciences, National Academy of Sciences, National Research Council: Postoperative wound infections: The influence of ultraviolet irradiation of the operating room and various other factors. Ann Surg 160(suppl):1–81, 1964.

Ali MZ, Goetz MB: A meta-analysis of the relative efficacy and toxicity of single daily dosing versus multiple daily dosing of aminoglycosides. Clin Infect Dis 24:796–809, 1997.

Belliveau PP, Nicolau DP, Nightingale CH, et al: Once-daily gentamicin: Experience in one hundred eighteen patients with post-partum endometritis. J Infect Dis Pharmacother 1:11–18, 1995.

Bhatia NN, Karram MM, Bergman A: Role of antibiotic prophylaxis in retropubic surgery for stress urinary incontinence. Obstet Gynecol 74:637–639, 1989.

Bhattacharya S, Parkin DE, Reid TMS, et al: A prospective randomised study of the effects of prophylactic antibiotics on the incidence of bacteraemia following hysteroscopic surgery. Eur J Obstet Gynaecol Reprod Biol 63:37–40, 1995.

Dellinger EP, Gross PA, Barrett TL, et al: Quality standard for antimicrobial prophylaxis in surgical procedures. Clin Infect Dis 18:422–427, 1994.

Garner JS, Jarvis WR, Emori TG, et al: CDC definitions for nosocomial infections, 1988. Am J Infect Control 16:128–140, 1988.

Garvey JM, Buffenmyer C, Rycheck RR, et al: Surveillance for postoperative infections in outpatient gynecologic surgery. Infect Control 7:54–58, 1986.

Horan TC, Gaynes RP, Martone WJ, et al: CDC definitions of

nosocomial surgical site infections, 1992: A modification of CDC definitions of surgical wound infections. Am J Infect Control 20:271–274, 1992.

Lepine LA, Hillis SA, Marchbanks PA, et al: Hysterectomy surveillance—United States 1980–1993. MMWR 46:1–15, 1997.

Letterie GS, Hibbert M: The role of antibiotic prophylaxis for tubal microsurgery. Arch Gynecol Obstet 253:193–196, 1993.

Mitra AG, Whitten MK, Laurent SL, et al: A randomized, prospective study comparing once-daily gentamicin versus thrice-daily gentamicin in the treatment of puerperal infection. Am J Obstet Gynecol 177:786–792, 1997.

Nicolau DP, Freeman CD, Belliveau PP, et al: Experience with a once-daily aminoglycoside program administered to 2,184 patients. Antimicrob Agents Chemother 39:650–655, 1995.

Pyper RJD, Ahmet Z, Houang ET: Bacteriological contamination during laparoscopy with dye injection. Br J Obstet Gynaecol 95:367–371, 1988.

Sawaya GF, Grady D, Kerlikowske K, et al: Antibiotics at the time of induced abortion: The case for universal prophylaxis based on a meta-analysis. Obstet Gynecol 87:884–890, 1996.

Tulkens PM, Clerckx-Braun F, Donnez J, et al: Safety and efficacy of aminoglycosides once-a-day: Experimental data and randomized, controlled evaluation in patients suffering from pelvic inflammatory disease. J Drug Dev 1(suppl):71–82, 1988.

# OBSTETRICS

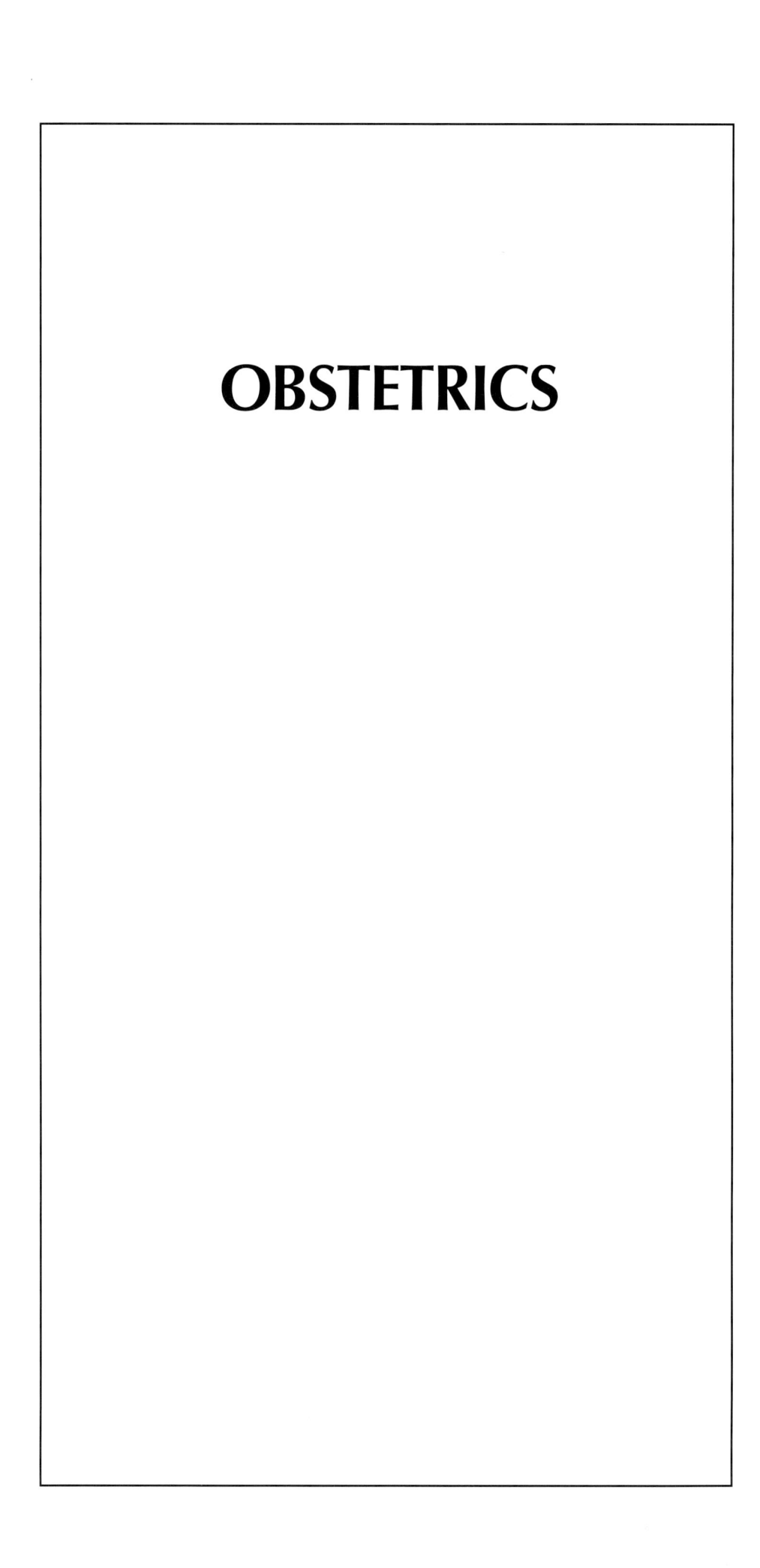

# 19

# Overview of Routine Prenatal Care

MARK W. TOMLINSON

Pregnancy is generally expected to end with a healthy mother delivering a normal infant. However, a variety of either maternal or fetal conditions may interfere, resulting in less than the anticipated outcome. Prenatal care is considered essential if the desired result is to be achieved. Numerous publications have reported a beneficial association between prenatal services and perinatal outcome. Critical review of the relationship between birth outcome and prenatal care has questioned the validity of these conclusions as well as the overall cost-effectiveness of antenatal care. Nevertheless, the present concept of prenatal care is firmly in place, and it will remain so until more definitive research is available to suggest alternative approaches for the care of pregnant women. As such, the relatively short course of gestation mandates planning, dedication, and considerable effort to provide high-quality care. This, combined with the fact that there are nearly 4 million annual births in the United States, makes obvious the public health implications of prenatal care.

## Definition

In 1989, a multidisciplinary expert panel was charged by the Department of Health and Human Services with evaluating the available evidence to determine the efficiency and effectiveness of current practices. The panel began the task by establishing a working definition. Prenatal care was defined as consisting of "... health promotion, risk assessment, and intervention linked to the risks and conditions uncovered. These activities require the cooperative and coordinated efforts of the woman, her family, her prenatal care providers, and other specialized providers. Prenatal care begins when conception is first considered and continues until labor begins. The objectives of prenatal care for the mother, infant, and family relate to outcomes through the first year following birth."

## Frequency and Timing of Prenatal Care

Despite the generally held belief that prenatal care improves pregnancy outcome, the optimal number of visits and the most beneficial content of each encounter are unknown. Traditionally, 14 prenatal visits have been recommended during the first 40 weeks of gestation for low-risk patients. The first visit is scheduled during the first trimester at approximately 8 weeks, with follow-up visits every 4 weeks until 28 weeks, then every 2 weeks until 36 weeks, and then weekly until delivery. Although this is common practice, there is very little evidence to suggest that this regime leads to improved outcomes. In an effort to increase both efficiency and effectiveness, an alternative schedule consisting of fewer visits was recommended by the Expert Panel on Prenatal Care. With this plan, 10 visits are scheduled for the nulliparous low-risk patient and 8 for her parous counterpart (Fig. 19–1). The initial visit is planned preconceptually, within 1 year of a considered pregnancy. After conception for the parous patient, visits occur at 8, 16, 24, 32, 36, 38, and 41 weeks of gestation. Nulliparous patients are also seen at 12 and 40 weeks. Both regimens advocate additional visits as clinical conditions demand. The panel's proposed schedule is attractive because of the potential to decrease resource utilization and cost. Both regimens may require modification for patients identified as high risk. Table 19–1 lists examples of factors that may increase the risk of an adverse maternal or fetal outcome. Patients identified to be at increased risk for adverse pregnancy outcome may require more frequent visits as well as additional education, surveillance, or intervention, depending on the specific risk factor or factors.

Since publication of the recommendations of the Expert Panel on Prenatal Care, reports have compared plans similar to that suggested by the panel with the traditional schedule. No increase in either maternal or fetal adverse outcomes was identified with two or three fewer visits, and patient satisfaction was maintained. The reduced number of visits did not lead to an increase in the use of other medical services. Investigations comparing traditional care with reduced visit frequency in other countries also identified a decrease in resource use without a compromise in outcome. Patient satisfaction, however, was not always maintained.

**Table 19–1** Examples of High-Risk Conditions Increasing the Potential for Adverse Maternal or Fetal Outcome

PRESENT BEFORE PREGNANCY
- Maternal medical complications (e.g., hypertension, diabetes, cardiac disease, renal disease, connective tissue disease)
- Extremes of maternal age (<18 or >35)
- Family history of birth defects, genetic disease, or chromosomal abnormalities
- Extremes of maternal weight (underweight or obese)
- Alcohol, drug, or substance abuse

DEVELOPING DURING PREGNANCY
- Inadequate weight gain
- Excess or inadequate fundal height growth
- Preterm labor
- Vaginal bleeding
- Gestational diabetes
- Pregnancy-induced hypertension
- Postdates
- Decreased fetal movement
- Maternal infectious disease (e.g., pyelonephritis, HIV, syphilis, rubella, genital herpes, varicella, parvovirus, cytomegalovirus, chorioamnionitis)

HIV = human immunodeficiency virus.

## Scope of Prenatal Care

The lack of objective data identifying the optimal number of prenatal visits is compounded by the fact that even less information is available to define the most effective or efficient scope of care. Early and continuing risk assessment is considered a key component of prenatal care despite a lack of definitive data supporting its role. The assessment begins during the first visit with a detailed history, physical examination, and basic laboratory testing. Based on the findings of the initial evaluation, a plan can be established for follow-up and further evaluation, if necessary. Ideally, the first assessment would take place preconceptually. Several standard prenatal forms are commercially available from several sources, including the American College of Obstetricians and Gynecologists (ACOG), Hollister, and Problem Oriented Pregnancy Risk Assessment System (POPRAS). These forms present information in

Expert Panel Recommendations

| Gestational Age (wk) | Traditional Schedule | Nulliparous | Multiparous |
|---|---|---|---|
| Preconceptual |  | ● | ● |
| 8 | ● | ● | ● |
| 12 | ● | ● |  |
| 16 | ● | ● | ● |
| 20 | ● |  |  |
| 24 | ● | ● | ● |
| 28 | ● |  |  |
| 30 | ● |  |  |
| 32 | ● | ● | ● |
| 34 | ● |  |  |
| 36 | ● | ● | ● |
| 37 | ● |  |  |
| 38 | ● | ● | ● |
| 39 | ● |  |  |
| 40 | ● | ● |  |
| 41 | ● | ● | ● |
| Total | 15 | 10 | 8 |

**Figure 19–1** Schedule of prenatal care visits for nulliparous and multiparous women: Comparison of recommendations of The Expert Panel on Prenatal Care with the traditional schedule.

a uniform manner and can help guide the screening process, aid in interpretation, and simplify later review. Standardization may also assist in obtaining more complete data collection.

Since publication of results of the Expert Panel on the Content of Prenatal Care, investigators have begun to question the assumed cause-and-effect relationship between the traditional ritualistic approach to prenatal care and improved maternal and fetal outcomes. Probable reasons for the total lack of success of medical interventions alone is that present risk assessment schemes lack sensitivity in identifying common conditions, such as preterm delivery, preeclampsia, intrauterine growth restriction (IUGR), and shoulder dystocia. Even when an at-risk group is identified, effective preventive measures or treatments are often lacking. In addition, social or inherited risk factors may not be alterable through medical intervention alone. As more objective information becomes available, the manner and methods by which prenatal care is provided can be rationally analyzed and modified.

## History and Physical Examination

Many factors associated with an increased risk for maternal or fetal complications, such as pregnancy-induced hypertension (PIH), medical conditions or communicable diseases, preterm delivery, IUGR, congenital anomalies, and genetic conditions, can be identified during the history and physical examination.

Factors associated with an increased incidence of preeclampsia include nulliparity, extremes of reproductive age, low socioeconomic status, nonwhite race, change in paternity, increased prepregnancy body mass index (BMI), and higher diastolic or systolic blood pressure at the time of examination. Additional risks include preeclampsia during a previous pregnancy, a positive family history of PIH, and underlying chronic hypertension or renal disease. Many of these same factors may be associated with uteroplacental insufficiency leading to IUGR.

Prospective identification of patients at risk for preterm delivery is difficult when the only significantly predictive factor is a history of a previous preterm delivery. Tobacco and substance abuse are also related to both preterm delivery and growth restriction. Past medical or family history, ethnic background, or age may prompt screening for specific genetic conditions or congenital anomalies. Table 19–2 displays conditions and associated risk factors that are amenable to prenatal screening and diagnosis.

**Table 19–2** Examples of Genetic or Fetal Conditions That Can Be Detected Preconceptually and Indications for Testing

| Fetal Condition | Indication for Testing |
| --- | --- |
| Down's syndrome, other trisomies | Maternal age >35, previously affected child, strong family history, abnormal multiple marker screen |
| NTD | Abnormal MS-AFP screen, family history |
| Hemoglobinopathy (sickle cell anemia, thalassemia) | At-risk ethnic groups |
| Tay-Sachs disease | Jewish descent |
| Inherited conditions (e.g., hemophilia, cystic fibrosis, muscular dystrophy, fragile X syndrome, skeletal dysplasias, Huntington's disease) | Family history |

MS-AFP = maternal serum alpha-fetoprotein; NTD = neural tube defect.

## Standard Laboratory Evaluation

When prenatal care is initiated, several laboratory tests are routinely performed for screening or general health maintenance, along with the history and physical examination. These include blood type, Rhesus (Rh) factor, antibody screen, hemoglobin and hematocrit values, rubella titer, the two syphilis screens either Venereal Disease Research Laboratory (VDRL) or rapid plasma reagin (RPR), hepatitis B surface antigen (HBsAg) level, human immunodeficiency virus (HIV) antibody, and urine culture. Cervical samples can be obtained for gonorrhea and *Chlamydia* DNA probe or culture. When indicated, tuberculosis should be screened for with the PPD (purified protein derivative) skin test (Table 19–3). An annual Papanicolaou smear should also be performed. Tests that should be ordered in patients who have genetic susceptibility include Tay-Sachs screening and hemoglobin electrophoresis. Although hemoglobin solubility tests, such as the Sickledex, are commonly used to screen for hemoglobinopathy, they can miss

**Table 19–3** Patient Risk Factors Requiring Skin Test Screening for Tuberculosis

Low socioeconomic status
Immigrants from high-prevalence countries
Close contact with a known infectious case
HIV-infected patients
Medical diseases that increase the risk of tuberculosis
Alcoholics and substance abusers

HIV = human immunodeficiency virus.

several clinically important hemoglobin abnormalities and are considered inadequate for assessing genetic risks. Additional evaluations, such as an ultrasonographic examination, multiple marker screen, karyotype analysis, diabetes screening, and group B streptococcal culture may be obtained at specified times throughout pregnancy, as indicated. Still other tests, such as antibody screen, hemoglobin and hematocrit levels, diabetes screen, VDRL/RPR, gonorrhea and *Chlamydia* specimens may need to be repeated, depending on patient risk. Table 19–4 outlines a schedule for obtaining the various prenatal laboratory tests.

Blood type, Rh factor, and antibody screen are obtained to identify patients at risk for erythroblastosis fetalis. If the antibody screen is positive for anti-D or atypical antibodies, further evaluation can be carried out to identify the fetus at risk for complications. Those fetuses found to be at risk can then be referred for appropriate therapy. Patients who have a negative antibody screen in early gestation may become sensitized during pregnancy, particularly during the third trimester. To screen for and subsequently prevent antepartum Rh sensitization, a repeat antibody screen is obtained at 28 weeks of gestation in Rh-negative women. If the screen is negative for antigen D, Rh immune globulin is given. This regimen has been shown to reduce the incidence of Rh sensitization from 3.4:1000 Rh-negative births to 2.2:1000 Rh-negative births with postpartum administration alone. Antibodies other than anti-D (atypical antibodies) can also cause erythroblastosis fetalis. The relative importance of atypical antibodies has increased, whereas the incidence of Rh disease has decreased since Rh immune globulin became available during the 1960s. The incidence of sensitization to atypical antibodies during pregnancy is approximately 1.3:1000 births, with more than half occurring after 28 weeks of gestation. Because of this, a repeat antibody screen in Rh-positive women obtained between 34 and 36 weeks has been suggested to identify these patients.

Hemoglobin and hematocrit values are determined at the initial visit. Severe anemia has been associated with low birth weight and preterm delivery. Although nearly all causes of anemia are encountered during pregnancy, iron deficiency is the most common etiology. Despite its frequency, routine iron supplementation has not been shown to be of value. In patients who have hemoglobinopathy, such as thalassemia or sickle cell disease, it may even lead to iron overload. Thus, screening allows timely identification of anemia and initiation of an appropriate diagnostic evaluation. Hemoglobin electrophoresis should be obtained in patients at risk (Table 19–5) for hemoglobinopathy or in the presence of significant anemia. If a carrier of a hemoglobinopathy or the disease state itself is identi-

**Table 19–4** Timing of Prenatal Laboratory Screening

| Laboratory Screening Test | Gestational Age at Prenatal Visit (Testing Range in wk) |  |  |  |  |
|---|---|---|---|---|---|
|  | Initial/Preconceptual Visit | 12 | 16 | 28 | 36 |
| Blood type | • |  |  |  |  |
| Antibody screen | • |  |  | •† |  |
| Hemoglobin | • |  |  | • |  |
| Rubella titer | • |  |  |  |  |
| HBsAg | • |  |  |  |  |
| VDRL (RPR) | • |  |  |  | • |
| HIV | • |  |  |  |  |
| Urine culture | • |  |  |  |  |
| Papanicolaou smear | • |  |  |  |  |
| MS-AFP/multiple marker screen |  |  | • (15–20) |  |  |
| Diabetes screen (1 hr glucola) | •‡ |  |  | • (24–28) |  |
| Group B Streptococcus screen* |  |  |  |  | • (35–37) |
| Gonorrhea* | • |  |  |  | • |
| *Chlamydia** | • |  |  |  | • |
| PPD* | • |  |  |  |  |
| Hgb electrophoresis* | • |  |  |  |  |
| Tay-Sachs disease* | • |  |  |  |  |
| Karyotype*§ |  | • (10–14) | • (14–22) |  |  |

*Optional tests as indicated.
†Rh-negative patients.
‡Patients who have risk factors
§Chorionic villus sampling (CVS) at 10–14 weeks or amniocentesis at 14–22 wk
HBsAG = hepatitis B surface antigen; Hgb = hemoglobin; HIV = human immunodeficiency virus; MS-AFP = maternal serum alpha-fetoprotein; PPD = purified protein derivative; VDRL (RPR) = Venereal Disease Research Laboratories/rapid plasma reagin (test).

Table 19-5  Hemoglobinopathies and Populations at Risk

| Hemoglobinopathy | At-Risk Groups |
| --- | --- |
| Sickle cell anemia | African |
| β-Thalassemia | Mediterranean, North African, Indian, Southeast Asian |
| α-Thalassemia | Asian |
| Hemoglobin C | African, Mediterranean |

fied, genetic counseling should be provided. Fetal diagnosis is available for many hereditary forms of anemia, if desired. If nutritional deficiency is identified, it can be treated with appropriate supplementation of iron, folate, or other vitamins, as indicated.

Congenital rubella infection is a rare but potentially devastating condition. Because the infection is preventable with immunization strategies that provide population protection, the Healthy People 2000 initiative has set as one of its goals the elimination of rubella and congenital rubella syndrome by the year 2000. Screening for rubella immunity with an immunoglobulin G (IgG) antibody titer identifies susceptible women and allows either preconceptual or postpartum vaccination. Rubella vaccine is a live attenuated virus that is contraindicated during pregnancy because of theoretical concerns about fetal infection. It is important to note, however, that no adverse fetal effects have been identified when accidental vaccination has occurred during early gestation. Hepatitis B viral infection is common and represents a major public health concern. Although perinatal cases make up a small percentage of all hepatitis B infections, 70 to 90% become chronic. Because of the severity of the perinatal disease and the failure of selective screening based on risk factors to identify many seropositive individuals, universal screening of all pregnant women has been recommended since 1988. In 1991, routine vaccination of all newborns was added to the recommendation. Susceptible women at risk for hepatitis B infection may be safely vaccinated during pregnancy.

With the recent approval of an effective varicella vaccine, consideration should be given to screening for this viral infection as well. Although varicella screening has not been routinely incorporated into standard prenatal care, potential maternal and fetal complications make pregnancy a particularly risky time to become infected. Primary varicella infection in adults is associated with significantly more morbidity and mortality than infection during childhood. There is also a suggestion that pregnant women may be at greater risk for complications than nonpregnant adults. In addition, maternal infection during the first 20 weeks of gestation can result in the congenital varicella syndrome in 2% of cases. Peripartum infection can also lead to severe neonatal infection. Although no consensus protocol has been put forth to date, a reasonable approach would be to screen by history. Patients who confirm a past infection can be reliably assumed to be immune. Those who have a negative history are found to be immune in more than 80% of cases. These patients may have susceptibility confirmed by measuring a varicella titer before vaccination, or they may simply be vaccinated in the postpartum period. In adults, the initial dose is followed by a second dose after 1 month. As with rubella, the vaccine for varicella is a live attenuated vaccine that should not be given during pregnancy. Susceptible patients exposed to varicella during pregnancy should be considered for vaccination with varicella immune globulin (VZIG) within 96 hours of exposure. This may result in reduction of maternal complications.

Syphilis is a reportable sexually transmitted disease with potential long-term devastating consequences for mother and fetus. Although treatment of patients who have early infection is effective, syphilis is often asymptomatic and undiagnosed during the initial stages. Routine screening should be performed using nontreponemal antibody tests, such as RPR or VDRL. A positive screen should be confirmed with fluorescent treponemal antibody absorption test (FTA-ABS) to exclude false-positive results caused by inflammatory conditions resulting from intravenous drug abuse or connective tissue disease. In patients at risk, a repeat screen in the third trimester may be prudent to exclude an infection occurring during pregnancy or to identify the rare individual who has a very early primary infection not detected at the initial screening.

Prenatal screening of women for HIV is complicated by both social and privacy issues. Despite the concerns, routine screening of all patients at the start of prenatal care is recommended. Several potential benefits may be realized through such a strategy. More infected patients are likely to be identified, because attempts to screen based on risk factors alone failed to identify nearly half of those who were infected. Transmission from mother to fetus can be reduced by roughly 65% from a baseline rate of 25% with zidovudine treatment. In addition, women who are found to be infected with HIV may begin obtaining comprehensive care at an earlier stage of disease than they otherwise would. Women whose test is negative may benefit from counseling aimed at changing behaviors associated with an increased risk of seroconversion. (See Chapter 40 on HIV Infection in Pregnancy.)

Screening and treatment for patients who have asymptomatic bacteriuria has been shown to decrease the incidence of pyelonephritis. The cost-effectiveness of this practice has been questioned, however.

The presence of asymptomatic bacteriuria has also been associated with increases in the incidence of preterm delivery and low birth weight. Identification and treatment of asymptomatic bacteriuria have been found to reduce the occurrence of these complications.

Maternal genital infections, such as gonorrhea and *Chlamydia*, can lead to neonatal infections. Cervical culture or antibody screens for these organisms allow identification and treatment as a means of preventing associated complications. Screening for tuberculosis should be obtained in high-risk (see Table 19–3) and symptomatic patients. Treatment of patients who have active disease can be started safely during pregnancy. In recent conversions of previously negative test to positive test, prophylactic isoniazid therapy should also be initiated during pregnancy. In patients who have a positive screening test for tuberculosis, no history suggestive of recent exposure, and a negative chest radiograph, prophylactic therapy may be postponed until after delivery.

# Prenatal Care Visits

Prenatal care visits after the initial history and physical examination and laboratory screening have been completed, provide the opportunity for continued assessment of maternal and fetal well-being. Several activities are routinely repeated during subsequent visits. Because many activities are dependent on gestational age, not all are performed at every visit. As with other components of prenatal care, there is limited objective evidence to support the value of many of these activities in improving maternal-fetal outcome in low-risk populations.

The gestational age at each prenatal visit should be routinely recorded and fetal well-being is assessed by confirming maternally perceived fetal movements and hearing fetal heart tones. Heart tones can initially be auscultated using Doppler instruments between 10 and 12 weeks of gestation and by the DeLee fetoscope between 18 and 20 weeks. In addition to documenting fetal viability, both of these techniques can be used as adjunctive criteria for confirming gestational age. Fetal movement is usually first appreciated near 18 weeks of gestation. There is considerable individual variation, however, with parous patients tending to feel movement earlier than nulliparous patients. During the third trimester, quantitative assessment of fetal movement may serve as a sensitive but nonspecific tool for fetal surveillance.

Fundal height measurement can serve as a screen for fetal growth abnormalities, polyhydramnios, and multiple gestation. Routine measurement should begin at 20 weeks of gestation. The fundus is typically felt at the umbilicus at this time. After 20 weeks, the fundal height should measure approximately 1 cm for each week of gestation. A discrepancy of ±3 cm in comparison with the gestational age should prompt referral for ultrasonographic examination and antenatal testing, if necessary. A difference of 3 cm larger than expected for the date is associated with a large for gestational age fetus, polyhydramnios, or multiple gestation; likewise, a fundal height 3 cm smaller than expected for the date can be seen with IUGR or oligohydramnios. Available evidence suggests fundal height screening achieves a relatively good specificity and moderate sensitivity in detecting the aforementioned conditions. Fetal presentation should be routinely ascertained beginning at 35 to 36 weeks or earlier if preterm labor or premature rupture of membranes is encountered. Before this time, fetal presentation frequently changes and is often nonvertex. Knowledge of a nonvertex presentation after 35 weeks, or when preterm delivery is anticipated, is helpful for several reasons:

1. A patient at risk for cord prolapse can be identified.
2. The mode of delivery can be planned.
3. External cephalic version can be attempted, if appropriate.

In the latter portion of the second trimester, the presence or absence of symptoms of preterm labor should be elicited. These include not only contractions but also menstrual-like cramps, low back pain, pelvic pressure, and increased vaginal discharge. Because many of these symptoms are commonly encountered during uncomplicated gestations, a cervical examination should be considered. Although not practical on a routine basis, ultrasonographic evaluation of the cervix has been suggested as a better predictor of preterm birth than digitally determined cervical dilatation.

Blood pressure, edema, urine protein, and weight gain are all monitored to screen for preeclampsia. Unfortunately, in a low-risk population, none of these measures is particularly sensitive for predicting preeclampsia. Although nulliparous patients who have early blood pressure elevation are at increased risk for preeclampsia, there is tremendous overlap with uncomplicated pregnancies. Edema, particularly dependent, is frequent in normal gestation because of a decrease in colloid osmotic pressure coupled with an increase in hydrostatic pressure. Although it is routinely obtained, dipstick measurement of urine protein in the absence of other risk factors or clinical signs has not been found to be a useful screen. Similarly, poor sensitivity and specificity are observed when rapid maternal weight gain is encountered. Routine weight measurement may be useful as an indicator of ongoing maternal nutrition, however. Maternal weight gain during gestation has been related to neonatal birth weight. Table 19–6 displays recommended weight gain based on prepregnancy BMI. Although not related to pre-eclampsia, urine glucose level is often routinely checked. The correlation between urine and blood glucose during pregnancy is poor, but in early pregnancy the presence of glucosuria can prompt earlier screening and diagnosis of gestational diabetes. After 24 to 28 weeks of gestation, when routine diabetes screening is performed, there is no clinical benefit in performing urine glucose monitoring.

## Additional Screening Evaluations

During scheduled prenatal care visits, additional testing may be indicated to screen for other potentially complicating conditions. These tests include ultrasonographic examination, genetic testing, multiple marker screen or alpha-fetoprotein, diabetes screen, and group B Streptococcus culture. How to make the most effective use of these screening procedures is often debated. This is particularly true of ultrasonography. There is no question that the availability of this testing modality has revolutionized obstetrics. It allows noninvasive access to the fetus and as such is invaluable for evaluation of a number of clinical situations (Table 19–7). However, the benefit of routine ultrasonography is controversial. In the Helsinki Ultrasound trial, a lower perinatal mortality rate was found as a result of increased detection of major malformations, which in turn led to elective pregnancy termination. On the other hand, the Routine Antenatal Diagnostic Imaging With Ultrasound (RADIUS) trial, a large randomized study involving 15,530 women, could identify "...no clinically significant benefit" with the use of routine screening ultrasonography in a low-risk population. Between the experimental group (who received routine ultrasonographic testing) and the control group (who did not receive such testing) no difference in perinatal outcome was observed in pregnancies that were complicated by postdates, multiple gestation, or small-

**Table 19–6** Recommended Gestational Weight Gain Based on Prepregnancy BMI

| BMI Category | Prepregnancy BMI (kg/m²) | Recommended Weight Gain (lb) |
| --- | --- | --- |
| Low | <19.8 | 28–40 |
| Average | 19.8–26.0 | 25–35 |
| High | 26.1–29.0 | 15–25 |
| Obese | >29.0 | <15 |

BMI = body mass index.

**Table 19–7** Indications for Obstetric Ultrasonography

**Indication**

Establish or confirm gestational age
Confirm fetal viability
Pelvic mass
Abnormal MS-AFP
History of previous fetal anomaly
Size-date discrepancy
Preterm labor or premature rupture of membranes
Third-trimester localization of the placenta when placenta previa was previously identified
Vaginal bleeding of unknown etiology
Evaluation of fetal growth in pregnancies at risk for IUGR
Antenatal fetal testing (biophysical profile)

IUGR = intrauterine growth restriction; MS-AFP = maternal serum alpha-fetoprotein.

for-gestational age infant. The outcome variables of the RADIUS study were preterm delivery rate, birth-weight distributions, induced abortion rates, total hospital stay, performance of amniocentesis, antenatal testing, external cephalic version, induction of labor, and cesarean section. One of the disappointing findings of the study was the unexpectedly low rate of detection of anomalies. In part, this appeared to be related to the levels of skill and experience of those performing and interpreting the examinations. It is also important to understand that if routine ultrasonography were not performed, the majority of pregnant women would still require clinically indicated ultrasonography. Sixty-one percent of the women screened for the trial were ineligible for participation because of the presence of additional clinical situations indicating the need for ultrasonographic examination. Of patients randomized to the control group (routine ultrasonography not performed), 45% required at least one examination during pregnancy.

The option for genetic testing of the fetus should be made available following the initial history-taking and parental laboratory screening when established risk factors are identified. Fetal karyotype determination is indicated in the presence of an increased risk for Down's syndrome or other chromosomal abnormality. Testing was originally limited to women who were of advanced maternal age, typically defined as older than 35 years of age, or mothers who had a previously affected child. The knowledge that differences exist between normal fetuses and those with Down's syndrome in multiple biochemical markers present in the maternal serum has allowed screening to include all pregnant women regardless of age or past history. Markers used in clinical practice today include maternal MS-AFP and human chorionic gonadotropin (hCG), with the addition of estriol in some protocols. The risk of Down's syndrome is increased with a pattern of decreased MS-AFP, de-

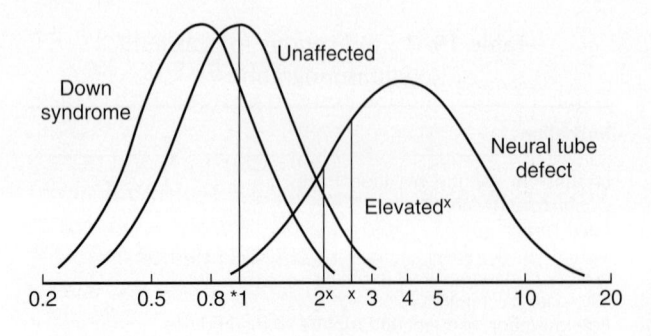

**Figure 19–2** Relative distribution of maternal serum α-fetoprotein (MS-AFP) values in fetuses with neural tube defects and Down syndrome compared with unaffected fetuses at the time of midtrimester screening.

creased serum estriol, and elevated serum hCG between 15 and 20 weeks of gestation. Several other potential serum markers are presently being investigated to improve sensitivity or allow earlier detection.

The primary diagnostic techniques used to obtain specimens for genetic testing are amniocentesis and chorionic villus sampling (CVS). The main practical difference between these two procedures is the gestational age at which they are performed. CVS obtains chorionic villi by either the transvaginal or the transabdominal route between 9 and 13 weeks of gestation, whereas amniocentesis is usually performed after 14 completed weeks of gestation. An additional advantage of amniocentesis is the ability to measure amniotic fluid AFP, which is used to aid in the diagnosis of neural tube defects (NTDs) (Fig. 19–2). These same procedures can also be used to obtain specimens for DNA or other biochemical testing for prenatal diagnosis of a number of other genetic conditions. The number of diseases amenable to prenatal diagnosis is rapidly increasing, and identification of a pregnancy at risk for an inheritable condition should prompt referral to a genetic counselor with access to up-to-date information on the availability of prenatal diagnosis. Helix is a national database that also provides such information. It can be accessed by telephone at (206) 527-5742 or via the Internet at www.genetests.org.

MS-AFP is also used as a screen for detecting NTDs. Alpha-fetoprotein is synthesized initially in the yolk sac and later in the fetal gastrointestinal (GI) tract and liver. It is excreted into the amniotic fluid in the fetal urine. Small amounts traverse the placenta and can be measured in maternal serum. Concentrations of alpha-fetoprotein in the maternal, fetal, and amniotic compartments are dependent on gestational age. The membrane covering the neural tube is permeable to alpha-fetoprotein, thus increasing the amniotic fluid concentration and subsequently the MS-AFP concentration in cases of neural tube defects. Levels exceeding 2.0 to 2.5 multiples of the median (MOM) are considered elevated.

A number of other conditions can result in elevated MS-AFP levels (Table 19–8). The most common explanation is assignment of incorrect gestational age. Several different mechanisms lead to elevated levels in other abnormalities. The amniotic fluid concentration can be increased by increased renal loss, such as occurs in congenital nephrosis, decreased by removal caused by GI tract obstruction, or increased by leakage through nonepithelialized surfaces in abdominal wall defects. Rising amniotic fluid levels lead to higher levels in the maternal serum by way of an increased concentration gradient. With normal amniotic fluid levels, elevated maternal serum levels are likely caused by increased placental permeability. In this situation, no fetal abnormality is identified and the MS-AFP elevation is termed unexplained. With unexplained elevations in MS-AFP levels, there is a greater risk of IUGR, preterm labor, and stillbirth, presumably related to an abnormality in placentation.

Screening for gestational diabetes mellitus (GDM) is also an integral part of prenatal care risk assessment. The condition affects approximately 3% of pregnancies and is associated with a greater incidence of macrosomia, cesarean delivery, birth trauma, and neonatal metabolic disturbances. Screening can be

**Table 19–8** Conditions Associated With Elevated MS-AFP

| Clinical Condition |
|---|
| Incorrect dating |
| Unexplained elevation |
| NTD |
| Abdominal wall defect |
| Multiple gestation |
| Renal agenesis |
| Congenital nephrosis |
| GI obstruction (e.g., congenital diaphragmatic hernia, esophageal/duodenal atresia) |
| Sacrococcygeal teratoma |
| Fetal demise |
| Oligohydramnios |
| Placental tumors |
| Fetomaternal hemorrhage |
| Maternal ovarian or liver tumor |

based on either historical risk factors or universal serum screening. Factors associated with an increased risk of GDM include maternal age older than 25 years, obesity, family history, previous stillbirth, macrosomia, and congenital anomalies. The incidence of GDM increases with advancing gestational age. With selective screening, patients are evaluated based on identified risk factors alone. Testing is typically performed early in gestation and repeated as clinically indicated. If universal screening is performed, high-risk patients are also tested early in pregnancy and again at 24 to 28 weeks of gestation. All low-risk women are also tested at this time. Screening for GDM is considered positive if after a standardized 50-g oral glucose load, serum glucose exceeds the range of 135 to 140 mg/dl. Positive screens are followed by a 3-hour glucose tolerance test (GTT) for the diagnosis of gestational diabetes as discussed in Chapter 35. Normal results for the 3-hour GTT are most commonly defined as a fasting level of <105 mg/dl, a 1-hour level of <190 mg/dl, a 2-hour level of <165 mg/dl, and a 3-hour level of <145 mg/dl. GDM is present when two abnormal values are identified.

Group B streptococcus (GBS) screening is a relatively recent addition to routine antepartum and intrapartum care. The known association between significant neonatal mortality and serious morbidity has focused considerable attention on identifying and implementing more effective management strategies. Present schemes are based on selective chemoprophylaxis of high-risk mothers during labor, or universal screening with treatment available to all patients who are found to have a positive screening culture. Management options will probably evolve further as additional tools, such as reliable rapid antigen tests and vaccines, become available in the future.

Several epidemiologic facts must be considered when approaching the problem of preventing neonatal GBS sepsis. The bacteria are known to colonize the vagina in 15 to 30% of patients. Neonatal disease occurs in 1 to 3:1000 overall births. The risk of neonatal infection is considerably higher in infants born to mothers who have prolonged rupture of membranes, fever, or chorioamnionitis, and to infants born preterm. Prophylactic treatment of colonized patients with penicillin during labor can significantly reduce the number of infants who develop GBS sepsis. Antibiotic use earlier in pregnancy can effectively eliminate vaginal colonization at the time of treatment; however, the GI tract serves as a reservoir, and recolonization frequently occurs. Based on this information, the Centers for Disease Control have published guidelines outlining two acceptable approaches for the prevention of neonatal GBS sepsis. The first involves a combined routine vaginal and rectal culture obtained between 35 and 37 weeks and incubated in a selective culture medium (Todd-Hewitt broth). Patients who are at high risk for neonatal infection with a positive culture receive intrapartum chemoprophylaxis. Although treatment is not mandatory in low-risk patients who are found to have GBS colonization during universal screening, antibiotic prophylaxis should be discussed and offered to these patients as well. Patients who demonstrate risk factors and who are likely to deliver before culture results are available should also receive chemoprophylaxis. The second alternative treatment is based on risk factors alone and avoids routine culture. At present, clinical data are not yet available to indicate that one regimen is superior to the other.

## Patient Education and Counseling

The importance of health promotion through patient counseling and education as components of prenatal care was stressed in the report by the expert panel on the content of prenatal care. As with other aspects of prenatal care, these activities would ideally begin during a preconceptual visit. Information on contraception, safe sex, and family planning are provided. The value of early prenatal care is also emphasized. Nutritional counseling, including the use of preconceptual folate supplementation (0.4 mg daily) should be provided. All patients should be introduced to or reminded of the adverse effects of tobacco, alcohol, and substance use and abuse. Because during pregnancy many women are motivated to change undesirable behaviors to prevent fetal harm, smoking cessation and alcohol or drug treatment programs may be more successful at this time. Screening for at-risk patients is thus important. An example of a simple screen for problem alcohol use is the Tolerance, Annoyed, Cutdown, Eye Opener (T-ACE) questionnaire. It consists of four questions (Table 19–9) and has been found to be more sensitive to identifying patients with increased alcohol use than a routine history. The possi-

**Table 19–9** T-ACE Questionnaire for Alcohol Screening

How many drinks does it take to make you feel high?

Have people annoyed you by criticizing your drinking?

Have you felt you ought to cut down on your drinking?

Have you ever had a drink first thing in the morning to steady your nerves or get rid of a hangover?

The response of "3 or more drinks" to the first question, or a positive response to 2 of the other 3 questions, indicates a positive screen, indicating that the patient requires further evaluation for risk drinking.
T-ACE = Tolerance Annoyed Cutdown Eye Opener

bility of domestic violence should be routinely explored. If the patient is not seen before pregnancy, counseling and education should be introduced at the first prenatal care visit.

At the first prenatal visit, additional topics to be addressed include an outline of the timing and content of prenatal visits, physiologic and emotional changes occurring during pregnancy, exercise, and fetal growth and development. At subsequent visits, relevant issues already discussed should be reviewed and reinforced. Maternal seatbelt use is encouraged. Beginning in the second trimester, preterm labor signs and symptoms are explained. In the third trimester, childbirth and parenting classes should be made available. Near term, labor precautions need to be reviewed. The trend toward shorter postpartum hospital stays increases the importance of providing information relating to postpartum issues, such as neonatal circumcision and infant car seat safety. Education on breast-feeding is also very important, with the Healthy People 2000 initiative calling for significant increases in the number of women who breast-feed. Breast milk supplies not only a balance of nutrients but also growth factors, enzymes, hormones, and immunoglobulins. Despite the importance placed on health education and counseling by the expert panel in 1989, these activities have yet to be routinely incorporated into many prenatal care settings. As with other aspects of prenatal care, the benefit provided by the additional counseling and education in relation to maternal and fetal outcome has been questioned.

In addition to the educational issues outlined above, patients are often curious about the impact and safety of everyday activities on pregnancy outcome. In patients at low risk for preterm delivery, most work and exercise programs can be continued at pre-pregnancy levels with little risk of preterm delivery or low birth weight. Jobs that require standing for more than 8 hours per day may be an exception, with a modest increase in the rate of preterm delivery. High-impact activities and initiation of a new, strenuous exercise program should, however, be postponed until after the postpartum period. Care should also be taken to avoid falls because the growing fundus alters balance. Sexual intercourse can be continued with little concern in patients at low risk for preterm delivery.

Physiologic changes associated with pregnancy result in several common clinical symptoms. Discussion of these conditions in advance allows the patient to anticipate them and may reduce anxiety. Nausea and vomiting are very frequent in the first trimester. The problem typically resolves early in the second trimester and usually requires little more than reassurance. In the second trimester, sharp, fleeting pains in the lower abdomen are common and often are attributed to stretching of the round ligaments. Changing position frequently relieves the discomfort, and as the uterus grows and becomes less mobile, the pains disappear. Constipation, acid reflux, and heartburn are common GI complaints accompanying smooth muscle relaxation, which can be treated symptomatically as necessary. The growth of the uterus leads to increased urinary frequency and can result in supine hypotension. Although no treatment is necessary for frequency of urination in the absence of a urinary tract infection, the patient should avoid lying on her back later in pregnancy.

# Preconceptual Care

Initiation of prenatal care prior to conception was emphasized by the expert panel document on the content of prenatal care and has been mentioned throughout this chapter. Several maternal and fetal benefits could potentially be realized by routinely beginning care before pregnancy. The comprehensive history and physical examination typically performed at the initial prenatal visit could be performed during this encounter. Many of the routine laboratory tests could also be obtained. The patient education and counseling outlined previously could also begin at this time, with the hope of a meaningful reduction in modifiable risk factors, such as poor nutrition and use or abuse of tobacco, alcohol, and substances.

Patients who have medical conditions can be identified and counseled concerning both the effects of their disease on pregnancy and the effect of pregnancy on the disease itself. Medical management may be optimized before conception to minimize adverse pregnancy outcome, or, in extreme situations, even discourage pregnancy. There are several well-documented situations in which such an approach is beneficial. With improved preconceptual control of diabetes, the fetal anomaly rate is reduced. Because many vital organ systems are already developing when the menstrual period is missed, efforts to improve control in the early first trimester are too late. In cases of maternal epilepsy, optimizing the anticonvulsant regime, if possible, can also decrease the risk of anomalies. Switching from warfarin to heparin preconceptually or in early pregnancy in conditions requiring chronic anticoagulation can reduce the increased incidence of spontaneous abortion as well as fetal anomalies attributed to warfarin. Connective tissue disease, chronic hypertension, chronic renal disease, and cardiac disease are other medical conditions in which maternal and fetal outcomes may be improved by optimizing the maternal condition before conception. Pregnancy should be avoided in disease states in which poor maternal health cannot be materially improved, such as severe pulmonary fibrosis in scleroderma, primary pulmonary hypertension, or congestive heart failure.

Persons who have a family history of an inheritable genetic disease can be screened before conception and informed of the risk of passing on the condition to their offspring. A few examples of diseases for which parent carrier status can be screened include cystic fibrosis, sickle cell disease, Tay-Sachs disease, hemophilia, and fragile X syndrome. The incidence of recurrent NTDs can be reduced by high-dose folic acid supplementation (4.0 mg/d), but this must be started preconceptually to be effective. The incidence of NTDs also appears to be decreased with lower doses of folic acid (0.4 mg/d) initiated before pregnancy in the general population.

Maternal health should be optimized preconceptually. Anemia can be identified, its etiology can be determined, and appropriate treatment can be instituted. Abnormal Papanicolaou smears can be properly evaluated and treated without the typical delay associated with pregnancy. Patients who are not immune to rubella or varicella can be identified and vaccinated before pregnancy, thereby eliminating any risk to the fetus. Individuals infected with—or at risk of acquiring—sexually transmitted diseases can be identified, treatment can be given, and counseling about safe sex practices can be provided.

Despite the advantages of preconceptual initiation of prenatal care, only a small percentage of patients actually take advantage of the opportunity. Several factors probably contribute to lack of utilization. Many pregnancies are unplanned. Both patients and physicians may be unaware of the availability and potential benefits of prepregnancy evaluation and counseling. Improved family planning strategies, wider dissemination of the recommendations of the expert panel on the content of prenatal care, and public education are necessary before significant increases in the number of patients receiving preconceptual care are seen.

## Access and Use of Prenatal Care

Even with effective and efficient prenatal care, the ultimate goal of optimal maternal and neonatal outcome cannot be realized without improved utilization. Over the past decade, several states have attempted to decrease financial barriers by significantly increasing the number of women eligible for Medicaid or other publicly funded prenatal care programs. In addition, presumptive eligibility programs (plans whereby patients are able to begin care while applications are being processed) have been instituted in several states. Despite greater access, only modest increases have been noted in the rates of those receiving care, with no improvement in rates of early initiation of care. Other factors that limit use of prenatal care services include fear of the health-care system, lack of understanding that care is of value, or belief that prenatal care is not important. In addition, difficulty in arranging appointments, lack of transportation, weather, illness, fatigue, and simple inconvenience also contribute to failure to obtain adequate prenatal care. Attempts to improve utilization services by providing pregnant mothers with various incentives have failed to overcome these barriers. Although elimination of financial barriers is important in improving access to prenatal supervision, this alone will not resolve the problem of inadequate care. Other limiting social factors must be overcome if significant improvement is to be realized.

## Summary

Despite a clear association between prenatal care and improved perinatal outcome, controversy exists concerning the content and quantity of care necessary to achieve optimal results. This chapter has outlined a traditional program for prenatal care in low-risk pregnancies. Analysis of the efficacy of many of today's common practices has been presented along with some additional and alternative approaches. It is evident that the psychosocial environment is an important aspect of the patient's health behavior that requires greater integration into present programs. In addition, recent efforts to broaden access to prenatal care must be coupled with an improved understanding of patient motivation leading to participation and to increased utilization. Quality prenatal care is still the cornerstone of maintaining maternal and child health. As research adds to our understanding of what quality prenatal care means, flexible programs should allow for incorporation of new information and approaches.

### REFERENCES

ACOG Technical Bulletin: Hepatitis in pregnancy. The American College of Obstetricians and Gynecologists, No. 174, Washington, DC, 1992.

ACOG Committee Opinion: Genetic screening for hemoglobinopathies. The American College of Obstetricians and Gynecologists, No. 168, Washington, DC, 1996.

ACOG Educational Bulletin: Maternal serum screening. The American College of Obstetricians and Gynecologists, No. 154, Washington, DC, 1996.

Adams MM, Sarno AP, Harlass FE, et al: Risk factors for preterm delivery in a healthy cohort. Epidemiology 6:525, 1995.

Allen ST, Dubner MS, Mockler ND: Routine prenatal screening for atypical antibodies. Am J Obstet Gynecol 99:274, 1967.

The American Academy of Pediatrics, The American College of Obstetricians and Gynecologists: Guidelines for Perinatal Care,

4th ed. Washington, DC, The American College of Obstetricians and Gynecologists, 1997.

The American College of Obstetricians and Gynecologists: Standards for Obstetric-Gynecologic Services, 7th ed. Washington, DC, The American College of Obstetricians and Gynecologists, 1989.

Amini SB, Catalano PM, Mann LI: Effect of prenatal care on obstetrical outcome. J Matern Fetal Med 5:142, 1996.

Balcazar H, Hartner J, Cole G, et al: The effects of prenatal care utilization and maternal risk factors on pregnancy outcome between Mexican Americans and non-Hispanic whites. J Natl Med Assoc 85:195, 1993.

Barbacci M, Repke JT, Chaisson RE: Routine prenatal screening for HIV infection. Lancet 337:709, 1991.

Barros H, Tavares M, Rodrigues T: Role of prenatal care in preterm birth and low birthweight in Portugal. J Public Health Med 18:321, 1996.

Belizán JM, Barros F, Langer A, et al: Impact of health education during pregnancy on behavior and utilization of health resources. Am J Obstet Gynecol 173:894, 1995.

Berenson AB, Wilkinson GS, Lopez LA: Effects of prenatal care on neonates born to drug using women. Subst Use Misuse 31:1063, 1996.

Bergsjo P, Villar J: Scientific basis for the content of routine antenatal care. II. Power to eliminate or alleviate adverse newborn outcomes; some special conditions and examinations. Acta Obstet Gynecol Scand 76:15, 1997.

Binstock MA, Wolde-Tsadik G: Impact of reduced visit frequency, focused visits and continuity of care. J Reprod Med 40:507, 1995.

Blankson ML, Goldenberg RL, Keith B: Noncompliance of highrisk pregnant women in keeping appointments at an obstetric complications clinic. South Med J 87:634, 1994.

Blondel B, Dutilh P, Delour M, et al: Poor antenatal care and pregnancy outcome. Eur J Obstet Gynecol Reprod Biol 50:191, 1993.

Bowell PJ, Allen DL, Entwistle CC: Blood group antibody screening tests during pregnancy. Br J Obstet Gynaecol 93:1038, 1986.

Bowman JM, Pollock J: Rh immunization in Manitoba: Progress in prevention and management. Can Med Assoc J 129:343, 1983.

Braveman P, Bennett T, Lewis C, et al: Access to prenatal care following major Medicaid eligibility expansions. JAMA 269:1285, 1993.

Burton BK, Dillard RG: Outcome in infants born to mothers with unexplained elevations of maternal serum α-Fetoprotein. Pediatrics 77:582, 1986.

Burton BK: Outcome of pregnancy in patients with unexplained elevated or low levels of maternal serum alpha-fetoprotein. Obstet Gynecol 72:709, 1988.

Campbell-Brown M, McFadyen IR, Seal DV, et al: Is screening for bacteriuria in pregnancy worthwhile? BMJ 294:1579, 1987.

Centers for Disease Control: Rubella vaccination during pregnancy—United States, 1971–1981. MMWR CDC Surveill Summ 31:477, 1982.

Centers for Disease Control: Prevention of perinatal transmission of Hepatitis B virus: Prenatal screening of all pregnant women for Hepatitis B surface antigen MMWR CDC Surveill Summ 37:341, 1988.

Centers for Disease Control: Hepatitis B Virus: A comprehensive strategy for eliminating transmission in the United States through universal childhood vaccination. Recommendations of the Immunization Practices Advisory Committee (ACIP): MMWR CDC Surveill Summ 40(No. RR-13):1, 1991.

Centers for Disease Control: Prevention of varicella: Recommendations of the Advisory Committee on Immunization Practices (ACIP). MMWR CDC Surveill Summ 45(No. RR-11):1, 1996.

Centers for Disease Control: 1993 Sexually Transmitted Diseases Treatment Guidelines. MMWR CDC Surveill Summ 42(RR-14):1, 1993.

Centers for Disease Control: Core Curriculum on Tuberculosis, 2nd ed. New York, The American Lung Association, 1991.

Centers for Disease Control: Prevention of perinatal group B streptococcal disease: A public health perspective. MMWR CDC Surveill Summ 45(No. RR-7), 1996.

Chang G, Wilkins-Haug L, Berman S, et al: Alcohol use and pregnancy: Improving identification. Obstet Gynecol 91:892, 1998.

Choo PW, Donahue JG, Manson JE, et al: The epidemiology of varicella and its complications. J Infect Dis 172:706, 1995.

Chu DC, Hsu C, Wenstrom KD, et al: Insulin-like growth factor binding protein-3 in the detection of fetal Down syndrome pregnancies. Obstet Gynecol 91:192, 1998.

Committee on Nutritional Status During Pregnancy and Lactation: Nutrition during pregnancy. Part I, weight gain: Part II, nutrient supplements. Washington, DC, National Academy Press, 1990.

Connor EM, Sperling RS, Gelber R, et al: Reduction of maternal-infant transmission of human immunodeficiency virus type I with zidovudine treatment. N Engl J Med 331:1173, 1994.

Coria-Soto IL, Bobadilla JL, Notzon F: The effectiveness of antenatal care in preventing intrauterine growth retardation and low birth weight due to preterm delivery. Int J Qual Health Care 8:13, 1996.

Damm P, Molsted-Pedersen L: Significant decrease in congenital malformations in newborn infants of an unselected population of diabetic women. Am J Obstet Gynecol 161:1163, 1989.

Delgado-Escueta AV, Janz D: Consensus guidelines: Preconception counseling, management, and care of the pregnant woman with epilepsy. Neurology 42:149, 1992.

Enders G, Miller E, Cradock-Watson J, et al: Consequences of varicella and herpes zoster in pregnancy: Prospective study of 1739 cases. Lancet 343:1547, 1994.

Ewigman BG, Crane JP, Frigoletto FD, et al: Effect of prenatal ultrasound screening on perinatal outcome. N Engl J Med 329:821, 1993.

Fiscella K: Does prenatal care improve birth outcomes? A critical review. Obstet Gynecol 85:468, 1995.

Freed GL: Breast-feeding: Time to teach what we preach. JAMA 269:243, 1993.

Gomez R, Galasso M, Romero R: Ultrasonographic examination of the uterine cervix is better than cervical digital examination as a predictor of the likelihood of premature delivery in patients with preterm labor and intact membranes. Am J Obstet Gynecol 171:956, 1994.

Gribble RK, Meier PR, Berg RL: The value of urine screening for glucose at each prenatal visit. Obstet Gynecol 86:405, 1995.

Gribble RK, Fee SC, Berg RL: The value of routine urine dipstick screening for protein at each prenatal visit. Am J Obstet Gynecol 173:214, 1995.

Haas JS, Berman S, Goldberg AB, et al: Prenatal hospitalization and compliance with guidelines for prenatal care. Am J Public Health 86:815, 1996.

Institute of Medicine: Nutrition during pregnancy. Part I. Weight gain. Washington, DC, National Academy Press, 1990.

Ion HW, Litt (Oxon) B: Can what counts be counted? Reflections on the content, costs, benefits, and impacts of prenatal care. Womens Health Issues 5:143, 1995.

Johnson JL, Primas PJ, Coe MK: Factors that prevent women of low socioeconomic status from seeking prenatal care. J Am Acad Nurse Pract 6:105, 1994.

Jones KL, Johnson KA, Chambers CD: Offspring of women infected with varicella during pregnancy: A prospective study. Teratology 49:29, 1994.

Kitzmiller JL, Gavin LA, Gin GD, et al: Preconception care of diabetes. JAMA 265:731, 1991.

Klebanoff MA, Shiono PH, Carey JC: The effect of physical activity during pregnancy on preterm delivery and birth weight. Am J Obstet Gynecol 13:894, 1990.

Kogan MD, Alexander GR, Kotelchuck M, et al: Comparing mothers' reports on the content of prenatal care received with recommended national guidelines for care. Public Health Rep 109:637, 1994.

Kogan MD, Alexander GR, Kotelchuck M, et al: Relation of the content of prenatal care to the risk of low birth weight. JAMA 27:1340, 1994.

Laken MP, Ager J: Using incentives to increase participation in prenatal care. Obstet Gynecol 85:326, 1995.

LeFevre ML, Bain RP, Ewigman BG, et al: A randomized trial of prenatal ultrasonographic screening: Impact on maternal management and outcome. Am J Obstet Gynecol 169:483, 1993.

Locksmith GJ, Duff P: Preventing neural tube defects: The importance of periconceptual folic acid supplements. Obstet Gynecol 91:1027, 1998.

McDuffie RS Jr, Beck A, Bischoff K, et al: Effect of frequency of prenatal care visits on perinatal outcome among low-risk women. JAMA 275:847, 1996.

McDuffie RS Jr, Bischoff KJ, Beck A, et al: Does reducing the number of prenatal office visits for low-risk women result in increased use of other medical services? Obstet Gynecol 90:68, 1997.

Meikle SF, Orleans M, Leff M, et al: Women's reasons for not seeking prenatal care: Racial and ethnic factors. Birth 22:81, 1995.

Moore TR, Piacquadio K: A prospective evaluation of fetal movement screening to reduce the incidence of antepartum fetal death. Am J Obstet Gynecol 160:1075, 1989.

Munjanja SP, Lindmark G, Nyström L: Randomized controlled trial of a reduced-visits programme of antenatal care in Harare, Zimbabwe. Lancet 348:364, 1996.

Oian P, Maltau JM, Noddeland H, et al: Oedema-preventing mechanisms in subcutaneous tissue of normal pregnant women. Br J Obstet Gynaecol 92:1113, 1985.

Oian P, Maltau JM: Calculated capillary hydrostatic pressure in normal pregnancy and preeclampsia. Am J Obstet Gynecol 157:102, 1987.

Pastuszak AL, Levy M, Schick B, et al: Outcome after maternal varicella infection in the first 20 weeks of pregnancy. N Engl J Med 330:901, 1994.

Peoples-Sheps MD, Hogan VK, Ng'andu N: Content of prenatal care during the initial workup. Am J Obstet Gynecol 174:220, 1996.

Piper JM, Mitchel EF Jr, Ray WA: Presumptive eligibility for pregnant Medicaid enrollees: Its effects on prenatal care and perinatal outcome. Am J Public Health 84:1626, 1994.

Piper JM, Ray WA, Griffin MR: Effects of Medicaid eligibility expansion on prenatal care and pregnancy outcome in Tennessee. JAMA 264:2219, 1990.

Poland ML, Ager JW, Olson KL, et al: Quality of prenatal care; selected social behavioral, and biomedical factors; and birth weight. Obstet Gynecol 75:607, 1990.

Public Health Service Expert Panel on Prenatal Care: Caring for our future: The content of prenatal care. Washington, DC, Public Health Service/Health and Human Services, 1989.

Romero R, Oyarzun E, Mazor M, et al: Meta-analysis of the relationship between asymptomatic bacteriuria and preterm delivery/low birth weight. Obstet Gynecol 73:576, 1989.

Rosen MG, Merkatz IR, Hill JG: Caring for our future: A report by the expert panel on the content of prenatal care. Obstet Gynecol 77:782, 1991.

Saari-Kemppainen A, Karjalainen O, Ylöstalo P, et al: Ultrasound screening and perinatal mortality: Controlled trial of systematic one-stage screening in pregnancy. The Helsinki Ultrasound Trial. Lancet 336:387, 1990.

Sacks DA, Abu-fadil S, Karten GJ, et al: Screening for gestational diabetes with the one-hour 50-g glucose test. Obstet Gynecol 70:89, 1987.

Shapiro CN: Epidemiology of hepatitis B. Pediatr Infect Dis J 12:433, 1993.

Sibai BM, Ewell M, Levine RJ, et al: Risk factors associated with preeclampsia in healthy nulliparous women. Am J Obstet Gynecol 177:1003, 1997.

Sikorski J, Wilson J, Clement S, et al: A randomized controlled trial comparing two schedules of antenatal visits: The antenatal care project. BMJ 312:546, 1996.

U.S. Department of Health and Human Services, Public Health Service: Immunization and Infectious Disease 20. *In* Healthy People 2000. Boston, Jones and Bartlett, 1992.

U.S. Department of Health and Human Services, Public Health Service: Maternal and Infant Health 14. *In* Healthy People 2000. Boston, Jones and Bartlett, 1992.

Van Allen MI, Fraser FC, Dallaire L, et al: Recommendations on the use of folic acid supplementation to prevent the recurrence of neural tube defects. Can Med Assoc J 149:1239, 1993.

Ventura SJ, Martin JA, Curtin S, et al: Report of final natality statistics, 1995. Mon Vital Stat Rep 45:1, 1997.

Villar J, Bergsjo P: Scientific basis for the content of routine antenatal care. I. Philosophy, recent studies, and power to eliminate or alleviate adverse maternal outcomes. Acta Obstet Gynecol Scand 76:1, 1997.

Waller DK, Lustig LS, Cunningham GC, et al: Second-trimester maternal serum alpha-fetoprotein levels and the risk of subsequent fetal death. N Engl J Med 325:6, 1991.

Wenstrom KD, Owen J, Chu DC, et al: α-Fetoprotein, free β-human chorionic gonadotropin, and dimeric inhibin A produce the best results in a three-analyte, multiple-marker screening test for fetal Down syndrome. Am J Obstet Gynecol 177:987, 1997.

# — 20 —

# Genetic Counseling, Screening, and Diagnosis

MARK I. EVANS

MARK PAUL JOHNSON

The 1970s saw the emergence of prenatal diagnosis as a possibility. In the 1980s, the expansion of available technology made offering prenatal diagnosis the standard of care for patients who had defined indications, such as advanced maternal age. As the number of physicians and facilities who could deal with such patients rapidly increased, the specifics of the indications were liberalized. For example, the magic number for offering genetic amniocenteses fell from the original maternal age of 40 to age 38 and then 35 or even lower. The development of other technologies, such as biochemical and ultrasonographic screening, added further flexibility to the indications for offering prenatal diagnosis.

## Prepregnancy Counseling

In an ideal world, patients would receive the facts about pregnancy, its risks to the mother, and the risk of genetic or congenital disorders before conception. Such prepregnancy planning would reduce the shock and panic often experienced by high-risk patients when they realize problem situations at the last possible moment. Given the inverse relationship between socioeconomic status and gestational age at the first prenatal visit, it is even more important before conception to discuss issues of maternal disease in pregnancy with patients who would ordinarily be unlikely to come early for prenatal care. Likewise, genetic risks and options are best discussed beforehand so that patients have the option of being tested in the first rather than the second trimester.

## Indications for Offering Prenatal Diagnosis

### ADVANCED MATERNAL AGE

At a bare minimum, patients who will be 35 years of age at delivery must be offered the opportunity of having either genetic amniocentesis or chorionic villus sampling (CVS). While it is most common that patients seeking prenatal diagnosis are concerned about Down syndrome, in reality, Down syndrome—although the most common genetic diagnosis made—represents only about 50% of the abnormalities that are detected. Thus, counseling should be directed at the total risk of chromosomal abnormalities for the maternal age, as listed in Table 20–1.

Table 20-1 Chromosome Risks by Maternal Age at Midtrimester and at Term Delivery

| Maternal Age | Trisomy 21 Mid-trimester | Trisomy 21 Term | All Aneuploidy Mid-trimester | All Aneuploidy Term |
|---|---|---|---|---|
| 20–21 | 1/1167 | 1/1167 | 1/368 | 1/526 |
| 22–23 | 1/1000 | 1/1429 | 1/350 | 1/500 |
| 24–25 | 1/875 | 1/1250 | 1/333 | 1/476 |
| 26 | 1/823 | 1/1176 | 1/333 | 1/476 |
| 27 | 1/778 | 1/1111 | 1/319 | 1/455 |
| 28 | 1/737 | 1/1053 | 1/304 | 1/435 |
| 29 | 1/700 | 1/1000 | 1/292 | 1/417 |
| 30 | 1/666 | 1/952 | 1/269 | 1/385 |
| 31 | 1/636 | 1/909 | 1/269 | 1/385 |
| 32 | 1/538 | 1/769 | 1/225 | 1/322 |
| 33 | 1/437 | 1/602 | 1/222 | 1/286 |
| 34 | 1/350 | 1/485 | 1/182 | 1/238 |
| 35 | 1/270 | 1/378 | 1/143 | 1/192 |
| 36 | 1/206 | 1/289 | 1/115 | 1/156 |
| 37 | 1/160 | 1/224 | 1/91 | 1/127 |
| 38 | 1/123 | 1/173 | 1/72 | 1/102 |
| 39 | 1/96 | 1/136 | 1/57 | 1/83 |
| 40 | 1/74 | 1/106 | 1/46 | 1/66 |
| 41 | | 1/82 | | 1/53 |
| 42 | | 1/63 | | 1/42 |
| 43 | | 1/49 | | 1/33 |
| 44 | | 1/38 | | 1/26 |
| 45 | | 1/30 | | 1/21 |
| 46 | | 1/23 | | 1/16 |
| 47 | | 1/18 | | 1/13 |
| 48 | | 1/14 | | 1/10 |
| 49 | | 1/11 | | 1/8 |

## PREVIOUS CHILD WITH CHROMOSOME ABNORMALITIES

Several studies have looked at the risk of having a second baby with a chromosome abnormality. Although there are certain subsets of populations in which one of the parents has a balanced translocation that can raise the risk in subsequent pregnancies to the range of 10 to 15%, in cases in which both parents are found to have normal chromosomes, the risk for abnormalities in a subsequent pregnancy is approximately 1%, which is equivalent to the risk level of a 38-year-old woman. Therefore, all patients who have had a previous child with Down syndrome or any other chromosomal abnormality should be offered prenatal diagnosis regardless of age.

## HISTORY OF MULTIPLE MISCARRIAGES

Several studies have addressed the issue of increased risk of having a live, aneuploid child after multiple miscarriages. From our own data and those of others, it would appear that women who have had two or more spontaneous losses that were not attributable to a specific factor (e.g., inadequate luteal phase), are at a somewhat increased risk of having abnormalities in a third or subsequent pregnancy. Therefore, we believe (although this is not a universally held opinion) that women who have had two or more miscarriages should be offered amniocentesis or CVS. Our own experience has indicated an approximately 1% detection rate of abnormalities in such women, again consistent with the risk rate for a 38-year-old patient.

## HISTORY OF NEURAL TUBE DEFECTS

The incidence of neural tube defects (NTDs), such as spina bifida and anencephaly vary by ethnic group (Table 20–2). To obtain a definitive diagnosis for a patient at high risk, amniocentesis should be performed to measure alpha-fetoprotein (AFP) and sometimes acetylcholinesterase. However, the vast majority (i.e., about 95%) of all babies born with NTDs are born to couples who have had no reason to suspect they are at any increased risk. Thus, inherent in a program to detect the vast majority of NTDs is the necessity of testing all pregnancies. Clearly, it is impossible to offer amniocentesis to all patients. Thus, the concept of maternal serum alpha-fetoprotein (MS-AFP) screening was developed in the mid-1970s. For NTDs approximately 3% of patients either have one very significantly elevated maternal serum alpha-fetoprotein (MS-AFP) value (higher than 4 multiples of the median [MOM]) or two values

Table 20-2 United States Ethnic Group Variation in Neural Tube Defects

| | |
|---|---|
| White | 1:700 |
| African-American | 1:1000 |
| Asian | 1:1200 |

higher than 2.5 MOM. For these patients, ultrasonography can detect an obvious explanation for the elevations in approximately half the cases: twins, anencephaly, severe NTD, or—most commonly—incorrect dates. The remaining 1.5% of patients are offered a genetic amniocentesis. In most large programs, including our own at Hutzel Hospital/Wayne State University, the pickup rate for abnormalities is approximately 5% of patients who undergo amniocentesis. It should be noted that even in a top-quality ultrasonography unit, approximately 10 to 15% of all defects may not be detected by the ultrasonographic screening. These data support the contention that although risk predictions can be lowered, amniocentesis is appropriate even if the ultrasonogram appears normal. Amniotic fluid AFP and acetylcholinesterase remain the most sensitive tests available for detection of defects in these patients.

## LOW MATERNAL SERUM ALPHA-FETOPROTEIN VALUES

In 1983, a chance association revealed that babies born with chromosome anomalies, such as Down syndrome, tended to have lower than normal MS-AFP values. This discovery led to a re-evaluation of genetic risk. Only 20% of babies who have chromosome abnormalities are born to women 35 years of age or older. Thus, despite the fact that for any given younger woman the risk of having a baby with a chromosome anomaly is lower than for an older woman, in total numbers, the vast majority of babies who have chromosome abnormalities are born to women who have no presumed risk factors. The calculation of low MS-AFP values, however, enabled us for the first time to alter the risk for younger women, allowing selective populations to receive prenatal diagnosis. Maternal age counseling became a two-function equation, using a priori risk at a given maternal age and how low the AFP was. In most programs, a low MS-AFP value was defined as the risk equivalent to that of a 35-year-old woman (i.e., approximately 1:200). Not surprisingly, the incremental increase required for a 32-year-old woman to have the equivalent rate of a 35-year-old is reached with a "less low" MS-AFP value than would be required of a 26-year-old. Thus different cutoff points for different maternal ages were used. Experience has also shown that MS-AFP values need to be adjusted according to multiple factors (Table 20–3).

## Multiple Markers

The potential benefits of mass screening for chromosomal abnormalities are obvious. If amniocentesis and

**Table 20–3** Adjustment Factors for Alpha-Fetoprotein

Maternal weight
Gestational age
Race
Diabetes
Multiple gestation

chorionic villus sampling (CVS) were offered only to women 35 years of age and older only about 20% of chromosome abnormalities would be detected in theory. In practice, only about 12% were detected in the 1980s; when properly performed, MS-AFP raised the detection rate to between 40 and 50%.

In an effort to increase the detection rate beyond 40 to 50%, additional serum markers have been investigated and introduced. One such combination, first proposed in 1988, is AFP + β-human chorionic gonadotropin + unconjugated estriol (triple screening). Wald and associates suggested that perhaps as many as 60% of Down syndrome cases could be identified by this combination. In their study, they developed a likelihood ratio based upon maternal age, the degree of diminishment of MS-AFP, elevation of β-hCG, and diminished unconjugated estriol. Some patients who might have a normal MS-AFP might be found to be at risk because of the triple screen findings, whereas others, who had a low MS-AFP, might not be considered to be at risk.

Multiple studies over the past several years have shown conclusively that of the three markers, hCG is unquestionably the best, with the mean AFP in Down syndrome being about 0.72 MOM, $E_3$ 0.73 MOM, and hCG 2.05 MOM. Because AFP is already used in the United States and most of the world for NTD screening, and because hCG is the best detector of Down syndrome, the remaining questions are how much—if at all—does estriol add to the sensitivity, and at what cost?

Throughout the 1990s, several studies attempted to answer these questions, with conflicting results. Approximately half the studies suggested that estriol ($E_3$) may increase sensitivity by 3 to 8%, whereas the other half suggested that it did no good or even lowered sensitivity; moreover, the $E_3$ test is relatively expensive. We believe a double-screen approach using the ratio of hCG/AFP MOMs is the best criterion at the lowest cost. Although there is debate about which is the best algorithm, there is no debate about the fact that multiple markers are far superior to AFP alone, and that offering AFP alone is no longer acceptable practice.

Extensive promotional and marketing strategies have been devised for the double and triple screening programs, and some of them have been misleading.

For example, some claims have been made for as much as an 80% detection rate. This could be true if only women older than 35 years of age were included, but some marketing information implies that detection frequencies are the same in younger women; this is clearly not the case. For example, Wald's data showed that one third of anomalies were detected in 20-year-old women; one half in 30-year-old women and two thirds in 35-year-old women. In other words, in the case of a 35-year-old woman, in whom 100% detection is possible and standard by invasive testing, one third of chromosomal anomalies would be missed if biochemical screening were relied upon to determine who would be offered invasive testing.

Another relevant issue concerns the type of β-hCG analysis. β-hCG can be measured in five ways:

1. Intact
2. Free
3. Nicked
4. Free nicked
5. Degradation core

The free and nicked (a structurally abnormal β is more likely to appear in Down syndrome) are both relatively unstable, and, therefore, the interval from blood draw to laboratory test can alter the result.

Other markers are constantly being evaluated, and it is reasonable to assume that there will be a continual evolution of markers that vary in sensitivity, specificity, and optimal gestational age at testing. Inhibin appears to be an excellent marker and does not vary with gestational age. Data suggest that neutrophil alkaline phosphatase (NAP) may be very sensitive. Pregnancy-associated plasma protein A (PAPPA) appears to be very good in the first trimester but useless in the second. The search for fetal cells that leak through to the maternal circulation has suggested that these cells can at least be isolated and characterized by fluorescence in situ hybridization (FISH) probes. However, there is still much more to be done before this can be accepted as a protocol.

Identification of patients at risk for chromosome abnormalities has acquired a new dimension with the discovery of the so-called nuchal translucency, which can be observed in the first trimester of pregnancy via ultrasonography as an outpouching at the back of the neck (Fig. 20–1). This marker, which probably represents fluid buildup, can be measured with reasonable accuracy. Several studies have shown that the presence of a nuchal translucency confers a considerably increased risk of an aneuploid fetus. In regard to our patients who come for other indications, aneuploidy was detected in over 40% of our patients when the nuchal translucence marker was present. In low-risk patients, Nicolaides and associates in London have detected a frequency of approximately 70% for 5% of patients at risk. However, the screening must be done in a standardized fashion between 10 and 12 weeks of gestation. The combination of nuchal translucency and first-trimester markers, such as free β-hCG and PAPPA, appears very promising, and we believe that there will be a shift in thinking away from either biochemical or biophysical screening to a combination of the two.

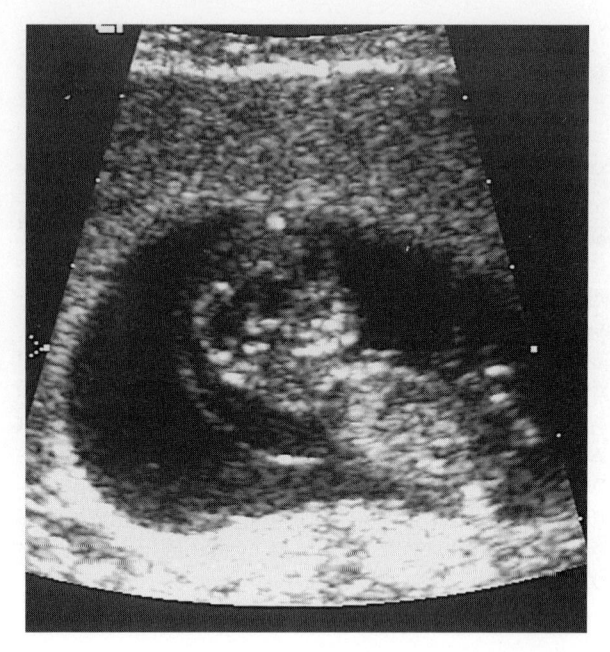

**Figure 20–1** Ultrasonographic scan showing large nuchal translucency located on the back of the neck in a fetus shown to have 47,XY + 21 karyotype by chorionic villus sampling (CVS).

## Procedures

### SECOND-TRIMESTER AMNIOCENTESIS

Midtrimester amniocentesis has been the mainstay of prenatal diagnosis for 15 years. As the number of physicians who are trained in performing the technique and the number of laboratories that can handle specimens have increased, the safety and efficacy of testing have similarly mushroomed. As performed by highly experienced physicians, genetic amniocentesis probably carries a procedure-related risk of no more than approximately 1:300. When it is performed by physicians who have less training, the risks may be considerably higher. Use of sophisticated ultrasonography for guided needle entry has been a major determinant in reducing the risks of the procedure. Baselines for AFP and other biochemical measurements have usually been worked out in large numbers of patients, thus allowing appropriate biochemical determinations.

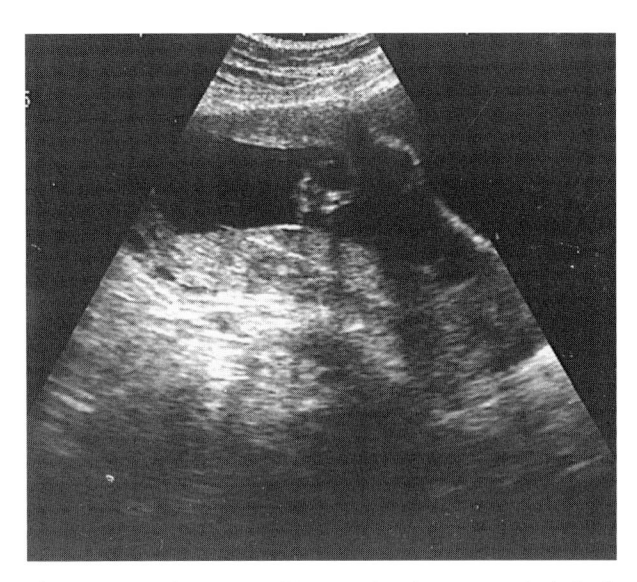

**Figure 20–2** Ultrasonographic scan showing transcervical chorionic villus sampling (CVS) procedure with a catheter passing from the lower right upward and left through the placenta.

## CHORIONIC VILLUS SAMPLING

CVS is a first-trimester alternative to second-trimester amniocentesis and has several major theoretical advantages (Fig. 20–2). These include the earlier stage at which the test is done, a usually shorter turnaround time for obtaining results, and the fact that the test is done so early in pregnancy that the patient is not visibly pregnant, which allows privacy of reproductive decisions for the couple. If an abnormality is detected and termination is elected by the couple, first-trimester procedures are safer, easier, quicker, simpler, and cheaper than second-trimester procedures that use either induction of labor by prostaglandin or dilatation and extraction. To date, over 200,000 CVS procedures have been done worldwide. A very experienced physician can obtain a usable sample in greater than 99% of cases. The ability to capture appropriate chromosomal spreads approaches 100%. In most centers, CVS is performed as a transvaginal transcervical ultrasonograph-guided placental aspiration, although an increasing number of procedures are now done transabdominally. In our experience, the transcervical route has produced faster, easier, and larger specimens and is the method of choice. However, taking into consideration such factors as placental location, stenosis of the cervix, vaginal infection, or fibroids hindering the path of the catheter, we can and do use the transabdominal approach reliably about 10 to 15% of the time. Some programs perform over half of these cases abdominally. There were some allegations in the early 1990s that CVS might be associated with an increased incidence of limb reduction defects. The overwhelming data refute this association if the procedure is performed at 10+ weeks and if operators are experienced. At extremely early gestational age (i.e., 6 to 8 weeks), there may be a small increased risk.

Either transabdominal or transcervical CVS seems to have a slightly higher complication rate than that of amniocentesis in the second trimester. It has been suggested that the procedure-related complication rate of CVS may be approximately 0.5 to 1%. Data from the largest centers around the country suggest that it may, in fact, be somewhat less than that. There does appear, however, to be a significant learning curve for the physician in both acquiring the ability to obtain a sample and in handling the procedure-related risk.

## FIRST-TRIMESTER AMNIOCENTESIS

Traditionally, amniocentesis has not been performed before 15 or 16 weeks of gestation. With advances in ultrasonography and laboratory testing that have allowed more efficient growth of cells in a culture, we are now able to perform amniocentesis even earlier. In our experience, successful procedures have been performed as early as 10 weeks of gestation, although the majority of cases are done at 12 to 13 weeks. As with CVS, it is possible to obtain a specimen in virtually 100% of cases and to receive a laboratory result in approximately 99%. Theoretical advantages of early amniocentesis include the ability to measure AFP for NTDs. At present, baselines for normal values are being worked out for earlier gestational ages. A disadvantage of performing first-trimester amniocentesis is that the numbers of cells in the amniotic fluid that are suitable for cytogenic biochemical, or molecular cultures, are somewhat diminished; consequently, it takes longer to obtain results than when midtrimester amniocentesis is performed. At comparable early gestational ages, CVS appears to have a lower loss rate than that of amniocentesis. In 1998, a Canadian collaborative study found a 17% risk of clubfoot in babies born after early amniocentesis at less than 12 weeks of gestation. Most authorities now believe that except in unusual circumstances, amniocentesis should not be performed before 12 weeks of gestation.

# Molecular Diagnosis

The ability to obtain fetal tissue in the second and even in the first trimester has provided tremendous advantages in early prenatal diagnosis of many disorders. There are now multiple approaches to the laboratory evaluation of molecular medicine.

## MUTATIONS AND POLYMORPHISMS

Many types of mutations can affect a gene. DNA within the gene contains information for the final sequencing of a protein as well as signals for the correct expression and processing of messenger ribonucleic acid (mRNA). If the actual coding region is altered, then the resultant protein may be changed. These alterations can take the form of deletions (many kilobases or as small as a single base), inversions, translocations (no net nucleotide changes but potential or actual protein changes), or single-base changes. Even a change at the junction of a coding or a noncoding region can result in abnormal mRNA formation. Defects in the promoter region may result in too little or too much expression of mRNA, which will be reflected in an abnormal protein synthesis. A deletion of all or part of the gene almost always results in the disruption of normal gene expression. An example of molecular pathology is the incidence of Tay-Sachs disease in the Ashkenazi Jewish population. In the severe infantile type of this disease, a mutation at an exon-intron splice site in the α-subunit has been identified (G to C transversion); another mutation is a four-base insertion in exon 11 of the α-subunit, causing a frame shift mutation and marked reduction in mRNA. Another example that has been identified is the mutation most commonly found in individuals of northern European ancestry who have cystic fibrosis (CF). There is a phenylalanine deletion in the cystic fibrosis transmembrane regulator (CFTR) protein at a critical adenosine triphosphate (ATP) binding site, arising from the deletion of three amino acids, two of which determine the code for phenylalanine. This ΔF 508 mutation accounts for approximately 70% of CF mutations in individuals of northern European ancestry, with the remaining 30% of cases caused by a heterogeneous assortment of other mutations.

Mutations may occur at practically all loci. Genes not found to be associated with mutations in vivo include those whose products are so vital that any change would probably result in death early in development ("housekeeping genes"). Possible examples of this type include enzymes coded by nuclear—or possibly mitochondrial—DNA catalyzing critical steps in aerobic metabolism. Genes that are not associated with clinical mutation include those whose protein products are coded by repetitive DNA, whereby the remaining DNA can compensate. For example, ribosomal RNA genes are so abundant that if deletion occurs with fusion of acrocentric chromosomes, as in a robertsonian translocation, it has no phenotypic effect. Other mutations unassociated with clinical disease can occur in noncoding areas such as introns, or in other unexpressed areas of the genome, such as pseudogenes, which are duplicated sequences similar to normally expressed genes but containing no introns.

A variety of approaches have been used to detect mutations. Optimally, determination of cDNA structure and sequence, followed by elucidation of gene structure and organization in the normal allele are completed before beginning a search for specific defects. However, only about 5 to 10% of clinically significant mutations are caused by gross alterations in gene structure detectable by Southern blot analysis of genomic DNA, leaving the remaining 90% unknown. The problem is compounded by normal variation in the nucleotide sequence (polymorphisms). Thus, when variations from the normal sequence are found, additional analysis is required before these changes can be construed as being a disease-causing mutation.

**Linkage Analysis.** Linkage analysis is a very powerful technique that can be used to follow genetic disorders throughout a family and to localize specific genes by closer mapping of linked markers to a putative disease gene. Linkage analysis can be used for genetic diagnosis when the precise nucleotide mutations are not known. A given trait can manifest a variety of genetic differences among individuals. These are called polymorphisms and are spread throughout the entire human genome. The functions of these polymorphisms are not always known.

The degree of linkage can be described mathematically by a number called an *LOD score*, developed in 1955 by Morton. LOD stands for *l*ogarithm of the *od*ds, which can be thought of as the likelihood that two given traits are linked. It can be derived from recombinations observed between clinical or biochemical traits from pedigree analysis or, more recently, from molecular polymorphisms. The probability of recombination between two loci during meiosis is quantified by a term called the recombination fraction ($\theta$ or q), the maximum being 0.5. The LOD score is derived from various values of $\theta$. Viewed simplistically, the higher the LOD score, the higher the likelihood of linkage. Because this number is used on a logarithmic scale, each integer increase reflects a 10-fold increase in likelihood of linkage.

**Restriction Fragment Length Polymorphism Analysis.** Bacteria possess enzymes that recognize and cleave DNA at specific sites. Presumably, these enzymes evolved as a defense against hostile invading DNA, as might occur with bacteriophages. Since these cleavage sites are quite specific, that is, *restricted* to specific palindromic sequences of 4 to 10 nucleotides in length, these enzymes have been termed *restriction endonucleases*. When these enzymes are added to eukaryotic DNA, the resultant mixture contains a variety of DNA fragments of different sizes, which can be separated by gel electrophoresis and transferred for analysis by Southern blotting. Each enzyme cuts an individual's DNA according to the positions of the cleavage sites, with every individual having his or her own unique pattern of cleaved DNA fragments. Thus, individuals are polymorphic for the resulting lengths of DNA fragments, which vary with different restrictor enzymes that are used and distribution of cleavage sites. Many of these recognition site polymorphisms are neutral and represent normal inherited variability. These characteristics have given rise to the term "restriction fragment length polymorphisms" (RFLPs), which refers to the polymorphic patterns observed in specific nucleotide sequences that are cleaved by bacterial restriction enzymes. The resultant mixture of DNA fragments can be separated and further characterized by gel electrophoresis, Southern blotting, and oligonucleotide probes.

## Molecular Diagnostic Techniques

Because DNA is present in each cell nucleus, any nucleated cell is theoretically suitable for DNA analysis regardless of whether the gene in question is being transcribed and expressed. Thus, white blood cells, amniocytes, and chorionic villi are all candidate cells for DNA analysis. RFLP analysis was described previously. Several other methods are also used for DNA diagnosis, including Southern blotting, oligonucleotide probe, and polymerase chain reaction. Northern blotting is used for RNA analysis.

**Southern Blotting.** Southern blotting is a standard method of DNA analysis used in both clinical and basic science settings. In the Southern blotting technique—named after the investigator Edwin Southern—double-stranded DNA is digested by a restriction endonuclease (see later) that is chosen because of its ability to detect a DNA polymorphism, which may or may not have any clinical significance. After endonuclease digestion, the resulting DNA fragments are separated by gel electrophoresis. The DNA in the gel is then denatured to generate single-stranded DNA molecules. DNA fragments are transferred from the gel to nylon filter blotting paper, where specific filter-bound DNA fragments can be detected by hybridization. A radiolabeled DNA or RNA probe that has sequence homology to the DNA fragment of interest is used, usually 200 to 2000 bases long. Subsequent autoradiography produces a film with banding patterns. These patterns indicate the hybridization locations on the filter, which reflects the fragment sizes of DNA sequences that are homologous to a particular probe.

**Oligonucleotide Probe Analysis.** Oligonucleotide probe analysis is similar to Southern blotting analysis because DNA is digested and electrophoresed in a gel. It differs by having a shorter probe, termed an oligonucleotide probe, which is used for hybridization. Each oligonucleotide probe is biochemically synthesized and is about 20 bases in length. Because of their short length, these probes do not hybridize to genomic DNA sequences that differ by even a single nucleotide from the probe sequence. Thus, these probes are useful because they can detect very subtle variations in genomic sequences if the specific nucleotide alterations in genomic DNA are known.

This approach to mutation detection was used before introduction of the polymerase chain reaction involved direct DNA analysis using sequence-specific oligonucleotides. These specific oligonucleotides were first used for detection of single-base mutations found in sickle-cell disease, the first "molecular" disease described. For purposes of routine mutation screening, this method is useful only if the gene for the disorder under consideration has been sequenced and is caused by a small number of mutant alleles. This is important, because the oligonucleotides, which are complementary and specific for the mutation in question, must be synthesized before testing. These nucleotide sequences can be synthesized to recognize the normal gene sequence or those that have specific nucleotide changes. Therefore, if a normal oligonucleotide sequence fails to recognize and hybridize to the gene in question, a change in its sequence must be present. In contrast, if the oligonucleotide probe is constructed to complement a specific mutation, recognition and hybridization of this probe imply that the mutation is present in that gene. Some diseases that can be detected in this manner include sickle-cell disease, CF, β-thalassemia, Tay-Sachs disease, and Gaucher's disease. In these diseases, the nucleotide abnormalities of the more commonly occurring mutations are already known.

**Polymerase Chain Reaction.** The polymerase chain reaction (PCR) has revolutionized the field of molecular genetics. This procedure allows in vitro amplification of minute amounts of DNA. This DNA generates sufficient quantities of signal to make detection possible by more traditional methods. This procedure makes use of a relatively heat-stable bacterial enzyme, *Thermus aquaticus* (Taq I) which is derived from a thermoacidophilic bacterium. If the target nucleotide sequence is known, a specific set of oligonucleotides, called primers, can be synthesized to encompass the target sequence. The target DNA, oligonucleotide primers, Taq I polymerase, and free nucleotides are placed in solution. This reaction mixture is heated further to allow already denatured DNA to anneal with the oligonucleotides, between which the polymerase synthesizes complementary strands. Repeated cycles of heating and cooling result in cyclic primer sequence synthesis, which leads to annealing and amplification of the target sequence, because each set of DNA strands gives rise to two additional sets of sequence templates in each cycle of the reaction. This process can be automated to allow 20 to 30 cycles, which can produce more than a million-fold duplication of the target sequence within hours. Modifications of this process can be performed to allow the following:

1. Analysis of RNA
2. Analysis of multiple DNA areas (multiplex PCR)
3. Selective amplification of one strand instead of both (asymmetric PCR)
4. Simultaneous use of one primer set within another to increase specificity (nested PCR)

or

5. Simultaneous use of two different primer sets, one of which selects a normal sequence and the other a mutant sequence (competitive oligonucleotide priming)
6. Simultaneous use of a known amount of a second, easily identified target DNA to measure the amount of original DNA (semiquantitative PCR).

Many technical difficulties must be addressed to eliminate both false-positive and false-negative results. Problems with reagent and reactant contamination can lead to false-positive results and require that appropriate control methods be simultaneously performed to verify positive PCR results. Other problems, such as primer (instead of target) amplification or nonspecific amplification, must be recognized and eliminated.

**Northern Blotting.** Northern blotting is used for RNA analysis. The general principles of the technique are similar to those used in Southern blotting. RNA analysis requires prompt specimen processing and committed laboratory reagents and instruments because of ubiquitous ribonucleases (RNases), present even on finger surfaces. Examination of the size and amount of an mRNA transcript is a useful initial step in evaluating mutations of genes that are expressed in cells or tissues, especially those that are expressed clinically. Fibroblasts and lymphocytes are good sources of mRNA. Hepatic or muscle tissue is useful if available. Placental tissue can be used if maternal cell contamination can be avoided. Of the cell's total RNA, only 1 to 2% is made up of mRNA, which is highly unstable at room temperature because of tissue RNases. The remainder of RNA is mainly ribosomal RNA (rRNA) and transfer RNA (tRNA). Once isolated, the mRNA is denatured, separated by agarose gel electrophoresis, transferred to a membrane filter, and analyzed by hybridization of a specific fluorescent or radiolabeled probe.

For most diseases studied at the molecular level, about 5 to 10% of patients have no detectable mRNA for the gene product in question; 10 to 20% have reduced but detectable amounts of normal mRNA, and about 5% have some alteration in mRNA size. The remaining approximately 50% have normal amounts of normalized mRNA. Given this information, it is possible to deduce the general type of mutation at the DNA level, such as large or total gene deletions (suggested by a total absence of mRNA), mutations in promoter regions (suggested by reduced amounts of normal mRNA), mutations at exon-intron junctions (suggested by changes in mRNA size), or point mutations (suggested by normal-sized mRNA but abnormally functioning proteins).

## Prenatal Diagnosis: Molecular Biology

Prenatal diagnosis has been successfully accomplished by analysis of fetal DNA extracted from a variety of samples. In the initial cases, the fetus was at risk for having a hemoglobinopathy, such as sickle-cell anemia or thalassemia, in which defects of the specific protein, mRNA, and DNA were known. Since that time, the number of genetic disorders in which DNA technology can be applied for prenatal diagnosis has continued to grow geometrically. In addition to the hemoglobinopathies, a partial list of other potentially prenatally diagnosable defects that can be evaluated by molecular genetic techniques include Duchenne muscular dystrophy (DMD), CF, fragile X syndrome, infantile myotonic dystrophy, hemophilias A and B, congenital adrenal hyperplasia (CAH), Tay-Sachs disease, neurofibromatosis type 1 (NF-1), and ornithine transcarbamylase (OTC) deficiency.

If the molecular abnormality of the abnormal gene is known, RFLP analysis or oligonucleotide probes can be used. PCR can also be used to amplify known regions and the resultant product can be analyzed by Southern blotting. PCR is especially useful when using milligram amounts of clinical material obtained at the time of CVS, amniocentesis, tissue culture, or cordocentesis. If the exact gene abnormality and location are not known, linkage analysis with RFLPs can be performed as an indirect method if family members are cooperative; this means that an affected family member must be available and willing to be tested. Occasionally, a patient may have a previously undescribed molecular pathology; in such a case, standard probes and markers are not helpful. This situation invariably lengthens the amount of time needed to make a diagnosis. Other difficult situations arise when a disease appears in a family of a particular ethnic group, in which the molecular pathology differs from other ethnic groups with known molecular pathology. An example of this situation is an African-American couple who have a child who has CF, in whom studies for the ΔF 508 mutation most commonly found in northern Europeans, are negative. Despite these problems, as more genes are cloned and more chromosomal markers are identified, this approach to prenatal diagnosis will become increasingly common.

## Prenatal Diagnosis: Biochemistry

Biochemical assays remain an important aspect of prenatal diagnostic testing, even with the tremendous advances in molecular genetics. These assays include an assessment of gene products, such as enzymes, receptors, transport proteins, and metabolites, such as amino acids, organic acids, vitamins, and hormones. Prenatal diagnosis of biochemical defects may be made by assay of fetal tissue, fetal cells, or tissue culture supernatant if the particular product is produced solely or primarily by the gene in question, and if the product is already known to be expressed in the fetal specimen to be analyzed. Enzyme assays can be performed using tissue, extracts from cultured fetal cells, or live cells kept in tissue culture. Biochemical tests for the diagnosis of metabolic disorders consist of identification of abnormal metabolite(s) or abnormal levels of metabolite(s) that reflect a metabolic block. Ultimately, the goal is identification, quantification, and characterization of the defective or deficient gene product that is responsible for the metabolic block. When the underlying biochemical defect is known and is expressed in accessible fetal tissue (chorionic villi, fetal muscle, or liver) or cells (trophoblasts, amniocytes, fetal erythrocytes, and leukocytes), prenatal diagnosis can be approached by analysis of the enzyme or other protein product that has been shown to be primarily involved.

Definitive biochemical diagnosis of an inherited metabolic disorder must be based on a clear-cut distinction between the values of affected and unaffected fetuses. In genetic disorders, there is potential for overlap between the normal and heterozygous ranges of enzyme activities. This arises mainly as a result of the wide variation found in the activity of almost any biologic enzyme in the normal population. Because variability stems from different mutations and because different genomic backgrounds exist among families, additional testing of leukocytes or cultured skin fibroblasts from presumably unaffected parents and siblings can provide valuable information. In addition to benefiting the interpretation of prenatal results, such studies may provide a reliable means for identification of other carriers among members of the extended family.

The fetus can also be indirectly assessed by determination of maternal serum enzyme activities during pregnancy. For example, the normal increase in serum hexosaminidase A that occurs in pregnancy appears to be of fetal origin. Therefore, unchanged levels in pregnancies at risk for Tay-Sachs disease may indicate an affected fetus.

For many inherited metabolic disorders or inborn errors of metabolism, biochemical methods of prenatal diagnosis are available or are theoretically possible. For an autosomal recessive disease, the assay employed should discriminate among homozygous affected, heterozygous unaffected, and homozygous normal fetuses. Assays for detection of autosomal dominant diseases, such as some of the porphyrias, are usually capable of identifying affected homozygotes but sometimes fail in conclusively differentiating affected heterozygotes from unaffected fetuses. X-linked disorders present unique difficulties in heterozygote detection, which arise because of random X inactivation. Depending on the ratio of active mutant X to normal X in tissues involved in the pathogenesis of the disease, a female who is heterozygous for an X-linked disorder may be clinically normal or may have mild or even severe disease manifestations. To complicate matters further, measured enzymatic activities also vary depending on the ratio of mutant to normal X chromosomes that are active in the analyzed specimen, such as chorionic villi. Occasionally, the activity levels in chorionic villi may not correlate with clinical expression. Males, on the other hand, have only one X chromosome and are hemizygous affected with deficient enzyme activity or hemizygous normal with activity in the normal range. Thus, prenatal biochemical assessment of X-linked disorders is less complicated if the fetus is male.

## Molecular and Biochemical Testing: Carrier Screening

Carrier screening is usually limited to populations or ethnic groups at increased risk for a diagnosable disease. The ultimate benefit of carrier detection programs is identifying couples who are at risk before they have an affected child, empowering them with reproductive choices. For example, carrier detection for Tay-Sachs disease is routinely offered to all individuals of Ashkenazi Jewish (northeastern Europe) descent in whom the combined frequency for the two common mutations in the α-subunit gene of hexosaminidase is 1 in 31. Hexosaminidase A levels can be assayed enzymatically in serum, plasma, or leukocytes and compared to a constant value of thermostabile hexosaminidase B. Pregnant women should have only the leukocyte assay performed because of problems with false-negative or indeterminate results in serum or plasma. Screening is also offered to individuals of French-Canadian background who have a disease that is similar to Tay-Sachs disease with a high carrier frequency but a different mutation (7.6 kb deletion in the α-subunit).

In individuals of African descent, sickle-cell screening is routinely offered. Sickle-cell screening is usually performed by a biochemical assay assessing hemoglobin solubility; positive results are followed up with electrophoresis to characterize the hemoglobin type. In unusual cases, the exact nucleotide defect can be characterized using techniques described above.

Biochemical screening programs for Tay-Sachs disease and sickle-cell disease, when coupled with appropriate counseling, are generally well received by patients. In contrast, the discovery of the molecular and biochemical characterization of the defect found in CF has not resulted in widespread implementation of screening programs, even though CF is a common genetic disease (1 in 2000 to 3000) with a relatively high heterozygote frequency in the Caucasian population of the United States (1 in 25). The controversy surrounding widespread implementation of CF screening stems from a variety of factors. First, approximately 70% of carriers are positive for the most common mutation (ΔF 508). Therefore, screening is required for multiple mutations, and this is performed at present with PCR and oligonucleotide probes specific for known CF mutations. Using probes for 32 mutations, approximately 90% of carriers can be identified. Over 600 mutations are known. If screening were to be implemented, there is no consensus on who should be screened and when the screening should take place. Some options include testing the fetus at the time of genetic testing for other indications, testing the mother alone, or testing both parents. Another factor affecting implementation of screening programs is the clinical variability of the disorder. In contrast to the infantile form of Tay-Sachs disease, CF morbidity can range from debilitating pulmonary disease and death in childhood to minimal symptoms and survival into adulthood, which correlates with the type and magnitude of the molecular defect. Also to be considered is the increased clinical burden on existing genetic services for appropriate counseling before and after testing. A final objection is the potential counseling difficulty arising when the fetus is found to have only one positive allele for a known CF mutation, and linkage analysis cannot be applied because there is no index case. Although the likelihood of an affected fetus is low, the possibility cannot be entirely ruled out, and the parents are left with an ambiguous result.

Pilot studies are under way examining different screening approaches and the resultant impact on patient choices along with their understanding of counseling and implications of screening. Some centers already offer parental and fetal CF screening to all patients who receive genetic counseling and procedures for other indications. Despite the difficulties outlined earlier; it is our personal belief that maternal (and possibly fetal) antenatal screening for CF, using PCR and oligonucleotide probes to detect multiple mutations, will eventually become a routine practice because of heightened public awareness and continued improvements in molecular technology.

Molecular cytogenetic analysis by FISH provides another valuable adjunct to traditional cytogenetic analysis by allowing the rapid detection of common chromosomal trisomies and sex chromosome aneuploidies in interphase cells. Technologic improvements to the nonisotopic methods for in situ hybridization have increased the diagnostic capabilities in clinical cytogenetics by providing a new screening test that allows the rapid detection of some prenatal chromosome aberrations in interphase cells. Chromosome-specific centromeric probes, that allow the detection of chromosomal aneuploidies in cells by simply counting the number of signals present in cultured or uncultured amniotic fluid cells are available. The ability to study uncultured cells or a small number of nondividing cells can provide valuable diagnostic information from a sample that otherwise would not be adequate for routine cytogenetic analysis. However, probes are not available for all chromosomes. Only 13, 18, 21, X, and Y probes are generally available; therefore, abnormalities of other chromosomes would be missed. Our data show that one third of abnormalities are not detectable. FISH is not a substitute for karyotyping but rather an addition.

"Chromosome-painting" probes, which can cover a specific region or an entire chromosome, are being developed. These allow detection of structural chromosomal rearrangements in interphase and mitotic cells. Clearly, these techniques will have a major clinical impact in the near future because they effectively extend the resolution of cytogenetic analysis. Significant improvements will facilitate rapid screening of large numbers of cells to rule out low-level mosaicism. Screening interphase and mitotic cells for structural rearrangements will be important in oncology as well as prenatal diagnosis. In addition, the ability to map human genes precisely and to detect submicroscopic deletions or even the loss of a single gene will provide a powerful new role for clinical molecular cytogenetics.

## REFERENCES

Ben-Yoseph Y: Biochemical genetics. *In* Evans MI (ed): Reproductive Risks and Prenatal Diagnosis. Norwalk, CT, Appleton & Lange, 1992, pp 251–263.

The Canadian Early and Mid-Trimester Amniocentesis Trial

(CEMAT) Group: Randomised trial to assess safety and fetal outcome of early and midtrimester amniocentesis. Lancet 351:242–247, 1998.

Caskey CT, Rossiter BJF: Molecular genetics. *In* Evans MI (ed): Reproductive Risks and Prenatal Diagnosis. Norwalk, CT, Appleton & Lange, 1992, pp 265–274.

Cole LA, Kardana A, Park SY, et al: The deactivation of hCG by nicking and dissociation. J Clin Endocrinol Metab 76:704–710, 1993.

Crossley JA, Aitken DA, Connor JM: Prenatal screening for chromosome abnormalities using maternal serum chorionic gonadotrophin, alpha-fetoprotein, and age. Prenat Diagn 11:83–101, 1991.

Drugan A, Dvorin E, Koppitch FC, et al: Counseling for low maternal serum alpha-fetoprotein should emphasize all chromosome anomalies, not just Down Syndrome! Obstet Gynecol 73:271–274, 1989.

Drugan A, Johnson MP, Evans MI: Inheritance. *In* Evans MI (ed): Reproductive Risks and Prenatal Diagnosis. Norwalk, CT, Appleton & Lange, 1992, pp 3–23.

Drugan A, Johnson P, Hume RF, et al: Amniocentesis. *In* Evans MI, Johnson MP, Moghissi KR (eds): Invasive Outpatient Procedures in Reproductive Medicine. Philadelphia, Lippincott-Raven, 1997, pp 3–13.

Evans MI, Chik L, O'Brien JE, et al: MOMs and DADs: Improved specificity and cost effectiveness of biochemical screening for aneuploidy with DADs. Am J Obstet Gynecol 172:1138–1147, 1995.

Evans MI, Chik L, O'Brien JE, et al: Logistic regression generated probability estimates for trisomy 21 outcomes from serum AFP and bHCG: Simplification with increased specificity. J Matern Fetal Med 5:1–6, 1996.

Firth HV, Boyd PA, Chamberlain PF, et al: Analysis of limb reduction defects in babies exposed to chorionic villus sampling. Lancet 343:1069–1071, 1994.

Froster UG, Jackson L: Limb defects and chorionic villus sampling: Results from an international registry, 1992–94. Lancet 347:489–494, 1996.

Ganshirt-Ahlert D, Borjesson-Stoll R, Burschyk M, et al: Detection of fetal trisomies 21 and 18 from maternal blood suing triple gradient and magnetic cell sorting. Am J Reprod Immunol 30:194–201, 1993.

Hecht CA, Hood EB: The imprecision in rates of Down syndrome by 1-year maternal age intervals: A critical analysis of rates used in biochemical screening. Prenat Diagn 14:729–738, 1994.

Isada NB, Johnson MP, Drugan A, et al: Chorionic villus sampling. *In* Evans MI, Johnson MP, Moghissi KR (eds): Invasive Outpatient Procedures in Reproductive Medicine. Philadelphia, Lippincott-Raven, 1997, pp 15–33.

Johnson MP, Johnson A, Holzgreve W, et al: First trimester simple hygroma, cause and outcome. Am J Obstet Gynecol 168:156–161, 1993.

Macri JN, Kasturi RV, Krantz DA, et al: Maternal serum Down syndrome screening: Unconjugated estriol is not useful. Am J Obstet Gynecol 162:672–675, 1990.

Martin LS, Evans MI: Molecular genetics. *In* Gleisher N, Buttino L, Elkayam U, (eds): Principles and Practices of Medical Therapy in Pregnancy, 3rd ed. Norwalk, CT, Appleton & Lange, 1999.

Merkatz IR, Nitowsky HM, Macri JN: An association between low maternal serum alpha-fetoprotein and fetal chromosomal abnormalities. Am J Obstet Gynecol 148:886–889, 1984.

Pandya PP, Snijders RJ, Johnson SP, et al: Screening for fetal trisomies by maternal age and fetal nuchal trasnslucency thickness at 10 to 14 weeks of gestation. Br J Obstet Gynaecol 102:957–2, 1995.

Tafas T, Evans MI, Cuckle HS, et al: An automated image analysis method for the measurement of neutrophil alkaline phosphatase in the prenatal screening of Down syndrome. Fetal Diagn Ther 11:254–260, 1996.

Wald NJ, Cuckle HS, Densem JW, et al: Maternal serum screening for Down syndrome in early pregnancy. BMJ 297:883–888, 1988.

White MB, Krueger LJ, Holsclaw DS, et al: Detection of three rare frameshift mutations in the cystic fibrosis gene in an African American (CF444delA), an Italian (CF2522insC), and a Soviet (CF3821delT). Genomics 10:266–269, 1991.

# 21

# Fetal Assessment

ANTHONY W. OPIPARI
TIMOTHY R. B. JOHNSON

Broadly considered, fetal assessment provides information on intrauterine behavior, development, genetic potential, and biochemical physiology. With this information, the pregnant woman and her care provider can act to decrease risks of morbidity and mortality faced by the fetus. Attention in this chapter is directed specifically to the assessment of parameters that indicate the physiologic well-being of the fetus. Other chapters in this text deal with fetal assessment directed to determine morphologic characteristics, pulmonary maturity, and genetically inherited disease.

The primary objective of antenatal testing is to avoid fetal death. Testing procedures were developed to identify premorbid fetal cardiorespiratory compromise. Ideally, abnormal test results trigger obstetric intervention to prevent imminent fetal mortality. Contemporary use of antenatal testing has a broader secondary objective that goes beyond reducing fetal mortality to improving perinatal outcome. This broader objective is appropriate. Fetal assessment would be of no practical value if it only replaced intrauterine death with neonatal death and long-term morbidity. Although this broader objective is appealing, it must be recognized that all current forms of antenatal testing were designed simply to predict and avoid fetal death.

As a general note, the benefit derived from testing is dependent not only on the performance of the test, but also on the effectiveness of the therapy available for responding to the abnormal test. Therapeutic responses on behalf of the compromised fetus are limited (e.g., delivery, corticosteroids, occasionally antiarrhythmic drugs). Hence, although antenatal testing has become more reliable, the full potential clinical benefit awaits advancement of therapeutic options. This chapter presents methods of antenatal testing, evidence to support the clinical use of these tests, and guidelines for testing based on specific risk factors that are supported by findings from clinical trials.

## What Is the Scope of the Problem?

Vital statistics record the occurrence of fetal and infant death using various measures. Table 21–1 displays mortality rate definitions as standardized by the National Center for Health Statistics. The direct comparison of data on perinatal mortality from international sources must account for the definition used by the World Health Organization, which includes fetuses from a gestational age of 22 weeks.

Data from the National Vital Statistics System have documented that in 1991, a total of 35,926 perinatal deaths occurred, yielding a perinatal mortality rate

Table 21-1  Mortality Rate Definitions

| Measurement | Description |
| --- | --- |
| Fetal mortality rate | Fetal deaths after 20 wk of gestation per 1000 births |
| Perinatal mortality rate (I) | Fetal deaths after 28 wk plus deaths in the first 6 d of life per 1000 births |
| Perinatal mortality rate (II) | Fetal deaths after 20 wk plus deaths in the first 27 d of life per 1000 births |
| Neonatal mortality rate | Deaths in the first 27 d of life per 1000 live births |

(I)* of 8.7.[1] This rate is a record low for the United States, and marks a 19% decline over the preceding 6 years. Considering all fetal and neonatal deaths combined (a total of 53,138 deaths), 17,101 deaths (32%) occurred in utero after 28 weeks. This percentage, in particular, represents perinatal mortality that can be influenced by antenatal testing. The McGill Obstetrical Neonatal Database classified the primary cause of 278 fetal deaths occurring between 1978 and 1985. When lethal anomalies and unexplainable deaths are excluded from this series, more than 30% of fetal deaths are attributable to pathophysiologic processes that could potentially be detected by fetal assessment and treated by expedited delivery. Overall, uteroplacental insufficiency is estimated to account for 20 to 40% of perinatal deaths.

Perinatal mortality rates are related to the presence of maternal disease and complications during pregnancy and delivery. It is helpful to understand the distribution of perinatal death as it relates to these factors in order to appreciate the magnitude of risk, associated with conditions common in an obstetric population. Perinatal mortality data from the Swedish Medical Birth Registry classified according to maternal disease and obstetric complication, are summarized in Table 21-2. These data were collected between 1977 and 1978, which accounts for an overall mortality rate higher than the current rate in the United States. From this comparison, it is clear that perinatal mortality occurs quite frequently among certain subpopulations. Even if the overall rate of eight deaths per thousand births is considered an acceptable standard, the elevated mortality rates in various subgroups clearly testify to a significant problem.

A single perinatal death can cause immeasurable grief and despair. This problem must be understood in personal terms to fully determine the social and psychological costs associated with perinatal loss. Patient expectations of childbirth can be unrealistic, partly, because they do not have a sense of the risk of mortality faced by a fetus or neonate. Any fetal or perinatal death is devastating for both the patient and the obstetric care team. Perinatal loss is a significant stress that can cause deterioration in a patient's mental health.

## Who Is at Risk for Perinatal Death?

Assessing the risk of a pregnancy ending in an adverse outcome is a fundamental component of prenatal care. Risk assessment identifies pregnancies that are at increased risk for a poor outcome; thus, special care can be provided to reduce morbidity and mortality. Although fetal or perinatal death can occur in any pregnancy, epidemiologic evidence defines identifiable factors associated with an increased risk of poor pregnancy outcome. Petitti has presented an extensive list of these factors. When multiple risk factors are present, the outcome depends on each individual factor and the complex interplay between factors.

A high-risk pregnancy is one in which the chance of a poor outcome is greater than the overall risk of the population. Recent Scandinavian data from a multicenter collaborative study on birth outcomes demonstrate the high prevalence of these risk factors. Approximately 40% of parous gravid patients are at high risk on the basis of having one or more risk factors associated with poor birth outcome. In the high-risk group, the rate of fetal death was twice that of the low-risk group (relative risk [RR] 2.0; 95% confidence interval [CI] 1.2–3.4).

Table 21-2  Perinatal Mortality by Maternal and Obstetric Complication

| Complication | Number of Births | Perinatal Mortality Rate |
| --- | --- | --- |
| All births | 189,228 | 9.6 |
| No complications | 125,440 | 6.0 |
| Diabetes | 727 | 41.3 |
| Blood incompatibility | 857 | 22.2 |
| Renal disease | 263 | 38.0 |
| Preeclampsia and eclampsia | 15,099 | 14.1 |
| Previa/abruption | 2061 | 98.5 |
| Dystocia | 7335 | 7.2 |
| Malpresentation of fetus | 2969 | 17.9 |
| Prolonged labor | 14,276 | 7.8 |
| Uterine rupture | 51 | 215.7 |
| Complications of the umbilical cord | 391 | 97.2 |
| Fetal complications | 11,703 | 6.0 |

From Bakketeig LS, Hoffman HJ, Oakley AR: Perinatal mortality. In Bracken MB (ed): Perinatal Epidemiology. New York, Oxford University Press, 1984, pp 130–131.

---

*Calculation of perinatal mortality rate (I): (number of deaths of infants younger than 7 days of age + number of fetal deaths after gestation of at least 28 weeks)/(number of live births + number of fetal deaths after gestation of at least 28 weeks) ×1000.

## Which Patients Should Undergo Fetal Testing?

Ideally, testing should be administered to patients who are likely to benefit based on well-controlled studies. Unfortunately, fetal testing procedures became part of routine practice before appropriate use was established and before such trials could be performed. In contemporary practice, fetal testing is performed in pregnancies that have identifiable risk factors for fetal and perinatal death. Although clinical studies have not substantiated a benefit from testing in most specific high-risk conditions, antenatal testing of patients who have these conditions is, nevertheless, part of routine practice. Some of the risk factors that prompt testing are likely associated with causes of death that do not alter uteroplacental function or fetal behavior; in these cases testing is likely to be of no benefit. Without clinical trials, however, the complexity of pathophysiologic processes makes it impossible to predict accurately that a particular high-risk subgroup would not benefit, and, therefore, it is impractical to withhold testing that is already commonplace. Given the current practice climate, clinical trials could be used to improve standard practice by revealing risk groups that derive no benefit from a specific test. Thus, unnecessary (and potentially harmful) use of testing could be curtailed.

It must be recognized that the ability of antenatal testing procedures to ascribe a probability of either fetal compromise or fetal well-being (i.e., positive or negative predictive values) depends on the prevalence of disease in the population being tested. It follows that in populations with a higher prevalence of fetal compromise, testing has a higher positive predictive value. Therefore, selecting the correct population for testing increases the benefit derived per test performed, decreases the number of unnecessary and potentially harmful interventions performed in response to false-positive tests, and supports efforts to distribute medical resources rationally.

## What Methods Can Be Used to Assess Fetal Well-being?

### MATERNAL ASSESSMENT OF FETAL MOVEMENT

Historically, maternal perception of fetal movement has been an important sign of intrauterine life. Mothers perceive 88% of the fetal movements detected by Doppler imaging. The physiologic basis for using movement as an indicator of fetal well-being is that a motor response reflects intact cortical nerve function, which in turn depends on adequate fetal cardiovascular and uteroplacental function. Moreover, fetal movements are coupled with fetal heart rate responses that independently indicate fetal well-being. During normal fetal development, patterns of movement evolve predictably according to gestational age.

---

**BOX 21–1  MATERNAL ASSESSMENT OF FETAL MOVEMENT**

*Definite Indications*
- None

*Weaker Indications*
- Any pregnancy irrespective of risk

*Appropriate Gestational Age*
- Beyond 24 wk

*Testing Frequency*
- Daily

*Abnormal Test Indicates Immediate Delivery If*
- Other tests cannot reassure fetal well-being

---

**Methodology.** Systematic monitoring of maternally perceived fetal movements offers a screening technique that can be universally applied and is independent of technologic cost. Various methods to systematize fetal movement reporting have been used. The Cardiff count-to-10 method was validated and used in the study by Moore and Picquadio. Beginning at 28 weeks of gestation, the patient is asked to record the time interval it takes to appreciate 10 fetal movements. The patient is asked to conduct the assessment in the evening while lying comfortably on her left side. A patient who does not perceive 10 movements within 2 hours is asked to present immediately for evaluation.

**Response.** The patient presents for further antenatal testing if fetal movement is below the threshold value of 10 movements in 2 hours. The patient is evaluated with a nonstress test and screened for evidence of ruptured membranes, labor, oligohydramnios or polyhydramnios, and preeclampsia.

**Limitations.** Two prospective, controlled studies suggest a benefit to maternal monitoring of fetal movement in low-risk populations. Neldam has reported on more than 3000 patients alternately assigned to either a specific monitoring group or a control group not instructed to monitor activity. Three times as many fetal deaths occurred in the unmonitored group. Moore and Piacquadio compared fetal mortality between a historical control group composed of 2519 deliveries and 1864 patients who monitored fetal activity. Four times as many fetal deaths occurred in the control group.

The largest and most convincing study reported to date includes 68,000 women randomized to compare formalized fetal movement counting with standard care in the overall obstetric population. This trial did not identify any improvement in perinatal outcome with formal daily movement monitoring in the low-risk population. Given the proper design and large sample size of this trial, daily movement monitoring is not a recommended screening practice for all pregnancies. Sizable clinical trials to evaluate this test in high-risk populations have not been performed. Without direct evidence in the literature, there continues to be speculation that this method is a reasonable adjunct to use with regularly scheduled fetal tests in the high-risk population.

## NONSTRESS TEST

The nonstress test (NST) is the most frequently used technique for fetal assessment. Depending on the test result and clinical situation, it is used both as a screening test to base further evaluation and as a diagnostic test to decide intervention. Historically, this method of testing evolved from early observations by Kennedy in 1833, which associated an ominous fetal outcome with the slow return of the fetal heart rate (FHR) to baseline after a uterine contraction. Conversely, fetal well-being was predicted by the presence of FHR accelerations during contraction activity. Analysis of the FHR during uterine *inactivity* (nonstressed state) demonstrated a similar correlation between spontaneous accelerations and good fetal outcome.

---

### BOX 21–2  NONSTRESS TEST

**Definite Indications**
- Decreased fetal movement
- Diabetes requiring insulin
- Rh incompatibility
- Trauma
- Hyperthyroidism
- Postdates

**Weaker Indications**
- Many risk factors

**Appropriate Gestational Age**
- Beyond 30 wk

**Testing Frequency**
- Twice weekly
- Trauma—up to 24 hr of continuous monitoring

**Abnormal test indicates immediate delivery if**
- Other tests cannot reassure fetal well-being

**False-negative rate**
- 3–5 fetal deaths per 1000 normal tests

**False-positive rate**
- Exceeds 50%

---

**Methodology.** The NST is simple, noninvasive, and easy to perform. FHR is determined with the patient lying on her left side, usually using electronic monitoring equipment to generate a cardiotocographic display. An NST is interpreted as being either reactive (reassuring) or nonreactive (nonreassuring) based on the presence of accelerations. The period of observation for an NST is usually 20 minutes. After 20 minutes, 76% of term fetuses have reactive tests, compared with 98% after 80 minutes. The length of time required to demonstrate reactivity does not correlate with fetal status. Testing is typically instituted at 30 to 32 weeks of gestation and is performed twice a week.

**Interpretation.** Interpretation of the NST is primarily based on the presence of FHR accelerations. At the University of Michigan Medical Center, criteria for a reactive tracing include the presence of two or more accelerations with an amplitude of at least 15 beats per minute above baseline and a duration of at least 15 seconds (baseline to baseline). No attempt is made to record fetal movement or correlate it with accelerations. Any tracing not demonstrating these findings during a 20-minute observation period is deemed nonreactive, and the patient is subsequently further assessed. Additionally, to be considered reactive, the tracing must have a baseline rate between 120 and 160 beats per minute and be without decelerations after spontaneous uterine contractions.

**Response.** Nonreactive NST results are followed up with immediate further testing. The subsequent testing is usually a biophysical profile, but ultrasonography for assessing growth, Doppler velocimetry, and, occasionally, hospital admission for continuous fetal monitoring are appropriate. If an ominous tracing (e.g., repetitive, late decelerations) is uncovered in a mature fetus, immediate delivery is appropriate.

**Limitations.** As a screening test for predicting perinatal mortality, the NST has a low false-negative rate (less than 2%), but a false-positive rate between 50 and 80% (based on a comprehensive review by Thacker and Berkelman). From the same review, *the sensitivity of the NST was less than 50%* in 9 of 19 studies. Data from four published randomized trials demonstrate no clinical benefit of NSTs in improving high-risk pregnancy outcome; however, the statistical power of these studies was insufficient to detect clinically relevant differences. It must be emphasized that the high false-positive rate associated with a nonreactive test obligates confirmation of fetal jeopardy by other means before definitive treatment is begun.

Reactive patterns characteristically develop as gestational age advances. The relationship between reactivity and gestational age has been explored in high-risk pregnancies. At 24 to 28 weeks of gestation, 45% of tests are reactive; between 28 and 32 weeks of gestation, approximately 85% of tests are reactive; beyond this gestational age, 95% of tests are reactive. Intriguingly, behavior analysis of fetuses less than 28 weeks of gestation has revealed that 97% of the FHR changes are *decelerations* and that the majority of these are associated with fetal movement. The baseline FHR declines with advancing gestation and partially accounts for fewer accelerations attaining an amplitude of 15 beats per minute in gestational ages between 24 and 28 weeks of gestation. Given these confounding influences, the predicative value of the nonreactive NST for pregnancy before 32 weeks has not been established.

## BIOPHYSICAL PROFILE

The high false-positive rate of the NST precludes its use as a test on which to base definitive intervention. Before the availability of real-time ultrasonography, nonreassuring NST results were followed up with a contraction stress test (CST). The NST-CST combination still resulted in an unacceptably high false-positive rate, approaching 75%. Additionally, the very nature of the CST poses a significant risk of aggravating many obstetric conditions. The biophysical profile was developed as a testing method that would have a lower false-positive rate than the NST, as well as a sufficiently high positive predictive value on which to base therapeutic decisions.

The biophysical profile (BPP) has been likened to a physical examination of the fetus in the intrauterine environment, with access provided by real-time ultrasonographic imaging. With consideration of the principles underlying Apgar scoring of the newborn infant, the BPP was designed to measure five similar biophysical variables: breathing, muscle tone, movements, FHR, and amniotic fluid volume. Because these parameters can be affected by hypoxemia, hypercapnia, and acidosis, the BPP is expected to detect fetal disease states that involve asphyxia. Even though asphyxia is not the primary pathophysiologic problem underlying many fetal diseases (e.g., infections and congenital malformations), nearly all disease processes that lead to a moribund fetus eventually result in asphyxia. This infers an additional role for the BPP in ruling out a moribund condition in pregnancies that are at high risk from diseases that are primarily nonasphyxiant in nature.

**Methodology.** At the University of Michigan, the most common reason a BPP is performed is to further evaluate a patient after a nonreactive NST. As described by Manning, real-time ultrasonographic imaging is used to measure biophysical variables. The observations are then scored according to the criteria outlined in Table 21–3. The period of observation for

**Table 21–3** Criteria for Scoring the Biophysical Profile

| Variable | Minimal Criteria | Points if Criteria Met |
|---|---|---|
| NST | Reactive pattern | 2 |
| Fetal breathing | 1 episode lasting at least 30 seconds | 2 |
| Gross body movement | 3 body/limb movements | 2 |
| Fetal muscle tone | 1 episode of extension with return to flexion | 2 |
| Amniotic fluid | 1 pocket at least 2 cm in vertical depth | 2 |

NST = nonstress test.

a BPP is set at 30 minutes. Any variable not meeting criteria within this time period is scored as abnormal. The NST component can be omitted when all other biophysical variables are normal. When used as the primary method of testing in a high-risk pregnancy, the BPP can be performed weekly, twice weekly, or daily, depending on the clinical situation.

---

**BOX 21–3  BIOPHYSICAL PROFILE**

*Definite Indications*
- Nonreactive nonstress test

*Weaker Indications*
- Many risk factors

*Appropriate Gestational Age*
- Beyond 24 wk

*Testing Frequency*
- Weekly after normal test
- Twice weekly after abnormal test

*Abnormal test indicates immediate delivery if*
- Score is 4 or lower
- Fetus is at term
- Other tests cannot reassure fetal well-being

*False-negative rate*
- 0.6 fetal deaths per 1000 normal tests

*False-positive rate (by score):*
- 6: 60%, 4: 37%, 2: 27%, 0: 0%

---

**Interpretation.** Observational studies have convincingly demonstrated a correlation between BPP score and perinatal mortality, establishing the ability of this test to predict adverse perinatal outcome. Perinatal morbidity and mortality data were collected by Manning on a subset of 26,780 high-risk fetuses assessed by BPP testing. Table 21–4 summarizes the mortality data from this study. Scores of 8 or 10 are associated with lower perinatal mortality than expected in the overall population and, on this basis, are considered

**Table 21–4** BPP Score With Associated Corrected Mortality Rate

| Score | Number of Fetuses | Fetal Mortality Rate | Perinatal Mortality Rate |
|---|---|---|---|
| 8 or 10 | 12,307 | 1.38 | 1.54 |
| 6 | 512 | 3.90 | 9.76 |
| 4 | 228 | 17.5 | 26.3 |
| 2 | 117 | 51.3 | 94 |
| 0 | 28 | 178.5 | 285.7 |

From Manning FA, Harman CR, Morrison I, et al: Fetal assessment based on intrauterine (IU) fetal biophysical profile scoring. An analysis of perinatal morbidity and mortality. Am J Obstet Gynecol 162:703–709, 1990.

reassurances of fetal well-being. On the other hand, the high mortality rate associated with scores of 6 or less allows these scores to proxy fetal compromise.

**Response.** No universal response to a given score can be outlined, because other factors affecting neonatal survival (gestational age, presence of fetal anomalies, availability of an expertly staffed neonatal intensive care unit [NICU] must be considered before obstetric intervention is decided. Nevertheless, a few generalizations can be made. Beginning at the gestational age at which neonatal treatment can reasonably be expected to rescue the moribund fetus, expedited or immediate delivery is indicated with scores of 4 or lower. At the University of Michigan, this qualification is currently met by pregnancies between 24 and 25 weeks of gestation. At term, or with documented fetal lung maturity, a score of 6 is an indication to deliver the fetus. When factors preclude delivery of a preterm fetus with a score of 6 points, repeat testing is indicated within 24 hours. At term or after the expected due date, a score of 8, derived from testing that allots zero points for amniotic fluid, is an indication for delivery.

**Limitations.** Manning and others have found a significantly better positive predictive value for the BPP compared with the NST, along with a trend toward improved sensitivity. Nonetheless, the sensitivity and positive predictive value of the BPP are not high enough to justify use in screening a low-risk population. Although observational studies have strongly suggested a link between BPP score and outcome, there are limited data supporting a beneficial effect on outcome in pregnancies exposed to BPP testing. Disappointingly, a meta-analysis of the randomized trials evaluating BPP found *no evidence that this testing decreased adverse outcomes* in high-risk pregnancies to any greater extent than did standard fetal cardiography.

## MODIFIED BIOPHYSICAL PROFILE

The modified biophysical profile is composed of an NST along with an ultrasonographically determined amniotic fluid index (AFI). With this combination of tests, both acute and chronic problems are expected to be manifest. The tests should reveal the fetal heart rate reflecting the *instantaneous* cardiorespiratory status of the fetal-placental unit and the amniotic fluid volume indexing *chronic* fetal and placental perfusion.

Observational studies have demonstrated that the modified BPP is an effective means of predicting fetal mortality. Miller and associates reported on the use of the modified BPP as the primary antepartum testing method in 15,482 high-risk pregnancies. In this study, the false-negative rate (defined as the incidence of fetal death within 1 week of normal testing) was 0.8 per 1000 patients. The false-negative rate is comparable to that achieved with the complete BPP (0.6 per 1000 patients). The false-positive rate has been reported to range from 41 to 60%. By way of comparison, these values are clearly superior to those associated with the NST.

---

**BOX 21–4   MODIFIED BIOPHYSICAL PROFILE**

*Definite Indications*
- Decreased fetal movement
- Diabetes requiring insulin
- Postdates

*Weaker Indications*
- Many risk factors

*Appropriate Gestational Age*
- Beyond 30 wk

*Testing Frequency*
- Usually twice weekly

*Abnormal test indicates immediate delivery if*
- Amniotic fluid index (AFI) <5 and gestation beyond 37 wk
- Other tests cannot reassure fetal well-being

*False-negative rate*
- 0.8 fetal deaths per 1000 normal tests

*False-positive rate*
- 40–60%

---

**Methodology.** The NST is performed as detailed previously. After the NST has been performed, with the patient in the same position, amniotic fluid volume is assessed with real-time ultrasonography. The frontal plane of the uterus is divided into four equal-sized quadrants. Each of the quadrants is scanned to visualize the amniotic fluid pocket within each quadrant having the largest anterior to posterior dimension. By convention, only pockets of fluid not containing umbilical cord can be considered. Measurements of the vertical depth (anterior to posterior distance in centimeters) of the largest fluid pocket in each quadrant are recorded. The AFI is calculated as the sum of the four quadrant measurements.

**Interpretation.** The NST component is considered reactive according to the criteria described earlier. The AFI is considered normal at values greater than or equal to 5. Having either a nonreactive NST or an AFI below 5 makes the modified BPP test nonreassuring.

**Response.** With a normal test result (reactive NST, AFI ≥5), testing is repeated within 1 week. If only the NST component is abnormal, a complete BPP should be performed immediately and used as a base for further management.

When the AFI is less than 5 but the NST is reactive, management hinges on gestational age. Beyond 37 weeks of gestation, immediate delivery should be considered. Before 37 weeks, further evaluation should include a complete BPP, an ultrasonogram for checking growth, a Doppler study of the umbilical artery, and other tests, as clinically indicated, for evaluation of oligohydramnios.

If both NST and AFI are abnormal and the patient is beyond 37 weeks, immediate delivery is indicated. At gestational ages less than 37 weeks, management should include an immediate complete BPP, an ultrasonogram for checking growth, a Doppler study of the umbilical artery, and hospitalization for continuous fetal monitoring until delivery or repeat testing becomes reassuring.

**Limitations.** Although its predictive ability has been established, the modified BPP has not yet been evaluated for its ability to improve perinatal outcome in comparative trials.

The primary advantage of this method compared with the complete BPP lies in the time and effort saved by abbreviating the ultrasonographic examination. Conversely, in a modified BPP the NST is mandatory, and this test alone requires a minimum of 20 minutes to complete. Because the NST can be omitted from a complete BPP when all other parameters are normal, the modified BPP may actually require more time. Given the comparable performance of these tests in clinical trials, factors such as personnel experience and equipment availability often determine the method favored by a testing unit.

## DOPPLER VELOCIMETRY OF THE UMBILICAL ARTERY

Doppler ultrasonography has been applied to the study of fetal cardiovascular function, including assessment of fetal blood flow within the umbilical artery. As flow through the umbilical artery is affected by downstream characteristics of the placental vascular tree, this technology was evaluated for its potential in predicting fetal outcome in pregnancies complicated by abnormal placental function. Early studies suggested that flow through the umbilical artery was different in fetuses that were compromised by complicated pregnancies compared with that of fetuses in normal gestations.

The umbilical artery Doppler waveform is used to determine the peak systolic frequency shift value (S), the peak diastolic value (D), and the mean value (M) over one cardiac cycle. From these measurements, the ratio of S/D and the pulsatility index ([S-D]/M) are calculated. Absence and reversal in the direction of diastolic flow can also be detected. Using statistical methods, normal values have been established from measurements taken during uncomplicated pregnancies. In the course of normal pregnancy the S/D ratio and the pulsatility index decrease as the gestational age advances.

Increased values of the S/D ratio and pulsatility index correlate with abnormal histomorphology of the placental bed. A prospective multicenter trial demonstrated the significance of absent or reversed diastolic flow in 459 high-risk pregnancies complicated with hypertension, fetal growth restriction, or both. In this high-risk population, the odds ratio for perinatal mortality with absent diastolic flow was 4.0; with reversed flow, it was 10.6. Many other observational studies support this relationship between abnormal flow and poor outcome in pregnancies complicated by chronic hypertension, preeclampsia, or growth restriction.

Unlike the testing methods described previously, controlled clinical trials *have* preceded the widespread adoption of this technology into practice. In aggregate, more than 9000 patients have been included in the controlled, comparative studies reported in the literature. In general, these studies suggest that *the addition of Doppler results to the information provided by other testing methods improves perinatal outcome.* In Maulik's review of 8 published randomized controlled trials 6 studies (involving 6022 patients) showed significant clinical benefit from the addition of Doppler testing. A meta-analysis of 11 carefully selected randomized trials by the Cochrane Database reported that Doppler testing in complicated pregnancies is associated with a 29% reduction in the risk of perinatal death. In this same analysis, trends toward fewer labor inductions and fewer cesarean sections were also identified.

**Methodology.** The patient is placed in a recumbent position with a comfortable amount of left lateral displacement. Real-time ultrasonography is used to allow identification of a loop of cord located nearer to the placenta than to the fetus and also to exclude the presence of concurrent fetal breathing activity. Although fetal breathing movements can alter the waveform, other fetal movements do not compromise Doppler results. We apply a 4-MHz continuous wave transducer and position it so as to achieve the maximum amplitude of the systolic wave shift. Doppler waveforms are captured on an attached video monitor, and from a representative cycle, the peak systolic shift, diastolic shift, S/D ratio, and direction (or absence) of end-diastolic flow is determined. For each study, these measurements are made three separate times. The S/D values are reported separately along with their mean. Absent or reversed diastolic flow is only reported when it is a consistent finding with each measurement. The report includes the corresponding normal values (mean, 5th, and 95th percentiles), according to gestational age derived from uncomplicated pregnancies as presented in Table 21–5.

**Table 21–5** Normal Range for S/D Values According to Gestational Age

| Gestational Age (wk) | S/D (Mean) | 5th Percentile | 95th Percentile |
|---|---|---|---|
| 20 | 3.94 | 2.73 | 7.04 |
| 24 | 3.46 | 2.56 | 5.35 |
| 28 | 3.15 | 2.47 | 4.37 |
| 30 | 2.79 | 2.11 | 4.08 |
| 32 | 2.70 | 2.08 | 3.85 |
| 34 | 2.57 | 1.90 | 3.95 |
| 36 | 2.25 | 1.77 | 3.09 |
| 38 | 2.16 | 1.74 | 2.85 |
| 40 | 2.07 | 1.72 | 2.60 |

Mean values, as well as 5th and 95th percentile values were calculated from data presented by Thompson and associates. All values were based on normal reference values for the Pourcelot ratio (PR) according to the formula S/D = 1/(1 − PR).

---

**BOX 21–5 UMBILICAL ARTERY DOPPLER VELOCIMETRY**

*Definite Indications*
- Hypertensive disorders, fetal growth restriction

*Weaker Indications*
- Postdates
- Many risk factors, excluding White class A–D diabetics

*Appropriate Gestational Age*
- Beyond 24 wk

*Testing Frequency*
- Weekly after normal test
- Twice weekly after abnormal test

*Abnormal test indicates immediate delivery if*
- Absent or reversed diastolic flow reported
- Fetus is at term
- Other tests cannot reassure fetal well-being

*False-negative rate*
- Not reported

*False-positive rate (by score)*
- Not reported

---

**Interpretation and Response.** Fetuses demonstrating absent or reversed end-diastolic flow are at significant risk for perinatal mortality, independent of gestational age. The risk of intrauterine death is 14% with absent flow and 24% with reversed flow; therefore, immediate delivery is advised for either of these findings once the fetus has reached the earliest gestational age that can be supported by the available NICU.

Finding an S/D value above the 95th percentile prompts immediate delivery of the term fetus. For the preterm fetus with an elevated S/D ratio, twice weekly testing, including umbilical artery Doppler ultrasonograms and amniotic fluid determination, is indicated. In addition, for fetuses within this group that are less than 34 weeks of gestational age, antenatal corticosteroids to accelerate fetal maturity should be strongly considered.

**Limitations.** Although data compiled in controlled trials clearly support the use of umbilical artery Doppler ultrasonography for improving perinatal outcome in high-risk pregnancy, differences in the methodology among the comparative studies limit direct extrapolation to clinical practice. Most significantly, *no particular response algorithm was established by these trials as being the appropriate treatment after an abnormal test.* Moreover, it is unclear from these reports whether testing should be limited to hypertensive and growth restricted pregnancies or whether the overall high-risk population would benefit from this testing. It is equally uncertain whether the S/D ratio or simply the presence and direction of end-diastolic flow is the more appropriate criterion on which to base the assessment.

## Guidelines for Indication-Specific Fetal Testing

Most studies supporting the diagnostic efficacy and the clinical benefit of antenatal testing have used populations of high-risk patients that are heterogeneous for risk factors. For example, in the studies reported by Manning and associates, based on their experience with the BPP, more than 20 different primary indications for testing were identified among the high-risk pregnancies evaluated. These indications are diverse, including conditions such as hypertension, twins, premature labor, congenital fetal heart disease, and Rh disease. The pathologic processes associated with these various clinical indicators are

**Table 21–6** Indication-Specific Fetal Assessment

| Indication | Appropriate Testing |
|---|---|
| Postdates | AFI, NST, BPP |
| Growth restriction, hypertension, vascular disease, antiphospholipid syndrome | Doppler, AFI, NST, BPP, Fetal ultrasound for growth |
| Insulin-dependent diabetes | NST, BPP |
| Insulin-dependent diabetes (class F-R) | NST, BPP, Doppler |
| Premature rupture of membranes | BPP, NST, AFI |
| Vaginal bleeding | NST, BPP |
| Decreased fetal movements | NST, BPP |
| Rh disease | Maternal fetal movement counts, Fetal ultrasound to rule out heart failure, BPP |
| Nonimmune fetal hydrops | BPP, NST |
| Fetal arrhythmia | Fetal ultrasound to rule out heart failure, BPP |
| Maternal hyperthyroidism | NST, Fetal ultrasound for growth |
| Low-risk pregnancies | ? |

AFI = amniotic fluid index; NST = nonstress test; BPP = biophysical profile.
From Vintzileos APM: Antepartum fetal surveillance. Clin Obstet Gynecol 38:1, 2, 1995.

thought to be different. Because a particular test measures only certain pathophysiologic effects, the efficacy of any test varies, depending on the indication. With the present availability of several alternative testing technologies, this notion logically suggests that testing should be specific to the indication. Vintzileos has supported the need for indication-specific testing and outlined appropriate tests for various common indications. His recommendations are presented in Table 21–6. It is important to realize that although indication-specific testing is a future direction in the field of fetal assessment, recommendations based on solid evidence cannot yet be made for most specific risk factors.

## GENERAL HIGH-RISK APPROACH

If high-risk patients have disease or risk factors for which no convincing evidence exists to specifically direct testing, we implement a general approach outlined in the following algorithm. As early as 26 to 28 weeks of gestation, the patients are instructed on maternal fetal movement monitoring according to the Cardiff method. Beginning at 30 to 32 weeks of gestation, patients are scheduled for twice weekly testing with either the NST or the modified BPP. The choice of method is left to the preference of the attending physician. According to the protocol, if either test is abnormal, a complete BPP is performed immediately. Consideration is also given to whether useful information would be provided by umbilical artery Doppler imaging, an ultrasonogram for checking growth, or admission for continuous fetal monitoring. Decisions are made using the test results in the context of the level of fetal maturity, the rate of disease progression, and the understanding of other comorbid factors. The information obtained from antenatal testing is only one supportive element in the management of patients who have high-risk pregnancies.

## REFERENCES

Alfirevic Z, Neilson JP: Biophysical profile for fetal assessment in high risk pregnancies. In Neilson JP, Crowther CA, Hodnett ED, et al (eds): Pregnancy and Childbirth Module of The Cochrane Database of Systematic Reviews, [updated June, 6 1996]. Available in The Cochrane Library [database on disk and CD ROM]. The Cochrane Colloboration; Issue 2. Oxford: Update Software; 1996, pp 1–8. Available from: BMJ Publishing Group, London.

Ananth CV, Smulian JC, Vintzileos AM: Epidemiology of antepartum fetal testing. Curr Opin Obstet Gynecol 9:101–106, 1997.

Brown R, Patrick J: The nonstress test: how long is enough? Am J Obstet Gynecol 141:646–649, 1981.

Clark SL, Sabey P, Jolley K: Nonstress testing with acoustic stimulation and amniotic fluid assessment: 5973 tests without unexpected fetal death. Am J Obstet Gynecol 160:694–697, 1989.

Cohn HE, Sacks EJ, Heymann MA, Rudolph AM: Cardiovascular responses to hypoxemia and acidemia in fetal lambs. Am J Obstet Gynecol 120:817–824, 1974.

Druzin ML, Fox A, Kogut E, Carlson C: The relationship of the nonstress test to gestational age. Am J Obstet Gynecol 153:386–389, 1985.

Forouzan I, Cohen AW, Arger P: Measurement of systolic-diastolic ratio in the umbilical artery by continuous-wave and pulsed-wave Doppler ultrasound: Comparison at different sites. Obstet Gynecol 77:209–212, 1991.

Fox HE, Steinbrecher M, Ripton B: Antepartum fetal heart rate and uterine activity studies. Am J Obstet Gynecol 126:61–69, 1976.

Fretts RC, Usher RH: Causes of fetal death in women of advanced maternal age. Obstet Gynecol 89:40–45, 1997.

Grant A, Elbourne D, Valentin L, Alexander S: Routine formal fetal movement counting and risk of antepartum late death in normally formed singletons. Lancet 2:345–349, 1989.

Hoyert DL: Perinatal mortality in the United States, 1985–91. National Center for Health Statistics. Vital Health Stat 20:1–20, 1995.

Isaksen CV, Laurini RN, Jacobsen G: Pre-pregnancy risk factors of small-for-gestational-age births and perinatal mortality. Acta Obstet Gynecol Scand 76:44–49, 1997.

Janssen HJ, Cuisinier MC, Hoogduin KA, de Graauw KP: Controlled prospective study on the mental health of women following pregnancy loss. Am J Psychiatry 153:226–230, 1996.

Johnson TRB, Jordan ET, Paine LL: Doppler recordings of fetal movement II. Comparison with maternal perception. Obstet Gynecol 76:42–43, 1990.

Kaar K: Antepartal cardiotocography in the assessment of fetal outcome. Acta Obstet Gynecol Scand 94(suppl):1, 1980.

Karsdorp VHM, van Vugt JMG, van Geijn HP, et al: Clinical significance of absent or reversed end diastolic velocity waveforms in umbilical artery. Lancet 344:1664–1668, 1994.

Lavin JP Jr, Modovnik M, Barden TP: Relationship of non-stress test reactivity and gestational age. Obstet Gynecol 63:338–344, 1984.

Lee CY, DiLoreto PC, Logrand B: Fetal activity acceleration determination for the evaluation of fetal reserve. Obstet Gynecol 48:19–27, 1976.

Manning FA, Platt LD: Maternal hypoxemia and fetal breathing movements. Obstet Gynecol 53:758–764, 1979.

Manning FA, Platt LD, Sipos L: Antepartum fetal evaluation:

development of a fetal biophysical profile. Am J Obstet Gynecol 136:787–795, 1980.
Manning FA, Lange IR, Morrison I, Harman CR: Fetal biophysical profile score and the nonstress test: a comparative trial. Obstet Gynecol 64:326–331, 1984.
Manning FA, Morrison I, Lange IR, et al: Fetal assessment based on fetal biophysical profile scoring: experience in 12,620 referred high-risk pregnancies. I. Perinatal mortality by frequency and etilogy. Am J Obstet Gynecol 151:343–350, 1985.
Manning FA, Morrison I, Lange IR, et al: Fetal biophysical profile scoring: Selective use of the nonstress test. Am J Obstet Gynecol 156:709–712, 1987.
Manning FA, Harman CR, Morrison I, et al: Fetal assessment based on fetal biophysical profile scoring IV. An analysis of perinatal morbidity and mortality. Am J Obstet Gynecol 162:703–709, 1990.
Manning FA: Dynamic ultrasound-based fetal assessment: The fetal biophysical profile score. Clin Obstet Gynecol 38:26–44, 1995.
Maulik D: Doppler ultrasound velocimetry for fetal surveillance. Clin Obstet Gynecol 38:91–111, 1995.
Miller DA, Rabello YA, Paul RH: The modified biophysical profile: Antepartum testing in the 1990s. Am J Obstet Gynecol 174:812–817, 1996.
Moore TR, Piacquadio K: A prospective evaluation of fetal movement screening to reduce the incidence of antepartum fetal death. Am J Obstet Gynecol 160:1075–1080, 1989.
Natale R, Nasello C, Turliuk R: The relationship between movements and accelerations in fetal heart rate at twenty-four to thirty-two weeks' gestation. Am J Obstet Gynecol 148:591–595, 1984.
Neilson JP, Alfirevic Z: Doppler ultrasound in high-risk pregnancies. In Neilson JP, Crowther CA, Hodnett ED, et al (eds): Pregnancy and Childbirth module of The Cochrane Database of Systematic Reviews, [updated 6 June 1996]. Available in The Cochrane Library [database on disk and CD ROM]. The Cochrane Colloboration; Issue 2. Oxford: Update Software; 1996, pp 1–5. Available from: BMJ Publishing Group, London.
Neldam S: Fetal movements. A comparison between maternal assessment and registration by means of dynamic ultrasound. Danish Med Bull 29:197–206, 1982.
Petitti DB: The epidemiology of fetal death. Clin Obstet Gynecol 30:253–258, 1987.
Platt LD, Walla CA, Paul RH, et al: A prospective trial of the fetal biophysical profile versus the nonstress test in the management of high-risk pregnancies. Am J Obstet Gynecol 153:624–633, 1985.
Thacker SB, Berkelman RL: Assessing the diagnostic accuracy and efficacy of selected antepartum fetal surveillance techniques. Obstet Gynecol Surv 41:121–141, 1986.
Thompson RS, Trudinger BJ, Cook CM, Giles WB: Umbilical artery velocity waveforms: Normal reference values for A/B ratio and Pourcelot ratio. Br J Obstet Gynaecol 95:589–591, 1988.
van Eyck J, Wladimiroff JW, Noordam MJ, et al: The blood flow velocity waveform in the fetal internal carotid and umbilical artery: Its relation to fetal behavioural states in the growth retarded fetus at 37–38 weeks gestation. Br J Obstet Gynaecol 95:473–477, 1988.
Vintzileos AM: Antepartum fetal surveillance. Clin Obstet Gynecol 38:1–2, 1995.
Voigt HJ, Becker V: Doppler flow measurements and histomorphology of the placental bed in uteroplacental insufficiency. J Perinatol Med 20:139–147, 1992.
Ware DJ, Devoe LD: The nonstress test: Reassessment of the "gold standard." Clin Perinatol 21:779–796, 1994.

# 22

# First-Trimester Ultrasonography

MARJORIE C. TREADWELL

Improvements in ultrasonography have resulted in increasing use of this modality for management of both obstetric and gynecologic patients. Obstetricians have access to office-based transvaginal sonography, which has increased the frequency of scanning in the first trimester of gestation. Obstetricians are thus required to gain familiarity with early fetal development and with potential markers for normal and abnormal pregnancy outcomes. Because of the increased ultrasonographic frequencies used in transvaginal scanning and the improved resolution that results, this chapter focuses on transvaginal vs. transabdominal ultrasonography for evaluation of the first trimester of pregnancy.

## Location of the Pregnancy

At approximately 4.5 weeks of gestation (based on the last menstrual period), an intradecidual sac may be seen via ultrasonography. The trophoblastic ring appears echogenic and is usually eccentrically located within the endometrial cavity. Definite identification of intrauterine pregnancy is possible as early as 29 to 35 days of gestation. The discriminatory zone refers to the β-human chorionic gonadotropin (β-hCG) level at which an intrauterine pregnancy can be identified with certainty. There is some variation between ultrasonographic units regarding the exact titer to use for the discriminatory zone, but a conservative β-hCG level of 2000 mIU/ml, First International Reference Preparation, minimizes the likelihood of labeling normal intrauterine pregnancy as abnormal and accounts for the increased β-hCG that is present in multiple gestation.

Initial identification of the gestational sac is made with the double ring or double decidua sign. This refers to the interface between the decidua and the chorion and appears as two distinct layers of the wall of the gestational sac. Although this is an early sign, it is not always reliable and false-positive test results do occur. Confirmation of an intrauterine pregnancy with 100% certainty is aided by identification of structures (yolk sac, fetal pole) within the gestational sac. Although a heterotopic pregnancy is unusual, the diagnosis should still be considered if the patient has clinical symptoms of an ectopic pregnancy despite identification of an intrauterine pregnancy.

If no intrauterine pregnancy is identified, it becomes more important to look for signs of ectopic pregnancy, especially if the β-hCG is greater than 2000 mIU/ml. Early in gestation, the endometrium appears prominent. Development of a pseudogestational sac may occur before or after onset of vaginal bleeding as the decidua begins to slough. The differentiation between a pseudogestational sac—or pseudosac—and an early intrauterine gestational sac is important. The pseudosac tends to be centrally located in the uterus and may be irregularly shaped. There are no structures present within the pseudosac, and the double ring sign, which signifies the chorion and decidua interface, is absent. Definitive diagnosis of ectopic pregnancy with visualization of an embryo outside the uterus may occur in fewer than 15% of ectopic pregnancies. More common findings include a cystic or complex adnexal mass or free fluid in the pelvis. The combination of a noncystic mass and free fluid in the cul-de-sac is found in 22% of all ectopic gestations. Correlation with patient history and clinical information is helpful.

## Determining Viability

Once a pregnancy has been determined to be intrauterine, serial ultrasonographic findings may be more helpful than repeated β-hCG measurements to determine progress of the pregnancy. The mean gestational sac size is determined by measuring the sac in three planes and averaging the values. The yolk sac should be visualized when the mean gestational sac size is larger than 12 mm. When the gestational sac reaches an average 17-mm diameter, the embryo should be identifiable in a normal pregnancy (Table 22–1). These findings have 100% specificity for a nonviable pregnancy as well as 100% positive predictive value and can lead to identification of 73% of nonviable pregnancies. Location of the gestational sac low in the uterus, a deformed gestational sac, or a limited decidual reaction is a less accurate sign of a nonviable gestation. Knowing that the gestational sac should increase in diameter by 1.1 mm per day allows appropriate scheduling of follow-up ultrasonograms for confirmation of viability. Structures may certainly be identified earlier, when the sac sizes are smaller than those related previously, but these provide standards of comparison by which a pregnancy may be deemed abnormal (Table 22–1). The presence of an amniotic sac without a fetus has been dubbed the empty amnion sign and is also diagnostic of a nonviable pregnancy.

**Table 22–1** Ultrasonographic Findings and Determining Viability

| Measurement | Expected Ultrasonographic Findings |
| --- | --- |
| Gestational sac >12 mm | Yolk sac seen |
| Gestational sac >17 mm | Embryo seen |
| Crown-rump ≥5 mm | Cardiac activity identified |

**Table 22–2** Gestational Age Assignment by Crown-Rump Length

| CRL (mm) | GA (weeks) |
| --- | --- |
| 2 | 5 0/7 |
| 3 | 5 2/7 |
| 4 | 5 4/7 |
| 5 | 5 6/7 |
| 6 | 6 1/7 |
| 10 | 7 0/7 |
| 17 | 8 0/7 |
| 25 | 9 0/7 |
| 34 | 10 0/7 |
| 45 | 11 0/7 |
| 57 | 12 0/7 |

CRL = crown-rump length; GA = gestational age.

Once a fetal pole has been identified by scanning, it should be examined for the presence of cardiac activity. Frequently, fetal cardiac activity can be identified before or as soon as the fetal pole can be measured. The initial heart rate may be slow, with a mean of 110 beats per minute at 5 weeks of gestation. This rate gradually becomes higher with advancing gestation. In 95% of normal pregnancies cardiac activity is detected when the fetal pole is less than 3 mm in length. The pregnancy should not be called abnormal unless absence of cardiac activity is noted when the crown-rump length is 5 mm or more. In the asymptomatic patient, ultrasonographic findings can be used to assess the risk of subsequent miscarriage. Once a gestational sac is identified, an 11.5% loss rate is reported; the presence of a yolk sac decreases the loss rate to 8.5%; if an embryo is seen, the loss rate is 7.2% provided the crown-rump length is more than 5 mm (0.5% for embryos larger than 10 mm).

## Dating the Pregnancy

The axiom that scans performed earlier in pregnancy are more accurate for dating is certainly true after 6 weeks of gestation. Dating a first trimester pregnancy by ultrasonography is most accurately done by crown-rump length; gestational sac size is not as accurate. Table 22–2 lists gestational age assignment based on crown-rump length. The crown-rump length is most accurate between 7 and 12 weeks of gestation because small differences in caliper placement very early in gestation may affect gestational age assignment. Curvature of the fetus is more pronounced as the pregnancy progresses, limiting the accuracy of crown-rump length measurement after 12 weeks of gestation. Fetal biparietal diameter and femur length measurements can be ascertained after 12 weeks and are more appropriate measurements for age assignment when obtainable.

Pitfalls encountered in early pregnancy dating include mistakenly measuring the yolk sac as part of the fetal pole. For patients whose dating is precise, (e.g., plotted on an ovulation detection chart), it is important to realize that abnormal pregnancies may exhibit early growth restriction. In multiple gestations discrepancies can also be detected that may herald twin-twin transfusion syndrome or congenital abnormalities. Dating can be enhanced by looking at the development of structures that are detected by ultrasonography.

## Anatomy

Understanding the development of normal anatomy during the first trimester of pregnancy aids in assignment of correct gestational age and facilitates evaluation of the normal and the abnormal fetus. Table 22–3 outlines the gestational age at which different structures are able to be identified. In patients in whom the size of the embryo does not correlate with the expected gestational age, the presence of these structures may help to confirm correct gestational age assignment.

It is important to recognize normal development. The brain structures appear as a single ventricle 7 weeks after the last menstrual period, and the falx can be identified between 9 and 10 weeks of gestation. Abnormalities, such as holoprosencephaly cannot be determined before this stage of the pregnancy. The extracoelomic space can be seen up to 10 weeks and possibly beyond and should not be mistaken for a cystic hygroma or abnormal membrane. Finally, recognition of physiologic midgut herniation up to 12 weeks of gestation prevents misinterpretation of the presence of an omphalocele in these patients.

## Early Markers for Abnormalities

During the first trimester, the use of markers to identify fetuses at increased risk for chromosomal anomalies is very exciting. Nuchal lucency or early cystic hygroma has been identified as such a marker (Fig. 22–1). The presence of a nuchal lucency measuring 3 mm or more is associated with an 18.6 to 35% risk of chromosomal abnormalities. In the United Kingdom, more intensive screening programs using the presence or absence of nuchal lucency and combined with maternal age have reported a sensitivity of 85% with a 5% false-positive rate for identification of fetuses with trisomy 21.

Pitfalls include mistaking the normal amnion for a nuchal lucency. Measurement of the echolucent space between the skin and the membrane should be recorded. If the initial positioning does not allow this differentiation from the amnion. It is important to observe the fetus during movement to ensure that the hygroma moves along with the fetus and is truly attached to the dorsum.

## Multiple Gestation

The increasing incidence of multifetal pregnancies requires appropriate evaluation of the number of fetuses. This is most easily accomplished in the first trimester. Subchorionic hematomas and fluid collections may be mistaken for gestational sacs; therefore, it is important to identify structures within the gestational sac before diagnosing multifetal pregnancies. An apparent gestational sac that contains a yolk sac or a fetal pole with cardiac activity may be correctly identified, and requiring the presence of these structures before labeling a gestation can avoid many mistakes. Follow-up of the pregnancy is important because of the increased first-trimester loss rate associated with multiple gestations. If two gestational sacs are identified, the probability of a twin birth is 52 to 63%. If viable embryos are identified, the probability of delivering twins is 84 to 90%. The first and early second trimesters provide an excellent opportunity for evaluating the chorionicity of a multiple gestation. This opportunity may not be present later in pregnancy and can potentially impact management of these high-risk patients. As part of the evaluation, the location of all placentas should be

**Table 22–3** Gestational Age and Structures Visualized by Transvaginal Ultrasonography

| Gestational Age (Menstrual Wk) | Structures Visualized |
|---|---|
| 5 | Gestational sac, yolk sac |
| 6 | Fetal pole, cardiac activity |
| 7 | Lower limb buds, physiologic midgut herniation |
| 8 | Upper limb buds, stomach |
| 9 | Spine, falx, choroid plexus |

(Data from Timor-Tritsch IE, Farine D, Rosen MG: A close look at early embryonic development with the high-frequency transvaginal transducer. Am J Obstet Gynecol 159:676–681, 1988; Blaas HG, Eik-Nes SH, Kiserud T, et al: Early development of the abdominal wall, stomach and heart from 7 to 12 weeks of gestation: A longitudinal study. Ultrasound Obstet Gynecol 6:240–249, 1995.)

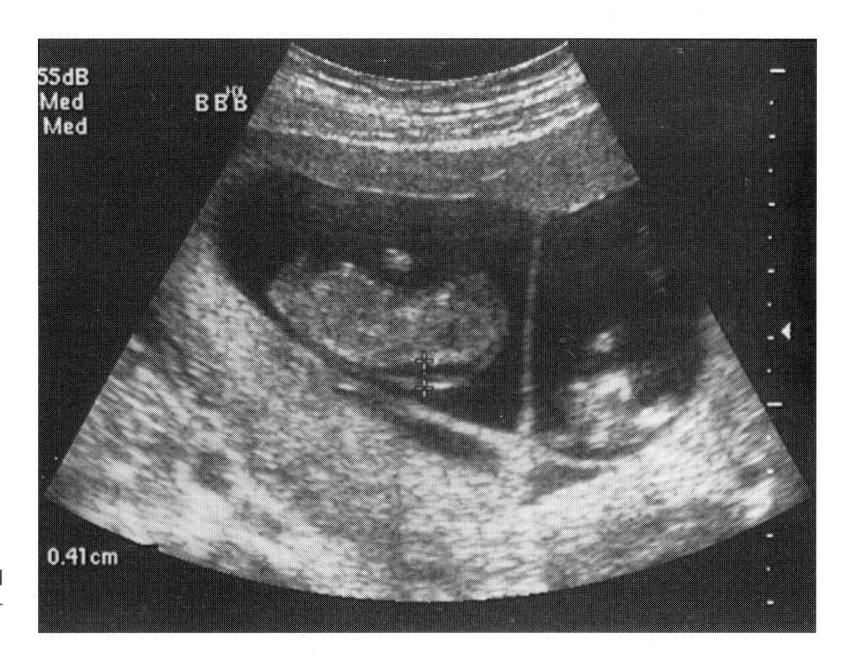

**Figure 22–1** Nuchal membranes identified in the first trimester and associated with increased risk of chromosomal abnormalities.

determined. Obviously, separate placental structures identify dichorionic pregnancies. Although fetuses of different genders are diagnostic for dichorionic gestations, fetal gender is not always ascertained in the first trimester. For placentas that are contiguous or fused, the "twin peaks" or "lambda" signs have been described to diagnose dichorionic pregnancies. Because chorionicity—not zygosity—is closely linked to the risk of complications, this information is clinically relevant. Presence or absence of placental tissue extending into the membranes between two gestational sacs is very reliable for identification of chorionicity (Fig. 22–2), and this can be accomplished after 7 weeks of gestation. The inability to identify a membrane separating the fetuses is also important and should be noted when patients are counseled regarding the outcome of the pregnancy.

## Subchorionic Hematomas

Although there is some controversy in the literature regarding the prognosis of subchorionic hematomas, the volume of the hematoma does seem to correlate with pregnancy outcome. Although small and moder-

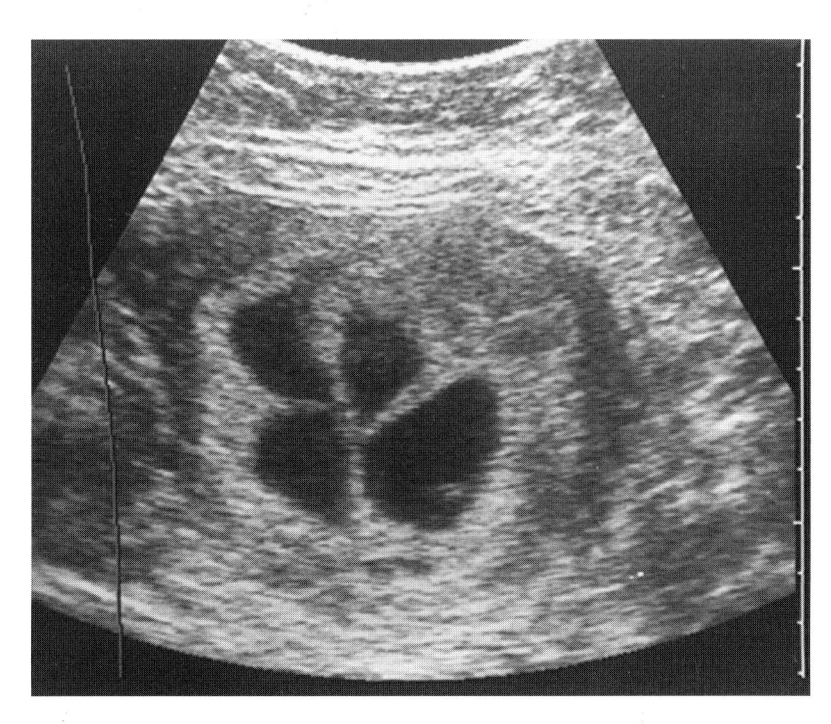

**Figure 22–2** Dichorionic placentas in a quadruplet pregnancy with placental tissue extending between membranes.

ate hematomas do not significantly increase the risk of spontaneous abortion, a large hematoma (defined as having a circumference large enough to elevate two thirds of the chorionic sac) is associated with an approximately threefold increased risk of spontaneous abortion. This risk is modified by maternal age and gestational age at the time of the scan. In patients who have bleeding less than or equal to that of an 8-week gestation, the abortion rate is 13.7% vs. 5.9% if the patient is past 8 weeks of gestation. Identification of a large hematoma in any patient warrants close surveillance.

## REFERENCES

Bennett GL, Bromley B, Lieberman E, et al: Subchorionic hemorrhage in first-trimester pregnancies: Prediction of pregnancy outcome with sonography. Radiology 200:803–806, 1996.

Blaas HG, Eik-Nes SH, Kiserud T, et al: Early development of the abdominal wall, stomach and heart from 7 to 12 weeks of gestation: A longitudinal ultrasound study. Ultrasound Obstet Gynecol 6:240–249, 1995.

Brambati B, Cislaghi C, Tului L, et al: First-trimester Down's syndrome screening using nuchal translucency: A prospective study in patients undergoing chorionic villus sampling. Ultrasound Obstet Gynecol 5:9–14, 1995.

Brown DL, Emerson DS, Felker RE, et al: Diagnosis of early embryonic demise by endovaginal sonography. J Ultrasound Med 9:631–636, 1990.

Dickey RP, Olar TT, Curole DN, et al: The probability of multiple births when multiple gestational sacs or viable embryos are diagnosed at first trimester ultrasound. Hum Reprod 5:880–882, 1990.

Fossum GT, Davajan V, Kletzky OA: Early detection of pregnancy with transvaginal ultrasound. Fertil Steril 49:788–791, 1988.

Goldstein SR, Snyder JR, Watson C, et al: Very early pregnancy detection with endovaginal ultrasound. Obstet Gynecol 72:200–204, 1988.

Hill LM, Chenevey P, Hecker J, et al: Sonographic determination of first trimester twin chorionicity and amnionicity. J Clin Ultrasound 24:305–308, 1996.

Kurjak A, Zalud I, Volpe G: Conventional B-mode and transvaginal color Doppler in ultrasound assessment of ectopic pregnancy. Acta Med Iugoslavica 44:91–103, 1990.

Levi CS, Lyons EA, Zheng XH, et al: Endovaginal US: Demonstration of cardiac activity in embryos of less than 5.0 mm in crown-rump length. Radiology 176:71–74, 1990.

Nicolaides KH, Azar G, Mansur BD, et al: Fetal nuchal translucency: Ultrasound screening for chromosomal defects in first trimester of pregnancy. BMJ 304:867–869, 1992.

Nicolaides KH, Brizot ML, Snijders RJ: Fetal nuchal translucency: Ultrasound screening for fetal trisomy in the first trimester of pregnancy. Br J Obstet Gynaecol 101:782–786, 1994.

Nyberg DA, Hill LM: Normal early intrauterine pregnancy: Sonographic development and hCG correlation. In Nyberg DA, Hill LM, Bohm-Velez M, et al (ed): Transvaginal Ultrasound. St. Louis, Mosby, 1992 pp 65–84.

Nyberg DA, Mack LA, Harvey D, et al: Value of the yolk sac in evaluating early pregnancies. J Ultrasound Med 7:129–135, 1988.

Rempen A: Diagnosis of viability in early pregnancy with vaginal sonography. J Ultrasound Med 9:711–716, 1990.

Romero R, Kadar N, Castro D, et al: The value of adnexal sonographic findings in the diagnosis of ectopic pregnancy. Am J Obstet Gynecol 158:52–55, 1988.

Sepulveda W, Sebire NJ, Hughes K, et al: The lambda sign at 10–14 weeks of gestation as a predictor of chorionicity in twin pregnancies. Ultrasound Obstet Gynecol 7:421–423, 1996.

Tadmor O, Nitzan M, Rabinowitz R, et al: Prediction of second trimester intrauterine growth retardation and fetal death in a discordant twin by first trimester measurements. Case report and review of the literature. Fetal Diagn Ther 10:17–21, 1995.

Tongsong T, Wanapirak C, Srisomboon J, et al: Transvaginal ultrasound in threatened abortions with empty gestational sacs. Int J Obstet Gynecol 46:297–301, 1994.

Timor-Tritsch IE, Farine D, Rosen MG: A close look at early embryonic development with the high-frequency transvaginal transducer. Am J Obstet Gynecol 159:676–681, 1988.

Weissman A, Achiron R, Lipitz S, et al: The first-trimester growth-discordant twin: An ominous prenatal finding. Obstet Gynecol 84:110–114, 1994.

# 23

# Second-Trimester Ultrasonography

DONNA D. JOHNSON
J. PETER VANDORSTEN

Ultrasonography is arguably the most important technologic advance introduced into modern obstetrics. Its use has revolutionized prenatal detection of fetal structural anomalies, growth aberrations, multiple gestations, and placental location. Today, 80% or more of pregnant women in the United States undergo sonographic evaluation of their fetuses. Some advantages of real-time ultrasonography include its relatively low cost, biosafety for fetus and mother, observation of in utero behavior, and noninvasive evaluation of fetal anatomy and gestational age.

## Types of Ultrasonographic Evaluation

Three types of fetal ultrasound evaluation are recognized by the American College of Obstetrics and Gynecology (ACOG). The examination that is chosen by the physician depends on the information that is sought. The first type of fetal sonographic evaluation, a limited ultrasonogram, is appropriate when the information needed is urgent or very specific. For example, limited ultrasonography may be useful in labor and delivery to confirm an intrauterine fetal demise, localize the placenta, or determine the fetal presentation. In addition, a limited ultrasonogram may be a useful adjunct to procedures such as external cephalic version, amniocentesis, or fetal biophysical profile. The information obtained from limited ultrasonography is not specifically defined but should be dictated by the clinical scenario.

The second type of fetal sonographic evaluation, a basic ultrasonogram, is sufficient for most obstetric patients in the second trimester. The basic sonographic evaluation should include fetal number and presentation, confirmation of fetal cardiac activity, placental location, and assessment of amniotic fluid. The maternal pelvis should be scanned for adnexal or uterine pathology. Measured fetal biometry determines gestational age and estimated fetal weight. Finally, the fetus should be surveyed for gross malformations. This anatomic survey should include cerebral ventricles, four-chamber view of the heart (including its position in the thorax), spine, stomach, renal areas, urinary bladder, and umbilical cord insertion. Additionally, the American Institute of Ultrasound in Medicine (AIUM) Educational Guidelines stipulate that the umbilical cord, placental appearance, and posterior fossa should be included.

The third type of evaluation of the fetus, comprehensive ultrasonographic examination, is indicated for the patient who is at increased risk of a fetal malformation based on maternal history, physical examination, or a previous ultrasonographic examination. The major difference between the basic examination and the comprehensive examination of the fetus is the level of expertise required of the sonographer. Whereas the basic examination can be performed or reviewed by most obstetrician-gynecologists, the comprehensive examination should be performed by a physician with specific expertise in sonographic evaluation of the fetus. In general, the comprehensive examination should include a more detailed anatomic survey than that performed in a basic examination. The at-risk organ system should be specifically targeted.

## Assessment of Gestational Age

Accurate assessment of fetal gestational age is one of the most important aspects of the second-trimester evaluation. Twenty percent of pregnant women are uncertain of the time of their last menstrual period. The most commonly used parameters for determining gestational age are the biparietal diameter (BPD), the head circumference (HC), the abdominal circumference (AC), and the femur length (FL). Numerous articles have touted the advantage of one or more of these parameters. However, all authors note increased variability of these parameters as pregnancy advances. In general, gestational age assessment in the second trimester is more accurate between 14 and 20 weeks. To overcome the pitfalls of a single measurement, a composite fetal age based on the average of these four measurements is preferable in clinical practice. This technique results in the greatest accuracy (lack of systematic bias), greatest precision (lowest range of variability), and smallest maximum of observed errors.

To reduce variability, the sonographer must obtain accurate measurements of the BPD, the HC, the AC, and the FL. When measuring the BPD and the HC, the fetal head should ideally be imaged in a transverse axial section. Intracranial landmarks should include the falx cerebri, cavum septum pellucidi, and the thalamic nuclei. By convention, BPD is recorded from the outer skull edge nearest the transducer to the inner edge on the opposite side of the skull table. This is not a true anatomic measurement because the distal skull plate and scalp are omitted. Nevertheless, it is very reproducible.

The HC is measured at the same level as BPD, but the measurement is taken from the outer perimeter of the calvarium. The HC can be traced directly by either a light pen or a digitalizer or can be calculated using the occipitofrontal diameter and the BPD. The sonographer should be aware that the HC is less shape-dependent than the BPD.

The femur is the easiest fetal long bone to visualize and measure. To measure the femur, the transducer should be aligned along the long axis of the bone. Ideally, the beam from the transducer should perpendicular to the shaft. The measured ends of the bone should be blunt rather than pointed. Other bones of the upper and lower extremity may be measured using the same technique. However, the addition of another measurement does not improve the accuracy of the composite age.

The AC should be obtained from a true transverse plane perpendicular to the longitudinal axis of the fetus just below the cross-sectional view of the heart and preferably at the level of the junction of the left and right portal veins. The image should be as round as possible, and care should be taken not to compress the abdomen with the transducer. Like the HC, the AC can be traced along its outer margin with either a light pen or a digitalizer or calculated using the anteroposterior and transverse diameters. AC is the most useful parameter for evaluating fetal growth aberrations and knowledge of this is necessary to estimate fetal weight.

The composite gestational age determined by these sonographic measurements should be compared with the menstrual dates. When the menstrual dates fall within the confidence limits of the sonographic dates, the estimated date of confinement (EDC), derived from the date of the last menstrual period, is confirmed. In general, when the menstrual dates fall outside the confidence limits of the sonographic dates, the EDC should be based on the ultrasonographic measurements. If the ultrasonographic measurements are used to establish fetal age, the sonographer must assume that the fetus is normally grown. If there is uncertainty about fetal growth, the sonographic measurements should be examined carefully for consistency and a follow-up scan for interval fetal growth should be considered.

## Basic Anatomic Survey

To avoid critical omissions, the sonographer should develop a systematic approach to recording the data obtained from the biometric and anatomic surveys in the second trimester. Documentation of the examination is essential. Images should be labeled clearly with the patient's name and identification number. A report of the biometric and anatomic surveys should be available in the patient's record. When structures cannot be well visualized for valid reasons, such as maternal habitus, unrevealing fetal position, or low amniotic fluid, the report should document that an attempt was made to image the structure, and it was not well visualized.

The shape of the fetal head is normally elliptical. An abnormal shape of the calvarium may provide important diagnostic information. For example, a cloverleaf skull can often be seen in a fetus with thanatophoric dwarfism. An abnormal concavity of the frontal bones may be seen; this finding, known as a lemon sign, has been associated with neural tube defects (NTDs). An absent cranial vault is highly suggestive of anencephaly. The shape of the fetal head can be easily evaluated in the same plane in which the HC and the BPD are measured.

An enlarged HC or BPD may suggest hydrocephalus. However, the lateral ventricles should be carefully examined in all fetuses to exclude more subtle ventriculomegaly because enlargement of the ventricles often precedes cranial enlargement. Two methods have been proposed for assessing the ventricular system: a ratio of the lateral ventricle width to the hemispheric width, or measurement of lateral ventricular atrium width. The latter method is the simpler of the two because only one measurement is necessary and its upper limit—10 mm—is constant throughout gestation. If the choroid occupies the atrium of the lateral ventricle, a lateral ventricular atrial measurement is not necessary during a basic scan (Fig. 23–1). However, if the choroid is separated from the medial wall of the lateral ventricle or appears to be dangling, a measurement should be obtained (Fig. 23–2). If ventriculomegaly is detected, the patient should be referred for a comprehensive examination because this condition is often associated with other anomalies.

During the evaluation of the ventricles, the choroid should be examined closely for the presence of cysts (see Fig. 23–1). The majority of choroid plexus cysts are benign and resolve spontaneously by 24 weeks of gestation, but these cysts have been known to be

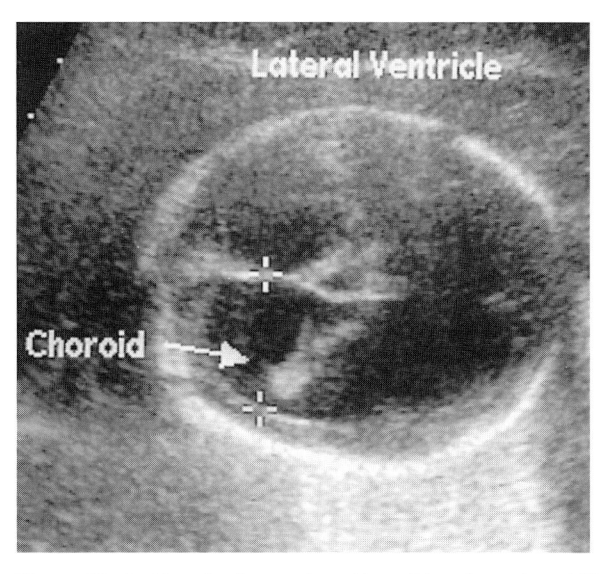

**Figure 23–2** Ventriculomegaly with a "dangling choroid" *(arrow)*. Although the lateral ventriculomegaly nearest the transducer is often difficult to evaluate because of artifacts, ventriculomegaly is presumed to be bilateral unless the sonographer can demonstrate otherwise.

associated with chromosomal abnormalities. The most common abnormal karyotypes are trisomy 18 and, to a lesser extent, trisomy 21. Attempts to characterize the cyst further (e.g., by size) have not been informative. Offering the patient amniocentesis remains controversial. On one hand, trisomy 18 is commonly associated with other malformations that are readily identifiable by sonography. If amniocentesis were performed in all fetuses with choroid plexus cyst, two normal fetuses would be lost for every trisomy 18 detected. On the other hand, the false-negative rate for detection of trisomy 18 is 28% between 14 and 24 weeks of gestation and even higher for trisomy 21. At the very least, a fetus identified with a choroid plexus cyst should be referred for comprehensive ultrasonography and genetic counseling.

The fetal cerebellum and cisterna magna should be imaged (Fig. 23–3). Although anomalies (e.g., Dandy Walker malformation) can be diagnosed, one of the most compelling reasons for examining the posterior fossa is that it may contain important clues about the presence of an NTD. In a fetus with an NTD, the normal contour of the cerebellum is lost and the posterior cerebellar surface becomes more flattened (i.e., the banana sign). In addition, the cisterna magna is often obliterated or effaced. These changes, which are found in the posterior fossa, are associated with Chiari type II malformation. Although NTDs can be difficult to identify, examination of the cerebellum and the cisterna magna greatly enhances their detection. The sensitivity of cranial signs in spina bifida exceeds 99%.

The spine should also be carefully examined when

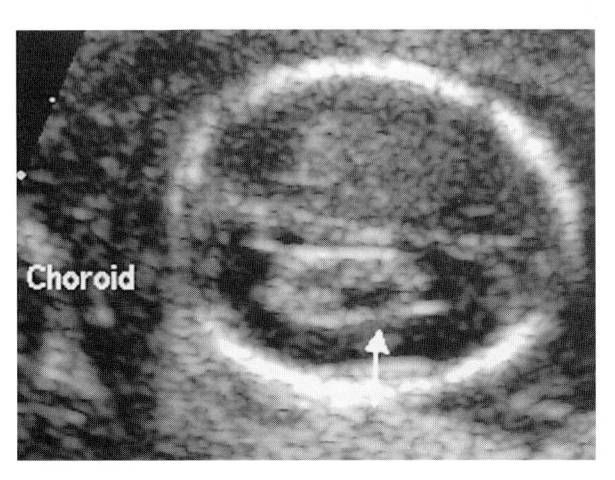

**Figure 23–1** Normal ventricle with a correctly positioned choroid. However, a choroid plexus cyst *(arrow)* is present.

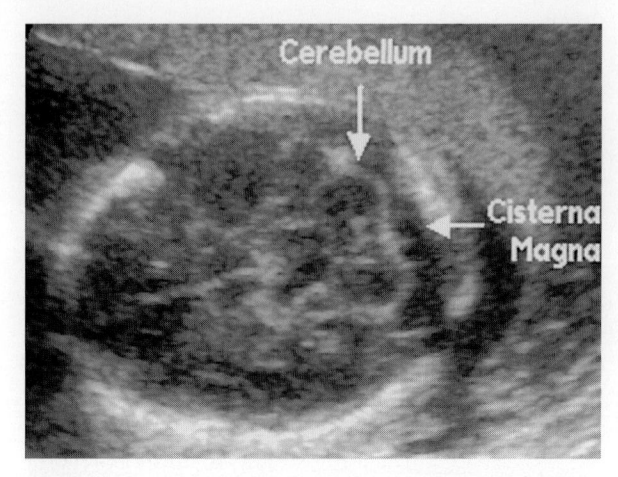

**Figure 23–3** The cerebellum and cisterna magna of a normal fetus.

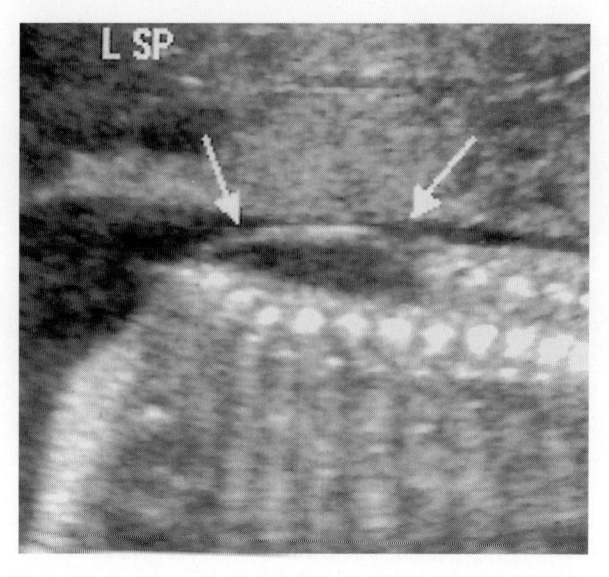

**Figure 23–5** Parasagittal view of the lumbosacral spine (LSP) in a fetus with a neural tube defect. Notice that the posterior elements *(arrows)* are missing.

a basic scan is performed in the second trimester. Three scanning planes are used to assess the spinal anatomy. In the parasagittal plane, the normal spine appears as two parallel lines converging in the sacrum (Figs. 23–4 and 23–5). The two parallel lines represent the posterior elements of the vertebrae and the vertebral body. From the coronal view, two parallel lines can be seen, which represent the lateral processes of the posterior element. The transverse view shows the spinal canal as a closed circle composed of three ossification centers. The anterior ossification center is that of the vertebral body, and the two posterior ossification centers are those of the posterior elements.

The four-chamber view of the fetal heart is an integral part of the basic second-trimester sonogram. This view is accessed from the transverse plane of the fetal chest. Knowing the orientation of the heart in the fetal chest is essential to the sonographer. The normal fetal heart is located on the left side of the chest. The axis of the interventricular septum is 45 degrees to the left of the anteroposterior axis of the fetus. The right ventricle is the chamber that is closest to the anterior chest wall. The left atrium is the most posterior chamber and closest to the fetal spine (Fig. 23–6). Important cardiac landmarks are the apex of the heart, the base, the interventricular septum, the interatrial septum, the tricuspid and mitral valves, and the four cardiac chambers delineated by these structures. The right and left ventricles should have practically the same width in the four-chamber view. Finally, fetal cardiac activity should be documented.

The four-chamber view alone detects approxi-

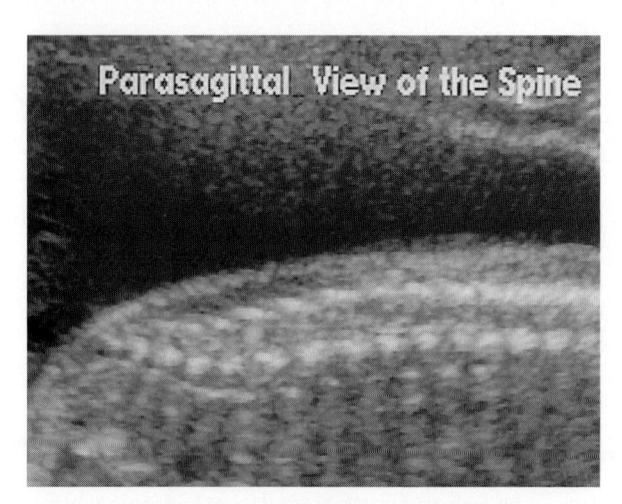

**Figure 23–4** Normal parasagittal view of the lumbosacral spine. The posterior elements and the vretebral body form parallel lines that converge in the sacrum.

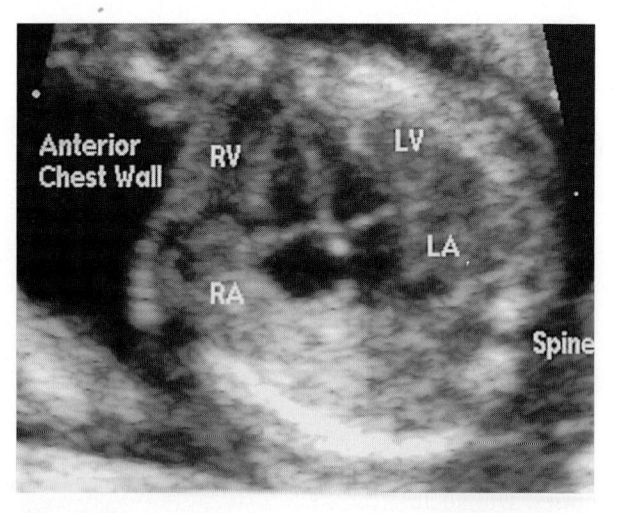

**Figure 23–6** A normal four-chamber view of the fetal heart in the second trimester. The right ventricle (RV) is closest to the anterior chest wall and the left atrium (LA) is closest to the spine. Both ventricles are located in the left thoracic cavity.

mately two thirds of fetal cardiac anomalies. Echocardiography examines the fetal heart more extensively and increases the detection rate of cardiac anomalies. For this reason, any fetus that is at risk for congenital heart disease should be referred for a fetal echocardiogram. Risk factors include a family history of congenital heart disease, maternal diseases (e.g., diabetes), certain teratogenic exposures, fetal abnormalities, nonimmune hydrops, and fetal cardiac arrhythmias. Although a normal fetal echocardiogram should reassure the obstetrician and the patient, it does not detect all fetal cardiac anomalies in utero. Diagnostic errors can result because of technical factors, such as maternal obesity or polyhydramnios. Furthermore, the diagnostic limits may preclude the diagnosis of small atrial or ventricular septal defects. Other defects, such as mild coarctation of the aorta or secundum atrial septal defects, may be impossible to detect because of the normal physiology of blood flow through the fetal heart. Finally, some cardiac lesions are not apparent until later in pregnancy.

Although examination of the fetal lungs is not an element of the basic scan, a sonographer often visualizes the fetal lungs in search of the four-chamber view of the heart. The fetal lungs produce homogeneous midrange echoes in the second trimester. Sonolucent, highly echogenic, or heterogeneous echoes should alert the examiner to be aware of a potential thoracic abnormality. In addition, some intrathoracic masses cause deviation of the fetal heart from its normal position.

The fetal abdomen contains several structures that must be visualized during performance of a basic second-trimester ultrasonogram. The fetal stomach appears as an echolucent area in the left upper quadrant of the fetal abdomen and is often visualized on the plane in which AC is measured. This "stomach bubble" could be seen in 98% of fetuses during the second trimester. If the stomach could not be visualized, 55% of fetuses had an abnormality. If the stomach bubble is not visualized by 20 weeks, most—if not all—fetuses have an abnormality. These anomalies include the following:

1. Mechanical obstruction, such as esophageal atresia
2. Depressed swallowing because of neuromotor problems or central nervous system abnormalities
3. Ectopic stomach with congenital diaphragmatic hernia.

Like the stomach, the bladder appears as a sonolucent structure in the fetal pelvis. By 14 weeks of gestation, the bladder can be visualized in 94% of fetuses. Unlike an absent stomach bubble, nonvisualization of the bladder on an otherwise normal sonogram is usually not clinically significant. In contrast, nonvisualization of the urinary bladder in the setting of oligohydramnios suggests a severe bilateral renal anomaly. Because the bladder normally fills and partially or completely empties every 25 minutes, the examination should be carried out for at least 30 minutes.

Because visualization of the fetal bladder does not exclude the presence of renal defects, the fetal kidneys should be imaged. In the early second trimester, the fetal kidneys may be difficult to visualize because of the lack of contrast between the kidneys and the surrounding structures. However, by the midsecond trimester, the fetal kidneys should be visible. Visualization of the kidneys can detect intrinsic renal lesions (e.g., multicystic dysplastic kidney, infantile polycystic kidney disease) and obstructive lesions that cause dilatation of the renal pelvis. Unless an obstructive uropathy is moderate to severe, the ureters and urethra are difficult to visualize and are not part of a routine examination.

While examining the intra-abdominal organs, the sonographer may note hyperechoic bowel in the second-trimester fetus. A strict definition of hyperechoic bowel does not exist, but most authors agree that the echogenic bowel is brighter than the liver density. Although an echogenic bowel may be normal, this finding in the second trimester warrants further investigation and genetic counseling. An echogenic bowel has been associated with cystic fibrosis, chromosomal abnormalities, intrauterine infection, and adverse perinatal outcome (e.g., intrauterine growth restriction and fetal death).

Examination of the umbilical cord insertion helps to exclude or differentiate between two of the most common abdominal wall defects: gastroschisis and omphalocele. Gastroschisis is a paraumbilical defect that is usually found to the right of a normal abdominal cord insertion site (Fig. 23-7 and 23-8). Small loops of bowel eviscerate through the abdominal wall defect. These loops of bowel are free-floating in the amniotic fluid because they are not covered by a membrane. In an omphalocele, the umbilical cord is inserted into a membrane-covered midline abdominal mass that may contain intestines, liver, or both. Differentiation between abdominal wall defects is essential because an omphalocele is strongly associated with other malformations, including chromosomal defects, and indicates a poor prognosis for the fetus.

Although documentation of fetal gender is not a requirement of the anatomic survey for basic second-trimester ultrasonography, determination of fetal gender is often an expectation of the parents. Accurate sonographic assessment of fetal gender requires perineal visualization to distinguish between female and male external genitalia. After adequate visualization of the perineum, fetal gender is incorrectly assigned in 1% of cases. Only documentation of testes within the scrotum is 100% accurate in gender assessment.

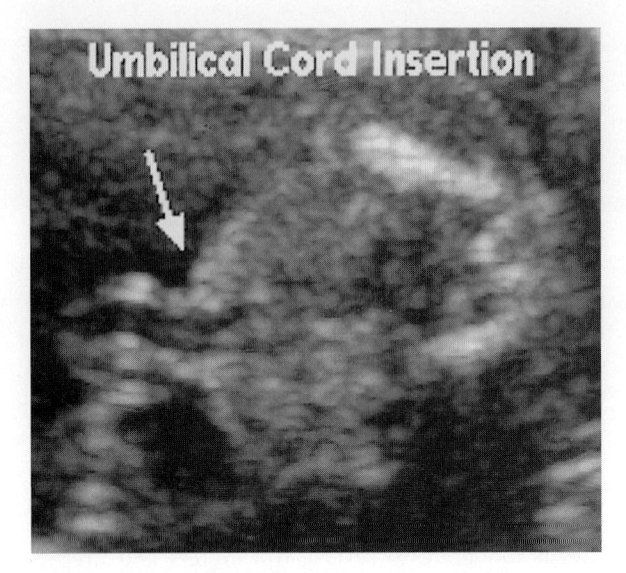

**Figure 23–7** A normal cord insertion into the anterior abdominal wall.

However, the testes do not descend into the scrotum until the third trimester. If the sonographer determines the fetal sex during performance of a second-trimester ultrasonogram and informs the parents of the findings, the parents should be cautioned about the limitations of sonography.

Examination of the placenta and umbilical cord is included in the basic second-trimester scan. The placenta is a relatively echogenic discoid mass of tissue and should be distinguished from intramyometrial masses, such as contractions or fibroids. To rule out placenta previa, it is important to assess the relationship of the placenta to the internal cervical os. The incidence of placenta previa is much higher during the second trimester than at term. Technical factors, such as an overdistended maternal bladder or focal uterine contraction, may contribute to a false-positive diagnosis of a placenta previa in the second trimester. If technical factors are corrected and the placenta previa persists on a second-trimester scan, a follow-up ultrasonogram is warranted in the third trimester.

An assessment of the amniotic fluid should be performed. Although subjective assessment of the amniotic fluid volume may be an appropriate screening method in the second trimester, the person interpreting the scan is often different from the person who performed the scan, and the former may not have been present while the scanning took place. Measurement of the amniotic fluid index offers a reproducible and quantitative technique for assessing amniotic fluid abnormalities. An amniotic fluid index is performed by dividing the uterus into four quadrants, longitudinally in the midline and transversely in the midsection. The sum of the deepest vertical pocket in each quadrant is equal to the amniotic fluid index.

## Ultrasonography of Multifetal Pregnancy

In addition to the biometric and anatomic surveys performed for each individual fetus, second-trimester sonography in multiple gestations should determine the type of placentation. In this chapter, only twins are discussed. However, higher orders of multiple births generally follow the same principles as apply to twin gestations. Three types of placentations are possible in a twin gestation: diamniotic dichorionic (DiDi), diamniotic monochorionic (DiMo), or monoamniotic monochorionic (MoMo). Dizygotic twins are always dichorionic (DiDi). Monozygotic twins most commonly have a monochorionic diamniotic (DiMo) placenta. Dichorionic (DiDi) placentation occurs in 20 to 30% of monozygotic twins. Only 1% of monozygotic twins have monoamniotic placentation (MoMo). Perinatal mortality is highest for monoamniotic (MoMo) twins and lowest for dichorionic (DiDi) twins. The incidence of congenital anomalies, which is higher in twin gestation, follows a pattern similar to that of perinatal mortality.

To determine the placentation of twins, the sonographer should use a systematic approach. The sex of the fetuses should be determined first. If the sexes are different, the placentation must be dichorionic (DiDi). If the sexes are the same, the sonographer must examine the placenta and membranes to determine the chorionicity. If two placentas are clearly present, the placentation is dichorionic (DiDi). If a single placental mass is present, the membranes must

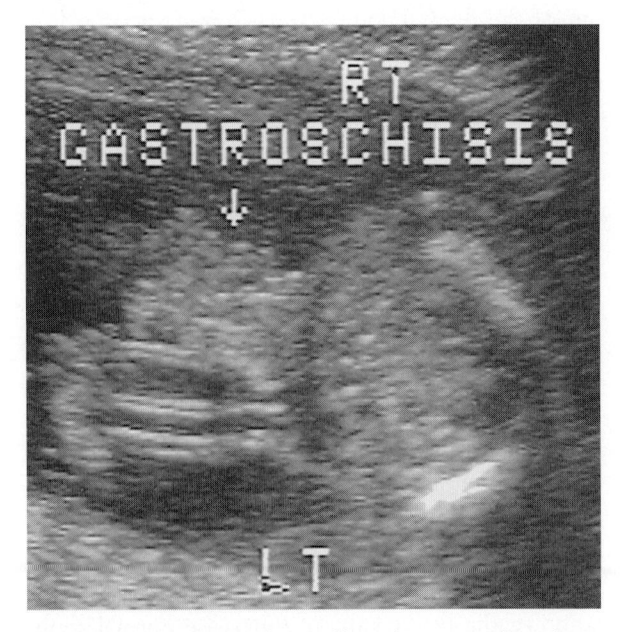

**Figure 23–8** Free-floating loops of bowel *(arrow)* to the right (RT) of a normal cord insertion. This finding is compatible with a gastroschisis. LT is left.

be examined, because a single placental mass may represent two fused placentas or a single placenta. Where the membranes meet the placenta, the sonographer should look for a twin peak sign, which is a projection of tissue similar in echogenicity to the placenta that extends into the dividing membrane. This tissue represents proliferating placental villi that grow into the interchorionic space of the two placentas. Sonographically, the twin peak sign appears as a triangle, with the base at the chorionic surface of the placenta and the point of the triangle in the intertwin membrane. The twin peak sign appears to be focal and does not extend along the entire junction of the membrane and the placenta. If the twin peak sign is present, the placentation is dichorionic (DiDi). However, absence of the twin peak sign does not confirm a monochorionic (DiMo) placentation. If a twin peak sign cannot be seen, the thickness of the membranes should be assessed. The dividing membrane in dichorionic (DiDi) twins is four layers and relatively thick, compared with two layers in monochorionic (DiMo) twins. A qualitative assessment of the dividing membrane as thick or thin has an 83% positive predictive value in both dichorionic (DiDi) and monochorionic (DiMo) twins. However, the positive predictive value decreases as gestational age advances and the membranes become more attenuated. A quantitative measurement of the membrane thickness may also be performed. A membrane measuring more than 2 mm is consistent with dichorionic (DiDi) twins. This measurement has a postive predictive value of 95% for dichorionic (DiDi) twins and 82% for monochorionic (DiMo) twins. If a dividing membrane cannot be visualized, the placentation is monoamniotic (MoMo). The sonographer should use caution when making this diagnosis because the intervening membrane of monochorionic (DiMo) twins can be difficult to see. If a monoamniotic placentation is suspected, the umbilical cords should be examined for entanglement (Fig. 23-9).

The safety of diagnostic ultrasonography in the second trimester of pregnancy has been well validated. Studies of clinical outcomes of infants exposed to ultrasonography have not demonstrated any resultant congenital abnormalities or adverse effects on birth weight. Long-term studies of children exposed to diagnostic ultrasonography 8 or 9 years earlier have not demonstrated different overall cognitive skills from those exhibited by controls. Nevertheless, the sonographer should use the lowest possible ultrasonic exposure time and intensity for each examination.

## Controversy Over Use of Routine Sonograms

Today, the use of indicated ultrasonography in obstetrics is undisputed. However, much controversy exists over the use of routine screening ultrasonography. At the center of the ongoing debate in this country is the Routine Antenatal Diagnostic Imaging with Ultrasound (RADIUS) study. In this study, 15,151 low-risk patients were randomized to a screening ultrasonogram between 15 and 22 weeks and between 31 and 35 weeks or to a control group whose members received an ultrasonogram only when clinically indicated. The rate of adverse pregnancy outcome was 5% in the screened group and 4.9% in the control group. A subanalysis was performed in women who had postdated pregnancies, multiple gestations, and small-for-gestational-age infants. Again, no significant differences were noted in the two groups. The authors concluded that routine use of ultrasonography did not improve perinatal outcome compared with the use of sonography only when clinically indicated.

The RADIUS study has often been compared with a European meta-analysis that included 15,935 patients who were allocated to either routine screening sonography or indicated scanning. The perinatal mortality rate was significantly lower in the screened group than in the control group. The reduction was largely attributed to the contribution of the Helsinki study in which perinatal mortality decreased by 49% from 9.0 to 4.6 per 1000. The investigators believed that the reduction of perinatal mortality was caused by the early detection of fetal malformations that led to pregnancy termination.

One of the main criticisms of the RADIUS study

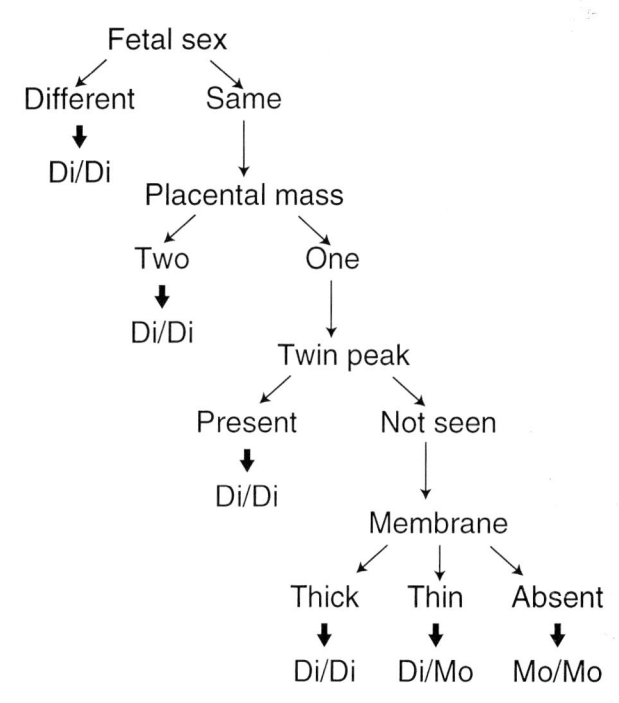

**Figure 23-9** Systematic approach to determine the type of placentation in twins. (Di/Di: diamniotic, dichorionic; Di/Mo: diamniotic, monochorionic; Mo/Mo: monoamniotic, monochorionic).

Table 23–1  Comparison of Sensitivities in Studies Evaluating Fetal Anomaly Detection Rate

| Author | No. Fetuses Screened | Yr Study Conducted | Sensitivity (%) |
| --- | --- | --- | --- |
| Levi | 16,072 | 1984–1989 | 40 |
| Chitty | 8432 | 1989–1990 | 74 |
| Shirley | 6183 | 1989–1990 | 61 |
| Crane (RADIUS) | 7685 | 1987–1991 | 17 |
| Luck | 8523 | 1988–1991 | 85 |
| Anderson | 7880 | 1991–1993 | 60 |
| VanDorsten | 2031 | 1993–1996 | 75 |

concerns the accuracy of the anomaly detection rate. In the 7685 patients scanned, 2.4% had a fetal anomaly. The sensitivity for the detection of a fetal anomaly in the RADIUS study was 17%. The overall sensitivity was much higher for ultrasonographically detectable fetal malformations in tertiary care centers (35%) than in nontertiary care centers (13%). However, both sensitivities are lower than those reported in most articles (Table 23–1). Furthermore, once a fetal abnormality was detected in the RADIUS study, very few patients chose to terminate their pregnancy. Importantly, sonography can only impact perinatal mortality if the majority of parents opt for termination of the pregnancy. In the future, as fetal surgery becomes more refined, new treatment options may reduce perinatal mortality.

One of the biggest considerations in the use of routine ultrasonography in low-risk pregnancies is cost-effectiveness. VanDorsten and associates examined the cost of routine ultrasonography in 1611 low-risk patients. The reimbursement for the combined professional and technical fees was $155,268. Of the 11 women in whom anomalous fetuses were detected, 4 out of 11 terminated their pregnancies. The projected combined hospital and professional costs for short-term newborn care of 3 fetuses that were aborted were $213,696. The projected short-term cost savings for newborn care more than offset the expense of the screening ultrasonographic program in a low-risk population. When long-term direct medical costs and indirect losses are evaluated, such as educational expenses and lost productivity, screening ultrasonograms become even more cost-effective. The benefit of parental reassurance in light of a normal ultrasonogram cannot be factored into cost-effectiveness, but undoubtedly this is also a major benefit of screening ultrasonography.

Currently, no technology exists that is more effective for anomaly detection than ultrasonography. The only current alternative is the multiple serum marker screen. Devore has calculated the total cost of identifying an abnormal fetus by maternal serum alpha-fetoprotein screening in California as being $10,805, which is more expensive than identifying an abnormal fetus by ultrasonography. Furthermore, sonography detects a wider range of anomalies than the serum screening program.

## Three-Dimensional Ultrasonography

Newer sonographic applications are on the horizon. With the introduction of three-dimensional ultrasonography into clinical medicine, we are now able to capture more lifelike images of the fetus in utero. The medical profession—and, more importantly, the expectant parents—may be dazzled by the fetal images created with three-dimensional technology. However, its clinical application in prenatal diagnosis must be defined. Early investigators have shown that three-dimensional ultrasonography is clearly applicable in prenatal diagnosis.

Three-dimensional ultrasonography differs from the current technology in the display of the ultrasonographic images. Fetal data are acquired in volumes that contain many images. The volume data are displayed in three arbitrary planar images that can be manipulated with an interactive display. The images can be interpreted at this point, or a three-dimensional image may be constructed from a subvolume of images in the volume data using computer software. The three-dimensional image may be displayed alone or with the three-planar images.

Viewing fetal structures with three-dimensional images has multiple advantages. First, the three-dimensional rendered image allows the physician to view complex structures in a single image. The physician does not depend on mental reconstruction of ultrasonographic images to define a defect. This feature may be particularly useful for less experienced operators. Second, the three-dimensional rendered image may serve as a reference; therefore, the exact location on the planar image is well defined. Third, the volume data can be reviewed many times after the ultrasonographic examination is complete. This feature enables the physician to teach residents and sonographers without needing the patient to be present. The volume can be reviewed millimeter by millimeter in any plane without concern for fetal movement. This feature may be a more effective teaching tool than viewing a videotape from two-dimensional sonography, because an abnormality may be viewed in three planes at once. Second opinions are easily achieved. Fourth, the three-dimensional image is one that most families can comprehend. Unlike the abstract images obtained with conventional technology, three-dimensional ultrasonography provides a realistic presentation of the fetus. This feature better allows the family to view normal as well as abnormal features of their unborn child.

In one of the largest studies published to date, Merz and associates examined 242 normal fetuses and 216 anomalous fetuses via two- and three-dimensional ultrasonography. Using only the display of the three planar images simultaneously, they found a diagnostic advantage with three-dimensional ultrasonography in 46% of cases. The three-dimensional rendered image alone provided additional information in 64% of cases. The largest diagnostic advantage (72%) resulted when the three-dimensional image was displayed together with the planar images. This type of display may improve our ability to evaluate the fetus, because fetal structures can be examined in planes that are unavailable with traditional technology.

In a similar study, Merz and associates evaluated 204 fetuses with anomalies. They found that three-dimensional ultrasonography was more advantageous than two-dimensional ultrasonography in diagnosing and defining the extent of congenital malformations in 62% of their population. Three-dimensional ultrasonography provided the same information in 36% of cases and less information in 2% of cases. Pretorius and associates published similar findings in 63 fetuses with 103 malformations. Three-dimensional ultrasonography provided additional diagnostic information in 51% of anomalies, was equivalent to conventional technology in 45%, and was disadvantageous in 4% of malformations. In these two studies, three-dimensional ultrasonography was inferior to two-dimensional technology in detecting cases of cardiac defects (because of motion artifacts) and in depicting complex anomalies (because of gross disruption of normal landmarks).

As in conventional technology, three-dimensional ultrasonography has limitations. Fetal volume data cannot be acquired during fetal movement because of motion artifacts. Once a set of volume data is acquired, the display of the planar images is rapid. However, the construction of a three-dimensional image is time-consuming. As computer technology advances, reconstruction time will continue to improve. Although this newer technology may be a useful teaching modality, three-dimensional ultrasonography does not immediately improve sonographic skills. Most importantly, the resolution of commercially available three-dimensional technology is not currently superior to that of existing technology. Poor scanning conditions, such as maternal habitus or oligohydramnios, are still problematic with both technologies.

In conclusion, it must be acknowledged that ultrasonography is a remarkable diagnostic tool. Its ability to determine gestational age, detect multifetal gestations, assess fetal growth and fetal well-being, and detect fetal anomalies has revolutionized obstetric care.

## REFERENCES

American College of Obstetricians and Gynecologists: Technical Bulletin, #187, 1993.
American Institute of Ultrasound in Medicine Educational Guidelines, 1994.
Anderson N, Boswell O, Duff G: Prenatal sonography for the detection of fetal anomalies: Results of a prospective study and comparison with prior series. AJR Am J Roentgenol 165:943–950, 1995.
Baba K, Satoh K, Sakamoto S, et al: Development of an ultrasonic system for three-dimensional reconstruction of the fetus. J Perinat Med 17:19–24, 1989.
Benacerraf BR, Harlow B, Frigoletto FO: Are choroid plexus cysts an indication for second trimester amniocentesis. Am J Obstet Gynecol 162:1001–1006, 1990.
Benirschke K, Kaufmann P: Pathology of the Human Placenta, 3rd ed. New York, Springer-Verlag, 1995, pp 719–725.
Birnholz JC: Determination of fetal sex. N Engl J Med 309:942–945, 1983.
Bromley B, Estroff JA, Sanders SP, et al: Fetal echocardiography: Accuracy and limitations in a population of high and low risk for heart defects. Am J Obstet Gynecol 166:1473–1481, 1992.
Bucher HC, Schmidt JG: Does routine ultrasound improve outcome in pregnancy? Meta-analysis of various outcome measures. BMJ 307:13–17, 1993.
Budorick NE, Pretorius DH, Nelson TR: Sonography of the fetal spine: Technique, imaging findings, and clinical implications. AJR Am J Roentgenol 164:421–428, 1995.
Cardoza JD, Goldstein RB, Filly RA: Exclusion of fetal ventriculomegaly with a single measurement: The width of the lateral ventricular atrium. Radiology 169:711–714, 1988.
Chitty LS, Hunt GH, Moore J, Lobb MO: Effectiveness of routine ultrasonography in detecting fetal structural abnormalities in a low risk population. Br Med J 303:1165–1169, 1991.
Clautice-Engle T, Pretorius DH, Budorick NE: Significance of nonvisualization of the fetal urinary bladder. J Ultrasound Med 10:615–618, 1991.
Comstock CH: Normal fetal heart axis and position. Obstet Gynecol 70:255–259, 1987.
Crane JP, LeFevre ML, Winborn RC, et al: A randomized trial of prenatal ultrasonographic screening: Impact on detection, management, and outcome of anomalous fetuses. Am J Obstet Gynecol 171:392–399, 1994.
DeVore GR: The routine antenatal diagnostic imagine with ultrasound study: Another perspective. Obstet Gynecol 84:622–626, 1994.
Dewhurst CJ, Beazley JM, Campbell S: Assessment of fetal maturity and dysmaturity. Am J Obstet Gynecol 113:141–149, 1972.
Dicke JM, Crane JP: Sonographically detected hyperechogenic fetal bowel: Significance and implications for pregnancy management. Obstet Gynecol 80:778–782, 1992.
Ewigman BC, Crane JP, Frigoletto FD, et al: Effect of prenatal ultrasound screening on perinatal outcome. N Engl J Med 329:821–827, 1993.
Finberg NJ: The "twin peak" sign: Reliable evidence of dichorionic twinning. J Ultrasound Med 11:571–577, 1992.
Goldstein RB, Filly RA: Sonographic estimation of amniotic fluid: Subjective assessment versus pocket measurements. J Ultrasound Med 7:363–369, 1988.
Hadlock FP, Deter RL, Harrist RB, et al: Estimating fetal age: Computer assisted analysis of multiple fetal growth parameters. Radiology 152:497–501, 1984.
Hadlock FP, Harrist RB, Martinez-Poyer J: How accurate is second trimester fetal dating? J Ultrasound Med 10:557–561, 1991.
Hughey M, Sabbagha RE: Cephalometry by real-time imaging: A critical evaluation. Am J Obstet Gynecol 131:825–830, 1978.
Hill LM, Guzick D, Hixson J, et al: Composite assessment of gestational age: A comparison of institutionally derived and pub-

lished regression equations. Am J Obstet Gynecol 166:551–555, 1992.

Kirbach D, Whittingham TA: 3D ultrasound—the Kretztechnik Voluson approach. Eur J Ultrasound 1:85–89, 1994.

Kuo HC, Chang FM, Wu CH, et al: The primary application of three-dimensional ultrasonography in obstetrics. Am J Obstet Gynecol 166:880–886, 1992.

Kupfermine MJ, Tamura RK, Sabbagha RE, et al: Isolated choroid plexus cyst(s): An indication for amniocentesis. Am J Obstet Gynecol 171:1068–1071, 1994.

Levi S, Jyjazi Y, Schaaps JP, et al: Sensitivity and specificity of routine antenatal screening for congenital anomalies by ultrasound: The Belgian multicentric study. Ultrasound Obstet Gynecol 1:102–110, 1991.

Luck CA: Value of routine ultrasound scanning at 19 weeks: A four year study of 8849 deliveries. Br Med J 304:1474–1478, 1992.

Merz E, Bahlmann F, Weber G, et al: Three-dimensional ultrasound in prenatal diagnosis. J Perinat Med 23:213–222, 1995.

Merz E, Bahlmann F, Weber G: Volume scanning in the evaluation of fetal malformations: A new dimension in prenatal diagnosis. Ultrasound Obstet Gynecol 5:222–227, 1995.

Moore RM, Jeng LL, Kacmarek RG, et al: Utilization of diagnostic imaging procedures and fetal monitoring devices in the medical care of pregnant women. Public Health Rep 105:471–475, 1990.

Moore TR, Cayle JE: The amniotic fluid index in normal human pregnancy. Am J Obstet Gynecol 162:1168–1173, 1990.

Nyberg DA, Kramer D, Resta RG, et al: Prenatal sonographic findings of trisomy 18. Review of 47 cases. J Ultrasound Med 12:103–113, 1993.

Nyberg DA, Dubinsky T, Resta RG, et al: Echogenic fetal bowel during the second trimester: Clinical importance. Radiology 188:527–531, 1993.

Pretorius DH, Gosink BB, Clautice-Engle T, et al: Sonographic evaluation of the fetal stomach: Significance of nonvisualization. AJR Am J Roentgenol 151:987–989, 1988.

Pretorius DH, Drose JA, Manco-Johnson ML: Fetal lateral ventricular ratio determination during the second trimester. J Ultrasound Med 5:121–124, 1986.

Pretorius DH, Nelson TR, Jaffe JS: 3-Dimensional sonographic analysis based on color flow Doppler and gray scale image data: A preliminary report. J Ultrasound Med 11:225–232, 1992.

Pretorius DH, Richards RD, Budorick NE, et al: Three-dimensional ultrasound in evaluation of fetal anomalies. Radiology 205(suppl):245, 1997.

Rabinowitz R, Peters MT, Vya S, et al: Measurement of fetal urine production in normal pregnancy by real time sonography. Am J Obstet Gynecol 161:1264–1266, 1989.

Riccabona M, Pretorius DH, Nelson TR, et al: Three-dimensional ultrasound: Display modalities in obstetrics. J Clin Ultrasound 25:157–167, 1997.

Rizos N, Doran TA, Miskin M, et al: Natural history of placenta previa ascertained by diagnostic ultrasound. Am J Obstet Gynecol 133:287–291, 1979.

Saari-Kemppainen A, Karjalainen O, Ylostalo P, et al: Ultrasound screening and perinatal mortality: Controlled trial of systematic one-stage screening in pregnancy. Lancet 338:387–391, 1990.

Salvesen KA, Bakketeig LS, Eik-Nes SH, et al: Routine ultrasonography in utero and school performance at age 8–9 years. Lancet 339:85–89, 1992.

Scioscia AL, Pretorius DH, Budorick NE, et al: Second trimester echogenic bowel and chromosome. Am J Obstet Gynecol 167:889–894, 1992.

Shields LE, Uhrich SB, Easterling TR, et al: Isolated fetal choroid plexus cysts and karyotype analysis: Is it necessary? J Ultrasound Med 15:389–394, 1996.

Shirley IM, Bottomley F, Robinson VP: Routine radiographer screening for fetal abnormalities by ultrasound in an unselected low risk population. Br J Radiol 65:564–569, 1992.

Stark C, Orleans M, Haverkamp A, et al: Short- and long-term risk after exposure to diagnostic ultrasound in utero. Obstet Gynecol 63:194–200, 1984.

Steiner H, Staudach A, Spitzer D, et al: Three-dimensional ultrasound in obstetrics and gynecology: Technique, possibilities and limitations. Hum Reprod 9:1773–1778, 1994.

Townsend RR, Laing FC, Nyberg DA, et al: Technical factors responsible for "placental migration": Sonographic assessment. Radiology 160:105–108, 1986.

Townsend RR, Simpson GF, Filly RA: Membrane thickness in ultrasound prediction of chorionicity of twin gestations. J Ultrasound Med 7:327–332, 1988.

VanDorsten JP, Hulsey TC, Newman RB, et al: Fetal anomaly detection by second-trimester ultrasonography in a tertiary center. Am J Obstet Gynecol 178:742–749, 1998.

Watson WJ, Cheschier NC, Katz VL, et al: The role of ultrasound in the evaluation of patients with elevated MSAFP: A review. Obstet Gynecol 78:123–128, 1991.

Winn HN, Gabrielli S, Reece EA, et al: Ultrasonographic criteria for the prenatal diagnosis of placental chorionicity in twin gestations. Am J Obstet Gynecol 161:1540–1542, 1989.

# 24

# Premature Rupture of Fetal Membranes (PROM)*

NEIL ATHAYDE
ELI MAYMON
PERCY PACORA
ROBERTO ROMERO

Premature or prelabor rupture of the fetal membranes (PROM) refers to membrane rupture before the onset of labor. The term preterm PROM refers to rupture of membranes before the 37th week. The latency period refers to the interval between rupture of membranes and spontaneous onset of labor. Prolonged PROM is a term to describe a latency period that is longer than 24 hours.

The overall incidence of PROM is 10%. Preterm PROM occurs in 2 to 3.5% of all pregnancies and is the leading identifiable cause of preterm delivery. Of all preterm neonates, 30 to 40% are born to women who have PROM. PROM is a risk factor for perinatal morbidity and mortality particularly when it occurs before 32 weeks. The main maternal risks associated with PROM are chorioamnionitis and puerperal infection. The incidence of chorioamnionitis increases from between 0.5 to 1% in the general obstetric population to 3 to 31% in women who have PROM.

## Etiology

Under normal circumstances and in the absence of intervention, the fetal membranes remain intact during pregnancy and spontaneous rupture occurs in the advanced first stage of labor (≥7 cm) or during the second stage of labor. The fetal membranes are formed by the apposition of amnion and chorion. Most of the strength of the fetal membranes has been attributed to the amnion. Chorion and amnion contain a cellular component as well as a strong extracellular matrix, which provides the tensile strength of membranes.

Fetal membranes produce enzymes that degrade extracellular matrix components. Histologic studies of membranes from patients with term PROM indicate that histologic abnormalities in the spongy layer amnion include decrease in the number of collagen fibers, disruption of the normal wavy pattern of these

---
*This chapter is in the public domain.

**Table 24–1** Risk Factor: Previous Preterm Delivery

| First Pregnancy | Second Pregnancy | |
| --- | --- | --- |
| | Preterm PROM (%) | Term PROM (%) |
| Preterm PROM | 21 | 17 |
| Preterm, no PROM | 10 | 13 |
| Term PROM | 7 | 26 |
| Term, no PROM | 4 | 17 |

PROM = premature rupture of membranes.
From Naeye RL: Factors that predispose to premature rupture of the fetal membranes. Obstet Gynecol 60:93, 1982. Reprinted with permission from the American College of Obstetricians and Gynecologists.

fibers, and deposit of amorphous material between fibers. It is unclear if these abnormalities are the cause or consequence of PROM. However, the histologic changes described earlier have been noted in membranes apposed to the cervix and obtained from patients not in labor who underwent elective cesarean sections. This implies that the changes responsible for PROM begin before labor.

**Matrix Degradation.** Total collagen content is reduced in the amnion of women with preterm PROM. Collagens are broken down by collagenases, which are members of the matrix metalloproteinase (MMP) family of enzymes. Increased protease activity caused by an increase in MMP activity, mainly MMP-2 and MMP-9, has been reported in membranes in cases of PROM when compared with membranes of women delivering preterm for other complications. Microbial invasion of the amniotic cavity (MIAC) is associated with a significant increase in MMP activity in amniotic fluid.

## WHO IS AT RISK FOR PROM?

The most significant risk factor for PROM is a history of this complication in a previous pregnancy (Table 24–1). Table 24–2 displays other clinical risk factors for preterm PROM; smoking and vaginal bleeding are the most significant. Most evidence indicates that sexual intercourse is not a risk factor for PROM. The incidence of PROM is increased in patients who have inherited disorders of collagen metabolism. In a retrospective study of the birth characteristics of patients with Ehlers-Danlos syndrome, the rate of prematurity was 77% (14 of 18); preterm PROM occurred in 92% (13 of 14) of those delivered preterm. Patients with a history of cervical conization have been considered at risk for preterm PROM, although the literature is controversial.

## DO DIGITAL EXAMINATIONS DURING PREGNANCY CAUSE PROM?

Lenihan reported a randomized prospective trial in which women at 37 weeks of gestation were randomized to weekly pelvic examinations vs. no pelvic examinations. PROM was more common in women who underwent repeated pelvic examinations than in the control group (18% [32 of 174] vs. 6% [10 of 175], $P < .001$). This observation is at variance with that reported by McDuffie and associates who conducted a prospective randomized trial comparing weekly cervical examinations from 37 weeks of gestation with no examinations and found no differences in the rates of PROM, chorioamnionitis, or neonatal infectious morbidity. Main and associates randomized women at risk for preterm delivery to either biweekly pelvic examinations or standard obstetric care. No difference in the incidence of PROM was noted between the two groups (50% [8 of 16] vs. 28.6% [4 of 14]). This observation was subsequently confirmed with a larger sample size. Holbrook and associates, in a retrospective review of patients enrolled in the Preterm Birth Prevention Program in California who received weekly cervical examinations, found no increase in the rates of preterm PROM, chorioamnionitis, or postpartum endometritis. Therefore, most evidence does not seem to support an etiologic role for digital examination in patients with PROM.

**Table 24–2** Clinical Risk Factors for Preterm Premature Rupture of the Membranes (PROM) Multivariate Analysis

| Risk Factors | Odds Ratio | 95% CI |
| --- | --- | --- |
| Previous preterm delivery | 2.48 | 1.40–2.48 |
| Cigarette smoking | 1.08 | 1.37–3.13 |
| No bleeding during pregnancy | 1.00 | — |
| First-trimester bleeding | 2.38 | 1.47–3.86 |
| Second-trimester bleeding | 4.42 | 1.62–12.03 |
| Third-trimester bleeding | 6.44 | 1.81–22.91 |
| Bleeding during more than one trimester | 7.43 | 2.16–25.60 |

CI = confidence interval.
From Harger JH, Hsing AW, Tuomala RE, et al: Risk factors for preterm premature rupture of fetal membranes: A multicenter case-control study. Am J Obstet Gynecol 163:130, 1990.

## THE ROLE OF INFECTION IN MEMBRANE RUPTURE

Intrauterine infection is detected in one third of all women with PROM (term and preterm) and has been implicated as a causal factor of ROM. Microorganisms and their products could weaken the membrane directly or through the effect of host (maternal fetal or both) by the production of proinflammatory cytokines and activation of enzymes that degrade the extracellular matrix (MMP). Lower genital tract colonization with *Chlamydia trachomatis* (CT) or *Neisseria gonorrhoeae* (NG) or *Trichomonas vaginalis* but not with group B streptococcus (GBS) is a risk factor for PROM.

**Chlamydia trachomatis (CT).** In a prospective observational study of women who had positive cultures (8% of women enrolled), PROM (term and preterm) was more common in those with positive serum immunoglobulin (IgM) (antichlamydial antibody titers of 1:32 or higher) than in those who had negative IgM (7 of 17 vs. 4 of 53, $P < .01$). In a case-control study, Alger and associates found that CT was isolated more frequently from women who had preterm PROM than from women in the control group (44 [23 of 52] versus 15% [13 of 84], $P < .01$). These observations indicate that PROM occurs not in patients who have infection with CT but in those who have a host response as judged by the IgM response. Two retrospective studies showed that patients who were successfully treated for CT had significantly lower rates of PROM compared with untreated or unsuccessfully treated women.

**Neisseria gonorrhoeae (NG).** Amstey and associates screened 5065 women at the time of the initial visit and at 36 weeks of gestation and found a positive cervical culture for NG in 4.4% of patients (222 of 5065). PROM was more common in women who had positive cultures than in women who had negative cultures (26% [52 of 198] vs. 19% [799 of 4246], $P < .01$). Edwards and associates reported that PROM was more common in women who had cervical gonorrhea at delivery than in women who had negative cultures (63% [12 of 19] vs. 29.3% [12 of 41], $P < .05$). However, the prevalence of PROM was not higher in women who had positive cervical cultures during pregnancy compared with a matched control group (28.1% [50 of 178] vs. 25.4% [98 of 386]). Prolonged PROM (more than 24 hours) has been reported to be significantly more common in women who have positive endocervical, endometrial, or placental cultures for NG than in women who have negative cultures (75% [9 of 12] vs. 37% [18 of 49], $P < .05$). Routine screening for NG is part of standard obstetric practice in the United States in centers where its prevalence justifies this policy.

**Group B Streptococcus (GBS).** Regan and associates reported that PROM was more common in women who had cervical colonization of GBS at the time of delivery than in noncarriers (15.3 [134 of 877] vs. 7% [409 of 5829], $P < .005$). In a study of 718 patients who had vaginal cultures for GBS monthly (starting at 24 weeks) and at the time of admission for labor, PROM that resulted in the delivery of a low birth weight infant was more common in carriers than in noncarriers (6% [4 of 71] vs. 2% [11 of 637], $P < .05$). However, the Vaginal Infection and Prematurity Study Group, who conducted the largest study to date that addressed this question, failed to demonstrate that colonization with GBS was a risk factor for PROM.

**Bacterial Vaginosis (BV).** Several case control studies link the presence of BV to PROM and preterm delivery, but the interpretation of these studies is made complex by the frequent coexistence of preterm labor and PROM. However, the association between BV and PROM has not been confirmed by the study conducted by the Vaginal Infection and Prematurity Study Group. This cohort study of 10,397 pregnant women who had no medical risk factors for preterm delivery could not demonstrate any significant association between BV and PROM.

***Trichomonas Vaginalis.*** In a prospective study of vaginal flora, Minkoff and associates cultured 233 patients at the time of their first prenatal visit (mean $13.8 \pm 3.6$ weeks) for *Trichomonas*, *Mycoplasmas*, and aerobic and anaerobic bacteria. The overall incidence of positive cultures for *Trichomonas* was 14.6% (34 of 233). Women who subsequently developed PROM had a higher rate of positive cultures than women who did not develop this complication (27.5% [11 of 40] vs. 12.8% [19 of 148], $P = .03$). Stepwise logistic regression analysis (including patient characteristics, such as parity, maternal age, preterm birth, and the effect of 12 different microorganisms) showed that colonization with *Trichomonas* was associated with a relative risk of developing PROM of 1.42 ($P < .05$), but no association between colonization and preterm PROM was found.

## Consequences of PROM

ROM has different implications in the preterm and the term gestation. Spontaneous labor follows ROM in the majority of cases. Consequently, the complications of prematurity are the major fetal risk in preterm gestation. The second major complication of PROM is infection, including chorioamnionitis, endometritis, septic pelvic thrombophebitis, wound infection, and maternal and neonatal sepsis. Oligohydramnios associated with preterm PROM may lead to clinical features of the oligohydramnios sequence, including pulmonary hypoplasia, pneumothorax, and skeletal deformities. Other obstetric complications of PROM are cord prolapse, placental abruption, and fetal distress during labor. These are responsible, in part, for the higher rate of cesarean sections in patients who have preterm PROM.

# Preterm PROM

## NATURAL HISTORY

Studies of the natural history of PROM are important for counseling patients about perinatal outcome without intervention. Three studies have addressed the natural history of preterm PROM.

Cox and associates looked at 298 patients who had preterm PROM and who were managed without steroids, tocolytics, or prophylactic antibiotics. Of the 267 patients who gave birth to infants weighing ≥750 g, 76% (204 of 267) were either in active labor when they were admitted to the hospital or spontaneously began labor within 12 hours of admission. Five percent of patients underwent delivery because of complications, including hypertension, fetal death, and diabetes. The remaining 19% (50 of 267) were managed expectantly. Sixty percent of these patients went into spontaneous labor within 48 hours of hospital admission. Thus, only 7% of the original 267 patients did not undergo delivery for more than 48 hours. Chorioamnionitis developed in 10.6% of cases, breech presentation occurred in 18%, twin gestation was present in 6.7%, and the incidence of cesarean section was 40%. Of the 284 infants who had birth weights of 750 g or more, there were 12 stillbirths (all before hospital admission) and 18 neonatal deaths (neonatal death rate 6.6%). The causes of death were complications of prematurity (N=12), malformations (N=3), hypoplastic lungs (N=1), and neonatal sepsis (N=2).

Wilson and associates reported on the outcome of 143 patients who had preterm PROM managed conservatively. Eighteen percent of patients had not given birth after 1 week of hospital admission. Maternal febrile infectious morbidity (antepartum and postpartum) occurred in 10% of patients, 18.6% (27 of 145) of neonates were born in breech presentation, and the incidence of cesarean section was 22% (31 of 143). The neonatal death rate was 12.4% (17 of 137). Nelson and associates reported on 511 women who had preterm PROM and singleton pregnancies that were managed without tocolytics, antibiotics, or steroids. Within 48 hours, 52.2% gave birth and 12.9% had not given birth after 1 week. The perinatal death rate was 8.4% (43 of 511), with 35 deaths occurring in cases of PROM before 28 weeks of gestation (death rate in this group was 35 of 82, or 42.7%). Maternal infection occurred in 21.7% of cases. Maternal infection increased the risk of neonatal death; the neonatal mortality rate was 46.6% (14 of 30) in patients who had preterm PROM at less than 28 weeks of gestation, and 1.2% (1 of 81) when PROM occurred after 28 weeks of gestation. The cesarean section rate was 20.5% (105 of 511). Another prospective observation study compared the outcome of patients managed expectantly with bed rest alone with another group managed with tocolytics and antibiotics. Women who were in labor at the time of admission were excluded. Fifty percent of patients in the expectant group gave birth within 48 hours of admission and 88% within 7 days.

## MICROBIAL INVASION OF THE AMNIOTIC CAVITY (MIAC)

The overall prevalence of positive cultures in fluid obtained by amniocentesis from patients with PROM is 36.1%. However, labor status is a major determinant of the rate of MIAC. Patients with preterm PROM who are in preterm labor when they are admitted to the hospital have a higher incidence of positive amniotic fluid cultures than those who are not in labor (39% vs. 26%, $P<.05$).

The microorganisms isolated from the amniotic fluid of women with PROM are similar to those normally found in the lower genital tract in 76% of cases, an observation which has been interpreted to support the concept that MIAC follows an ascending pathway. *Mycoplasmas* (*M. hominis* and *Ureaplasma urealyticum*) are the most frequently isolated organisms, followed by GBS, other streptococci, *Bacteroides* species, and *Gardnerella vaginalis*. Polymicrobial infection has been found in 26.7% (43 of 161) patients. An inoculum size of more than $10^5$ colony-forming units was found in 23% (6 of 26) and more than $10^4$ in 66.9% (6 of 9).

Patients who have MIAC are more likely to develop chorioamnionitis, endometritis, and neonatal sepsis than patients who have negative amniotic fluid culture at hospital admission. Table 24-3 shows the rate of these complications in studies in which antibiotics were not used before delivery.

It is of considerable interest that the microorganisms isolated from septic newborns are similar to those found in the amniotic fluid. In a study of 221 patients who had preterm PROM, we found six cases of culture-proved neonatal sepsis. In 5 of these cases, the microorganisms were the same as those found in the amniotic fluid; in the remaining case, the amniotic fluid culture was negative 48 hours before delivery. The practical implication of this observation is that amniocentesis performed before delivery may provide microbiologic information helpful in guiding antibiotic choice for treatment of the newborn infant.

Traditionally, it was believed that MIAC was the consequence of the membrane rupture. However, a growing body of evidence suggests that PROM may be the result of subclinical infection and inflammation. First, the prevalence of histologic chorioamnionitis is significantly higher in women who have

Table 24-3  Rate of Infectious Complications in Premature Rupture of the Membranes (PROM)

| Main Author | MIAC Number | CA (%) | Endometritis (%) | DNS (%) | No MIAC Number | CA (%) | Endometritis (%) | DNS (%) |
|---|---|---|---|---|---|---|---|---|
| Garite | 9 | 66.6 | 33.3 | 22.2 | 21 | 4.7 | 4.7 | 0 |
| Vintzileos | 20 | 55 | 25 | 25 | 66 | 7.5 | 1.5 | 3.0 |
| Broekhuizen | 15 | 20 | 33 | 7 | 38 | 0 | 3 | 3 |
| Cotton | 6 | 100 | * | 17 | 35 | 9 | * | 0 |
| Feinstein | 12 | 17 | NA | 17 | 38 | 5 | NA | 0 |
| Zlatnik | 9 | 66.6 | * | 1.1 | 20 | 15 | * | 0 |

MIAC = microbial invasion of the amniotic cavity; CA = chorioamnionitis; DNS = documented neonatal sepsis; NA = not available.
*Inclusive of chorioamnionitis and endometritis.

PROM. Naeye and Peters reported that patients who had PROM 1 to 4 hours before the onset of labor had a higher prevalence of histologic chorioamnionitis than patients who delivered preterm without PROM. Several lines of evidence suggest that the most likely cause of histologic chorioamnionitis is subclinical infection. Bacteria have been recovered from 72% of placentas with histologic chorioamnionitis. Furthermore, Romero and associates demonstrated a strong correlation between a positive amniotic fluid culture for microorganisms and histologic chorioamnionitis. Neonates born to women who have PROM have increased levels of IgM, IgA, and interleukin-6 (IL-6), suggesting that the fetal immune system has had time to respond to a pre-existing infection of some duration.

## ABRUPTIO PLACENTAE

Abruptio placentae occurs more frequently in patients who have preterm PROM than in the general obstetric population (0.8%). Ananth and associates reported that women who had PROM were three times more likely to develop placental abruption than those who did not have PROM (odds ratio [OR]: 3.05; 95% confidence interval [CI]: 2.16–4.32). The mechanisms responsible for separation of the placenta in preterm PROM have not been determined. Nelson and associates proposed that leakage of fluid after PROM may lead to a disproportion between the placental and uterine surfaces that in turn may lead to placental separation. An alternative etiopathogenetic hypothesis to explain the relationship between abruptio placentae and preterm PROM postulates that a disorder of decidual homeostasis leads to separation of the membranes from the decidua, with subsequent compromise of their nutritive support. Weakening of the membranes eventually may lead to rupture.

## PULMONARY HYPOPLASIA

Pulmonary hypoplasia refers to a condition in which the number of lung cells and alveoli are decreased. The perinatal mortality resulting from pulmonary hypoplasia is about 70% in most series. Pulmonary hypoplasia is associated with an increased risk of neonatal death and other complications, such as pneumothorax and persistent pulmonary hypertension. Two studies have looked specifically at pulmonary hypoplasia in the context of PROM. Vergani and associates performed a prospective study of patients with PROM at 28 weeks of gestation or less who were managed conservatively. Pulmonary hypoplasia was diagnosed at autopsy or by clinical or radiologic findings. The frequency of pulmonary hypoplasia was 28% (15 of 54). Gestational age at the time of PROM and presence of oligohydramnios were independent predictors of occurrence of pulmonary hypoplasia, whereas duration of latency period was not significantly associated with pulmonary hypoplasia. Rotschild and associates in a retrospective study examined the outcome of 88 infants born to women with PROM at less than 28 weeks of gestation and with a latency period of at least 1 week and used logistic regression to determine the risk factors for the development of pulmonary hypoplasia. Gestational age at the time of PROM but not duration of latency period or severity of oligohydramnios was associated with pulmonary hypoplasia. The incidence of pulmonary hypoplasia was 16% (14 of 88). It appears that the risk of pulmonary hypoplasia when PROM occurs at 19 weeks is 50%, whereas it is only 10% if the membranes rupture at 25 weeks.

## FETAL COMPRESSION SYNDROME

This syndrome includes limb position deformities and craniofacial deformities that are thought to result from the limitation of fetal growth and movement.

Nimrod and associates reported an incidence of 12% in women with preterm PROM, most occurring when the latency period was longer than 5 weeks. Blott and Greenough found that 14 of 30 (46.7%) infants born after prolonged membrane rupture (>4 weeks) had limb abnormalities. Studies of second-trimester PROM reported an overall incidence of less than 1%. Rotschild and associates used multiple logistic regression to show that the duration of the latency period and the severity of oligohydramnios was most predictive of skeletal deformities. McIntosh and associates reported that 25 of 117 (21.6%) infants born after PROM had deformities. The median duration of rupture in the group with deformities was 28 days, compared with 9 days in infants without deformities.

## Diagnosis

Evaluation of the patient who has suspected PROM begins with a sterile speculum examination. Visualization of a vaginal pool or obvious leakage of fluid from the cervix into the posterior fornix is strong evidence supporting the diagnosis of ruptured membranes. A sterile swab of fluid should be obtained from the posterior fornix and placed on a clean glass slide and on nitrazine paper. Amniotic fluid, if allowed to dry, shows arborization (ferning) under the microscope at low magnification. Meconium has no effect on ferning and blood inhibits ferning only at very high concentrations. Ferning has an overall accuracy in the diagnosis of PROM of 96%. False-positive results are rare and have been described by contamination with semen and cervical mucus. False negatives (5 to 10%) may be caused by dry swabs or by contamination with blood. The glass slide should be evaluated after at least 10 minutes of drying to decrease the false-negative rate. Nitrazine paper changes color (yellow to blue) when exposed to any alkaline fluid (i.e., pH of 7.0 or more). The normal pH of the vagina is 4.5 to 5.5, whereas that of the amniotic fluid is 7.0 to 7.5. The Nitrazine test has an overall accuracy of 93.3% in the diagnosis of PROM. False-positive results range from 1 to 17% and can result from alkaline urine, blood, semen, vaginal discharge in cases of bacterial vaginosis, or *Trichomonas* infection.

Oligohydramnios detected by an ultrasonographic examination increases the index of suspicion that rupture of the membranes has occurred but other causes of oligohydramnios, such as severe fetal growth retardation or fetal urinary tract anomalies, must be carefully ruled out. Conversely, a normal amount of amniotic fluid does not exclude the diagnosis of PROM. Occasionally, the diagnosis is so uncertain that amniocentesis is required for final diagnosis. Transabdominal injection of dye (phenazopyridine hydrochloride [Pyridium], phenolsulfonphthalein, Evans blue, fluorescein, and indigo carmine) is the method of choice. Methylene blue should not be used, because it may cause fetal methemoglobinemia, hemolytic anemia, and hyperbilirubinemia. A sterile tampon in the vagina can document subsequent leakage in cases of PROM.

Performing a digital examination to determine cervical status in patients with PROM who are not in labor is not justified. This information can be obtained adequately by examination with a sterile speculum and visual examination of the cervix. Two prospective studies have shown a reasonable correlation in the assessment of cervical status (dilatation and effacement) between digital and speculum examination when examinations were performed by the same examiner. Three studies indicate that a digital examination reduces the duration of the latency period, probably by increasing the likelihood of ascending intrauterine infection. Therefore, we believe that digital examinations should be avoided. The diagnosis of cord prolapse can be made by an examination using a sterile speculum.

## Management of Preterm PROM

The initial evaluation of a patient with preterm PROM includes assessment of gestational age and fetal weight, presentation, evaluation of the risk of infection, lung maturity, and fetal well-being. Ultrasonographic examination is performed to determine fetal presentation, biometry, the volume of amniotic fluid, and fetal well-being. Sonographic estimates of fetal weight have been shown to have a tendency to underestimate the real weight by 2 to 20%.

### ASSESSMENT OF THE RISK OF INTRAUTERINE INFECTION

#### Amniocentesis

This procedure is widely used for the evaluation of the microbiological state of the amniotic cavity and of fetal lung maturity in the patient with preterm PROM. Results of amniotic fluid analysis provide a rational approach to management of preterm PROM. Patients without evidence of infection and lung immaturity are managed expectantly. Those who have evidence of infection at 32 weeks of gestation (estimated fetal weight [EFW] >1500 grams) are given antibiotics and their infants are delivered. Determining the optimal management of patients who have

MIAC and a gestational age earlier than 30 weeks is a challenge. Extensive discussion with the patient is required. One approach is delivering the infants of all patients who have microbial invasion regardless of gestational age. However, this carries the risk of extreme prematurity and its consequences in the neonate. An alternative approach is to attempt eradication of microbial invasion with antibiotic therapy.

How effective is this approach? Ogita and associates first reported the successful treatment of established chorioamnionitis with antibiotic treatment via a transcervical catheter. Subsequently, Romero and associates reported that in a mother who had preterm PROM at 29 weeks of gestation and an amniotic fluid culture positive for *Bacteroides bivius*, *Veillonella parvula*, and *Peptococcus* without clinical signs of chorioamnionitis, treatment with antibiotics resulted in eradication of the microbial invasion of the amniotic cavity. In a second case, Romero and associates were successful in eradicating *U. urealyticum* from the amniotic cavity with antibiotic treatment. These observations demonstrate that antibiotic treatment may alter the progression of microbial invasion of the amniotic cavity. However, the safety and efficacy of this technique has not been established.

How successful is amniocentesis? Retrieval rates of amniotic fluid vary from 49 to 96%. The wide disparity in retrieval rates is probably attributable to differences in policy regarding patient selection in different institutions. As experience with ultrasonography and invasive techniques of prenatal diagnosis grow, the success rate of amniotic fluid retrieval in patients with PROM is likely to increase. Only one small randomized clinical trial has examined the value of amniocentesis in the setting of preterm PROM. Forty-seven patients (at 26 to 34 weeks of gestation who had an accessible amniotic fluid pocket) were randomized to amniocentesis or no amniocentesis. Indications for induction of labor included positive Gram's stain of amniotic fluid or mature fetal lungs, as determined by a lecithin/sphingomyelin (L/S) ratio greater than 2.0 or positive phosphatidylglycerol (PG). Neonates born to women who underwent amniocentesis had a lower incidence of fetal distress during labor (as judged by fetal heart rate tracing) and a shorter hospital stay than those born to women randomized not to have amniocentesis (fetal distress: 4% [1 of 24] vs. 32% [7 of 22], $P<.05$; hospital stay: median 8.5 days vs. 22 days, $P<.01$). No difference in the rate of neonatal sepsis, maternal chorioamnionitis, or endometritis was noted between the two groups. Although the rate of neonatal sepsis was threefold higher in the control group, the difference was not statistically significant (14% [3 of 22] vs. 4% [1 of 22]). However, the power of this study to detect differences in neonatal morbidity was small. Thus, these data are insufficient to determine whether amniocentesis is beneficial in the management of PROM.

The optimal laboratory method for detecting microorganisms in amniotic fluid has not been determined. Amniotic fluid cultures are considered the gold standard but may take several days to yield results. Therefore, rapid, sensitive, and simple tests must be developed to detect microbial invasion of the amniotic cavity. In practice, we use a combination of Gram's stain of amniotic fluid as well as amniotic fluid white blood cell count. Gram's stain has a sensitivity of less than 50% in the detection of microorganisms.

Table 24–4 summarizes the diagnostic criteria and predictive values of different amniotic fluid tests in detection of positive amniotic fluid cultures in patients with preterm PROM. Amniotic fluid (AF) IL-6 performed best in detecting MIAC as well as in identifying patients at risk for impending preterm delivery and neonatal complications. We have shown that AF IL-6 is a sensitive test for the prospective diagnosis of acute histologic chorioamnionitis (IL-6 >17ng/ml had a sensitivity of 79%, 23 of 29, and specificity of 100%, 21 of 21) and significant neonatal morbidity (sepsis, respiratory distress syndrome [RDS], pneumonia, intraventricular hemorrhage [IVH], bronchopulmonary dysplasia [BPD] and necrotizing enterocolitis [NEC]) and mortality (IL-6 >17ng/ml sensitivity 69%, 18 of 26, and specificity 79%, 19 of 24). Other rapid tests on amniotic fluid reported for the detection of MIAC include:

1. Amniotic fluid (AF) catalase (sensitivity of 90% [19 of 21], specificity of 93% [15 of 16], positive predictive value of 95% [19 of 20] and negative predictive value of 88% [15 of 17]).
2. Leukocyte amebocyte lysate (LAL) test: Hazan and associates found that a combination of Gram's stain and LAL test had a sensitivity of 51.7% (15 of 29), specificity of 95.1% (58 of 61), positive predictive value of 83.3% (15 of 18) and negative predictive value of 80.6% (58 of 72) in detecting MIAC. The LAL test had the worst performance in detection of *Mycoplasma* species.
3. Bacterial PCR: This technique may prove to be of great value. Using primers for amplification of the 16S ribosomal DNA from all known human bacteria, including *U. urealyticum*, Jalava and associates found PCR positive in 5 of 20 women with PROM, whereas cultures were positive in 2 of 20.

The risk of amniocentesis has been addressed by Yeast and associates, who studied 91 patients in whom amniocentesis had been performed in the setting of PROM. A retrospective review of the neonatal records uncovered no evidence of fetal trauma in any case. A hematoma of the broad ligament was noted

Table 24–4 Diagnostic Indices and Predictive Values of Different Amniotic Fluid Tests in the Detection of Positive Amniotic Fluid Culture in Patients With Preterm Premature Rupture of the Membranes (PROM)

| | Sensitivity % (N) | Specificity % (N) | PPV % (N) | NPV % (N) |
|---|---|---|---|---|
| Gram's stain | 23.8 (10/42) | 98.5 (67/68) | 90.9 (10/11) | 67.8 (67/99) |
| IL-6 ≥ 7.9 ng/ml | 80.9 (34/42) | 75.0 (51/68) | 66.7 (34/51) | 86.4 (51/59) |
| White blood count (≥30 cell/mm$^3$) | 57.1 (24/42) | 77.9 (53/68) | 61.5 (24/39) | 74.6 (53/71) |
| White blood cell (≥50 cells/mm$^3$) | 52.4 (22/42) | 83.8 (57/68) | 66.7 (22/33) | 74 (57/77) |
| Glucose (<10 mg/dl) | 57.1 (24/42) | 73.5 (50/68) | 57.1 (24/42) | 73.5 (50/68) |
| Glucose (<14 mg/dl) | 71.4 (30/42) | 51.5 (35/68) | 47.6 (30/63) | 74.5 (35/47) |
| Gram's stain + white blood cell (≥30 cell/mm$^3$) | 61.9 (26/42) | 77.9 (53/68) | 63.4 (26/41) | 76.8 (53/68) |
| Gram's stain + glucose (<10 mg/dl) | 66.7 (28/42) | 73.5 (50/68) | 60.9 (28/46) | 78.1 (50/64) |
| Gram's stain + IL-6 (≥7.9 ng/dl) | 80.9 (34/42) | 75 (51/68) | 66.7 (34/51) | 86.4 (51/59) |
| Gram's stain + glucose (<10 mg/dl) + white blood cell (≥30 cell/mm$^3$) | 76.2 (32/42) | 60.3 (41/68) | 54.2 (32/59) | 80.4 (41/51) |
| Gram's stain + white blood cell (≥30 cell/mm$^3$) + IL-6 ≥ 7.9 ng/ml | 85.7 (36/42) | 61.8 (42/68) | 58.1 (36/62) | 87.5 (42/48) |
| Gram's stain + glucose (<10 mg/dl) + IL-6 > 7.9 ng/ml | 85.7 (36/42) | 52.9 (36/68) | 52.9 (36/68) | 85.7 (36/42) |
| Gram's stain + white blood cell (≥30 cell/mm$^3$) + glucose (<10 mg/dl) + IL-6 ≥ 7.9 ng/ml | 92.9 (39/42) | 47.1 (32/68) | 52 (39/75) | 91.4 (32/35) |

NPV = negative pressure ventilation; PPV = positive pressure ventilation.
From Romero R, Yoon BH, Mazor M, et al: A comparative study of the diagnostic performance of amniotic fluid glucose, white blood cell count, interleukin-6 and Gram stain in the detection of microbial invasion in patients with preterm rupture of membranes. Am J Obstet Gynecol 169:846, 1993.

in one patient who had a cesarean section for an indication unrelated to amniocentesis. This study also found that the incidence of spontaneous labor in patients who underwent amniocentesis was no different from that of patients who did not undergo amniocentesis secondary to oligohydramnios or an anterior placenta.

## EVALUATION OF LUNG MATURITY

Lung maturity can be assessed from the amniotic fluid obtained by amniocentesis or from the vaginal pool. Three studies have reported neonatal outcome and L/S ratio results in preterm PROM. In two of the studies, a mature L/S ratio was an indication for delivery. In the third study, PG presence was used as an indication for delivery. The data are quite consistent: With a mature L/S ratio, the risk of RDS is extraordinarily small. Sbarra and associates demonstrated that cervical and vaginal washings are generally devoid of lecithin and sphingomyelin (9 of 10 cases) and thus, these secretions are unlikely to alter L/S results. Two studies determined that introduction of amniotic fluid (obtained by transabdominal amniocentesis) into the vagina results in little change in the L/S ratio.

A mature phospholipid study has been demonstrated in about 50% of patients with preterm PROM at gestational ages earlier than 34 weeks. Garite and associates reported that none of the neonates with an L/S ratio greater than or equal to 1.8 developed RDS. The incidence of this complication in neonates with immature L/S was 33% (5 of 15).

What is the optimal management of patients with a mature phospholipid profile? Three randomized clinical trials have addressed this question. The first had 47 patients with preterm PROM (earlier than 36 weeks of gestation) and mature amniotic fluid indices. Patients were randomized to either prompt delivery (N = 26) or expectant management (N = 21). A mature test was defined as an L/S ratio greater than 2 or a foam stability index (FSI) of 47 or more. There were no differences in perinatal mortality between the two groups. There were no cases of RDS in the expectant management group, but there were 2 in the delivery group. One baby died from severe hyaline membrane disease (birth weight 900 g, vaginal FSI = 48), whereas the other infant survived (birth weight 1700 g, vaginal L/S = 2.0). There was no difference in the rate of neonatal sepsis or other neonatal complications in the two groups. However, the only 2 cases of intraventricular hemorrhage (grade not stated) occurred in the delivery group. Maternal chorioamnionitis was more common in the expectant management group than in the delivery group (38% [8 of 21] vs. 8% [2 of 26], P = .02). The predictive value of a mature test was 97%.

Mercer and associates reported the second study, in which 93 women with mature AF phospholipid studies between 32 and 36 weeks of gestation (vaginal or transabdominal amniocentesis FSI ≥47) were randomized to induction of labor with oxytocin or bed rest and expectant management. Clinical chorioamnionitis was more frequent in the expectant group (13 of 47 vs. 5 of 46). There were no significant differences in the cesarean section rate (3 of 47 vs. 4 of 46) or in the incidence of confirmed neonatal sepsis (2 of

47 vs. 3 of 46). Suspected sepsis was higher in neonates born to women in the expectant group (28 of 47 vs. 13 of 46). However, neonatologists were not blinded to treatment allocation. There were no cases of neonatal deaths, RDS, IVH, or NEC in either group. Of the 106 women who had amniocentesis, only 13 had immature AF phospholipid studies. Cox and associates conducted a randomized trial of expectant management vs. delivery in PROM between 30 and 34 weeks of gestation in 129 women. Corticosteroids were not used and fetal lung maturity was not assessed. Chorioamnionitis was higher in the group managed expectantly [14.7 (10 of 68) vs. 1.6% (1 of 61)]. The cesarean section rate was lower in the expectant group [11.7 (8 of 68) vs. 23% (14 of 61); $P > 0.05$). There was 1 stillbirth due to *Escherichia coli* sepsis in the expectant group. In total, there were 3 neonatal deaths, all in the delivery group (2 caused by sepsis and 1 caused by pulmonary hypoplasia). No differences were seen in the incidence of RDS, IVH, NEC, or neonatal sepsis.

A limitation of these trials is that the status of microbial invasion of the amniotic cavity does not appear to have been part of the decision-making process. However, the results of these trials appear to indicate that intervention, simply because there is lung maturity, may not be uniformly beneficial to the neonate. Recent evidence indicates that neonates born to women with clinical chorioamnionitis are at risk for IVH, periventricular leukomalacia, and seizures within the first 24 hours of life. These data suggest that the presence of clinical chorioamnionitis may have substantial implications for the welfare of the neonate who is smaller than 1500 g, and that detection of infection may be a crucial part of obstetric management to prevent neurologic injury in utero.

## EVALUATION OF FETAL WELL-BEING

Antepartum surveillance of the patient with PROM has been undertaken with the nonstress test (NST) or the biophysical profile (BPP). The rationale is to detect fetal compromise caused by either hypoxia or infection. This section provides a critical review of available data on the reliability of these tests.

Vintzileos and associates have demonstrated that each component of the BPP contains useful information for the prediction of infectious outcome (defined as maternal chorioamnionitis, possible neonatal sepsis, and proved neonatal sepsis) in patients with PROM. A BPP of 7 or below performed 24 hours before delivery had a sensitivity of 94% (15 of 16), a specificity of 97% (36 of 37), a positive predictive value of 94% (15 of 16), and a negative predictive value of 97% (36 of 37) in a population with a prevalence of infectious outcome of 30% (16 of 53). In this study, the BPP was not used for patient management.

Subsequently, Vintzileos and associates compared the outcome of pregnancy in patients managed with serial BPPs compared with two historical control groups: one managed expectantly without BPP or amniocentesis, and the other managed with a single amniocentesis on admission. A score of 7 or below on two examinations 2 hours apart was used as an indication for delivery. An abnormal score required a nonreactive NST and absence of fetal breathing. The results of this study indicated that patients managed with daily BPPs had a lower rate of overall neonatal sepsis (suspected and culture-proved) than patients in the no amniocentesis and single amniocentesis groups. However, this study did not provide the frequency of other indices of neonatal morbidity (RDS, IVH, duration of mechanical ventilation) in the different groups. This issue is important because 14 patients whose infants were delivered because of a low BPP score showed no evidence of neonatal infection (false positives). If intervention were not associated with an increased rate of other neonatal complications, management with serial BPPs would seem a reasonable approach. Vintzileos and associates have also reported the results of a study in which 111 fetuses whose mothers had preterm PROM were followed with daily BPPs. The lower the BPP score, the higher was the incidence of infection. Although some studies have found no association between the BPP score and infectious morbidity related to infection, it is possible that these results were caused by the fact that BPPs were not performed daily and thus the test could not detect rapid changes in fetal status.

## NONSTRESS TEST (NST)

The differential diagnosis of a nonreactive NST in the preterm gestation includes lack of reactivity because of prematurity, infection, or hypoxia. A few studies have demonstrated that fetuses whose mothers had preterm PROM between 24 and 37 weeks of gestation had a significantly higher incidence of reactive tracings than gestational age-matched counterparts with intact membranes. Possible theories for explaining the increased fetal heart rate (FHR) reactivity in preterm PROM include, first, accelerated fetal central nervous system (CNS) maturation and, second, umbilical vein compression with resulting FHR acceleration. Thus, lack of reactivity should not be ascribed to prematurity without further testing. Isolated FHR decelerations have frequently been described in NSTs of patients with PROM. Their occurrence seems to be related to the amniotic fluid volume, because the amniotic fluid index is lower in patients with decelerations than in patients without them (4.32/1.67 vs. 6.47/3.59, $P < 0.01$). Overall, most studies support an association between nonreactive NST and infectious outcome. Three studies have found the NST to be an insensitive predictor of infectious outcome, and with the high false-positive rate, overall about 35%, it is inappropriate to make clinical decisions based solely on the results of this test. For this reason, we advocate the use of the BPP for antepartum surveillance in patients with PROM.

## AMNIOTIC FLUID VOLUME

Membrane rupture is not necessarily associated with oligohydramnios. Vintzileos and associates reported that 65.5% (59 of 90) of patients with PROM had a vertical pocket of amniotic fluid greater than 2 cm, 15.5% (14 of 90) had a vertical pocket between 1 and 2 cm, and only 19% (17 of 90) had a vertical pocket of less than 1 cm. There have been a number of studies that have looked at the relationship between oligohydramnios and outcomes in PROM. Vintzileos reported that patients who had a vertical amniotic fluid pocket of less than 1 cm had a shorter latency period and a higher incidence of chorioamnionitis and neonatal sepsis than patients who had a vertical pocket greater than 2 cm. A similar set of findings was reported by Gonik and associates in a study of 39 patients. Women with a vertical amniotic fluid pocket of less than 1 cm had a higher incidence of chorioamnionitis and endometritis than those with an amniotic fluid pocket greater than 1 cm. No difference in the duration of the latency period between the two groups was found in this study.

## FETAL BREATHING MOVEMENTS

Preterm PROM is associated with a significant and prolonged reduction of fetal breathing movements lasting approximately 2 weeks. This phenomenon seems to be related to ROM per se rather than to infection, hypoxia, or intrauterine growth retardation. The mechanisms responsible for the reduction in breathing movements are unknown. Membrane rupture leads to reduction in intra-amniotic pressure and thus favors loss of lung fluid. Teleologically, a reduction in fetal breathing may be a mechanism of protection against lung fluid loss and pulmonary hypoplasia.

## FETAL BODY MOVEMENTS

The number and the duration of fetal body movements are lower in patients with preterm PROM and positive amniotic fluid cultures than in patients with negative amniotic fluid cultures. Decreased fetal motion in the context of infection may be the counterpart of the reduction in motor behavior observed during the course of febrile illnesses in adults and children.

## CONCLUSION

We believe that the best approach to monitoring patients with preterm PROM is a combination of amniocentesis and BPP. Amniocentesis is performed on admission to assess the initial risk of infection, lung maturity, and fetal well-being. In the absence of demonstrable infection, patients can be followed with serial BPP. A decrease in the BPP below 7 is an indication that amniocentesis should be performed to screen for microbial invasion of the amniotic cavity. In centers where amniocentesis is not performed, management could rely on the findings of the BPP and maternal clinical signs of infection. The onset of preterm labor should be considered as evidence of subclinical intrauterine infection, and, therefore, efforts to delay delivery should be avoided. The end point for expectant management of patients with preterm PROM is controversial. An acceptable approach is to deliver the infant after 34 completed weeks of gestation because the risk of complications of prematurity is low.

# Management Issues in Preterm PROM

Three controversial issues in the management of preterm PROM are the use of tocolysis, antibiotics, and steroids. We will review the pertinent literature and provide our view on these issues.

## TOCOLYSIS

Meta-analysis of four clinical trials indicates that tocolysis does result in prolongation of pregnancy of no more than 48 hours. Moreover, no study has shown an improvement in maternal or neonatal outcome after tocolysis administration. Thus, at present there is insufficient evidence to justify the use of tocolytic agents in patients with PROM.

## ANTEPARTUM ANTIBIOTICS

One third of patients with preterm PROM have a positive amniotic fluid culture at the time of admission to the hospital; further, the onset of labor in preterm PROM is associated with microbial invasion of the amniotic cavity in about 70% of patients. Consequently, several investigators have conducted randomized clinical trials to examine the potential benefits of antibiotic administration. Several meta-analyses of these randomized clinical trials have been published. Mercer and Arheart, in their meta-analysis, looked at studies that used intravenous antibiotics in patients for at least 24 hours followed by oral therapy for at least 1 week or until delivery occurred; they found a significant improvement in pregnancy prolongation and reduction in chorioamnionitis and postpartum febrile morbidity in the antibiotic-treated groups.

The largest trial was reported by Mercer and associates. Overall, administration of antibiotics to patients resulted in pregnancy prolongation of 7 days and reduction in the rate of clinical chorioamnionitis and neonatal sepsis. There is controversy as to whether antibiotic administration to patients may reduce the rate of IVH and RDS. Based upon these data, antibiotic administration can be justified in patients with preterm PROM before 32 weeks of gestation. Our choice is ampicillin (2 g every 6 hours) and erythromycin (250 mg every 6 hours) for 48 hours followed by oral amoxycillin (250 mg every 8 hours) and erythromycin (333 mg every 8 hours) for 5 days, because this combination was used in the clinical trial reported by Mercer and associates. An alternative to erythromycin is azithromycin given as a single dose of 500 mg the first day and then 250 mg per day. However, the selection of antibiotics and the duration of therapy remain open issues. Table 24–5 displays the antibiotics used in the different trials. The adverse effects of antibiotics have not been systematically addressed. Most studies have found antibiotic use to be safe, well tolerated by patients, and not associated with the emergence of resistant strains. However, McDuffie and associates reported on the development of resistant *Enterobacteriaceae* (three *E. coli* and one *Klebsiella pneumoniae*) in 4 infants born after PROM whose mothers had completed between 25 and 35 weeks of gestation and who were treated antepartum with ampicillin or amoxycillin. Three infants died of fulminant sepsis.

## STEROID ADMINISTRATION

The use of steroids in PROM has been controversial. Evidence of an effect of PROM on fetal lung maturation is conflicting. When considered individually, most studies have failed to demonstrate a significant reduction in the incidence of RDS with steroid administration. However, meta-analyses of randomized trials showed that steroid administration resulted in a significant reduction in the incidence of RDS. Ohlsson's meta-analysis included only five randomized clinical trials and demonstrated a reduction in the incidence of RDS (relative risk [RR] 0.63, 95% CI 0.5–0.81, $P < .01$). Steroid treatment was associated with a modest yet significant increase in the risk of puerperal endometritis (RR 2.42, 95% CI 1.38–4.24) but no significant increase in neonatal sepsis. The 1994 NIH Consensus Conference recommended the use of corticosteroids in pregnancies complicated by preterm PROM with expected delivery between 24 and 30 to 32 weeks of gestation. This recommendation was based largely on data suggesting that the incidence of IVH was lower in neonates exposed to corticosteroids. The modest increased risk of puerperal infection can be easily managed with modern

Table 24–5  Randomized Clinical Trials of Antibiotic Therapy in Preterm (PROM)

| Author | Year | N | Antibiotics |
| --- | --- | --- | --- |
| Lebherz et al | 1963 | 332 | Tetracycline |
| Dunlop et al | 1986 | 48 | Cephalexin |
| Amon et al | 1988 | 43 | Ampicillin |
| Morales et al | 1989 | 78 | Ampicillin |
| Johnston et al | 1990 | 95 | Metronidazole/ampicillin |
| McGregor et al | 1991 | 55 | Erythromycin |
| Christmas et al | 1992 | 94 | Ampicillin/clindamycin/gentamycin |
| Kurki et al | 1992 | 101 | Penicillin |
| McCaul et al | 1992 | 84 | Ampicillin |
| Mercer et al | 1992 | 220 | Erythromycin |
| Blanco et al | 1993 | 186 | Ceftizoxime |
| Lockwood et al | 1993 | 75 | Piperacillin |
| Owen et al | 1993 | 117 | Ampicillin/erythromycin |
| Ernest and Givner | 1994 | 77 | Penicillin |
| Guinn et al | 1995 | 44 | Ampicillin/erythromycin |
| Lovett et al | 1997 | 112 | Ampicillin/sulbactam Amoxicillin/clavulanate |
| Mercer et al | 1997 | 614 | Ampicillin/erythromycin Amoxicillin/erythromycin |

antibiotic therapy. However, neonates should be closely followed for laboratory and clinical signs of infection. Leitich and associates published the results of two meta-analyses comparing the outcome of treatment with antibiotics and steroids vs. antibiotic treatment without steroids. Steroid administration diminished the beneficial effects of antibiotics in treatment of patients who had chorioamnionitis, endometritis, neonatal sepsis, or IVH. We interpret this evidence as calling for careful follow-up of infants born to mothers who have had microbial invasion of the amniotic cavity and who have been exposed to steroids.

## Term PROM

Women who have suspected PROM at term should be examined to establish the diagnosis of PROM. These women should be screened for infection, cord prolapse should be excluded, and fetal well-being should be evaluated. Relevant management issues include induction, or expectant management; when induction should be undertaken and by what means?

### NATURAL HISTORY

Of all women who have PROM at term, 90% are in spontaneous labor by 24 hours. Nulliparous women seem to have a longer latency period than multiparous women. Wagner and associates found that 38% of patients who had an unfavorable cervix and who were not in labor within 6 hours of ROM did not begin labor by 24 hours and, thus, represented a management dilemma.

The largest trial of different management strategies in term PROM included 5041 women. This international trial was conducted by Hannah and associates. Patients were randomly allocated to four groups: a group who had immediate induction with oxytocin; a group who were expectantly managed with oxytocin (induction with oxytocin after 4 days); a group who received induction vaginal dinoprostone (PGE$_2$) (1 to 2 mg of PGE$_2$ repeated once and followed by intravenous oxytocin if not in labor 4 hours after the second dose of PGE$_2$); and a group who were expectantly managed with PGE$_2$ (induction as for the PGE$_2$ group if not in labor by 4 days). The results from this trial showed that induction with oxytocin or PGE$_2$ resulted in similar rates of cesarean section and neonatal sepsis. Induction with oxytocin was associated with a lower rate of maternal chorioamnionitis and a lower frequency of neonatal antibiotic treatment. Women preferred induction (either with oxytocin or PGE$_2$) to expectant management.

A meta-analysis of 23 studies (7493 patients) of term PROM that compared expectant management vs. induction of labor with oxytocin or prostaglandins, demonstrated that induction was superior to expectant management. The meta-analysis compared three policies: immediate oxytocin induction; expectant management, which included delayed induction with oxytocin; and induction of labor with vaginal or endocervical prostaglandin E$_2$ gel, suppositories, or tablets. Chorioamnionitis and endometritis were significantly lower in patients who underwent immediate induction of labor with oxytocin than in those managed expectantly (OR 0.67, 95%, CI 0.52–0.85, and OR 0.71, 95% CI, 0.51–0.99, respectively). Of interest is that the rate of chorioamnionitis was significantly higher in those who received vaginal prostaglandin than in the group who received immediate oxytocin but lower than in those in the expectant management group (OR 1.55, 95%, CI, 1.09–2.21, and OR 0.68, 95%, CI, 0.51–0.91, respectively). The rates of cesarean deliveries and neonatal infections were not different among the three management schemes (Table 24–6). We endorse a policy of immediate induction of labor in patients with term PROM. Antibiotic administration is justified before cesarean section for obstetric indications or carriers of GBS.

## Special Management Issues

### CERVICAL CERCLAGE

Cerclage removal has been advocated to reduce the risk of infection-related complications in patients

**Table 24–6** Pooled ORs and CIs for Three Treatment Policies of Term Premature Rupture of the Membranes (PROM) and Outcome Variables of Interest

|  | Chorioamnionitis |  | Endometritis |  | Cesarean Section |  | Neonatal Infection |  |
|---|---|---|---|---|---|---|---|---|
|  | OR | CI | OR | CI | OR | CI | OR | CI |
| Oxytocin vs. conservative | 0.91 | (0.51–1.62) | 0.78 | (0.50–1.21) | 1.24 | (0.89–1.73) | 0.73 | (0.47–1.13) |
| Prostaglandins vs. conservative | 0.68 | (0.51–0.91) | 0.81 | (0.53–1.23) | 0.95 | (0.76–1.20) | 1.06 | (0.67–1.66) |
| Prostaglandins vs. oxytocin | 1.55 | (1.09–2.21) | 0.78 | (0.23–2.62) | 0.67 | (0.34–1.29) | 1.50 | (0.91–2.45) |

CI = confidence interval; OR = odds ratio; PROM = premature rupture of fetal membrane.
From Mozurkewich EL, Wolf FM: Premature rupture of membranes at term: A meta-analysis of three management schemes. Obstet Gynecol 89:1035, 1997. Reprinted with permission from the American College of Obstetricians and Gynecologists.

with preterm PROM. On the other hand, leaving the cerclage in place has been recommended to favor pregnancy prolongation. Four studies have addressed this problem. Yeast and Garite reported the results of a case-control study in which the outcomes of patients with cervical cerclage removed after preterm PROM were compared with those of patients with PROM of a similar gestational age. There was no difference in the incidence of chorioamnionitis or other infectious complications and neonatal outcomes between the two groups. The interval between PROM and delivery was not significantly different between patients with and without cerclage. Similar findings were reported by Blickstein and associates after comparing the outcome of 32 patients with cerclage and 76 without it. In contrast, Goldman and associates compared the outcomes of 46 patients with preterm PROM in whom the cerclage was not removed with those of 46 women with preterm PROM without cerclage. Patients with cerclage had a significantly shorter PROM-to-delivery interval and lower gestational age at delivery than patients without the cerclage. However, the rates of chorioamnionitis, other infection-related complications, and neonatal outcomes were not different between the two groups. Ludmir and associates evaluated the role of immediate cerclage removal in preterm PROM in 30 women. In 20 women, the cerclage was removed immediately after the diagnosis of ruptured membranes was made, and in 10 women the cerclage was retained after the membranes ruptured. A greater proportion of women with retained cerclages delivered their babies within 48 hours (9 of 10 vs. 10 of 20). Perinatal morbidity (7 of 10 vs. 2 of 20) was significantly higher in infants born to women in whom cerclages were retained. Sepsis was the cause of the neonatal morbidity in 71% of cases. Our approach is to perform an amniocentesis to determine whether infection is present. If microbial invasion of the amniotic cavity is documented, we remove the cerclage and begin antibiotic treatment. If amniotic fluid analysis is negative, the options are discussed with the patient, who is informed that infections in patients with cervical cerclage have led to maternal sepsis and rarely requirement of hysterectomy. If lung maturity is documented, the benefits of maintaining the cerclage are probably minimal, and, therefore, removal is appropriate.

## HUMAN IMMUNODEFICIENCY VIRUS (HIV) AND PROM

Intrapartum events may play a role in the likelihood of vertical transmission of HIV-1. In a retrospective study, Minkoff and associates found that women with low CD4 counts (<20%) were significantly more likely to transmit the virus if rupture of the membranes occurred 4 or more hours before delivery (RR 4.53, 95% CI 1.14–1.81). This association was not seen in women with CD4 counts of more than 20%. The mode of delivery did not affect the risk of transmission. Data from the Women and Infants Transmission Study showed that duration of membrane rupture longer than 4 hours before delivery was associated with a transmission rate of 25% compared with 14% if membranes ruptured 4 hours or less before delivery. After multivariate analysis, presence of ruptured membranes of more than 4 hours nearly doubled the risk of transmission of the virus (OR 1.82, 95% CI 1.1–3.0) regardless of the mode of delivery.

In a recent meta-analysis of 15 prospective cohort studies, the relationship between elective cesarean section and vertical transmission of HIV-1 was evaluated. The results of the meta-analysis suggest that elective cesarean section before the onset of labor and rupture of membranes reduces the risk of transmission of HIV-1 from mother to child independently of the effect of treatment with zidovudine. The likelihood of vertical transmission in women with rupture of membranes was lower with elective cesarean section than with other modes of delivery (odds ratio, 0.55; 95% CI, 0.40 to 0.77; $P<0.001$ among women with ROM less than 1 hour before delivery; odds ratio, 0.53; 95% CI, 0.40 to 0.71; $P<0.001$ among women with ROM less than 4 hours before delivery). However, current recommendations are for multiple antiviral therapy with HIV infection to reduce vertical transmission (see Chapter 40). There are currently no data to indicate that cesarean section is protective when multiple antiviral drugs are used for prophylaxis.

## HERPES SIMPLEX GENITALIS

Preterm PROM complicated by maternal genital herpes is a clinical dilemma: The risk of prematurity must be balanced against the risk of potential exposure of the neonate to intrauterine herpes. At the time of this writing, this issue had been examined in one study. Major and associates reported the outcomes of 18 patients who had preterm PROM between 24 and 32 weeks of gestation and concomitant recurrent genital herpes who were managed expectantly. None of the babies had any clinical or laboratory evidence of neonatal herpes. Six patients received antenatal acyclovir. The results of this study would seem to justify expectant management in patients who have this complication.

## REFERENCES

Alexander JM, Gilstrap LC, Cox SM, et al: Clinical chorioamnionitis and the prognosis for very low birth weight infants. Obstet Gynecol 9:725, 1998.

Alger LS, Lovchik JC, Hebel JR, et al: The association of *Chlamydia trachomatis*, *Neisseria gonorrhoeae*, and group B streptococci with preterm rupture of the membranes and pregnancy outcome. Am J Obstet Gynecol 159:397, 1988.

Amon E, Lewis SV, Sibai BM, et al: Ampicillin prophylaxis in preterm premature rupture of the membranes: A prospective randomized study. Am J Obstet Gynecol 159:539, 1988.

Amstey MS, Steadman KT: Asymptomatic gonorrhea and pregnancy. J Am Ven Dis Assoc 33:14, 1976.

Ananth C, Santz D, William M: Placental abruption and its association with hypertension and prolonged rupture of membranes: A methodologic review and metaanalysis. Obstet Gynecol 88:309, 1996.

Ananth CV, Guise JM, Thorp JM Jr: Utility of antibiotic therapy in preterm premature rupture of membranes: A meta-analysis. Obstet Gynecol Surv 51:324, 1996.

Artal R, Burgeson RE, Hobel CJ, et al: An in vitro model for the study of enzymatically mediated biomechanical changes in the chorioamniotic membranes. Am J Obstet Gynecol 133:656, 1979.

Atkinson M, Goldenberg R, Gaudib F, et al: Maternal corticosteroid and tocolytic treatment and morbidity and mortality in very low birth weight infants. Am J Obstet Gynecol 173:299, 1995.

Blickstein I, Katz Z, Lancet M, et al: The outcome of pregnancies complicated by preterm rupture of the membranes with and without cerclage. Int J Gynaecol Obstet 28:237, 1989.

Blott M, Greenough A: Neonatal outcome after prolonged rupture of the membranes starting in the second trimester. Arch Dis Child 63:1146–1150, 1988.

Broekhuizen FF, Gilman M, Hamilton PR: Amniocentesis for Gram stain and culture in preterm premature rupture of the membranes. Obstet Gynecol 66:316, 1985.

Brookes C, Shand K, Jones WR: A reevaluation of the ferning test to detect ruptured membranes. Aust N Z J Obstet Gynaecol 26:260, 1986.

Brown C, Ludwizak M, Blanco J, et al: Cervical dilation: Accuracy of visual and digital examinations. Obstet Gynecol 81:215, 1993.

Carroll S, Papaioannou S, Ntumach I, et al: Lower genital tract swabs in the prediction of intrauterine infection in preterm premature rupture of the membranes. Br J Obstet Gynaecol 103:54, 1996.

Carroll S, Papaioannou S, Nicolaides K: Assessment of fetal activity and amniotic fluid volume in prediction of intraamniotic infection in preterm premature rupture of the membranes. Am J Obstet Gynecol 172:1427, 1995.

Cederqvist L, Francis L, Zervoudakis I, et al: Fetal immune response following prematurely ruptured membranes. Am J Obstet Gynecol 126:321, 1972.

Christensen KK, Christensen P, Ingemarsson I, et al: A study in complications in preterm deliveries after prolonged premature rupture of the membranes. Obstet Gynecol 48:670, 1976.

Christmas J, Cox S, Andrews W, et al: Expectant management of preterm ruptured membranes: Effects of antimicrobial therapy. Obstet Gynecol 80:754, 1992.

Cohen J, Valle J, Calkins B: Improved pregnancy outcome following successful treatment of chlamydia infection. JAMA 263:3160, 1990.

Cotton DB, Gonik B, Bottoms SF: Conservative versus aggressive management of preterm rupture of membranes: A randomized trial of amniocentesis. Am J Perinatol 1:322, 1984.

Cotton DB, Hill LM, Strassner HT, et al: Use of amniocentesis in preterm gestation with ruptured membranes. Obstet Gynecol 63:38, 1984.

Coultrip L, Grossman J: Evaluation of rapid diagnostic tests in the detection of microbial invasion of the amniotic cavity. Am J Obstet Gynecol 167:1231, 1992.

Cowett RM, Hakanson DO, Kocon RW, et al: Untoward neonatal effect of intra-amniotic administration of methylene blue. Obstet Gynecol 48:74s, 1976.

Cox S, Leveno K: Intentional delivery versus expectant management with preterm ruptured membranes at 30–34 weeks gestation. Obstet Gynecol 86:875, 1995.

Cox SM, Williams ML, Leveno KJ: The natural history of premature ruptured membranes: What to expect of expectant management. Obstet Gynecol 71:558, 1988.

Daikoku NH, Kaltreider DF, Khouzami VA, et al: Premature rupture of membranes and spontaneous labor: Maternal endometritis risks. Obstet Gynecol 59:13, 1982.

David J, Permezel M: Pregnancy outcomes following preterm premature rupture of the membranes at less than 26 weeks' gestation. Aust N Z J Obstet Gynaecol 32:120, 1992.

DelValle G, Joffe G, Isquierdo L, et al: The biophysical profile and the non stress test. Poor prediction of chorioamnionitis and fetal infection in prolonged preterm premature rupture of the membranes. Obstet Gynecol 80:106, 1992.

Diaz Garzon J: Indigo carmine test of preterm rupture of membranes. Rev Colomb Obstet Gynecol 20:373, 1969.

Draper D, McGregor J, Hauth J, et al: Elevated protease activity in human amnion and chorion correlates with preterm premature rupture of the membranes. Am J Obstet Gynecol 173:1506, 1995.

Dudley J, Malcolm G, Ellwood D: Amniocentesis in the management of preterm premature rupture of the membranes. Aust N Z J Obstet Gynaecol 31:531, 1991.

Dunlop P, Crowley P, Lamont R, et al: Preterm ruptured membranes, no contractions. J Obstet Gynecol 7:92, 1986.

Edwards LE, Barrada MI, Hamann AA, et al: Gonorrhea in pregnancy. Am J Obstet Gynecol 132:637, 1978.

Egarter C, Leitich H, Karas H, et al: Antibiotic treatment in preterm premature rupture of membranes and neonatal morbidity. A meta analysis. Am J Obstet Gynecol 174:589, 1996.

Ekwo E, Gosselink C, Moawad A: Unfavourable outcome in penultimate pregnancy and premature rupture of membranes in successive pregnancy. Obstet Gynecol 80:166, 1992.

Ernest JM, Givner LB: A prospective randomized placebo-controlled trial in preterm PROM. Am J Obstet Gynecol 170:516, 1994.

Fayez JA, Hasan AA, Jonas HS, et al: Management of premature rupture of the membranes. Obstet Gynecol 52:17, 1978.

Feinstein SJ, Vintzileos AM, Lodeiro JG, et al: Amniocentesis with premature rupture of membranes. Obstet Gynecol 68:147, 1986.

Font G, Gauthier D, Meyer W, et al: Catalase activity as a predictor of amniotic fluid culture results in preterm labor or preterm premature rupture of the membranes. Obstet Gynecol 85:656, 1995.

Fortunato S, Welt S, Eggleston M, et al: Active expectant management in very early gestations complicated by premature rupture of the fetal membranes. J Reprod Med 39:13, 1994.

Friedman ML, McElin TW: Diagnosis of ruptured fetal membranes: Clinical study and review of literature. Am J Obstet Gynecol 104:544, 1969.

Fujimoto S, Kishida T, Sagawa T, et al: Clinical usefulness of the dye injection method for diagnosing premature rupture of the membranes in equivocal cases. J Obstet Gynecol 21:215, 1995.

Gardner M, Goldenberg R: Use of antenatal corticosteroids for fetal maturation. Curr Opin Obstet Gynecol 8:106, 1996.

Garite TJ, Freeman RK, Linzey E, et al: The use of amniocentesis in patients with premature rupture of membranes. Obstet Gynecol 54:226, 1979.

Garite TJ, Freeman RK: Chorioamnionitis in the preterm gestation. Obstet Gynecol 59:539, 1982.

Garite TJ, Keegan KA, Freeman RK, et al: A randomized trial of ritodrine tocolysis versus expectant management in patients with premature rupture of membranes at 25 to 30 weeks of gestation. Am J Obstet Gynecol 157:388, 1987.

Gauthier D, Meyer W, Bieniarz A: Biophysical profile as a predictor of amniotic fluid culture results. Obstet Gynecol 80:102, 1992.

Gauthier D, Meyer W, Bieniarz A: Expectant management of premature rupture of the membranes with positive cultures for *Ureaplasma urealyticum* alone. Am J Obstet Gynecol 170:587, 1994.

Gibbs RS, Castillo MS, Rodgers PJ: Management of acute chorioamnionitis. Am J Obstet Gynecol 136:709, 1980.

Gibbs RS, Blanco JD: Premature rupture of the membranes. Obstet Gynecol 60:671, 1982.

Golde SH: Use of obstetric perineal pads in collection of amniotic fluid in patients with rupture of the membranes. Am J Obstet Gynecol 146:710, 1983.

Goldman JM, Greene MF, Tuomala RE, et al: Outcome of expectant management in preterm premature rupture of membranes with cervical cerclage in place (Abstract). Presented at the Tenth Annual Meeting of the Society of Perinatal Obstetricians, Houston, Texas, 1990.

Goldstein I, Romero R, Merrill S, et al: Fetal body and breathing movements as predictors of intra-amniotic infection in preterm premature rupture of membranes. Am J Obstet Gynecol 159:363, 1988.

Gonick B, Bottoms SF, Cotton DB: Amniotic fluid volume as a risk factor in preterm premature rupture of the membranes. Obstet Gynecol 65:456, 1985.

Guinn DA, Goldenberg RL, Hauth JC, et al: Risk factors for the development of preterm premature rupture of the membranes after arrest of preterm labor. Am J Obstet Gynecol 173:1311, 1995.

Gunn CS, Mishell DR, Morton DG: Premature rupture of the fetal membranes. Am J Obstet Gynecol 106:469, 1970.

Hagskog K, Nisell H, Sarmam I, et al: Conservative ambulatory management of prelabor rupture of the membranes at term in nulliparas. Acta Obstet Gynecol Scand 73:765, 1994.

Handsfield HH, Hodson WA, Holmes KK: Neonatal gonococcal infection: Orogastric contamination with *Neisseria gonorrhoeae*. JAMA 225:697, 1973.

Hannah M, Ohlsson A, Favine D, et al: Induction of labor compared with expectant management for prelabor rupture of membranes at term. N Engl J Med 334:1005, 1996.

Harger JH, Hsing AW, Tuomala RE, et al: Risk factors for preterm premature rupture of fetal membranes: A multicenter case-control study. Am J Obstet Gynecol 163:130, 1990.

Harger JH: Comparison of success and morbidity in cervical cerclage procedures. Obstet Gynecol 56:543, 1980.

Harrison HR, Alexander ER, Weinstein L, et al: Cervical *Chlamydia trachomatis* and mycoplasmal infections in pregnancy. JAMA 250:1721, 1983.

Hauth J, Goldenberg R, Andrews W, et al: Reduced incidence of preterm delivery with metronidazole and erythromycin in women with bacterial vaginosis. N Engl J Med 333:1732, 1995.

Hazan Y, Mazor M, Horowitz S, et al: The diagnostic value of amniotic fluid Gram stain examination and Limulus amebocyte assay in patients with preterm birth. Acta Obstet Gynecol Scand 74:132, 1995.

Hibbard J, Hubbard M, Ismail M, et al: Pregnancy outcome after expectant management of premature rupture of membranes in the second trimester. J Reprod Med 38:945, 1993.

Hillier S, Nugent R, Eschenbach D, et al: Association between bacterial vaginosis and preterm delivery of a low-birth weight infant. N Engl J Med 333:1737, 1995.

Holbrook R, Falcon J, Hemass M, et al: Evaluation of the weekly cervical examination on a preterm birth prevention program. Am J Perinatol 4:240, 1987.

The International Perinatal HIV Group: The mode of delivery and the risk of vertical transmission of human immunodeficiency virus type I. N Engl J Med 340:977–987, 1999.

Jalava J, Mantymaas M, Ekblad U, et al: Bacterial 16 S DNA polymerase chain reaction reaction in the detection of intraamniotic infection. Br J Obstet Gynaecol 103:664, 1996.

Johnson JW, Daikoku NH, Niebyl JR, et al: Premature rupture of the membranes and prolonged pregnancy. Obstet Gynecol 57:547, 1981.

Johnston MM, Sanchez-Ramos L, Vaughn AJ, et al: Antibiotic therapy in preterm PROM: A randomized prospective double-blind trial. Am J Obstet Gynecol 163:743, 1990.

Kanayama N, Terao T, Kawashima Y, et al: Collagen types in normal and prematurely ruptured amniotic membranes. Am J Obstet Gynecol 153:899, 1985.

Keirse MJNC, Ohlsson A, Treffers PE, et al: Prelabour rupture of the membranes preterm. *In* Chalmers I, Enkin M, Keirse MJNC (eds): Effective Care in Pregnancy and Childbirth. Vol. 4: Pregnancy, Parts I–V. Oxford, England, Oxford University Press, 1989, p 666.

Kivikoski AI, Amon E, Vaalamo PO, et al: Effect of third-trimester premature rupture of membranes on fetal breathing movements: A prospective case-control study. Am J Obstet Gynecol 159:1474, 1988.

Knudsen FU, Steinrud J: Septicaemia of the newborn, associated with ruptured fetal membranes, discoloured amniotic fluid or maternal fever. Acta Paediatr Scand 65:725, 1976.

Kurki T, Hallman M, Zilliacus R, et al: Premature rupture of the membranes: Effect of penicillin prophylaxis and long term outcome of the children. Am J Perinatol 9:11, 1992.

Landsmann S, Kalish L, Burns D, et al: Obstetrical factors and the transmission of human immunodeficiency virus type I from mother to child. The Women and Infants Transmission Study. N Engl J Med 334:1617, 1996.

Lauria M, Gonik B, Romero R: Pulmonary hypoplasia: Pathogenesis, diagnosis and antenatal prediction. Obstet Gynecol 83:466, 1995.

Lebherz TB, Hellman LP, Madding R, et al: Double-blind study of premature rupture of the membranes. Am J Obstet Gynecol 87:218, 1963.

Leitich H, Egarter C, Reisenberger K, et al: Concomitant use of glucocorticoids: A comparison of two metaanalyses on antibiotic treatment in preterm premature rupture of membranes. Am J Obstet Gynecol 178:899, 1998.

Lenihan JP: Relationship of antepartum pelvic examination to premature rupture of the membranes. Obstet Gynecol 63:33, 1984.

Lewis DF, Major CA, Towers CV, et al: Effects of digital vaginal exams on latency period in preterm premature rupture of membranes. Obstet Gynecol 80:630, 1992.

Lockwood C, Costigan K, Ghidini A, et al: Double blind placebo controlled trial of piperacillin prophylaxis in preterm membrane rupture. Am J Obstet Gynecol 169:970, 1993.

Lodeiro JG, Hsieh KA, Byers JH, et al: The fingerprint, a false-positive fern test. Obstet Gynecol 73:873, 1989.

Lovett SM, Weiss JD, Diogo MJ, et al: A prospective, double-blind, randomized, controlled clinical trial of ampicillin-sulbactam for preterm premature rupture of membranes in women receiving antenatal corticosteroid therapy. Am J Obstet Gynecol 176:1030, 1997.

Ludmir J, Bader T, Chen L, et al: Poor perinatal outcome associated with retained cerclage in patients with premature rupture of membranes. Obstet Gynecol 84:823, 1994.

Main DM, Gabbe SG, Richardson D, et al: Can preterm deliveries be prevented? Am J Obstet Gynecol 151:892, 1985.

Main DM, Richardson DK, Hadley CB, et al: Controlled trial of a preterm labor detection program: Efficacy and costs. Obstet Gynecol 74:873, 1989.

Major C, Kitzmuller J: Perinatal survival with expectant management of mid trimester rupture of membranes. Am J Obstet Gynecol 163:838, 1990.

Major CA, Towers CV, Lewis DF, et al: Expectant management of patients with both preterm premature rupture of membranes and genital herpes (Abstract). Am J Obstet Gynecol 164:248, 1991.

Matsuda Y, Ikenoue T, Hokanishi H: Premature rupture of membranes. Aggressive versus conservative approach: Effect of tocolysis and antibiotic therapy. Gynecol Obstet Invest 36:102, 1993.

Mc Enerney J, Mc Enerney L: Unfavourable neonatal outcomes after intraamniotic injection of methylene blue. Obstet Gynecol 61(Suppl):351, 1983.

McCaul JF, Perry KG Jr, Moore JL Jr, et al: Adjunctive antibiotic treatment of women with preterm rupture of membranes or preterm labor. Int J Gynaecol Obstet 38:19, 1992.

McDuffie R, McGregor J, Gibbs R: Adverse perinatal outcome and resistant enterobacteriaceae after antibiotic usage for premature rupture of the membranes and group B streptococcus carriage. Obstet Gynecol 82:487, 1993.

McDuffie R, Nelson G, Osborn C, et al: Effect of routine weekly examinations at term on premature rupture of the membranes: A randomized controlled trial. Obstet Gynecol 79:219, 1992.

McGregor J, French J, Seo K: Antimicrobial therapy in preterm premature rupture of membranes: Results of a prospective double blind placebo controlled trial of erythromycin. Am J Obstet Gynecol 165:632, 1991.

McGregor J, French J, Seo K: Premature rupture of the membranes and bacterial vaginosis. Am J Obstet Gynecol 169:463, 1993.

McGregor JA, French JI, Lawellin D, et al: Bacterial protease-induced reduction of chorioamniotic membrane strength and elasticity. Obstet Gynecol 69:167, 1987.

McGregor JA, Johnson S: "Fig-leaf" ferning and positive nitrazine testing: Semen as a cause of misdiagnosis of premature rupture of membranes (Letter). Am J Obstet Gynecol 151:1142, 1985.

McIntosh N, Harrison A: Prolonged premature rupture of membranes in the preterm infant: A seven year study. Eur J Obstet Gynecol 57:1, 1994.

Mercer B, Arheart K: Antimicrobial therapy in expectant management of preterm premature rupture of membranes. Lancet 346:1271, 1995.

Mercer B, Crocker L, Boe N, et al: Induction versus expectant management in premature rupture of membranes with mature amniotic fluid at 32–36 weeks. A randomized trial. Am J Obstet Gynecol 169:775, 1993.

Mercer B, Moretti M, Prevost R, et al: Erythromycin therapy in preterm premature rupture of the membranes: A prospective randomized trial of 220 patients. Am J Obstet Gynecol 166:794, 1992.

Mercer BM, Miodovnik M, Thurnau GR, et al: Antibiotic therapy for reduction of infant morbidity after preterm premature rupture of the membranes. A randomized controlled trial. JAMA 278:989, 1997.

Meyer B, Gonik B, Creasy R: Evaluation of phenazopyridine hydrochloride as a tool in the diagnosis of premature rupture of the membranes. Am J Perinatol 8:297, 1991.

Mills JL, Harlap S, Harley EE: Should coitus late in pregnancy be discouraged? Lancet i:136, 1981.

Minkoff H, Burns D, Landsmann S, et al: The relationship of the duration of ruptured membranes to vertical transmission of HIV. Am J Obstet Gynecol 158:106, 1988.

Minkoff H, Grunebaum AN, Schwarz RH, et al: Risk factors for prematurity and premature rupture of membranes: A prospective study of vaginal flora in pregnancy. Am J Obstet Gynecol 150:965, 1984.

Morales W, Talley T: Premature rupture of membranes at <25 weeks: A management dilemma. Am J Obstet Gynecol 168:503, 1993.

Morales WJ, Angel JL, O'Brien WF, et al: Use of ampicillin and corticosteroids in premature rupture of membranes: A randomized study. Obstet Gynecol 73:721, 1989.

Morales WJ, Lazar AJ: Expectant management of rupture of membranes at term. South Med J 79:955, 1986.

Moretti M, Sibai BM: Maternal and perinatal outcome of expectant management of premature rupture of membranes in the midtrimester. Am J Obstet Gynecol 159:390, 1988.

Mozurkewich EL, Wolf FM: Premature rupture of membranes at term: A meta-analysis of three management schemes. Obstet Gynecol 89:1035, 1997.

Munson LA, Graham A, Koos BJ, et al: Is there a need for digital examination in patients with spontaneous rupture of the membranes? Am J Obstet Gynecol 153:562, 1985.

Naeye RL, Peters EC: Causes and consequences of premature rupture of fetal membranes. Lancet 1:192, 1980.

Naeye RL: Factors that predispose to premature rupture of the fetal membranes. Obstet Gynecol 60:93, 1982.

Nelson DM, Stempel LE, Zuspan FP: Association of prolonged, preterm premature rupture of the membranes and abruptio placentae. J Reprod Med 31:429, 1986.

Nelson L, Anderson R, O'Shea M, et al: Expectant management of preterm premature rupture of membranes. Am J Obstet Gynecol 171:350, 1994.

NIH Consensus Conference: Effect of corticosteroids for fetal maturation on perinatal outcome. JAMA 273:413, 1995.

Nimrod C, Varela-Gittings F, Machin G, et al: The effect of very prolonged membrane rupture on fetal development. Am J Obstet Gynecol 148:540, 1984.

Ogita S, Imanaka M, Matsumoto M, et al: Premature rupture of the membranes managed with a new cervical catheter. Lancet 1:1330, 1984.

Ohlsson A: Treatments of preterm premature rupture of the membranes: A meta-analysis. Am J Obstet Gynecol 160:890, 1989.

O'Keeffe DF, Garite TJ, Elliott JP, et al: The accuracy of estimated gestational age based on ultrasound measurement of biparietal diameter in preterm premature rupture of the membranes. Am J Obstet Gynecol 151:309, 1985.

Owen J, Groome L, Hauth J: Randomized trial of prophylactic antibiotic therapy after preterm amnion rupture. Am J Obstet Gynecol 169:976, 1993.

Pankuch GA, Appelbaum PC, Lorenz RP, et al: Placental microbiology and histology and the pathogenesis of chorioamnionitis. Obstet Gynecol 64:802, 1984.

Parry S, Strauss JF: Premature rupture of fetal membranes. N Engl J Med 338:664, 1998.

Phillippe M, Acker D, Torday J, et al: The effects of vaginal contamination on two pulmonary phospholipid assays. J Reprod Med 5:283, 1982.

Raio L, Ghezzi F, Di Naro E, et al: Duration of pregnancy after carbon dioxide laser conization of the cervix: Influence of cone height. Obstet Gynecol 90:978, 1997.

Reece EA, Chervenak FA, Moya FR, et al: Amniotic fluid arborization: Effect of blood, meconium, and pH alterations. Obstet Gynecol 64:248, 1984.

Regan JA, Klebanoff MA, Nugent RP, et al: Colonization with group B streptococci in pregnancy and adverse outcome. VIP Study Group. Am J Obstet Gynecol 174:1354, 1996.

Regan JA, Chao S, James LS: Premature rupture of membranes, preterm delivery, and group B streptococcal colonization of mothers. Am J Obstet Gynecol 141:184, 1981.

Rhydstrom H, Ingermarsson I: No benefit from conservative management in nulliparous women with premature rupture of the membranes (PROM) at term. Acta Obstet Gynecol Scand 70:543, 1991.

Rib D, Sherer D, Woods J: Maternal and neonatal outcome associated with prolonged premature rupture of membranes below 26 weeks' gestation. Am J Perinatol 10:369, 1993.

Roberts AB, Goldstein I, Romero R, et al: Fetal breathing movements after preterm premature rupture of membranes. Am J Obstet Gynecol 164:821, 1991.

Romero R, Emamian M, Quintero R, et al: The value and limitations of the Gram stain examination in the diagnosis of intraamniotic infection. Am J Obstet Gynecol 159:114, 1988.

Romero R, Gomez R, Ghezzi F, et al: A fetal systemic inflammatory response is followed by the spontaneous onset of preterm parturition. Am J Obstet Gynecol 179:186, 1998.

Romero R, Hagay Z, Nores J, et al: Eradication of *Ureaplasma urealyticum* from the amniotic fluid with transplacental antibiotic treatment. Am J Obstet Gynecol 166:618, 1992.

Romero R, Quintero R, Oyarzun E, et al: Intra-amniotic infection and the onset of labor in preterm rupture of the membranes. Am J Obstet Gynecol 159:661, 1988.

Romero R, Ray J, Sepulveda W, et al: Evidence of active forms of 72 kDa and 92 kDa type IV collagenases in human parturition. 39th annual meeting of the Society for Gynecologic Investigation, San Antonio, TX, 1992.

Romero R, Salafia C, Athanassiadis A, et al: The relationship between acute inflammatory lesions of the preterm placenta and amniotic fluid microbiology. Am J Obstet Gynecol 166:1382, 1992.

Romero R, Scioscia AL, Edberg SC, et al: Use of parenteral antibiotic therapy to eradicate bacterial colonization of amniotic fluid in premature rupture of membranes. Obstet Gynecol 67(Suppl):15, 1986.

Romero R, Yoon BH, Mazor M, et al: A comparative study of the diagnostic performance of amniotic fluid glucose, white blood cell count, interleukin-6 and Gram stain in the detection of microbial invasion in patients with preterm rupture of membranes. Am J Obstet Gynecol 169:846, 1993.

Rosemond RL, Lombardi SJ, Boehm FH: Ferning of amniotic fluid contaminated with blood. Obstet Gynecol 75:338, 1990.

Rotschild A, Ling EW, Puterman ML, et al: Neonatal outcome after prolonged preterm rupture of the membranes. Am J Obstet Gynecol 162:4, 1990.

Russell KP, Anderson GV: Aggressive management of ruptured membranes. Am J Obstet Gynecol 83:930, 1962.

Ryan G, Abdella T, McNeely S, et al: *Chlamydia trachomatis* infection in pregnancy and effect of treatment on outcome. Am J Obstet Gynecol 162:34, 1990.

Sachs M, Baker TH: Spontaneous premature rupture of the membranes. Am J Obstet Gynecol 97:888, 1967.

Sagot P, Canot Y, Winer N, et al: Obstetrical prognosis for carbon dioxide laser conization of uterine cervix. Eur J Obstet Gynecol Reprod Biol 58:53, 1995.

Sbarra AJ, Blake G, Cetrulo CL: The effect of cervical/vaginal secretions on measurements of lecithin/sphingomyelin ratio and optical density at 650 nm. Am J Obstet Gynecol 139:214, 1981.

Schutte MF, Treffers PE, Kloostermen GJ, et al: Management of the premature rupture of the membranes: A risk of vaginal examination to the fetus. Am J Obstet Gynecol 146:395, 1983.

Skinner SJM, Campos GA, Liggins GC: Collagen content of hu-

man amniotic membranes: Effect of gestation length and premature rupture. Obstet Gynecol 57:487, 1981.
Smith CV, Greenspoon J, Phelan JP, et al: Clinical utility of the nonstress test in the conservative management of women with preterm spontaneous premature rupture of the membranes. J Reprod Med 32:1, 1987.
Smith RP: A technique for the detection of rupture of the membranes: A review and preliminary report. Obstet Gynecol 48:172, 1976.
Spinnato JA, Shaver DC, Bray EM, et al: Preterm premature rupture of the membranes with fetal pulmonary maturity present: A prospective study. Obstet Gynecol 69:196, 1987.
Sukcharaen N, Vasuratria A: Effects of digital cervical examinations on duration of latency period, maternal and neonatal outcomes in preterm premature rupture of membranes. J Med Assoc Thai 76:203, 1993.
Taylor J, Garite TJ: Premature rupture of membranes before fetal viability. Obstet Gynecol 64:615, 1984.
Toohey JS, Lewis DF, Harding JA, et al: Does amniotic fluid index affect the accuracy of estimated fetal weight in preterm premature rupture of membranes? Am J Obstet Gynecol 165:1060, 1991.
Troche BI: The methylene blue baby. New Engl J Med 320:1756, 1989.
Verber IG, Pearce JM, New LC, et al: Prolonged rupture of the fetal membranes and neonatal outcome. J Perinat Med 17:469, 1989.
Vergani P, Ghidini A, Locatelli A, et al: Risk factors for pulmonary hypoplasia in second trimester premature rupture of membranes. Am J Obstet Gynecol 170:1359, 1994.
Vintzileos A, Knuppell R: Fetal biophysical assessment. Clin Obstet Gynecol 38:45, 1995.
Vintzileos AM, Bors-Koefoed R, Pelegano JF, et al: The use of fetal biophysical profile improves pregnancy outcome in premature rupture of the membranes. Am J Obstet Gynecol 157:236, 1987.
Vintzileos AM, Campbell WA, Nochimson DJ, et al: The fetal biophysical profile in patients with premature rupture of the membranes: An early predictor of infection. Am J Obstet Gynecol 152:510, 1985.
Vintzileos AM, Campbell WA, Nochimson DJ, et al: Degree of oligohydramnios and pregnancy outcome in patients with premature rupture of the membranes. Obstet Gynecol 66:162, 1985.
Vintzileos AM, Campbell WA, Nochimson DJ, et al: Qualitative amniotic fluid volume versus amniocentesis in predicting infection in preterm premature rupture of the membranes. Obstet Gynecol 67:579, 1986.
Vintzileos AM, Campbell WA, Nochimson DJ, et al: The use of the nonstress test in patients with premature rupture of the membranes. Am J Obstet Gynecol 155:149, 1986.
Wagner M, Chin V, Peters C, et al: A comparison of early and delayed induction of labor with spontaneous rupture of the membranes at term. Obstet Gynecol 74:93, 1989.
Weiner CP, Renk K, Klugman M: The therapeutic efficacy and cost-effectiveness of aggressive tocolysis for premature labor associated with premature rupture of the membranes. Am J Obstet Gynecol 159:216, 1988.
Wenstrom K: Pulmonary hypoplasia and deformations related to premature rupture of membranes. Obstet Gynecol Clin North Am 19:397, 1992.
Wilson JC, Levy DL, Wilds PL: Premature rupture of the membranes prior to term: Consequences of nonintervention. Obstet Gynecol 71:558, 1988.
Yeast JD, Garite TJ, Dorchester W: The risks of amniocentesis in the management of premature rupture of the membranes. Am J Obstet Gynecol 149:505, 1984.
Yeast JD, Garite TR: The role of cervical cerclage in the management of preterm premature rupture of the membranes. Am J Obstet Gynecol 158:106, 1988.
Yoon B, Romero R, Kim C, et al: Amniotic fluid interleukin-6: A sensitive test for antenatal diagnosis of acute inflammatory lesions of preterm placentas and prediction of perinatal morbidity. Am J Obstet Gynecol 172:960, 1995.
Zeevi D, Sadovsky E, Younis J, et al: Antepartum fetal heart rate characteristics in cases of premature rupture of membranes. Am J Perinatol 5:260, 1988.
Zlatnik F, Cruikshank D, Petzold CR, et al: Amniocentesis in the identification of inapparent infections in preterm patients with premature rupture of the membranes. J Reprod Med 29:656, 1984.
Zlatnik F: Management of premature rupture of membranes at term. Obstet Gynecol Clin North Am 19:353, 1992.

# 25

# Normal and Abnormal Labor

KENNETH J. LEVENO

The rate of cesarean delivery in the United States is among the highest for developed nations (Centers for Disease Control, 1995). Consequently, a national health objective for the year 2000 is to reduce the overall cesarean rate. The leading reason for the escalated incidence of cesarean deliveries is the increased diagnosis of abnormal labor, or dystocia. Indeed, the dramatic rise in the diagnosis of dystocia in the United States during the past two decades suggests that American women have suddenly developed a reproductive disadvantage, or that dystocia is being incorrectly diagnosed. To address this national health issue, the Centers for Disease Control and Prevention has published recommendations for reducing the cesarean rate, which include the implementation of standardized protocols for labor management (Centers for Disease Control, 1995).

Dystocia—literally, difficult labor—is characterized by abnormally slow progress of labor with a variety of causes (Table 25-1). It is the consequence of four distinct abnormalities that may exist singly or in combination:

1. Abnormalities of the expulsion, with uterine forces insufficiently strong or inappropriately coordinated to efface and dilate the cervix (i.e., uterine dysfunction), or inadequate voluntary muscle effort during the second stage of labor
2. Abnormalities of presentation, position, or development of the fetus
3. Abnormalities of the maternal bony pelvis (i.e., pelvic contraction)
4. Abnormalities of the birth canal (other than those of the bony pelvis) that obstruct fetal descent.

Pelvic contraction is often accompanied by uterine dysfunction, and the two together constitute the most common cause of dystocia. Similarly, faulty presentation or unusual fetal size or shape may be accompanied by uterine dysfunction. As a generalization, uterine dysfunction is common if there is disproportion between the presenting part of the fetus and the birth canal.

Dystocia is the most common contemporary indi-

**Table 25-1** Causes of Dystocia

Expulsive forces insufficient
    Uterine contractions infrequent
    Voluntary muscle fatigue or inadequate muscle effort in the second stage of labor
    Related to epidural analgesia
Fetal malpresentations
    Presentations such as breech, face, or brow
    Positions such as occiput posterior or transverse
    Malformations such as fetal hydrocephalus
Inadequate pelvic dimensions (midpelvic most common)
Obstructed descent
    Examples include uterine leiomyomas and benign ovarian tumors

cation for primary cesarean delivery. Notzon and associates (1994) found that 12% of American women who had no history of cesarean section were diagnosed in 1990 with dystocia that required abdominal delivery, the rate had increased from 7% in 1980. Inevitably, methods of labor management are receiving renewed interest as obstetricians grapple with means of controlling escalating cesarean delivery rates. Dystocia is very complex, and although its definition—abnormal progress in labor—seems simple, there is no consensus as to what "abnormal progress" means. Thus, it seems prudent to attempt a better understanding of normal labor, including diagnosis, to determine any departure from the norm.

## Labor Diagnosis

The greatest impediment to understanding normal labor is recognizing its commencement. The strict definition of labor—*uterine contractions that bring about demonstrable effacement and dilatation of the cervix*—does not easily aid the clinician in determining when labor has actually begun, because this diagnosis is confirmed only after the event. Several options may be used to deal with this dilemma. One is to instruct the woman to quantify contractions for some specified period and subsequently define labor onset as the clock time when painful contractions become regular. This is very subjective and frequently causes considerable frustration for both obstetrician and patient. Indeed, uterine irritability that causes discomfort but does not represent true labor may develop at any time during pregnancy.

A second option is to define the onset of labor as the time of admission to the labor unit. At the National Maternity Hospital in Dublin, efforts have been made to codify admission criteria, after which labor management is standardized (O'Driscoll and colleagues 1993). These criteria at term require painful uterine contractions accompanied by any one of the following:

1. Ruptured membranes
2. Bloody "show"
3. Complete cervical effacement.

In the Irish scheme, the duration of labor is determined by the amount of time elapsed from admission to delivery, whereas, in the United States, admission for labor is frequently based on the extent of dilatation accompanied by painful contractions. When the woman arrives at the labor unit with intact membranes, cervical dilatation of 3 to 4 cm or more is presumed to be a reasonably reliable threshold for diagnosis of labor. In this case, onset of labor commences with the time of admission. This presumptive method of diagnosing true labor obviates many of the uncertainties in diagnosing labor during earlier stages of cervical dilatation.

## Normal Labor

Assuming that the diagnosis has been confirmed, what are the expectations for progress of normal labor? Historically, this was usually described by simple elapsed time, with the realization that normal labor could be diagnosed only after the fact. A scientific approach to the study of labor was begun in 1954 by Friedman, who described a characteristic sigmoid pattern for statistically analyzed labor and then graphed cervical dilatation against time.

As shown in Figure 25–1, the progress of labor in nulliparous women has particular significance, because these curves all reveal a rapid change in the slope of cervical dilatation between 3 and 4 cm. That is, the active phase of labor, in terms of most rapid rates of cervical dilatation, consistently begins when the cervix is 3 to 4 cm dilated. These rather remarkable similarities serve to define active labor and provide useful guideposts for its management. That is, cervical dilatation of 3 to 4 cm or more in the presence of uterine contractions can be taken to represent reliably the threshold of active labor. Similarly, these curves permit the clinician to ask—given that labor

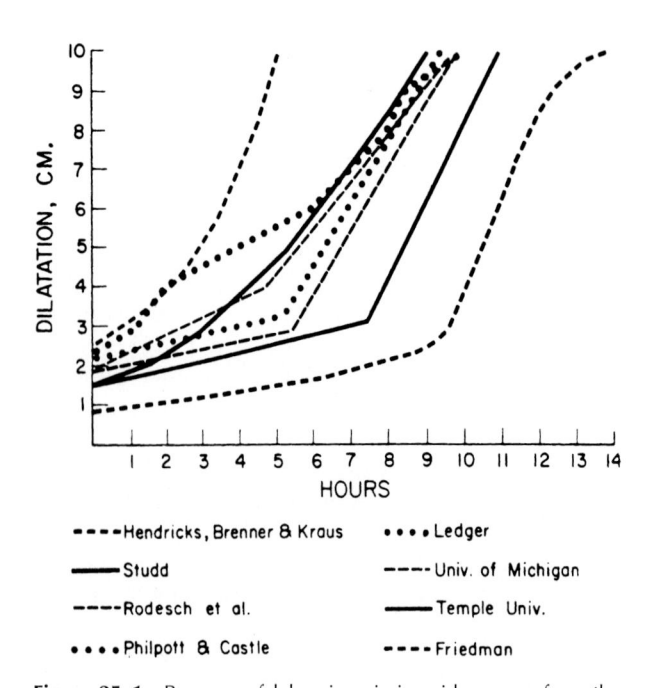

**Figure 25–1** Progress of labor in primigravid women from the time of hospital admission. When the starting point on the abscissa begins with admission to the hospital, there is no latent phase observed. (From O'Connor TCF, Woods RE, Cavanaugh D: Indications for the stimulation of labor. *In* Parke-Davis & Company: Oxytocin-Induced Labor. Greenwich, CT, CPC Communication, 1976, p 10.)

can be reliably diagnosed to have commenced—how much time should elapse in normal active labor?

Turning again to Friedman's work (1955), the mean duration of active-phase labor in nulliparous women was 4.9 hours. The standard deviation (SD) of 3.4 hours is quite large, however. Hence, the active phase was reported to have a statistical maximum of 11.7 hours (mean + 2 SD), with considerable variation in the duration. Indeed, rates of cervical dilatation ranged from 1.2 to 6.8 cm per hour. Thus, when the rate of dilatation considered normal for active phase labor in the nulliparous woman is reported to be 1.2 cm per hour, this is the minimum—not the maximum—normal rate. Multiparous women progress somewhat faster in active-phase labor, with a minimum normal rate of 1.5 cm per hour (Friedman, 1978).

Another feature shared by the several labor curves (see Figure 25–1) is the remarkable tendency for similar durations of active labor. Specifically, nulliparous women who enter the active phase at 3 to 4 cm of dilatation can reliably be expected to reach 8 to 10 cm of dilatation within 3 to 4 hours. This observation may have potential usefulness. For example, if cervical dilatation reaches 4 cm, the clinician can expect complete dilatation to be achieved in approximately 4 hours if spontaneous labor is normal. Abnormalities in the active-labor phase, however, are quite common. Sokol and associates (1977) reported that 25% of nulliparous women had labors complicated by active-phase abnormalities, and 15% of multigravid women developed this problem. Indeed, active-phase disorders are the most common abnormalities of labor.

Kilpatrick and Laros (1989) reported that the mean length of first- and second-stage labor combined was approximately 9 hours in nulliparous women who received no regional analgesia, and that the 95th percentile upper limit was 18.5 hours. Corresponding times for multiparous women were a mean of about 6 hours, with a 95th percentile of 13.5 hours. They defined labor onset as the time when the woman recalled regular, painful contractions every 3 to 5 minutes, which led to a cervical change. Cervical dilatation at admission is not stated.

## SUMMARY

Normal human labor is characterized by brevity, considerable biologic variation, and less complexity than anticipated based on contemporary graphic statistical interpretations. Active labor can be reliably diagnosed when cervical dilatation is 3 cm or more in the presence of uterine contractions. Once this cervical dilatation threshold is reached, normal progress to delivery can be expected, depending on parity, in the ensuing 4 to 6 hours.

# Dystocia

The Greek antonym for *eutocia*, or normal labor, is *dystocia* to signify abnormal labor or difficult childbirth. Dystocia can result from several distinct abnormalities involving the cervix, the uterus, the fetus, other obstructions in the birth passageway, or the maternal bony pelvis. Quite often, combinations of these interact to produce dysfunctional labor. Today, expressions such as *cephalopelvic disproportion* and *failure to progress* are often used to describe dysfunctional labors that require cesarean delivery (Table 25–2).

The expression *cephalopelvic disproportion* came into use before the 20th century to describe obstructed labor caused by disparity between the dimensions of the fetal head and the maternal pelvis, such as to preclude vaginal delivery. This term, however, originated at a time when the main indication for cesarean delivery was overt pelvic contracture resulting from rickets (Olah and Neilson, 1994). Such true cephalopelvic disproportion is now rare, and most disproportions are attributable to malposition of the fetal head—asynclitism, or extension of the bony diameters of the fetal head—or ineffective uterine contractions.

It has become obvious that true cephalopelvic disproportion is a tenuous diagnosis, because two thirds or more of women who were variously diagnosed to have this disorder and who delivered by cesarean section subsequently delivered even larger infants vaginally. Experience with attempted vaginal birth after cesarean section can also provide insights into clinical findings consistent with bona fide dystocia. Hoskins and Gomez (1996) confirmed that two thirds of unselected women who had undergone previous cesarean sections for dystocia could subsequently deliver vaginally, but they found that women who had had cesarean sections for dystocia in the second stage of labor accomplished vaginal birth in only 13% of

Table 25–2 Imprecise Terms or Diagnoses for Dystocia Requiring Cesarean Delivery

**Cephalopelvic Disproportion (CPD)**

Originally meant overt pelvic contracture caused by rickets
Now tenuous because $2/3$ of women who have cesareans for CPD can subsequently deliver vaginally

**Failure to Progress (FTP)**

Increasingly popular diagnosis
Used to convey lack of progressive cervical dilatation or lack of fetal descent
Diagnosis often made before active phase of labor and, therefore, before an adequate trial of labor has been achieved

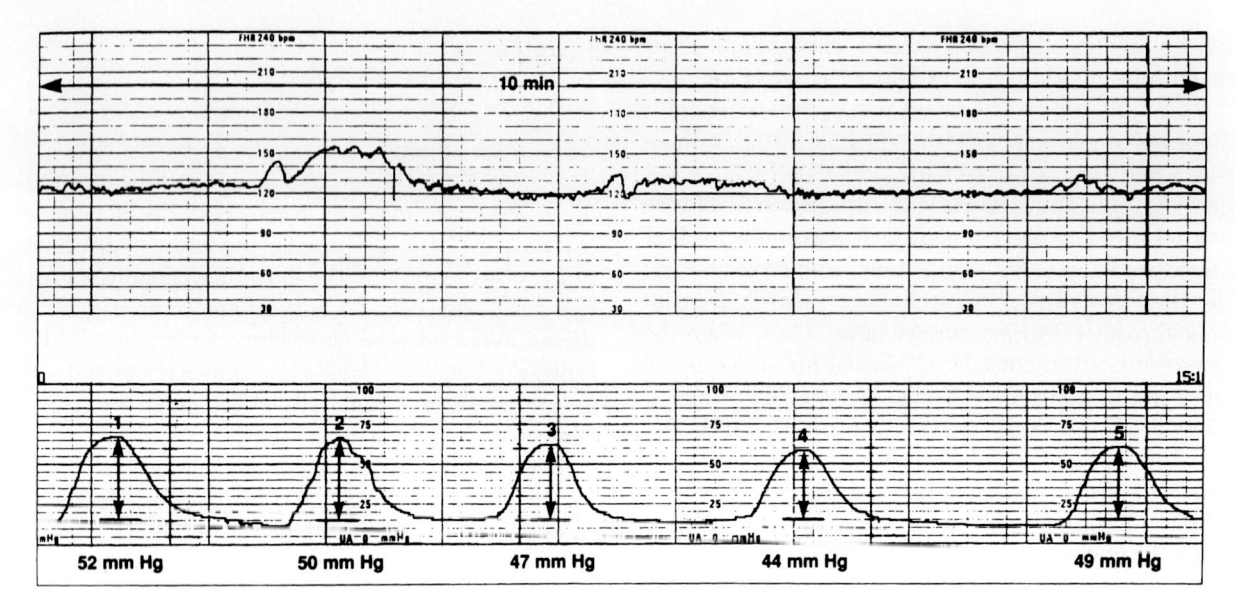

**Figure 25–2** Montevideo units are calculated by subtracting the baseline uterine pressure from the peak contraction pressure for each contraction in a 10-minute window and adding the pressures generated by each contraction. In the example shown, five contractions occurred, producing pressure changes of 52, 50, 47, 44, and 49 mm Hg, respectively. The sum of these five contractions is 242 Montevideo units.

attempts. Thus, inability to achieve vaginal delivery after reaching complete dilatation is a significant marker of true dystocia because it is likely to recur.

*Failure to progress* in either spontaneous or stimulated labor has become an increasingly popular description of ineffectual labor. This term includes lack of progressive cervical dilatation or lack of descent. Often, the diagnosis is made before the active phase of labor has begun, and, therefore, before an adequate trial of labor has been achieved. Olah and Neilson (1994) concluded that failure to progress was not a diagnosis but an observation. According to the American College of Obstetricians and Gynecologists (ACOG) (1995), neither failure to progress nor cephalopelvic disproportion are precise terms. They conclude that a more practical classification is to divide labor abnormalities into either slower than normal labor (protraction disorder) or complete cessation of progress (arrest disorder). The woman must be in the active phase of labor (cervix dilated 3 to 4 cm or more) for either of these disorders to be diagnosed.

Handa and Laros (1993) diagnosed active-phase arrest (no dilatation for ≥ 2 h) in 5% of term nulliparous women. Interestingly, this incidence has not changed since the 1950s (Friedman, 1978). Inadequate uterine contractions, defined as less than 180 Montevideo units (Fig. 25–2), were diagnosed in 80% of women who had active-phase arrest. Protraction disorders have been less well described, probably because the time interval required before making a diagnosis of slow progress is undefined. Said another way, how many hours must elapse before deciding that less than 1.2 cm per hour (Table 25–3) of cervical dilatation has occurred? The World Health Organization (1994) proposed a labor management "partograph" in which protraction is defined as less than 1 cm per hour of cervical dilatation *for a minimum of 4 hours.*

## OVERDIAGNOSIS

It is generally agreed that dystocia leading to cesarean delivery is overdiagnosed in the United States and elsewhere. Factors leading to increased use of cesarean delivery for dystocia, however, are controversial. Those implicated have included obstetrician convenience, incorrect diagnosis of dystocia, and fear of litigation (Fraser and associates, 1987).

Variability in the criteria for diagnosis is likely a major determinant of the increase in cesarean deliver-

**Table 25–3** Criteria for Diagnosis of Abnormal Labor Caused by Arrest or Protraction Disorders

| Labor Pattern | Nullipara | Multipara |
|---|---|---|
| **PROTRACTION DISORDER** | | |
| Dilatation | <1.2 cm/hr | <1.5 cm/hr |
| Descent | <1.0 cm/hr | <2.0 cm/hr |
| **ARREST DISORDER** | | |
| Dilatation | >2 hr | >2 hr |
| Descent | >1 hr | >1 hr |

From the American College of Obstetricians and Gynecologists (ACOG): Dystocia and the Augmentation of Labor. (Technical Bulletin No. 218). Washington, DC, © ACOG, 1995.

ies for dystocia. Stewart and associates (1990) from Ottawa reported that 30% of 3740 women in labor were given a diagnosis of dystocia. Cesarean delivery for dystocia was performed during all phases of labor, but the largest number (40%) took place in latent phase. They concluded that many cesarean deliveries were, therefore, performed for dystocia without a trial of labor. Similarly, Cartmill and Thornton (1992) claimed that labor progress graphs—because they included the latent phase—appeared flat and portrayed long labor; this depiction erroneously influenced early diagnosis of dystocia. DeMott and Sandmire (1992) reported that obstetricians who had the lowest cesarean delivery rates for dystocia used higher dosages of oxytocin to stimulate labor, used oxytocin for longer durations, and started administration of oxytocin at more advanced cervical dilatations. King (1993) found that cesarean sections performed for dystocia in private patients in the United Kingdom were related to office hours and surgery schedules, whereas the timing of procedures for fetal distress were evenly distributed throughout the day.

## DIAGNOSIS OF ACTIVE-PHASE LABOR DISORDERS

The current criteria recommended by the ACOG (1995) for diagnosis of protraction and arrest disorders are shown in Table 25–3. These criteria are adapted from Cohen and Friedman (1983).

Hauth and associates (1986, 1991) reported that to induce or augment labor with oxytocin effectively, most women (90%) achieve between 200 and 225 Montevideo units, and 40% achieve at least 300 Montevideo units (see Fig. 25–2). These results suggest that there are certain minimums of uterine activity that should be achieved before performing cesarean delivery for dystocia. Accordingly, the ACOG (1989b) has suggested that before the diagnosis of arrest during first-stage labor is made, both of these criteria should be met: the latent phase has been completed, with the cervix dilated 4 cm or more and a uterine contraction pattern of 200 Montevideo units or more in a 10-minute period has been present for 2 hours without cervical change. It is also important to emphasize that epidural analgesia can slow labor.

# Labor Management Protocols

O'Driscoll and colleagues (1984) at the National Maternity Hospital in Dublin pioneered the concept that a disciplined, standardized labor management protocol reduced cesarean deliveries for dystocia. The approach advocated by O'Driscoll and others is now referred to as *active management of labor*. Its components, or at least two of them—amniotomy and oxytocin—have been widely used, especially in English-speaking countries outside the United States (Thornton and Lilford, 1994).

## ACTIVE MANAGEMENT OF LABOR

This term describes a codified approach to labor diagnosis and management. Labor is diagnosed when painful contractions are accompanied by complete cervical effacement, bloody show, or ruptured membranes. Women who have such findings are committed to delivery within 12 hours. Pelvic examination is performed each hour for the next 3 hours, and thereafter at 2-hour intervals. Progress is assessed for the first time 1 hour after admission. When dilatation has not increased by at least 1 cm, amniotomy is performed. Progress is again assessed at 2 hours and high-dose oxytocin infusion is started unless significant progress (i.e., 1 cm/hr) is documented. Women are constantly attended by midwives.

If membranes rupture before admission, oxytocin is begun for no progress at the 1-hour mark. No special equipment is used either to dispense oxytocin or to monitor its effects; that is, electronic uterine contraction monitoring is not used. Oxytocin is dispensed by gravity and regulated by a personal nurse. The solution contains 10 units of oxytocin in 1 liter of dextrose and water; the total dose may not exceed 10 units and the infusion rate may not exceed 60 drops per min (15 to 20 drops = 1 ml). Scalp blood sampling is used as the definitive test of fetal distress.

López-Zeno and associates (1992) prospectively compared active management with the traditional approach to labor management as practiced at Northwestern Memorial Hospital in Chicago. In an unblinded fashion, they randomized 705 uncomplicated nulliparous women who were in spontaneous labor at term. The cesarean rate was 10.5% with active management and 14.1% with the traditional approach. More recently, Frigoletto and associates (1995) reported a randomized trial of active management in 1934 nulliparous women whose babies were delivered at Brigham and Women's Hospital in Boston. Although they found that such management somewhat shortened labor, it did not affect the rate of cesarean sections that were performed.

## WORLD HEALTH ORGANIZATION PARTOGRAPH

A *partogram* was designed for use in developing countries (Dujardin and associates, 1992). This divides labor into a latent phase, which should last no longer than 8 hours, and an active phase starting at 3 cm of dilatation, the rate of which should be no slower than 1 cm per hour. A 4-hour wait (lag time) is recommended before intervention when the active phase is slow. Labor is graphed and analysis includes use of *alert and action* lines. The protocol was found to be beneficial in Southeast Asia (World Health Organization, 1994).

## PARKLAND HOSPITAL LABOR MANAGEMENT PROTOCOL

During the 1980s, the obstetric volume at Parkland Hospital doubled to approximately 15,000 births per year. In response, a second delivery unit designed for women who had uncomplicated term pregnancies was developed. This provided a unique opportunity to implement and evaluate a standardized protocol for labor management. The design was based upon the labor management approach that had evolved at the University of Texas Southwestern Medical Center up to that time, which emphasized the implementation of specific sequential interventions when abnormal labor was suspected. This approach is currently used in both complicated and uncomplicated pregnancies.

Women at term are admitted when active labor—defined as cervical dilatation of 3 to 4 cm or more in the presence of uterine contractions—is diagnosed or ruptured membranes are confirmed. Management guidelines stipulate that pelvic examinations should be performed approximately every 2 hours. Ineffective labor is suspected when the cervix does not dilate within about 2 hours of admission. Amniotomy is then performed, and labor progress is checked at the next 2-hour evaluation. Women whose labors do not progress receive intrauterine catheter placement to evaluate uterine function. Hypotonic contractions and no cervical progress after an additional 2 to 3 hours result in stimulation of labor using the high-dose oxytocin regimen described later in this chapter. Uterine activity of 200 to 250 Montevideo units is expected for 2 to 4 hours before dystocia is diagnosed. Dilatation rates of 1 to 2 cm per hour are accepted as evidence of progress after satisfactory uterine activity has been established with oxytocin. This can require up to 8 hours or more before cesarean delivery is performed for dystocia. Probably the cumulative time required to effect this stepwise management approach permits many women the time necessary to establish effective labor. This management protocol has been evaluated in more than 20,000 women who had uncomplicated pregnancies. Cesarean delivery rates in nulliparous and parous women were 8.7% and 1.5%, respectively. Importantly, these labor interventions and the relatively infrequent use of cesarean delivery did not jeopardize the fetus.

## OXYTOCIN STIMULATION OF LABOR

Synthetic oxytocin is one of the most commonly used medications in the United States. Virtually every parturient receives oxytocin after delivery, and many also receive this drug to induce or augment labor. According to the National Center for Health Statistics (Ventura and associates, 1995), 14% of women who delivered in the United States during 1993 received oxytocin for labor augmentation and another 13% were induced with either oxytocin, amniotomy, or both. In total, it is estimated that more than 1 million American women were given oxytocin to stimulate labor.

Two questions must be answered before a treatment plan using oxytocin or any other method to stimulate labor can be formulated: First, has the woman actually been in active labor? If there has been rhythmic uterine activity of sufficient intensity to produce some discomfort and the cervix has undergone distinct changes in effacement and dilatation to 3 or 4 cm, it is correct to conclude that there has been real labor. Second, is there cephalopelvic disproportion? Uterine dysfunction is often protective against some degree of pelvic contraction or abnormalities of fetal size or presentation. Fortunately, the uterus does not typically persist in spontaneous activity that would lead to rupture. Instead, the usual forces of labor are replaced by hypotonic dysfunction.

Most often, once the diagnosis of active labor followed by hypotonic dysfunction has been made and the head is well fixed in the pelvis, the membranes, if intact, should be ruptured. Ideally, an intrauterine catheter and fetal scalp electrode are placed. Close observation may be employed for 30 to 60 minutes to see if the amniotomy improves contractions. A decision must then be made whether to stimulate labor with oxytocin or to effect cesarean delivery. For many years, the choice to augment labor has been an empiric decision based largely upon clinical judgment as to fetal size, presentation, and position, as well as clinical assessment of pelvic size and fetal condition.

*Induction* of labor implies stimulation of contractions before spontaneous onset of labor, with or without ruptured membranes. *Augmentation* refers to stimulation of contractions when spontaneous contractions are considered inadequate, with resultant failure of progressive dilatation or descent. Some consider augmentation to include stimulation of contractions after spontaneous rupture of membranes without labor.

## TECHNIQUE FOR INTRAVENOUS OXYTOCIN

Oxytocin was the first synthesized polypeptide hormone, and the Nobel Prize in chemistry was awarded in 1955 for this achievement to DuVigneaud and associates. A variety of methods for stimulation of contractions with this synthetic posterior pituitary hormone have been employed. Seitchik and associates (1984) studied the pharmacokinetics of synthetic oxytocin and found that a uterine response occurs with 3 to 5 minutes of infusion and that a steady state is reached in plasma within approximately 40 minutes. Response depends on pre-existing uterine activity, sensitivity, and cervical status, which are related to individual biologic differences and to the pregnancy duration. Caldeyro-Barcia and Poseiro (1960) reported that uterine response to oxytocin increases slowly from 20 to 30 weeks and is unchanged from 34 weeks until term, at which time sensitivity rapidly increases. Satin and associates (1992) studied factors affecting the dose response to oxytocin for labor stimulation in 1773 pregnancies. Important predictors of oxytocin dosage included cervical dilatation, parity, and gestational age. The mother should be continually monitored while oxytocin is being infused. The goal is to effect uterine activity that is sufficient to produce cervical change and fetal descent while avoiding uterine hyperstimulation and fetal distress. Contractions must be evaluated continuously and oxytocin discontinued if they exceed five in a 10-minute period or last longer than 1 minute, or if the fetal heart rate decelerates significantly. With hyperstimulation, immediate discontinuation of oxytocin nearly always corrects the disturbances. The oxytocin concentration in plasma falls rapidly because its mean half-life is approximately 5 minutes.

Synthetic oxytocin is usually diluted into 1000 ml of a balanced salt solution that is administered by infusion pump. Administration by any other route is not recommended for labor stimulation. To avoid bolus administration, the infusion should be inserted into the mainline intravenous line close to the venipuncture site. A typical oxytocin infusate consists of 10 units, USP (equivalent to 10,000 mU), mixed into 1000 ml of lactated Ringer's solution, resulting in an oxytocin concentration of 10 mU per ml. According to the ACOG (1995), any of the oxytocin regimens shown in Table 25–4, as well as others are appropriate for labor stimulation.

## PARKLAND HOSPITAL PROTOCOL

At Parkland Hospital, approximately 30% of labors are induced or augmented using oxytocin, and from 1991 to 1995, 21,602 women were given oxytocin according to the following protocol:

1. Constant bedside attendance is provided by trained nursing personnel.
2. Continuous electronic monitoring of fetal heart rate and uterine activity is conducted.
3. Oxytocin is generally not administered in cases of abnormal fetal presentations and marked uterine overdistention, such as pathologic hydramnios, an excessively large fetus, or multiple fetuses.
4. Women of high parity (6 or more children) are generally not given oxytocin because it could increase the risk of uterine rupture, which occurs more readily in these patients. Oxytocin is usually withheld from a woman who has a previous uterine scar and a live fetus.
5. Fetal condition must be good, as evidenced by heart rate and lack of thick meconium in amniotic fluid. A dead fetus is not a contraindication unless there is overt fetopelvic disproportion.

In late 1990, we changed the protocol to a high-dose oxytocin regimen (Satin and associates, 1992, 1994). A standard low-dose regimen was compared with a flexible high-dose protocol in nearly 5000 pregnancies, and the new protocol was found to be superior. Oxytocin infusion is commenced at 6 mU per min, and this is increased as needed every 40 minutes by 6 mU per minute, not to exceed a maximum of 42 mU per minute. Hyperstimulation occurs in approximately half of cases and is managed by oxytocin discontinuation followed by resumption, if indicated, at half the stopping dosage. Thereafter, the dosage is increased to 3 mU per minute every 40 minutes. If hyperstimulation persists, 1 mU per minute increments every 40 minutes are used. Labor augmentations were more than 3 hours shorter if this flexible high-dose regimen was used, and there were fewer cesarean deliveries for dystocia. Inductions failed less frequently, but cesarean delivery for fetal distress was increased to 6 vs. 3% with the flexible high-dose regimen. No adverse fetal effects were observed, however, in either group. Xenakis and associates (1995) reported similar benefits for a high-dose oxytocin regimen in which the starting dose was 4 mU per minute with 4 mU per minute increments every 15 minutes.

# Effects of Epidural Analgesia on Labor

Epidural analgesia is widely used in the United States to relieve pain during childbirth. Reported usage rates vary greatly, but in some centers up to 90% or more of laboring women receive epidural analgesia. Im-

**Table 25–4** Examples of Low-Dose and High-Dose Oxytocin Regimens for Stimulation of Labor

| Oxytocin Regimen | Starting Dose (mU/min) | Incremental Increase (mU/min) | Dosage Interval (min) | Maximum Dose (mU/min) |
|---|---|---|---|---|
| Low Dose | 0.5–1 | 1 | 30–40 | 20 |
|  | 1–2 | 2 | 15 | 40 |
| High Dose | ≈6 | ≈6 | ≈15 | ≈40 |
|  | 6 | 6,* 3, 1 | 20–40 | 42 |

*The incremental increase is reduced to 3 mU/min in the presence of recurrent hyperstimulation.

portantly, usage of epidural analgesia during labor has increased greatly during the past two decades coincident with significant escalation in the national cesarean birth rate (Taffel and associates, 1990). There is general agreement that epidural analgesia increases the chances of the mother's requiring an instrumental delivery with forceps or vacuum extraction because of prolonged second-stage labor (Chestnut, 1994; Thorp and Breedlove, 1996). There has been controversy concerning the influence of epidural analgesia on cesarean delivery rates with some investigators suggesting a direct relationship between increasing epidural use and excessive cesarean births (Thorp and Breedlove, 1996; Morton and associates, 1994).

In contrast, Sharma and associates (1997) randomized 358 women in labor who had uncomplicated term pregnancies to receive epidural analgesia or patient-controlled (via pump) intravenous meperidine, and cesarean rates were not affected by the type of analgesia used.

Inhibition of voluntary skeletal muscle function necessary to accomplish expulsion of the infant may be related to the prolonged second stage of labor commonly attributed to the effect of epidural analgesia. There seems to be consensus about this side effect of epidural analgesia during labor, and we observed this effect in our investigations. Acknowledgment of this effect is implicit in the ACOG guidelines, which define a prolonged second stage of labor differently if epidural analgesia is used (ACOG, 1989a). Specifically, an additional hour is added to the obstetric time permitted for management of the second stage of labor when epidural analgesia is in use. Similar attention has not heretofore generally been focused on the epidural effects during the first stage of labor. Alexander and associates (1998) and other investigators (Chestnut, 1994; Thorp and Breedlove, 1996) have observed that the first stage of labor is increased by 1 or 2 hours when epidural analgesia is used. Moreover, the amount of oxytocin required during labor stimulated with epidural analgesia is significantly increased (Alexander and associates, 1998). These first-stage labor effects of epidural analgesia have considerable potential significance in labor management. Perhaps, obstetric management during the first stage of labor, as in the case of the second stage of labor, should be modified to permit a longer first stage when epidural analgesia is used.

## REFERENCES

Alexander JM, Lucas MJ, Ramin SM, et al: The course of labor with and without epidural analgesia. Am J Obstet Gynecol 178:516, 1998.

American College of Obstetricians and Gynecologists (ACOG): Dystocia and the Augmentation of Labor. Technical Bulletin No. 218. Washington, DC, ACOG, 1995.

American College of Obstetricians and Gynecologists on Obstetrics (ACOG): Maternal and Fetal Medicine. Obstetrics Forceps. Committee Opinion No. 71. Washington, DC, ACOG, 1989a.

American College of Obstetricians and Gynecologists (ACOG): Dystocia. Technical Bulletin No. 137. Washington, DC, ACOG, 1989b.

Caldeyro-Barcia R, Poseiro JJ: Physiology of the uterine contraction. Clin Obstet Gynecol 3:386, 1960.

Cartmill RS, Thornton JG: Effect of presentation of partogram information on obstetric decision-making. Lancet 339:1520, 1992.

Centers for Disease Control: Rates of cesarean delivery—United States, 1993. MMWR 44:303, 1995.

Chestnut DH: Effect on the progress of labor and method of delivery. In Chestnut DH (ed): Obstetric Anesthesia: Principles and Practices. St. Louis, Mosby–Year Book, 1994, pp 403–419.

Cohen W, Friedman EA (eds): Management of Labor. Baltimore, University Park Press, 1983.

DeMott RK, Sandmire HF: The Green Bay cesarean section study. II. The physician factor or a determinant of cesarean birth rates for failed labor. Am J Obstet Gynecol 166:1799, 1992.

Dujardin B, DeSchampheleire I, Sene H, et al: Value of the alert and action lines on the partogram. Lancet 339:1336, 1992.

DuVigneaud V, Ressler C, Swan JM, et al: The synthesis of oxytocin. J Am Chem Soc 75:4879, 1953.

Fraser W, Usher RH, McLean FH, et al: Temporal variation in rates of cesarean section for dystocia: Does "convenience" play a role? Am J Obstet Gynecol 156:300, 1987.

Friedman EA: Primigravid labor. A graphicostatistical analysis. Obstet Gynecol 6:567, 1955.

Friedman EA: Labor: Clinical Evaluation and Management, 2nd ed. New York, Appleton-Century-Crofts, 1978.

Frigoletto FD, Lieberman E, Lang JM, et al: A clinical trial of active management of labor. N Engl J Med 333:745, 1995.

Handa VL, Laros RK: Active-phase arrest in labor: Predictors of cesarean delivery in a nulliparous population. Obstet Gynecol 81:758, 1993.

Hauth JC, Hankins GD, Gilstrap LC III, et al: Uterine contraction pressures with oxytocin induction/augmentation. Obstet Gynecol 68:305, 1986.

Hauth JC, Hankins GD, Gilstrap LC III: Uterine contraction pressures achieved in parturients with active phase arrest. Obstet Gynecol 78:344, 1991.

Hoskins IA, Gomez JL: Correlation between maximum cervical dilatation at c/section and subsequent VBAC success rate. Am J Obstet Gynecol 174:480, 1996.

Kilpatrick SJ, Laros RK: Characteristics of normal labor. Obstet Gynecol 74:85, 1989.

King JF: Obstetric intervention and the economic imperative. Br J Obstet Gynaecol 100:1063, 1993.

López-Zeno JA, Peaceman AM, Adashek JA, et al: A controlled trial of a program for the active management of labor. N Engl J Med 326:450, 1992.

Morton SC, Williams MS, Keeler EB, et al: Effect of epidural analgesia for labor on the cesarean delivery rate. Obstet Gynecol 83:1045, 1994.

Notzon FC, Cnattinguis S, Bergsjo P, et al: Cesarean section delivery in the 1980s: International comparison by indication. Am J Obstet Gynecol 17:495, 1994.

O'Driscoll K, Meagher D, Boylan P: Diagnosis of labor. Active Management of Labor, 3rd ed. London, Mosby–Year Book, 1993, p 43.

O'Driscoll K, Foley M, MacDonald D: Active management of labor as an alternative to cesarean section for dystocia. Obstet Gynecol 63:485, 1984.

Olah KSJ, Neilson JP: Failure to progress in the management of labour. Br J Obstet Gynaecol 101:1, 1994.

Satin AJ, Leveno KJ, Sherman ML, et al: Factors affecting the dose response to oxytocin for labor stimulation. Am J Obstet Gynecol 166:1260, 1992.

Satin AJ, Leveno KJ, Sherman ML, et al: High-dose oxytocin: 20- versus 40-minute dosage interval. Obstet Gynecol 83:234, 1994.

Seitchik J, Amico J, Robinson AG, et al: Oxytocin augmentation of dysfunctional labor. IV. Oxytocin pharmacokinetics. Am J Obstet Gynecol 150:225, 1984.

Sharma SK, Sidawi JE, Ramin SM, et al: Cesarean delivery: A randomized trial of epidural versus patient-controlled meperidine analgesia during labor. Anesthesiology 87:487, 1997.

Sokol RJ, Stojkov J, Chik L, et al: Normal and abnormal labor progress: I. A quantitative assessment and survey of the literature. J Reprod Med 18:47, 1977.

Stewart PJ, Dulberg C, Arnill AC, et al: Diagnosis of dystocia and management with cesarean section among primiparous women in Ottawa-Carleton. Can Med Assoc J 142:459, 1990.

Taffel SM, Placek PJ, Moien M: 1988 U.S. cesarean-section at 24.7 per 100 births—a plateau? N Engl J Med 323:99, 1990.

Thornton JG, Lilford RJ: Active management of labour: Current knowledge and research issues. BMJ 309:366, 1994.

Thorp JA, Breedlove G: Epidural analgesia in labor: An evaluation of risks and benefits. Birth 23:63, 1996.

Ventura ST, Martin JA, Taffel SM, et al: Advance report of final mortality statistics, 1993. National Center for Health Statistics, Monthly Vital Statistics Report, 44 (suppl), 1995.

World Health Organization: Partographic management of labour. Lancet 343:1399, 1994.

Xenakis EMJ, Langer O, Piper JM, et al: Low-dose versus high-dose oxytocin augmentation of labor—a randomized trial. Am J Obstet Gynecol 173:1874, 1995.

# 26

# Obstetric Anesthesia

COLLEEN DARGIE
H. MICHAEL MARSH

Anesthesia and analgesia are now accepted as essential elements in advanced obstetric practice in the United States and most of the Western world. In 1992, The American College of Obstetricians and Gynecologists (ACOG) and the American Society of Anesthesiologists (ASA) drafted and issued a joint statement on pain in labor that states "Labor results in severe pain for many women. There is no other circumstance where it is considered acceptable for a person to experience severe pain amenable to safe intervention, while under a physician's care. Maternal request is a sufficient justification for pain relief during labor" (Norris, 1993).

This was not always the case. In 1591, Dame Euphanie MacAlyane of Edinburgh was burnt at the stake by order of James VI of Scotland, who later became James I of England, for attempting secretly to bribe Agnes Samson, a midwife, to relieve the pains of her labor. This was judged to be impious and contrary to the Scriptures (Genesis 3:12–14, 16).

In that same city, on January 19, 1847, James Young Simpson first administered diethyl ether to a woman in labor. He preferred chloroform and began to use it in November of that same year, and this use continued because of chloroform's superiority for the purpose of brief analgesia with each contraction. The first recipient of obstetric anesthetic administered in the United States was Fanny Appleton Longfellow, the wife of the poet. The anesthetic was administered by Nathan Cooley Keep in Cambridge, Massachusetts, on April 7, 1847. Analgesia for labor finally became fashionable when chloroform was administered to Queen Victoria on April 7, 1853, for the delivery of her seventh child, Prince Leopold. John Snow was the attending anaesthetist. He wrote "With regard to the cases of labor in which chloroform may be employed, it will readily be conceded that, in cases where the pain is not greater than the patient is willing to bear cheerfully, there is no occasion to use chloroform....The benefits arising from chloroform in severe cases of labor are experienced in a lesser degree in favorable cases; and the patient may fairly be allowed to have a voice in this."

Today, neuraxial analgesia is the preferred technique for pain relief during labor (Bader, 1993), using bolus and continuous infusion of dilute local anesthetics and narcotics, administered epidurally, intrathecally, or by both routes (Brownridge, 1988). Alternative strategies, such as the Read or Lamaze methods, and patient-controlled analgesia (PCA) still suffice for 30 to 40% of uncomplicated deliveries. The most controversial factor reducing the universal application of epidural analgesia in every delivery is the belief that epidural analgesia increases the duration of labor and the cesarean section rate (Thorp, 1993). Although epidural anesthetics do have a small rate of complications, it is comparable to the rates of other means of analgesia that might be employed (Auroy,

1997; Eisenach, 1997). There is, unfortunately, no large controlled trial to prove or disprove the contention that the cesarean rate is increased through the use of epidural anesthesia (Birnbach, 1997; Chestnut, 1997).

The aims of this chapter are to outline the mechanisms and pain pathways relevant to labor; to discuss analgesia and sedative techniques, including neuraxial blocks used in labor and delivery; and, finally, to review the anesthetic management of the patient in whom surgical intervention may be indicated during pregnancy and confinement.

## Pain and Its Mechanisms in Labor

Uterine pain is mediated through afferents that accompany the sympathetic nerves in the uterovaginal and pelvic plexuses. These sympathetic nerves pass through the inferior hypogastric plexus, the hypogastric nerve, the superior hypogastric plexus, the lower aortic plexus, and the lower lumbar splanchnic nerves. They join the sympathetic trunk from L4 to S1 and then proceed to spinal nerves T11 and T12 and through these nerves to the spinal cord. During the first stage of labor, pain starts in the uterus and its adnexa and is generated by the following five stimuli:

1. Pressure on nerve endings between the muscle fibers of the uterus.
2. Contraction of an ischemic myometrium and cervix
3. Vasoconstriction secondary to sympathetic hyperactivity
4. Inflammatory change in the uterine muscle as labor progresses
5. Dilation of the lower uterine segment and cervix

Pain stemming from cervical dilation and the upper vagina is mediated through the pelvic splanchnic nerves to spinal nerves S2, S3, and S4; simultaneously, somatic afferents from the lower vagina and perineum running along the pudendal nerves also travel to S2, S3, and S4 to mediate pain from these structures. As labor progresses, pain sensation from uterine contractions may involve T10 and L1 in addition to T11 and T12. In the second and third stages of labor, after the cervix is fully dilated and thus not generating pain, pain is mainly caused by increasing pressure from the presenting fetal part on pain-sensitive structures in the pelvis and the perineum. Referred pain may be noted in the back during the first stage, whereas some parturients may notice aching, burning, or cramping in the thighs or legs during the later stages of labor. This late-stage pain arises from traction on the pelvic parietal peritoneum and the uterine ligaments; stretching and tension in the bladder, urethra, and rectum; and stretching and tension of ligaments, fascia, and muscles of the pelvic cavity. Pressure on one or more of the roots of the lumbosacral plexus may also contribute to the pain, either as an isolated cause or in conjunction with other late-stage pain sources.

Labor pain ranks among the most severe forms of physical discomfort and has been described as intolerable by about 30% of women. Benjamin Rush, who advised bleeding to relieve labor pain, believed that removing three pints would reduce both the severity of the pain and its adverse effects. In reality, this old-fashioned remedy would only exacerbate the stress induced by the pain of parturition as outlined in Figure 26–1. Prevention of this stress is mandatory in high-risk pregnancies and preferable in most deliveries when it can be achieved at little risk to the mother or fetus.

## Anesthetic Risk in Obstetrics

The risks inherent to any use of analgesic or anesthetic technique are compounded during pregnancy because of the physiologic changes that are taking place, because of the nonelective timing, because the mother frequently has a full stomach, and because risks to both mother and fetus must be considered. To optimize the outcome (Hood, 1988), these risks must be balanced against those arising from the stress of the situation in which the patient is placed. Frequent and effective communication between the obstetric and anesthetic teams is essential in providing optimal care for mother and fetus.

### MATERNAL MORBIDITY AND MORTALITY

Statistical data regarding maternal mortality rates have been maintained in the United States since 1915. Initially, there were 600 maternal deaths per 100,000 live births. In 1933, the New York Academy of Medicine examined these deaths and declared that 60% were preventable. In 1978, the rate had declined to 8.5 to 15 per 100,000, but 40 to 90% were still regarded as preventable. The leading causes of maternal mortality in the United States, England, and Wales in 1978 were similar and included embolism (thrombotic and amniotic fluid) 3 per 100,000; preeclampsia or eclampsia 2.2 per 100,000; obstetric hemorrhage 1.8 per 100,000; obstetric infection 1.1 per 100,000; analgesia or anesthesia 1.1 per 100,000; and cerebrovascular accidents 1.1 per 100,000 maternal deaths per live births. There has been little change over the last 20 years in these risks.

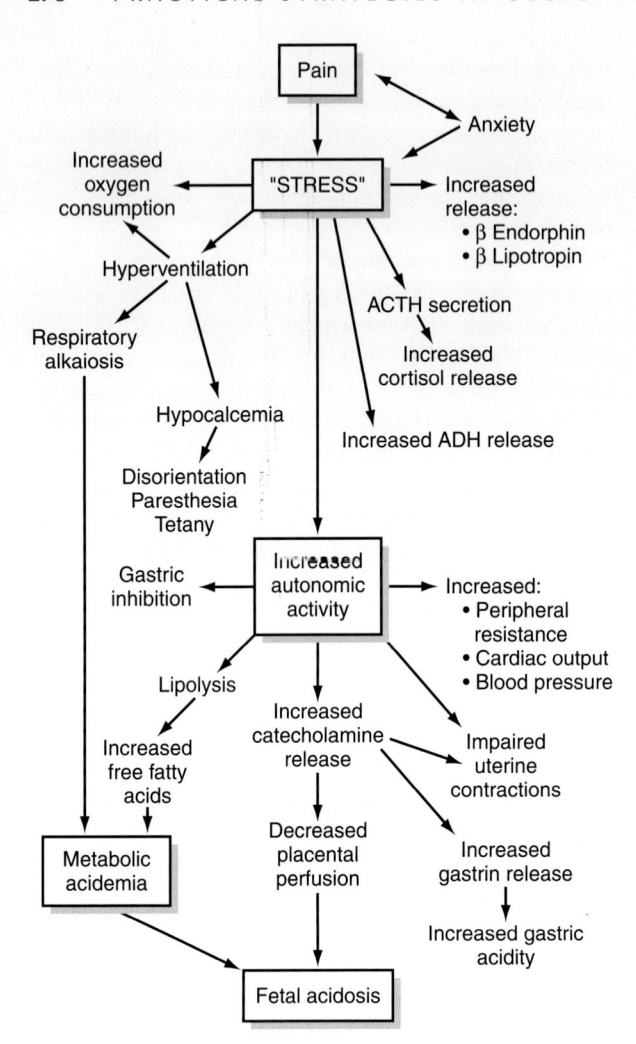

**Figure 26–1** Pathophysiologic changes secondary to pain in labor and delivery. (From Brownridge P, Cohen SE: Neural blockade for obstetrics and gynecologic surgery. From Cousins MJ, Bridenbaugh PO [eds]: Neural Blockade in Clinical Anesthesia and Pain Management. Philadelphia, JB Lippincott, 1988, pp 593; 634.) ACTH = adrenocorticotrophic hormone; ADH = antidiuretic hormone.

Cesarean section carries about a 12-fold higher risk to the mother than vaginal delivery, with an emergency cesarean section carrying an even higher risk than an elective operation. The leading causes of maternal death after a cesarean section are pulmonary embolism, sepsis, hemorrhage, and anesthesia complications. The most common avoidable factors associated with anesthesia relate to aspiration of gastric contents. Preventive measures include administration of clear, nonparticulate antacids (Bicitra or Gold Alka-Seltzer), $H_2$ receptor blockers (ranitidine [Zantac], cimetidine [Tagamet]), and drugs that increase gastric motility (e.g., metoclopramide [Reglan]) immediately before induction. Mismanagement of a difficult airway, misuse of drugs, equipment accidents, and mismanagement of hemorrhage, often compounded by inexperience on the part of the anesthetic provider, are also related to poor outcomes.

Maternal morbidity may be associated with use of analgesic techniques. Postdural puncture headache, backache related to use of neuraxial blocks, possible delay of progress of labor, or surgical intervention for delivery must be considered, as must maternal respiratory depression and acidosis and the possibility of fetal depression when systemic narcotics are used. When natural childbirth methods are used, inadequate pain relief and complications of stress, with secondary fetal effects from decreased uteroplacental flow, must be considered.

## PERINATAL MORBIDITY AND MORTALITY

Perinatal mortality is usually defined as fetal death after 20 or more weeks of gestation and neonatal death at less than 7 days after birth. Few studies address the influence of anesthetic events on perinatal outcome (Rawlings, 1995). Although the major concern for the outcome of the neonate rests with the neonatologist, management of the mother during the progress of labor, monitoring of the fetus, and appropriate steps to avoid prolonged fetal asphyxia are direct concerns for the obstetric and anesthesia teams. Rapid and appropriate resuscitation of the newborn is responsible for improved outcome (Iams, 1998).

Appropriate prenatal care is a fundamental requirement for establishing a situation in which prematurity is regarded as a preventable complication (Lieberman, 1995). This topic is more fully discussed in Chapter 33, Preterm Birth.

# Pharmacologic and Nonpharmacologic Pain Relief

The options open to women in labor for pain relief include both pharmacologic and alternative methods. Among alternative methods are the prepared childbirth techniques developed by Read, Lamaze, and Leboyer, which feature hypnosis, acupuncture, or biofeedback. Transcutaneous electrical nerve stimulation (TENS) is also used, either alone or in conjunction with one of the other prepared childbirth techniques. The birth experience using these methods may still be extremely painful and often requires addition of narcotics or anesthetics in as many as 30 to 40% of women who attempt completely natural childbirth.

## NONPHARMACOLOGIC TECHNIQUES

Prepared childbirth stresses three major elements: first, educating the mother in the process of labor and setting appropriate expectations, with training in appropriate techniques of deep breathing and pushing for the advancing phases of labor; second, training in relaxation techniques; and, finally, preparing the husband or other supportive lay companion (the duola) who will be present during labor and delivery to provide coaching and reassurance to the mother. Studies suggest that this final element—the presence of a well-trained coach—ensures a more rested mother after delivery and one who is more ready to bond with her infant (Norris, 1993).

## PHARMACOLOGIC AIDS

Conscious sedation and analgesia may be added to the prepared childbirth techniques to calm the mother and enhance the benefits from correct breathing. This approach may suffice for a proportion of women. However, up to 30% of women may require neuraxial techniques for adequate pain relief in labor, and up to 80% of primiparous women do request these aids when they receive adequate instruction about the benefits and risks.

# Obstetric Emergencies and Anesthesia

From the anesthesiologist's point of view, obstetric emergencies can be classified into four groups: those that are *related to the fetus*, including fetal distress, asphyxia, malpresentation, or multiple birth; those *related to the chorioamnion*, including intra-amniotic infections and pre-eclampsia or eclampsia; those *related to the mother*, including a difficult airway or coexisting disease that may complicate the delivery or labor; and, finally, those that are *direct anesthetic or obstetric complications*, such as obstetric hemorrhage, aspiration, intraoperative hypotension, or other postoperative complications. The anesthetic team must be prepared and equipped to deal effectively with all these emergencies.

# Diagnostic Considerations

When the pregnant patient comes into the labor ward, she should be seen and assessed by the anesthesia team and the obstetrician. This anesthesia assessment should encompass the airway, any coexisting diseases, or any potential for emergencies. If these risks are apparent during prenatal care visits, a formal anesthesiology consultation could be beneficial to allow development of an adequate plan for a potentially complicated delivery.

## MATERNAL PHYSIOLOGIC CHANGES OF PREGNANCY

The physiologic changes that occur in the mother during pregnancy carry implications for anesthetic management. These include changes in the respiratory system, the cardiovascular system, the nervous and endocrine systems, the gastrointestinal system, and the urinary system, as shown in Table 26–1. Preparation should be made to handle a difficult airway; to provide adequate oxygenation and gas exchange in the face of altered mechanics in the lung during the phases of pregnancy and parturition; to manage possible fluid shifts; to control bleeding during and after delivery; and to counter the risks of aspiration of gastric contents, which are associated with pregnancy. All these possibilities must be controlled by the anesthetic team for safe management.

## MOST COMMON COEXISTING DISEASES

The most common coexisting diseases present during pregnancy—which may become exacerbated during

**Table 26–1** Maternal Physiologic Changes in Pregnancy—Systems Review

| Respiratory System | Possible Treatment Elements |
|---|---|
| *Engorged mucosa in airway | Phenylephrine HCl (Neo-Synephrine) spray to nasal mucosa |
| 20% ↑ $O_2$ consumption<br>70% ↑ alveolar ventilation<br>↓ $PaCO_2$ between 30–32 mm Hg<br>↓ Lung volumes secondary to diaphragmatic displacement<br>↓ $PaO_2$ secondary to ↑ CC (late gestation) contrasts with early stage ↑ $PaO_2$<br>*Rapid desaturation with ↓ FRC<br>*Possible airway compromise | Preoxygenation, positioning, CPAP<br>ASA algorithm for difficult airway |
| **Cardiovascular System** | |
| 35% ↑ blood volume, 45% ↑ plasma volume<br>40% ↑ cardiac output (30% ↑ SV; 15% ↑ HR)<br>↓ MAP and ↓ TPR (15%)<br>CVP unchanged<br>*Aortocaval compression<br>*High output states | Positioning<br>Epidural analgesia |
| **Gastrointestinal System** | |
| ↑ Acid and liquid volume in stomach<br>Stomach shifted upward, altered G-E function angles<br>*Acid aspiration | Nonparticulate antacid, $H_2$ block, metoclopramide |
| **Other Systems** | |
| Renal ↓ serum creatinine<br>    ↑ urinary volume/frequency<br>*Neuroendocrine changes underlie some of these features<br>*Mass effect accounts for others | Epidural analgesia<br>Positioning |

*Points for particular attention in anesthetic management.
ASA = American Society of Anesthesiologists; CC = closing capacity; CPAP = continuous positive airway pressure; CVP = central venous pressure; FRC = functional reserve capacity; G-E = gastroesophageal; HR = heart rate; MAP = mean arterial pressure; SV = stroke volume; TPR = total peripheral vascular resistance.

the third trimester and complicate provision of analgesia or anesthesia—are hypertension, including pregnancy-induced hypertension and pre-eclampsia or eclampsia; diabetes mellitus or pregnancy-induced diabetes; heart disease, including valvular disease; neuromuscular diseases, including multiple sclerosis, myasthenia gravis, and others; sexually transmitted diseases, including human immunodeficiency virus (HIV); substance abuse; massive obesity; liver disease; pulmonary embolism; asthma; and cerebrovascular disease that may lead to stroke.

## ASSESSING THE AIRWAY

Each prospective parturient's airway must be assessed to prevent an unanticipated difficulty if emergency anesthesia is needed during delivery. Problems of airway access may arise from pre-existing anatomic abnormalities or as a consequence of changes during pregnancy. Examination of the mouth and airway reveals anatomic abnormalities and allows assignment of a Mallampatti score (from 0 [no difficulty] to 3 [potentially very difficult]) (Norris, 1993). The examination is completed by checking the range of motion of the neck and jaw and ensuring access to the anterior neck for laryngoscope placement and manipulation, because access is sometimes impeded by breast engorgement or obesity. If difficulty is anticipated, plans should be made with provision for potential use of fiberoptic intubation, a lightwand, or intubation through a combitube or temporary laryngeal mask airway. The availability of help for performance of cricothyrotomy or tracheostomy should be ascertained. Each case must be evaluated with consideration given to the institution's own difficult airway algorithm as it applies to the particular patient.

Analgesia is managed differently if the patient has a difficult airway. Early use of neuraxial techniques and cautious titration of both narcotics and local anesthetics is mandatory. The difficult airway may become a partial indication for semielective use of cesarean delivery under regional anesthesia.

## AVOIDING THE MOST FREQUENT COMPLICATIONS

Adequate preoperative preparation makes it possible to avoid the dire consequences of most of the complications of pregnancy and delivery. Careful screening of coexisting diseases, as outlined previously, and preparation for the difficult airway (see Anesthesia Society of America [ASA] algorithm), blood loss, neonatal resuscitation, and subsequent critical care for the neonate must all be planned and ready to be carried out.

Drug abuse is also a potential problem that may complicate delivery. Usually, a mother who is a drug abuser is unprepared for childbirth and has avoided seeking prenatal care for herself and for the infant she will bear. Thus, on entry of this type of parturient into the labor ward, careful assessment by both the obstetric team and the anesthesiologist is mandatory and can usually prevent the most serious potential complications from developing.

# Management of Uncomplicated Cases

There are many recent reviews of techniques for management of uncomplicated vaginal delivery (Bader, 1993; Norris, 1993). The choice of technique must address the needs of both mother and fetus.

## ANALGESIA FOR LABOR—PRACTICAL ASPECTS

For providing pain relief during vaginal delivery, there are three major sets of techniques that can be chosen. First, there is so-called natural childbirth using nonpharmacologic techniques of reassurance and relaxation, as described previously.

Second, parenteral medications can be used for pain relief and sedation. These can be administered by inhalation (as in the original work of Simpson and Snow) or by intravenous (IV) or intramuscular (IM) routes. There must be a clear awareness that these agents can potentially affect the fetus. Intravenously administered narcotics, using patient-controlled analgesia (PCA) are the drugs most commonly used in this category. Other drugs include tranquilizers, such as benzodiazepines, phenothiazines, barbiturates, ketamine, and scopolamine.

Morphine (PCA: loading dose of 2 mg repeated × 5 every 10 minutes, then 1 mg/15 minutes lockout) was in the past, the primary agent chosen as an IV narcotic for use during labor. Fentanyl (PCA: 1 to 2 μg/kg, then 1 μg/kg per 1-hour lockout) may now be used in low doses. Nalbuphine (PCA: 2–5 mg + 1 mg/15-minute lockout) and butorphanol (PCA: 0.2–0.3 mg/5 to 15 minutes lockout), partial agonist-antagonist drugs, are now being used with increasing frequency because of the potential ceiling effect on respiratory depression that is thought to be achieved with these agents.

Meperidine (PCA: 10 to 50 mg/load + 5–10 mg/ 15 minutes lockout) is currently the most commonly used narcotic for labor analgesia. It is given in doses of 10 to 50 mg IV or 50 to 100 mg IM. The major concern with use of narcotics is neonatal respiratory depression. If meperidine is given IM less than 1 hour or more than 3 hours before delivery, neonatal respiratory depression is said to be minimized.

A secondary concern is that IV agents given in this way provide maximal narcosis and sedation, and some mothers believe that this creates a loss of control and decreased participation in the delivery.

Many mothers prefer other techniques that would allow them to be conscious but pain-free, and thus neuraxial techniques have proved superior. Regional anesthesia techniques have great advantages for vaginal delivery (Sharma, 1997). At present, local appropriately delivered anesthetics can provide complete pain relief while the mother is awake, alert, and cooperative. This gives the mother a feeling of control and decreases stress; therefore, this is probably the ideal technique. Common regional anesthetic techniques include pudendal block as well as spinal and epidural anesthetics. Paracervical blocks are still used occasionally but they carry the risk of inadvertent injection into the fetus. Potential disadvantages of neuraxial techniques include increased risk for instrumental delivery and, possibly, an increased rate of cesarean sections. There is also the risk of postdural puncture headache. There are theories that labor may proceed more slowly with use of epidural anesthesia than without it, but proof of poorer outcomes is lacking.

## CONTROVERSIAL ISSUES IN TIMING INTERVENTIONS

At present, epidural anesthesia (see Tables 26–2 and 26–3) is the most frequently used and popular technique for pain relief in labor. It is usually administered when labor is well established and the patient is committed to proceed to delivery. Controversy exists about the use of epidural analgesia during prolonged labor and as to whether its use causes an increased rate of cesarean sections. The patient must provide informed consent for the technique to be employed, and the risks should be explained fully. These include possible dural puncture with postdural puncture headache (Choi, 1996), total spinal anesthesia, hypotension secondary to the use of local anesthetics and narcotics, rare epidural or intrathecal infections, rare nerve damage, occasional persistent backache, pruri-

**Table 26–2** Techniques for Epidural and Spinal Anesthesia and Analgesia

| Technique for Epidural Anesthesia | Technique for Spinal Anesthesia |
|---|---|
| The medical history, obstetric history, and physical status of the parturient are evaluated. Absolute contraindications to the use of epidural anesthesia include the presence of a coagulopathy, severe hypovolemia, or active infection over the lumbar area. The obstetrician is consulted to ensure that labor is well established and that fetal heart rate (FHR) pattern is normal. <br><br> Adequate intravenous access is ensured, and the patient is hydrated acutely with 500 to 1000 ml of balanced salt solution. <br><br> Thirty ml of a nonparticulate antacid, sodium citrate (Bicitra) are administered. <br><br> The block may be administered in the labor room, where oxygen and wall suction are available and resuscitation equipment is present on the anesthesia cart. A nurse is present to assist with patient positioning, to record vital signs, and to monitor the FHR pattern. <br><br> A blood pressure cuff is placed and baseline vital signs are obtained. <br><br> The patient is placed in either the right lateral or left lateral decubitus position. Sitting position may be required if placement is technically difficult because of obesity or anatomic abnormalities. <br><br> After sterile preparation and subcutaneous infiltration, the epidural needle with stylet in place is inserted at the level of L2–3 or L3–4 until the tissue resistance of the interspinous ligament is felt. <br><br> The needle is always advanced with the bevel direction either cephalad or caudad; otherwise, threading of the catheter may be difficult. At this point, the stylet is removed and the epidural space is identified by one of the following methods: Hanging drop technique: A drop of saline is placed into the hub of the advancing needle. When the ligamenta flava is pierced, the drop is sucked into the needle by a negative pressure in the epidural space. This sign may not be completely reliable and is usually confirmed with one of the methods described below. Loss of resistance to air or saline: 3 ml of either air or saline are placed in a glass syringe and connected to the epidural needle. The needle is advanced with continuous pressure on the syringe, and as the needle enters the epidural space, a loss of resistance is felt. <br><br> A test dose of 3 ml of local anesthetic is injected into the epidural space through the needle, and the patient is monitored for signs of inadvertent intravascular or subarachnoid injection. <br><br> The epidural catheter is placed into the space to a distance of about 2 cm. The needle is then removed, and the distance the catheter extends into the space is recorded. <br><br> The catheter is checked by both gravity and aspiration to ensure that it does not contain either cerebrospinal fluid (CSF) or blood. <br><br> A second test dose is given through the catheter, and the patient is monitored as indicated previously. <br><br> The catheter is taped in place, and the patient placed with a wedge in the semilateral position. The patient's blood pressure and heart rate are monitored frequently over the next 20 minutes, and hypotension is treated promptly with fluids and ephedrine. <br><br> The patient receives a local anesthetic in 3- to 4-ml increments until the desired sensory level is achieved. This generally requires a total of 10 to 15 ml of drug administered over a 10- to 15-minute period. | The medical and obstetric history and the physical status of the parturient are evaluated. Absolute contraindications to the use of spinal anesthesia include the presence of a coagulopathy, severe hypovolemia, or active infection over the lumbar area. <br><br> Adequate intravenous access is ensured, and the patient is hydrated acutely with at least 1000 ml of a balanced salt solution. <br><br> Thirty ml of a nonparticulate antacid (Bicitra) are administered. <br><br> The patient is taken to the delivery room, where the anesthesia machine, medication cart, and resuscitation equipment are available. <br><br> Electrocardiograph, blood pressure cuff, and pulse oximeter are placed and baseline values obtained. Oxygen is administered via face mask. <br><br> The patient is placed either in the right lateral decubitus or sitting position. <br><br> After sterile preparation and subcutaneous infiltration, a 26- or 27-gauge needle is placed through an introducer into the subarachnoid space at the level of L2–3 or L3–4. Medication is not injected during uterine contraction because this may result in a higher sensory level than desired. Should administration of the spinal anesthetic prove difficult and excessive time be required, an FHR monitor should be available so that the well-being of the fetus is ensured. <br><br> After injection, the patient is placed supine with left uterine displacement. <br><br> Blood pressure is monitored every 30 seconds for the first few minutes and then every 2 or 3 minutes. <br><br> Blood pressure should be maintained near baseline with intravenous fluid infusion and 5-mg boluses of ephedrine. |

Data from Bader AM, Datta S: Anesthesia for Obstetrics. In Tinker JH, Rogers MC, Covino BG, (eds): Principles and Practice of Anesthesiology. St. Louis, Mosby–Year Book, 1993, pp 2065–2103.

tus, nausea, and potential difficulty with micturition (Auroy, 1997). The drugs usually chosen include bupivacaine or ropivacaine and low doses of fentanyl. Other agents can be chosen and are well described in other more detailed sources (Bader, 1993; Brownridge, 1988). Mild disadvantages of the epidural technique include the need for the patient to be relatively quiet during the placement of the catheter, and the potential for delayed onset of motor block after prolonged infusion of these agents, together with an instance of failed or patchy block.

Intrathecal (spinal) analgesia, using only narcotics, is also a choice. In some instances, it is used in conjunction with epidural analgesia (Nageotte, 1997). The advantages of intrathecal introduction of narcotic before using a mixture of local anesthetic and narcotic for epidural analgesia, include quick onset of pain relief and absence of motor block. The disadvan-

Table 26-3  Continuous Infusion Protocols for Epidural Analgesia

|  | Plain Bupivacaine | Bupivacaine-Fentanyl | Bupivacaine-Butorphanol | Bupivacaine-Sufentanil | Ropivacaine-Fentanyl |
|---|---|---|---|---|---|
| **LOADING DOSE** | | | | | |
| Bupivacaine | 0.25–0.5% | 0.125–0.25% | 0.125–0.25% | 0.0625–0.125% | 0.1% |
| Narcotic | None | Fentanyl 2.5–5 µg/ml | Butorphanol 0.2 mg/ml | Sufentanil 1–2 µg/ml | Fentanyl 2.5–5 µg/ml |
| Volume | 10–15 ml | 10 ml | 10 ml | 10 ml | 10 ml |
| **INFUSION** | | | | | |
| Bupivacaine | 0.125–0.25% | 0.0625–0.125% | 0.0625–0.125% | 0.031–0.125% | 0.1% |
| Narcotic | None | Fentanyl 2 µg/ml | Butorphanol 0.1 mg/ml | Sufentanil 0.2/0.3 µg/ml | Fentanyl 2 µg/ml |
| Rate | 10–20 ml/hr | 8–12 ml/hr | 8–12 ml/hr | 6–10 ml/hr | 6–10 ml/hr |

From Naulty JS: Continuous infusions of local anesthetics and narcotics for epidural anesthesia in the management of labor. Int Anesthesiol Clin 28:17, 1990.

tages of intrathecal introduction of drugs include possible postdural puncture headache, hypotension, a higher incidence of pruritus and nausea if narcotics are used without leaving an epidural catheter in place, and less flexibility in the timing of the delivery, because this is a one-shot technique. It has also been suggested that fetal bradycardia may be induced with the use of intrathecal sufentanil. The so-called "walking epidural," which is either an intrathecal narcotic or an ultralow dose of local anesthetic for epidural analgesia, does not produce motor block; therefore; the mother can ambulate. The use of combined spinal and epidural anesthesia has increased the popularity of this option by replacing the one-shot technique with a more flexible approach.

The choice of labor analgesia technique depends on the interaction and preferences of the patient, the obstetrician, and the anesthesiologist. Dosages of drugs for analgesia and combinations of drugs for analgetic effect need to be tailored to the stage of labor and the patient's coexisting medical conditions. No single technique is appropriate for all patients.

In summary, epidural analgesia is the most commonly chosen technique for pain relief during an uncomplicated vaginal delivery. Concern exists about the potential effects of epidural anesthesia on the course of labor. Epidural anesthesia is usually requested only after labor is well established. The overall effect on the first stage of labor is minimal with use of combinations of epidural narcotics and dilute concentrations of local anesthetics. The second stage of labor, from full dilatation to delivery, has been shown to be slightly prolonged by use of regional anesthesia. However, the incidence of instrumental delivery can be minimized by use of lower concentrations of local anesthetics and narcotics in combination with effective coaching. Addition of narcotics to local anesthetics allows more dilute concentrations of the latter drugs. The results are lower systemic levels of drugs and lower incidence of motor block together with fewer complications and a more rapid labor.

Episiotomy and retained placenta may complicate a normal delivery. Local infiltration with lidocaine is usually sufficient for episiotomy repair. Manual removal of retained products of conception and curettage can frequently be accomplished with use of IV sedation. The choice of anesthetic technique in this situation is dependent on several factors: the patient's volume status; whether a regional anesthetic was used during the delivery; whether the patient has an infection; and the choice made by the obstetrician, the anesthesiologist, and the patient. Inhalational agents cause uterine relaxation; therefore, bleeding may become a problem with prolonged use of these agents.

## ANESTHESIA FOR POSTPARTUM TUBAL LIGATION

Postpartum tubal ligation (PPTL) can be performed under spinal, epidural, or general anesthesia. There is controversy concerning the optimal timing of PPTL. Immediate performance of PPTL is commonly elected if an epidural anesthetic has been used for labor. The potential difficulty of obtaining informed consent from an anesthetized patient is an ethical issue that must be addressed on an individual basis.

In the past, waiting 24 to 48 hours after delivery for a planned PPTL under general anesthesia was usual. This is no longer considered crucial. The most significant problem in deciding how long to wait before PPTL is performed relates to the ethics of obtaining informed consent, particularly if the patient received sedation or narcosis during labor.

## ANESTHESIA FOR CERCLAGE

The goal of anesthesia for cerclage is to minimize exposure of the fetus to pharmacologic agents. This can usually be accomplished by block techniques, but cerclage can also be performed under general anesthesia.

# Management of Complicated Cases

Several coexisting medical conditions can potentially create a high-risk situation for parturient and the fetus (Norris, 1993). These include hypertensive disorders of pregnancy, diabetes mellitus, heart disease, certain neuromuscular diseases, coexisting infectious diseases (including human immunodeficiency virus [HIV]), drug abuse, morbid obesity, and potential embolism and stroke. Each of these conditions will be discussed in more detail in other parts of this text; we will comment briefly in this section on the anesthesiologist's concerns for management of delivery in these particular patients.

## MEDICAL COMPLICATIONS OF PREGNANCY AND LABOR

### Hypertension and Eclampsia

Pregnancy-induced hypertension occurs in about 3 to 7% of parturients and is a major cause of maternal morbidity and mortality (see Chapter 37). Specific anesthetic issues include the presence of generalized edema which may involve the airway, causing unexpected difficulties. Assessment of the patient's volume status is extremely important because the patient may have peripheral edema but intravascular volume status may be reduced; therefore, the patient may react to potential drug-induced drops in blood pressure. Such a patient is also sensitive to catecholamines.

Epidural analgesia is the preferred technique if it is feasible because it provides adequate pain relief, and if urgent cesarean section is required, it can be used as an anesthetic method of choice. Regional anesthesia may be contraindicated by coagulopathy, which is a frequent complication of pre-eclampsia and eclampsia. The patient's platelet counts must be checked and surveillance must be maintained to detect other features of the HELLP syndrome (hemolysis, elevated liver enzymes, and a low platelet count).

It is important to optimize the patient's condition medically before administering an epidural anesthetic. Blood pressure should be controlled with such antihypertensive agents as hydralazine or labetalol. Magnesium sulfate should be administered. Prehydration may be needed if the patient is intravascularly depleted, and the presence of a central venous line or a pulmonary artery catheter may be required for adequate monitoring. The use of thromboelastography to monitor clotting function may be advisable.

### Diabetes Mellitus

Morbidity and mortality are increased in the diabetic parturient and fetus. Hectic blood glucose levels may occur during labor and can be exacerbated by general anesthesia. Frequent blood glucose estimations and management with insulin infusion may be necessary. During labor and delivery, maintaining blood glucose levels at or below 120 mg/dl for prevention of neonatal hypoglycemia is an important goal while the patient is anesthetized.

Uteroplacental blood flow has been shown to be compromised, even in cases of mild gestational diabetes, and close attention to monitoring of the fetal heart rate and alertness to fetal distress after any anesthetic intervention is mandatory.

### Heart Disease

The choice of technique for administering analgesia to the pregnant patient who has heart disease must be tailored to the pathophysiology of the specific lesion. The most common acquired cardiac lesion that manifests during pregnancy is mitral stenosis, often secondary to rheumatic heart disease. The increase in cardiac output during labor and delivery is reduced by lumbar epidural analgesia, and this is the technique of choice for labor analgesia in these patients. Mitral value prolapse occurs in 5 to 10% of childbearing women. The great majority of these patients are asymptomatic and require no special consideration other than antibiotic prophylaxis.

Aortic stenosis, when present, may contraindicate any intervention that would lower peripheral vascular resistance and further compromise diastolic coronary blood flow. Thus, regional anesthesia techniques may be relatively contraindicated. Other techniques may be required for other cardiac disease states. A well-conducted regional anesthetic is appropriate for many of these patients because it reduces the catecholamine release that occurs in labor.

### Neuromuscular Disease

Patients who have multiple sclerosis, myasthenia gravis, paraplegia, or lumbar disk disease who desire vaginal delivery should no longer be denied neuraxial anesthesia, if this is indicated. A documented neurologic exam should be performed immediately before placement of an epidural catheter or spinal anesthetic and the patient should be observed for any changes after the anesthetic wears off, but the use of these techniques is not absolutely contraindicated by these diseases.

Patients who have intracranial disease, including

cranial arterial aneurysms, arteriovenous malformations (AVMs), and increased intracranial pressure with brain tumors or benign intracranial hypertension (pseudotumor cerebri) may also require anesthesia for delivery (Kittner, 1996). Aneurysms and AVMs respond well to the use of neuraxial anesthesia, which may be relatively contraindicated in the presence of increased intracranial pressure. A well-conducted regional anesthetic in conjunction with forceps delivery and absence of pushing, or institution of Valsalva maneuvers, may be useful in managing patients who have cranial aneurysms. It is important to prevent rises in blood pressure in these patients.

## Human Immunodeficiency Virus (HIV) Infections

A substantial proportion of perinatally acquired infections in patients who have HIV occur at or near delivery, suggesting that obstetric factors may have an important influence on transmission of the virus from mother to infant (see Chapter 40). Although obstetricians have the major responsibility for managing these patients, it is mandatory that the anesthesia team be well informed about the situation (Bryson, 1995; Landesman, 1996; McIntosh, 1995). This is a situation in which a variety of factors may increase the risk of transmission of HIV from mother to infant (O'Brien, 1998; Schreiber, 1996). Reducing this risk is a responsibility of the team managing the labor.

## Obesity

The obese parturient carries an increased risk for prolonged labor, a higher rate of maternal complications—including hypertension, pre-eclampsia, and diabetes—and a high cesarean delivery rate (Wolfe, 1998). Weight greater than 90 kg complicates approximately 6 to 10% of pregnancies and occurs more commonly in older women of higher parity.

With use of regional anesthesia, landmarks may be difficult to palpate, and in the obese patient, the gravid uterus and abdominal fat pad both contribute to caval compression. Hypotension is a likely complication of poor positioning. If general anesthesia is contemplated, the situation may become complex because of difficult intubation, high rate of pulmonary aspiration of gastric contents, rapid onset of hypoxia associated with a decreased functional residual capacity, and somewhat unpredictable drug dose requirements. (Cnattingius, 1998). The use of continuous spinal anesthetics for labor in the morbidly obese is a possible means of management. A continuous spinal anesthetic provides very reliable control of pain. Because obese patients have an increased incidence of coexisting diseases and a high rate of cesarean sections, the reliability of this technique may be very useful.

## Asthma

Asthma occurs uncommonly during labor and delivery; however, when treatment is required, one must bear in mind the potential effects of bronchodilator agents on uterine tone. Epidural analgesia is useful and has been shown to improve pulmonary function. Oxytocin infusions may be needed to maintain labor in the face of sympathomimetic drug use. Prostaglandin $F_2$ can cause bronchoconstriction in the asthmatic patient; prostaglandins $E_2$ or $E_1$ may be safe to use. (See Chapter 36.)

## Embolism

Venous thromboembolism is five times more common in pregnant women than in nonpregnant woman of similar age. Venous thromboembolism occurs in 1 of 1000 to 2000 pregnancies (Toglia, 1996). The risk of venous thrombosis is greatest during the third trimester and immediately postpartum. The presence of factor V deficiencies carries a sevenfold increased risk of venous thromboembolism. If venous thromboembolism precedes labor and delivery, anticoagulant therapy may have been commenced. It is usual to instruct patients to discontinue heparin at the start of regular uterine contractions, although subcutaneous doses may be continued throughout labor. The decision for use of regional anesthesia must be made on an individual basis because there is a small but definite risk of spinal hematoma. It has been shown that blood loss at the time of cesarean section is not markedly increased. Protamine can be used if coagulation status is monitored carefully. Pregnancy is recognized as initiating a hypercoagulable state that encompasses a period of 10 to 11 months. The amount of heparin required may be greater than previously recognized. Low molecular weight heparin shows promise for the future.

Amniotic fluid embolism is rare but is associated with a very high rate of morbidity and mortality. The true incidence of amniotic fluid embolism has been hard to determine because making an exact diagnosis may be difficult. If peripartum pulmonary embolus is associated with profoundly disseminated intravascular coagulation and cardiovascular collapse, the patient should be managed supportively and a presumptive diagnosis of amniotic fluid embolism made.

## Liver Disease in Pregnancy

Liver disease is uncommon in pregnancy but may have profound effects. The liver diseases of late preg-

**Table 26–4** Antepartum Hemorrhage—Causes

|  | Placenta Previa | Abruptio Placentae | Uterine Rupture |
|---|---|---|---|
| Incidence | 0.1–1.0% | 0.2–2.4% | 0.08–0.1% |
| Presenting symptoms | Painless vaginal bleeding | Painful vaginal bleeding; abnormalities in FHR; irritable uterus | Pain with or without vaginal bleeding; abnormalities in FHR; irritable uterus |
| Predisposing condition | Previous pregnancy with placenta previa | Hypertension, uterine abnormalities, history of cocaine abuse | Previous uterine surgery, prolonged intrauterine manipulation |
| Associated complications | Potential for massive blood loss | Potential for massive blood loss; blood loss may be concealed; DIC; renal failure | Potential for massive blood loss |

DIC = Drug Information Center; FHR = fetal heart rate.
Data from Badter AM, Datta S: Anesthesia for Obstetrics. In Tinker JH, Rogers MC, Covino BG (eds): Principles and Practice of Anesthesiology. St. Louis, Mosby–Year Book, 1993, pp 2065–2103.

nancy include acute fatty liver, pre-eclampsia or eclampsia with hepatic involvement, and the HELLP syndrome associated with pre-eclampsia. About 50% of patients who have acute fatty liver of pregnancy (AFLP) also have evidence of pre-eclampsia or eclampsia and may have laboratory test results characteristic of the HELLP syndrome. Differential diagnosis is based on full analysis of test results and liver biopsy (Knox, 1996). However, liver biopsy is unnecessary to confirm a classic presentation of AFLP or to distinguish it from AFLP with severe pre-eclampsia, because both conditions require the same management, supportive care, and rapid delivery. The use of regional anesthesia in these patients is dependent on their clotting status.

## RISKS OF TRANSFUSION

Transfusion is an indispensable part of medical therapy and may be required during the peripartum period. Postpartum hemorrhage is the condition most likely to necessitate transfusion at or near the time of delivery. However, antepartum hemorrhage (Table 26–4) may also occur and can lead to fetal compromise or death and predispose to postpartum hemorrhage. To date, serious risks from blood components given to patients are smaller than those from underlying disease (Holland, 1996; Sloand, 1995). More than 80% of the blood supply in the United States comes from volunteer donors who make multiple donations. The risk of transmission of viral disease by transfusion is calculated to be 1 in 641,000 for human T-cell lymphotropic virus (HTLV), 1 in 103,000 for hepatitis C virus (HCV), and 1 in 63,000 for hepatitis B virus (HBV). The risk of infection with HIV, the danger of greatest concern to transfusion recipients, has been estimated between 1 in 450,000 and 1 in 660,000. The aggregate risk of transmission of any of these viruses is 1 per 34,000 units of blood administered and is remarkably low when one recalls that not many years ago the risk of HCV infection alone was 1 per 200 units administered (Conry-Cantilena, 1996). One would conclude that the risk of transmitting HIV, HCV, HBV, or HTLV by the transfusion of screened blood is currently very small (Etchason, 1995; Rutherford, 1995).

## DRUG ABUSE

There is in the United States an epidemic use of cocaine. Polydrug abuse, which involves abuse of, and dependence on, cocaine as well as alcohol, opiates, and nicotine, appears to be increasing in subgroups of the population, including minority women of childbearing age. One prevalent pattern is the concurrent use of cocaine and heroin. In 1993 and 1994, abusers of intravenous (IV) cocaine and heroin accounted for a major new group of persons with HIV infection in several large metropolitan areas in the United States. In 1992, 4.5 million Americans used cocaine, with 1.3 million reporting cocaine use at least monthly. Concurrent cigarette smoking and cocaine use may also have serious adverse effects on cardiac function.

Effective medication for the treatment of cocaine overdose and addiction is a major unmet need (Leshner, 1996). In contrast to heroin, for which there are effective medications to treat overdose (naloxone) and addiction (methadone), there are no pharmacologic treatments for any aspect of cocaine addiction (Mendelson, 1996). The molecular mechanism underlying cocaine addiction appears to be related to its effects on the dopamine-reuptake transporter and the level of dopamine in synapses centrally. Cocaine binds strongly to the dopamine-reuptake transporter and blocks reuptake after normal neuronal activity. Dopamine remains at high concentrations in the synapse and continues to affect adjacent neurons. Knockout mice, who lack the gene encoding the dopamine transporter, did not respond to cocaine biochemically or behaviorally. There are multiple dopamine receptors, and it is suggested that the $D_1$ dopamine receptor system is a potential target for medications to treat cocaine addiction. However, at present, no drug therapy is uniquely effective in treating cocaine abuse and dependence. Cocaine-dependent persons who take the drug by inhalation often have major psychosocial, cognitive, and legal problems. The most seriously ill are those who use the drug intravenously. Use of cocaine in pregnancy is associated with abruptio placentae and decreased birth weight, but it fails to shorten labor, contrary to a popular myth among users (Dombrowski,1991). From an anesthetic viewpoint, the risk of its use in proximity to anesthesia lies in interactions with other drugs, particularly sympathomimetics.

# Obstetric Complications

The indications for surgical delivery, placental removal, and hysterectomy to control bleeding are well outlined elsewhere in this text. The anesthesia concerns are discussed here.

## ELECTIVE CESAREAN SECTION

Elective cesarean section can be managed using any of the three major forms of anesthesia: general, spinal, or epidural (Table 26–5). Most anesthesiologists and patients prefer regional anesthetics for cesarean section so that the mother can be alert and able to participate in the delivery as well as recognize and bond with her infant. There may be reduced risk of complications if endotracheal intubation and general anesthesia can be avoided; however, studies focusing on conclusive outcome are lacking.

The major concern if spinal anesthesia is the chosen technique is hypotension. Fluids and pressors can be used to prevent or reverse this problem. It is important to use positioning to avoid caval compression as a cause of hypotension and decreased uteroplacental flow. Spinal anesthesia is optimally administered to achieve a T4 analgetic level. In comparison with epidural anesthesia, spinal anesthesia has the advantages of ease in technique, dense quality of block, and increased reliability. Local anesthetics (Table 26–6) can be supplemented with narcotics (e.g., fentanyl) for short-term potentiation of the block. Intrathecal morphine can be introduced for prolonged postpartum pain relief.

Epidural anesthesia can also be used, with the advantages that the block is established more slowly and there is a decreased risk of hypotension. Epidural anesthesia or analgesia can be continued for pain management into the postpartum period.

## EMERGENCY CESAREAN SECTION

Traditionally, emergency cesarean sections were performed using general anesthesia and a rapid-sequence intubation technique. Surgery would not begin until anesthesia was established and a secure airway obtained. IV medications were normally not given for induction until the surgeon was ready, with the abdomen prepared to minimize the effects of these agents on the fetus. The goal was to provide the shortest induction-to-delivery interval.

If the patient receives epidural analgesia during labor, it can be dosed with quick-acting agents, such as 3% 2-chloroprocaine, or 2% bicarbonated lidocaine which establish anesthesia between 5 and 10 minutes (McMahon, 1996). At all times one should be prepared to move ahead with rapid general anesthesia and endotracheal intubation if this becomes necessary because of the conditions encountered or because of a failed block. Rapid single-shot spinal anesthesia may also be used for less urgent situations.

## EMERGENCY UTERINE RELAXATION

Retained placenta, uterine inversion, and head in breech position may necessitate administration of anesthesia for surgical management and uterine relaxation. General, spinal, or epidural anesthesia may be used. Uterine relaxation can be accomplished with IV nitroglycerin (50-μg bolus or 0.5 μg/kg per min), a uterine smooth muscle relaxant; in the past, amylnitrite was inhaled for this purpose. Volatile anesthetic agents, such as halothane or isoflurane, can produce marked uterine relaxation. Preparation must be made to control potential uterine bleeding, and oxytocin and ergot alkaloids may be required.

Table 26–5 Local Anesthetics for Epidural Anesthesia for Cesarean Section

| | 3% 2-Chloroprocaine | 2% Lidocaine With Epinephrine |
|---|---|---|
| Dose | 15–25 ml | 15–25 ml |
| Onset of action | 3–5 min | 5–15 min |
| Duration of action | 40–50 min | 60–75 min |

Table 26-6  Local Anesthetic for Subarachnoid Block for Cesarean Section

| Dose According to Height (cm) | Lidocaine 5% in 7.5% Dextrose (mg) | Tetracaine 1% in Equal Volume of 10% Dextrose (mg) | Bupivacaine 0.75% in 8.25% Dextrose (mg) | Ropivacaine 0.75% in 8.25% Dextrose (mg) |
|---|---|---|---|---|
| 150–160 | 70 | 8 | 8 | 8 |
| 160–182 | 75 | 9 | 10 | 10 |
| 182 and taller | 85 | 10 | 12 | 12 |
| Onset (min) | 1–3 | 3–5 | 2–4 | 5–20 |
| Duration (min) | 45–75 | 120–180 | 120–180 | 120–240 |

Data from Bader AM, Datta S: Anesthesia for Obstetrics. *In* Tinker JH, Rogers MC, Covino BG (eds): Principles and Practice of Anesthesiology. St. Louis, Mosby–Year Book, 1993, pp 2065–2103.

## RUPTURED UTERUS AND HYSTERECTOMY

The major problem for the anesthesia team when uterine rupture or hysterectomy is indicated is resuscitation from hypovolemia caused by blood loss. Massive transfusion may be needed. General anesthesia is usually preferred for these types of surgery, and induction of general anesthesia may be necessary, even if regional anesthesia was the primary anesthetic for the preceding delivery.

## Fetal Resuscitation—The Anesthesiologist's Role

Resuscitation of the baby begins with fetal monitoring and in utero maneuvers. Left uterine displacement to avoid caval compression, appropriate oxygenation of the mother, and maintenance of maternal blood pressure may improve placental flow in utero and contribute to improved neonatal status immediately after delivery.

Once the baby is delivered and the anesthesia team have discharged their primary responsibility for care of the mother in a safe way, members of the team may assist in neonatal resuscitation. Teams for neonatal resuscitation are constructed in various ways, depending on the institution in which the delivery takes place. If there is more than one anesthesia provider, they are not infrequently called on to take responsibility for portions of fetal resuscitation. Familiarity with algorithms for care of the neonate is mandatory, and these should receive close attention from the obstetric anesthesiologist.

## Summary

Pregnancy, labor, and delivery are associated with physiologic changes involving many organ systems. These changes require specific considerations for anesthesia care. Anesthesia drug dose requirements may be changed during pregnancy. Up to 25% less local regional anesthetic may be required than is needed for a comparable nonpregnant patient. Inhalation agents may also be effective at lower doses. It must be borne in mind that drugs enter the fetal circulation and that the fetus is exposed to many of the drugs that are given to the mother. Narcotics remain the most commonly used agents, with meperidine as the narcotic most frequently used for maternal pain relief. Maternally administered narcotics may produce neonatal depression related to the total dose and to the time interval between administration and delivery. Maximal depression occurs within 1 to 3 hours after intramuscular injection.

Neuraxial techniques are now preferred for labor analgesia and elective cesarean sections because they avoid the sedative effects of systemic medications, give excellent pain relief, and usually provide excellent conditions for the fetus as well. If general anesthesia is used for cesarean section, the time from induction to delivery of the infant should be minimized because of the potential effects of inhaled anesthetic agents on the neonate.

The anesthesiology team must be fully versed in managing potential complications and coexisting diseases that may occur in association with pregnancy. They must also be prepared to deal with resuscitation if it should be required for the mother, the newborn infant, or both.

## ACKNOWLEDGMENTS

*The authors wish to acknowledge discussion and review by Dr. A. Betel and Dr. M. Dombrowski.*

## REFERENCES

Auroy Y, Narchi P, Messiah A, et al: Serious complications related to regional anesthesia. Anesthesiology 87:479–486, 1997.

Bader AM, Datta S: Anesthesia for Obstetrics. In Tinker JH, Rogers MC, Covino BG, (eds): Principles and Practice of Anesthesiology, 2nd ed. St Louis, Mosby–Year Book, 1993, 2065–2103.

Birnbach DJ: Analgesia for Labor. N Engl J Med 337:1764–1766, 1997.

Brownridge P, Cohen SE: Neural blockade for obstetrics and gynecologic surgery. In: Cousins MJ, Bridenbaugh PO (eds): Neural Blockade in Clinical Anesthesia and Management of Pain, Philadelphia, JB Lippincott, 1998, pp 593–634.

Bryson YJ, Pang S, Wei LS, et al: Clearance of HIV infection in a perinatally infected patient. N Engl J Med 332:833–838, 1995.

Chestnut DH: Epidural analgesia and the incidence of cesarean section: Time for another close look—editorial. Anesthesiology 87:472–476, 1997.

Choi A, Laurito CE, Cunningham FE: Pharmacologic management of postdural puncture headache. Ann Pharmacother 30:830–831, 1996.

Cnattingius S, Bergstrom R, Lipworth L, et al: Prepregnancy weight and the risk of adverse pregnancy outcomes. N Engl J Med 338:147–152, 1998.

Conry-Cantilena C, VanRaden M, Gibble J, et al: Routes of infection viremia, and liver disease in blood donors found to have hepatitis C virus infection. N Engl J Med 334:1691–1696, 1996.

Dombrowski MP, Wolfe HM, Welch RA, et al: Cocaine abuse is associated with abruptio placentae and decreased birth weight, but not shorter labor. Obstet Gynecol 77:139–141, 1991.

Eisenach JC: Regional anesthesia: Vintage Bordeaux (and Napa Valley). Anesthesiology 87:467–469, 1997.

Etchason J, Petz L, Keeler E, et al: The cost-effectiveness of preoperative autologous blood donations. N Engl J Med 332:719–724, 1995.

Holland PV: Viral infections and the blood supply. N Engl J Med 334:1734, 1735, 1996.

Hood DD, Dewan DM: Obstetric anesthesia. *In* Brown DL: Risk and Outcome in Anesthesia. Philadelphia, JB Lippincott, 1992, pp 310–362.

Iams J: Prevention of preterm birth—editorial. N Engl J Med 338:54–56, 1998.

Kittner SJ, Sloan BJ, Feeser BR, et al: Pregnancy and the risk of stroke. N Engl J Med 335:768–774, 1996.

Knox TA, Olans LB: Liver disease in pregnancy. N Engl J Med 335:569–576, 1996.

Landesman SH, Kalish LA, Burns DN: Obstetrical factors and the transmission of human immunodeficiency virus type 1 from mother to child. N Engl J Med 334:1617–1623, 1996.

Leshner AI: Molecular mechanisms of cocaine addiction. N Engl J Med 335:128–129, 1996.

Lieberman E: Low birth-weight—not a black and white issue. N Engl J Med 332:117, 118, 1995.

McIntosh K, Burchett SK: Clearance of HIV—lessons from newborns. N Engl J Med 332:883–884.

McMahon MJ, Luther ER, Bowes WA, et al: Comparison of a trial of labor with an elective second cesarean section. N Engl J Med 335:689–695, 1996.

Mendelson JH, Mello NK: Management of cocaine abuse and dependence. N Engl J Med 334:965–972, 1996.

Nageotte MP, Larson D, Rumney PJ, et al: Epidural analgesia compared with combined spinal-epidural analgesia during labor in nulliparous women. N Engl Med 337:1715–1719, 1997.

Norris MC: Obstetric Anesthesia. Philadelphia, JB Lippincott Company, 1993.

O'Brien TR, Goedert JJ: Chemokine receptors and genetic variability—another leap in HIV research. JAMA 279:317, 318, 1998.

Rawlings JS, Rawlings VB, Read JA: Prevalence of low birth-weight and preterm delivery in relation to the interval between pregnancies among white and black women. N Engl J Med 332:69–74, 1995.

Rutherford CJ, Kaplan HS: Autologous blood donation—can we bank on it?—editorial. N Engl J Med 332:740–742, 1995.

Schreiber GB, Busch MP, Kleinman SH. The risk of transfusion-transmitted viral infections. The retrovirus. Epidemiology Donor Study. N Engl J Med 334:1685–1690, 1996.

Sharma S, Sidawi JE, Ramin SM, et al: A randomized trial of epidural versus patient-controlled meperidine analgesia during labor. Anesthesiology 87:487–494, 1997.

Sloand EM, Pitt E, Klein HG: Safety of the blood supply. JAMA 274:1368–1372, 1995.

Thorp JA, Hu DH, Albin RM, et al: The effect of intrapartum epidural analgesia on nulliparous labor: A randomized, controlled, prospective trial. Am J Obstet Gynecol 169:851–585, 1993.

Toglia MR, Weg JR: Venous thromboembolism during pregnancy. N Engl J Med 335:108–114, 1996.

Wolfe H: High prepregnancy body-mass index—A maternal-fetal risk factor—editorial. N Engl J Med 338:191, 192, 1998.

# 27

# Vaginal Delivery, Operative and Breech

KAROLINE S. PUDER
MITCHELL P. DOMBROWSKI

Pregnancy concludes with a vaginal delivery in the majority of women. At term, 95% of fetuses are in the vertex presentation. During a normal vaginal delivery, the fetus undergoes the cardinal movements of labor, which are engagement, descent, flexion, internal rotation, extension, external rotation, and expulsion. Although listed as a sequence, they may occur throughout labor and some may occur simultaneously. The cardinal movements are the result of uterine and voluntary maternal expulsive forces, whereas the fetus is essentially passive. The movements allow an irregularly shaped fetus to successfully negotiate an irregularly shaped pelvis with the least amount of difficulty.

Engagement occurs when the largest diameter of the fetal head descends below the pelvic inlet. This may occur during the first or second stage of labor but is frequently completed before the onset of labor in nulliparous women. Descent of the fetus occurs mainly during the end of the first stage of labor and throughout the second stage. The remaining steps happen in concert with the descent. Flexion of the fetal head allows the smallest possible head diameter to traverse the pelvis. The fetal head may be flexed before the onset of labor, but complete flexion, resulting in the fetal chin resting on the chest, occurs during labor. Internal rotation takes place when the fetal head turns, usually from the transverse position to the anteroposterior orientation. In general, this brings the fetal occiput from the transverse position to an occipitoanterior position under the symphysis pubis although sometimes the rotation is to the occipitoposterior position. Again, this allows the fetus to pass through the bony pelvis most effectively. Extension of the fetal head proceeds once the fetus is crowning. At this point, the fetal occiput pivots under the pubic symphysis as the birth canal turns anteriorly. The fetal head is delivered over the perineum by extension. After the head is delivered, the shoulders of the fetus are in the anteroposterior diameter of the pelvis and, therefore, the fetal head returns, or restitutes, to its natural position before internal rotation. Further rotation of the head to a transverse position occurs as external rotation. The fetal shoulders then follow a mechanism similar to that of the head, with the anterior shoulder rotating under the symphysis, after which expulsion of the remainder of the fetus usually happens rapidly.

## Normal Vaginal Delivery

Vaginal delivery is commonly assisted by a birth attendant. The purpose of an assisted delivery is to prevent uncontrolled expulsion of the fetus, limit maternal and neonatal trauma, and provide support to the neonate.

## PREPARATION

Although it is common for women to deliver in the dorsal lithotomy position, there are many positions in which delivery may be accomplished with the assistance of an attendant. For example, the parturient may lie on her side, squat, be on all fours, or be sitting upright. There are also options for using the delivery bed or table that can be individualized to meet the needs of each mother and her fetus. Therefore, the foot of the bed can remain in place, be lowered, or be removed. Similarly, the use of stirrups or foot rests is not mandatory, and their use varies by situation. Presurgical preparation of the perineum need not be done. If foreign matter or stool needs to be removed, cleansing with tap water and soap is adequate. Repeated povidone-iodine washing and perineal shaving are not indicated. Draping the patient may be done to maintain a clean area, but a vaginal delivery is always considered a contaminated procedure.

It is important to consider the needs of each patient and her fetus when preparing for delivery. Patient preferences and desires should be taken into account, but it is the attendants' responsibility to ensure the health of both patients. Therefore, the course of the labor, potential complications, parity, estimated fetal weight, and medical history should be considered carefully in addition to psychological and social factors. The role of the accoucheur is to improve the conduct of an otherwise natural process to achieve the best outcome.

## PROCEDURES

Episiotomy is the surgical incision of the perineum that is performed to enlarge the vaginal outlet at delivery. The most common indications for an episiotomy are to prevent perineal lacerations and to shorten the second stage of labor. The incision is usually made with straight Mayo scissors, although a scalpel may be used. It is commonly performed when the head is distending the perineum and separating the labia. The head (or other presenting part) should be protected by the operator's fingers to prevent fetal trauma. For a median episiotomy, the incision is made in the midline of the perineum for about one half its length. The incision is then extended for several centimeters along the vaginal mucosa, carefully avoiding the rectum posteriorly. A mediolateral episiotomy may also be performed, with an incision that begins at the posterior fourchette and extends at a 45-degree angle from the midline. The length of the incision is determined by the amount of room needed and is not limited by the length of the perineum.

Delivery of the fetal head occurs by extension, as described previously. As the mother pushes with each contraction, it is the role of the accoucheur to control and assist the delivery. Gentle counterpressure is often applied to the head to allow the perineal tissues to stretch and to limit lacerations. Delivery of the fetal head may also be assisted by the use of the modified Ritgen maneuver, in which the fetal chin is first identified through the perineum; then a towel-covered hand is used to grasp and lift the chin, thereby causing extension. After delivery of the head, the nares and oropharynx are cleared of mucus with a bulb syringe. If meconium-stained amniotic fluid is present, more thorough suctioning should be performed with a DeLee suction device to decrease the risk of meconium aspiration syndrome. Next, a finger may be slid along the neonate's neck to check for the presence of a loop of cord. If a loose loop of cord is found, it should be slipped over the head, but if the cord is wrapped too tightly to be reduced, it should be doubly clamped and then divided between the clamps.

Restitution and external rotation should occur while the suctioning and cord check are being performed. To deliver the shoulders, the assistant should place both hands on the parietal bones with the fingertips towards the neonate's mouth. With a maternal push, gentle downward pressure should be exerted to deliver the anterior shoulder. Once the anterior shoulder has cleared the pubic symphysis and appeared at the introitus, the gentle pressure should be directed upward to deliver the posterior shoulder over the perineum. At this point, the remainder of the infant's body should be delivered easily by uterine and maternal forces. One hand of the attendant should support the infant's head and the other its body. The neonate may be held by the attendant or placed on the mother's abdomen to be dried, suctioned, and have the cord doubly clamped and cut between the clamps. A segment of cord from the placental side may be clamped and divided to use for blood gas determination.

The process is completed by checking the cervix, the vagina, and the perineum for lacerations or episiotomy extensions and repairing them, and by delivering the placenta. Delivery of the placenta is most commonly managed by early clamping of the cord and controlled gentle traction on the umbilical cord once signs of placental separation have occurred; however, given time, the placenta delivers on its own by uterine force. Signs of placental separation include a gush of blood from the uterus, lengthening of the cord, and the movement of the uterus, which feels globular, up into the abdomen. While gentle traction is placed on the umbilical cord, the operator's other hand is used to maintain suprapubic pressure, which prevents uterine inversion. After the placenta is delivered, the fundus should be massaged to promote uterine contraction and limit postpartum blood loss. Uterotonic agents, such as oxytocin, are typically used to ensure that the uterus contracts well and that bleeding is minimized.

## Shoulder Dystocia

### DEFINITION

Shoulder dystocia occurs when there is a disproportion between the bisacromial diameter of the fetus and the anteroposterior diameter of the maternal pelvic inlet. The anterior shoulder is lodged behind the pubic symphysis and the posterior shoulder behind the sacral promontory. The diagnosis should be suspected when the delivered fetal head retracts against the perineum (turtle sign) and gentle downward traction fails to deliver the anterior shoulder under the pubic symphysis. Although risk factors for shoulder dystocia have been identified, they are poor predictors when used prospectively (Diani, 1997; Blickstein, 1998; Nocon, 1993). When shoulder dystocia is identified, it is important to assemble the necessary personnel rapidly and be prepared to perform the maneuvers required to relieve this obstruction to limit maternal and neonatal morbidity. Fetal trauma may include brachial plexus injury (Erb's and Klumpke's palsies), fetal acidosis, paralysis of the diaphragm, fracture of the clavicle or humerus, or death. Maternal complications include postpartum hemorrhage, lacerations and hematomas of the vaginal wall, and uterine rupture.

Although most risk factors for shoulder dystocia are associated with fetal macrosomia, only about half of all cases happen in neonates weighing more than 4000 g. These factors include maternal obesity and diabetes, fetal macrosomia, previous delivery of a macrosomic infant, prolonged gestation, multiparity, prolonged deceleration phase, prolonged second stage of labor, and midpelvic delivery (American College of Obstetricians and Gynecologists [ACOG], 1991). Currently, the ACOG notes that it may be reasonable to offer cesarean delivery to patients who have an estimated fetal weight of more than 5000 g or more than 4500 g in the presence of diabetes (ACOG, 1994).

### PROCEDURES

Every member of the delivery team needs to be familiar with the maneuvers to relieve shoulder dystocia. It is especially important that each accoucheur be prepared for this rare emergency and have a plan in mind for management of its occurrence. Different authors have recommended various sequences for the following maneuvers, but it appears that it is the timely and orderly application of a well-learned routine that is most important (Nocon, 1993).

The first step is to call for any assistants who may be needed. These may include two other experienced members of the delivery team as well as personnel from the pediatric and anesthesia departments. As in any other emergency operation, experienced team members, be they physicians, midwives, or nurses, are the key to success. If it has not already been performed, an episiotomy should be done. This helps to relieve any soft tissue component of the dystocia and also allows room for any intravaginal manipulation that may be needed. Pushing the anterior shoulder toward the fetal chest may reduce a mild degree of shoulder dystocia. This facilitates delivery of the anterior shoulder by decreasing the bisacromial diameter and bringing it into an oblique diameter with the maternal pelvis.

If these initial attempts are not successful, the McRoberts maneuvers may be attempted next. This is successful in about 50% of patients (Gherman, 1997). To accomplish this maneuver, the aid of two assistants and the mother's cooperation are required. The mother should flex her hips and knees, which will cause her thighs to rest on her abdomen. This position straightens the lumbosacral angle and rotates the symphysis cephalad, changing the anatomic relationship of the fetus to the pelvis and freeing the impacted shoulder. Gentle traction should be attempted to determine whether this maneuver has been successful.

Suprapubic pressure may also relieve a shoulder dystocia. A knowledgeable assistant should apply pressure correctly. The pressure should not be applied directly downward but on an angle toward the fetal chest, with the intent of rotating the fetal shoulders out of the direct anteroposterior diameter. Fundal pressure should not be exerted because it has been associated with a higher incidence of maternal and neonatal injuries and, perhaps, a worsening of the impaction.

If delivery is not effected using these maneuvers, the Woods screw maneuver may be performed next. The operator should place his or her hand into the vagina and push the posterior shoulder toward the infant's chest. This brings the bisacromial diameter into an oblique diameter of the pelvis, which may allow the anterior shoulder to advance. The pressure may be continued until the posterior shoulder becomes the anterior shoulder, which should have moved past the area of obstruction.

If the Woods screw maneuver fails, delivery of the

posterior arm may be attempted. The operator's hand is placed into the vagina along the infant's thorax. Pressure is applied in the antecubital fossa. As the elbow flexes, the posterior forearm is grasped and delivered, thereby bringing the posterior shoulder past the sacral promontory and allowing the anterior shoulder to slip under the pubic symphysis. If delivery still cannot be completed, the shoulders can be rotated as previously described.

Performance of the above maneuvers may result in a spontaneous fracture of the infant's clavicle or humerus. This usually heals without significant sequelae. Intentional clavicular fracture may be attempted to decrease the bisacromial diameter and allow delivery of the shoulders when the other maneuvers have been unsuccessful. In practice, it is difficult to accomplish, however. The Zavanelli maneuver, which involves cephalic replacement and abdominal delivery, may be used as a last resort. Results have been mixed, and the procedure is much more difficult in practice than it is in theory (O'Leary, 1992; Gallaspy, 1991; Graham, 1992). If even this is unsuccessful, emergency symphysiotomy has been described, although lack of experience hinders its usefulness in the United States (Goodwin, 1997). After delivery, the cervix and the vagina should be carefully inspected for lacerations or hematomas and the uterus explored for rupture.

## Forceps Delivery

The proper role of forceps, especially midforceps, in modern obstetrics has been a source of continuing controversy. There has been extensive discussion of indications, associated risk factors, anticipated outcome, and the possibility of brain damage, particularly with the use of midforceps, but such discussion is beyond the scope of this chapter.

### DEFINITIONS

Forceps deliveries are classified by the station at which they are performed and the degree of rotation of the fetal head. In the United States, station is classified as centimeters above and below the ischial spines (from −5 to +5 cm). In 1988, forceps operations were redefined by the ACOG and published in ACOG Committee Opinion #196. These definitions are listed in Table 27–1. Note that there is no classification of high forceps because they are no longer considered appropriate tools in the practice of modern obstetrics. In addition, current recommendations include preparation for cesarean delivery with mid-

**Table 27–1** Forceps Classification

| | |
|---|---|
| Midforceps | 0 or +1 station |
| Low forceps | +2 station or below, rotation of <or>45 degrees |
| Outlet forceps | Head is crowning or on the perineum, <45 degrees from direct occiput anterior or posterior |

forceps in the event that the forceps-assisted procedure is unsuccessful.

Forceps include either classic (standard cephalic and pelvic curves) or special instruments (designed for specific problems, such as Barton forceps for deep transverse arrest in the flat pelvis and Piper forceps for the after-coming head of a breech presentation). Typically, forceps are named after the physician who invented the modification.

### PROCEDURES

At least eight conditions should be met before forceps are used and these are listed in Table 27–2. To accomplish an appropriate forceps application, the blades must be applied precisely over the parietal bones of the fetal head. If an appropriate cephalic application cannot be attained, the forceps procedure should be abandoned. A detailed description of the technique for application of forceps in various situations is beyond the scope of this chapter. It is best learned from experienced operators in the delivery room and from detailed texts devoted to this subject.

### CHOICE OF FORCEPS

For traction to the anterior or posterior occiput, most clinicians prefer to use either Simpson or Elliot forceps. Simpson forceps have a longer cephalic curve than that of Elliot forceps, and are therefore more

**Table 27–2** Conditions for Forceps Application

Uterine cervix must be fully dilated.
The vertex should be presenting. The exception is use of Piper forceps for delivery of the after-coming head in vaginal breech delivery.
The vertex should be engaged. Application of forceps with the vertex above 0 station is no longer considered appropriate in current obstetric practice.
The amniotic membranes should be ruptured.
The position of the vertex should be carefully determined and known with certainty.
There should be no disproportion.
The patient should receive adequate analgesia.
The bladder should be empty.

appropriate for delivery of the nulliparous patient, a situation in which there is likely to be more molding of the fetal head. Elliot forceps tend to be more appropriate for use in the multiparous patient. Traction may be created with the operator's hands alone or with an axis traction handle such as the Bill handle. It is important to exert traction that follows the path of the pelvis, which follows a curve. To create manual axis traction, the handles of the forceps should rest in the upturned palm of the operator's dominant hand while the other hand exerts downward force on the shanks.

For procedures that involve rotation of more than 45 degrees (occiput posterior or occiput transverse to the occiput anterior position), many obstetricians prefer Kielland forceps because they lack a pelvic curve. Classic instruments, such as Simpson forceps, may be used, although their handles require rotation through a large arc to avoid damage to the maternal pelvis by the tips of the forceps blades. For a transverse arrest in a platypoid pelvis, the Barton forceps may be used, although they have fallen out of favor. If Simpson forceps or another classic forceps is used for rotation from the posterior to anterior occiput, it is typically reapplied once the occipitoanterior position has been attained. Traction is then applied for delivery. This combination is termed the Scanzoni maneuver. After rotation with Kielland forceps, many operators replace it with a different instrument for traction and delivery.

Although forceps deliveries are associated with a greater risk of episiotomy, third- and fourth-degree lacerations, vaginal lacerations, and postpartum hemorrhage than spontaneous vaginal delivery (Yancey, 1991; Poen, 1997), the morbidity is considerably lower than that of cesarean delivery (Bashore, 1990). There is, therefore, an associated longer hospital stay for patients delivered by the abdominal route than for patients whose babies are delivered by forceps. There is no increased risk of neonatal morbidity or mortality in infants delivered by low or outlet forceps (Yancey, 1991; Hagadorn-Freathy, 1991; Carmona, 1995). The conclusion regarding midforceps is not as clear in the literature, and it appears that if there is any relationship of midforceps delivery to adverse neurologic outcomes, it is, in fact, very small (Nilsen, 1984; Seidman, 1991; Menticoglou, 1995; Wesley, 1993). Even if the relative risk of an adverse outcome associated with midforceps is relatively high, the absolute risk is probably quite low. A large majority of infants delivered with midforceps can be expected to be normal. The wise accoucheur uses these procedures with careful judgment and patient selection and shows the willingness to abandon the procedure if excessive force is needed. With this in mind, vaginal delivery with midforceps may well be less traumatic and yield a better chance of normal maternal and infant outcome than cesarean delivery.

The new classification of forceps is better able to differentiate procedures that have a minimal risk from those that have an increased risk of morbidity. In studies of the new classification, the risk of vaginal lacerations was greater with midforceps and the use of low forceps and a rotation greater than 45 degrees. Under the new classification, umbilical pH lower than 7.2 (36.5%), and neonatal injury (19.0%) (e.g., facial nerve palsy, brachial plexus palsy, clavicular fracture, or hematoma) were significantly increased among the cohort delivered by midforceps (Hagadorn-Freathy, 1991).

Issues to remember for decreasing the risk to mother, neonate, and accoucheur are as follows:

1. Carefully assess the patient's overall condition, her labor curve, estimated fetal weight, clinical pelvimetry, and fetal position.
2. Review the indications for the procedure and the available options.
3. Be prepared to abandon an attempted operative delivery if forceps cannot be applied properly or if greater force than expected is required.
4. Be prepared to perform a cesarean delivery immediately when performing midforceps procedures (Boyd, 1986; Lowe, 1987; Revah, 1997).

## Vacuum Delivery

Vaginal delivery assisted by the use of vacuum extraction is an operative delivery, and, as such, it is recommended that the conditions necessary for conducting forceps delivery also be met. Both metal and soft-cup devices are used (Kuit, 1992), and suction may be created by either an electric or a hand-held pump. It is important to know the recommended vacuum pressure for the instrument being used to maximize its utility and minimize its adverse effects. With appropriate patient selection and indication, safe vacuum delivery can be performed (Vintzileos, 1996) with the same caution that is used for forceps delivery.

### PROCEDURES

The operator should first evaluate the instrument to be sure that it is in correct working order. The device is then carefully placed in the vagina and positioned in the midline over the fetal occiput. Knowing the position of the fetal head and the correct placement of the cup are not trivial matters, because incorrect placement of the cup may cause deflexion or asynclitism of the fetal head and thereby doom what might otherwise be a successful procedure. Care must be taken to ensure that no maternal vaginal or cervical tissue is caught between the vacuum cup and the vertex. Vacuum force of about 200 mm Hg should be created and the placement of the cup should be rechecked. If it is appropriate, the vacuum should be increased to about 600 mm Hg with a contraction, and then traction should begin in the axis of the pelvis while the mother pushes. The operator's nontraction hand can be used to monitor movement of the fetal head as well as to detect any evidence that the cup is not properly applied. The vacuum should be released between contractions and the same process repeated with each contraction, although continuous vacuum may be used without any increased morbidity (Bofill, 1997; Lim, 1997). As with forceps deliveries, there should be detectable descent with each traction effort. If progress does not occur or if the cup has detached twice, it is prudent to abandon the procedure.

Vacuum delivery has a lower risk of maternal genital tract trauma than forceps delivery, although the risk of vaginal and cervical lacerations still exists. The risk of neonatal trauma is greater, with an increased risk of cephalhematoma, subgaleal hematoma, intracranial hemorrhage, retinal hemorrhage, and neonatal jaundice (Williams, 1991; Williams, 1991; Williams, 1993; Johanson, 1993). Although there has been concern that retinal hemorrhage may correlate with poor neurobehavioral development, there has been no confirmation of that relationship, and the significance of retinal hemorrhage remains unclear.

Based upon the available literature, there appears to be little difference in outcome for patients for whom either forceps or vacuum extraction delivery is indicated (Bofill, 1996; Williams, 1991; Johanson, 1993). Therefore, the decision between these two instruments should be based on the experience and competence of the operator as well as the practice setting.

## Vaginal Breech Delivery

Breech presentation is found in about 3 to 4% of term pregnancies, although the frequency is inversely related to gestational age. By definition, breech presentation is a longitudinal fetal lie, with the fetal buttocks as the main presenting part. There is further classification based upon the position of the legs:
- Frank breech—hips are flexed and knees are extended
- Complete breech—both hips and knees are flexed
- Footling breech—one or both feet or knees appear below the buttocks.

There is an increased risk of adverse outcome associated with breech presentation, regardless of the mode of delivery. This risk is, for the most part, related to the etiology of the presentation, such as prematurity, fetal anomaly, or, possibly, pre-existing neurologic abnormality. Despite the fact that the majority of infants in the breech position are delivered by cesarean section in the United States, this risk has not decreased. Whether to attempt a vaginal breech delivery for a preterm infant remains a controversial decision, and the recommendations are continually changing. It is unclear whether there is any increased risk in attempting vaginal breech delivery in the well-selected term patient, because available studies are all limited by selection bias. Another alternative for management of the breech presentation is external cephalic version. Detailed discussion of this technique, its risks, and its benefits is beyond the scope of this chapter. The evidence suggests that there is a small increase in neonatal morbidity and mortality associated with vaginal breech delivery vs. cesarean section (Koike, 1996), just as there remains an increase in maternal morbidity and mortality with cesarean section vs. vaginal delivery.

Several recommendations for choosing appropriate candidates for vaginal breech delivery have been made. Those suggested by the ACOG are listed in Table 27–3 (ACOG, 1986). Even if the patient is selected appropriately, it is still important to counsel her and obtain her informed consent. Use of oxytocin for labor abnormalities remains controversial, but there does not appear to be any contraindication to administration of epidural anesthesia during labor.

## PROCEDURES

If progress is normal during the first and second stages of labor, the following description outlines a technique that may be used for a vaginal breech delivery. The delivery should occur in a delivery or operative suite, so that, if necessary, abdominal delivery can be performed rapidly without excessive confusion. The support of pediatric specialists should be available in the delivery room, and a second experienced operator should be present to assist in the

**Table 27–3** Criteria for Vaginal Breech Delivery

Facility capable of performing an emergency cesarean delivery
Obstetrician experienced in performing breech deliveries
Available anesthesia support
Frank breech of less than 4000 g estimated fetal weight; Fetal head is not hyperextended or macrocephalic
Adequate pelvis
Adequate progress through the first and second stages of labor

From American College of Obstetricians and Gynecologists: Management of the breech presentation. ACOG Technical Bulletin #95. Washington, DC, ACOG, 1986.

delivery. The patient should be allowed to push with contractions until the umbilicus has reached the introitus. This allows the fetal body to maintain cervical dilatation and avoids head entrapment resulting from a deflexed fetal head. In addition, early traction may increase the risk of nuchal arms. The decision to perform an episiotomy remains with the operator and is based on the usual considerations. Some recommend an episiotomy for all vaginal breech deliveries because the largest part of the fetus, the head, comes last. Once the fetus has delivered to the level of the umbilicus, check to make sure there is no tension on the umbilical cord. Following this, the operator should deliver the fetal legs. The operator should run a finger along the posterior surface of the fetal thigh to the level of the knee. This causes flexion of the knee and abduction of the thigh, resulting in delivery of the leg. The process should be repeated on the other side. At this point, many operators wrap the fetal legs and buttocks in a warm, wet towel to aid in traction. Delivery continues with downward traction on the fetus, with the thumbs on the fetal sacrum and the fingers on the iliac crests. The position of the fingers is important, because pressure placed on the abdomen may cause traumatic rupture or damage to the abdominal organs, such as the liver. Downward traction and maternal expulsive efforts allow delivery of the shoulders. As one shoulder becomes visible, the fetus should be gently rotated away from that side. The operator can deliver that arm by placing a thumb on the scapula and sliding a finger along the humerus; this causes the elbow to flex, and the arm may be swept across the fetal chest. After the first arm is delivered, the fetus is rotated in the opposite direction and the procedure is repeated for the other arm.

At this point, only the head is not delivered. An assistant should provide suprapubic pressure to maintain flexion of the fetal head. Some obstetricians feel that the use of Piper forceps for the after-coming head is appropriate in all breeches, whereas others believe in more limited use. Employing these forceps is preferable to placing excessive traction on the fetal neck, which can cause neurologic damage. When Piper forceps are used, an assistant is needed to hold the body of the fetus in a horizontal (not vertical) plane while the forceps are applied. If forceps are not used, the head may be delivered using the Mauriceau-Smellie-Viet maneuver. While an assistant maintains suprapubic pressure, one hand of the operator is placed under the fetal body and a finger on either side of the fetal maxilla to maintain flexion of the head. The other hand is placed on top of the body, with one finger on either side of the neck, and gentle traction is exerted. It is important to note that this maneuver does not involve placing fingers into the infant's mouth and using traction on the mandible.

After the delivery of the head, the remainder of the delivery is otherwise unremarkable.

## Conclusion

Although the debate about whether anyone should have a vaginal delivery under any circumstances continues, it remains clear that for most mothers and neonates this method is safe. Current literature supports vaginal delivery as causing less maternal morbidity and mortality than cesarean delivery; therefore, the techniques involved in both normal and operative vaginal deliveries remain important to teach and learn.

### REFERENCES

American College of Obstetricians and Gynecologists: Management of the breech presentation. ACOG Technical Bulletin 95. Washington, DC, ACOG, 1986.

American College of Obstetricians and Gynecologists: Fetal macrosomia. ACOG Technical Bulletin 159. Washington, DC, ACOG, 1991.

American College of Obstetricians and Gynecologists: Operative vaginal delivery. ACOG Technical Bulletin 196. Washington, DC, ACOG, 1994.

American College of Obstetricians and Gynecologists: Diabetes and pregnancy. ACOG Technical Bulletin 200. Washington, DC, ACOG, 1994.

Bashore RA, Phillips WH, Brinkman CR: A comparison of the morbidity of midforceps and cesarean delivery. Am J Obstet Gynecol 162:1428, 1990.

Blickstein I, Ben-Arie A, Hagay ZJ: Antepartum risks of shoulder dystocia and brachial plexus injury for infants weighing 4,200 g or more. Gynecol Obstet Invest 45:77, 1998.

Bofill JA, Rust OA, Schorr SJ, et al: A randomized trial of two vacuum extraction techniques. Obstet Gynecol 89:758, 1997.

Bofill JA, Rust OA, Schorr SJ, et al: A randomized prospective trial of the obstetric forceps versus the M-cup vacuum extractor. Am J Obstet Gynecol 175:1325, 1996.

Boyd MK, Usher RH, McLean FH, et al: Failed forceps. Obstet Gynecol 68:779, 1986.

Carmona F, Martinez-Romain S, Manau D, et al: Immediate maternal and neonatal effects of low-forceps delivery according to the new criteria of The American College of Obstetricians and Gynecologists compared with spontaneous vaginal delivery in term pregnancies. Am J Obstet Gynecol 173:55, 1995.

Diani F, Venanzi S, Zanconato G, et al: Fetal macrosomia and management of delivery. Clin Exp Obst & Gyn XXIV:212, 1997.

Gallaspy JW, Dunnihoo DR, DeGueurce JC, et al: Cephalic replacement in severe shoulder dystocia. South Med J 84:1373, 1991.

Gherman RB, Goodwin TM, Souter I, et al: The McRoberts' maneuver for the alleviation of shoulder dystocia: How successful is it? Am J Obstet Gynecol 176:656, 1997.

Goodwin TM, Banks E, Millar LK, et al: Catastrophic shoulder dystocia and emergency symphysiotomy. Am J Obstet Gynecol 177:463, 1997.

Graham JM, Blanco JD, Wen T, et al: The Zavanelli maneuver: A different perspective. Obstet Gynecol 79:883, 1992.

Hagadorn-Freathy AS, Yeomans ER, Hankins GD: Validation of the 1988 ACOG forceps classification system. Obstet Gynecol 77:357, 1991.

Johanson RB, Rice C, Doyle M, et al: A randomised prospective study comparing the new vacuum extractor policy with forceps delivery. Br J Obstet Gynaecol 100:524, 1993.

Koike T, Minakami H, Sasaki M, et al: The problem of relating fetal outcome with breech presentation to mode of delivery. Arch Gynecol Obstet 258:119, 1996.

Kuit JA, Wallenburg HCS, Huikeshoven FJM: Current cup designs for obstetric vacuum extraction. Br J Obstet Gynaecol 99:933, 1992.

Lim FTH, Holm JP, Schuitemaker NWE, et al: Stepwise compared with rapid application of vacuum in ventouse extraction procedures. Br J Obstet Gynaecol 104:33, 1997.

Lowe B: Fear of failure: A place for the trial of instrumental delivery. Br J Obstet Gynaecol 94:60, 1987.

Menticoglou M, Perlman M, Manning FA: High cervical spinal cord injury in neonates delivered with forceps: Report of 15 cases. Obstet Gynecol 86:589, 1995.

Nilsen ST: Boys born by forceps and vacuum extraction examined at 18 years of age. Acta Obstet Gynecol Scand 63:549, 1984.

Nocon JJ, McKenzie DK, Thomas LJ, et al: Shoulder dystocia: An analysis of risks and obstetric maneuvers. Am J Obstet Gynecol 168:1732, 1993.

O'Leary JA, Cuva A: Abdominal rescue after failed cephalic replacement. Obstet Gynecol 80:514, 1992.

Poen AC, Felt-Bersma RJF, Dekker GA, et al: Third degree obstetric perineal tears: Risk factors and the preventive role of mediolateral episiotomy. Br J Obstet Gynaecol 104:563, 1997.

Revah A, Ezra Y, Farine D, et al: Failed trial of vacuum or forceps—Maternal and fetal outcome. Am J Obstet Gynecol 176:200, 1997.

Seidman DS, Laor A, Gale R, et al: Long-term effects of vacuum and forceps deliveries. Lancet 337:1583, 1991.

Vintzileos AM, Nochimson DJ, Antsaklis A, et al: Effect of vacuum extraction on umbilical cord blood acid-base measurements. J Matern Fetal Med 5:11, 1996.

Wesley BD, van den Berg BJ, Reece EA: The effect of forceps delivery on cognitive development. Am J Obstet Gynecol 169:1091, 1993.

Williams MC, Knuppel RA, O'Brien WF, et al: Obstetric correlates of neonatal retinal hemorrhage. Obstet Gynecol 81:688, 1993.

Williams MC, Knuppel RA, O'Brien WF, et al: A randomized comparison of assisted vaginal delivery by obstetric forceps and polyethylene vacuum cup. Obstet Gynecol 78:789, 1991.

Williams MC, Knuppel RA, Weiss A, et al: A prospectively randomized comparison of forceps and vacuum assisted vaginal delivery. Am J Obstet Gynecol 164:323, 1991.

Yancey MK, Herpolsheimer A, Jordan GD, et al: Maternal and neonatal effects of outlet forceps delivery compared with spontaneous vaginal delivery in term pregnancies. Obstet Gynecol 78:646, 1991.

# 28

# Cesarean Section

MARK B. LANDON

Cesarean section accounts for approximately one million major operations performed annually in the United States. Nearly 23% of women have their babies delivered by cesarean section, which is the most common major surgical procedure undertaken today, compared with approximately 5% more than 30 years ago. The rise in cesarean section rates has prompted increased interest in the indications, complications, and techniques involved with this procedure. Despite clear documentation of the prevalence of cesarean section, there is remarkably little prospectively gathered information concerning a variety of issues related to abdominal delivery. The overwhelming economic burden of this surgery on health-care delivery has focused considerable effort on strategies aimed at reducing cesarean delivery rates. Because cesarean section carries with it a well-recognized risk for uncommon complications, such as maternal mortality and, more often, infectious complications, data now are being employed to reflect overall quality of care for many obstetric services. It follows that increased use of a trial of labor (TOL) in women who have had previous cesarean sections has become a focus for providers and payers of obstetric care as well. This chapter reviews indications for cesarean section, as well as techniques and complications of the procedure.

## Definition

Cesarean section has classically been defined as delivery of a fetus via a surgically created incision in the anterior uterine wall. As cesarean and section both refer to an incision, some prefer the term cesarean delivery or cesarean birth to describe the procedure.

## Cesarean Delivery Rates

Cesarean delivery rate describes the percentage of women undergoing cesarean delivery among all women giving birth during a specific time period. The cesarean rate may be further subdivided into primary (first-time operation) and repeat cesarean rates. Cesarean delivery rates have risen in the United Stated in a dramatic fashion from approximately 5% in 1965 to a peak of 24% in 1990. A modest decline to 22% was observed in 1995. For more than 30 years, an increase in international cesarean rates has been documented, although for most European nations, the overall rate remains 10 to 15%.

Given the discrepancy in cesarean rates between the United States and other countries without a perceivable benefit in neonatal outcomes, health policy groups have critically evaluated this issue, including its cause and possible solutions. In 1981, the National Institutes of Health published a report prepared by a task force on cesarean childbirth. It was recognized that the increase in cesarean section rates was caused almost wholly by repeat operations, dystocia, and fetal distress (Table 28–1). With expanding indications for cesarean delivery and little enthusiasm for TOL before 1980, it was obvious that previous cesarean sec-

**Table 28–1** Factors Responsible for Increased Cesarean Rates

- Increased diagnosis of cephalopelvic disproportion
- Elective repeat operations
- Increased diagnosis of fetal distress with fear of litigation
- Declining use of operative vaginal delivery
- Declining vaginal breech delivery

tion had become a major indication. Dystocia was also being diagnosed more frequently through the 1970s and 1980s, along with a parallel decline in operative vaginal delivery rates. Fear of litigation was recognized as liberalizing the indications for cesarean section, particularly with respect to the diagnosis of fetal distress. Despite the fact that electronic monitoring of the fetal heart rate has not been shown to reduce the risk of metabolic acidosis, birth asphyxia, or cerebral palsy compared with intermittent auscultation, its widespread use was cited as a factor in increasing the diagnosis of fetal distress and thus of cesarean delivery. The conferees concluded that both dystocia and elective repeat cesarean deliveries clearly required further study and institution of strategies to reduce their contribution to the overall rise in cesarean delivery. This recommendation was appealing because these two categories represented the greatest contributions to the increased performance of cesarean section and would also likely be the most amenable to a reduction, because physician practice patterns greatly influence these categories of cesarean delivery.

It is not possible to determine an optimal cesarean rate, because an ideal rate must be a function of multiple clinical factors that vary according to population and level of obstetric care provided. In spite of this, third-party payors continue to rely on expert opinion concerning optimal cesarean rates without benefit of risk stratification. It follows that institutions involved in tertiary obstetric care, that manage a large number of preterm deliveries and maternal complications, should have higher cesarean rates than primary care facilities. It has been suggested that an overall cesarean rate of 15% is a reasonable target by the year 2000. This figure may be low considering Quilligan's optimal ranges for cesarean by indication as follows: cephalopelvic disproportion (2 to 4%); repeat cesarean (2 to 6%); abnormal bleeding (1.3 to 3.5%); and bleeding (1%).

## Indications for Cesarean Delivery

Cesarean delivery is employed if labor is contraindicated, vaginal delivery represents substantial maternal or fetal risk, or fetal condition deteriorates to the extent that awaiting vaginal delivery would result in a less favorable outcome than proceeding with cesarean section. Indications for cesarean delivery are listed in Table 28–2. Clearly, some indications are purely maternal or fetal, whereas others represent a benefit to both. It is recognized that short of placenta previa, almost every indication for cesarean delivery has been challenged, and controversy exists for most of the listed diagnoses.

### MATERNAL INDICATIONS

Maternal indications for cesarean delivery are relatively few and can be considered as medical or mechanical in nature. Although somewhat debatable, certain maternal cardiac conditions (e.g., ischemic coronary disease, dilated aortic root with Marfan's syndrome) could be considered indications for cesarean section. Central nervous system abnormalities in which increased intracranial pressure would be undesirable would also mandate cesarean section. Mechanical vaginal obstruction caused by pelvic masses (e.g., lower segment myomas, massive condylomata) would require cesarean section as well.

### FETAL INDICATIONS

Fetal indications are primarily recognizable distress with potential for long-term consequences of metabolic acidosis. Somewhere between 1 and 3% of women undergo cesarean section for a nonreassuring fetal heart rate pattern. Other fetal indications include risk of transmission of infection or fetal trauma. Examples of these categories include active maternal herpes infection and breech delivery in which head entrapment is a possibility. Excessive fetal size or suspected macrosomia has been increasingly designated as an indication for cesarean delivery, although

**Table 28–2** Indications for Cesarean Delivery

- **Maternal**
  Specific cardiac disease
  CNS disease with increased intracranial pressure
  Vulvar obstruction for condylomata
  Vaginal obstruction resulting from pelvic masses
- **Fetal**
  Nonreassuring FHR pattern
  Rise of infection (herpes)
  Risk of trauma from excessive size of anatomic congenital defects
- **Maternal-Fetal**
  Placenta previa
  Abruption
  Dystocia

CNS = central nervous system; FHR = fetal heart rate.

few data exist to support this approach in the nondiabetic woman. Cesarean section has been traditionally mandated for certain birth defects (e.g., hydrocephalus with macrocephaly, neural tube defect) but insufficient data exist to make this an absolute indication. Less convincing data exist for use of cesarean section with abdominal wall defects (e.g., omphalocele, gastroschisis).

**MATERNAL-FETAL INDICATIONS**

The majority of cesarean deliveries are performed for conditions that might pose a threat to both mother and fetus if vaginal delivery occurred. Placenta previa and placental abruption with potential for hemorrhage are clear examples of such conditions. Dystocia presents a direct risk of fetal and maternal trauma and it may also compromise fetal oxygenation and metabolic status. Cephalopelvic disproportion (CPD) is a diagnosis that is generally made on a relative basis after a sufficient TOL, often with oxytocin augmentation. The criteria for CPD remain subjective, and at present norms for progress in labor are under challenge. Although failure to make sufficient progress in the active phase of labor has been attributed to deficiencies in uterine activity, it may also occur in response to the physician's approach to the management of labor itself. In protraction disorders, the proper length of time for an adequate TOL with oxytocin stimulation is undefined, with most practitioners allowing "a few hours." Because it has been shown that in many cesareans performed for dystocia oxytocin has not been employed at all, it can be concluded that inadequate trials of oxytocin stimulation may be a significant factor in the performance of some unnecessary operative deliveries.

Blumenthal and associates found a large difference between the incidence of dystocia in public and private patients and concluded that the difference probably resulted from differences in criteria used for the two groups. However, they were unable to determine whether the differences resulted from excessive intervention in the private group or from less than optimal intervention in the public group. Haynes de Regt and associates similarly demonstrated an overall cesarean section rate of 17.1% in clinic patients vs. 21.4% in private patients. In this study, a private patient giving birth to a first child was significantly more likely than a comparable clinic patient to undergo cesarean delivery if dystocia, malpresentation, or fetal distress were diagnosed. Unfortunately, this large retrospective study could not provide detailed information concerning criteria used to diagnose both dystocia and suspected fetal compromise.

Understanding that physician characteristics may affect cesarean rates, Berkowitz and associates analyzed 6327 deliveries performed by 48 different practitioners between 1983 and 1985. Although no significant differences were found according to gender or practice setting of the physicians, those who were older and more experienced performed significantly fewer cesarean sections for dystocia and instead had higher percentages of forceps deliveries and breech extractions. This finding is of great interest inasmuch as Frigoletto and associates noted that between 30 and 40% of primary cesarean deliveries at both Brigham and Women's Hospital and Northwestern University are performed during the second stage of labor in contrast to less than 5% at the National Maternity Hospital in Dublin. Confirmation of this finding could provide insight into potential strategies to further reduce cesarean deliveries performed for dystocia.

# Technique

**SITE PREPARATION**

Preparation of the skin is performed to reduce the risk of wound infection by decreasing the amount of skin flora and contaminants at the incision site. Incision site preparation is accomplished in the operating room through application of a surgical scrub that generally includes an antimicrobial agent. Before applying a scrub solution, hair is removed from the operative site. Use of a razor for removal may actually increase the risk of infection by causing breaks in the skin and allowing entry of bacteria. For this reason, some advocate clipping the hair before surgery. In either case, only enough hair should be removed to allow good reapproximation of skin edges. Cesarean incisions are considered to be clean contaminated wounds. In both this type of wound and a clean incision, the type of surgical scrub and the duration of scrubbing have not been associated with any change in the frequency of wound infections. Some surgeons employ a scrub for several minutes, whereas others apply a single swab of bactericidal solution, which takes less than 1 minute. The rate of wound infection following cesarean delivery is approximately 5% and is not influenced by preparation technique.

# Prophylactic Antibiotic Administration

Prophylactic antibiotics are clearly of benefit in reducing the frequency of postcesarean endomyometritis. This is particularly true for cases of prolonged labor and ruptured membranes. Some physicians administer prophylaxis to women scheduled for cesarean delivery without TOL, although the benefit of this approach is debatable. The preferred agent for prophylaxis is a first-generation cephalosporin, such as cefazolin, 1–2 g, administered intravenously after the cord is clamped. A second dose is given 4 hours later if surgery is prolonged or other high-risk factors are present. There is no apparent prophylactic advantage in using a broader spectrum antibiotic, and use of these agents adds expense and limits their efficacy for subsequent treatment. Patients who are allergic to penicillin may receive a single dose of metronidazole, 500 mg. For women who have clinical chorioamnionitis, treatment with combination antibiotic therapy supplants the need for prophylaxis. This therapy should be instituted promptly (before delivery) and continued until the patient has responded clinically.

## Incision Type

The surgeon has a choice of a vertical or transverse skin incision, with the transverse Pfannenstiel incision being the most commonly employed type. Factors that influence this decision include the urgency of the delivery, previous incision type, and the potential need to explore the upper abdomen for nonobstetric pathology. Although some surgeons prefer a vertical incision in emergency stat situations, Pfannenstiel's incision may actually add relatively little extra operative time, particularly in a nonobese individual. The previous incision type is usually repeated in most cesarean deliveries. There is a continuing debate about the surgical merits of a transverse skin incision. Although these incisions are more cosmetic and less painful, it is unclear whether subsequent herniation and postoperative pulmonary complications are influenced by incision type. This author prefers Pfannenstiel's incision in most cases in which a transverse incision is to be made. Occasionally, a transverse incision of the rectus sheath and muscles (Maylard incision) is necessary for proper exposure and room to deliver the fetus. In such a case, only the medial half of the muscle is incised to avoid lacerating the deep epigastric vessels. The Cherney incision allows complete transection of the rectus muscles, which requires identification of the epigastric vessels and bilateral ligation.

If a transverse skin incision is employed, it is made approximately 3 cm above the symphysis in the midline and extended laterally in a slight curvilinear manner. In obese individuals, the incision should not be made in the underside of the panniculus. The length of the incision should be based on the estimated fetal size and can be enlarged after deeper dissection. The subcutaneous tissue can then be bluntly pushed away to identify the underlying fascia. In repeat operations, sharp dissection of the subcutaneous adipose tissue is generally required. The fascia is incised and dissected in a curvilinear manner bilaterally. It should be tented with the surgeon's forceps to separate it from the underlying muscle and identify perforating vessels that require ligation or coagulation. The fascia is then grasped in the midline bilaterally and separated from the underlying fascia superiorly and inferiorly from the median raphe by blunt and sharp dissection. Once this is accomplished, the rectus muscles are gently separated in the midline to reveal the posterior rectus sheath and the peritoneum, which are incised sharply. The peritoneum is tented and palpated for underlying bowel and then entered with a scalpel or scissors. The point of entry should be as superior as possible to avoid bladder injury, particularly in repeat operations.

## UTERINE INCISION

A low transverse incision is employed in more than 90% of cases. It is preferred because it does not compromise the upper uterine segment and it is easier to perform and repair. It is also associated with less blood loss. This type of incision provides the option of a subsequent trial of labor because it has the lowest rate of rupture.

A vertical incision is either low or classic and should have clear indications. A vertical incision is performed if the lower uterine segment is poorly developed or if the fetus is in a backdown transverse lie. Some prefer a vertical incision for preterm breech delivery as well. This approach is prudent unless the lower segment is extremely well developed. A vertical incision should also be strongly considered for a complete anterior previa or for leiomyomas that obstruct the lower segment, as well as certain fetal anomalies, such as massive hydrocephalus or very large sacrococcygeal teratoma.

The classic uterine incision includes the upper uterine segment. The decision to use this incision depends on the need to extend a vertical cut; as in cases of anterior previa. The disadvantages of a classic incision are its tendency for greater adhesion formation and a greater risk of rupture with subsequent pregnancies.

Following full entry into the peritoneal cavity, the surgeon should palpate the uterus for fetal presentation and alignment and then place a bladder retractor to expose the lower uterine segment. The uterus is often dextrorotated, and this must be appreciated to plan the incision site. The vesicouterine serosa is picked up with smooth forceps and incised in the midline with Metzenbaum scissors. The incision is carried out laterally in a curvilinear manner. The vesicouterine fold is then tented with forceps or a pair of hemostats, which allow direct visualization as the bladder flap is bluntly created using the index and middle fingers of the surgeon's hand. Sharp dissection may be necessary, particular in repeat operations. The surgeon then bluntly sweeps out laterally on each side to allow just enough room for insertion of the bladder blade. A Richardson retractor is then inserted laterally, and continuous suction is made available for preparation for the uterine incision.

In the cases of a low transverse incision, the entry is begun at least 2 cm above the bladder margin. Suction is applied, as is tamponade, with sponges if considerable bleeding is encountered. This allows better visualization and minimizes the risk of fetal lacerations. The incision is extended laterally and superiorly at the angles by either sharp dissection or blunt spreading using the index fingers. The latter method is best suited for well-developed lower segments, although the choice is made by the operator based on experience with the goal to avoid lateral extension into the uterine vessels and broad ligament. The likelihood of extension is not influenced by choice of technique as much as by the stage of labor at which the cesarean section is performed.

The low vertical incision depends on downward displacement of the bladder to confine the incision to the true lower segment. The incision is begun as inferiorly as possible and extended cephalad with bandage scissors. If the thick myometrium of the upper segment is incised, the incision becomes classic and should be described as such.

Once an adequate uterine incision has been completed, the fetal head is extracted by elevation and flexion using the operator's hand as a fulcrum. If the head is not easily delivered, the uterine incision may be extended. Rarely, a T-incision is made to facilitate delivery. In cases in which the vertex is wedged in the maternal pelvis, an assistant may need to vaginally displace the presenting part. Vacuum extraction or short Simpson forceps may be applied, although this is rarely necessary if the previously mentioned steps may be taken. After nasal and oropharyngeal suction have been performed, fundal pressure is applied to extract the fetal body. The cord is clamped and cut and the infant is passed from the field.

After delivery of the infant, prophylactic antibiotics may be administered along with intravenous oxytocin, 20 units/L. Removal of the placenta may be accomplished by either manual extraction or spontaneous expulsion with gentle cord traction. A prospective randomized trial has demonstrated greater blood loss and a higher rate of endometritis with the manual extraction method.

Uterine repair may be greatly facilitated by lifting the fundus and delivering the uterus through the abdominal incision. This facilitates better visualization of the extent of the incision to be repaired as well as the adnexae. The disadvantage of elevation of the uterus is that it may increase patient discomfort or nausea or vomiting. There is no apparent increased risk for either blood loss or infection with exteriorization of the uterus. Bleeding along the incision line is temporarily controlled by using Ring clamps because these produce less trauma than other instruments. The uterus is then manually curetted with a moistened sponge, and all obvious placental fragments or membranes are teased away from the uterine wall.

The uterine incision should be carefully inspected before closure. The lateral aspects of the incision may encroach upon the ascending branch of the uterine artery, making palpation of its pulse a requirement before suturing. Any inferior extensions of the incision should be visualized and repaired separately before closure. The lower uterine incision may be closed as either a single layer of running locking suture or a second imbricating (nonlocking) running layer. The locking of the primary layer of closure facilitates hemostasis and may not be necessary if the incision is fairly hemostatic before closure. This author prefers to use No. 1 chromic gut sutures; however, a synthetic suture of similar gauge is acceptable. The single layer of closure method has gained great popularity because it significantly decreases operating time, with less extra hemostatic suturing required and no difference in the rate of prospective infection. It is unknown whether the risk of subsequent uterine rupture is affected by single- vs. double-layer closure technique.

A vertical uterine incision generally requires a two-layer closure technique. This may be accomplished by first running a locking continuous layer. This author prefers a second interrupted layer in which each side is sutured twice before securing the knot. The myometrium is gathered laterally with this method, and the needle is placed parallel to the uterus while incorporating the myometrium. The serosa is not pierced with the needle. The assistant then pinches each segment for the surgeon tying the knot. This technique is somewhat more time-consuming than a second continuous layer; however, it is often more hemostatic and leads to better tissue approximation.

The vesicouterine serosa may be approximated with a 2–0 or 3–0 suture; however, most surgeons today omit this step because reperitonealization occurs spontaneously over several days.

The uterine incision is inspected for hemostasis before returning it to the peritoneal cavity. Individual bleeding points are ligated with as little suture placement as possible. Superficial bleeding can be controlled with electrocoagulation. The adnexa are inspected and tubal ligation is performed, if desired.

After return of the uterus, the pelvis is irrigated with warm saline solution.

The rectus fascia is closed with either a continuous nonlocking or an interrupted technique. A suture with good tensile strength and relatively delayed absorption is preferred; synthetic braided or monofilament sutures are the best choice. In closing the fascia, placement of the sutures should be a minimum of 1.5 cm from the margin of the incision. In most cases of wound disruption, the suture remains intact but has cut through the fascia as a result of placement too close to the cut margin. Patients at risk for wound disruption may benefit from either the Smead-Jones closure technique or interrupted figure-of-eight sutures, both of which employ delayed absorption suture material, such as monofilament polyglycolic acid. Sutures are placed at 1-cm intervals. In most instances, a running continuous monofilament propylene suture suffices for a transverse incision. The Smead-Jones closure technique is preferred for vertical incisions in high-risk cases. A figure-of-eight far-near, near-far placement, which passes through the anterior rectus fascia and adjacent subcutaneous adipose tissue and then crosses the midline to pick up the medial edge of the rectus fascia and then the opposite side similarly before returning to the far margin contralaterally, accomplishes this technique.

The subcutaneous tissue is not closed unless it facilitates skin closure. Subcutaneous drainage through a separate stab site is employed in obese individuals if the incision is not perfectly hemostatic, although its benefit has not been established. The skin is closed with either a staple device or a subcutaneous closure for transverse incisions.

# Operative Complications

Maternal morbidity and mortality are increased in cesarean delivery compared with vaginal birth, even when controlling for conditions that might predispose to cesarean section. Given the infrequent nature of maternal death arising from cesarean delivery, it is not surprising that the attributable death rate has ranged from 6:100,000 to 22:100,000. The relative risk for maternal death as a result of cesarean delivery compared with vaginal birth range from several-fold higher to more than 10 times as likely an event.

The principal causes of morbidity related to cesarean section are infectious and thromboembolic disease. Anesthesia-related morbidity and mortality have been substantially reduced through wider use of regional anesthesia and employment of awake intubation for patients who require general anesthesia and who may have a suboptimal airway.

# Infectious Complications

## ENDOMYOMETRITIS

Postcesarean endomyometritis is the most common complication of cesarean delivery despite a reduced frequency with the use of prophylactic antibiotic regimens. Primary cesarean section with labor is associated with an average rate of endometritis of 30 to 40% without administration of prophylaxis. In indigent populations, rates of postcesarean infection as high as 75% have been reported. Labor, prolonged rupture of membranes, and lower socioeconomic status appear to be the factors that most influence the incidence of this complication. Before the institution of protocols using broad-spectrum antibiotic coverage that included possible anaerobic bacteria, severe complications (e.g., hysterectomy, superimposed septic thrombophlebitis) were encountered in a small percentage of refractory cases. The general perception is that these severe complications have been reduced, although there is little improvement in available outcome data to demonstrate this.

The majority of endomyometritis cases arise from ascending infection that develops from cervicovaginal flora. Infections that are found past the deepest part of the uterine incision may extend to the uterine musculature, and, if not adequately treated, may produce peritonitis, abscess, or septic phlebitis. The diagnosis of endomyometritis is often based on clinical risk factors in association with a febrile postoperative patient. The presence of chorioamnionitis, prolonged labor, and ruptured membranes should especially prompt early treatment in suspected cases. The utility of endometrial cultures is limited because of contamination with vaginal flora; therefore, these are often omitted, and treatment is based on clinical findings, including uterine tenderness, leukocytosis, and fever.

The patient should be treated with parenteral antibiotics employing a regimen directed against possible anaerobic infection. This author prefers to use clindamycin and an aminoglycoside, such as gentamycin or a single-agent, penicillin-based regimen using β-lactamase inhibition to allow for anaerobic coverage. Ampicillin/sulbactam (Unasyn) has been shown to have success rates comparable to the combined approach using clindamycin and gentamycin.

For women who fail to respond to antibiotic therapy over 2 to 3 days, an alternative source of fever, such as wound infection, deep abscess, hematoma, or septic pelvic thrombophlebitis, should be considered. On occasion, significant mastitis may contribute to the febrile state.

## WOUND INFECTION

Wound infection complicates approximately 5% of cesarean deliveries. Most cesarean sections are considered clean contaminated wounds because of the interface with the lower reproductive tract. Emergency cesarean deliveries, or those associated with chorioamnionitis, are considered contaminated and have higher wound infection rates.

The diagnosis of wound infection is usually straightforward, with patients manifesting tenderness, erythema, or discharge. Early wound infection (first 2 days) is often a result of streptococcal infection, whereas later wound infection is generally caused by overgrowth of *Staphylococcus* or mixed aerobic and anaerobic bacterial infection. Extreme wound discoloration or anesthesia of the surrounding tissue should prompt consideration of necrotizing fasciitis, particularly if the patient is very ill with a marked leukocytosis.

Discharge from the wound should be sent for culture before instituting therapy. The infected portion of the wound should be opened, inspected, irrigated, and débrided as necessary. In most cases, this alone suffices for therapy, and the wound is left to close by secondary intention. If extensive infection, discoloration, gangrene, or bullae are encountered, the would should be inspected and débrided under general anesthesia. Tissue analysis may aid in establishing a diagnosis of necrotizing infection, in which all nonviable tissue should be removed. For such cases, consultation with an experienced surgeon is recommended. Antibiotic coverage, which is rarely necessary for simple wound infection, should be instituted promptly for advanced serious would disruptions.

## THROMBOEMBOLIC DISEASE

Deep venous thrombosis is not uncommonly encountered during pregnancy secondary to higher levels of clotting factors and venous stasis. The puerperal period is a time of high risks, with cesarean section contributing further to this phenomenon. Other risk factors are immobility, obesity, advanced age, and parity. An untreated deep venous thrombosis can progress to a life-threatening pulmonary embolism in up to 25% of cases. Prompt treatment with anticoagulation substantially reduces this risk.

Deep venous thrombosis (DVT) is suggested by the presence of unilateral leg pain and swelling. A significant difference in the calf or thigh diameter may be present; however, error with this measurement is possible. A strongly positive Homans' sign (pain with foot dorsiflexion) is often present if the calf is involved. Many cases of DVT appear as pulmonary embolus (PE), particularly in the postoperative patient. Tachypnea, dyspnea, tachycardia, and pleuritic pain are the classic symptoms, with cough and specific pulmonary auscultatory findings less common.

If DVT is a consideration, Doppler studies may be useful for the diagnosis of proximal disease but are less sensitive for the diagnosis of calf thrombosis. Impedance plethysmography is also useful in the diagnosis of proximal disease; however, it is of limited value in the diagnosis of pelvic thrombosis. If DVT is highly suspected and the previously mentioned studies are inconclusive, a venogram should be obtained. The workup for suspected PE includes an arterial blood gas level and chest radiograph. A ventilation and perfusion study should be performed. Oxygen should be administered and heparin begun if clinical PE appears likely. An indeterminate perfusion scan requires pulmonary angiography to establish or rule out the diagnosis of pulmonary embolism.

## SEPTIC PELVIC THROMBOPHLEBITIS

It is likely that less than 1% of women who have endomyometritis will develop septic pelvic thrombophlebitis; however, accurate figures for the frequency of this condition in current practice are lacking. Septic pelvic thrombophlebitis is most often a diagnosis of exclusion established in refractory cases of women being treated for endomyometritis. Pelvic computed tomograph (CT) scan may aid in the diagnosis, although the sensitivity and specificity of this technique are clearly difficult to establish. In practice, postcesarean section patients who fail to respond to appropriate broad-coverage antibiotic therapy for suspected uterine infection are begun on full-dose heparin therapy, which is continued for several days after a clinical response. Long-term anticoagulation is not prescribed. Patients who have septic pelvic phlebitis may have spiking nocturnal fever and chills, although these findings may be absent and a persistent febrile state may be all that is present. In cases in which there is no response to anticoagulation therapy, radiologic imaging for possible abscess or hematoma is indicated. Refractory cases may require laparotomy to rule out an abscess.

# Vaginal Birth After Cesarean Section (VBAC)

It has been concluded that primary emphasis should be placed on reducing performance of cesarean section for dystocia and repeat operations because these two indications have increased the rate of cesarean section far beyond any other indications. The modest decline in cesarean delivery over the past few years has been largely the result of an increased TOL rate in women who had previous cesarean sections. At the present time, approximately 30% of women who have had previous cesarean sections undergo a TOL in the United States. It has been established that two thirds of women who have had previous cesarean deliveries are actually candidates for a TOL. Thus, between 50 and 65% of repeat operations may be unnecessary and are often influenced by physician discretion. A comparison of TOL rates between the United States and several European nations reveals significant underutilization of TOL in this country.

The overall success rate of VBAC is approximately 75%. Given this information and the fact that 8 to 10% of the obstetric population have had previous cesarean deliveries, more widespread use of TOL has the potential to decrease the overall cesarean section rate by approximately 5%. In 1988, the American College of Obstetrics and Gynecology (ACOG) published "Guidelines for Vaginal Delivery After a Previous Cesarean Birth," recommending VBAC-TOL because it was clear that this procedure was safe and not associated with excessive perinatal morbidity compared with elective cesarean delivery. They recommended that each hospital develop its own protocol for the management of VBAC patients and that a woman who had had one previous low transverse cesarean section should be counseled and encouraged to attempt labor in the absence of a contraindication, such as a previous classic incision. More recently, the ACOG published a practice pattern on the management of VBAC-TOL patients. This document used evidence-based criteria to present clinical guidelines for obstetricians and patients regarding appropriate care. Like the 1988 committee opinion, the 1995 practice patterns endorsed VBAC-TOL as being safe in women who have had a single primary low transverse incision. It thus established that most women who have had previous cesarean sections are candidates for TOL, and that the only contraindication for TOL is a previous classic incision because of the high rate of uterine rupture in such cases. The document did acknowledge that insufficient data existed to provide counseling for patients who have had previous low vertical incisions, multiple gestations, breech presentations, or estimated fetal weights greater than 4000 g (Table 28–3). Administration of oxytocin was

**Table 28–3** ACOG Practice Patterns on VBAC-TOL

- **Limited Data**
  Multiple cesarean sections
  Macrosomia
- **Insufficient Data**
  Previous low vertical scar
  Unknown scar
  Twins
  Breech
  Prior myomectomy

**Table 28–4** Risks of VBAC—Trial of Labor

| Risk | (%) |
| --- | --- |
| Uterine rupture | 0.2–1.0 |
| Fetal death (with ruptured uterus) | 2.0–15.0 |
| Maternal mortality (with ruptured uterus) | Nearly zero |

deemed safe for patients, although its use appears to be associated with a decreased success rate of TOL. Although the ACOG document states that the use of oxytocin is not associated with an increase in perinatal mortality, a case-control study found that excessive infusion rates increased the risk of uterine rupture or dehiscence. Because of limited data available, meta-analysis has been employed to address the safety of oxytocin use in TOL patients. Using this method, Rosen reported that oxytocin use does not appear to influence the risk of a dehiscence or rupture.

## RISKS OF VBAC-TOL

The principal risk of VBAC-TOL is uterine rupture. Older literature failed to differentiate between uterine rupture and dehiscence. This distinction is clinically important because dehiscence most often represents an occult scar separation observed via laparotomy in a woman who has had previous a cesarean section. The serosa of the uterus is intact, and hemorrhage, with its potential sequelae for mother and fetus, is absent. In contrast, uterine rupture is a complete disruption of all uterine layers with consequences of hemorrhage, fetal distress, stillbirth, significant maternal morbidity, and potential for mortality. The risk of uterine rupture varies between 0.5 and 1.0% and has remained the same for more than the 20 years. The risk of perinatal mortality with rupture has been cited as 13.6% (3 of 22 cases of rupture) in the meta-analysis of Rosen and associates. More recent analysis of outcomes after uterine rupture suggests a lower risk of perinatal death and asphyxia, although data on the latter are clearly lacking. Published literature has revealed a risk of neonatal death, subsequent neurologic injury, or both to be as high as 23% (6 of 26) in cases of uterine rupture. Maternal mortality as a result of uterine rupture with planned VBAC-TOL is extremely rare, with one case being reported in the American literature over a 15-year period (Table 28–4). The most common maternal risks associated with TOL compared with planned repeat operations are infectious morbidity and operative injuries in those who fail a TOL and require cesarean section. Because the overwhelming majority of complications represent postpartum endomyometritis—a treatable condition—VBAC-TOL continues to be an option for many women.

## PREDICTORS OF VBAC-TOL SUCCESS

The overall success rate of VBAC appears to be between 70 and 80% according to published reports. The indication of previous cesarean delivery clearly impacts on the likelihood of successful VBAC. A history of previous vaginal birth or a nonrecurring condition, such as previous breech position or fetal distress, is associated with the highest success rates for VBAC (Table 28–5). In contrast, previous operative delivery for cephalopelvic disproportion is associated with a success rate as high as 67%. In such women, oxytocin is frequently required in subsequent labor, and failure to maximize uterine stimulation may lower the success of VBAC. Although many reports have attempted to predict the success of VBAC based on previous labor characteristics, such scoring systems are at best only moderately successful. The length of previous labor has been universally linked to subsequent VBAC success, but the maximal cervical dilatation reached in a previous attempt has not been predictive of successful VBAC. Conflicting data are also present with regard to macrosomia and success rates in women who have had previous CPD.

Despite acknowledgment of the safety of VBAC in women who have had one previous cesarean section, there is apparent reluctance to offer TOL to women who have had multiple previous operations. In a large series conducted between 1983 and 1992, TOL was employed in 80% of women who had one previous cesarean delivery, in 54% who had two, and in 30% who had three or more. These figures are among the highest TOL rates reported and far exceed the practice in nontertiary care settings. The overall success rate of TOL in women who have had more than one previous cesarean delivery is approximately 65%, a figure that is slightly lower than that of woman who had one previous cesarean delivery. Meta-analysis of 29 studies has confirmed a lower likelihood of successful VBAC with more than one previous cesarean section (odds ratio [OR] = 0.7).

The ACOG states that "present data are insufficient to predict success rates" in women who have had multiple previous cesarean sections. Most studies concerning women with multiple previous cesarean sections include less than 100 cases, yet a single large series from Los Angeles County (LAC) University of Southern California (USC) Medical Center included 1827 cases. The success rate was confirmed to be lower with two or more previous cesarean sections (OR = 0.61, 95% confidence interval [CI] 0.52-0.69). Most interesting was the finding of a significantly greater risk of uterine rupture (1.7%) in women who had two or more prior cesarean sections compared with women with only one previous operation (0.5%). These authors concluded that although TOL is a reasonable option in women who have two or more low transverse incisions, it is best reserved for motivated patients who understand and accept the *increased* risk of uterine rupture and the decreased likelihood of success.

**Table 28–6** Indications for Cesarean Hysterectomy

- Placenta accreta/percreta
- Uterine atony
- Hemorrhage
- Uterine rupture

## Cesarean Hysterectomy

Cesarean hysterectomy refers to the removal of the uterus at the time of a planned or unplanned cesarean delivery. Postpartum hysterectomy encompasses both cesarean hysterectomy as well as removal of the uterus following vaginal delivery. In most cases of hysterectomy following vaginal birth, the indication for the procedure is uterine atony with uncontrolled hemorrhage that has failed to respond to conservative measures. In contrast, placenta accreta is the most common indication for postcesarean hysterectomy (Table 28–6). There appears to be an increasing trend of cesarean hysterectomy as a result of an increased frequency of previous cesarean birth, which is a risk factor for placenta accreta. Nearly 25% of women who have placenta previa and who had previous cesarean delivery develop placenta accreta, which in most cases requires hysterectomy to control bleeding. With two or more previous cesarean births and existing placenta previa, the risk of cesarean hysterectomy approaches 50%. Although placenta accreta itself poses a risk for peripartum hysterectomy, its association with previous uterine scarring (incision) is responsible for the 50- to 100-fold increased risk of hysterectomy after cesarean section compared with

**Table 28–5** Likelihood of Successful VBAC According to Indication for Previous Cesarean Section

| Indications | (%) |
| --- | --- |
| Cephalopelvic disproportion; failure to progress | 50–77 |
| Breech presentation | 90 |
| Fetal distress | 85 |

that after vaginal delivery. A history of previous cesarean section is now present in 67% of women undergoing peripartum hysterectomy.

Most cesarean hysterectomies are emergency procedures performed to control hemorrhage when conservative measures have failed. Occasionally, cesarean hysterectomy is planned for the treatment of cervical cancer or large myoma. The most common indications for emergency cesarean hysterectomy are placenta accreta, uterine atony, and uterine rupture. Together, these account for over 95% of the procedures performed in the United States.

Before the introduction of effective oxytocics, such as prostaglandin $F_2\alpha$, uterine atony was the most common indication for cesarean hysterectomy. Improved oxytocics, coupled with a rising cesarean rate, which again has increased the frequency of abnormal placentation, have resulted in placenta accreta becoming the most common indication for cesarean hysterectomy. In two reports from LAC-USC Medical Center over an 18-year period, placenta accreta accounted for 30% of peripartum hysterectomies initially and later was associated with 45% of procedures. The frequency of atony associated with peripartum hysterectomy fell from 43 to 20% between 1978 and 1990.

In the previously mentioned series, uterine rupture accounted for 11 to 13% of peripartum hysterectomies. In most cases of symptomatic rupture, the uterus can be preserved if so desired. The decision to proceed with hysterectomy ultimately depends on the ability to satisfactorily repair the uterus with hemostasis as well as the future childbearing desires of the patient. Small dehiscences discovered at cesarean section or following successful VBAC are generally not an indication for cesarean hysterectomy.

## TECHNIQUE AND COMPLICATIONS

A peripartum hysterectomy, including cesarean hysterectomy, may be subtotal (supracervical) or total depending upon the clinical circumstances. In most planned procedures, a total hysterectomy is performed, whereas a subtotal hysterectomy may be preferable in cases in which emergency surgery is necessary for life-threatening hemorrhage and dissection of the cervix is difficult. Subtotal hysterectomy is a faster procedure and has been suggested in unstable patients, but a comparison of this procedure with total hysterectomy was not associated with less blood loss, operative time, or morbidity. However, selection bias is probable, because women who have significant bleeding from atony or accreta are more likely to undergo subtotal hysterectomy. Subtotal hysterectomy is more likely to be performed in fact in cases of atony. In one series of 30 cases of peripartum hysterectomy for atony, a subtotal procedure was accomplished in 77% of individuals. Subtotal hysterectomy is less often performed in cases of placenta previa or accreta, because lower uterine segment bleeding with these conditions often requires a total hysterectomy to control hemorrhage.

The operative technique for cesarean hysterectomy consists of the same general surgical protocols for the procedure as those that are performed in the nonpregnant individual. Specific considerations include adequate inferior displacement of the bladder, if possible, before hysterectomy, because taking the bladder down may be difficult after uterine incision and delivery of the infant. Additionally, care must be taken to avoid bladder and ureteral injury, which appears to be relatively common with peripartum hysterectomy. Cystotomy has been reported to occur in up to 4 to 5% of procedures. Ureteral injury is observed in 1:200 operations. The ureter is particularly vulnerable to injury if broad ligament bleeding occurs, and lateral clamping is necessary to control this. If ureteral injury is suspected, the dome of the bladder may be incised and retrograde stenting of the uterus performed. Intravenous injection of indigo carmine may also be useful in identifying ureteral injury or suspected ligature.

The sequence of maneuvers for cesarean hysterectomy is not the same as the sequence of maneuvers in the the procedure for the nonpregnant woman. As mentioned previously, efforts to displace the bladder inferiorly before delivery are advised. After delivery and removal of the placenta, the uterine incision is frequently reapproximated, or attention is given to securing hemostasis by ligating the utero-ovarian anastomosis bilaterally. The bladder should be inspected and mobilized by blunt and sharp dissection. In most cases, the ovaries are left intact, although the adnexa in the pregnant patient are vulnerable to hematoma formation, which has necessitated salpingo-oophorectomy in as many as 17% of emergency procedures. The avascular portion of the broad ligaments is incised and the uterine vessels are identified, clamped, and suture-ligated. Clamps are placed tightly along the lateral aspect of the uterus to prevent injury to the ureter and formation of a hematoma. This is often the point at which the decision is made whether to proceed with subtotal or total hysterectomy. In most instances, a total procedure is performed unless the patient is unstable, and bleeding can be adequately controlled by the subtotal approach. If the cervix is amputated, it is closed with figure-of-eight sutures and reperitonealization may or may not be performed. If total hysterectomy is to be accomplished, the cervical stump is elevated with traction and is separated from the cardinal and uterosacral ligaments by clamping and ligature. The vagina is then entered anteriorly or at the lateral angle above a curved clamp. An effort should be made to be certain the cervix is completely removed, although in surgery performed after labor, this may be difficult. Excess portions of the superior vagina, however, should not be excised. To minimize complications, some surgeons prefer to insert a finger through an incision in the lower uterine segment before excision of the cervix to identify the cervicovaginal junction. The vaginal cuff is supported by approximation to the cardinal and uterosacral ligament pedicles. The cuff may be left open or closed with an interrupted (or running), locking, continuous suture. If significant bleeding is a concern, the cuff is better left open for dependent drainage or placement of a drain. Reperitonealization has fallen out of favor and been replaced by many surgeons with fixation of the ovarian pedicles to the round ligaments; this reduces the risk of adhesion to the vaginal cuff. The principal complications of cesarean hysterectomy are urologic injury, as discussed, and hemorrhage. The average blood loss varies, with a range of 500 to 1000 ml in excess of blood lost in a routine cesarean delivery. In many cases, the indication for hysterectomy is hemorrhage itself, with extensive pre-existing blood loss before hysterectomy is performed. Febrile morbidity is common, particularly in unplanned cesarean hysterectomy, with infection rates of 25 to 30% despite prophylactic antibiotic administration. Because pelvic tissue is friable and because coagulopathy often precedes the surgery, postsurgical bleeding is observed with increased frequency after peripartum hysterectomy. Re-exploration has thus been reported in 2 to 4% of cases.

## REFERENCES

Alexander JW, Fischer JE, Bovajian M, et al: The influence of hair removal methods on wound infections. Arch Surg 118:347–353, 1983.
Alexander JW, Aerni S, Plettner JP: Development of a safe and effective one minute preoperative skin preparation. Arch Surg 120:1357–1361, 1985.
American College of Obstetrics and Gynecology: Guidelines for Vaginal Delivery after a Previous Cesarean Birth. Committee Opinion No. 64, 1988.
American College of Obstetrics and Gynecology: Practice Patterns: Clinical Practice Guidelines for Issues in Obstetrics and Gynecology. Vaginal birth after previous cesarean birth. ACOG, 1995.
Berkowitz GS, Fiarman GS, Mijicca MA, et al: Effect of physician characteristics on the cesarean birth rate. Am J Obstet Gynecol 161:146–151, 1989.
Blumenthal NJ, Harris RS, O'Conner MC, et al: Changing cesarean section rates. Experience at a Sydney obstetric teaching hospital. Aust N Z J Obstet Gynaecol 24:246–251, 1984.
Bottoms SF, Rosen MG, Sokol RJ: The increase in the cesarean birth rate. N Engl J Med 302:559–563, 1980.
Clark SL, Yeh S-Y, Phelan JP, et al: Emergency hysterectomy for postpartum hemorrhage. Obstet Gynecol 64:376–382, 1984.
Eisenkop SM, Richman R, Platt LD, et al: Urinary tract injury during cesarean section. Obstet Gynecol 60:591–598, 1982.
Farmer RM, Kirschbaum T, Potter D, et al: Uterine rupture during a trial of labor after previous cesarean section. Am J Obstet Gynecol 165:996–1001, 1991.
Flamm BL, Newman LA, Thomas SJ, et al: Vaginal birth after cesarean delivery: Results of a 5 year multicenter collaborative study. Obstet Gynecol 76:750–755, 1990.
Flamm BL, Goings JR, Lin Y, et al: Elective repeat cesarean delivery versus trial of labor: A prospective multicentered study. Obstet Gynecol 83:927–932, 1994.
Frigoletto FD, Lieberman E, Lang JM, et al: A clinical trial of active management of labor. N Engl J Med 338:745–750, 1995.
Gibbs RS: Clinical risk factors for puerperal infection. Obstet Gynecol 55:1785–1790, 1980.
Gibbs RS, Sweet RL: Maternal and fetal infections. In Creasy RK, Resnik R (eds) Maternal-Fetal Medicine: Principles and Practice, 3rd ed. Philadelphia, WB Saunders, 1994; p 652.
Haynes de Regt RH, Minkoff HL, Feldman J, et al: Relation of private or clinic care to the cesarean birth rate. N Engl Med 315:619–626, 1986.
Leung AS, Farmer RM, Leung EK, et al: Risk factors associated with uterine rupture during trial of labor after cesarean delivery: A case controlled study. Am J Obstet Gynecol 186:1358–1364, 1983.
Magann EF, Dodson MK, Albert JR, et al. Blood loss at time of cesarean section by method of placental removal and exteriorization versus in situ repair of the uterine incision. Surg Gynecol Obstet 177:389–394, 1993.
McCurdy CM, Magann EF, McCurdy CJ, et al: The effect of placenta management at cesarean delivery on operative blood loss. Am J Obstet Gynecol 167:1363–1367, 1992.
McMahon ML, Luther E, Bowes W, et al: Comparison of trial of labor with elective second cesarean section. N Engl J Med 35:689–695, 1996.
Mickal A, Begneaud WP, Hawes TP: Pitfalls and complications of cesarean hysterectomy. Clin Obstet Gynecol 12:660–668, 1969.
Miller DA, Diaz FG, Paul RH: Vaginal birth after cesarean: A 10-year experience. Obstet Gynecol 84:255–261, 1994.
Nielson TF, Hokegard KH: Cesarean section and intraoperative surgical complications. Acta Obstet Gynaecol Scan 63:103–106, 1984.
NIH Consensus Development Statement on Cesarean Childbirth. The Cesarean Birth Task Force. Obstet Gynecol 57:537–545, 1981.
Ollendorff DA, Goldberg JM, Minogue JP, et al: VBAC for arrest of labor: Is success determined by maximal cervical dilatation during the prior labor? Am J Obstet Gynecol 159:636–641, 1988.
Paul RH, Phelan JP, Yeh S: Trial of labor in the patient with a prior cesarean birth. Am J Obstet Gynecol 151:297–301, 1985.
Phelan JP, Eglinton GS, Horenstein JM, et al: Previous cesarean birth: Trial of labor in women with macrosomic infants. J Reprod Med 29:36–42, 1984.
Pietrantoni M, Parsons MT, O'Brien WF, et al: Peritoneal closure or non-closure at cesarean. Obstet Gynecol 77:293–297, 1991.
Placek PJ, Taffel SM, Kappel KG: Maternal and infant characteristics associated with cesarean section delivery. HHS Pub. No. 844. National Center for Health Statistics, 1983.
Porreco RP, Thorp JA: The cesarean birth epidemic: Trends, causes, and solutions. Am J Obstet Gynecol 175:369–379, 1996.
Porter TF, Clark SL, Esplin MS, et al: Timing of delivery and neonatal outcome in patients with clinically overt uterine rupture during VBAC. SPO Abstract #73, 1998.
Quilligan EJ: Making inroads against the C-section rate. Contemp Obstet Gynecol 21:221–225, 1983.
Rosen MG, Dickinson JC, Westhoff C: VBAC: A meta-analysis of morbidity and mortality. Obstet Gynecol 7:465–467, 1991.
Rouse DJ, Owen J, Hauth J. Active phase of labor arrest: Two hours of oxytocin augmentation is not enough. SPO Abstract #8, 1998.
Sachs BP, Yeh J, Acker D, et al: Cesarean section-related maternal mortality in Massachusetts, 1954–1985. Obstet Gynecol 71:385–392, 1988.
Stanco LM, Schrimmer DB, Paul RH, et al: Emergency peripar-

tum hysterectomy and associated risk factors. Am J Obstet Gynecol 168:879–885, 1993.

Sweet RL, Gibbs RS: Infectious diseases of the female genital tract. Baltimore, Williams & Wilkins, 1990, pp 356–340.

US Department of Health and Human Services: Healthy Children 2000. DHHS Pub No. HRSA-M-CH 91–2.

Weinstein D, Benshushan A, Tanos V, et al: Predictive score for vaginal birth after cesarean section. 174:1992–1998, 1996.

Wessler S: Medical management of venous thrombosis. Ann Rev Med 37:313–319, 1976.

Zelop CM, Harlow BL, Frigletto FD, et al: Emergency peripartum hysterectomy. Am J Obstet Gynecol 1993; 168:1443–1449, 1993.

# 29

# Obstetric Hemorrhage

YORAM SOROKIN

In this chapter, we discuss practical aspects of the most common causes of obstetric hemorrhage: placenta previa, abruptio placentae, and uterine atony.

Hemorrhage is ranked third among causes of direct maternal mortality in advanced gestation. In Massachusetts, a reduced incidence of uterine atony and timely use of transfusions were secondary to an observed reduction in hemorrhage-related maternal death over a 30-year period (1954 to 1985). Hemorrhage was a contributing factor in 13% of maternal deaths between 1982 and 1985.

Stones and associates evaluated risk factors for obstetric hemorrhage in 37,497 deliveries in 1 region during 1 year. They found 498 cases (1.33%) complicated by hemorrhage of 1000 ml or more. The study confirmed the significance of known risk factors (e.g., abruptio placentae, placenta previa, cesarean delivery, multiple pregnancy) and suggested that more attention should be drawn to the risk of hemorrhage associated with obesity, retained placenta, induced labor, and delivery of a large baby.

Evaluation of the patient with obstetric hemorrhage must include a careful history and physical examination concurrently with initial resuscitative measures. Assessment of blood volume deficit is more difficult in pregnant women. With 40% volume expansion during pregnancy, women do not usually demonstrate the expected early signs of volume depletion.

Hemorrhage is divided into four classes:

1. Class I: modest bleeding: 15% or less of circulating volume is lost; there are few hemodynamic changes, with only a slight tachycardia (pulse 80 to 110 span) and a negative tilt test.
2. Class II: modest bleeding: 20 to 25% of circulating blood volume is lost; there is tachycardia (pulse 100 to 130 span); a rise in diastolic pressure; decreased pulse pressure; moderate tachypnea; positive tilt test; and cool, moist, pale skin
3. Class III: severe bleeding: 30 to 35% of circulating volume is lost; there is marked tachycardia (pulse 120 to 160 span); hypotension; tachypnea (30 to 50 breaths/min); oliguria; and cold, clammy, pallid skin.
4. Class IV: severe bleeding: 40 to 45% of circulating volume is lost; patient is in profound shock with profound hypotension; it is difficult to obtain peripheral blood pressure, and ankle and wrist pulses are not palpable; there is marked tachycardia; circulatory collapse; and oliguria or anuria.

Treatment of class I and II hemorrhaging usually includes rapid intravenous crystalloid infusions while crossmatching for blood. When blood loss is severe or bleeding continuous, the patient usually needs treatment with blood and blood products.

## Antepartum Hemorrhage

Antepartum bleeding occurs in 3 to 5% of pregnancies beyond 22 weeks of gestation. The bleeding can

**Table 29–1** Known Causes of Bleeding >20 Weeks of Gestation

| Nonuterine | Uterine |
|---|---|
| Sexual intercourse | Placental abruption |
| Trauma | Placenta previa |
| Varicose veins | Vasa previa |
| Vulvar/vaginal tears and lacerations | |
| Vaginal infections | |
| Foreign bodies | |
| Cervical polyp | |
| Cervical erosions | |
| Cervicitis | |
| Cervical carcinoma | |
| Hematuria | |

be minimal (e.g., spotting) or profuse. At initial evaluation, nonuterine and uterine causes can be diagnosed (Table 29–1). The three main known causes of antepartum uterine bleeding are abruptio placentae, placenta previa, and vasa previa. Unexplained antepartum uterine bleeding is a risk factor for poor outcome; at term, it is an indication for delivery. Midtrimester antepartum bleeding is a risk factor for abruptio placentae, placenta previa, late abortion, preterm delivery, and perinatal mortality.

## Abruptio Placentae

Premature separation of the normally implanted placenta from the uterine wall is called abruptio placentae. External bleeding, uterine hyperactivity, and fetal stress or distress are clinical findings indicating abruptio placentae. The incidence of abruptio placentae is 0.4 to 1.2%. Most cases occur before onset of labor. Variations in incidence are probably related to several factors (e.g., no uniform criteria for definition, variations in lower limit of gestational age in definition, recent recognition of milder forms of the disease, referral hospitals rather than treatment centers). A Swedish survey of nearly 850,000 births found 3959 (0.44%) cases of abruptio placentae.

### PERINATAL MORTALITY

The perinatal mortality associated with abruptio placentae is 20 to 35%. In the data of the National Hospital Discharge Survey (400 hospitals and 200,000 deliveries each year), stillbirths were 11 times more common among women with placental abruption, for a rate of 7.1%, with nearly 10% of all stillbirths occurring among women with abruptio placentae. In Washington State during 1980 and 1981, the stillbirth rate in pregnancies with abruptio placentae was 15.5%, and the combined perinatal mortality rate was 21%. Spinillo and associates found that moderate to severe abruptio placentae in infants of low birth weight is associated with increased risk of intraventricular hemorrhage, neonatal mortality, and subsequent cerebral palsy when compared with controls. Rate of normal outcome tended to decrease with increased severity of abruptio placentae.

### ETIOLOGY, RECURRENCE, CLASSIFICATION

The etiology of abruptio placentae is unknown in the majority of pregnancies. Occasionally, the etiology is obvious (e.g., direct abdominal trauma). Several risk factors are known to be associated with abruptio placentae (Table 29–2). Naeye and associates reviewed abruptio placentae in the Collaborative Perinatal Project of The National Institute of Neurological and Communicative Disorders and Stroke. They confirmed the importance of maternal hypertension and found that short umbilical cord, hydramnios, and abdominal trauma explain only a few cases. Ananth and associates conducted a meta-analysis of published studies on placental abruption and concluded that it is strongly associated with chronic hypertension, premature rupture of membranes (PROM), previous abruptio placentae, and pre-eclampsia. Maternal hypertension, vascular disease, and pre-eclampsia have the strongest association with abruptio placentae. The overall perinatal outcome of women experiencing abruptio placentae is not significantly different whether they are normotensive or hypertensive. External trauma is implicated in a small but increasingly important number of patients who have been involved in motor vehicle accidents, with maternal battering accounting for most of the cases. There is an association between cigarette smoking, cocaine abuse, or both and abruptio placentae.

The largest single study of placental abruption found a 10-fold increased risk from 0.4% in the first pregnancy with abruptio placentae to 4% in subsequent pregnancies. In a recent review of the world literature, the average recurrence risk was 10 to 15%. The reports had striking variation in the baseline and

**Table 29–2** Risk Factors— Abruptio Placentae

| | |
|---|---|
| Maternal hypertension | Uterine anomaly |
| Maternal vascular disease | Uterine tumors |
| Trauma | Preterm rupture of membranes |
| Parity | Chorioamnionitis |
| Sudden uterine decompression | External cephalic version |
| Cigarette smoking | Circumvallate placenta |
| Cocaine use | Maternal age |

Table 29–3  Abruptio Placentae Classification

| Grade | Features |
|---|---|
| 0 | No symptoms or signs diagnosed when placenta is examined after delivery. |
| 1 | External bleeding present. Uterine tetany and tenderness may or may not be present. No fetal distress. No shock. |
| 2 | External bleeding may or may not be present. Concealed hemorrhage is present. Uterine tetany and tenderness develop. Fetal distress is usually present. Fetal death in utero may occur. No maternal shock. |
| 3 | External bleeding usually is present. Marked uterine tetany. Fetal demise is present. Maternal shock is present. A coagulation defect may be present. |

recurrence risks of abruptio placentae. After a second pregnancy with abruption, there is a 25% recurrence rate. Subsequent episodes are usually more severe than the first.

The severity of abruptio placentae is most commonly classified according to clinical criteria (Table 29–3). The detachment may be complete or partial. In the latter instance, only the placental margin may be involved; this is referred to as marginal sinus bleeding or marginal sinus rupture. Concealed hemorrhage may be associated with retroplacental bleeding when margins are adherent.

## CLINICAL PRESENTATION AND DIAGNOSIS

In a prospective study, Hurd and associates found the following symptoms and signs at clinical presentation: vaginal bleeding (78%), uterine tenderness or back pain (66%), fetal distress (60%), high frequency of contractions (17%), uterine hypertonia (17%), preterm labor (22%), and fetal death (15%). Ultrasonographic confirmation of clinical diagnosis occurred in 1 of 59 (1.7%) cases. In another study, ultrasonographic confirmation by visualization of a blood clot occurred in 25% of cases with clinical placental abruption. In the few patients with concealed hemorrhage, evidence of retroplacental clot made the diagnosis. Absence of a clot on ultrasonography does not rule out abruption but ultrasonography can rule out placenta previa and is useful to confirm fetal death.

The amount and character of external vaginal bleeding or pain do not always correlate with the severity of the abruption. There are unsuspected or silent abruptions that are more common in posterior placentas. External bleeding may be profuse, but the separation of the placenta may not compromise the fetus. There may be no external bleeding with complete separation of the placenta and fetal death.

The presence of sharp pain of sudden onset usually indicates extravasation of blood into the myometrium. Other symptoms may be nausea, vomiting, restlessness, faintness, and decreased or absent fetal movement. Labor is the most common precipitating factor for placental separation, and nearly 50% of patients with abruptio placentae are in established labor at clinical presentation. With significant blood loss, signs of shock are present, for example, weak, thready pulse, tachycardia, pallor, and cold, clammy skin. In patients who have disseminated intravascular coagulation (DIC), there is an absence of clotting in vaginal blood. Diagnosis is made on clinical grounds and is usually focused on the triad of pain, bleeding, and uterine tonicity. Patients who have concealed hemorrhage often have uterine contractions that are unresponsive to tocolysis.

## DIFFERENTIAL DIAGNOSIS

The diagnosis of abruptio placentae is often made by exclusion of other causes of symptoms. The differential diagnoses of patients who have vaginal bleeding include placenta previa, labor, and vasa previa (see Table 29–1). Ultrasonography is helpful in excluding the diagnosis of placenta previa, and history and physical examination are helpful in excluding most other diagnoses. Presence or absence of pain or contractions is not always helpful. In patients with placenta previa, presence of labor may cause pain. Some patients have silent abruption, and many times the cause of bleeding is clarified only at delivery, or it may remain unclear even after delivery.

## PATHOLOGY

A firmly adherent retroplacental clot attached to the cotyledons in areas of hemorrhagic infarction and depression or disruption of the underlying placental tissue are hallmark findings in abruptio placentae. Most placental beds of patients with abruptio placentae show vascular malformations that may result from trophoblastic invasion and may be the site of vessel rupture.

The initial event is hemorrhage into the basal decidua from pathologically altered small arterial vessels. The hemorrhage splits the decidua, leaving a thin layer attached to the placenta. The decidual hematoma grows with further separation, compression, and obliteration of the intervillous space. There is destruction of the placental tissue in the area.

In some patients with abruptio placentae the process is self-limited, with no consequences to the pregnancy. In other patients, the bleeding continues. There may be continued dissection and separation in the decidua and extravasation into the myometrium through the peritoneal surface, resulting in a Couvelaire uterus. A Couvelaire uterus may be complicated by uterine atony.

## MANAGEMENT

Patients with suspected abruptio placentae are hospitalized. A rapid maternal and fetal evaluation is performed. Management is highly dependent on maternal and fetal status and gestational age.

**Mild Abruption.** In patients with mild abruption (grade 1), blood volume loss is greater than 15%, and vital signs and urine output are within normal limits. If the fetus is mature, delivery should be accomplished with induction or augmentation of labor as long as the mother and fetus are stable. In addition to the history and physical examination, the patient should have an ultrasonographic examination, and a large-bore intravenous line should be established. Blood for a complete blood (cell) count (CBC) level, with platelets, electrolytes, and fibrinogen is drawn. If the possibility of DIC is present, prothrombin time (PT), partial thromboplastin time (PTT), and fibrin degradation products are ordered. These do not change until after the fibrinogen level falls. If the fetus is immature, the mother and fetus are observed closely. If the mother has signs of preterm labor and is in stable condition with a normally developed fetus, no abnormalities are revealed by fetal heart rate (FHR) monitoring, and the gestational age is less than 34 weeks, the risks and benefits of betamethasone and tocolysis should be considered. In selected cases of minor abruption and extreme prematurity, tocolysis with magnesium sulfate may be appropriate. In most patients with abruptio placentae, tocolysis is of no value. If the patient is not in labor with an immature fetus, she is observed as an inpatient and later evaluated for ambulatory follow-up.

**Moderate Abruption.** Patients with moderate abruption (grade 2) have mild to moderate vaginal bleeding. Maternal tachycardia is common, along with slight uterine tenderness and an irritable or tetanic uterus. Typically, fetal distress either is present or may develop during labor, but the patient does not have maternal shock.

Once the diagnosis is established, baseline laboratory testing (CBC, platelets, electrolytes, and fibrinogen) results are obtained and cardiovascular resuscitation is under way. The method of delivery should be planned. Usually fetal distress is present and delivery is by cesarean section. If the FHR is reassuring and there is uterine relaxation between contractions, vaginal delivery may be attempted. Amniotomy is helpful, and oxytocin augmentation may be necessary. Amniotomy may reduce extravasation of blood into the myometrium and stimulate labor; it also allows placement of a fetal scalp electrode, and an intrauterine pressure catheter. Cesarean delivery should be performed for signs of fetal distress or for uterine hypertonia during labor. Very few patients with moderate abruption (i.e., a very immature and stable fetus and stable mother) could be considered for transfusions and conservative management.

**Severe Abruption.** Patients with severe abruption have moderate to severe bleeding, marked uterine tenderness, tetany, and unstable vital signs, with tachycardia, tachypnea, and orthostatic changes.

The mother is typed and crossmatched for four units of packed red blood cells. The mother has an indwelling Foley catheter for accurate assessment of urine output. Maternal vital signs, urine output, laboratory values, and clotting parameters are followed on a flow sheet.

**Live Fetus.** Plans should be made for a cesarean delivery unless special circumstances are present (e.g., previable fetus, maternal shock, or both). When the mother is stable and blood products are being infused, a cesarean delivery should be performed. In circumstances of relatively slow rate of blood loss, management is influenced by fetal status. When there is massive external bleeding necessitating intensive resuscitation with electrolyte solutions and blood products, rapid delivery is necessary for maternal and fetal indications.

**Dead Fetus.** The mother usually has significant risk of hypovolemia and consumptive coagulopathy (30%). It is critical to provide adequate fluid and blood replacement therapy before delivery. Vaginal delivery is preferred, unless there are contraindications or maternal hemorrhage cannot be managed with vigorous blood replacement. Adequate amounts of blood and crystalloids are given to achieve a hematocrit (HCT) of more than 30, and urine output of more than 30 ml/hr. Coagulopathy should be treated. If necessary, a Swan-Ganz catheter and arterial lines may be placed for hemodynamic monitoring.

## CONSUMPTIVE COAGULOPATHY

Infusion of thrombin-rich decidual tissue into the maternal circulation can result in DIC. Intravascular fibrinogen is converted to fibrin by activation of the extrinsic clotting cascade.

Significant coagulopathy is encountered in only 10% of cases of abruption, but it is much more common (30%) in severe abruption marked by massive hemorrhage or fetal death. Serious coagulopathy is usually evident by the time a symptomatic woman seeks care.

Screening for clinically significant coagulopathy is effected either by observing clot formation in a 5-ml clot tube without added anticoagulant or by performing laboratory measurement of fibrinogen concentrations. If the blood fails to clot within 6 minutes, a very marked coagulopathy is present, and the usual coagulation studies are grossly abnormal. If there is no clotting, an order for blood replacement products (cryoprecipitate and fresh frozen plasma) need not await confirmatory test results.

Fibrinogen depletion is the predictable consequence. Normal maternal fibrinogen concentration is 450 mg/dl. With fibrinogen levels lower than 300 mg/dl, significant coagulation is usually present, and patients usually require blood transfusions for maintenance of adequate circulating volume. When the fibrinogen level is less than 150 mg/dl the patient has lost approximately 30% of blood volume. In 30% of women with placental abruption severe enough to kill the fetus, there is overt hypofibrinogenemia—less than 150 mg/dl of plasma. Decreased plasma fibrinogen is present together with elevated levels of fibrinogen-fibrin degradation products, D-dimer concentration, and decreases in other coagulation factors.

Management of severe coagulopathy is controversial, but the mainstay of therapy is restoration of blood volume and coagulation status. Fresh frozen plasma, cryoprecipitate, or both are useful in replacing fibrinogen and clotting factors, especially if cesarean section or an episiotomy is performed. The goal is to achieve a fibrinogen level over 125 mg/dl. Platelet transfusions may be needed before performance of cesarean delivery. Vaginal delivery without episiotomy may be performed even with very low levels of clotting factors. The ultimate treatment of abruptio placentae complicated by DIC is delivery of the fetus and placenta. Spontaneous resolution of the coagulopathy occurs after delivery. Fibrinogen levels rise faster than platelet count. Initial management must be geared toward replacing lost blood volume and lost or consumed clotting factors. Such replacement may fuel further DIC and fibrinolysis, but it is necessary until the uterus is emptied.

## Placenta Previa

### DEFINITION

Placenta previa is an abnormal location of the placenta in close proximity to the internal cervical os. The placenta develops within the zone of dilatation and effacement of the low segment, enabling the placenta to precede the fetus at delivery. There are four categories of placenta previa:
1. Total—the entire internal cervical os is covered by placenta
2. Partial—the internal cervical os is partially covered by placenta
3. Marginal—the edge of the placenta lies adjacent to the internal os of the cervix
4. Low-lying—the placenta is located very near, but not directly adjacent to, the internal os

### ETIOLOGY

Abnormal vascularization has been proposed as a mechanism for abnormal placentation. Risk factors for placenta previa include increased age, parity, previous induced abortion, previous cesarean delivery, black race, smoking, cocaine use, large placenta (e.g., multiple pregnancies, erythroblastosis), endometritis, and congenital malformation.

The most important obstetric risk factor for placenta previa is previous cesarean delivery. Nielsen and associates in a study of nearly 25,000 deliveries found a fivefold increased incidence of placenta previa in women with previous cesarean delivery. Miller and associates found a threefold increased risk of placenta previa in a study of 150,000 pregnancies with previous cesarean delivery. In a review by Ananth and associates of 36 studies identifying 3.7 million pregnant women, of whom 13,992 patients had placenta previa, women who had at least one previous cesarean delivery were at 2.6 times greater risk for development of placenta previa in subsequent pregnancies. The risk increased with the number of previous cesarean deliveries.

### INCIDENCE

The incidence of clinically evident placenta previa at delivery is between 0.28% and 2.0%, or approximately 1 in 200 deliveries. A large series reports 0.3% to 0.5%.

Incidence of placenta previa is affected by gestational age at time of diagnosis. In midtrimester, the incidence is 5.3%. By term, at least 90% of these cases convert to a normal placental location, giving rise to the concept of placental migration. Placentas that do not cover the internal os in the second or early third trimester have a low likelihood of persistence of placenta previa at term. If an ultrasonogram demonstrates placenta previa beyond 28 weeks, it has a high likelihood of persistence. Recurrence rate of placenta previa is 4 to 8%.

## CLINICAL PRESENTATION

Vaginal bleeding is the most common symptom and is usually painless. Up to 70% of pregnancies with placenta previa demonstrate painless vaginal bleeding, and 20% have uterine activity with vaginal bleeding. The average gestational age at the time of the first bleeding episode is 29 to 30 weeks. The peak incidence is at 34 weeks of gestation. The bleeding may be substantial, but it almost always ceases spontaneously. Maternal death in the first bleeding episode is very rare. The bleeding results from separation of part of the placenta from the lower uterine segment and the cervix. It may be a result of uterine activity. The bleeding occurs suddenly without warning, and it is maternal in origin. In pregnancies with low-lying placenta, the bleeding occurs only at the onset of labor.

There is an increased rate of abnormal fetal presentation in the presence of placenta previa. Most transverse lies are associated with placenta previa.

## DIAGNOSIS

The diagnosis is based on ultrasonographic demonstration of placental location relative to the internal cervical os. Transabdominal ultrasonography provides 93 to 97% accuracy. Overdistention of the urinary bladder, myometrial contractions, uterine fibroids, blood clots, late placental migration, and a posterior placental location are causes of diagnostic errors. Transvaginal sonography, which improves diagnostic accuracy, can be conducted safely with no risk of bleeding and transperineal sonography gives excellent diagnostic results. In a small number of patients, a double set up examination for delivery may be necessary for definitive diagnosis.

## MANAGEMENT

The management of pregnancies with vaginal bleeding resulting from placenta previa includes hospitalization, hemodynamic stabilization, and expectant management until fetal maturity occurs. After initial hospitalization with bed rest, care as an outpatient is considered if the patient is motivated, can comply with restriction of activity, has assistance, and has emergency transportation. Expectant management, combined with blood transfusion and cesarean delivery, has reduced maternal and perinatal mortality. Maternal mortality as a consequence of placenta previa has dropped from 5% to 0.1% with the introduction of conservative management. The degree of bleeding and fetal lung maturity are the most important considerations in management. When bleeding is severe, the patient is resuscitated with Ringer's lactated solution administered intravenously, blood replacement, and, if necessary, fresh frozen plasma, platelets, and cryoprecipitate. Urine output and measurements from a Swan-Ganz catheter may help in fluid management. Delivery is by cesarean section.

When bleeding is moderate and the acute episode subsides, gestational age and pulmonary maturity are important considerations. Term pregnancies with placenta previa that never had vaginal bleeding should be delivered by elective cesarean section. In pregnancies more advanced than 36 weeks of gestation with uterine activity, persistent bleeding, and diagnosis of placenta previa, cesarean delivery is preferred after resuscitation has been begun. Perinatal mortality is directly related to gestational age at delivery. Most episodes of bleeding in pregnancies with placenta previa are self-limited and not fatal to mother or fetus in the absence of labor. Most women who have placenta previa and preterm vaginal bleeding are treated expectantly with an aggressive approach. However, 20% of women with placenta previa are delivered earlier than 32 weeks of gestation. It is prudent to check pulmonary maturity and perform cesarean delivery if there is a moderate amount of vaginal bleeding and if gestational age is between 33 and 36 weeks. If there is heavy persistent vaginal bleeding, delivery is performed after stabilization of the patient. Pregnancies that are less than 32 weeks and accompanied by moderate bleeding that has stopped are observed; tocolysis with magnesium sulfate may be used for uterine irritability, and steroids are given if there are no contraindications. Rh-immunoglobulin should be given to all at-risk patients with third trimester bleeding who are Rh-negative and not sensitized. A Kleihauer-Betke test to detect fetomaternal hemorrhage greater than 30 ml should be performed on Rh-negative women. Antepartum expectant management is appropriate for the majority of preterm gestations. In selected preterm patients with placenta previa who are hospitalized for vaginal bleeding that has ceased, there seems to be no benefit to inpatient rather than outpatient management.

# Placenta Accreta

Placenta accreta is characterized by invasive placental implantation with abnormally firm adherence to the uterine wall. In placenta previa accreta, the poorly formed decidua of the lower uterine segment offers little resistance to trophoblastic invasion. The degree of myometrial invasion distinguishes placenta accreta (placental villi are attached to the myometrium) from placenta increta (villi invade the myometrium) and placenta percreta (villi penetrate the entire myometrial wall). Uterine wall scar from prior cesarean section, as well as other uterine surgery, is the most important risk factor associated with placenta accreta. Incidence of placenta accreta is 4% in pregnancies with placenta previa and no previous cesarean delivery, and 10 to 35% in pregnancies with placenta previa and previous cesarean deliveries. Most patients with placenta previa and placenta accreta require hysterectomy. In some cases, placenta accreta may be managed successfully by placing interrupted sutures through and through in a circular pattern surrounding the bleeding implantation site. Placenta accreta has been diagnosed prenatally with ultrasonography and magnetic resonance imaging. Angiographically guided selective embolization may be used before surgical treatment in clinical settings of postpartum and post cesarean hemorrhage. The therapy is relatively noninvasive, highly effective, and underutilized. An intra-arterial catheter may be placed prophylactically in the preoperative period in patients with placenta previa and suspected placenta accreta who are undergoing cesarean delivery. It is placed with stable coagulation indices and may theoretically reduce the risk of maternal morbidity or mortality.

## Vasa Previa

In vasa previa, the umbilical cord inserts into the membranes of the placenta rather than into the central mass of the placental tissue. Fetal vessels cross the membranes beneath the presenting part of the fetus, adjacent to the internal os of the cervix. If one of the vessels ruptures, fetal bleeding occurs. Vasa previa is primarily associated with velamentous insertion of the umbilical cord or vessels into a succenturiate lobe of the placenta. Because of the low blood volume of the fetus, a seemingly insignificant amount of blood loss may place the fetus in jeopardy.

Bleeding caused by vasa previa is a fetal obstetric emergency. Rupture of the membranes before delivery may cause disruption of the blood vessels and fetal hemorrhage. This is a rare event, occurring in 0.1 to 1.8% of all pregnancies, with a true incidence closer to 0.1%. The incidence is much higher in twins (6 to 10%) compared with that in singletons (0.25%). The hemorrhage is small and usually occurs after spontaneous rupture of membranes. Sudden FHR changes (tachycardia followed by bradycardia) occurring with hemorrhage must raise a high index of suspicion. A diagnosis must be made rapidly, and immediate cesarean delivery is the only option available. There is not always enough time to confirm the clinical diagnosis by detecting fetal red cells with the aminophenylthioether (APT) test. In the APT test, one part of bloody vaginal fluid is mixed with 5 to 10 parts of tap water. The mixture is centrifuged for 2 minutes, and the supernatant must be pink in color to proceed. Five parts of supernatant are then mixed with one part of 1% sodium hydroxide (NaOH) and centrifuged for 2 minutes. A pink color indicates fetal blood; whereas a yellow-brown color indicates maternal blood. The APT test distinguishes fetal blood from maternal blood on the basis of marked resistance to pH changes in fetal red cells compared with the friable nature of adult red cells in the presence of a strong base (NaOH). Perinatal mortality is very high (50%) in vasa previa resulting from a tear or rupture with fetal exsanguination. In addition to the APT test, examination of the blood for nucleated red blood cells (RBCs), electrophoresis, or both may help in the diagnosis. Abnormalities in FHR are common with sinusoidal pattern, tachycardia, and late or prolonged decelerations. Emergency cesarean delivery is the appropriate treatment.

## Postpartum Hemorrhage

### DEFINITION, INCIDENCE, ETIOLOGY

There is no universally accepted definition of postpartum hemorrhage. Traditionally, blood loss of more than 500 ml after vaginal delivery was defined as postpartum hemorrhage. It is defined in the American College of Obstetrics and Gynecology (ACOG) Educational Bulletin as a decrease of 10 points or more in HCT level between admission and the postpartum period, or a need for erythrocyte transfusion. A decrease of 10 points or more corresponded to the 97th percentile of HCT change in vaginal deliveries and the 92nd percentile in cesarean deliveries. The mean postpartum decrease in HCT level was 2.6% ± 4.3% in vaginal deliveries, and 4.0% ± 4.2% in cesarean deliveries. Vaginal delivery has been associated with a 3.9% incidence and cesarean delivery with a 6.4% incidence of postpartum hemorrhage. One third of vaginal deliveries had no decline or an increase in HCT level, and 20% had no decline after cesarean delivery. Early postpartum hemorrhage occurs during the first 24 hours after delivery. Late postpartum hemorrhage occurs after the first 24 hours but before 6 weeks postpartum. Early postpartum hemorrhage is caused by excessive bleeding from the placental implantation site (uterine atony, retained placental tissue, placenta accreta) or trauma to the genital tract (lacerations, extensions of episiotomy, ruptured uterus, uterine inversion, hereditary coagulopathies). Late postpartum hemorrhage is much less common than early postpartum hemorrhage and it is caused by excessive bleeding from the placental implantation site (subinvolution, retained placental tissue), endometritis, and hereditary coagulopathy. In women who deliver vaginally, risk factors for postpartum hemorrhage include prolonged third stage of labor, preeclampsia, episiotomy, uterine overdistention (hydramnios, multiple gestation), use of oxytocin, preterm and post-term delivery, abnormal labor (very rapid or prolonged), high parity, use of uterine relaxing agents (terbutaline, magnesium sulfate, halogenated anesthetic agents, nitroglycerin), chorioamnionitis, previous postpartum hemorrhage, conduction anesthesia, soft tissue lacerations, instrumental vaginal delivery, obesity, and Asian or Hispanic ethnicity. Risk factors for hemorrhage after cesarean delivery include classic uterine incision, chorioamnionitis, preeclampsia, abnormal labor, and use of general anesthesia.

## PROTRACTED THIRD STAGE OF LABOR

In over 12,000 singleton vaginal deliveries without manual removal of the placenta, the median third stage duration was 6 minutes, with 3.3% lasting more than 30 minutes. Several measures of postpartum hemorrhage are blood loss greater than 500 ml, change in HCT level greater or equal to 10%, dilatation and curettage (D&C), transfusions, and third stage of labor longer than 30 minutes. The duration of the third stage of labor is prolonged in preterm deliveries. In a retrospective analysis of over 45,000 singleton deliveries of greater than or equal to 20 weeks of gestation, Dombrowski and associates found that the duration of the third stage of labor and the frequencies of hemorrhage and manual removal of placentas decreased with increasing gestational age. The frequency of retained placentas was markedly increased among gestations less than or equal to 26 weeks (25.4%) compared with that of term gestations (1.6%). Manual removal of placentas shortened the duration of the third stage of labor.

## MANAGEMENT

Recognizing risk factors for postpartum hemorrhage after vaginal or cesarean birth and applying proven methods to limit blood loss after delivery can prevent some cases of postpartum hemorrhage. A randomized trial comparing active management and expectant management of the third stage of labor found that active management reduced the incidence of postpartum hemorrhage and shortened the third stage of labor. Active management included prophylactic administration of oxytocin, cord clamping within 30 seconds of delivery, and gentle cord traction. Patients at significant risk for postpartum hemorrhage should have adequate intravenous access and blood sent for HCT and type and screen.

Fortunately, the major risk factors for postpartum hemorrhage are known and the causes are few. When hemorrhage occurs after vaginal delivery, concurrent steps should be taken to evaluate and treat the patient. The etiology of the bleeding is determined by a physical examination, including uterine palpation to rule out atony, inspection of the lower genital tract for laceration, and inspection of the placenta. Manual or instrumental curettage, or both, are used to remove retained placenta. Sometimes bleeding may have several causes (e.g., both atony and trauma). Initial management includes documentation of vital signs, administration of supplemental oxygen, placement of a urinary catheter, and initial laboratory tests (CBC, platelet concentration, type and screen; fibrinogen, fibrinogen split products [FSP], PT, PTT). Pulmonary artery catheterization is not usually indicated.

## UTERINE ATONY

Risk factors for uterine atony include advanced maternal age, high parity, use of oxytocin or uterine relaxing agents in labor, macrosomia, chorioamnionitis, prolonged third stage of labor, and uterine overdistention. In most pregnancies with intractable uterine atony, known risk factors can be identified and the problem should be anticipated. Atony is initially managed by bimanual uterine massage and compression, which may involve prolonged periods of intermittent uterine massage and observation. Medical treatment starts with intravenous oxytocin (40 U/L with rapid infusion). The patient also receives rapid crystalloid infusion and blood products are ordered. Methylergonovine (0.2 mg intramuscularly) may be used to stimulate uterine contractility, but it is contraindicated in the presence of hypertension and is not known to be superior to oxytocin. Today, with the availability of highly effective prostaglandin, the use of ergonovine is less frequent. If initial treatment with uterine massage and oxytocin, ergonovine, or both are unsuccessful, synthetic prostaglandin derivatives—15-methyl-prostaglandin $F_{2\alpha}$ ($PGF_{2\alpha}$) (carboprost tromethamine)—should be useful. In a multicenter study by Oleen and Mariano, prostaglandin derivatives have been shown to have a very high success rate when used alone (88%) or in combination (95%) with oxytocin agents; the 12 (5%) women in whom drug treatment failed required surgical intervention. 15-methyl-$PGF_{2\alpha}$ is usually given intramuscularly, 0.25 mg, every 15 to 90 minutes, not to exceed 8 doses. It may be given directly into the myometrium (transabdominally or transvaginally), but it is not clear that route of administration is important. 15-methyl-PGF$_{2\alpha}$ has side effects (e.g., diarrhea, hypertension, vomiting, fever, flushing, and tachycardia), few women develop hypotension, and it is associated with pulmonary airway and vascular constriction that may cause oxygen desaturation. Prostaglandin E$_2$ (PGE$_2$), 20 mg suppository, is useful in patients who have heart or lung disease and in whom 15-methyl-PGF$_{2\alpha}$ is contraindicated. PGF$_{2\alpha}$ is usually preferable, since PGE$_2$ may cause vasodilatation and exacerbation of hypotension. In most patients who have uterine atony, only uterine massage and oxytocin agents are necessary. Blood transfusions are usually necessary when uterine massage, oxytocin, and prostaglandins fail to control the bleeding. However, it is not uncommon for a patient to experience intermittent atony that requires repeated uterine massage and pharmacologic intervention. If medical therapy for uterine atony fails, re-evaluation for lacerations and retained placental tissue, as well as exploratory laparotomy, should be considered.

If bleeding persists, the patient should have two large-bore intravenous lines inserted, and she will probably need packed RBC transfusions and manual exploration of the uterine cavity. Uterine curettage is performed for removal of suspected retained placental tissue. If the uterine bleeding is not responsive to medical therapy, no placental fragments are present in the uterus, and there are no vulvar, vaginal, or cervical lacerations, surgical exploration is necessary.

Uterine artery ligation (ascending branches of the uterine arteries) at the level of the vesicouterine peritoneal reflection is useful for hemorrhage secondary to atony. If necessary, the blood flow to the uterus from the infundibulopelvic ligament is interrupted by ligation of the anastomosis of the ovarian and uterine arteries, located high on the fundus, just below the utero-ovarian ligament. Several uncontrolled series had 25 to 60% success rates in attempts to employ bilateral internal iliac artery ligation for control of otherwise intractable postpartum hemorrhage and for avoidance of hysterectomy. Ureteral injury, blood loss, and operative cardiac arrest caused by blood loss were increased in pregnancies in which patients underwent bilateral internal iliac ligation when compared with patients who underwent emergency hysterectomy. Bilateral internal iliac (hypogastric) artery ligation is technically more difficult and is reserved for hemodynamically stable patients of low parity for whom future childbearing is of paramount importance.

Hysterectomy is a life-saving procedure in patients who have postpartum hemorrhage when other treatments are unsuccessful. Most common indications for hysterectomy in pregnancies with postpartum hemorrhage are uterine atony, placenta accreta, and uterine rupture.

Logothetopulos described a pelvic pressure pack as a tamponade for persistent posthysterectomy hemorrhage. Several reports of modified pelvic packs suggest this technique for uncontrolled obstetric hemorrhage after hysterectomy, with or without bilateral internal iliac ligation. The mushroom-shaped pack is placed in the pelvis and brought out through the vagina by means of traction. The pack is removed 24 to 48 hours later.

Selective embolization with small particles of Gelfoam is effective in controlling postpartum, postcesarean, and posthysterectomy hemorrhaging. Bilateral internal iliac ligation reduces access for arterial embolization. The need for skilled interventional radiologists and the requirement of transferring the bleeding patient to the radiology suite make this technique less useful. This is particularly a problem in the acutely hemorrhaging postpartum patient. In pregnancies with placenta previa and antepartum placenta accreta (detected ultrasonographically), the prophylactic preoperative placement of an intra-arterial catheter may be appropriate.

## REFERENCES

Abdella TN, Sibai BM, Hayes JM, et al: Perinatal outcome in abruptio placentae. Obstet Gynecol 63:365, 1984.

Ajayi RA, Soothill PW, Campbell S, et al: Antenatal testing to predict outcome in pregnancies with unexplained antepartum haemorrhage. Br J Obstet Gynaecol 99:122, 1992.

Alvarez M, Lockwood CJ, Ghidini A, et al: Prophylactic and emergent arterial catheterization for selective embolization in obstetric hemorrhage. Am J Perinatol 9:441, 1992.

American College of Obstetricians and Gynecologists: Diagnosis and Management of Postpartum Hemorrhage. ACOG Educational Bulletin No. 143. Washington, DC, ACOG, 1990.

American College of Obstetricians and Gynecologists. Postpartum Hemorrhage. ACOG Educational Bulletin No. 243. Washington, DC, ACOG, 1998.

Ananth CV, Savitz DA, Williams MA: Placental abruption and its association with hypertension and prolonged rupture of membranes: A methodologic review and meta-analysis. Obstet Gynecol 88:309, 1996.

Ananth CV, Smulian JC, Vintzileos AM: The association of placenta previa with history of cesarean delivery and abortion: A meta-analysis. Am J Obstet Gynecol 177:1071, 1997.

Baker R: Evaluation and management of critically ill patients. Obstet Gynecol Annu 6:295, 1977.

Benedetti TJ: Obstetric hemorrhage. *In* Gabbe SG, Niebyl JR, Simpson JE (eds): Obstetrics. Normal & Problem Pregnancies, 3rd ed. New York, Churchill Livingstone, 1996, pp 499–529.

Bowie JD, Rochester D, Cadkin AV, et al: Accuracy of placental localization by ultrasound. Radiology 128:177, 1978.

Cho JY, Kim SJ, Cha KY, et al: Interrupted circular suture: Bleeding control during cesarean delivery in placenta previa accreta. Obstet Gynecol 78:876, 1991.

Chou MM, Ho ES: Prenatal diagnosis of placenta previa accreta with power amplitude ultrasonic angiography. Am J Obstet Gynecol 177:1523, 1997.

Clark SL, Koonings PP, Phelan JP: Placenta previa/accreta and prior cesarean section. Obstet Gynecol 66:89, 1985.

Clark SL, Phelan JP, Yeh SY: Hypogastric artery ligation for obstetric hemorrhage. Obstet Gynecol 66:353, 1985.

Clark SL, Yeh SY, Phelan JP, et al: Emergency hysterectomy for obstetric hemorrhage. Obstet Gynecol 64:376, 1984.

Combs CA, Laros RK: Prolonged third stage of labor: Morbidity and risk factors. Obstet Gynecol 77:863, 1991.

Combs CA, Murphy EL, Laros RKL Jr: Factors associated with hemorrhage in cesarean deliveries. Obstet Gynecol 77:77, 1991.

Combs CA, Murphy EL, Laros RKL Jr: Factors associated with postpartum hemorrhage with vaginal birth. Obstet Gynecol 77:69, 1991.

Comeau J, Shaw L, Marcell C, et al: Early placenta previa and delivery outcome. Obstet Gynecol 61:577, 1983.

Cotton D, Ead J, Paul R, et al: The conservative aggressive management of placenta previa. Am J Obstet Gynecol 17:687, 1980.

Cunningham FG, MacDonald PC, Gant NF, et al (eds): Williams Obstetrics, 20th ed. Stamford, Connecticut, Appleton & Lange, 1997, pp 745–782.

Dombrowski MP, Bottoms SF, Saleh AA, et al: Third stage of labor: Analysis of duration and clinical practice. Am J Obstet Gynecol 172:1729, 1995.

Dombrowski MP, Wolfe HM, Welch RA, et al: Cocaine abuse is associated with abruptio placentae and decreased birth weight, but not shorter labor. Obstet Gynecol 77:139, 1991.

Dommisse J, Tiltman A: Placental bed biopsies in placental abruption. Br J Obstet Gynaecol 99:651, 1992.

Drost S, Keil K: Expectant management of placenta previa: Cost-benefit analysis of outpatient treatment. Am J Obstet Gynecol 170:1254, 1994.

Farine D, Fox HE, Jakobson S, et al: Vaginal ultrasound for diagnosis of placenta previa. Am J Obstet Gynecol 159:566, 1988.

Finberg H, Williams J: Placenta accreta: Prospective sonographic diagnosis in patients with placenta previa and prior cesarean section. J Ultrasound Med 11:333, 1992.

Hallak M, Dildy GA III, Hurley TJ, et al: Transvaginal pressure pack for life-threatening pelvic hemorrhage secondary to placenta accreta. Obstet Gynecol 78:938, 1991.

Hankins GDV, Berryman GK, Scott RT Jr, et al: Maternal arterial desaturation with 15-methyl prostaglandin $F_2$ alpha for uterine atony. Obstet Gynecol 72:367, 1988.

Hankins GDV, Clark SL, Cunningham FG, et al (eds): Operative Obstetrics, 1st ed. Norwalk, Connecticut: Appleton & Lange, 1995, pp 475–492.

Heppard MCS, Garite TJ: Antepartum hemorrhage. In Heppard MCS, Garite TJ (eds): Acute Obstetrics: A Practical Guide. St. Louis, Mosby-Year Book, 1992, pp 151–174.

Hertzberg BS, Bowie JD, Carroll BA, et al: Diagnosis of placenta previa during the third trimester. Role of transperineal sonography. AJR 159:83, 1992.

Hurd WW, Miodovnik M, Hertzberg V, et al: Selective management of abruptio placentae: A prospective study. Obstet Gynecol 61:467, 1983.

Iyasu S, Saftlas AK, Rowley DL, et al: The epidemiology of placenta previa in the United States. 1979 through 1987. Am J Obstet Gynecol 168:1424, 1993.

Karegaard M, Gennser G: Incidence and recurrence rate of abruptio placentae in Sweden. Obstet Gynecol 67:523, 1986.

Kaunitz AM, Hughs JM, Grimes DA, et al: Causes of maternal mortality in the United States. Obstet Gynecol 65:605, 1985.

King DL: Placental migration demonstrated by ultrasonography. Radiology 109:167, 1973.

Knab DR: Abruptio placentae: An assessment of the time and method of delivery. Obstet Gynecol 52:625, 1978.

Konje JC, Walley RJ: Bleeding in late pregnancy. In James DK, Steer PJ, Weiner CP, et al (eds): High Risk Pregnancy: Management Options. Philadelphia, WB Saunders, 1984, pp 119–136.

Krohn M, Voigt L, McKnight B, et al: Correlates of placental abruption. Br J Obstet Gynaecol 94:333, 1987.

Leetentveld RA, Gilberts ECAM, Arnold MJCWJ, et al: Accuracy and safety of transvaginal sonographic placental localization. Obstet Gynecol 76:759, 1990.

Lipitz S, Admon D, Menczer J, et al: Midtrimester bleeding: Variables which affect the outcome of pregnancy. Gynecol Obstet Invest 32:24, 1991.

Logothetopulos K: Eine absolut sichere blutstillungsmethode bei vaginalen und abdominalen gynakologischen operationen. Zentralbl Gynakol 50:3202, 1926.

Miller DA, Diaz FG, Paul RH: Incidence of placenta previa with previous cesarean. Am J Obstet Gynecol 174:345, 1996.

Morgan MA, Berkowitz KM, Thomas SJ, et al: Abruptio placentae: Perinatal outcome in normotensive and hypertensive patients. Am J Obstet Gynecol 170:1595, 1994.

Mouer JR: Placenta previa: Antepartum conservative management, inpatient versus outpatient. Am J Obstet Gynecol 170:1683, 1994.

Naeye RL: Abruptio placentae and placenta previa: Frequency, perinatal mortality, and cigarette smoking. Obstet Gynecol 55:701, 1980.

Naeye R, Harkness W, Utts J: Abruptio placentae and perinatal death: A prospective study. Am J Obstet Gynecol 128:740, 1977.

Nielsen TF, Hagberg H, Ljungblad U: Placenta previa and antepartum hemorrhage after previous cesarean section. Gynecol Obstet Invest 27:88, 1989.

Notelovitz M, Bottoms SF, Dase DF, et al: Painless abruptio placentae. Obstet Gynecol 53:270, 1979.

O'Leary JA: Stop of hemorrhage with uterine artery ligation. Contemp Ob/Gyn 28:13, 1996.

Oleen MA, Mariano JP: Controlling refractory atonic postpartum hemorrhage with Hemabate sterile solution. Am J Obstet Gynecol 162:205, 1990.

Page EW, King EB, Merrill JA: Abruptio placentae: Dangers of delay in delivery. Obstet Gynecol 3:385, 1954.

Prendiville WJ, Harding JE, Elbourne DR, et al: The Bristol third stage trial: Active versus physiological management of third stage of labour. BMJ 297:1295, 1988.

Pritchard JA, Brekken AL: Clinical and laboratory studies on severe abruptio placentae. Am J Obstet Gynecol 97:681, 1967.

Pritchard JA, Cunningham FG, Pritchard SA, et al: On reducing the frequency of severe abruptio placentae. Am J Obstet Gynecol 165:1345, 1991.

Rizos N, Doran TA, Miskin M, et al: Natural history of placenta previa ascertained by diagnostic ultrasound. Am J Obstet Gynecol 133:287, 1979.

Rochat RW, Loonin LM, Atrash HK, et al: Maternal mortality collaborative: Maternal mortality in the United States: Report from the Maternal Mortality Collaborative. Obstet Gynecol 72:91, 1988.

Sachs BP, Brown DAJ, Driscoll SG, et al: Hemorrhage, infection, toxemia, and cardiac disease, 1954–85: Causes for their declining role in maternal mortality. Am J Public Health 78:671, 1988.

Saftlas AF, Olson DR, Atrash HK, et al: National trends in the incidence of abruptio placentae. 1979–1987. Obstet Gynecol 78:1081, 1991.

Sanderson DA, Milton PJD: The effectiveness of ultrasound screening at 18–20 weeks' gestational age for prediction of placenta previa. J Obstet Gynaecol 11:320, 1991.

Sholl JS: Abruptio placentae: Clinical management in nonacute cases. Am J Obstet Gynecol 156:40, 1987.

Slutsker L: Risks associated with cocaine use during pregnancy. Obstet Gynecol 79:778, 1992.

Smith RS, Lauria MR, Comstock CH, et al: Transvaginal ultrasonography for all placentas that appear to be low-lying or over the internal cervical os. Ultrasound in Obstet Gynecol 9:22, 1991.

Spinillo A, Fazzi E, Stronati E, et al: Severity of abruptio placentae and neurodevelopmental outcome in low birth weight infants. Early Hum Dev 35:44, 1993.

Stones RW, Paterson CM, Saunders NJ: Risk factors for major obstetric hemorrhage. Eur J Obstet Gynecol Reprod Biol 48:15, 1993.

Thorp JM Jr, Councell RB, Sandridge DA: Antepartum diagnosis of placenta previa percreta by magnetic resonance imaging. Case reports. Obstet Gynecol 80:506, 1991.

Townsend RR, Laing FC, Jeffrey RB: Placental abruption associated with cocaine abuse. AJR 150:1339, 1988.

Vendantham S, Goodwin SC, McLucas B, et al: Uterine artery embolization: An underused method of controlling pelvic hemorrhage. Am J Obstet Gynecol 176:938, 1997.

Voigt LF, Hollenbach KA, Krohn MA, et al: The relationship of abruptio placentae with maternal smoking and small for gestational age infants. Obstet Gynecol 75:771, 1990.

Williams MA, Lieberman E, Mittendorf R, et al: Risk factors for abruptio placentae. Am J Epidemiol 134:965, 1991.

Wing DA, Paul RH, Millar LK: Management of symptomatic placenta previa: A randomized, controlled trial of inpatient versus outpatient expectant management. Am J Obstet Gynecol 174:305, 1996.

# 30

# Postpartum Management

ROBERT H. HAYASHI
MARY ANN ZETTELMAIER

Assessment of the mother and her newborn during the postpartum period is important to ensure the appropriate and uneventful transition to normal physiologic functioning and successful psychological adjustment to birth and motherhood. A woman is routinely evaluated on two occasions in the postpartum period: while she is still in the hospital or at home 2 or 3 days later for those in an early discharge program, and during the follow-up office visit, usually at 6 weeks post partum. Thorough assessment and instruction should be provided to the new mother, and these may help to identify abnormal events quickly. Most dysfunctions that occur in the postpartum period can be managed successfully if they are identified and treated early.

The purpose of this chapter is to describe contemporary concepts regarding the postpartum period and efficient methods of caring for the postpartum woman and her newborn (from the obstetrician's perspective). We will first discuss general principles and concepts of postpartum care as formulated by the health-care team. These are divided into early and late postpartum periods. The last portion of this chapter will be directed toward more specific postpartum management by the physician.

## Early Postpartum Period

Giving the most efficient care for the postpartum period requires a coordinated effort by the physician and nurse care providers, to educate the patient and offer support targeted to the early postpartum period. Because of shortened hospital stays, this process necessarily begins in the prenatal period during the third-trimester prenatal visits. In the past, when hospital stays were longer, thorough education could be provided before discharge, either at the bedside or through postpartum classes taught by nurses over several days. Now, postpartum education is primarily conveyed by assessment and validation of parental competence in self- and infant care in preparation for discharge, usually within the first 24 to 48 hours after delivery. Therefore, the majority of teaching and information transfer must take place in the prenatal period. This is most efficiently accomplished by identifying and sequencing critical components, so that nurses can work with patients to achieve identified goals in an appropriate time frame. A checklist of topics, competencies, and skills facilitates the educational process and helps focus the patient on mastery. An example of such a checklist is presented in Table 30–1.

Some topics are best covered in group class sessions, such as breastfeeding, baby care, and self-care. Additionally, time is well spent in the late prenatal period reviewing what to expect during the inpatient experience, for cesarean as well as vaginal delivery, because one out of every five deliveries is a cesarean birth. An organized hospital tour, especially for first-time parents, usually serves to allay anxiety. In the

**Table 30–1**  Information and Skills Checklist for Going Home

**SELF-CARE**

_____ I can locate my uterus and evaluate whether it is making the normal and expected changes after delivery.
_____ I can evaluate whether the flow from my vagina is normal in amount and appearance.
_____ I can take my own temperature and know if it is normal.
_____ I can identify the following problems and contact my physician or midwife if they occur:
  Pain anywhere, but especially in my abdomen, chest, legs, bladder, or breasts.
  Fever, which means a temperature, taken by mouth, of 100.4°F, or higher, especially within the first 10 days after delivery.
  Excessive vaginal bleeding.
  Problems with mood changes beyond those related to normal adjustment (blues).
_____ I know what to do about breast engorgement (milk coming in) whether or not I am breastfeeding.
_____ I am satisfied that I have the information I need about birth control and resumption of sexual activity after delivery.

**BABY CARE**

_____ I can hold my baby safely and comfortably at least two different ways.
_____ I know how my baby should be laid down safely.
_____ I can tell differences in my baby's behavior and what those differences usually mean.
_____ I can tell when my baby is hungry.
_____ I know at least two or three different ways to console my baby when he or she is fussy or crying.
_____ I can bathe and dress my baby, including changing diapers.
_____ If I am breastfeeding, I can tell if my baby is breastfeeding correctly.
_____ If I am bottle-feeding, I know what kind of formula to feed my baby and how much.
_____ I know how often to feed my baby.
_____ I know how to take my baby's temperature under the arm and rectally, and I can read the thermometer.
_____ I can take care of my baby's cord.
_____ I can take care of my baby boy's circumcised or uncircumcised penis.
_____ I can use a bulb syringe to clear out my baby's nose and throat.
_____ I have an infant car seat; I know how to place it in the car correctly, and I can put my baby into it correctly.
_____ I can identify the following problems and contact my baby's doctor if they occur:
  My baby is getting jaundiced (the skin or eyes are turning yellow).
  My baby has a fever (underarm temperature higher than 99°F; rectal temperature higher than 100.4°F).
  My baby's temperature is too low (underarm temperature lower than 97.6°F; rectal temperature lower than 98°F).
  My baby isn't urinating enough (less than 6 wet diapers a day).
  My baby has diarrhea.
  My baby's behavior has changed (too sleepy; too upset or jittery).
  The cord isn't healing or looks infected.
  The circumcision is bleeding or isn't healing.
  My baby's skin is turning blue.

SIGNATURE _____

---

group session, parents' questions and concerns about the assessment and admission process, what to bring to the hospital, and what services and facilities are provided for parents, can be addressed.

A brief review of fundamentals of newborn care is desirable in the late prenatal period. Before delivery, parents should also be encouraged to select and meet with the pediatrician who will provide care to their newborn. Typical discussion topics are philosophy and logistics of either maternal-newborn or rooming-in care, newborn eye prophylaxis, cord care, newborn screening tests for treatable metabolic disorders, and circumcision (including social and medical indications or absence thereof, anesthesia, timing of circumcision, and required care).

Additional topics to be addressed include how to identify postpartum and newborn complications, use of medication for relief of maternal pain, other typical postpartum problems (e.g., constipation, mild anemia), return to activities of daily living, perineal care, contraception, and resumption of sexual activity. The couple should be encouraged to develop a strategy for help at home after discharge, because rest and recovery are of major importance to the new mother. A guideline of 2 weeks of relatively limited activity and major focus on establishing successful breastfeeding is appropriate for most women. Identification of community resources, as well as a discussion of posthospital care, can be part of the information conveyed before delivery. All topics can then be reinforced after delivery and before discharge.

A relatively controversial issue has been popularized in the lay literature regarding early discharge for mothers from the hospital. Many obstetric hospital programs have developed shortened postpartum stay programs coupled with prenatal education and a posthospital visiting nurse home care program. A recent review of the literature examined the consequences of early postpartum discharge. It reveals limited information and points out the need for rigorous studies of sufficient size to examine the impact of different lengths of hospital stay and different postdischarge practices on a range of outcomes for mothers and newborns in diverse populations and settings. This review concludes that discharge planning should be made cautiously. Nevertheless, many major hospitals are using home visiting nursing care after an early postpartum-newborn discharge. Such a program is in use at the University of Michigan. After an uncomplicated vaginal or cesarean delivery, a normal newborn course, and focused prenatal preparation, the mother completes a nursing checklist of skills and information (see Table 30–1), at or about 24 hours postpartum following a vaginal delivery and 48 hours following a cesarean delivery, and then she and her newborn are discharged. A first contact by phone from the visiting nurse service is made on the first day at home, to assess the condition of mother and the newborn and to arrange a home visit on the second or third day at home. The home visit is about 2 hours long and includes physical examination of both mother and infant and instruction in response to the parents' identified needs. Because approximately 75% of women are discharged breastfeeding, and the home visit usually coincides with onset of lactation, a great deal of breastfeeding instruction and support occurs at the home visit. A final contact is made by telephone the next day, which concludes this extended care program. If problems are identified at any contact point, care providers are notified immediately.

A recent case-control study of the participants in this program was compiled and demonstrated no significant increase in readmission for complications. As more acceptance of these programs occurs and reimbursement is made by third-party sources, the early discharge programs may become the norm and may be considered more efficient and effective than a more prolonged hospital stay because of the actual extension of postpartum care into the home.

## Late Postpartum Care

A 2-week postpartum visit to clinic or office is used to follow up an at-risk pregnancy (e.g., maternal hypertension, diabetes, anemia, infectious complication, or other medical diseases). The health-care provider can check on the medical condition of the patient and arrange for follow-up care by other specialty providers, if necessary.

In the increasingly competitive health-care marketplace, patient satisfaction is important. Many health-care programs are initiating a routine 2-week postpartum visit to assess the patient's psychological well-being and to perform a wound check (abdominal or perineal). The newborn's postnatal visit to the pediatrician's office usually occurs within the first 2 weeks after birth. Pediatric colleagues often find that questions about maternal postpartum issues are addressed to them, suggesting a need for a 2-week postpartum visit.

The usual 6-week postpartum visit brings closure to the postpartum management period. A brief physical examination is performed, focusing especially on assessment of breast, abdomen, and pelvis. A discussion of family planning and method of birth control is appropriate, as well as discussion of plans to return to work, resumption of prepregnancy physical activity, or both. In the United States, the usual amount of time for maternity leave from work is 6 to 8 weeks. In Europe, the medical leave is much more beneficent and reasonable (3 months or more).

## Postpartum Adjustment and Role Transition Issues

A transient depressed mood, or postpartum "blues," is reported by 50 to 70% of women, beginning on the third or fourth day after delivery. Symptoms of postpartum blues include insomnia (70%), tearfulness (66%), depressed mood (54%), anxiety (51%), headache (35%), poor concentration (29%), and confusion (21%). These symptoms usually resolve without sequelae in 1 to 2 weeks. It would be helpful in coping with postpartum blues if the patient were forewarned of this transient syndrome. Less common is a more severe and protracted syndrome of nonpsychotic postpartum depression, occurring in 15 to 20% of women.

Symptoms of depression include insomnia or somnolence, loss of interest in everyday activities, extreme anxiety, extreme tearfulness, inability to eat or tendency to overeat for at least 2 weeks. Even suicidal ideation may occur. Management of this syndrome requires professional help. The risk of sequelae, especially in relation to mother-child interaction, is significant. Finally, 2 out of 1000 women may require psychiatric admission after delivery because of psychosis. The vast majority of these psychotic episodes are affective disorders (e.g., manic or depressive psychosis). A history of a bipolar disorder is a major risk factor.

Also, the postpartum period is a time when there may be transient thyroid dysfunction. In about 6% of women, postpartum autoimmune thyroiditis may occur. Signs and symptoms of hyperthyroidism manifest between 3 and 6 months post partum and may persist up to 3 months. A transient subsequent hypothyroid phase occurs that may lasts 1 to 3 months. Treatment depends upon severity of symptoms. The syndrome can recur in subsequent pregnancies. Thus, the puerperal patient should be warned to report any symptoms of thyroid dysfunction that persist beyond the 6-week postpartum visit.

## Postpartum Management

In this section we review specific physician issues in the early postpartum period. When the patient arrives on the postpartum floor, the physician should spend an important few minutes reviewing her chart. Under vital signs, a slow pulse rate predicts a favorable outcome, whereas tachycardia is a red flag that should alert the clinician to look for peripartum urinary tract infection (UTI), upper respiratory infection (URI), anemia, or excessive blood loss. A mild temperature elevation soon after delivery could be related to dehydration, epidural anesthesia, or a peripartum UTI or URI. A significant temperature elevation is defined as higher than 100.4°F on two occasions during and beyond the first 24 hours post partum. The clinician should consider possible etiologies for investigation: wind, water, wound, and womb (rule of the W's). A review of prenatal laboratory tests is important for the ongoing care of mother and newborn. The Rh status, if negative without antibodies, and an Rh-positive newborn requires an injection of Rh (D) immunoglobulin. Most blood bank laboratories make a quantitative estimate based on samples of cord and maternal blood to determine how much immunoglobulin is needed to protect the mother from being sensitized. The risk of a large fetomaternal hemorrhage at delivery is increased by manual removal of the placenta or abruption of the placenta. If the mother is rubella nonimmune, she may receive rubella vaccine before discharge. In the event of a hepatitis antigen–positive prenatal finding, the newborn will receive an injection of the immune globulin and hepatitis B vaccine within 12 hours of birth, and a follow-up program will be instituted. All parents should be offered the option of beginning the newborn's hepatitis B vaccination program before discharge. A discharge checklist is presented in Table 30–2.

A routine postpartum complete blood count has not been found cost-effective and, in many hospitals, it is no longer performed. A review of previous medications will dictate whether orders should be written for continuance of any of them in the postpartum period. Other routine medications to order will include oral medication for treatment of pain and stool softeners.

It is very reassuring for the recent parturient to have her clinician visit her and ask, "How are you feeling?" and spend time listening to her. A brief physical examination includes locating the uterine fundus by abdominal palpation, auscultation of bowel sounds, visual inspection of the wound (abdominal or perineal), and checking calf or groin tenderness to reassure the patient.

## Circumcision

It is usually the obstetrician who performs the newborn's circumcision. The use of various anesthetic techniques has now become a routine practice. There is some evidence that the pain and suffering of the procedure put the newborn at some risk. Studies of altered vital signs and behavior support this notion. Dorsal penile nerve block is the most popular technique. A circumferential subcutaneous placement of local anesthetics about mid-shaft provides adequate anesthesia. Also, putting granulated sugar on a pacifier and giving it to the newborn just before and during the procedure provides some alleviation of discomfort for him.

## Summary

From an administrative perspective, the early postpartum discharge program provides cost-per-patient savings. When the cost of a home nursing visit is compared with the cost of an additional day in the hospital, the home care compares favorably and affords the patient exclusive time with a nurse without institutional overhead costs. Under any circumstances, the guiding principle for location of care is to provide the most appropriate care in the most appropriate place. For a stable mother and newborn, there is a benefit to be derived from extending early

**Table 30–2** Discharge Checklist

| Mother | Baby |
|---|---|
| _____ Discharge order written | _____ Discharge order written |
| _____ Discharge summary signed/complete | _____ Band cut/custody signed |
| _____ Discharge envelope with registration card, Rx, baby physical examination | _____ Newborn screen info |
| _____ Rubella ordered/given | _____ Circumcision done |
| _____ RhoGAM ordered/given | _____ Cord clamp off |
| _____ Discharge supplies | _____ Hepatitis B vaccine given |
| _____ Name on Visiting Nurse Association referral list | _____ Discharge supplies |

postpartum and newborn care into the home between 3 and 5 days post partum. There also tends to be a high level of patient satisfaction with a home care program. Administrators are necessarily paying more attention to keeping obstetric patients happy, because safe, satisfying maternal-newborn care leads to long-term use of a health-care system.

## REFERENCES

Amino N, Mori H, Iwatani Y, et al: High prevalence of transient postpartum thyrotoxicosis and hypothyroidism. N Engl J Med 306:849, 1982.

Braveman P, Egerter S, Pearl M, et al: Early discharge of newborns and mothers: A critical review of the literature. Pediatrics 96:716, 1995.

Fontaine P, Dittberner D, Scheltema KE: The safety of dorsal penile nerve block for neonatal circumcision. J Fam Pract 39:243, 1994.

Herschel M, Khoshnood B, Ellman C, et al: Neonatal circumcision. Randomized trial of a sucrose pacifier for pain control. Arch Pediatr Adolesc Med 152:279, 1998.

Lander J, Brady-Fryer B, Metcalf JB, et al: Comparison of ring block, dorsal penile nerve block and topical anesthesia for neonatal circumcision: A randomized controlled trial. JAMA 278:2157, 1997.

Luke B, Zettelmaier MA, Avni M, et al: Comprehensive prenatal care: Effects on maternal and neonatal morbidity and costs (abstract). Am J Obstet Gynecol 178:S124, 1998.

O'Hara MW, Neunaber DJ, Zeloski EM: Prospective study of postpartum depression: Prevalence, course and predictive factors. J Abnorm Psychol 93:158, 1984.

Taddio A, Katz J, Ilersich AL, et al: Effects of neonatal circumcision on pain response during subsequent routine vaccination. Lancet 349:599, 1997.

Wellington N, Rieder MJ: Attitudes and practices regarding analgesia for newborn circumcisions. Pediatrics 92:541, 1993.

Young D, Early discharge—whose decision, whose responsibility? Birth 23:2, 1996.

# 31

# Fetal Growth Disorders: Diagnosis and Management

CHUKWUMA I. ONYEIJE

MICHAEL Y. DIVON

Abnormal fetal growth is a common clinical dilemma. Fetal growth patterns at either end of the spectrum can present various problems for both fetus and mother. Fetal growth restriction (FGR), results in an infant who is small for gestational age, and who carries a substantial risk for perinatal morbidity and mortality, as well as long-term neurologic complications. The infant who is large for gestational age (LGA, macrosomia) is likewise at increased risk. Shoulder dystocia, birth asphyxia, trauma, intrauterine death, and the development of non–insulin-dependent diabetes in later life have all been described. Important clinical considerations involved with aberrant fetal growth are further complicated by the fact that mothers of infants with either insufficient or excessive growth are themselves at risk for a number of conditions that have implications not only on their pregnancies, but also on their health (e.g., chronic hypertension, diabetes mellitus).

The etiology, diagnosis, and management of abnormally grown fetuses have been the focus of many articles. This chapter summarizes current advances in the field of abnormal fetal growth and presents the practitioner with a management algorithm for cases in which fetal growth is suspected to be above or below the norm.

The physiology of fetal growth regulation is unique. In addition to factors that control growth in postnatal life, the fetus must cope with factors such as placental blood flow, physical restrictions imposed by the shape and volume of the uterus, and, above all maternal factors that may inhibit or enhance fetal growth potential. Furthermore, certain determinants of fetal growth which be manipulated during prenatal life, may theoretically reduce the risk of an abnormally grown fetus.

The etiologies of abnormal fetal growth can be related to aberrations in growth determinants that may affect the fetus, the mother, the placenta, or other factor in the uterine environment. Table 31–1 outlines factors known to be related to normal fetal growth.

## Fetal Growth Restriction

To fully understand the causes of FGR, it is important to have an unambiguous definition of this condition.

**Table 31–1** Determinants of Normal Fetal Growth

| |
|---|
| *Fetal Factors* |
| Genetic |
| Fetal hormones |
| Multifetal pregnancy |
| Congenital malformations |
| *Maternal Factors* |
| Obesity |
| Height |
| Prolonged pregnancy |
| Weight gain in pregnancy |
| Abnormal nutrition |
| Drug use |
| Smoking |
| *Placental Factors* |
| Uterine constraints |

From a statistical standpoint, if we view all birth weights of infants at a particular gestational age along the distribution of a normal gaussian curve, only infants whose weight is more than two standard deviations below the mean would be considered abnormally grown. Clinically, this definition of FGR is problematic; data demonstrate that the complications of fetal growth restriction are found in more than just the 2.3% of fetuses identified by this definition. For this reason, most clinical classifications for fetal growth restriction use birth weight at less than the 10th percentile using population-based specific birth weights for gestational age. Interpretation of gestational age-specific growth curves should also be viewed with caution because prematurely born fetuses are more likely to be growth restricted. Some authors have suggested that one third of preterm deliveries could be associated with FGR. Furthermore, it is important to remember that growth curves should be population specific. This is highlighted by the observation that the application of the Colorado birth weight for gestational age data to newborns in Vermont resulted in a 2% incidence of birth weight less than the 10th percentile and a 34% incidence of birth weight greater than the 90th percentile.

## FETAL FACTORS

Intrauterine growth restriction has been reported in karyotypic abnormalities, such as trisomy 13, 18, or 21, as well as the 45X/46Xi variant of Turner's syndrome. Such abnormalities of fetal chromosomes account for approximately 5% of fetal growth restriction. A variety of conditions causing autosomal recessive dwarfism, such as Bloom, Seckel's, and Donohue's syndromes, have also been associated with growth restriction. As would be expected, fetuses with congenital anomalies, such as dysplastic kidneys, cardiovascular malformations, or significant neural tube defects, are unable to attain and maintain normal growth and are, therefore, growth restricted at birth. Multiple gestation may also be associated with impaired fetal growth resulting from abnormal placentation, fetal infection, physical restraints, shared fetal circulation, or any of the other conditions known to result in FGR in a singleton pregnancy.

## MATERNAL FACTORS

Fetal growth restriction caused by maternal factors may be subdivided into conditions related to maternal nutrition, maternal illness, drug use, or demographic parameters. Although the association between adequate maternal nutrition during pregnancy and fetal growth seems intuitive, several epidemiologic studies performed during periods of famine or widespread maternal starvation in pregnancy have not shown a diminution of fetal growth that corresponds to maternal dietary deprivation, except in extreme cases. What appears to be more important as an index of fetal growth is the mother's pregestational dietary status and weight gain during pregnancy. Numerous recent studies have demonstrated an increased incidence of FGR among women of low body mass index (BMI) who have inadequate gestational weight gain. In 1990, the Institute of Medicine recommended target values for weight gain during pregnancy based on prepregnant BMI. Subsequent studies showed that mothers who had weight gain below these guidelines were at increased risk of delivering growth-restricted neonates.

Maternal drug use has been suggested as an etiology for FGR, possibly because of additional risk factors found in these patients, such as poor prepregnancy nutritional status or the inherent effects of certain drugs on maternal-fetal circulation. Cocaine, for example, has been implicated as a cause of vasoconstriction and placental abruption, both of which may contribute to inadequate fetal growth.

Chronic maternal illnesses that can lead to FGR are numerous and often have implications for the mother's long-term health (Table 31–2). Although a detailed analysis of the mechanisms involved in FGR with these maternal conditions is beyond the scope of this chapter, it should be recognized that the vast majority of these disorders can cause abnormal growth via an alteration of either uteroplacental blood flow or maternal (and in turn fetal) malnutrition and hypoxemia.

**Table 31–2** Maternal Conditions Associated with Fetal Growth Restriction

Hypertensive disorders
Diabetes mellitus
Cardiovascular disease
Renal disease
Collagen vascular diseases
Maternal hypoxemia

Although no medical conditions uniformly result in inadequate fetal growth, certain conditions are noteworthy because of to their contribution to the overall rate of FGR in pregnancy:

## Hypertensive Disorders

Chronic hypertension is associated with a twofold to threefold increase in the incidence of FGR. Furthermore, the severity of hypertension has been linked to increasing frequency of FGR. Animal models of the effect of hypertension on fetal growth have shown that microembolization of the uterine vasculature in sheep results in offspring with growth restriction. Although most hypotheses indicate that a diminution of uterine blood flow results in the increased prevalence of FGR in women who have chronic hypertension, attempts to decrease the incidence of FGR in these patients by the administration of antihypertensive medications or aspirin have not been uniformly successful. Other studies show that some of the agents used to control blood pressure in chronic hypertension (e.g., beta blockers) may themselves be associated with FGR when used chronically.

## Renal Disease

Maternal renal disease is associated with FGR in a significant but complex manner. Studies indicate that the rate of growth restriction is approximately 23% in mothers who have preexisting renal disease. A common clinical dilemma occurs in patients who demonstrate evidence of renal pathology during pregnancy with no known history of kidney disease. In such patients, it is often difficult to determine whether symptoms noted are caused by preeclampsia, hypertension, or pregnancy-associated renal deterioration. Regardless of the exact pathophysiology, the presence of FGR is more likely in these patients. The management paradigm of these patients includes assessment of fetal well-being and growth, prevention of maternal deterioration, and delivery of the fetus in a timely manner.

## Collagen Vascular Disorders

Antiphospholipid antibodies are the result of a fairly common group of autoimmune disorders that feature the production of antibodies directed against maternal cellular antigens. Patients who have systemic lupus erythematosus (SLE) are eight times more likely to deliver a growth-restricted infant than the general population; however, the reasons for this are still unclear. Furthermore, the incidence of FGR in patients with SLE is directly correlated to the extent of their disease at the time of conception, with an overall incidence of 23% in women who have inactive disease compared with a rate of 65% in women who have active disease. The correlation between SLE and FGR is so striking that it has been advised that all patients who have a pregnancy complicated by FGR be screened for the autoimmune antibodies that characterize SLE.

## Diabetes Mellitus

Insulin-requiring diabetes occurs in 1 of every 200 pregnancies and, as such, is one of the most common medical disorders encountered by the practicing obstetrician. The majority of patients who are noted to exhibit carbohydrate intolerance during pregnancy do not have pre-existing diabetes mellitus. As will be discussed, in such patients, maternal hyperglycemia often results in fetal hyperglycemia and hyperinsulinemia, which lead to increased fetal growth, enhanced subcutaneous fat deposition, and, thus, macrosomia. However, in patients who have long-standing diabetes mellitus (e.g., pregestational diabetes), the influence of maternal hyperglycemia on fetal growth is counteracted and eventually surpassed by the effect of maternal vascular disease, resulting in abnormal placental function and inadequate fetal growth.

## Maternal Hypoxemia

The effects of maternal oxygen-carrying capacity on fetal growth have been studied in mothers residing in areas of low oxygen partial pressure. Lichty and associates have found that birth weights among infants delivered at elevations of 10,000 feet are, on average, 250 g less than those of infants born at sea level. FGR is also commonly seen in patients who have cardiac and pulmonary disorders that result in chronic maternal hypoxia. Eisenmenger's complex and tetralogy of Fallot are two examples of infrequently encountered cyanotic cardiovascular diseases that may lead to FGR resulting from the combined effects of chronic maternal hypoxia and compromised hemodynamic status.

Asthma occurs in 3 to 4% of women of reproductive age and has also been shown to contribute to diminished fetal growth in extreme cases.

## Infectious Diseases

The role of maternal infectious diseases in the genesis of FGR has been studied extensively. Although the role of such protozoan infections as malaria, toxoplasmosis, and trypanosomiasis in FGR has been clearly demonstrated, the case for an association between bacterial infections and FGR is not as clear. However, an association has been established between FGR and some viral infections. Two mechanisms have been described. Rubella is thought to contribute to FGR by damaging endothelial capillaries during organogenesis, with a resultant overall decrease in the total number of cells in all organs and reduced growth potential. The mechanism of FGR induction by infection with cytomegalovirus is much more localized and results in fetal cytolysis and cellular necrosis.

## Demographic Variables

These include extremes of maternal age, maternal parity, maternal height and weight, and maternal and paternal race. Categorizing such infants as growth restricted is problematic because a small infant born to small parents may actually represent a constitutionally small but appropriate-for-gestational-age infant.

## DIAGNOSIS OF FETAL GROWTH RESTRICTION

Proper management of FGR involves identification of pregnancy at risk, making an accurate and timely diagnosis of FGR and then devising a plan of management that optimizes both maternal and fetal outcome.

## Identification of Pregnancies at Risk

Determination of an individual patient's risk of delivering an infant with growth restriction should take place at the first prenatal visit. In some patients, this assessment can take place before conception. It is possible that the propensity of chronic illnesses to result in growth restriction may be decreased if treated properly before pregnancy. Table 31–3 lists various risk factors for FGR and indicates when they may be detected during the course of preconceptual and prenatal care.

Traditionally, fetal growth has been monitored by measurement of the fundal height and maternal

**Table 31–3** Detection of Risk Factors for Fetal Growth Restriction

*Detectable Before Conception or at a First Prenatal Visit*

Previous fetal growth restriction
History of chronic medical illnesses
History of antiphospholipid syndrome
Low maternal body mass index
Substance abuse (including alcohol)
Maternal hypoxia

*Detectable During Pregnancy*

Elevated MSAFP/hCG
Drug ingestion (coumarin, hydantoin)
Vaginal bleeding
Placental abnormalities
Preterm labor
Twin gestation
Poor maternal weight gain

hCG = human chorionic gonadotropin; MSAFP = maternal serum alpha-fetoprotein.

weight gain. These parameters are easily obtainable and reproducible; however, when used alone, they are relatively poor predictors of fetal growth restriction.

Once fetal growth restriction is detected or suspected, ultrasonography becomes the primary modality for diagnosis and subsequent management of the fetus. The most common mode of sonographically assessing fetal size is the estimated fetal weight (EFW). Serial sonographic examinations are more informative than the "snapshot" afforded by a single examination. Serial examinations allow differentiation of a normally growing but small fetus—which may not be at increased risk for neonatal morbidity—from the pathologically small fetus. Clearly, the fetus that has shown an inadequate growth rate is at increased risk compared with a fetus of normal interval growth.

Discrepancies between growth curves of birth weight and estimated fetal weight growth curves exist in preterm gestations. This is due to the aforementioned increased incidence of FGR in preterm birth. Hence, ultrasonographically generated growth curves have consistently greater EFW in the preterm period than normograms generated with the use of birth weights.

An alternative to the use of serial ultrasonographic evaluations is the construction of individualized growth models popularized by Rossavik and associates in the 1980s. This method of fetal growth surveillance requires at least three ultrasonographic assessments; however, it has not been shown to be superior to commonly used techniques.

An acceptable management scheme for patients who have risk factors for FGR would be to perform an initial ultrasonographic assessment early in pregnancy to accurately establish gestational age and then to repeat the examination at 32 to 34 weeks of gestation. In selected cases, however, more stringent follow-up of fetal growth may be necessary. When fetal growth is evaluated serially, measurements are usually taken at 2- to 4-week intervals. Some authors have questioned this assumption of continuous fetal growth, noting the sporadic nature of postnatal growth and the underlying fact that the sonographic detection of growth may be limited not only by technical factors but also by the physiologic intervals of growth pulses in the fetus.

Because liver size has been shown to correlate directly with fetal nutritional status, measurement of the fetal abdominal circumference at the level of the umbilical portion of the left portal vein has been suggested as a means of identifying the growth-restricted fetus. We have previously reported a significant difference in the rate of growth of the fetal abdominal circumference between fetuses that are growth restricted and those that have grown appropriately. An increase in the fetal abdominal circumference of less than 10 mm in 14 days had a sensitivity of 85% for detection of the FGR.

Increased accuracy in the detection of fetal growth abnormalities may also be afforded by analysis of selected biometric ratios. One such parameter that has been subjected to intense study is the ratio of the head circumference to the abdominal circumference (HC/AC ratio). The HC/AC ratio is particularly useful in detection of a fetus that has asymmetric growth restriction. This is reflected by an abdominal circumference that is smaller than would be expected at a particular gestational age. When abnormalities of HC/AC ratio are added to traditional means of detecting growth restriction, sensitivity exceeds 85%. Because femur length is also spared in some cases of asymmetric growth restriction, the ratio of the femur length to the abdominal circumference is another useful tool in increasing the sensitivity of the diagnosis of FGR. In the normally grown fetus, the fetal length/abdominal circumference (FL/AC) ratio remains at approximately 22% from a gestational age of 21 weeks to term. We found that for the purposes of diagnosing FGR, a FL/AC ratio of >23.5% had a sensitivity of 55% and a specificity of 90%.

Doppler flow studies of the fetal vasculature are an additional modality used to assess the condition of a fetus thought to be growth restricted. Abnormalities of fetal growth patterns associated with FGR correlate with abnormal flow velocity waveforms of uteroplacental and fetal vessels. Studies by Wladimiroff and associates have demonstrated an increased pulsatility index of the umbilical artery in association with a reduced pulsatility index in the internal carotid artery in the growth-restricted fetus. This constellation of Doppler findings was described as "brain sparing" and mirrors the biometric changes seen with HC/AC ratios.

The pathophysiologic basis of abnormal Doppler indices in FGR is thought to be increased impedance to blood flow caused by obliteration of the small arterial vessels in the tertiary stem villi of the placenta. Systolic and diastolic ratios rise as the degree of FGR and its related hypoxia increase. In severe cases of hypoxia and acidemia in fetuses with FGR, a unique pattern of absent end diastolic flow representing a major placental abnormality may be noted. As fetal involvement increases, this pattern may worsen and is reflected by the appearance of reverse flow in the Doppler recordings.

Absent or reversed end-diastolic flow in the umbilical artery has been consistently associated with poor perinatal outcome including early delivery, growth restriction, oligohydramnios, pregnancy-induced hypertension, low Apgar scores, and cesarean delivery for fetal distress.

Nicolaides and associates have suggested that the response of fetal Doppler waveforms to maternal hyperoxygenation may be used as a prognostic tool in pregnancies complicated by FGR. In this study, fetuses demonstrating an improvement of waveform indices had better outcomes compared with those that did not show improvement. In terms of clinical management of fetuses with FGR, Doppler velocimetry allows identification of fetuses at greatest risk for neonatal morbidity and mortality.

In addition to determining fetal morphometric and Doppler measurements, ultrasonography allows quantitative assessment of amniotic fluid volume as an adjunct to the diagnosis of FGR. Oligohydramnios is a recognized sequela of FGR, and its presence has been used by various investigators to improve diagnostic accuracy and predict fetal compromise.

Manning and coworkers studied 120 pregnancies in which FGR was suspected and defined oligohydramnios as a largest pocket of less than 1 cm. This report gave a sensitivity of 84% and a specificity of 97% for diagnosing FGR. Although these results appear promising, this level of sensitivity for the detection of FGR has not been reported by other investigators. In any case, the presence of oligohydramnios in a pregnancy suspected of FGR in the absence of ruptured membranes or genitourinary anomalies, provides strong evidence of significant growth restriction and the potential for intrapartum complications.

## MANAGEMENT OF THE GROWTH-RESTRICTED FETUS

When dealing with a fetus suspected of being growth restricted, it is important to remember that a large number of these infants will be normally grown. In addition to normally grown infants erroneously suspected of being growth restricted, a significant number of supposed growth-restricted fetuses are actually constitutionally small. In both of these cases, no intervention is required. Unfortunately, diagnoses of the normally grown infant suspected of FGR and of the constitutionally small infant are often made retrospectively.

Another group of patients with FGR are symmetrically growth restricted as a result of an early fetal insult that is not amenable to antepartum therapy. This last group of patients have growth restriction noted before delivery as a result of placental disease or reduced uteroplacental blood flow. In these cases, antepartum fetal monitoring and timely intervention have been shown to improve neonatal outcome. Proper management of FGR requires identification of patients suitable for monitoring and limiting intervention in groups of patients that would not benefit from early delivery.

Certain maternal risk factors for FGR, such as smoking and alcohol ingestion, may be ameliorated by counseling or insight-oriented support groups. Although inadequate diet has not been conclusively shown to be related to FGR in the US population, dietary supplementation may be helpful in patients who have a low BMI or inadequate weight gain during pregnancy.

**Fetal Testing**

Once growth restriction is suspected, serial evaluations of fetal growth should be instituted. If at all possible, measurement of fundal height and assessment of approximate fetal weight should be performed at each visit by the same examiner.

Ultrasonographic examinations scheduled every 3 to 4 weeks appear to be an accurate and cost-effective method. At each ultrasonographic evaluation, particular attention should be placed on determination of the estimated fetal weight, biparietal diameter, HC/AC ratio, FL/AC ratio, amniotic fluid volume, and Doppler indices. Plotting biometric parameters on appropriate graphs allows visual assessment of changes in growth patterns. In particular, arrested head growth should prompt consideration of the plausibility of delivery.

Ultrasonography also allows the detection of lethal congenital anomalies associated with inadequate fetal growth. Growth restriction of the fetus in the presence of polyhydramnios is particularly suggestive of fetal aneuploidy. Delivery options should be discussed and clearly delineated for patients in whom fetal anomalies or chromosomal anomalies incompatible with life are diagnosed antenatally.

Amniocentesis for determination of fetal lung maturity is occasionally an important component of the decision-making process for growth-restricted infants. Infants suspected of growth restriction with very low lecithin-sphingomyelin ratios may actually be misdated and premature. In cases of symmetric growth restriction at term, amniocentesis may also be used to collect fluid for karyotype analysis.

Antenatal surveillance of the infant suspected of growth restriction primarily involves daily assessment of fetal movement, serial ultrasonography, and fetal testing when appropriate. The primary fetal assessment tool is the nonstress test (NST). The NST is generally performed in conjunction with the biophysical profile (BPP) or the contraction stress test (CST). A positive CST, the presence of oligohydramnios, or a BPP score of less than 4 should prompt consideration of delivery. If fetal head growth is maintained and testing is reassuring, no intervention is necessary.

A multidisciplinary management approach becomes important if delivery is contemplated in the preterm growth-restricted fetus. Fetal lung maturity testing is especially important in these situations. If testing is positive, delivery should be pursued in a setting where experienced neonatal care personnel are available. If fetal lung maturity testing is negative, consideration should be given to administration of steroids and continuous fetal heart monitoring until delivery.

The association between intrapartum late decelerations of the fetal heart and asphyxia is considerably stronger in growth-restricted than in normally grown infants. Delivery by cesarean section is appropriate for growth-restricted infants who have recurrent late decelerations remote from delivery as judged by cervical examination.

# Macrosomia

It is generally believed that macrosomia is associated with an increased risk to both mother and fetus. Unfortunately, there is no universal agreement regarding the definition of a macrosomic neonate. Two definitions have been suggested. The first is an arbitrary cut-off value of birth weight that is associated with increased risk for pregnancy complications. A review of the literature reveals that there are a number of such cut-off levels at which a newborn in considered to be macrosomic. These values range from 4000 g to 4500 g and quite often depend on the specific patients evaluated in a particular study. The second definition is a statistical construct based on birth weight for gestational age criteria. Most often, LGA is defined by a birth weight larger than the 90th percentile for gestational age. This nomenclature has advantages that are readily apparent when compared with the empirical standard. For example, an infant with a birth weight of 3800 g at 35 weeks of gestation would not be considered macrosomic by standard definitions, but would be considered LGA.

At present, a consensus has not been reached regarding obstetric management for macrosomia. This is due, in part, to the difficulty of prospectively identifing fetuses that are actually macrosomic and to differentiate which macrosomic infants are more prone to intrapartum and neonatal difficulties. However, proper assessment and identification of patients at risk may reduce the number of false diagnoses. The American College of Obstetricians and Gynecologists has concluded that the term *macrosomia* should be reserved for fetuses who weigh 4500 g or more.

The incidence of macrosomia varies by the population studied; in general, however, most large series have shown that between 5 and 7% of newborns weigh more than 4000 g and fewer than 1% weigh more than 4500 g.

## RISK FACTORS FOR FETAL MACROSOMIA

Women who deliver macrosomic infants are more likely to be obese, have excessive weight gain in pregnancy, or have prolonged gestation. Factors shown to be associated with fetal macrosomia are listed in Table 31–4. Of the known risk factors for macrosomia, the strongest correlations have been found with maternal diabetes mellitus, obesity, and prolonged gestation.

When large fetuses are considered as a group, it has been noted that certain variables (e.g., maternal diabetes) place a given infant at increased risk for adverse neonatal outcome when compared with other infants of similar birth weight. Therefore, an infant weighing 4250 g born to a mother who has diabetes mellitus is at a substantially higher risk for shoulder dystocia than an infant of the same size born to a mother who does not have diabetes. We have previously described the different types of growth patterns seen in large infants as being either constitutional or metabolic. The constitutionally large neonate is symmetrically grown and usually at lower risk for adverse outcome. The large infant born to a mother who has insulin-dependent mellitus (IDM) has organomegaly, increased fat deposition in the region of the shoulders and abdomen, and is at increased risk for shoulder dystocia.

## Maternal Diabetes

Growth potential of the developing fetus is regulated by the adequacy and nature of placental nutritional support. The Pederson hyperglycemia-hyperinsulinemia hypothesis states that maternal hyperglycemia results in fetal hyperglycemia. Glucose levels in the fetus remain at levels that are approximately 75% of those in the mother and stimulate fetal hyperinsulinism. Insulin in the fetus acts as a growth hormone and stimulates increased triglyceride synthesis in adipose cells as well as glycogen storage in the fetal liver. These lead to overgrowth and, hence, the characteristic macrosomic appearance of infants of diabetic mothers. Other investigators have hypothesized roles for other nutritional fuels and growth factors in addition to the original work of Pederson.

Women who have diabetes are more than 10 times more likely to deliver an infant weighing more than 4500 g than similar nondiabetic control subjects. Excessive (asymmetric) growth can predispose macrosomic infants of mothers who have diabetes to shoulder dystocia, traumatic birth injury, and asphyxia. Difficult vaginal deliveries in IDMs are thought to be directly related to the disproportionate increase in the size of the shoulder and trunk compared with the head.

Several authors have shown that the risks of macrosomia in IDMs can be decreased substantially by a regimen of tight antenatal maternal glycemic control. Studies by Jovanovic and associates have suggested that the degree of control of postprandial glucose correlates with risk of macrosomia. Other authors have implicated fasting glucose as the factor most suggestive of risk of macrosomia, suggesting that higher maternal glucose levels are associated with increased incidence of macrosomia.

## Maternal Obesity

Maternal obesity as a risk factor for fetal macrosomia has strong genetic and nutritional components. The association between obesity and macrosomia is clearly related to hereditary constitutional factors in the mother and is influenced by increased nutritional intake in obese women. However, even when these confounding variables are eliminated, there remains an increased risk of macrosomia in these women. When a pregnant woman weighs more than 300 pounds, her risk of delivering a macrosomic infant is approximately 30% higher than in the general population.

**Table 31–4** Risk Factors for Fetal Macrosomia

Maternal diabetes
Maternal obesity
Multiparity
Prolonged gestation
Large size of parents (constitutional)
Male fetus
Previous macrosomic fetus

Separate studies by Larsen and associates and Wolfe and associates on the effect of pregravid obesity on infant birth weight have shown a marked increase in macrosomia with maternal obesity independent of gestational age at delivery, diabetes, and duration of pregnancy.

## Prolonged Pregnancy and Macrosomia

Maternal, fetal, and neonatal complications increase as pregnancy progresses beyond 42 weeks of gestation.

The post-term pregnancy appears to be at substantial risk for excessive fetal growth. The increased size of the post-term fetus is a natural consequence of the extra time the fetus has spent in utero.

## Genetic Causes of Macrosomia

Although they are uncommon, inherited forms of macrosomia are an important subset of disorders that may be potentially detected antenatally and are, therefore, amenable to genetic counseling and determination of risk in selected couples. Beckwith-Wiedemann syndrome features large muscle mass, polyhydramnios, macroglossia, and omphalocele. Mental retardation is seen in some cases. As a result of fetal hyperinsulinemia and other metabolic disorders, many of these infants will be born with hypoglycemia and may experience seizures, apnea, or cyanosis.

Nesidioblastosis is a rare disorder caused by disseminated proliferation of pancreatic islet cells that are not sensitive to usual paracrine control. These infants are born with hyperinsulinemia and hypoglycemia. Surgical ablation of up to 95% of the pancreas is the only long-term treatment that has proved efficacious. Antenatal management is similar to that of an infant exposed to maternal diabetes mellitus. Although ultrasonographic diagnosis is difficult, some investigators have reported favorable diagnostic results by measuring amniotic fluid insulin levels.

Macrocephaly, dolichocephaly, and prognathism are the hallmarks of Soto's syndrome. Although the inheritance of this disorder is thought to be autosomal dominant, the majority of cases apparently represent new mutations. Moderate to severe mental retardation is present in 83% of these individuals, and endocrine abnormalities are generally absent. In general, when a rare cause of macrosomia is suspected, management should be guided by accurate assessment of fetal anatomy and size. Intervention is usually guided by the same principles that guide diabetic management, and elective operative delivery is reserved for excessively large infants who pose a substantial danger to maternal or neonatal well-being by vaginal delivery.

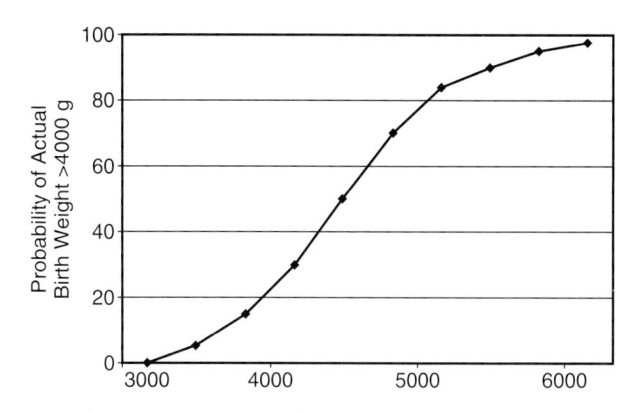

**Figure 31–1**  Sonographic estimates of fetal weight.

## DIAGNOSIS OF MACROSOMIA

Accurate diagnosis of fetal macrosomia would be helpful for making delivery plans as well as providing mothers with prognostic information before labor. However, present methods for determining the extent of excessive fetal growth are limited by poor sensitivity and predictive values. Numerous attempts have been made to improve the diagnostic accuracy of estimated fetal weight by ultrasonography, and although these formulas are often useful with the normal-sized fetus, their accuracy falls off substantially at extreme ranges of fetal size. The difficulty of assessing fetal weight by palpation of the maternal abdomen in suspected macrosomic fetuses is complicated by the high prevalence of obesity in mothers at risk.

The relationship between the probability of an actual birth weight being greater than 4000 g or 4500 g and a sonographic estimation of fetal weight is plotted in Figures 31–1 and 31–2. These data from

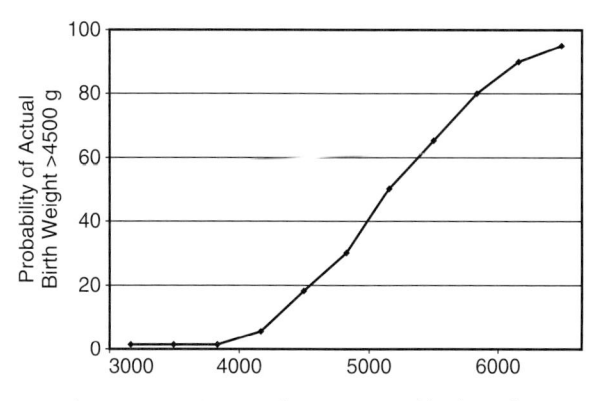

**Figure 31–2**  Sonographic estimates of fetal weight.

studies by Watson and Seeds show that when an EFW is 4000 g or 4500 g, there is only a 50% probability that the fetal weight will be equal to or greater than the estimate.

The use of other sonographically measured parameters to estimate fetal soft tissue distribution (e.g., the cheek-to-cheek diameter, the thickness of the fetal abdominal fat line, or three-dimensional ultrasound) has not resulted in substantial improvement in the prediction of fetal macrosomia.

Methods of population-specific, computer-generated statistical models may be used in addition to ultrasonography in determining a patient's risk of delivering a macrosomic neonate. In a preliminary study, we were able to achieve sensitivities of 85% and 83% for detecting birth weights of 4000 g and 4500 g, respectively, using ultrasonography and cut-off values generated by receiver operator characteristic curves.

Although decreasing the rate of macrosomia-related complications is an important goal, some authors have suggested that clinical decision-making based solely on ultrasonographic estimation of fetal weight only increases the rates of cesarean deliveries, while protecting relatively few infants. For this reason, ultrasonographic measurements should always be used in conjunction with clinical estimates of fetal size, maternal pelvic architechture, and careful consideration of maternal and fetal risk factors for excessive growth.

## MANAGEMENT OF FETAL MACROSOMIA

A rational approach to the management of the fetus suspected of having macrosomia should be guided by attempts to avoid major complications of macrosomia, such as fetopelvic disproportion and shoulder dystocia, while avoiding unnecessary intervention based solely on ultrasonographic findings. A careful assessment of maternal risk factors should begin at the first prenatal visit and should focus on the birth weights of previous infants, as well as the course and duration of labor in previous pregnancies. Unfortunately, up to 40% of patients who deliver macrosomic neonates do not exhibit any obvious risk factors for macrosomia during pregnancy.

Serial measurements of fundal height are an important part of prenatal care, and an abnormally large fundal height should prompt ultrasound evaluation for macrosomia, polyhydramnios, and multiple gestation. As with fetal growth restriction, serially recorded measurements of fetal size may be more useful than a single EFW recorded by ultrasonography.

Detection and treatment of maternal diabetes may substantially decrease the incidence of macrosomia. Maternal risk factors for diabetes, such as previous macrosomic infant, previous stillbirth, or a family history of diabetes mellitus, should prompt a screen test for diabetes, regardless of gestational age. All patients, however, should be screen tested for diabetes at 24 to 28 weeks of gestation.

Strategies for the management of diabetes in pregnancy primarily involve dietary interventions and the institution of insulin therapy when necessary. Whenever possible, this approach should be managed by a multidisciplinary team who have experience managing pregnancies in women who have diabetes.

Shoulder dystocia in the macrosomic infant and its associated risk of permanent brachial plexus injury are areas of concern in obstetrics. Thirty percent of brachial plexus injuries occur in infants who weigh more than 4000 g, although these infants account for fewer than 10% of all births.

Intrapartum management of the large fetus requires strict attention to the course of labor, because a prolonged first or second stage of labor have been associated with shoulder dystocia. Maneuvers for relief of the impacted shoulder in cases of shoulder dystocia are published in Chapter 27, and should be reviewed periodically by obstetric, anesthesic, and nursing staff.

Finally, the risks of a policy of liberal cesarean section for sonographically diagnosed fetal macrosomia was pointed out in an article by Rouse and associates. They calculated that in the nondiabetic population, 3695 cesarean deliveries would be necessary (at a cost of $8.7 million) to prevent one case of permanent brachial plexus injury resulting from shoulder dystocia if all of these patients were delivered by cesarean section. Furthermore, these authors suggested that such a policy would result in 1 maternal death for each 3.2 cases of permanent brachial plexus injury prevented. This evidence supports the management goals of the macrosomic fetus, which hold that delivery should be pursued in a manner that is safest for both mother and fetus. Although some infants with macrosomia require cesarean section for delivery, institution of such measures for all cases of presumed macrosomia would have detrimental effects on the well-being of mothers and benefit relatively few infants. Ongoing research into better methods of predicting which infants are at risk for complications of macrosomia may someday allow us to make this important distinction.

## REFERENCES

Abramowicz JS, Sherer DM, Woods JR: Ultrasonographic measurement of cheek to cheek diameter in fetal growth disturbances. Am J Obstet Gynecol 169:405, 1993.

Abrams BF, Parker JD: Maternal weight gain in women with good pregnancy outcome. Obstet Gynecol 76:1, 1990.

Abrams BF, Laros RK: Prepregnancy weight, weight gain, and birth weight. Am J Obstet Gynecol 154:503, 1986.

Acker DB, Sachs BP, Freidman EA: Risk factors for shoulder dystocia. Obstet Gynecol 66:762, 1985.

Adams JM, Gordon LP, Dutton RV, et al: Leprechaunism (Donohue's syndrome) in a low birth weight infant. South Med J 70:998, 1977.

American College of Obstetricians and Gynecologists: Dystocia: Technical Bulletin no. 37. ACOG, December 1989.

Bahar AM: Risk factors and fetal outcome in cases of shoulder dystocia compared with normal deliveries of a simialr birth weight. Br J Obstet Gynaecol 103:868, 1996.

Battaglia FC, Lubehenco LO: A practical classification of newborn infants by weight and gestational age. J Pediatr 71:159, 1967.

Berkowitz GS, Skovron ML, Lapinski RH, et al: Delayed childbearing and the outcome of pregnancy. N Engl J Med 322:659, 1990.

Bernstein IM, Meyer MC, Capeless EL: "Fetal growth charts:" Comparison of cross-sectional ultrasound examinations with birth weight. J Maternal Fetal Med 3:182, 1994.

Bernstein IM, Blake K: Evidence that normal fetal growth is not continuous. J Maternal Fetal Med 4:197, 1995.

Bernstein PS, Divon MY: Etiologies of fetal growth restriction. Clin Obstet Gynecol 40:723, 1997.

Bond AL, Chevernak F: Early screening: Genetic factors and fetal anomalies in intrauterine growth retardation and macrosomia. In Divon MY (ed): Abnormal Fetal Growth. New York, Elsevier, 1991, pp 111–127.

Boscherini B, Iannacione G, LaCauza C, et al: Intrauterine growth retardation. A report of two cases with bird-headed appearance, skeletal changes and peripheral GH resistance. Eur J Pediatr 137:237, 1981.

Boyd ME, Usher PH, McLean FH: Fetal macrosomia: Prediction, risks and proposed management. Obstet Gynecol 61:715, 1983.

Campbell S, Pearce JM, Hacket G, et al: Qualitative assessment of uteroplacental blood flow: early screening test for high risk pregnancies. Obstet Gynecol 68:49, 1986.

Chervenak JL: Macrosomia in the postdated pregnancy. Clin Obstet Gynecol 35:151, 1992.

Clapp JF: Etiology and pathophysiology of intrauterine growth retardation. In Divon MY (ed): Abnornmal Fetal Growth. New York, Elsevier, 1991, pp 83–97.

Clifford SH: Postmaturity—with placental dysfunction. J Pediatr 44:1, 1954.

Cooper LZ, Preblud SR, Alford CAJ: Rubella. In Remington JS, Klein JO (eds): Infectious Diseases of the Fetus and Newborn Infant. Philadelphia, WB Saunders, 1995, p 268.

Coustan DR: Management of gestational diabetes. Clin Obstet Gynecol 34:558, 1991.

Creasy RK, Barnett CT, deSwiet M, et al: Experimental intrauterine growth retardation in the sheep. Am J Obstet Gynecol 112:566, 1972.

Divon MY, Chamberlain PF, Sipos L, et al: Identification of the small for gestational age fetus with the use of gestational-age independent indices of fetal growth. Am J Obstet Gynecol 155:1197, 1986.

Divon MY, Guidetti DA, Braverman JJ, et al: Intrauterine growth retardation: A prospective study of the diagnostic value of real-time sonography combined with umbilical artery flow velocimetry. Obstet Gynecol 72:611, 1988.

Divon MY, Girz BA, Lieblich R, et al: Clinical management of the fetus with markedly diminished umbilical artery end diastolic flow. Am J Obstet Gynecol 161:1523, 1989.

Dombrowski MP: Pharmacologic therapy of asthma during pregnancy. Obstet Gynecol Clin North Am 24:559, 1997.

Eik-Nes SH, Grottum P, Persson PH, et al: Prediction of fetal growth by ultrasound biometry. I. Acta Obstet Gynecol 61:53, 1982.

Gabbe SG: Intrauterine growth retardation. In Gabbe SG, Niebyl JR, Simpson JL (eds): Obstetrics: Normal and Problem Pregnancies, 2nd ed. New York, Churchill Livingstone, 1991, p 923.

Gabbe SG, Mestman JH, Freeman RK, et al: Management and outcome of pregnancy in diabetes mellitus, classes B–R. Am J Obstet Gynecol 129:723, 1977.

Ghindini A: Idiopathic fetal growth restriction: A pathophysiologic approach. Obstet Gynecol Surv 51:376, 1996.

Giles WB, Trudinger BJ, Bard PJ: Fetal umbilical artery flow velocity waveforms and placental resistance: Pathological correlation. Br J Obstet Gynecol 92:31, 1985.

Golditch IM: The large fetus: Management and outcome. Obstet Gynecol 52:26, 1978.

Gonen O, Rosen DJ, Dolfin Z, et al: Induction of labor versus expectant management in macrosomia: A randomized study. Obstet Gynecol 89:913, 1997.

Guidetti DA, Divon MY, Braverman JJ, et al: Sonographic estimates of fetal weight in the intrauterine growth retardation population. Am J Perinatol 7:5, 1990.

Hadlock FP, Harrist RB, Martinez-Poyer J: In-utero analysis of fetal growth: A sonographic weight standard. Radiology 181:129, 1991.

Hickey CA, Cliver SP, Goldenberg RL, et al: Prenatal weight gain, term Birth Weight and fetal growth retardation among high risk multiparous black and white women. Obstet Gynecol 81:529, 1993.

Hirsch HJ, Loo S, Evans N, et al: Hypoglycemia of infancy and nesidioblastosis: Severe neonatal hypoglycemia in two families. J Pediatr 95:44, 1979.

Institute of Medicine: Subcommittee on Nutritional Status and Weight Gain During Pregnancy. Institute of Medicine. Nutrition During Pregnancy. Washington, DC, National Academy Press, 1990.

Jones KL: Beckwith-Wiedemann syndrome. In Smith's Recognizable Patterns of Human Malformation, 4th ed. Philadelphia, WB Saunders, 1988, p 136.

Jones KL: Sotos syndrome. In Smith's Recognizable Patterns of Human Malformation, 4th ed. Philadelphia, WB Saunders, 1988, pp 128–129.

Jovanovic L, Druzin M, Peterson CM: Effect of euglycemia on the outcome of pregnancy in insulin-dependent diabetic women as compared with normal control subjects. Am J Med 72:921, 1981.

Julkumen H, Jouhikainen T, Kaaja R, et al: Fetal outcomes in lupus pregnancy: A retrospective case control study of 242 pregnancies in 112 patients. Lupus 2:125, 1993.

Kalkhoff RK: Impact of maternal fuels and nutritional state on fetal growth. Diabetes 2(suppl) 61, 1991.

Katz AE, Davison JM, Hayslett JP, et al: Pregnancy in women with kidney disease. Kidney Int 18:192, 1980.

Kitzmiller J, Cloherty J, Younger MD, et al: Diabetic pregnancy and perinatal morbidity. Am J Obstet Gynecol 131:560, 1978.

Lampl M, Veldhuis JD, Johnson ML: Saltation and stasis: A model of human growth. Science 258:801, 1992.

Langer O: Fetal macrosomia: etiological factors. In Divon MY (ed): Abnornmal Fetal Growth. New York, Elsevier, 1991, pp 99–110.

Larsen CE, Serdula MK, Sullivan KM: Macrosomia: Influence of maternal overweight among a low-income population. Am J Obstet Gynecol 162(2):490–494, 1990.

Lechtig A, Yarbrough C, Delgado H, et al: Effect of moderate maternal malnutrition on the placenta. Am J Obstet Gynecol 123:191, 1975.

Lichty JA, Ting RY, Bruns PD, et al: Studies of babies born at high altitude. Am J Dis Child 93:666, 1957.

Lin CC, Moawan AH, Rosenow PJ, et al: Acid base characteristics of fetuses with intrauterine growth retardation during labor and delivery. Am J Obstet Gynecol 137:553, 1980.

Little BB, Snell LM, Klein VR, et al: Cocaine abuse during pregnancy: Maternal and fetal implications. Obstet Gynecol 74:157, 1989.

Llerena JC, Murer-Orlando M: Bloom syndrome and ataxia telangiectasia. Semin Hemat 28:95, 1991.

Long PA, Abell DA, Beischer NA: Fetal growth retardation and preeclampsia. Br J Obstet Gynaecol 87:13, 1980.

Low JA, Galbraith RS, Muir D, et al: Intrauterine growth retardation: A preliminary report of long-term morbidity. Am J Obstet Gynecol 130:534, 1978.

Mandruzzato GP, Bogatti P, Fischer L, et al: The clinical significance of absent or reverse end diastolic flow in the fetal aorta and umbilical artery. Ultrasound Obstet Gynecol 1:192, 1991.

Manning FA, Hill LM, Platt D: Qualitative amniotic fluid volume determination by ultrasound: Antepartum detection of intrauterine growth retardation. Am J Obstet Gynecol 139:254, 1981.

Martkainen AM, Heinonen KM, Saarikoski SV: The effect of

hypertension in pregnancy on fetal and neonatal condition. Int J Gynaecol Obstet 30:213, 1989.

McClure-Browne JC: Postmaturity. Am J Obstet Gynecol 85:373, 1963.

McGowan LM, Erskine LA, Ritchie K: Umbilical artery Doppler blood flow studies in the preterm small for gestational age fetus. Am J Obstet Gynecol 156:655, 1987.

Meizner I, Glezerman M: Cordocentesis in the evaluation of the growth-retarded fetus. Clin Obstet Gynecol 35:126, 1992.

Miller H, Merritt TA: Fetal growth in humans. Chicago, Year Book Medical Publishers, 1979.

Milner RDG: Amino acids and beta cell growth in structure and function. In Merkatz IR, Adam PAJ (eds): The Diabetic Pregnancy: A Perinatal Perspective. New York, Grune & Stratton, 1979, pp 145–153.

Mintz MC, Landon MB: Sonographic diagnosis of fetal growth disorders. Clin Obstet Gynecol 31:44, 1988.

Mintz G, Niz J, Gutierrez G, et al: Prospective study of pregnancy in systemic lupus erythematosus. Results of a multidisciplinary approach. J Rheumatol 13:732, 1986.

Modanlou HD, Dorchester WL, Thorosian A, et al: Macrosomia—maternal, fetal, and neonatal implications. Obstet Gynecol 55:420, 1980.

Modanlou HD, Komatsu G, Dorchester W, et al: Large-for-gestational age neonates: Anthropometric reasons for shoulder dystocia. Obstet Gynecol 60:417, 1982.

Neerhof MG: Causes of intrauterine growth restriction. Clin Perinatol 22:375, 1995.

Neigler R: Fetal macrosomia in the diabetic patient. Clin Obstet Gynecol 35:138, 1992.

Nicolaides KH, Campbell S, Bradley RJ, et al: Maternal oxygen therapy for intrauterine growth retardation. Lancet 1:942, 1987.

Ott WJ: Intrauterine growth retardation and preterm delivery. Am J Obstet Gynecol 168:1710, 1993.

O'Reilly-Green CP, Divon MY: Receiver operating characteristic curves of sonographic estimated fetal weight for prediction of macrosomia in prolonged pregnancy. Ultrasound Obstet Gynecol 9:403, 1997.

Parker JD, Abrams B: Prenatal weight gain advice: An examination of the recent prenatal weight gain recommendations of the Institute of Medicine. Obstet Gynecol 79:664, 1992.

Parks DG, Ziel HK: Macrosomia—a proposed indication for primary cesarean section. Obstet Gynecol 52:407, 1978.

Patterson RM, Prihoda TJ, Pouliot MR: Sonographic amniotic fluid measurement and fetal growth retardation: A reappraisal. Am J Obstet Gynecol 157:1406, 1987.

Patterson RM, Prihoda TJ, Gibbs CE, Wood RL: An analysis of birthweight percentile as a predictor of perinatal outcome. Obstet Gynecol 68:459, 1986.

Paz I, Gale R, Laor A, et al: The cognitive outcome of full-term small-for-gestational-age infants at late adolescence. Obstet Gynecol 85:452, 1995.

Pederson J: The Pregnant Diabetic and Her Newborn: Problems and Management. 2nd ed. Baltimore, Williams and Wilkins, 1977, pp 211–220.

Petrella R, Hirschhorn K, German J: Triple autosomal trisomy in a pregnancy at risk for Bloom's syndrome. Am J Med Genet 40:316, 1991.

Petrikovsky B, Gelertner N, Oleschuck C: Fetal abdominal fat line: Can macrosomia be diagnosed? Am J Obstet Gynecol 174:428, 1996.

Ramin SM, Cunningham FG: Obesity in pregnancy. In William's Obstetrics, 19th ed (suppl 13). East Norwalk, CT, Appleton & Lange, 1995.

Redman CRG, Beilin LJ, Bonnar J, et al: Fetal outcome in antihypertensive trial in pregnancy. Lancet 2:753, 1976.

Rosendahl H, Kivinen S: Detection of small for gestational age fetuses by the combination of clinical risk factors and ultrasonography. Eur J Obstet Gynecol Reprod Biol 39:7, 1991.

Rossavik IK, Deter RL: Mathematical modeling of fetal growth. I. Basic principles. J Clin Ultrasound 12:529, 1984.

Rouse DJ, Owen J, Goldenberg RL, et al: The effectiveness and costs of elective cesarean delivery for fetal macrosomia diagnosed by ultrasound. JAMA 276:1840, 1996.

Roversi GD, Gargiulo M: A new approach to the treatment of diabetic pregnant women. Am J Obstet Gynecol 135:567, 1979.

Schatz M, Zeiger RS, Hoffman CP: Intrauterine growth is related to gestational pulmonary function in pregnant asthmatic women. Kaiser Permanente Asthma and Pregnancy Study Group. Chest 98:389, 1990.

Scott KF, Usher R: Fetal malnutrition: Its incidence, causes and effects. Am J Obstet Gynecol 94:951, 1966.

Scott A, Moar V, Ounsted M: The relative contributions of different maternal factors in small-for-gestational-age pregnancies. Eur J Obstet Gynecol Reprod Biol 12:157, 1981.

Seeds JW: Impaired fetal growth: Definition and clinical diagnosis. Obstet Gynecol 64:303, 1984.

Sheilds LE, Huff RW, Jackson GM, et al: Fetal growth: A comparison of growth curves with mathematical modeling. J Ultrasound Med 5:271, 1993.

Shushan A, Ezra Y, Samueloff A: Early treatment of gestational diabetes reduces the rate of fetal macrosomia. Am J Perinatol 14:253, 1997.

Sickler GK, Nyberg DA, Sohaey R, Luthy DA: Polyhydramnios and fetal intrauterine growth restriction: Ominous combination. J Ultrasound Med 16:609, 1997.

Smith CA: Effects of maternal undernutrition upon the newborn infant in Holland (1944–1945). Am J Obstet Gynecol 30:229, 1947.

Spellacy WN, Miller S, Winegar A, et al: Macrosomia—maternal characteristics and infant complications. Obstet Gynecol 66:185, 1985.

Teberg AJ, Walther FJ, Pena IC: Mortality, morbidity and outcome of the small-for-gestational-age infant. Semin Perinatol 11:84, 1988.

Walle T, Hartikainen-Sorri AL: Obstetric shoulder injury: Associated risk factors, prediction and prognosis. Acta Obstet Gynecol Scand 72:450, 1993.

Watson W, Seeds J: Sonographic diagnosis of macrosomia. In Divon MY (ed): Abnormal Fetal Growth. New York, Elsevier, 1991, p 237.

Westgren M, Beall M, Divon MY, et al: Fetal femur length/abdominal circumference ratio in preterm labor patients with and without successful tocolytic therapy. J Ultrasound Med 5:243, 1986.

Wladimiroff JW, Wijngaard JAGW, Degani S, et al: Cerebral and umbilical arterial blood flow velocity waveform in normal and growth-retarded fetuses. Obstet Gynecol 69:705, 1987.

Wolfe HM, Zador IE, Gross TL, et al: The clinical utility of maternal body mass index in pregnancy. Am J Obstet Gynecol 164:1306, 1991.

Zulman JI, Alal N, Hoffman GS, et al: Problems associated with the management of pregnancies in patients with systemic lupus erythematosus. J Rheumatol 7:327, 1980.

# 32

# Multifetal Pregnancy

JASON O. GARDOSI

## Epidemiology

Multifetal pregnancy rates are subject to a variety of factors. They increase with maternal age and parity and vary between racial groups. The rate is approximately 1 to 2% in tertiary referral centers but has been on a steep increase in recent years because of fertility treatments and assisted reproduction techniques. Depending on the population, approximately one third of twins and three fourths of triplets and higher order multiples occur after assisted conception. Such pregnancies are also more likely at higher maternal age, which further adds to the likelihood of multiple pregnancy. Thus, most of the increase in multifetal pregnancies has occurred in a well-defined group, primiparous women who are older than 30.

These factors affect mainly dizygotic twinning rates, although assisted conception multiples also have a higher chance of additional spontaneous monozygotic twinning. In contrast, the rate of monozygotic twins is relatively constant (about 3 to 4:1000); therefore, approximately one third of all spontaneously conceived twin pregnancies are monozygotic.

More pregnancies are multifetal before viability is established. Multiples are more likely than singletons to abort before being clinically apparent, and after the pregnancy is confirmed, another 30 to 40% of twin pregnancies end with either a complete miscarriage or loss of one fetus (vanishing twin) by the end of the first trimester.

Perinatal mortality is 6 to 7 times higher in twins and 15 to 20 times higher in triplets than singletons. Among survivors, the relative risk of severe handicap compared with singletons is 1.7 for twins and 2.9 for triplets. Infants of multiple births have significantly lower mental and physical indices in early childhood; the worst effects occur in premature fetuses who are also growth retarded. The medical risks associated with multifetal pregnancies have also resulted in a considerable increase in health-care costs.

## Prematurity and Growth Restriction

The special problems of multifetal pregnancy are the increased likelihood of prematurity and growth restriction. In twins, perinatal mortality is more strongly associated with growth restriction than with prematurity. There is a larger increase across weight categories for a given gestational age than across gestational ages for a given birth weight.

Twins are almost 10 times more likely than singletons to have a low birth weight (<2500 g or <1500 g), and their mean birth weight is approximately 1000 g less than that of singletons (i.e., 2400 g vs. 3400 g). This weight difference compared with singletons is, in approximately equal measures, caused by slower growth and by birth at earlier gestations. Controlled for gestational age, twins weigh approximately 500 g less at term. They are also born on average 3 weeks earlier than singletons. The typical (i.e., modal) length of gestation for twins is 37 weeks, which includes spontaneous as well as induced deliveries. Thus, if one uses the singleton definition for premature birth (<37 weeks), half of all twin births are premature. For triplets, the typical length of gestation is another 3 weeks earlier (i.e., approximately 34 weeks).

Controlled for gestational age, preterm twins have a *lower* perinatal mortality rate than preterm singletons. However, although preterm twins are more likely to survive, there is an increased rate of cerebral palsy among survivors. The lowest perinatal mortality rate for twins is at 37 weeks, (i.e., 3 weeks earlier than for singletons). The mortality rate increases for twins at 39 weeks (as it does at 42 weeks for postterm singletons). Lung maturation in twins also occurs earlier than in singletons.

Considerations of normal gestation length are important when counseling a mother at the beginning of pregnancy, as Nägele's rule for determining the expected date of confinement does not apply in multifetal pregnancy. It is also relevant when determining a date for elective delivery by cesarean section, if this is indicated. If a date is set for 38 to 39 weeks, as is customary for singletons, then most twin pregnancies would have already commenced spontaneous labor at this gestational age, and a planned elective procedure is more likely to become an emergency procedure with its attendant increased risks. Based on these considerations, the optimal time to plan an elective cesarean section in twins is at about 36 weeks by sure dates based on an early dating scan.

## Diagnostic Strategies

Early diagnosis of multifetal pregnancies results in better outcome.

Multifetal pregnancy may be suspected if there is a personal or family history of multiple pregnancies. Of course, there is increased suspicion if the pregnancy follows fertility treatment.

The mother may complain of excessive weight gain or other pregnancy symptoms because all pregnancy hormones are increased. The uterine size may be unduly large for the period of amenorrhea. Later, there may also be a sensation of excessive fetal movements, or multiple parts felt on examination. In centers where early ultrasonographic scan is routine, most spontaneous multiple pregnancies are first detected on ultrasonography.

## IMAGING

Ultrasonography is essential in the initial assessment of multifetal pregnancies, as well as in subsequent antenatal surveillance. It has several important functions in early pregnancy:

1. *To establish plurality:* Even after assisted reproduction, when the number of replaced embryos is known, some may twin spontaneously, resulting in a mixed dizygotic/monozygotic multifetal pregnancy.
2. *To confirm viability of each fetus:* This is important in view of the increased number of miscarriages in multifetal pregnancies.
3. *To confirm structural normality:* There is an increased risk of congenital abnormality in multifetal pregnancies (see later). Serologic tests, such as alpha-fetoprotein, are of limited use, because normal limits are higher and wider. Early prenatal diagnosis allows the mother to make a decision. Selective termination of one twin is possible and considered a safe and effective option, provided monochorionicity has been excluded.
4. *To establish dates:* An accurate gestational age is an important prerequisite of adequate care in any pregnancy. Unless the exact date of conception is known, it is now well established that even a "certain" last menstrual period can have considerable error. This may result in wrong calculation of gestational age at potentially critical decision points during preterm gestation periods. Furthermore, the assessment of growth may be incorrect when the dates are wrong and the error becomes proportionately larger at preterm gestations. Accurate dates can establish an appropriate baseline for subsequent monitor-

**Table 32–1** Ultrasonography in Multiple Pregnancy

| 1st and 2nd Trimesters |
|---|
| Establish plurality |
| Viability; vanishing twin |
| Chorionicity; membranes; lambda sign; fetal sex |
| Dating the pregnancy |
| Structural (anomaly) scan |
| Early hydramnios IUGR, TTTS |

| 3rd Trimester |
|---|
| Amniotic fluid |
| Presentation and position |
| Monitoring growth |
| Estimation of fetal weight |
| Twin-twin discordance |

IUGR = intrauterine growth restriction; TTTS = twin-twin transfusion syndrome.

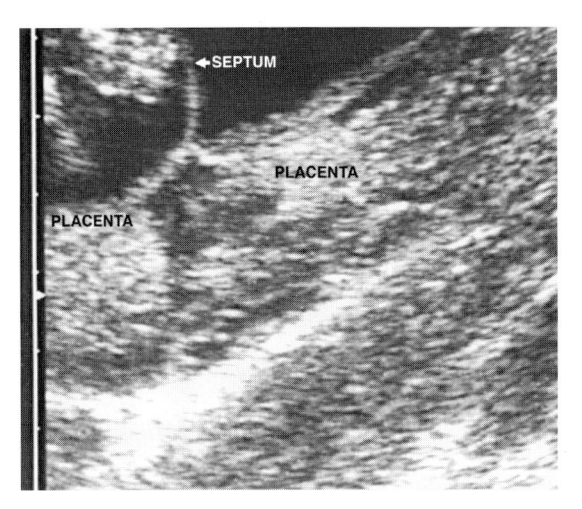

**Figure 32–1** Dichorionic pregnancy in second trimester, showing separate placentas, thick membrane, and lambda sign.

ing of fetal growth. Ultrasonographic dating is accurate in twins and triplets, as in singletons, and the same first- and second-trimester dating formulas can be used regardless of plurality.

5. *To establish chorionicity:* Unless it is clear that a twin pregnancy has unlike-sex fetuses, (i.e., is dizygotic), it is important to establish chorionicity and zygosity as early as possible. The number of placenta disks is not a reliable indicator for chorionicity. A single disk may represent a fused dichorionic placenta, because a small number of monochorionic placentas may have two disks or disks joined by bridges of parenchymal tissue. Large succenturate lobes of monochorionic placentas may be mistaken for dichorionic disks.

   The information about chorionicity is best provided from the septum between the embryos. This should be done in the first or early second trimester, preferably by vaginal ultrasonography. Rarely (1% of all twins) a monochorionic twin is also monoamniotic and no septum is seen. In most monochorionic twins, a thin septum consisting of amniotic membrane (i.e., two fused membranes) is seen, with a thickness of less than 2 mm. In dichorionic pregnancies, two single or fused chorionic layers are also seen between the amniotic membranes, with an overall thickness of 4 mm or more. A further sign is provided by the attachment of the septum to the placental plate. The two membranes of the intraseptal chorion can usually be seen to diverge here, forming a delta or lambda shape (Fig 32–1). These signs may be more difficult to assess later in pregnancy because of crowding, pressure effects from amniotic fluid, and resultant thinning of the membrane.

6. Early ultrasonography can also detect the presence of early, severe twin-twin transfusion syndrome (see later).

## Practical Strategies

Multiple pregnancies are high risk and require special provisions, policies, and expertise. In recent years, dedicated twin clinics have been set up in tertiary referral centers, but the principles can be applied in a variety of settings.

### CARE OF THE MOTHER

*Counseling* at the beginning of pregnancy needs to address special issues for multifetal pregnancy. The mother should be warned about increased pregnancy symptoms, more discomfort, more visits, shorter length of gestation, increased likelihood of rupture of membranes, and higher rate of operative delivery. Delivery should be planned at a center that has appropriate obstetric and neonatal backup.

*Rest* is important in multifetal pregnancies, but rou-

**Table 32–2** Increased Risks of Multifetal Pregnancy

| Fetus |
|---|
| Miscarriage; vanishing twin |
| Congenital abnormality |
| Cerebral palsy |
| Perinatal mortality |
| Oligohydramnios |
| Preterm delivery |
| Growth restriction |
| Twin-twin transfusion: donor (hypertensive, small) or recipient (hydrops) |
| Malpresentation |
| Cord prolapse |
| "Locked twins" |
| Intrapartum fetal injury |

| Mother |
|---|
| Excessive nausea and other pregnancy symptoms |
| Iron deficient or megaloblastic anemia |
| Edema, weight gain |
| Polyhydramnios |
| Pregnancy-induced hypertension and preeclampsia |
| Preterm labor |
| Antepartum hemorrhage |
| Cesarean section |
| Postpartum hemorrhage |
| Postnatal adjustment |

tine admission to the hospital is not warranted. Occupations that require prolonged standing should be discouraged. Prolonged standing has been shown to contribute to shortening and widening of the cervix. Alternatively, regular rest periods of at least 2 hours three times a day have been advocated.

*Anemia* is more likely to occur in multifetal pregnancy, but a low hemoglobin reading may also be the result of increased intravascular volume; therefore, the mean corpuscular hemoglobin concentration and ferritin levels are better indicators. Nevertheless, iron supplementation is often given prophylactically. Folic acid supplements are given in early pregnancy to cover the larger fetal demands, which together with poor nutrition, may result in megaloblastic anemia.

*Maternal weight gain* should be expected to be higher than in singleton pregnancies. The steepest rise is in early pregnancy and reflects the maternal hormonal response. In pregnancies with normal outcome, average maternal weight gained by the time of viability (24 weeks) is approximately 12 pounds in singleton pregnancy, 24 pounds in twins, and 36 pounds in triplets. Subsequently, for a mother of average weight, a weekly weight gain of 1.5 pounds is considered satisfactory in twin pregnancy. It is important that appropriate dietary advice is given and that malnutrition is corrected, if present. However, it is uncertain whether increasing the weight gain is of benefit, and in obese mothers it may be counterproductive.

*Pregnancy-induced hypertension*; it is important to have an early record of maternal blood pressure along with regular assessment and urinalysis. In twin pregnancies, the incidence of preeclampsia is about 5 times higher in primigravida and 10 times higher in multigravida than in their respective singleton counterparts.

*Antepartum hemorrhage*, the likelihood of bleeding during pregnancy, may be higher because of the larger surface area of the placental bed. In in vitro fertilization pregnancies, the incidence of low-lying placentas is significantly increased.

An important part of special counseling in multifetal pregnancy is instruction in early recognition of preterm labor. Home uterine monitoring for preterm labor is increasingly advocated, and there is some evidence that, at least in multiple pregnancies, it is effective and leads to improved outcome.

Cervical length can be assessed by repeat vaginal examinations or, better, by vaginal ultrasonography, which can quantify cervical length and the state of the internal os (funneling). A cervical length of more than 25 or 30 mm in the early third trimester and the absence of funneling at the internal os have been suggested to be useful in predicting progress to term in singleton pregnancies. However, efficacy in multiple pregnancy has not been proven, and further studies are awaited.

Fetal fibronectin has been established as a useful predictor of preterm delivery in singleton pregnancy and recent evidence suggests that it is equally effective in predicting early ($\leq 34$ weeks) delivery in multifetal pregnancy.

Past strategies against preterm labor in multifetal pregnancies have included prophylactic administration of β-mimetics or cervical cerclage. Neither has evidence of benefit. Cerclage may be beneficial in cases with evidence of cervical incompetence in the second trimester (decreased cervical length, increased dilatation, or funneling), but these findings were not based on randomized trials.

## FETAL SURVEILLANCE

### Prenatal Diagnosis

Multifetal pregnancies have a higher rate of congenital abnormalities. This excess is associated with monozygotic twins, whereas the rate in dizygotic twins is virtually the same as in singletons. Abnormalities may relate to the placenta with single or multiple vascular anastomoses, or the embryo, with localized defects in morphogenesis. These may affect any system, including the cardiovascular system, the central nervous system, or the gastrointestinal tract. Specific anomalies include septal defects, abnormalities of the diaphragm, tracheoesophageal fistulas, hernias, cystic kidneys, encephalocoele, and cleft lip and palate.

### Monitoring Growth

Twins and higher multiples are at increased risk of intrauterine growth restriction (IUGR). Fundal height measurements may assess abdominal girth and detect rapid increases associated with hydramnios, but are not indicative of fetal growth. In a normal twin pregnancy, the uterine size at 25 weeks is already close to that of a term singleton pregnancy. The slowing of growth is predominantly a third trimester phenomenon. At term, the median weight-for-gestation of twins is little over the 10th percentile for singletons.

The standard method of surveillance is by regular ultrasonographic scans. Various policies exist for serial scanning, but they should be done at least every 4 weeks and preferably every 2 to 3 weeks in the third trimester. The most sensitive measurements for detecting growth disturbances are fetal abdominal circumference and fetal weight assessment based on abdominal circumference, femur length, and head circumference.

Serial ultrasonographic studies confirm that abdominal circumference growth and weight gain are slower in multifetal pregnancies. It is a question of debate whether small-for-gestational age twin pregnancies are all growth restricted because they are smaller than singletons, or whether their slower growth is an adaptive, physiologic response. The latter concept would indicate a downward adjustment of the growth standard, which allows a better distinction between normal and pathologic multifetal pregnancies. Figure 32–2 shows curves for the median, 90th and 10th percentiles of optimal fetal growth for twins. It was derived from serial ultrasonographic estimations of fetal weight in twin A in 105 consecutive, normal-outcome twin pregnancies with early ultrasonographic dates. Normal outcome was defined as pregnancies reaching at least 34 weeks of gestation, spontaneous onset of labor, and intertwin weight discordance at birth of less than 15%.

Reports on the accuracy of weight prediction in twin pregnancies are mixed. Several studies suggest that the error is larger in twins than in singletons, whereas others have maintained that with appropriate methods and formulas, the range of error is similar. There is evidence, however, that the detection of intertwin discordance is often inaccurate. This may be related to problems with measuring abdominal circumference in a crowded intrauterine environment, oligohydramnios, and/or malposition.

The predominant cause of growth restriction in twins, as in singletons, is placental failure. Intertwin disparities exist in monochorionic and dichorionic twins. As most twin pregnancies are dichorionic, intertwin disparities are more likely to be caused by fetal growth restriction than by intertwin transfusion. Even in monochorionic twins who have weight discordance at birth, the smaller twin has polycythemia in only a third of cases, suggesting that the cause for discordance is more often uteroplacental dysfunction rather than twin-twin transfusion.

Surveillance of a fetus with slow growth requires further investigation, including Doppler velocimetry and biophysical profile, to establish the optimal time for delivery.

## Twin-Twin Transfusion Syndrome

About two thirds of monozygotic twins are monochorionic (i.e., about one fourth of all twins are monochorionic). Transplacental communications between the circulations of twins are almost always associated with monochorionic placentas. A variety of different anastomoses and shunts may develop, which may be single or multiple and located superficially or deep within the placenta. Superficial anastomoses are more likely to be arterial-arterial and venous-venous, whereas deep anastomoses are more likely to be arteriovenous shunts.

In an unselected population, such communications are thought to lead to twin-twin transfusion syndrome (TTTS) in about 10% of cases. The sequence may start with velamentous insertion of one cord, resulting in that twin being biophysically disadvantaged and hypertensive, which increases the likelihood of a net transfer of blood via vascular communications. The drainage of blood from one fetus to the other results in the donor fetus being growth restricted, with arterial hypoperfusion and vascular shutdown resulting in oligohydramnios. The recipient twin becomes hydropic and polycythemic with accompanying hydramnios.

Thus the antenatal features of TTTS are a monochorionic placenta, oligohydramnios, and weight discordance. In addition to oligohydramnios, the donor twin may have abnormal arterial and venous Doppler flows, and the recipient will have enlarged vessels and abnormal systemic arterial flow patterns. However, Doppler studies have not been reliably diagnostic in these circumstances. Cordocentesis may be indicated to investigate hematocrit of each fetus and to exclude congenital abnormalities or infection (cytomegalovirus or parvovirus), which may be implicated in 15% of cases of TTTS.

Management methods include serial therapeutic amniocentesis, whereby up to 1500 ml can be withdrawn each time. This is essential for maternal comfort and for the reduction of preterm labor, and has been shown to reduce perinatal mortality. Laparoscopic laser ablation of communicating vessels is currently being investigated. Vascular anastomoses may be superficial and visualized, or deep within the pla-

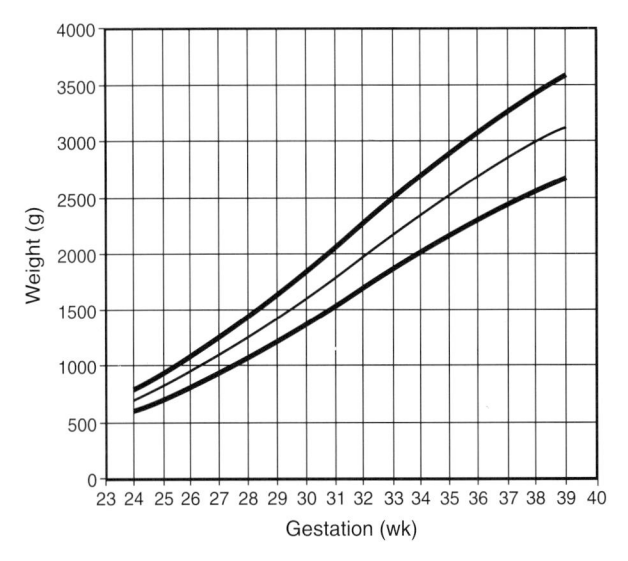

**Figure 32–2** Fetal growth curve for twins, with median and 10th and 90th percentiles. Derived from average individual log-polynomial curve fits of ultrasonographic fetal weight estimates of twin A, in 105 serially scanned pregnancies with normal outcome (defined as live birth after 34 weeks of gestation, spontaneous onset of labor, and no twin-twin discordance >15%).

centa, where they can be visualized by color Doppler flow imaging. For laser ablation, the afferent and efferent vessels need to be identified before they dip into the placenta to form arteriovenous shunts. Further details on these and other management options, such as selective fetocide, are outside the scope of this chapter. A pregnancy with suspected TTTS requires urgent referral to a maternal-fetal medicine unit.

## INTRAPARTUM CARE

The method of delivery depends on plurality, previous scars, and presentation. Triplets and higher multiples are usually delivered by elective caesarean section. For twins, the method of delivery is controversial, and evidence from randomized trials is scarce. Generally, an additional risk factor, such as previous uterine scar or nonvertex presentation of the first twin, is taken as an indication for cesarean section. A previous uterine scar may be unduly stressed during maneuvers for delivery of the second twin. With a breech first twin and a cephalic second twin, the possibility of interlocking twins exist, although this is rare.

Vaginal delivery is the method of choice if the first twin presents by the vertex, regardless of whether twin B is cephalic, breech, or transverse. However, there are advocates for cesarean section if twin B is noncephalic and estimated to weigh less than 1500 g, as intrapartum maneuvers may result in hypoxia. Data are insufficient to ascertain whether such a policy is justified.

Both twins should be monitored continuously throughout labor. It is easier to keep the two heart rates distinct by monitoring twin A directly with a scalp electrode. The mother should have a good intravenous line with a large-bore needle, blood grouped and saved, and an oxytocin infusion at the ready. Usually epidural analgesia is advised, which allows intrauterine assessment and manipulation. After delivery of the first twin, the position of twin B should be ascertained by abdominal palpation and internal examination. An ultrasonographic scanner should be used if there is doubt about the presentation.

If the second twin is cephalic, the head should be allowed to come down, aided if necessary, by an infusion of oxytocin if contractions are weak or infrequent. Controlled rupture of membranes can then be undertaken with a reduced chance of cord prolapse. If twin B is breech, the membranes should be ruptured and breech extraction undertaken. If twin B is transverse, the best option depends on examination findings and operator preference. Many advocate external cephalic version as the first option, followed by descent and judicious rupture of membranes. Others prefer internal podalic version. In this maneuver, the foot or both feet are identified and distinguished from a hand by the presence of the heel. The foot is pulled down to turn the baby to the breech position, followed by breech extraction. Internal podalic version can be attempted with the second membranes still intact.

### Postpartum Hemorrhage

The incidence of postpartum hemorrhage is significantly increased in multiple pregnancy, because of the larger placental mass, uterine overdistention, and predisposition to atony. Third stage should be managed actively after a stat dose of oxytocin with ergometrine. It is advisable to maintain an oxytocin infusion for 4 hours after delivery as prophylaxis against postpartum hemorrhage. Continued bleeding should be managed by uterine massage, investigation and removal of retained products, prostaglandin $F_{2\alpha}$, and blood transfusion as required.

## POSTNATAL CARE

Multifetal pregnancies require increased postnatal attention and care. The mother is likely to need a longer inpatient stay and additional assistance with care of the babies and breastfeeding. There are now various multiple pregnancy support groups, and links with one of them should be facilitated.

### REFERENCES

Arabin B, Aardenburg R, van Eyck J: Maternal position and ultrasonic cervical assessment in multiple pregnancy: Preliminary observations. J Reprod Med 42:719–724, 1997.

Blickstein I: The twin-twin transfusion syndrome. Obstet Gynecol 76:714–721, 1990.

Buekens P, Wilcox A: Why do small twins have a lower mortality rate than singletons? Am J Obstet Gynecol 168:937–941, 1993.

Callahan TL, Hall JE, Ettner SL, et al: The economic impact of multiple gestation pregnancies and the contribution of assisted reproduction techniques to their incidence. N Engl J Med 331:244–249, 1994.

**Table 32–3** Multifetal Pregnancy: Preferred Mode of Delivery

---

Previous cesarean section → elective cesarean section
Twin A vertex → vaginal delivery
  (1) Twin B vertex → ± oxytocin, controlled rupture of membranes
  (2) Twin B breech → rupture of membranes, breech extraction
  (3) Twin B transverse → external cephalic version and (1)
    or
    → internal podalic version and (2)
Twin A nonvertex → elective cesarean section
Triplets and higher multiples → elective cesarean section

Caravello JW, Chauhan SP, Morrison JC, et al: Sonographic examination does not predict twin growth discordance accurately. Am J Obstet Gynecol 89:529–533, 1997.

Chervenak FA, Johnson RE, Youcha S, et al: Obstet Gynecol 65:119–124, 1985.

Chervenak FA, Skupski DW, Romero R, et al: How accurate is fetal biometry in the assessment of fetal age? Am J Obstet Gynecol 178:678–687, 1998.

Crane JMG, van der Hof M, Armson BA, Liston R: Transvaginal ultrasound in the prediction of preterm delivery: Singleton and twin gestations. Obstet Gynecol 90:357–363, 1997.

DeLia JE, Cruickshank DP, Keye WR: Fetoscopic neodymium: YAG laser occlusion of placental vessels in severe twin-twin transfusion syndrome. Obstet Gynecol 75:1046–1053, 1990.

Derom C, Vlietinck R, Derom R, et al: Increased monozygotic twinning rate after ovulation induction. Lancet 1:1236–1237, 1987.

Dyson DC, Crites YM, Ray DA, et al: Prevention of preterm birth in high risk patients: The role of education and provider contact versus home uterine monitoring. Am J Obstet Gynecol 164:756–762, 1991.

Gardosi J, Mul T, Francis A, et al: Comparison of second trimester biometry in singleton and twin pregnancies conceived with assisted reproductive techniques. Br J Obstet Gynaecol 104:737–740, 1997.

Geirsson RT, Have G: Comparison of actual and ultrasound estimated second trimester gestational length in in-vitro fertilized pregnancies. Acta Obstet Gynecol Scand 72:344–346, 1993.

Keith L, Papiernik E: Multiple gestation. Clin Obstet Gynecol 41:1, 1998.

Kilpatrick SJ, Jackson R, Croughan-Minihane MS: Perinatal mortality in twins and singletons matched for gestational age at delivery at ≥30 weeks. Am J Obstet Gynecol 174:66–71, 1996.

Leveno KJ, Quirk G, Whalley PJ, et al: Fetal lung maturation in twin gestation. Am J Obstet Gynecol 148:405–411, 1984.

Luke B, Keith LG: The contribution of singletons, twins, and triplets to low birth weight, infant mortality, and handicap in the United States. J Reprod Med 37:661–666, 1992.

Luke B: The changing pattern of multiple births in the United States: Maternal and infant chanracteristics, 1973 and 1990. Obstet Gynecol 84:101–106, 1994.

Luke B, Minogue J, Witter FR, et al: The ideal twin pregnancy: Patterns of weight gain, discordancy, and length of gestation. Am J Obstet Gynecol 169:588–597, 1993.

Machin GA, Keith LG: An Atlas of Multiple Pregnancy, Biology and Pathology. New York, Parthenon, 1997.

Michaels WH, Schreiber FR, Padgett RJ, et al: Ultrasound surveillance of the cervix in twin gestations: Management of cervical incompetence. Obstet Gynecol 78:739–744, 1991.

Newman RB, Ellings JM: Antepartum management of the multiple gestation: The case for specialized care. Semin Perinatol 19:387–402, 1995.

Papiernik E, Richard A, Tafforeau J, Keith L: Social groups and prevention of twin births in a population of twin mothers. J Perinat Med 24:669–676, 1996.

Rabinovici J, Barhai G, Reichman B, et al: Internal podalic version with unruptured membranes for the second twin in transverse lie. Obstet Gynecol 71:428–430, 1988.

Reisner DP, Mahoney BS, Petty CN, et al: Stuck twin syndrome: Outcome in thirty-seven consecutive cases. Am J Obstet Gynecol 169:991–995, 1993.

Saari-Kemppainen A, Karjalainen O, Ylostalo P, et al: Controlled study of systematic one-stage screening in pregnancy. Lancet 336:387–391, 1990.

Sebire NJ, D'Ercole C, Soares W, et al: Intertwin disparity in fetal size in monochorionic and dichorionic pregnancies. Obstet Gynecol 91:82–85, 1998.

Suitor CW: Maternal weight gain: A report of an Expert Work Group. Arlington, VA, National Center for Education in Maternal and Child Health, 1997.

Ville Y, Hyett J, Hecher K, Nicolaides K: Preliminary experience with endoscopic laser surgery for severe twin-twin transfusion syndrome. N Engl J Med 332:224–227, 1995.

Wennerholm UB, Holm B, Mattsby-Baltzer I, et al: Fetal fibronectin, endotoxin, bacterial vaginosis and cervical length as predictors of preterm birth and neonatal morbidity in twin pregnancies. Br J Obstet Gynaecol 104:1398–1404, 1997.

Wenstrom KD, Tessen JA, Zlatnik FJ: Frequency, distribution, and theoretic mechanisms for hematology and weight discordance in monochorionic twins. Obstet Gynecol 80:257–261, 1992.

Westergaard T, Wohlfahrt J, Aaby P, et al: Population based study of rates of multiple pregnancies in Denmark, 1980–94. BMJ 314:775–779, 1997.

# 33

# Preterm Birth

DAVID F. COLOMBO
JAY D. IAMS

Premature birth is the single largest cause of perinatal mortality and morbidity in nonanomalous infants in all developed nations. In the United States, complications of prematurity account for more than 70% of fetal and neonatal deaths annually in infants without anomalies. The long-term sequelae of prematurity disproportionately contribute to developmental delay, visual and hearing impairment, chronic lung disease, and cerebral palsy. Fortunately, advances in the care of the neonate have significantly improved during the last 30 years and have led to a reduction in the mortality and long-term morbidity of the premature infant. However, despite a large amount of investigation, the actual rate of preterm delivery before 37 weeks of gestation has risen from 93 per 1000 live births in 1970 to 101 per 1000 live births in 1993.

Most of the emphasis in the study of preterm delivery has focused on the identification and treatment of a single etiology to explain all preterm births. Unfortunately, this methodology has met with little success. The current belief is that the pathway to premature delivery is a multifactorial process that is not completely understood. This chapter describes the basic terms used in discussing preterm birth, discusses the diagnoses of patients at risk for preterm delivery, and relates the current treatment modalities available for these patients.

# Definitions

The concept of prematurity is hampered by confusion and imprecise terminology. Multiple terms are used interchangeably in the literature to describe similar but not identical situations. This confusion seems to have evolved in an era when accurate determination of gestational age was not possible. Because of developments in sensitive serologic markers for pregnancy and in ultrasonography, in most cases we are now able to pinpoint gestational age within 1 to 2 weeks. With this new knowledge, we are more able to be specific in discussing the premature infant. When discussing the status of an infant, it is common to refer to gestational age, weight, and maturity.

## GESTATIONAL AGE

*Preterm delivery*: An infant is considered full term if he or she is born after the 37th week of gestation (259 days after the first day of the mother's last menstrual period or 245 days after conception).
*Term delivery*: A delivery between 37 and 42 weeks of gestation.
*Post-term (postdates) delivery*: A delivery after 42 weeks of gestation.

## WEIGHT

*Low birth weight*: Infant weighing less than 2500 g
*Very low birth weight*: Infant weighing less than 1500 g
*Extremely low birth weight*: Infant weighing less than 1000 g

## MATURITY

*Prematurity*: The condition used to describe any infant who is not capable of independent function after delivery (e.g., respiratory distress syndrome, necrotizing enterocolitis)

# Epidemiology of Spontaneous Preterm Birth

A large number of risk factors are associated with preterm birth. These can be grouped into three categories. The first group of risk factors includes isolated events that can occur in a given pregnancy and that are not necessarily prone to recurrence. These include items such as placenta previa, placental abruption, polyhydramnios, oligohydramnios, and multiple gestation. The second group of risk factors includes those over which the patient has no control, including African-American ethnicity, a history of preterm delivery, being younger than 18 years of age or older than 40 years of age, and having a uterine anomaly or an incompetent cervix. Finally, some risk factors associated with preterm delivery are modifiable, such as smoking, substance abuse, poor nutrition, the presence of sexually transmitted disease or other infection, poor socioeconomic status, excessive maternal activity, sexual activity, and low prepregnancy weight.

Although all of these risk factors are associated with preterm birth, it is imperative that the clinician note that more than half of the patients who deliver before 35 weeks of gestation have no identifiable risk factors. This fact has made prediction of preterm birth by history alone not practical. To date, the best attempt to produce a prematurity prediction scoring system was developed in 1980 by Creasy and associates. This system was able to predict two thirds of those who delivered prematurely in a middle-class population. However, when the same scoring system was used in a higher risk indigent population, the results were much less impressive.

# Possible Etiologies for Spontaneous Preterm Birth

Once risk factors for preterm birth are recognized, the logical next step is to link risk factors into pathways that attempt to explain why preterm birth occurs. The next section addresses current concepts for explaining preterm labor.

## DECIDUAL ISCHEMIA

Until recently, it was assumed that the fetus played little role in the process of preterm labor and birth. Data now suggest that the prevalence of preterm birth is increased in pregnancies with poor interuterine growth. Salafia and associates evaluated placentas from patients who delivered between 22 and 32 weeks of gestation and found decidual vascular abnormalities significantly more often than in control subjects (odds ratio = 4.1). Arias and associates performed a case-control study that found that placental vascular lesions were significantly more common in placentas from noninfected women who delivered after preterm labor (odds ratio = 3.8).

It has been postulated that the contribution of fetal stress to the onset of preterm labor may be mediated in part by the release of uteroplacental corticotropin-releasing hormone. This peptide is produced by the placenta and enhances prostinoid production in the amniochorion and decidua. These reports make it biologically plausible that abnormalities of the placenta or uterine blood flow could precipitate preterm labor and delivery.

## INFECTION AND PREMATURITY

Numerous studies have shown an association between preterm birth and infection. Early clinical evidence of this phenomenon was noted in a study that found that 20 to 30% of women who delivered prematurely had a positive amniotic fluid culture. In addition, the incidence of maternal and neonatal infections after preterm birth is significantly higher than that of patients who deliver at term. In fact, the association between clinical and histologic amnionitis increases as the gestational age decreases, especially before 32 weeks of gestation.

Microbiologic studies have observed an association between preterm birth and maternal vaginal colonization with various microflora. These include bacterial vaginosis, group B streptococci, *Chlamydia trachomatis*, and *Trichomonas*. Bacterial vaginosis has gained much attention as a causative factor in the increased risk of preterm birth. Rather than a specific infection, bacterial vaginosis is an alteration of the maternal vaginal flora, which is predominately *Lactobacillus*, to anaerobic bacteria such as *Gardnerella vaginalis*, *Bacteroides*, *Pervotella*, *Mobiluncus* species, and *Mycoplasma*. In a study by Gravett and associates, it was noted that women who tested positive for bacterial vaginosis in the second and third trimesters had an increased risk for preterm labor (odds ratio = 2.0), preterm premature rupture of the membranes (odds ratio = 2.0), and intra-amniotic infection (odds ratio = 2.7). It is believed that the bacteria isolated from women who have bacterial vaginosis may produce collagenases and proteases that are capable of injuring the fetal membranes.

Until the relationship between bacterial vaginosis and preterm labor becomes clear, the following recommendations are reasonable:

1. Screening for bacterial vaginosis should be considered in women at high risk for preterm labor.
2. Women who have symptoms of bacterial vaginosis should be treated with *oral* metronidazole.
3. It is unclear whether there is any benefit in screening women for bacterial vaginosis to prevent preterm labor.

# Diagnosis of Preterm Labor

The diagnosis of preterm labor (PTL) is traditionally made by the combination of persistent uterine contractions and a change in dilatation or effacement (or both dilatation and effacement) of the cervix as diagnosed by a digital examination. The *Guidelines for Perinatal Care* (fourth edition) published by the American College of Obstetricians and Gynecologists suggest the following criteria for diagnosis:

1. Gestational age of more than 20 weeks but less than 37 weeks
2. Persistent uterine contractions (4 every 20 minutes or 8 every 60 minutes)
3. Documented cervical change or cervical effacement greater than 80% with cervical dilatation greater than 1 cm.

Although the preceding criteria seem straightforward, they have been shown to have a poor sensitivity for diagnosing preterm delivery. Randomized clinical trials of tocolytic drugs have found that approximately 40% of subjects diagnosed by these criteria and treated with placebo went to full term before delivery. The continued use of these criteria for diagnosis has been justified by studies that have shown that 25 to 50% of women who are diagnosed with PTL have spontaneous rupture of the membranes or cervical dilatation greater than 3 cm. In either case, successful tocolysis is much less likely. The consequences of this approach are the unnecessary treatment of women who have only uterine activity and not PTL.

The current goal of obstetricians is to decrease the number of false-positive diagnoses of PTL without increasing the number of false-negative diagnoses. To improve the accuracy of the diagnosis of PTL in symptomatic women, two new methods of evaluation have been created. The first is transvaginal cervical sonography for measuring cervical length. The second is the screening for fetal fibronectin (fFN) in the vaginal vault.

## CERVICAL SONOGRAPHY

Several studies have shown that a clinician is able to assess cervical dilatation digitally with some degree of accuracy after the cervix is dilated at least 3 cm. However, assessment of cervical dilatation and effacement of the cervix dilated less than 3 cm is more subjective. One can certainly see how this fact would increase both the overdiagnosis and underdiagnosis of PTL.

The first studies that attempted to evaluate the cervix by ultrasonography used the transabdominal approach. However, this method was less than optimal because it was affected by factors such as maternal body habitus and degree of bladder fullness. The use of transvaginal sonography has allowed for accurate images in more than 95% of patients. In fact, the diagnostic accuracy of PTL has improved with this technique. A cervical length of 30 mm or greater is good evidence that significant cervical effacement has not occurred. (Previous studies have shown that 30 mm is the 25th percentile for length.) The power of this technique becomes clear when cervical length is combined with obstetrical history. Table 33–1 presents the probabilities of spontaneous delivery at less than 35 weeks of gestation as a function of gestational age and cervical length.

For a clinician to use the data in the literature regarding cervical length and preterm delivery prediction with any certainty, it is important to take an accurate image of the cervix. The following is a standard protocol that can be used to measure the cervix length consistently. The total examination time is usually between 5 and 10 minutes.

1. Ask the patient to void.
2. Insert the vaginal probe under direct visualization.

**Table 33–1** Probability of Spontaneous Delivery <35 Weeks of Gestation Based on Obstetric History and Cervical Length

| Gestational Age of Previous Birth | Cervical Length at 24 Wk of Gestation | | |
|---|---|---|---|
| | <25 mm (%) | 26–35 mm (%) | >36 mm (%) |
| 18 to 26 wk | 33 | 17 | 8 |
| 27 to 31 wk | 39 | 21 | 10 |
| 32 to 36 wk | 28 | 14 | 6 |
| Term delivery | 8 | 4 | 2 |

3. Identify bladder, amniotic fluid, and fetal presenting part. Be certain to identify any findings, such as placenta previa or absence of fetal heart motion.
4. Find the midline sagittal plane of the cervix and look in the proximal third for the internal os.
5. Pull back the probe until the lightest touch gives a good image of the cervical canal.
6. Angle the probe slightly to get the best long axis of the cervix.
7. Measure the cervical length three times by placing the calipers appropriately and recording the distance between the internal os and external os.
8. Record the measurement of the best image and make a hard copy of the image.
9. Make sure to record any evidence of funneling, dilatation, and membrane protrusion.
10. Apply gentle upward pressure on the lower uterine segment for approximately 15 seconds. Remeasure the cervix in the same manner as described previously if it shortens or if a funnel becomes apparent.

## FETAL FIBRONECTIN

fFN is an extracellular matrix protein that is normally found in the fetal membranes and decidua (choriodecidual junction). It can be easily distinguished from the adult form of fibronectin secondary to a unique region called the III-CS domain. Detection of the fFN is made possible with a monoclonal antibody to this III-CS domain called the FDC-6. Fetal fibronectin is normally found in the cervicovaginal fluid in the first 20 weeks of gestation. However, its presence in the vagina or cervix after 20 weeks indicates a disruption in the attachment of the membranes to the decidua. One possible etiology for the disruption of this extracellular matrix may be the presence of a localized inflammation of the fetal membrane-uterine interface. This inflammation might be caused by an occult ascending bacterial infiltration that could incite a maternal response, affecting the extracellular matrix.

The Food and Drug Administration (FDA) approved the clinical use of the fFN test in 1995 for evaluating the risk for preterm delivery. Before approval was granted, multiple studies were performed to assess the usefulness of the test. One of the larger studies was performed by Peaceman and associates who tested 763 women with symptoms of PTL. In this group, 129 women were clinically diagnosed with PTL and treated. In this subset, 86 of the women tested negative for fFN. Of those, only 3 delivered in the following 7 days, giving a negative predictive value of 96.5%. In the remaining 634 women who did not meet clinical criteria for diagnosis and treatment, only 9 women delivered within 7 days of the test. It is interesting to note that all 9 of these women tested positive for fFN. In a similar study by Iams and associates, 192 women who had symptoms of PTL were studied to evaluate fFN in the clinical diagnosis of PTL. In this population of symptomatic patients, an fFN test had a sensitivity of 93% and a specificity of 82% for predicting preterm delivery within 7 days of the test. In this group, the positive predictive value of fFN was 29% with a negative predictive value of 99%. In both of these examples, the endpoint of the study was 7 days. Other investigations have shown that a similar result is obtained when a 14-day endpoint is used. Based on all the data, it appears clear that the fFN test is most useful in a clinical setting as a test to rule out PTL and prevent overtreatment. Finally, all studies in which fFN was noted to be of clinical use were performed in a symptomatic population. There is no current clinical role for using fFN testing as a screening test to evaluate the risk of PTL in a low-risk population.

## Clinical Evaluation of Patients Who Have Possible Preterm Labor

The following is a sample protocol for evaluating a patient to rule out PTL. This protocol should be used for any patient who presents with persistent contractions (painless or painful), pelvic pressure, backache, increase or change in vaginal discharge, or vaginal spotting or bleeding.

1. The patient should be monitored for fetal heart tones and uterine contractions.
2. Take a careful obstetric history with care to note any previous preterm delivery or gynecologic procedures involving the cervix or uterus (including any cervical laceration during a previous delivery).
3. A sterile speculum examination should be performed to evaluate:
Vaginal pH
    Evidence of spontaneous rupture of the membranes (e.g., vaginal pool, fern test, nitrozine paper)
    Group B streptococcus (culture of the outer third of the vagina and perineum)
    Chlamydia (culture of the cervix)
    *Neisseria gonorrhoeae* (culture of the cervix)
    Fetal fibronectin (swab samples of the external cervical os and posterior vagina)
4. A transabdominal ultrasonogram should be obtained to evaluate placental location, amniotic

fluid volume, estimated fetal weight, and overall fetal well-being.
5. Perform a digital examination to evaluate the cervix for dilatation and effacement if preterm rupture of the membranes is ruled out.
   *Cervix >3 cm dilatation*: Diagnosis of PTL confirmed. Consider tocolysis (if not contraindicated).
   *Cervix 2 to 3 cm dilatation*: Diagnosis of PTL possible, but not confirmed. Obtain a transvaginal ultrasonogram to evaluate cervical length; if less than 30 mm, consider tocolysis. Repeat digital examination and transvaginal cervical sonography in 30 to 60 minutes. Consider tocolysis (if not contraindicated) if there is a cervical change, increase in contraction frequency, or fFN is positive.
   *Cervix <2 cm dilatation*: The diagnosis of PTL is uncertain. Monitor contraction frequency. Obtain a transvaginal ultrasonogram to evaluate cervical length; if less than 30 mm consider tocolysis. Repeat digital examination and transvaginal cervical sonography in 1 to 2 hours. Consider tocolysis (if not contraindicated) if there is a cervical change, increase in contraction frequency, or fFN is positive.
6. If patient is symptomatic with positive fFN:
   Begin parenteral tocolysis
   If patient is stable, transfer patient to a tertiary care center.
   Administer glucocorticoids. Betamethasone, 12 mg intramuscularly every 24 hours for two doses, or dexamethasone, 6 mg intramuscularly every 6 hours for four doses.
   Begin Group B streptococcus prophylaxis.

## Tocolytic Therapy

Tocolytic drugs are used to decrease or stop uterine activity primarily in an acute setting. They are relatively safe when used according to the published protocols. The choice of tocolytic requires careful consideration of the efficacy, risks, and side effects with regard to the individual patient. One must also evaluate the potential contraindications to tocolysis from a maternal and fetal standpoint (Table 33–2). The next section briefly describes the tocolytic agents available to the clinician.

### β-MIMETICS

The β-mimetic drugs have been the most commonly used tocolytics in the United States for the last 30 years. They are structurally similar to epinephrine and norepinephrine. This category of drugs includes ritodrine, terbutaline, albuterol, fenoterol, hexoprenaline, isoxsuprine, metaproterenol, nylidrin, orciprenaline, and salbutamol. Ritodrine and terbutaline are by far the most commonly used. Ritodrine is the only agent approved by the FDA for tocolysis. There is good evidence that β-mimetics act by stimulating β-receptors to cause smooth muscle relaxation. Side effects of the β-mimetics are related to stimulation of other β-receptors throughout the body. These include increased heart rate, increase in smooth muscle relaxation of the vasculature walls, and changes in hepatic glycogen production and insulin release from the islet cells.

**Table 33–2** Contraindications to the Use of Tocolytic Agents

| Maternal Contraindications to Tocolysis | Fetal Contraindications to Tocolysis |
|---|---|
| Significant hypertension | Gestational age >37 wk |
| Eclampsia | Estimated fetal weight >2500 g |
| Antepartum hemorrhage | Fetal demise or lethal anomaly |
| Cardiac disease | Chorioamnionitis |
| Allergy to a tocolytic agent | Fetal distress |
|  | Intrauterine growth restriction |

### MAGNESIUM SULFATE

Intravenous magnesium sulfate has been used in obstetrics for many years as seizure prophylaxis in preeclampsia. It was not until the 1970s that magnesium was used as a tocolytic. The exact mechanism of action of magnesium is not completely understood. One theory that has been proposed is that magnesium acts by competing with calcium at the motor endplate to reduce excitation or at the cell membrane to reduce the amount of calcium influx. Relatively few studies have compared magnesium with placebo for tocolysis; however, in several studies magnesium was found to be equivalent to β-mimetics for pregnancy prolongation.

Magnesium has relatively few side effects compared with the other tocolytic agents. Magnesium has been associated with nausea, flushing, vomiting, headache, generalized muscle weakness, shortness of breath, and pulmonary edema. At higher concentrations, magnesium has been associated with cardiac arrhythmias and coma.

There has been no therapeutic level set for magnesium to date. Mean serum levels are similar in patients who are successfully and unsuccessfully tocolysed. Magnesium sulfate is usually administered by starting with an intravenous bolus with 4 to 6 g in a 10 to 20% solution over 20 minutes. A maintenance dose of 2 g/hr is then begun. The maintenance dose is increased by 1 g/hr until tocolysis is obtained. The maximum maintenance dose is usually 4 to 5 g/hr. The patient must be carefully monitored for signs of magnesium toxicity. Urine output and serum creatinine must be closely monitored because magnesium is cleared renally. In addition, fluid intake and urine output must be carefully recorded, because the risk of pulmonary edema is increased.

## INDOMETHACIN

Prostaglandins are important mediators in the pathway for uterine muscle contraction. Prostaglandin synthesis inhibitors interfere with these effects and therefore have a theoretical appeal for tocolysis. The use of nonsteroidal anti-inflammatory drugs leads to reduced synthesis of prostaglandins by inhibition of cyclo-oxygenase, the enzyme that converts arachidonic acid to prostaglandins.

Indomethacin is an effective tocolyzing agent. Niebyl and associates found indomethacin superior to placebo in delaying delivery for 48 hours (80% vs. 33%). Zuckerman and associates found that 95% of indomethacin-treated patients were undelivered at 48 hours. In addition, 83% were undelivered at 7 days. This was significantly different from delivery in placebo controls, with 23% undelivered at 48 hours and 16% undelivered at 7 days.

The maternal side effects of indomethacin are relatively few. The contraindications to its use include patients who have renal disease, hepatic disease, severe hypertension, coagulation disorders, and peptic ulcer disease. In contrast, the side-effect profiles of the fetus are more extensive, and can be significant and life threatening. The most worrisome of the potential fetal effects include constriction of the ductus arteriosus, oligohydramnios, and neonatal pulmonary hypertension. It has been shown that these effects can be minimized if the drug is used only before 32 weeks of gestation and for less than 48 consecutive hours. Other agents, such as sulindac, may further decrease the risk of side effects, because there is less transplacental transfer of the drug. However, there have been only limited studies exploring the tocolytic efficacy of sulindac.

The recommended dose of indomethacin for tocolytic therapy is a 50 mg to 100 mg loading dose followed by 25 to 50 mg every 4 to 6 hours for 48 hours. As previously stated, use of indomethacin should be limited to patients whose gestations are earlier than 32 weeks and who have a normal amniotic fluid index.

## CALCIUM CHANNEL BLOCKERS

Inhibitors of intracellular calcium entry have potent effects on the contraction of smooth muscle. For this reason, they are useful as tocolytics. The primary effect of calcium channel blockers is to inhibit the voltage-dependent channels of calcium into the cell. Of all the calcium channel blockers, nifedipine is the most widely used tocolytic because of its relatively selective inhibition of uterine contraction. Nifedipine is quickly becoming the tocolytic of choice for many centers because of its relatively low maternal and fetal side-effect profile.

Nifedipine is usually given as a 10 to 20 mg oral dose every 6 hours. If the patient is actively contracting, a loading dose of 10 mg orally every 20 minutes for a total of three doses may be given.

## TREATMENT WITH MULTIPLE TOCOLYTICS

As stated previously, all tocolytics have significant failure rates. This is especially true in advanced PTL. Therapy with multiple agents has been studied to improve efficacy. However, patients with refractory contractions in PTL have an increased incidence of underlying conditions, such as amnionitis and abruptio placentae. Both these conditions must be ruled out before multiagent therapy is begun. A final vital consideration is that successful tocolysis does not require the absence of contractions. It is often acceptable to reduce the frequency of contractions to less than four to six per hour to prevent further cervical change.

The combination of β-mimetics and calcium channel blockers provides the most rapid cessation of contractions, usually within 30 minutes. Another combination of agents that has proven effective is that of magnesium and indomethacin; however, this combination may take 1 to 2 hours to be effective. Centers using magnesium as their primary tocolytic often use supplemental doses of subcutaneous terbutaline (0.25 mg). This approach is effective in the rapid reduction of contractions. One must be careful not to give more than one or two doses of terbutaline, because the risk of side effects such as pulmonary edema and cardiovascular symptoms significantly increases. This complication becomes evident when intravenous ritodrine is used in combination with magnesium. Another combination of agents that should be avoided is that of magnesium and calcium channel blockers. This combination has been associated with hypotension and potential cardiac ischemia.

## The Role of Antibiotics in the Treatment of Preterm Labor

There are two potential uses for the use of antibiotics in PTL. The first is in the treatment of prophylaxis of neonatal group B streptococcal infection. This intervention has been effective in repeated studies. The second is antibiotic therapy aimed at prolonging gestation in women with PTL by targeting a broad range of micro-organisms that have been implicated in the pathogenesis of PTL. Currently there appears to be no clinical advantage to the administration of antibiotics for women in PTL except for the treatment of a specific pathogen or for prophylaxis of group B streptococci.

## Cervical Incompetence

Reduced cervical competence is a clinical diagnosis marked by the gradual, painless dilatation and effacement of the cervix. This diagnosis is usually made by a history of short labor, with the delivery of an immature fetus or loss of a pregnancy at progressively earlier gestational ages in successive pregnancies. Until recently, objective criteria for diagnosing incompetent cervix in the absence of a typical history have been lacking. The use of dilators and balloons for determining cervical resistance and hysterosalpingograms for measuring the width of the cervical canal between pregnancies has not been successful in the diagnosis of incompetent cervix. Cervical sonography has provided a reproducible method of evaluating the cervix. The sonographic characteristic of reduced cervical competence is a short cervix with a length less than 20 mm, often accompanied by funneling at the internal cervical os. A funnel at the internal os may be considered to be effacement in progress.

To fully appreciate the changes associated with an incompetent cervix as seen by cervical sonography, one must understand the normal method by which the cervix shortens and dilates. The cervix seems to shorten from the inside out. For this reason, digital examination is of limited value in determining if a cervix is incompetent. In the early stages of cervical change, one may see a funneling of the amniotic membranes into the internal cervical os. This funnel moves caudad and broadens, causing the shoulders of the funnel to become more pronounced. During this time, one may first palpate a change in the cervical examination as a subtle softening of the lower uterine segment. Eventually, the shoulders of the funnel disappear, leaving a shortened cervical length. Finally, the funnel proceeds caudally until one sees a dilatation of the external cervical os. This process is identical to cervical change in PTL and in term labor, the only exception being the absence of contractions.

## Cerclage

Since the 1950s, obstetricians have sought an effective surgical technique to strengthen the cervix. In 1955, Shirodkar reported the successful management of cervical incompetence with the use of a submucosal band placed at the level of the internal os. This procedure could be performed during pregnancy; however, it required an extensive amount of submucosal dissection and the displacement of the bladder anteriorly. Cerclage involved the use of mersilene suture and was so difficult to remove that a cesarean section was often required for delivery of the infant. In 1957, McDonald described the use of a pursestring suture that involved four bites and required no dissection. In addition, this suture could be easily removed and allowed for vaginal delivery of the infant. The McDonald cerclage has proved to be as effective as the Shirodkar cerclage, and is now considered the method of choice. As to the suture material, there does not appear to be a consensus. At the Ohio State University, we use 5 Ethibond; however, any permanent suture should work equally well.

Prophylactic cerclage sutures are usually placed in women between the 10th and 14th week of gestation. We do not routinely use tolocolysis before placement of a prophylactic cerclage; however, we do treat patients who have a positive culture for group B streptococci with ampicillin. After the cerclage is placed, we recommend that the patient abstain from sexual intercourse and avoid prolonged standing and heavy lifting for the remainder of the pregnancy. We also routinely monitor the patient with serial cervical length assessments by transvaginal sonography. No additional restrictions are recommended as long as the cervix remains more than 25 mm long without the presence of a funnel. Some shortening of the cervix can be expected after 20 weeks of gestation. In fact, if the cervical length remains greater than 35 mm, the accuracy of the original diagnosis may be questioned.

In the event of a patient newly diagnosed with cervical incompetence, an emergency cerclage can be placed. This can be placed up to the 24th week of gestation. We do not recommend placement after this time, because the infant is periviable and we believe the risk of the procedure outweighs the potential benefits. If the diagnosis is made before cervical dilatation and the cervical length is still 10 to 15 mm, we admit the patient for approximately 24 hours before the procedure. During this time we administer broad-spectrum antibiotics and give the patient perioperative indomethacin. We routinely observe the patient for 48 to 96 hours after the procedure. If the patient has had cervical dilatation before cerclage placement, we routinely monitor the patient for 5 to 7 days and often longer after the cerclage has been placed.

## Risk of Cerclage

Cervical injury at the time of delivery is the most commonly reported morbidity from a McDonald cerclage. The formation of a fibrous band at the site of the cerclage has been reported, causing a prolonged labor curve; however, most patients will have normal labor after the cerclage has been removed. A fibrous band may rupture at the time of labor, causing a cervical laceration in 1 to 13% of patients or may prevent dilatation, requiring a cesarean birth in 2 to 5% of patients. Other risk factors include infection (1%) and displacement of the suture, requiring a second suture placement (3 to 12%). A second suture has a much lower success rate compared with a single suture placement.

## Summary

1. Preterm labor is a multifactorial process that is not completely understood.
2. Preterm delivery is the largest contributor to neonatal morbidity and mortality in the non-anomalous infant.
3. The ultimate prevention of preterm birth requires aggressive intervention to reduce the rate of PTL in patients considered to be at high risk.
4. Tocolytics, glucocorticoids, and antibiotics are all useful in decreasing the morbidity and mortality associated with prematurity; however, they will never be able to eliminate the complications associated with preterm delivery.
5. Inaccurate diagnosis of PTL has been one of the largest impediments to the evaluation of treatment strategies for premature labor. Newer diagnostic methods should aid in a more accurate diagnosis.

### REFERENCES

Adeza Biomedical: Presentation to the United States Food and Drug Administration. 1995.
Anonymous: Comparison of success and morbidity in cervical cerclage procedures. Obstet Gynecol 56:543, 1980.
Arias F, Rodriquez L, Rayne S, Kraus F: Maternal placental vasculopathy and infection: Two distinct subgroups among patients with preterm labor and preterm rupture of the membranes. Am J Obstet Gynecol 168:585, 1993.
Bobitt J, Hayslip C, Damato J: Amniotic fluid infection as determined by transabdominal amniocentesis in patients with intact membranes in preterm labor. Am J Obstet Gynecol 140:947, 1981.
Carlan S, O'Brian W, O'Leary T, et al: Randomized comparative trial of indomethacin and sulindac for the treatment of refractory preterm labor. Obstet Gynecol 79:223, 1992.
Creasy R, Gummer B, Liggins G: System for predicting spontaneous preterm birth. Obstet Gynecol 55:692, 1990.
Feinberg R, Kliman H, Lockwood C: Is oncofetal fibronectin a trophoblast glue for human implantation? Am J Pathol 138:537, 1991.
Gomez R, Galasso M, Romero R: Ultrasonic examination of the uterine cervix is better than cervical digital examinations as a predictor of the likelihood of premature delivery in patients with preterm labor and intact membranes. Am J Obstet Gynecol 171:956, 1994.
Gravett M, Nelson H, DeRouen T, et al: Independent association of bacterial vaginosis and *Chlamydia trachomatis* infection and adverse pregnancy outcome. JAMA 256:1899, 1986.
Guyer B, Strobino D, Venttura S: Annual summary of vital statistics—1994. Pediatrics 96:1029, 1995.
Hack M, Taylor H, Klein N: School-age outcomes in children with birth weight under 750 grams. N Engl J Med 331:756, 1994.
Harger J: Cervical ceclage: patient selection, morbidity, and success rates. Clin Perinatol 10:321, 1998.
Herron M, Katz M, Creasy R: Evaluation of a preterm birth prevention program: preliminary report. Obstet Gynecol 59:452, 1982.
Holcomb W, Smeltzer J: Cervical effacement: Variations in belief among clinicians. Obstet Gynecol 78:43, 1991.
Iams J, Casal D, McGregor J, et al: Fetal fibronectin improves the accuracy of diagnosis of preterm labor. Am J Obstet Gynecol 173:141, 1995.
Iams J, Paraskos J, Landon M: Cervical sonography in preterm labour. Obstet Gynecol 84:40, 1994.
Iams J, for the NICHD Maternal Fetal Medicine Unit Network BM: the Preterm Prediction Study: A model for estimation of risk of spontaneous preterm birth in parous women (Abstract). Am J Obstet Gynecol 176:S51, 1997.
Iams J: Preterm birth. *In* Gabbe S, Niebyl J, Simpson J (eds): Obstetrics: Normal and Problem Pregnancies, 3rd ed. New York, Churchill Livingstone, 1996, pp 764–765.
King J, Grand A, Keirse M: Beta mimetics in pre-term labour: An overview of a randomized controlled trials. Br J Obstet Gynaecol 95:211, 1988.
Krohn M, Hillier S, Lee M, et al: Vaginal *bacteroides* are associated with an increased rate of preterm delivery in women with preterm labor. J Infect Dis 164:88, 1991.
Lockwood C: The diagnosis of preterm labor and the prediction of preterm delivery. Clin Obstet Gynecol 38:675, 1995.
Matsuura H, Hakomori S: The oncofetal domain of fibronectin defined by the monoclonal antibody FDC-6: Its presence in fibronectins from fetal and tumor tissues and its absense from adult tissues and plasma. Proc Natl Acad Sci U S A 82:6517, 1985.
McDonald I: Suture of the cervix for inevitable abortion. J Obstet Gynaecol Br Emp 64:346, 1957.
Miller Y, Keane M, Horger E: A comparison of magnesium sulfate and terbutaline for the arrest of preterm labor. J Reprod Med 27:348, 1982.
Minkoff H: Prematurity: Infection as an etiologic factor. Obstet Gynecol 62:144, 1983.
National Center for Health Statistics: Monthly Vital Statistics Report, Advance Report of Final Natality Statistics for 1993. National Center for Health Statistics, 1993.
Niebyl J, Blake D, White R, et al: The inhibition of premature labor with indomethacin. Am J Obstet Gynecol 136:1014, 1980.
Peaceman A, Andrews W, Thorp J: Fetal fibronectin as a predictor of preterm birth in symptomatic patients: A multicenter trial. Am J Obstet Gynecol 174:303, 1996.

Romero R, Drum S, Dinarello C: Interleukin-1 stimulates prostaglandin biosynthesis by the human amnion. Prostaglandins 37:13, 1989.

Romero R, Sibai B, Caritis S, et al: Antiobiotic treatment of preterm labor with intact membranes: A randomized, double blind, placebo-controlled trial. Am J Obstet Gynecol 169:764, 1993.

Russell P: Inflammatory lesions of the human placenta: Clinical significane of acute chiorioamnionitis. Am J Diagn Gynecol Obstet 1:127, 1979.

Salafia C, Vogel C, Vintzeleos A, et al: Placental pathologic findings in preterm birth. Am J Obstet Gynecol 165:934, 1991.

Shirodkar V: A method of operative treatment for habitual abortions in the second trimester of pregnancy. Antiseptic 52:299, 1955.

Stubbs T, VanDOrsten J, Miller M: The preterm cervix and preterm labor: Relative risks, predictive changes, and change over time. Am J Obstet Gynecol 155:829, 1986.

The American College of Obstetrician and Gynecologists: Obstetric complications. *In* Hauth J, Merenstein G (eds): Guidelines for Perinatal Care, 4th ed. Dallas, TX, AAP/ACOG, 1997, pp 127–146.

The American College of Obstetrician and Gynecologists: Committee Opinion #198: Bacterial vaginosis screening for prevention of preterm delivery, Dallas, TX, ACOG, 1998.

Weissman A, Jakobi P, Zahi S, et al: The effect of cervical cerclage on the cource of labor. Obstet Gynecol 76:168, 1990.

Zuckerman H, Shalev E, Gilad G, et al: Further study of the inhibition of premature labor by indomethacin. Part 1. J Perinat Med 12:19, 1984.

# 34

# Post-Term Pregnancy

DAVID E. KAUFFMAN
STEVE CARITIS

Although much focus in perinatal medicine today centers on deliveries before term, post-term pregnancies—those extending beyond 294 days—are not without significance. In 1902, Ballantyne, a famous Scottish midwife, was one of the first persons in the modern era to address the issue of post-term pregnancies when he said that "The post-mature infant . . . has stayed so long in utero that his difficulty is to be born with safety to himself and his mother." It was not until the 1950s and 1960s, however, when Clifford first described in detail the "post maturity syndrome" and McClure Browne reported on the increased perinatal mortality rate in neonates delivered after 42 weeks of gestation, that the current ongoing debate about prolonged pregnancies was reborn.

## Background and Incidence

The length of a normal human pregnancy is 266 to 294 days (38 to 42 weeks) from the onset of the last menstrual period. A variety of terminology has been used, correctly or incorrectly, to describe pregnancies progressing beyond 42 completed weeks (294 days). The term *postdates* designates those pregnancies that have persisted beyond the patient's estimated date of confinement. The term *post-term* correctly refers to pregnancies that have completed 42 weeks of gestation (294 days) from the onset of the last menses. The term *postmature* is a pathologic term used to describe a specific subset of neonates born to women who have post-term pregnancies.

The incidence of post-term pregnancies had previously been difficult to assess because of poor gestational dating criteria in many older studies. With the advent of early prenatal care and ultrasound, the incidence of pregnancies extending beyond term has now been more clearly established. The incidence of pregnancies continuing beyond 42 completed weeks (294 days) is approximately 10% (range 4 to 14%), for those beyond 43 completed weeks (301 days) approximately 4% (range 2 to 7%), and for those extending to and beyond 44 completed weeks (308 days) 1%.

The most frequent cause of an apparently post-term pregnancy is error in gestational age assignment. Establishment of correct dates is the most critical aspect of post-term pregnancy management. Many suspected post-term pregnancies are, in fact, routine term pregnancies that have simply been poorly dated. Ultrasonography has developed as an essential tool in establishing a correct gestational age. In general, ultrasonography is accurate to within 3 to 5 days when performed at a gestational age of less than 12 weeks, 7 days at 12 to 20 weeks, 14 days from 20 to 30 weeks, and 21 days after 30 weeks.

Once an accurate due date has been established, the reason that some pregnancies truly persist beyond the normal range remains a mystery. Certainly, even in term pregnancies, the initiating events of labor remain for the most part unknown. Although our knowledge of term human labor has significantly increased over the last several decades, it is unlikely that we will understand why some gestations extend past 42 weeks until normal human parturition is better understood. Interestingly, however, certain specific clinical conditions have been associated with post-term gestations, and these have provided some insight into potential mechanisms of parturition. For example, fetuses with absent pituitary glands, isolated pituitary hypoplasia, or anencephaly with absent pituitary glands are commonly delivered post-term. Also, pregnancies complicated by placental sulfatase deficiency, which results in extremely low levels of estriol, frequently are prolonged. The reason that labor is delayed in these conditions is unknown. The fetal pituitary adrenal axis or changes in estrogen and progesterone ratios may play a role in the initiation of parturition.

## Fetal and Neonatal Risks

### OVERVIEW

It had long been suspected that post-term fetuses were at increased risk of adverse outcomes; however, few studies had formally addressed this until the mid-twentieth century. Using the National Birthday Trust in Britain, McClure Browne in 1962 published a report of nearly 17,000 births in England that were stratified according to gestational age during a 1-week period. He demonstrated a rise in perinatal mortality starting at 42 completed weeks (294 days), a doubling of the perinatal mortality rate by 43 completed weeks (301 days), and a tripling by 44 weeks (308 days). As a result of this publication, serious concern about post-term pregnancies arose. It is now better understood that the perinatal mortality initially quoted by McClure Browne is likely overestimated because both fetuses with lethal congenital anomalies and patients with underlying medical conditions were not excluded from his evaluation. Approximately 25% of the perinatal mortality in post-term pregnancies is related to lethal congenital anomalies. Therefore, if these patients are not excluded from analysis, perinatal mortality rates will be overestimated. Subsequent well-controlled studies have failed to demonstrate such a significant increase in perinatal mortality. Recently, Campbell and associates reported on the impact of post-term pregnancy using the Medical Birth Registry of Norway. This 10-year cohort spanning 1978 to 1987 included more than 65,000 post-term births. The authors were able to identify only a small increase in perinatal mortality in infants delivering beyond 42 completed weeks (294 days) compared with term controls (relative risk, 1.11; 95% confidence interval, 0.97, 1.27). It has become clear that patients who have identifiable risk factors, such as maternal medical complications (e.g., diabetes, hypertensive disorders) or fetal conditions, such as oligohydramnios or macrosomia, are indeed at higher risk of adverse pregnancy outcome if allowed to persist beyond 42 completed weeks (294 days). However, for the low-risk patient with normal fetal assessment, there is little or no increased risk of adverse perinatal outcome.

The etiology of an increase in perinatal morbidity and mortality in the post-term fetus at risk is in part due to progressive uteroplacental insufficiency, which subsequently leads to oligohydramnios, passage of meconium, loss of subcutaneous fat, and—in severe cases—meconium aspiration, asphyxia, and fetal death. There is also an increased incidence of macrosomia in post-term pregnancies, which carries its own particular fetal and maternal complications.

### MECONIUM PASSAGE AND ASPIRATION

As the fetus nears term and the gastrointestinal tract matures, passage of meconium into the amniotic fluid is common. In most neonates, the finding of meconium at delivery does not result in any significant sequelae. However, serious neonatal morbidity can occur when meconium is aspirated into distal fetal pulmonary airways. These infants with meconium aspiration syndrome suffer a chemical pneumonitis characterized by progressive hypoxemia, respiratory failure, pulmonary hypertension, and, occasionally, neonatal death. Persistent fetal circulation can also be a considerable complication in neonates with meconium aspiration syndrome. In these infants, abnormal muscularization of the small pulmonary arteries leads to persistent pulmonary hypertension and right to left shunting. This abnormal vascular pattern, demonstrable histologically, indicates that an insult must have occurred prenatally. The combination of both prenatal and perinatal insult to the pulmonary architecture contributes to the development of persistent fetal circulation and pulmonary hypertension in neonates who have meconium aspiration syndrome. Many studies have linked post-term pregnancies with meconium passage and meconium aspiration syndrome. In a retrospective review of well-dated post-term pregnancies between 1978 and 1986, Usher and associates demonstrated a doubling of meconium-stained amniotic fluid (31.5% vs. 15.3%, $P<.001$)

in pregnancies at or beyond 42 completed weeks compared with those delivered at term, and an eightfold increase in meconium aspiration syndrome. Additional studies have confirmed the increased incidence of meconium-stained amniotic fluid with or without an increase in meconium aspiration syndrome, with rates of meconium staining averaging 20 to 25% in the fetus delivered at 42 weeks compared with rates of 10 to 15% at term. The impact of meconium is compounded by the higher incidence of oligohydramnios in post-term pregnancies. With little amniotic fluid, meconium cannot be diluted. This results in a thicker, more tenacious material that is more difficult to clear from neonatal airways.

## OLIGOHYDRAMNIOS

As human gestation progresses beyond term, the amniotic fluid volume normally decreases, with a loss of approximately 12% each week in the post-term period. It has been well established that oligohydramnios, commonly defined as an amniotic fluid index of 5 cm or less, increases the risk of an adverse perinatal outcome regardless of gestational age. Low amniotic fluid volume is associated with meconium, fetal distress in labor, and increased cesarean section rate. Oligohydramnios as an independent marker of fetal risk is discussed in further detail later.

## POSTMATURITY SYNDROME

It was once thought that the postmaturity syndrome as described by Clifford was a frequent and dangerous complication of the post-term fetus. It is now believed that infants with these characteristics most likely represent growth restriction at term rather than a separate clinical entity. Although most neonates delivered post-term are normal in appearance, a subset display features of postmaturity or dysmaturity. These characteristics include absent vernix; dry, parchment-like skin; long nails; depletion of subcutaneous fat; meconium staining; and a wide-eyed, hyperalert appearance. The loss of adipose stores predisposes these neonates to hypoglycemia and hypothermia. The perinatal mortality rate is increased in neonates with postmaturity syndrome, as opposed to neonates delivered post-term without these characteristics. In one study, small for gestational age (SGA) post-term fetuses had a risk of perinatal death that was 5.7 times greater than that of non-SGA births. These postmature fetuses demonstrate an increased risk of fetal heart rate abnormalities in labor, meconium, cesarean delivery, and neonatal intensive care unit (NICU) admissions. Fortunately, the incidence of postmaturity is low in post-term pregnancies, averaging only about 20%. Oligohydramnios, in addition to poor growth, has been shown to be a sensitive marker for detection of these particular fetuses at risk.

## MACROSOMIA

Even though the placenta in pregnancies persisting beyond term may appear aged, the fetus continues to grow. This continued growth results in an increased incidence of macrosomia in post-term pregnancies. The incidence of birth weight greater than 4000 g in neonates delivered after 41 completed weeks (287 days) averages 23 to 40%; incidence of birth weight greater than 4500 g is 3 to 4%. The attendant complications associated with macrosomia, such as birth trauma, shoulder dystocia, and maternal injury, are seen with increased frequency as well. Unfortunately, although the incidence of macrosomia is significant, accurate means of detection remain elusive. The utility of ultrasonography in predicting macrosomia in the late third trimester is severely limited. Pollack and associates used ultrasonography to estimate birth weights in 519 post-term pregnancies, all of which were delivered within 1 week of the ultrasonographic study. The sensitivity and positive predictive value of an ultrasonographically estimated fetal weight of ≥4000 g were 56% and 65% respectively. Although these values improved somewhat for estimated weights of ≥4500 g, they still remained poor predictors of birth weight.

In summary, it does appear that the post-term fetus is at an increased risk for certain complications. Fortunately, with careful evaluation and management, most infants delivered post-term do not suffer significant sequelae.

# Surveillance

Because of the increased perinatal morbidity in some post-term pregnancies, several different testing strategies have been used in an attempt to modify fetal risk; however, care must be used with any of these testing schemes. While no form of surveillance has been shown to eliminate the risk of stillbirth completely, tests that have a high false-positive rate may lead to unnecessary interventions that are potentially hazardous to the patient. A balance must be established, therefore, in which truly at-risk fetuses can be identified without intervening for a high proportion of normal fetuses. The various testing schemes are reviewed later.

## NONSTRESS TEST

Several studies have addressed the utility of nonstress testing (NST), specifically in the setting of post-term pregnancies. Miyazaki and Miyazaki were among the first to question the value of nonstress testing in assessing the post-term pregnancy, and they found an unacceptably high false-negative rate. Subsequent studies have failed to confirm this high rate of poor outcomes. When the NST alone is used as a means of fetal surveillance, as opposed to NST's in combination with ultrasonographic evaluation, some fetuses at risk may not be identified. Additionally, the presence of variable decelerations, despite a reactive tracing otherwise, heightens the risk of an adverse outcome. Benedetti and Easterling surveyed several studies that used the NST as a means of fetal assessment. The corrected perinatal mortality rate in their review was 15 of 1000 if variable decelerations were present, and 5 of 1000 if the decelerations were absent. Therefore, despite its usefulness in other settings for prenatal surveillance, the NST is not recommended as the only method of testing fetal well-being beyond 42 weeks in the post-term pregnancy.

## CONTRACTION-STIMULATION TEST

Because of concern for impaired uteroplacental perfusion in the post-term pregnancy, the contraction-stimulation test (CST), which provides the best means to assess uteroplacental reserve, has also been used in assessing fetal well-being in pregnancies extending beyond 42 weeks. Several different studies have evaluated the CST in predicting perinatal complications; however, only one such trial was sufficiently large to provide any useful information. In this study, the CST was prospectively evaluated as a means of surveillance in 679 well-dated post-term pregnancies. There were no perinatal deaths in the post-term group, and only 10 patients had positive CSTs. Unfortunately, there were a large number of equivocal tests (28.4%), all of which required additional evaluation or intervention. In a review of several other trials using the CST as a means of fetal surveillance, Benedetti and Easterling demonstrated a corrected perinatal mortality rate of only 2.5 per 1000 and concluded that the CST appears to be a "good but not infallible" test for preventing perinatal death in post-term pregnancies.

## ULTRASONOGRAPHY

Ultrasonography has developed over the last several decades as an essential tool to evaluate pregnancies, whether normal or high risk. Assessment of fetal activity status, as well as amniotic fluid volume by ultrasonography, termed the *biophysical profile*, is effective in identifying fetuses at risk for adverse perinatal outcome. Use of the biophysical profile is also helpful in evaluating post-term pregnancies. Over a 3-year period, Johnson and associates prospectively evaluated the utility of the biophysical profile to identify fetuses at risk in 307 post-term pregnancies. In fetuses with an abnormal biophysical profile—defined as a score of 6 of 10 or 8 of 10 with an abnormal amniotic fluid volume—the incidence of perinatal morbidity (fetal distress requiring cesarean section, 5-minute Apgar score ≤6, meconium aspiration) was significantly higher than for those with normal biophysical assessments. Furthermore, the perinatal morbidity was highest in fetuses with the lowest amniotic fluid volume. Because of the small study size, no differences in perinatal mortality could be demonstrated.

As mentioned previously, ultrasonographic assessment of amniotic fluid volume has been studied in a variety of trials and has been shown to be valuable in evaluating the post-term pregnancy. Although oligohydramnios was defined in several different ways in these trials, the finding of low amniotic fluid volume in the post-term pregnancy is of concern. Fetuses with decreased amniotic fluid volumes have a higher rate of fetal heart rate decelerations in labor, meconium passage, fetal distress, need for neonatal resuscitation, cesarean delivery, and perinatal morbidity. In one study, as many as 30% of patients who had oligohydramnios required cesarean delivery, and 35% suffered from meconium aspiration syndrome. The corrected perinatal mortality rate was 6 of 1000 when a 1-cm vertical pocket of amniotic fluid was used as an indication for delivery, whereas if a 3-cm vertical pocket was used, the mortality rate fell to 1.8 per 1000. More significant, however, was the finding that intervention for oligohydramnios can improve perinatal outcome. Pregnancies with oligohydramnios that are induced have a lower perinatal morbidity rate than those that are managed expectantly.

Clearly, the type of antenatal surveillance in post-term pregnancies varies. Although the NST and CST do provide some measure of reassurance, they are certainly not perfect in prediction of adverse outcome. It does appear, however, that oligohydramnios indicates potential for significant fetal compromise. Unfortunately, a full ultrasonographic evaluation requires significant time and expense. The modified biophysical profile, however, in which an ultrasonographic estimation of amniotic fluid volume only is combined with an NST, may provide a compromise between these testing strategies. No prospective trials have used this approach in evaluating post-term pregnancies.

Not only does the type of antenatal surveillance stir controversy in the obstetric literature, but the gestational age at which to initiate testing is also debatable. Although most studies evaluating post-term pregnancies begin surveillance after 294 days, several studies have suggested that adverse fetal outcome may actually precede 42 weeks and, therefore, testing should begin earlier. Grausz and Heimler compared a cohort of normal infants with infants born with unexpected asphyxia, which was defined as the presence of persistent fetal tachycardia or bradycardia in the absence of other known etiology, loss of beat-to-beat variability, late or prolonged variable decelerations, or thick meconium. They found that the mean gestational age of neonates with unexpected asphyxia was 289 days, which was earlier than the expected 294 days. In a smaller study, Arias showed that the perinatal complication rate and incidence of macrosomia increased significantly at 41 weeks of gestation compared with term control neonates. Other studies have also suggested that testing beginning at 41 weeks may decrease the perinatal morbidity rates associated with post-term pregnancies.

## Management

The post-term pregnancy presents the practicing obstetrician with several challenges. Perinatal morbidity begins to rise at around 41 to 42 weeks, and despite close antenatal surveillance, adverse perinatal outcomes still occur. The question is, what is the optimal way to care for these patients?

Management issues in patients who have favorable cervices are not controversial. There is little information in the literature comparing expectant management with labor induction in the post-term patient who has a favorable cervix, because these patients are at low risk for complications related to the induction itself, but current obstetric practice favors induction. The real dilemma arises in the patient who has an unripe cervix. The central issue in these patients is whether induction and delivery by 42 weeks will reduce perinatal morbidity and mortality, or whether attempting an induction in a patient who has an unfavorable cervix may create additional problems. Because the overall perinatal mortality rate is so low in these patients, it is unlikely that any one trial will be able to assess differences in mortality. However, morbidities associated with post-term pregnancies can be addressed.

Several studies have attempted to answer this question. Unfortunately, many of these have shown contradictory results (Table 34–1). This discrepancy may have occurred because the study populations in these trials varied. Patients who had ripe cervices were included with those who had unfavorable cervices, cervical ripening agents were not used in some trials, patients were not uniformly selected for inclusion, and antepartum surveillance techniques were different. This makes comparisons between these studies less valid. However, two well-designed and well-executed studies, one in the United States and one in Canada, have provided useful information.

In 1992, Hannah and associates published the results of the Canadian Multicenter Post-Term Pregnancy Trial Group in which 3407 women who had uncomplicated, well-dated pregnancies at 41 completed weeks (287 days) were randomized to induction with cervical ripening or antenatal surveillance and expectant management. Patients whose cervices were dilated ≥3 cm were excluded. Women in the expectant management group were monitored with kick counts, thrice weekly NSTs, and amniotic fluid assessment two to three times weekly. Patients were induced for nonreassuring fetal heart rate tracings, oligohydramnios (defined as a pocket <3 cm), or when 44 completed weeks was reached. The trial group found that labor induction at 41 or more weeks in this patient population was not associated with any difference in perinatal mortality or neonatal morbidity compared with serial antenatal surveillance and expectant management. Specifically, no differences in Apgar scores, mean birth weight, birth weight of more than 4500 g, meconium aspiration, or NICU admissions were demonstrated. Sixty-seven percent of the patients in the expectant management group entered labor spontaneously, with the remainder requiring induction. The only significant differences identified were that patients in the expectant management group were more likely to have meconium staining of amniotic fluid (28.7% vs. 25.0%, $P$ = .015), fetal distress, and an increased cesarean section rate (24.5% vs. 21.2%, $P$ = .03). This increased operative delivery rate was attributable to an increased rate of cesarean sections performed for fetal distress intrapartum, a definition left to the attending physician, rather than for failed induction or dystocia.

Table 34–1  Comparison of Expectant Management vs. Induction Trials

|  | Cardozo et al, 1986 | Augensen et al, 1987 | Dyson et al, 1987 | Hannah et al, 1992 | NICHHD, 1994 |
| --- | --- | --- | --- | --- | --- |
| Cesarean section | *OR 0.73 (0.39, 1.36) | OR 1.63 (0.80, 1.20) | OR 2.22 (1.25, 3.96) | OR 1.22 (1.02, 1.45) | OR 0.85 (0.52, 1.38) |
| Meconium | OR 0.86 (0.49, 1.51) | OR 0.94 (0.56, 1.58) | OR 3.71 (2.21, 6.21) | OR 1.21 (1.04, 1.41) | OR 1.21 (0.80, 1.82) |
| Fetal distress | OR 0.56 (1.06, 3.41) | NA | OR 8.12 (2.75, 23.81) | OR 1.28 (1.03, 1.58) | NA |
| Macrosomia | NA | NA | OR 1.65 (0.96, 2.83) | OR 1.22 (0.90, 1.66) | OR 2.32 (0.64, 8.33) |

*Statistics presented in terms of odds ratio (OR) of expectant management compared with induction with 95% confidence intervals.
NA = not applicable; NICHHD = National Institute of Child Health and Human Development.

Table 34–2  Post-term Pregnancy Management Guidelines

| 41 wk (287 d) | 41 to 42 wk (287–294 d) | >42 wk (294 d) |
|---|---|---|
| Cervical examination<br>  Induction if favorable<br>  Surveillance if unfavorable | Surveillance<br>  NST or CST with AFV<br>  BPP or modified BPP<br>Induction<br>  Nonreassuring NST/CST<br>  Oligohydramnios<br>  Variable decelerations<br>  Favorable cervix | Continued expectant management with reassuring surveillance or scheduled elective induction |

NST = nonstress test; CST = contraction-stimulation test; AFV = amniotic fluid volume; BPP = biophysical profile.

A similar but smaller trial sponsored by the National Institute of Child Health and Human Development was published in 1994. This study was discontinued early because of a very low rate of perinatal complications. A comparable patient population of low risk, well-dated pregnancies at 41 completed weeks of gestation (287 days) were selected for randomization to either immediate induction with cervical ripening or expectant management with surveillance. Patients who had ripe cervices (Bishop score ≥7), oligohydramnios (largest pocket <2 cm), or decelerations on NST were excluded from randomization. Patients randomized to surveillance and expectant management received twice weekly NSTs, amniotic fluid volume assessments, and weekly cervical examinations. They were induced for a Bishop score >6, estimated fetal weight >4500 g, abnormal fetal heart rate tracing, amniotic fluid pocket <2.0 cm, or when they reached 44 weeks of gestation. The incidence of adverse perinatal outcome was no different between the two groups, and there were no fetal deaths in either group. Unlike the Canadian trial, in this study the cesarean section rate was not different between patients induced immediately and those who were randomized to expectant management.

These two trials support the conclusion that because of the low perinatal risks regardless of treatment arm, either expectant management with surveillance or immediate induction is an acceptable option for the low-risk post-term pregnancy.

## Summary

Pregnancies lasting beyond 41 to 42 completed weeks (287 to 294 days) present the obstetric community with a variety of controversial issues. Although it is clear that neonates in these pregnancies are at increased risk of meconium aspiration, macrosomia, cesarean delivery, and fetal distress, with modern means of fetal surveillance, these risks can be significantly modified. With proper evaluation, the post-term fetus with normal amniotic fluid volume and reassuring antenatal testing is at very low risk for significant perinatal morbidity. Current management guidelines for pregnancies at 41 to 42 completed weeks of gestation (287 to 294 days) include the following (Table 34–2):

1. An initial cervical assessment at approximately 41 completed weeks (287 days) with induction planned in patients who have favorable cervices.
2. Antenatal surveillance starting at 41 to 42 weeks with either the biophysical profile or the NST/CST used in conjunction with an amniotic fluid volume assessment.
3. Planned induction, regardless of cervical status, for oligohydramnios, nonreassuring fetal testing, or variable decelerations seen on NST or CST.
4. Either continued expectant management with surveillance or induction in patients reaching 42 completed weeks (294 days) with reassuring testing.

## REFERENCES

Arias F: Predictability of complications associated with prolongation of pregnancy. Obstet Gynecol 70:101, 1987.

Augensen K, Bergsjo P, Eikeland T, et al: Randomised comparison of early versus late induction of labour in post-term pregnancy. BMJ 294:1192, 1987.

Ballantyne JW: The problem of the postmature infant. J Obstet Gynaecol Br Emp 2:36, 1902.

Benedetti TJ, Easterling T: Antepartum testing in postterm pregnancy. J Reprod Med 33:252, 1988.

Bochner CJ, Williams J, Castro L, et al: The efficacy of starting postterm antenatal testing at 41 weeks as compared with 42 weeks of gestational age. Am J Obstet Gynecol 159:550, 1988.

Campbell MK, Ostbye T, Irgens L: Post-term birth: Risk factors and outcomes in a 10-year cohort of Norwegian births. Obstet Gynecol 89:543, 1997.

Cardozo L, Fysh J, Pearce JM: Prolonged pregnancy: The management debate. BMJ 293:1059, 1986.

Clifford SH: Postmaturity with placental dysfunction. Clinical syndromes and pathologic findings. J Pediatr 44:1, 1954.

Dyson DC: Fetal surveillance vs. labor induction at 42 weeks in postterm gestation. J Reprod Med 33:262, 1988.

Dyson DC, Miller PD, Armstrong MA: Management of prolonged pregnancy: Induction of labor versus antepartum fetal testing. Am J Obstet Gynecol 156:928, 1987.

Eden RD, Gergely RZ, Schifrin BS, Wade ME: Comparison of antepartum testing schemes for the management of the postdate pregnancy. Am J Obstet Gynecol 144:683, 1982.

Eden RD, Seifert LS, Winegar A, et al: Perinatal characteristics of uncomplicated postdate pregnancies. Obstet Gynecol 69:296, 1987.

Freeman RK, Garite TJ, Modanlou H, et al: Postdate pregnancy: Utilization of contraction stress testing for primary fetal surveillance. Am J Obstet Gynecol 140:128, 1981.

Grant JM: Induction of labour confers benefits in prolonged pregnancy. Br J Obstet Gynaecol 101:99, 1994.

Grausz JP, Heimler R: Asphyxia and gestational age. Obstet Gynecol 62:175, 1983.

Guidetti DA, Divon MY, Langer O: Postdate fetal surveillance: Is 41 weeks too early? Am J Obstet Gynecol 161:91, 1989.

Hannah ME, Hannah WJ, Hellmann J, et al: Multicenter Postterm Pregnancy Trial Group: Induction of labor as compared with serial antenatal monitoring in post-term pregnancy. N Engl J Med 326:1587, 1992.

Johnson JM, Harman CR, Lange IR, et al: Biophysical profile scoring in the management of the postterm pregnancy: An analysis of 307 patients. Am J Obstet Gynecol 154:269, 1986.

Johnson JM, Harman CR, Lange IR, et al: Biophysical profile scoring in the management of the postterm pregnancy: An analysis of 307 patients. Am J Obstet Gynecol 154:269, 1986.

Manning, FA: The use of sonography in the evaluation of the high-risk pregnancy. Radiol Clin North Am 28:205, 1990.

Mannio F: Neonatal complications of postterm gestation. J Reprod Med 33:271, 1988.

McClure Browne JC: Postmaturity. Am J Obstet Gynecol 85:574, 1963.

McLean FH, Boyd ME, Usher RH, et al: Postterm infants: Too big or too small. Am J Obstet Gynecol 164:619, 1991.

Miyazaki FS, Miyazaki BA: False reactive nonstress tests in postterm pregnancies. Am J Obstet Gynecol 140:269, 1981.

Moore TR, Cayle JE: The amniotic fluid index in normal human pregnancy. Am J Obstet Gynecol 162:1168, 1990.

Naeye R: Causes of perinatal mortality excess in prolonged gestations. Am J Epidemiol 108:429, 1978.

National Institute of Child Health and Human Development Network of Maternal-Fetal Medicine Units: A clinical trial of induction of labor versus expectant management in postterm pregnancy. Am J Obstet Gynecol 1994;170:716.

Phelan JP, Platt LD, Yeh SY, et al: The role of ultrasound assessment of amniotic fluid volume in the management of the postdate pregnancy. Am J Obstet Gynecol 151:304, 1985.

Pollack RN, Hauer-Pollack G, Divon MY: Macrosomia in postdates pregnancies: The accuracy of routine ultrasonographic screening. Am J Obstet Gynecol 167:7, 1992.

Rayburn WF, Motley ME, Stempel LE, et al: Antepartum prediction of the postmature infant. Obstet Gynecol 60:148, 1982.

Resnik R: Postterm gestation. J Reprod Med. 33:249, 1988.

Sachs BP, Friedman EA: Results of an epidemiologic study of postdate pregnancy. J Reprod Med 31:162, 1986.

Usher RH, Boyd ME, McLean FH, et al: Assessment of fetal risk in postdate pregnancies. Am J Obstet Gynecol 158:259, 1988.

# 35

# Diabetes in Pregnancy

ODED LANGER

Diabetes is a common medical complication in pregnancy that affects 250,000 women annually. Of these, 2.5 to 10% of pregnancies are complicated by gestational diabetes mellitus (GDM) and 0.4 to 5% by type 1 and type 2 diabetes. The prevalence of diabetes will increase in the near future due to the lowering of thresholds for the diagnostic criteria for both GDM and type 2 diabetes. The magnitude of the problem is reflected by the accompanying fetal morbidity and mortality in both GDM and pregestational diabetes mellitus (PGDM) and the maternal complications involving both type 1 and type 2 diabetes.

This chapter discusses the importance of GDM as a clinical entity and differentiates between the definitions offered by several governing bodies regarding screening and diagnosis of GDM. Readers will become aware of the use of nutritional guidelines and learn how to identify the patient who needs diet therapy. In addition, they will learn to recognize the criteria for insulin initiation in GDM and to understand the algorithm used with this treatment. Finally, they will understand the indications for elective delivery.

## Is Gestational Diabetes a Clinical Entity?

The association between maternal and neonatal mortality and morbidity and PGDM has been recognized since the 1920s. Complications, including ketoacidosis, hypoglycemia, and vascular complications, have led to the development of intensified management strategies for these gravida. The high rates of stillbirth, neonatal macrosomia, congenital anomalies, and additional metabolic complications were associated with poorly controlled diabetes. Of greater controversy in the past was the question if GDM, a condition of abnormal glucose tolerance first recognized in pregnancy, is a clinical entity. To classify a condition as a disease, two factors need to be established: demonstrated morbidity or mortality associated with the condition and the benefits of intervention override the risks.

Two measures are used to establish the increased morbidity associated with GDM (which can also be used to characterize PGDM). The short-term measure is perinatal mortality and morbidity. Although it is customary to assume that perinatal mortality is not increased in GDM, several reports in the last decade demonstrated a three to four fold higher rate of stillbirth in these patients when compared with a nondiabetic population with a current stillbirth rate of 3 to 4/1000 live births.

Macrosomia is defined by most researchers as birth weight greater than 4000 g. Most studies in the last decade report a rate of macrosomia of 15 to 30%, which is three to fourfold higher than the incidence in the nondiabetic population. A better characterization of the large fetus is achieved by using the term *large for gestational age* (LGA; birth weight >90th percentile). The incidence of LGA among GDM patients is reported to be 20 to 50% compared with 10% among nondiabetic patients. Recently, in several centers it has been proposed that diabetic infants should be delivered (including GDMs) at approximately 37 to 38 weeks gestation. Although most infants in this gestational age will not weigh 4000 g, substantial numbers will be LGA. It should be remembered that macrosomia is not only a weight definition but rather a diabetic fetopathy characterized by organomegaly. With the exceptin of the brain, most fetal organs, including the heart, spleen, liver, lungs, and subcutaneous fat, are affected by the fetal hyperinsulinemia resulting from maternal hyperglycemia. The extent of growth of the different organs may range from 150 to over 200% when compared with weight standard tables for nondiabetic infants.

Metabolic, hematologic, and respiratory complications affect 15 to 30% of pregnancies with poor glycemic control. Shoulder dystocia represents the main trauma complication, with an incidence increased five to sevenfold that of the general population (7% vs. 0.6%, respectively). Several studies demonstrated that within 3 to 15 years after the occurrence of gestational diabetes, 20 to 50% of gravida will develop overt diabetes, mainly type 2. Long-term complications affecting the neonate include child obesity, higher rates of diabetes in adolescence, and intellectual impairment related to abnormal diabetic metabolism.

Thus, in summary, diabetes in pregnancy is associated with substantial morbidity. Optimal results in decreased morbidity approach that of a nondiabetic patient. Therefore, the two components that define disease, morbidity, and benefit of treatment, are present in patients with GDM.

## Screening for Gestational Diabetes

A lack of consensus exists as to when diabetes should be screened during pregnancy. The American College of Obstetrics and Gynecology (ACOG) recommends that all women older than 29 and those with risk factors such as family history of diabetes; previous macrosomia, deformed, or stillborn fetus; obesity; hypertension; or glycosuria are screened during pregnancy. Screening should be performed at 24 to 28 weeks gestation with a 50-g glucose challenge test measuring the 1-hour plasma glucose. If the 1-hour glucose is at least 140 mg/dl, then a 3-hour 100-g diagnostic oral glucose tolerance test (OGTT) is performed.

The Second and Third International Workshop Conference on Gestational Diabetes Mellitus (sponsored by the American Diabetes Association, ACOG, and the American Academy of Pediatrics) advised universal screening for all pregnant women.

The Centers for Disease Control and Prevention recommend universal screening whenever possible. When this is not attainable, all gravidas older than 25 years of age should be screened and those under age 25 are screened with risk factors such as obesity, family history of diabetes (first degree), hypertension, history of delivery of stillbirth, an infant weighing more than 9 lb, or an infant with congenital malformation.

The report of the US Preventive Services Task Force (1996) recommends that all pregnant women should be screened for glucose intolerance. However, women with *all* of the following characteristics, age less than 25 years, normal body weight, no family history (i.e., first-degree relative) of diabetes mellitus, not a member of an ethnic group at increased risk for type 2 diabetes, need *not* be screened.

The Fourth International Workshop/Conference on GDM in March 1997 and the proceedings Report of the Expert Committee on the Diagnosis and Classification of Diabetes recommend *selective screening* for women aged 25 or older. However, they recommend that in women with obesity, previous history of gestational diabetes, macrosomia, specific ethnic groups at risk for developing type 2 diabetes (Hispanic American, African American, Native American, Asian American, Indian Subcontinent, Pacific islanders, and indigenous Australian), family history of diabetes, and presence of hypertension disorders, screening should be performed regardless of gestational age.

Screening of GDM should be through a 50-g glucose load administered between the 24th and 28th week, without regard to time of day or time of last meal. In the case of high-risk women, screening should be performed at the first office visit. Venous plasma glucose should be measured 1 hour after the glucose load. A value of at least 140 mg/dl indicates the need for a full 3-hour OGTT. However, it should be understood that the threshold value for screening abnormality can be modified according to the prevalence of GDM in a given geographic locale. In areas of high prevalence, lower threshold values will identify more patients at risk for developing GDM; this approach will still be cost effective. Thus, thresholds of 130 or 135 mg/dl are in use in different locations in the U.S. In the fasting state, the threshold of 140 mg/dl yields a sensitivity of 90%, whereas in the fed state, a threshold of 139 mg/dl yields a sensitivity of 83%.

A plasma glucose measurement of at least 200 mg/dl outside the context of a formal glucose challenge test or a truly fasting plasma glucose of 126 mg/dl suggests the diabetic state and warrants further investigation. The recommendation for universal testing at 24 to 28 weeks' gestation should not preclude earlier testing for women at high risk, including marked obesity, a strong family history of type 2 diabetes, a personal history of GDM, glucose intolerance, or glucosuria. The use of glycated hemoglobin or glycosylated proteins is not recommended because they are not sensitive for screening purposes. Capillary glucose meters are valuable in management but do not have the diagnostic accuracy for screening.

Historical risk factors for determining risk have merit but may lack sensitivity; 47% of GDM in O'Sullivan and Mahan's study did not have historical risk factors. In a population of 2077 pregnant women, 53.5% of the 30 GDM women did not have risk factors. The frequency of abnormal OGTTs was 1.5% among those women with traditional risk factors and 1.4% among those without risk factors. Among 434 obstetric patients, 50% of the 12 GDM women did not have risk factors. The frequency of abnormal OGTTs was 3.2% among those with risk factors and 2.4% among those without. Among 6216 pregnancies screened, 49% of the 126 GDM women (National Diabetic Data Group criteria) did not have historical risk factors. Therefore, the use of historical risk factors is a very insensitive method of screening for GDM.

Although maternal age has consistently been considered a criteria for screening, its inclusion as a prerequisite needs to be evaluated. O'Sullivan and Mahan found that 84% (16/19) of GDM women in a cohort of 752 were older than 25, yet 52% of their total population was less than 25 years old. Thus, universal screening for those older than 25 has been suggested. Marquette and colleagues found that 83% (10/12) of the GDM women in the population of 434 were older than 24 years; thus, universal screening for those older than 24 was suggested. Coustan reported an almost 50% decrease in the prevalence of diabetes under 30 years of age (Table 35–1).

At the University of Texas Health Science Center at San Antonio, low-risk patients are screened with a 1-hour 50-g OGTT at 24 to 28 weeks. For high-risk patients, a 1-hour 50-g OGTT is ordered at the initial visit. An abnormal result is a blood glucose level of at least 130 mg/dl. For high-risk patients with a positive screen but negative GTT at 24 to 28 weeks, the GTT is repeated at 34 weeks. High-risk patients for GDM are identified as follows: obesity (>20% ideal body weight by Metropolitan Life Table and/or body mass index >27 to 29 based on prepregnancy weight), previous gestational diabetes, high-risk ethnic group (e.g., Mexican American), previous macrosomic infant (≥4000 g), or fetus with congenital anomalies.

# Diagnosis

The definition of GDM is carbohydrate intolerance of variable severity with onset or first recognition during the current pregnancy. The definition applies irrespective of whether or not insulin is used for treatment or whether the condition persists after pregnancy. It does not exclude the possibility that the glucose intolerance may have antidated the pregnancy. The traditional criteria for diagnosis was devised by O'Sullivan and Mahan in the classic study in which a 100-g glucose load was administered to 754 consecutively selected women. The glucose analysis of whole blood was done by the Somogyi-Nelson technique, and the study group was followed for up to 8 years for subsequent development of diabetes mellitus. The rationale for selection of this diagnostic criteria was maternal outcome, not perinatal outcome.

In 1979, the National Diabetic Data Group (NDDG) modified the O'Sullivan criteria from whole blood to plasma by multiplying each value by 115%. Glucose concentration was determined in plasma or serum by a glucokinase or hexokinase method (whichever is the most widely used). Two or more abnormal values are considered diagnostic of GDM. The OGTT is performed with a 100-g glucose load in the morning after an overnight fast of more than 8 hours after 3 days of an unrestricted carbohydrate diet (>150 g). The NDDG criteria was altered by Carpenter and Coustan to account for the specific laboratory methodologies, resulting in a decrease of approximately 10 mg/dl for each determination.

Sacks and colleagues proposed a different modification with automated enzymatic glucose measurement. The study consisted of 995 patients undergoing an OGTT. Glucose was measured on each specimen by both Somogyi-Nelson (whole blood) and automated enzymatic method (plasma) results (for equivalency to original O'Sullivan and Mahan criteria) (Table 35–2).

Currently, the most widely used criteria for the diagnosis of GDM is the diagnostic criteria established by the NDDG (any two abnormal values): fasting more than 105 mg/dl, 1-hour more than 190

**Table 35–1** Prevalence of Gestational Diabetes by Maternal Age

| Age | No. | GDM (%) |
| --- | --- | --- |
| 25 | 2319 | 28 (1.2) |
| 25–29 | 2160 | 42 (1.9) |
| 30–34 | 1299 | 39 (3.0) |
| 35–59 | 397 | 15 (3.8) |
| >40 | 39 | 1 (2.6) |
| Total | 6214 | 125 (2.0) |

GDM = gestational diabetes mellitus.

**Table 35–2** 100-g Oral Glucose Tolerance Test Positive Diagnosis Criteria

|  | O'Sullivan* | NDDG | 4th International Workshop Carpenter/ Coustan† | Sacks† |
|---|---|---|---|---|
| Fasting | 90 mg/dl | 105 mg/dl | 95 mg/dl | 96 mg/dl |
| 1 hr | 165 mg/dl | 190 mg/dl | 180 mg/dl | 172 mg/dl |
| 2 hr | 145 mg/dl | 165 mg/dl | 155 mg/dl | 152 mg/dl |
| 3 hr | 125 mg/dl | 145 mg/dl | 140 mg/dl | 131 mg/dl |

*Whole blood: Somogyi-Nelson method.
†Plasma or serum: glucokinase or hexokinase method.
Note: The 4th International Workshop Conference on GDM also supported a one-step procedure for the detection of GDM using a 2-hour, 75-g OGTT (World Health Organization Criteria).

mg/dl, 2-hour more than 165 mg/dl, 3-hour more than 145 mg/dl. Recently, researchers questioned the ability of the OGTT to identify gravida at risk for delivering LGA infants. The identification of women at risk for adverse fetal outcome is critical. Several studies examined the patients who, although not meeting the criteria of two abnormal values during an OGTT, appear to have impaired glucose tolerance because of either high normal values or the presence of one abnormal value during the OGTT. Those women who remain untreated had a three-fold higher risk for LGA infants and macrosomia.

In a recent prospective randomized study, the hypothesis was tested that treatment of gravida with one abnormal OGTT value will reduce adverse outcomes. One hundred twenty-six women with one abnormal OGTT value and 146 women in the control group (normal OGTT values) participated in a prospective study during the third trimester of pregnancy. The subjects with one abnormal test result were randomized into treated (group I) and untreated (group II) groups. Group I subjects were treated with a strict diabetic protocol to maintain tight glycemic control by means of diet and insulin therapy. Group II subjects tested their capillary blood glucose for a baseline period. The study revealed that the level of glycemic control was similar before initiation of therapy between the treated and untreated groups. The overall incidence of neonatal metabolic complications was 4% in the treated group and 14% in the untreated group. Macrosomia was present in 7% of the treated women and 24% in the untreated women. Thus, women with one abnormal value are similar to patients with GDM (two abnormal values) in their glycemic control before therapy and rate of macrosomia (30%). Treatment of these women also will result in perinatal outcomes comparable with nondiabetic subjects. In contrast, a relatively flat OGTT curve is associated with small-for-gestational-age infants.

Thus, this suggests a metabolic subgroup within the intrauterine growth retardation population.

## UNIVERSITY OF TEXAS HEALTH SCIENCE CENTER AT SAN ANTONIO DIAGNOSIS PROTOCOL FOR PATIENTS WITH AN OGTT AT LEAST 130 mg/dl

A 3-hour 100-g glucol OGTT is performed after a 150- to 250-g per day carbohydrate load for 3 days before the test. Testing should occur after an overnight fast of 12 hours. Values for an *abnormal* 3-hour OGTT are fasting plasma glucose more than 104 mg/dl, 1 hour more than 189 mg/dl, 2 hour more than 164 mg/dl, and 3 hour more than 144 mg/dl. For the purpose of diagnosis, one or more abdominal values is considered GDM. If the patient does not tolerate the 100-g glucol because of nausea and vomiting, a 100-g lemonade glucol prepared by laboratory personnel should be administered.

# Treatment Rationale

Despite a significant decrease in perinatal mortality in the last decade, perinatal morbidity remains virtually unchanged, approaching a 10 to 50% rate. Approximately 15 to 50% of GDM women will be hyperglycemic despite dietary therapy, depending on criteria used and frequency of blood glucose testing. Glucose values currently accepted as satisfactory are fasting less than 95 mg/dl, postprandial less than 120 mg/dl, and mean blood glucose 95 to 100 mg/dl. The use of HbA1c as a measure of glycemic control is questionable. There is a weak correlation (r = 0.51) between fasting, postprandial, and mean blood glucose and HbA1c.

Glucose testing 4 to 7 times a day is optimal. At a minimum, the care provider should determine glucose levels at least three times a week: fasting, and postprandial. He or she should assume that the values on the day of testing are the best values of the week. Women who are found to have fasting hyperglycemia or abnormal carbohydrate tolerance in the first trimester may have pre-existing diabetes mellitus and should be treated in the same way as women who have type 2 diabetes.

The metabolic management of the pregnant diabetic woman, based on the need to lower maternal capillary glucose levels below 5.3 mmol/L (95 mg/dl) in the fasting state and 6.7 mmol/L (120 mg/dl) 1 to 2 hours after meals, can reduce the risk of excessive fetal growth to approximately that of the general population. Thus, the primary management strategy is based on maintaining maternal glucose levels below these thresholds for the prevention of macrosomia in women with GDM and PGDM (type 1 and type 2).

If management is targeted primarily at controlling maternal hyperglycemia, then self-glucose monitoring may detect elevated glucose warranting more intensive therapy beyond standard dietary management. Glucose monitoring should include postprandial testing. One- and 2-hour measurements are most commonly used. The use of self-monitoring reflectance meters that store results electronically provides ongoing validation of the accuracy of patient monitoring techniques. Patients who fail to achieve or maintain glycemic goals or who show signs of excessive fetal growth should receive insulin in addition to standard nutritional management. There is increasing data that demonstrate the cost effectiveness of insulin therapy to prevent fetal complications. It has been recommended that insulin administration is individualized to achieve glycemic goals. Human rather than porcine or bovine insulin preparations have been recommended to minimize the transplacental transport of anti-insulin antibodies. Regular aerobic exercise is also recommended because it has been shown to lower fasting and postprandial glucose concentrations in several studies of previously sedentary women. Even though the optimal frequency and intensity of exercise for lowering maternal glucose levels has not yet been determined, three exercise periods of more than 15 minutes' duration have been shown to help modify maternal glucose levels. Therefore, if appropriate, exercise may be used in conjunction with nutritional therapy to improve glucose levels.

Patients who have fasting plasma glucose greater than 95 mg/dl who fail to achieve the desired level of glycemia should be placed on insulin. In a review of national and international peer-reviewed literature, 40 to 60% of GDM women required insulin. This again demonstrates that the proper terminology for classification of diabetes should be based on an individualized pattern of diet or insulin requirements rather than a dogmatic classification of GDM, A1, or A2 diabetes.

We investigated the effect of intensified treatment of diabetes on patients' emotional status and compliance to treatment. Insulin administration and multiple glucose determinations had no adverse effect on the emotional profile of GDM women. The multiple determinations coupled with the glycemic control provided by the glucose meter may actually enhance patient empowerment to control and cope. Although women with GDM are coping with an acute disease that will resolve with the birth of the fetus, those with preexisting diabetes frequently develop specific coping mechanisms. The emotional profile was not associated with the severity of the disease, but the severity was associated with decreased compliance as measured by the rate of clinic visits and no-shows, in addition to an overall decreased compliance when compared with nondiabetic subjects. Customizing medical and behavioral goals for each patient should be the ultimate goal for care of the preexisting diabetic patient because it can maximize patient satisfaction and enhance the willingness and/or ability of the patient to comply.

Insulin requirements necessary to maintain desired glycemic control in GDM are approximately 90 ± 30 units per day (average of 1 to 1.5 units insulin/kg per actual body weight in pregnancy). The therapeutic algorithm is based on human insulin divided into three injections: regular and intermediate-acting insulin in the morning, regular at dinner, and intermediate acting at bedtime. The standard formula for the amount of insulin prescribed is two thirds of the dose in the morning (2:1, intermediate acting: regular) and one third in the evening (1:1, regular: intermediate acting). If after 3 days of self-monitoring blood glucose levels have not reached the glycemic goal (overall mean 85 to 95 mg/dl or postprandial <120 mg/dl), each insulin dose should be increased by 15 to 20%. This is repeated until glycemic control has been achieved. Thereafter, alteration in insulin dose is based on achievement of glucose target ranges for overall (85 to 95 mg/dl), fasting (60 to 80 mg/dl), preprandial (70 to 90 mg/dl), and postprandial (<120 mg/dl) levels.

The length of dietary therapy before insulin initiation was previously recommended to be two or more abnormal glucose values during a 1- to 2-week period. This recommendation was made before the extensive use of self-monitoring blood glucose in the management of these patients. We found that if patients failed to achieve good glycemic control within 2 weeks, allowing more time did not lead to success. This resulted in our program with the approach that a fasting plasma glucose greater than 95 mg/dl during an OGTT in obese patients will be sufficient to initiate insulin therapy. In contrast, nonobese GDMs will have a 2-week trial of diet before the decision to initiate insulin.

Dietary therapy is based on 30 to 35 kcal/kg of ideal body weight. In general, obese patients should receive 25 kcal/kg for current body weight and nonobese patients should be prescribed a diet of 35 kcal/kg body weight. The diet should be calculated according to the American Diabetes Association (ADA) recommendations (carbohydrate 45 to 55%, protein 20 to 30%, fat 25%) and should be synchronized with the insulin dose throughout the day. One hundred twenty-five grams of protein should be included in the diet to prevent extremes of glycemic excursions. Care providers should be sensitive to cultural preferences and habits.

Modification of dietary therapy should be based on the following: self-monitoring blood glucose—

glycemic control; weight gain—appropriate weight gain of 0.9 lb/wk in second and third trimester is not required in gestational diabetes, especially with obese patients; ketonuria—if present, blood ketones need to be tested; diet adjustment—calories should be adjusted in accordance with blood glucose level and presence of ketonuria. If caloric adjustment fails, insulin therapy should be initiated.

## Optimal Timing and Mode of Delivery

Delivery at term is indicated under the following conditions: obstetric indications, failure to achieve adequate glycemic control, patient noncompliance either because of missed appointments and/or inadequate self-monitoring blood glucose, if estimated fetal weight is at least 4250 g, previous stillbirth at term, and vasculopathy.

Before induction or cesarean delivery, maturity testing is recommended due to the delay in fetal lung maturation, which may result in respiratory distress syndrome (RDS). The interpretation of amniotic fluid should consider the following facts: poor glycemic control is associated with delayed lung maturity, good control is not associated with a delay in lung maturity; at 37 to 38 weeks gestation at approximately 20% will have immature lung test results but after 37 to 38 weeks RDS rarely occurs; lecithin/sphingomyelin ratio does not guarantee lung maturity in GDM, and when phosphatidylglycerol results are positive, lung disease will not occur; the risk of macrosomia or stillbirth must be balanced against the risk of hyaline membrane disease. The dilemma is the stillborn with mature lungs vs. a live neonate with immature lungs.

The method of delivery of the macrosomic infant remains controversial. A greater mean birth weight and an abnormal weight distribution per body composition puts the fetus of a diabetic mother at increased risk for shoulder dystocia. A higher proportion of shoulder dystocia occurs in macrosomic infants of diabetic mothers compared with nondiabetic patients. Ultrasonography estimated fetal weight facilitates determination of mode of delivery, such as cesarean section for patients at high risk for shoulder dystocia estimated fetal weight (>4250 g).

## Problems Related to Pregestational Diabetes

Several principles in the management of diabetes in pregnancy are similar for both GDM and PGDM

**Table 35–3** White Classification

Gestational diabetes
   Maintained by diet alone
   Insulin required
Pregestational class
   A   Euglycemia by diet alone, any duration, onset at any age
   B   Onset age 20 or older, duration <10 yr
   C   Onset during age 10–19 yr, or duration of 10–19 yr
   D   Onset at age <10 yr, duration of >20 yr, background retinopathy or hypertension (not PIH)
   R   Proliferative retinopathy or vitreous hemorrhage
   F   Nephropathy with proteinuria >500 mg/dl
   RF  Criteria for classes R and F
   H   Arteriosclerotic heart disease clinically evident
   T   Prior renal transplantation

PIH = pregnancy-induced hypertension.

patients (i.e., diet and insulin management and timing of delivery). PGDM is also characterized by maternal complications and an increased risk of congenital anomalies. Among the acute maternal complications of PGDM are ketoacidosis, hypoglycemia, hypertension (20 to 40% of cases), urinary tract infections, and polyhydramnios. There may be acceleration of microvascular, renal, ocular, and neural complications during pregnancy among poorly controlled diabetics. Maternal and fetal complications can result in frequent and extended hospitalizations. Type 1 diabetes is characterized by insulin deficiency, dependency on exogenous insulin, tendency to become ketoacidotic, lean body mass, and abrupt onset of symptoms, usually before 30 years of age. Type 1 patients are further stratified by the White classification system, which is based on the presence/absence and severity (organ involvement) of vascular complications.

The type 2 diabetic patient may be free of classic symptoms, may require exogenous insulin, are not prone to ketoacidosis, may have a family history of diabetes, is usually obese or has a history of obesity, and is usually diagnosed with diabetes after age 30. These patients also qualify for further stratification by the White classification (Table 35–3).

Recently, the NDDG recommended changes in the criteria for type 2 diabetes diagnosis (Table 35–4).

**Table 35–4** 1997 ADA Diagnostic Criteria

|  | FPG (mg/dl) | GTT (mg/dl) |
| --- | --- | --- |
| DM | ≥126 | 2 h ≥ 200 |
| IFG | ≥110 < 126 | — |
| IGT | — | 2 h ≥ 140 < 200 |

DM = diabetes mellitus; FPG = fasting plasma glucose; GTT = 75 g glucose tolerance test during nonpregnant state; IFG = impaired fasting glucose; IGT = impaired glucose tolerance.
From Report of the Expert Committee on the Diagnosis and Classification of Diabetes Mellitus. Diabetes Care 20:1183, 1997.

They concluded that to diagnose type 2 diabetes, the patient must have either diabetic symptoms (polyuria, polydipsia, and unexplained weight loss) plus casual (any time of day without regard to time since the last meal) plasma glucose concentration at least 200 mg/dl (11.1 mmol/l), fasting (no caloric intake for at least 8 hours) plasma glucose at least 126 mg/dl (7.0 mmol/l), or 2-hour plasma glucose at least 200 mg/dl during a 75-g OGTT in a nonpregnant individual. The test should be performed using a glucose load containing the equivalent of 75 g anhydrous glucose dissolved in water. Repeat testing on a different day is needed for confirmation using this diagnostic criteria. The NDDG further classified normality (nondiabetic state) as fasting plasma less than 111 mg/dl and 2-hour postglucose load of less than 141 mg/dl. A fasting glucose of 111 to 125 mg/dl and 2-hour postprandial at least 140 mg/dl but less than 200 mg/dl reflects impaired glucose tolerance. This change in criteria doubles the incidence of diabetes in the general population, turning some previously categorized GDM into type 2 patients.

Congenital anomalies are now the main contributors to perinatal morbidity and mortality among infants of diabetic mothers. The most common malformations are congenital heart disease and caudal regression syndrome, and both occur embryologically before 7 weeks' gestation. Congenital malformations occur at least three times more frequently than the 2 to 3% in the general population. The most widely accepted theory is that hyperglycemia, before and early in conception, plays the major role in abnormal organogenesis. Elevated levels of glycosylated hemoglobin during the first trimester are associated with an increased risk of major congenital anomalies. Animal studies confirmed these findings. Therefore, preconceptual enrollment into education and clinical programs may improve patient compliance; controlling glycemia can decrease the rate of malformations. However, evidence is inconclusive to support the concept of increased risk of congenital anomalies in GDM. As proposed by Freinkel, a "metabolic teratogen" induced by diabetes is a distinct possibility. Therefore, normalization of hyperglycemia among the few GDM mothers detected very early in pregnancy is desirable.

Diabetic ketoacidosis (DKA) is a severe metabolic decompensation characterized by uncontrolled hyperglycemia (generally >300 mg/dl), dehydration, depletion of potassium, metabolic acidosis (arterial blood pH, usually <7.30), and increased ketones (β-hydroxybutyric and acetoacetic acid) concentrations (>5 mM). The key diagnostic feature is the elevation of blood ketone concentration that is reflected in an increased anion gap.

Pregnant diabetic women may have severe DKA with minimal hyperglycemia due to volume expansion, increased glomerular filtration, and/or the continued use of glucose by the fetoplacental unit in the presence of insulin deficiency. This represents a nonhepatic explanation that can be characterized by lack of association between glucose and bicarbonate levels. Correction of fluid deficits is especially important because it promotes glucosuria and decreased release of insulin counterregulatory hormones that produce insulin resistance. Therefore, in diabetes in pregnancy, glucose-containing fluid must be initially administered when glucose concentrations are approximating 300 to 350 mg/dl. Patients are treated with insulin in addition to free water for the hyperglycemia and hypertonicity, sodium bicarbonate for the ketoacidosis, and potassium and sodium chloride for the fluid and electrolyte losses.

Fluid/electrolyte replacement and insulin management remain the basis of DKA therapy. Intravenous regular insulin corrects hyperglycemia and inhibits ketogenesis. Unless the insulin resistance is extremely severe, ketoacidosis responds to a 5- to 10-U/hr infusion of insulin. The metabolic acidosis is characterized by a decrease in the serum bicarbonate concentration. DKA patients with severe hypobicarbonatemia (<5 to 6 mEq/L) and a blood pH (<7.10 to 7.15) usually benefit most from bicarbonate therapy. When deciding to treat with bicarbonate, it is important to give only sufficient amounts of alkali to raise the serum bicarbonate level to 10 to 12 mEq/L.

Hypoglycemia is also a problem that adversely affects the quality of life. Severe hypoglycemia results in confusion, coma, and seizures. Patients need to be informed of the warning signs, including tingling of the tongue, numbness, sweating, and loss of level of concentration. Patients need to be taught to respond immediately by measuring capillary blood glucose and ingesting carbohydrates or milk. Recurrent mild or chemical hypoglycemia can accompany pregnancy because of the continuous glucose consumption by the fetus. In general, hypoglycemic episodes are more common in the pregnant woman during the first 20 weeks of pregnancy. We found that hypoglycemia (ranging from 50 to 30 mg/dl) may occur in 6 to 10% of women with GDM regardless of treatment modality (diet or insulin).

## REFERENCES

American College of Obstetricians and Gynecologists: Management of diabetes mellitus in pregnancy. ACOG Technical Bulletin, 1994.

Berkus MD, Stern MP, Mitchell BD, et al: Relationships between glucose levels and insulin secretion during glucose challenge test. Am J Obstet Gynecol 163:1818, 1990.

Berkus MD, Stern MP, Mitchell BD, et al: Does fasting interval affect the glucose challenge test? Am J Obstet Gynecol 163:1812, 1990.

Brustman L, Langer O, Engel S, et al: Verified self-monitored blood glucose data versus glycosylated hemoglobin and glycosylated serum protein as a means of predicting short and long term metabolic control in gestational diabetes. Am J Obstet Gynecol 155:635, 1986.

Buchanan TA, Catalano PM: The pathogenesis of GDM: Implications for diabetes after pregnancy. Diabetes Rev 3:584, 1995.

Carpenter MW, Coustan DR: Criteria for screening tests for gestational diabetes. Am J Obstet Gynecol 144:768, 1982.

Conway DL, Langer O: Elective delivery of infants with macrosomia in diabetic women: Reduced shoulder dystocia versus increased cesarean deliveries. Am J Obstet Gynecol 178:922, 1998.

Cousins L, Baxi L, Chez R: Screening recommendations for gestational diabetes mellitus. Am J Obstet Gynecol 165:493, 1991.

Coustan DR: Diagnosis of gestational diabetes: Are new criteria needed? Diabetes Rev 3:614, 1995.

Coustan DR: Pregnancy in diabetic women. N Engl J Med 319:1663, 1998.

Freinkel N: Of pregnancy and progeny. Diabetes 20:1023, 1980.

Hod M, Rabinerson D, Peled Y: Gestational diabetes mellitus: Is it a clinical entity? Diabetes Rev 3:602, 1995.

Kaplan A: The Conduct of Inquiry. CA, Chandler Publishing Company, 1964.

Kjos SL, Henry OA, Montoro M, et al: Insulin-requiring diabetes in pregnancy: A randomized trial of active induction of labor and expectant management. Am J Obstet Gynecol 169:611, 1993.

Kreisberg RA: Diabetic ketoacidosos: Revisited again [editorial]. Mayo Clin Proc 63:1144, 1988.

Langer N, Langer O: Emotional adjustment to diagnosis and intensified treatment of gestational diabetes. Obstet Gynecol 84:329, 1994.

Langer O: Is normoglycemia the correct threshold to prevent complications in the pregnant diabetic? Diabetes Rev 4:24, 1996.

Langer O: Gestational diabetes: A contemporary management approach. Endocrinologist 5:180, 1995.

Langer O: Management of gestational diabetes. Clin Perinatol 30:603, 1993.

Langer O: Diabetes in pregnancy. In Merkatz IR, Cherry S (eds): Medical, Surgical and Gynecologic Complications of Pregnancy, 4th ed. Baltimore, Williams & Wilkins, 1991.

Langer O: Prevention of macrosomia. In Oats N (ed): Diabetes in Pregnancy. London, WB Saunders, 1991, pp 333–347.

Langer O: Critical issues in diabetes and pregnancy: Early identification, metabolic control, and prevention of adverse outcome. In Merkatz IR, Thompson JE, Mullen PD, et al (eds): New Perspectives on Prenatal Care. Baltimore, Williams & Wilkins, 1991, pp 445–59.

Langer O: Scientific rationale for management of diabetes in pregnancy: Recent approaches with innovative computer-based technology. Diabetes Care 11:67–72, 1988.

Langer O, Anyaegbunam A, Brustman L, et al: Management of women with one abnormal oral glucose tolerance test value reduces adverse outcome in pregnancy. Am J Obstet Gynecol 161:593–599, 1989.

Langer O, Anyaegbunam A, Brustman L, et al: Pregestational diabetes: Insulin requirements throughout pregnancy. Am J Obstet Gynecol 159:616, 1988.

Langer O, Anyaegbunam A, Brustman L, et al: Gestational diabetes: Insulin requirements in pregnancy. Am J Obstet Gynecol 157:669, 1987.

Langer O, Berkus MD, Brustman L, et al: The rationale for insulin management in gestational diabetes mellitus. Diabetes 40(S2):186,1991.

Langer O, Berkus MD, Huff RW, et al: Shoulder dystocia: Should the fetus weighing >4000 grams be delivered by cesarean section? Am J Obstet Gynecol 165:831, 1991.

Langer O, Brustman L, Anyaegbunam A, et al: The significance of one abnormal glucose tolerance test value on adverse outcome in pregnancy. Am J Obstet Gynecol 157:758, 1987.

Langer O, Damus K, Maiman M, et al: A link between relative hypoglycemia-hypoinsulinemia during oral glucose tolerance tests and intrauterine growth retardation. Am J Obstet Gynecol 155:711, 1986.

Langer O, Gabbe S, Berkus M, et al: Diabetes and level of glycemic control: How normal is normal? Proceedings of the 39th Annual Meeting of the Society for Gynecologic Investigation, San Antonio, TX, 1992.

Langer O, Hod M: Management of gestational diabetes mellitus. Obstet Gynecol Clin North Am 23:137, 1996.

Langer O, Landon M, Gabbe S, et al: IDDM: The relationship between neonatal morbidity and glycemic control. San Antonio, TX, Proceedings of the 38th Annual Meeting of the Society for Gynecologic Investigation, 1991.

Langer O, Langer N, Piper JM, et al: Is cultural diversity a factor in self-monitoring blood glucose in gestational diabetes? JAAMP 6:73, 1995.

Langer O, Levy J, Brustman L, et al: Glycemic control in gestational diabetes mellitus. How tight is tight enough: Small for gestational age versus large for gestational age? Am J Obstet Gynecol 161:646, 1989.

Langer O, Mazze RS: The relationship between glycosylated haemoglobin and verified self-monitored blood glucose among pregnant and non-pregnant women with diabetes. Pract Diabetes 4:32, 1987.

Langer O, Mazze RS: Diabetes in pregnancy: Evaluating self-monitoring performance and glycemic control with memory-based reflectance meters. Am J Obstet Gynecol 155:635, 1986.

Langer O, Rodriguez DA, Xenakis EMJ, et al: Intensified vs. conventional management of gestational diabetes. Am J Obstet Gynecol 170:1036, 1994.

Lavin JP Jr: Screening of high-risk and general populations for gestational diabetes. Diabetes 35:24, 1985.

Marquette GP, Klein VR, Niebyl JR: Efficacy of screening for gestational diabetes. Am J Perinatol 2:7, 1985.

McFarland M, Berkus M, Conway D, et al: Can the need for insulin treatment in gestational diabetes be anticipated at the time of diagnosis? Chicago, Proceedings of the American Diabetes Association 4th International Workshop Conference on Gestational Diabetes Mellitus, 1997.

Mills JL, Baker L, Goldman AS: Malformations in infants of diabetic mothers occur before the seventh gestational week. Diabetes 28:292, 1979.

National Diabetes Data Group: Classification of diagnosis of diabetes mellitus and other categories of glucose intolerance. Diabetes 28:1039, 1979.

Naylor CD, Sermer M, Chen E, et al: Cesarean delivery in relation to birth weight and gestational glucose tolerance: Pathophysiology or practice style? JAMA 275:1165, 1996.

O'Sullivan JB, Mahan CM: Criteria for the oral glucose tolerance test in pregnancy. Diabetes 13:278, 1964.

Pendergrass M, Fazioni E, DeFronzo RA: Non–insulin-dependent diabetes mellitus and gestational diabetes mellitus: Same disease, another name? Diabetes Rev 3:566, 1995.

Piper JM, Samueloff A, Langer O: Outcome of amniotic fluid analysis and neonatal respiratory status in a population of diabetic and nondiabetic pregnancies. J Reprod Med 40:780, 1995.

Public health guidelines for enhancing diabetes control through maternal and child health programs. Department of Health & Human Services, PHS, CDD Publication 00–4906, 1986.

Reece EA, Pinter EA, Leranth CZ: Ultrastructural analysis of malformations of the embryonic neural axis induced by in vitro hyperglycemia conditions. Teratology 32:363, 1985.

Report of the Expert Committee on the Diagnosis and Classification of Diabetes Mellitus. Diabetes Care 20:1183, 1997.

Rouse DJ, Owen J, Goldenberg RL, et al: The effectiveness and costs of elective cesarean delivery for fetal macrosomia diagnosed by ultrasound. JAMA 276:1480–1486, 1996.

Sacks DA, Abu-Fadil S, Greenspoon JS, et al: Do the current standards for glucose tolerance testing in pregnancy represent a valid conversion of O'Sullivan's original criteria? Am J Obstet Gynecol 161:638, 1989.

Saider TW: Effects of maternal diabetes on embryogenesis: Hyperglycemia-induced exencephaly. Teratology 21:349, 1980.

Schwartz ML, Brenner WE: The need for adequate and consistent diagnostic classifications for diabetes mellitus diagnosed during pregnancy. Am J Obstet Gynecol 143:119, 1982.

Second International Workshop Conference on Gestational Diabetes Mellitus. Diabetes 34(S2), 1985.

Sokol R, Kazzi GM, Kalhan SC, et al: Identifying the pregnancy at risk for intrauterine growth retardation: Possible usefulness of the intravenous glucose tolerance test. Am J Obstet Gynecol 143:220, 1982.

Summary and Recommendations of the Third International Workshop—Conference on Gestational Diabetes Mellitus. Diabetes 40:197, 1991.

Tallarigo L, Giampietro O, Penno G, et al: Relation of glucose tolerance to complications of pregnancy in nondiabetic women. N Engl J Med 315:989, 1986.

US Preventive Services Task Force: Guide to Clinical Preventive Services, 2nd ed. VA, International Medical Publishers, 1996, pp 199–208.

# 36

# Asthma in Pregnancy

MITCHELL P. DOMBROWSKI

## Definition

Asthma is characterized by chronic airway inflammation with increased airway responsiveness to a variety of stimuli and airway obstruction that is partially or completely reversible.

In general, women of childbearing age are free of serious medical conditions. The exception is asthma, which may be the most common potentially serious medical complication of pregnancy. Approximately 4% of women of childbearing age have a history of asthma, but up to 10% of the population appears to have nonspecific airway hyper-responsiveness. In general, the prevalence, morbidity, and mortality from asthma are increasing. It is not known whether this is a function of environmental, immunologic, or other etiologies.

The obstetric management of asthma is problematic because maternal exacerbations can cause serious fetal sequelae, the efficacy of common medical therapies has not been well studied, and medications may have untoward fetal and maternal effects. Insight into the pathogenesis of asthma has changed with the recognition that airway inflammation is present in nearly all cases. The effects of pregnancy on asthma are controversial because previous studies have had conflicting results, but pregnancy may be associated with a worsening of more severe asthma. Asthma during pregnancy has been associated with considerable maternal morbidity. Mabie and associates reported that 42.5% pregnant women who had asthma required hospitalization, and an additional 18% had one or more emergency room visits for asthma exacerbations during pregnancy. Similarly, Perlow and associates reported a 46% rate of asthma exacerbations requiring hospital admission during pregnancy. In contrast, in a managed care setting with a higher socioeconomic population, Schatz and associates reported an emergency room visit rate of 12.6%, but a hospitalization rate of only 1.1% for asthma exacerbations during pregnancy.

Although birth weight has commonly been used as an outcome measure, few studies have controlled for factors known to affect birth weight, such as maternal race, height, weight, parity, nutrition, chronic hypertension, cigarette smoking, and corticosteroid therapy. Persons who have asthma have increased frequency of chronic hypertension, and maternal smoking, may also complicate the effects of other influences. Ethnicity may be a particularly important confounding factor in assessing the relationship between asthma and pregnancy outcomes, because African-Americans (aged 15 to 44 years) are five times more likely to die of asthma and are twice as likely to be hospitalized because of asthma compared with white Americans.

The mechanisms by which asthma may have adverse perinatal effects are not well defined. Poor control of asthma leading to chronic or episodic fetal hypoxia is thought to be important. Medications used in asthma treatment may also play a role, although the limited available data suggest minimal or no effects. However, corticosteroids may be associated with low birth weight and preeclampsia. A summary of possible maternal, fetal, and neonatal complications related to asthma and asthma therapy is presented in Table 36–1.

Studies have shown that patients who have more severe asthma may have the greatest risk for complications during pregnancy. Quantitating this risk is problematic because most studies have not categorized the severity of the asthma of their subjects. This problem is further complicated because there is no universally accepted definition of asthma severity during pregnancy. In 1993, the National Asthma Education Program (NAEP) working group defined mild, moderate, and severe asthma according to symptomatic exacerbations (wheezing, cough, dyspnea, or all three) and objective tests of pulmonary function. The most commonly used parameters are the peak expiratory flow rate (PEFR) and the forced expiratory volume in 1 second ($FEV_1$). The NAEP guidelines did not consider the need for regular medication to be a factor for classifying asthma severity (Table 36–2). However, it seems prudent to consider patients who require regular medications (β-agonist, theophylline, or inhaled corticosteroids) to have moderate asthma and those requiring regular systemic corticosteroids for control of asthma symptoms to have severe asthma.

## Asthma Management

The ultimate goal of asthma therapy is to maintain adequate oxygenation of the fetus by preventing hypoxic episodes in the mother. The effective management of asthma during pregnancy relies on four integral components.

**Table 36–1** Reported Effects of Asthma and Asthma Treatment Regimens

| Increased Maternal |
|---|
| Preeclampsia |
| Cesarean delivery |
| Asthma exacerbations |
| Preterm rupture of membranes |

| Increased Perinatal |
|---|
| Mortality |
| Prematurity |
| Low birth weight |
| Hypoxia/asphyxia |
| Hypoadrenalism |
| Theophylline toxicity |

**Table 36–2** Modified NAEP Asthma Severity Classification

| Mild Asthma |
|---|
| Brief (<1 hr) symptomatic exacerbations ≤ twice/wk |
| PEFR ≥80% of personal best |
| $FEV_1$ ≥80% of predicted when asymptomatic |

| Moderate Asthma |
|---|
| Symptomatic exacerbations >twice/wk |
| Exacerbations affect activity levels |
| Exacerbations may last for days |
| PEFR, $FEV_1$ range from 60 to 80% of predicted |
| Regular medications necessary to control symptoms |

| Severe Asthma |
|---|
| Continuous symptoms/frequent exacerbations limit activity levels |
| PEFR, $FEV_1$ <60% of expected, and are highly variable |
| Regular oral corticosteroids necessary to control symptoms |

$FEV_1$ = forced expiratory volume in the first second; PEFR = peak expiratory flow rate.

## OBJECTIVE MEASURES FOR ASSESSMENT AND MONITORING

Subjective measures of lung function by the patient and physician provide an insensitive and inaccurate assessment of airway hyper-responsiveness, airway inflammation, and asthma severity. The $FEV_1$ after a maximal inspiration is the single best measure of pulmonary function, however, measurement of $FEV_1$ requires a spirometer. The PEFR correlates well with the $FEV_1$ and can be measured reliably with inexpensive, disposable, portable peak flow meters. Because PEFR reflects only large airway functions, it may not be sufficient by itself to make a diagnosis or fully evaluate the severity of asthma. However, patient self-monitoring of PEFR provides valuable insight into the course of asthma throughout the day, assesses circadian variation in pulmonary function, and helps detect early signs of deterioration so that timely therapy can be instituted.

## AVOIDANCE OR CONTROL OF ASTHMA TRIGGERS

Limiting adverse environmental exposures during pregnancy is important for controlling asthma. Irritants and allergens that provoke acute symptoms also increase airway inflammation and hyper-responsiveness. Avoiding or controlling such triggers can reduce asthma symptoms, airway hyporesponsiveness, and the need for medical therapy. Association of asthma with allergies is common; 75 to 85% of patients who have asthma have positive skin tests to common allergens, including animal dander, house dust mites, cockroach antigens, pollens, and molds. Other common nonimmunologic triggers of asthma include tobacco smoke, strong odors, air pollutants, food additives (e.g., sulfites), and certain drugs, including aspirin and β-blockers. Another trigger can be strenuous physical activity. For some patients, exercise-induced asthma can be avoided with inhalation of a $β_2$-agonist, 5 to 60 minutes before exercise. Specific measures for avoiding asthma triggers are listed in Table 36-3.

## PATIENT EDUCATION

The patient should be made aware that controlling asthma during pregnancy is especially important for the well-being of the fetus. She should be made aware that she can reduce asthma triggers. The patient should have a basic understanding of the medical management of asthma during pregnancy, including self-monitoring of PEFRs and the correct use of inhalers.

## PHARMACOLOGIC THERAPY

The goal of asthma therapy is multiphasic:
1. Relieve bronchospasm
2. Protect the airways from irritant stimuli
3. Prevent the pulmonary and inflammatory response to an allergen exposure
4. Resolve the inflammatory process in the airways with resultant improved pulmonary function and reduced airway hyper-responsiveness.

Individual medications may be described with regard to their capacity to improve pulmonary function by bronchodilation or reduce hyper-responsiveness via anti-inflammatory properties. The NAEP working group guidelines emphasize the need to incorporate anti-inflammatory medications as first-line therapy in the treatment of patients with moderate or severe asthma. Specific therapies must be tailored to the needs and circumstances of individual patients.

**Table 36-3** Limiting Exposure to Asthma Triggers

Use plastic mattress and pillow covers
Wash bedding in hot water weekly
Control animal dander
    Bathe pet weekly
    Keep pets out of the bedroom
    Remove pet from the home
Control cockroaches
Avoid tobacco smoke
Inhibit mite and mold growth by reducing humidity
Do not be present when home is vacuumed

The step-care therapeutic approach includes increasing the number and frequency of medications in response to increasing asthma severity.

## Asthma Pharmacotherapy

Current medical treatment for asthma emphasizes treatment of airway inflammation to decrease airway hyper-responsiveness and prevent asthma symptoms. Although it is assumed that asthma medications are as effective in pregnant as in nonpregnant patients, differences in maternal physiology and pharmacokinetics may affect the absorption, distribution, metabolism, and clearance of medications during pregnancy. Published studied have not adequately compared treatment regimens during pregnancy, and it may not be valid to infer conclusions about optimal asthma treatment during pregnancy from studies with nonpregnant subjects.

Marked endocrinologic and immunologic changes during pregnancy include elevations in free plasma cortisol, possible tissue refractoriness to cortisol, and changes in cellular immunity. Although animal studies have indicated association of corticosteroids with increased risk of cleft palate and decreased fetal survival, human studies have failed to suggest any increased in facial clefts or other birth defects. However, the use of oral corticosteroids has been associated with low birth weight. Potential adverse effects of oral or high-dose inhaled corticosteroids include adrenal suppression, weight gain, impaired fetal growth, hypertension, diabetes, cataracts, and osteoporosis. Patients who have asthma, especially if they are receiving systemic corticosteroids, may be at increased risk for developing preeclampsia. Systemic corticosteroids may also potentiate the risk for weight gain and the development of gestational diabetes mellitus.

In the United States, only three classes of inhaled anti-inflammatory asthma medications are available: inhaled corticosteroids, nedocromil sodium, and cromolyn sodium. In separate controlled studies of nongravid subjects, use of inhaled corticosteroids or cromolyn sodium led to improvement in asthma symptoms, pulmonary function, nonspecific bronchial hyperactivity, emergency room relapses, and hospitalizations.

Typical dosages of commonly used asthma medications are listed in Table 36-4.

### INHALED CORTICOSTEROIDS

Airway inflammation is present in nearly all cases; therefore, inhaled corticosteroids have even been ad-

**Table 36–4** Typical Dosages of Common Asthma Medications

| | |
|---|---|
| Cromolyn sodium | 2 Inhalations qid |
| Beclomethasone | 2–5 Inhalations bid–qid |
| Theophylline | Maintain serum levels of 8–12 µg/ml. Decrease dosage by half if treated with erythromicin or cimetidine |
| Triamcinolone | 2 Inhalations tid–qid |
| Prednisone | 1 Wk 40 mg/d burst for active symptoms followed by 1-wk taper |
| Albuterol | 2 Inhalations q3–4hr |

vocated as first-line therapy for patients who have mild asthma. The use of inhaled corticosteroids among nonpregnant asthmatic women has been associated with a marked reduction in fatal and near-fatal asthma. In addition to their anti-inflammatory effect, corticosteroids increase the effectiveness of β-adrenergic drugs by inducing formation of new β-receptors.

Corticosteroids are the most potent anti-inflammatory agents available for the treatment of asthma. Inhaled corticosteroids produce clinically important improvements in bronchial hyper-responsiveness that appears dose related, can occur as early as a few weeks after start of treatment but take months to attain maximal effect, and includes prevention of increased bronchial hyper-responsiveness after seasonal exposure to allergens. Continued administration is also effective in reducing the immediate pulmonary response to an allergen challenge. Inhaled corticosteroids are also more effective than β-agonists, theophylline, nedocromil sodium, and cromolyn sodium in reducing airway hyper-responsiveness during maintenance treatment.

Several studies have focused on hypothalamic-pituitary-adrenal axis suppression. These studies show that the 24-hour excretion of free cortisol, 17-hydroxyglucocorticoids, baseline serum cortisol, and responses to ACTH (adrenocorticotropic hormone) and metyrapone administration are not different from those of control patients after long-term maintenance therapy with inhaled corticosteroids given in doses up to 800 µg/day. Although inhaled corticosteroids generally have been thought to be free of systemic effects, data from nonpregnant patients have suggested that systemic effects, including adrenal suppression, can be detected at commonly used dosages. Tabachnik and Zadik studied 10 children (10 to 14 years old) who had chronic asthma and who received beclomethasone dipropionate as a dose of 200 µg by aerosol twice daily (400 µg/day) for 3 months. There was a marked reduction in spontaneous diurnal cortisol secretion as measured by the 24-hour urinary excretion of cortisol and a decrease in the diurnal variation of cortisol after 3 months of beclomethasone therapy. The peak cortisol level in response to corticotropin administration, however, was normal.

Inhaled corticosteroids may have untoward effects in addition to hypothalamic-pituitary-adrenal axis suppression. Several studies have examined the effects of inhaled corticosteroids on bone metabolism. Abnormally low total body calcium levels, decline in hydroxyproline, creatinine ratios, decreased alkaline phosphatase, depressed osteocalcin levels, and decreased bone density have all been documented when inhaled corticosteroids were used. These changes are significantly less than those seen with systemic corticosteroids. The potential effects of corticosteroids on fetal bone development are unknown. There is concern that inhaled corticosteroids impair growth in children as measured by height or lower leg growth using a knenometer. Inhaled corticosteroids can cause thrush and hoarseness, problems that may be mitigated by the use of metered-dose inhalers with spacers.

Only about 10 to 20% of the inhaled dose of corticosteroid reaches the lungs; approximately 50% is deposited in the oropharynx. The use of spacers can increase delivery to the lungs and mouth rinsing after inhalation decreases oral absorption. Systemic bioavailability is affected by the first-pass metabolism of the drug; fluticasone propionate has a 99% hepatic first-pass metabolism compared with 89% for budesonide and approximately 70% for beclomethasone.

Given a general fear of any drug used during pregnancy, with specific concerns that side effects and adverse perinatal outcomes may result from any type of steroid, clinicians have been reluctant to prescribe inhaled corticosteroids to pregnant women. As a result, inhaled corticosteroids have been underused during pregnancy.

## Beclomethasone Dipropionate

The most commonly used inhaled corticosteroid in pregnancy is beclomethasone. The NAEP working group recommended the use of beclomethasone during pregnancy because more clinical studies have been conducted with this drug than with any other corticosteroids. Greenberger and Patterson reported the use of beclomethasone during 45 pregnancies among 40 women; there was a single cardiac malformation in a neonate of a woman who had diabetes and schizophrenia. Fitzsimons and associates reported the outcomes for 56 pregnancies among 51 women; there were no anomalies in this group. Neither of the two previous studies had a control group. In a case analysis of 12,301 nonpregnant asthmatics, Ernst and associates reported that use of beclomethasone for at least 1 year resulted in a significantly lower risk of fatal and near-fatal asthma compared with regimens that did not include inhaled corticosteroids. Wendel and associates in a study of 84 pregnant women, randomized subjects to receive either an oral corticosteroid taper or an oral corticosteroid taper plus inhaled beclomethasone. The cohort receiving inhaled beclomethasone had a reduced readmission rate, 33% vs. 12%, $P < .05$.

There are no prospective, randomized studies of beclomethasone therapy during human pregnancy. Tinkelman and associates conducted a randomized, prospective, double-blind study of inhaled beclomethasone (n = 102) vs. theophylline (n = 93) among children aged 6 to 17 years. They found that patients receiving beclomethasone used bronchodilators and systemic corticosteroids, significantly less than those treated with theophylline. There was a trend for decreased emergency visits among children treated with beclomethasone, but there were no significant differences in the number of physician visits, emergency room visits, or hospitalizations for asthma exacerbations among the two groups. Surprisingly, a significantly increased proportion of subjects withdrew from the study for a perceived lack of benefit among the group treated with beclomethasone (7.8%) compared with theophylline (1.1%). Of concern was the finding that growth velocity was significantly suppressed in the group treated with beclomethasone. It should be noted, however, that inhalation spacers were not used in this study population, and spacers may decrease systemic absorption of inhaled corticosteroids. The National Institute of Child Health and Human Development (NICHD) and the National Heart, Lung, and Blood Institute (NHLBI) are presently conducting a randomized, blinded, placebo-controlled trial comparing theophylline with inhaled beclomethasone. The primary outcome of this trial is frequency of maternal asthma exacerbations with secondary outcomes, including birth weight and spirometry measures.

Beclomethasone is identical to betamethasone except that the former drug has a chlorine at the 9-α position instead of a fluorine. This difference is significant because betamethasone is known to cross the placenta and enter fetal blood. The typical recommended starting dose of inhaled beclomethasone for adults is two inhalations, three or four times per day, or four inhalations twice a day; each inhalation delivers approximately 42 μg. High-dose beclomethasone is typically considered to be dosages of 1000 μg/day.

## Triamcinolone Acetonide

Data on inhaled triamcinolone use during pregnancy are limited to a single report of pregnancy outcomes for 15 women who were treated with inhaled triamcinolone, 14 treated with inhaled beclomethasone, and 25 who received oral theophylline therapy. There was a significantly lower incidence of hospital admissions for asthma exacerbations among gravidas receiving inhaled triamcinolone (n = 5, 33%) compared with those treated with inhaled beclomethasone cohort (n = 11, 79%; $P < .05$); but not compared with the theophylline cohort (n = 7, 28%; $P = NS$). The mean triamcinolone group birth weight was 502 g more than that of the beclomethasone group, and 316 g more than that of the theophylline group; however, these differences were not statistically significant. Several patients in the triamcinolone and beclomethasone groups also received theophylline, oral corticosteroids, or both. It is also possible that the three groups in this study had different levels of asthma severity. Therefore, the finding of a lower hospitalization rate and the trend for larger birth weights among the group treated with inhaled triamcinolone may be due to confounding factors.

Triamcinolone has been shown to have minimal systemic absorption after oral administration via metered-dose inhalers with spacers. Limited systemic absorption during pregnancy may have a positive impact on clinical efficacy and birth weight. Additional studies are needed to evaluate further the safety and efficacy of inhaled triamcinolone during pregnancy.

## Fluticasone Propionate and Flunisolide

Fluticasone propionate is a synthetic trifluorinated glucocorticoid inhalation aerosol that was recently approved for the treatment of asthma. Both fluticasone propionate and flunisolide (the fourth approved inhaled corticosteroid) are potent anti-inflammatory corticosteroids. There are no published studies of their use during human pregnancy.

## Cromolyn Sodium and Nedocromil Sodium

Given the potential for systemic effects of inhaled corticosteroids, even at low doses, it is important to identify nonsteroidal anti-inflammatory medications. At the present time, cromolyn sodium and nedocromil sodium are the only approved medications that fit into this category. Nedocromil sodium, a pyranoquinalone, exerts a number of anti-inflammatory effects in vivo and in vitro. Cromolyn sodium, which is virtually devoid of significant side effects, blocks both early and late phase pulmonary response to allergen challenge and prevents the development of airway hyper-responsiveness. Although the precise mechanism of action is unknown, cromolyn sodium may stabilize mast cells and have some suppressive effects on other inflammatory cells. Cromolyn sodium does not have any intrinsic bronchodilator or antihistaminic activity, making it the preferred anti-inflammatory agent in children because of its efficacy and long safety record. However, its role in adult asthma is limited because it is not as effective as inhaled corticosteroids. Compared with inhaled corticosteroids, the time to maximal clinical benefit is longer for cromolyn sodium, 4 weeks compared with 2 weeks. Nedocromil sodium and cromolyn sodium appear to be less effective than inhaled corticosteroids in reducing objective and subjective manifestations of asthma. There are no published reports of nedocromil sodium use during pregnancy.

## BRONCHODILATORS

In some respects, these medications are now viewed as supplementary to nonbronchodilator, antiasthma medications. An increased frequency of bronchodilator use could be an indicator of the need for additional anti-inflammatory therapy.

### Theophylline

Theophylline has been the most widely prescribed drug in pregnant women with asthma. It has been used for more than 50 years, and no increased risk of developmental problems has been identified. The NAEP Working Group on Asthma and Pregnancy recommended that theophylline should be considered a second-line drug for supplementing inhaled corticosteroids when control is not achieved. There have been concerns about clinical efficacy and adverse effects. High doses have been observed to cause jitteriness, tachycardia, and vomiting in mothers and neonates. Life-threatening complications, including seizures and cardiac arrhythmias, have been associated with severe toxicity (serum concentrations >30 μg/ml). New dosing guidelines have recommended that serum concentrations be maintained at 8 to 12 μg/ml during pregnancy. The recognized narrow window between efficacy and toxicity requires obtaining serum drug levels. Subjective symptoms of adverse theophylline effects, including insomnia, heartburn, palpitations, and nausea, may be difficult to differentiate from typical pregnancy symptoms. Theophylline can have significant interactions with other drugs, causing decreased clearance and resultant toxicity. Two commonly used drugs are cimetidine, which can cause a 70% increase, and erythromicin, which causes a 35% increase in theophylline serum levels.

Although theophylline is a weak bronchodilator compared with β-agonists, its main advantage is the long duration of action, 10 to 12 hours with the use of sustained-release preparations; this characteristic is especially useful in the management of nocturnal asthma. In its sustained-release form, it may be taken once or twice a day. Theophylline inhibits mast cell release of histamine, increases ciliary mucus clearance, and decreases respiratory muscle fatigue. Theophylline has moderate bronchoprotective effects in regard to exercise and histamine challenge and also attenuates the early and late phase pulmonary response to an allergen challenge. This may be related to potential anti-inflammatory properties, because it decreases microvascular leakage and macrophage activity. Theophylline does not protect against the increase in nonspecific bronchial hyperactivity after antigen challenge and, in long-term treatment, reduced bronchial hypcractivity only slightly.

Compared with inhaled corticosteroids, theophylline appears to be approximately equally effective in the control of asthma symptoms among nonpregnant subjects but has more toxicity. Theophylline therapy may be associated with less risk of prematurity, preeclampsia, and low birth weight. The primary use of theophylline should be as an additional therapy when β-agonists and inhaled anti-inflammatory agents do not control symptoms adequately. A study of nonpregnant subjects who had moderate asthma found that low-dose theophylline with a low-dose inhaled corticosteroid resulted in better control of bronchial hyper-responsiveness than high-dose inhaled corticosteroid therapy.

Theophylline is indicated only for chronic therapy and was ineffective for the treatment of acute exacerbations during pregnancy in a randomized, controlled study. The addition of intravenous aminophylline to a regimen including intravenous methylprednisolone did not shorten hospitalization duration compared with a cohort receiving only intravenous methylprednisolone.

### Inhaled β-Agonists

β-Agonists are currently recommended for use with all degrees of asthma during pregnancy. This group of medications has evolved from those that are relatively short acting (epinephrine, isoproterenol) to those of longer duration of action (albuterol, terbutaline, pirbuterol), but still lasting only 4 to 6 hours. Their greatest advantage is a rapid onset of effect in the relief of acute bronchospasm via smooth muscle relaxation. These medications are the treatment of choice for acute exacerbations of asthma and are indicated for the treatment of episodic bronchoconstriction. They are also excellent bronchoprotective agents for pretreatment before exercise, perhaps related to their effect of blocking release of mediators from mast cells. Before allergen exposure, they effectively block

the pulmonary response but are of insufficient duration of action to prevent the late-phase pulmonary response unless administered in high doses. They do not block the development of airway hyper-responsiveness.

Although β₂-agonists are associated with tremor, tachycardia, and palpitations, recent studies have found more serious complications, including an association with an increased risk of death with chronic use. As-needed use may be better than chronic use. Sears and associates performed a double-blind, placebo-controlled, randomized crossover trial involving 89 adult asthmatic patients excluding pregnant women. Their patients had better control when the bronchodilators were used on an as-needed basis rather than with regular bronchodilator therapy. Of great concern is the apparent failure of chronic β₂-agonist therapy to reduce airway hyper-responsiveness. Indeed, when an inhaled glucocorticoid, budesonide was compared with the inhaled β₂-agonist terbutaline, it was unclear whether routine use of the terbutaline could result in increased airway hyper-responsiveness.

### Emerging Therapies

Leukotrienes are arachidonic acid metabolites that have been implicated in transducing bronchospasm, mucus secretion, and increased vascular permeability. Bronchoconstriction associated with aspirin ingestion can be blocked by leukotriene receptor antagonists. Treatment with leukotriene-receptor antagonist has been shown to significantly improve pulmonary function as measured by $FEV_1$ (Knorr 1998). A leukotriene-receptor antagonist (zafirlukast) and a 5-lipoxygenase inhibitor (zileuton) were recently approved by the Food and Drug Administration. There are no data regarding the efficacy or safety of these agents during human pregnancy.

### STEP THERAPY

Specific therapies should be tailored to meet the needs and circumstances of the patient. Step-care therapeutic approach includes increasing the number and frequency of medications with increasing asthma severity (Table 36–5). The least number of medications needed to control asthma symptoms should be used. Oral corticosteroids should be considered for most patients with severe asthma. A burst of oral corticosteroids is indicated for exacerbations not responding to initial β-agonist therapy regardless of asthma severity. Additionally, patients who require increasing inhaled β₂-agonist therapy (more than 12 puffs per day) to control their symptoms may benefit

**Table 36–5** Step Therapy: Medical Management of Asthma

MILD
Inhaled β₂-agonist as needed*

MODERATE
Inhaled β₂-agonist as needed*
Inhaled corticosteroids (or cromolyn)
Theophylline for nocturnal asthma or increased symptoms

SEVERE
Inhaled β₂-agonist as needed*
Inhaled corticosteroids (or cromolyn)
Theophylline for nocturnal asthma or increased symptoms
Oral systemic corticosteroids

*Peak expiratory flow rate (PEFR) or forced expiratory volume in first second ($FEV_1$) <80%, asthma exacerbations, or exposure to exercise or allergens (oral corticosteroid burst if inadequate response to β₂-agonist regardless of asthma severity)

from oral corticosteroids. In such cases, a short course of oral prednisone, 40 to 60 mg/day for 1 week, followed by 7 to 14 days of tapering, may be effective.

## Antenatal Management

The obstetric management of asthma is complicated because maternal exacerbations can cause serious fetal sequelae, and asthma medications may have untoward fetal and maternal effects. Patients with mild, well-controlled asthma may not have increased risks of adverse pregnancy outcomes; however, those with moderate and severe asthma should be considered to have high-risk pregnancies. Coexistent medical complications increase the risk of pregnancy complications for patients with asthma. Adverse outcomes can be increased by underestimation of asthma severity and undertreatment of asthma exacerbations. A perinatologist should be consulted for a pregnant patient with uncontrolled asthma or other pregnancy complications.

In addition to routine obstetric and medical histories, the first prenatal visit also should include a detailed medical history with attention to medical conditions that could complicate the management of asthma. These include diabetes mellitus, hypertension, cardiac disease, adrenal disease, hyperthyroidism, human immunodeficiency virus, hemoglobinopathies, hepatic disease, and active pulmonary disease (cystic fibrosis, bronchiectasis, tuberculosis, sarcoidosis, recurrent sinopulmonary infections, bronchitis). The patient should be questioned about the presence and severity of symptoms, episodes of nocturnal asthma, the number of days of work missed because of asthma exacerbations, history of acute asthma emergency care visits, and smoking history. The type and amount of asthma medications, including the number of puffs of $\beta_2$-agonists used each day, should be recorded. Asthma severity should be determined (see Table 36-2).

Pregnant women who have mild, well-controlled asthma may receive routine prenatal care. Moderate and severe asthmatic patients should have prenatal visits based on clinical judgment. Most need prenatal visits at least every 2 weeks, then weekly at 36 weeks of gestation. In addition to routine care, each antenatal visit should include an evaluation of asthma severity and symptom frequency, including presence of nocturnal asthma; $FEV_1$ or PEFR; medications (assess compliance and dosage); and emergency visits and hospital admissions for asthma exacerbations.

Patients should be instructed on proper dosing and administration of their asthma medications. Specific therapies should be tailored to meet individual needs and circumstances Step-care therapeutic approach includes increasing the number and frequency of medications with increasing asthma severity (see Table 36-5). The least number of medications needed to control asthma symptoms should be used.

Patients should be instructed on proper peak flow meter technique; PEFR should be determined with peak flow meters before medications are taken in the morning and after dinner. At each of these times, the patient should make the measurement while standing, take a maximum inspiration, and note the reading on the instrument. Personal best PEFR should be determined and personalized green, yellow, and red zones should be established and explained (Table 36-6). Those who have moderate to severe asthma should be instructed to maintain an asthma diary containing daily assessment of asthma symptoms, including morning and evening peak flow measurements, symptoms and activity limitations, indication of any medical contacts initiated, and a record of regular and as needed medications taken.

As previously discussed, avoidance and control of asthma triggers (see Table 36-3) are particularly important in pregnancy because pharmacologic control of asthma potentially has adverse fetal effects. Specific recommendations should be made for appropriate environmental control subjects based on the patient's history of exposure and, when available, demonstrated skin test reactivity.

**Table 36-6** Individualized PEFR Zones

Establish personal best PEFR, then calculate:

1. Green zone >80% of personal best PEFR
2. Yellow zone 50–80% of personal best PEFR
3. Red zone <50% of personal best PEFR

(Typical PEFR = 380–550 L/min)

PEFR = peak expiratory flow rate.

Moderate and severe asthmatic patients require additional fetal surveillance by ultrasonographic examinations and antenatal fetal testing. Because asthma has been associated with intrauterine growth retardation and preterm birth, it is critical to establish pregnancy dating accurately. Ultrasonography can be invaluable for accurate pregnancy dating, and ultrasonograms performed early in gestation have greater precision. For this reason, first-trimester ultrasonogram may be optimal for patients with moderate and severe asthma. Ultrasonographic examinations also are needed to evaluate fetal viability, anatomy, amniotic fluid volume, placental location, and interval fetal growth. Repeat ultrasound examinations are recommended for patients with suboptimally controlled asthma and after asthma exacerbations to evaluate fetal activity, growth, and amniotic fluid volume.

The intensity of antenatal fetal surveillance should be based on the severity of the asthma. All patients should be instructed to be attentive to fetal activity and keep a record of fetal kick counts. In most cases, moderate and severe asthmatics should have fetal testing starting at 28 to 32 weeks of gestation at weekly or twice weekly intervals. Most commonly, antenatal testing primarily consists of nonstress testing but may also include biophysical profile testing, contraction stress testing, and Doppler studies of the umbilical arteries or other vessels.

Patients who have asthma, especially if they are receiving systemic corticosteroids, may have an increased risk for developing preeclampsia. Use of systemic corticosteroids may be associated with excessive weight gain and the development of gestational diabetes mellitus. Inhaled coticosteroids can cause thrush and hoarseness. Theophylline may cause nervousness, tremor, heartburn, palpitations, and nausea, side effects that may be difficult to differentiate from normal pregnancy symptoms.

## HOME MANAGEMENT OF ASTHMA EXACERBATIONS

An asthma exacerbation that causes no problems for the mother may have severe sequelae for the fetus. Indeed, abnormal fetal heart rate tracing may be the initial manifestation of an asthmatic exacerbation. A maternal $PO_2$ <60 mm Hg or hemoglobin saturation <90% may be associated with profound fetal hypoxia. Therefore, asthma exacerbations in pregnancy must be aggressively managed. An approach to administering rescue medications has been recommended by the NAEP working group. Patients should be given an individualized guide for decision making and rescue management. Albuterol should be used for the management of increasing symptoms or a decrease in PEFR that requires treatment.

Patients should be educated to recognize signs and symptoms of early asthma exacerbations, such as coughing, chest tightness, dyspnea, or wheezing, as well as a 20% decrease in their PEFR. This is important so that prompt home rescue treatment may be instituted to avoid maternal and fetal hypoxia. In general, patients should use inhaled albuterol, 2 to 4 puffs every 20 minutes for up to 1 hour. A good response is considered if symptoms (wheezing, chest tightness, cough, or breathlessness) are gone or become subjectively mild, normal activities can be resumed, and the PEFR is >70% of personal best. The patient should seek further medical attention if the response is incomplete or fetal activity is decreased (Table 36–7).

## HOSPITAL AND CLINIC MANAGEMENT

The principal goal should be the prevention of hypoxia. Continuous electronic fetal monitoring should be initiated if gestation has advanced to the point of potential fetal viability. In cases of severe exacerbations or incomplete response to therapy, a perinatal consultation should be obtained. The patient should be assessed for general level of activity, color, pulse rate, use of accessory muscles, and airflow obstruction determined by auscultation and $FEV_1$, PEFR, or both before and after each bronchodilator treatment. Measurement of oxygenation via pulse oximeter or arterial blood gases is essential. Arterial blood gases should be obtained if oxygen saturation remains <95%; chest radiograph studies are not commonly needed. It should be emphasized that treatment must be individualized based on the severity of symptoms, past asthma history, medications, patient reliability, and gestational age. Albuterol can be delivered by nebulizer (2.5 mg = 0.5 ml albuterol in 2.5 ml normal saline) driven with oxygen, and treatments should be given every 20 minutes. Occasionally, nebulized treatment is not effective because the patient is moving air poorly; in such cases, terbutaline, 0.25 mg, can be administered subcutaneously every 15 minutes for three doses. Terbutaline is preferred to epinephrine because of its more specific $\beta_2$ agonist effect. Guidelines for the management of asthma exacerbations are presented in Table 36–8.

**Table 36–7** Home Management of Acute Asthma Exacerbations

Use inhaled albuterol 2–4 puffs and check PEFR in 20 min

If PEFR <50% predicted or symptoms are severe, obtain emergency care

If PEFR is 50–70% predicted:
　Repeat albuterol treatment, check PEFR in 20 min if PEFR 50–70% predicted:
　　Contact caregiver or go for emergency care

If PEFR >70% predicted:
　Continue inhaled albuterol
　(2–4 puffs q3–4hr for 6–12 hr prn)

If decreased fetal movement:
　Contact caregiver or go for emergency care

PEFR = peak expiratory flow rate.

**Table 36–8** Emergency Assessment and Management of Asthma Exacerbations

INITIAL EVALUATION:
History, examination, PEFR, oximetry
Fetal monitoring if potentially viable

INITIAL TREATMENT
Inhaled $\beta_2$-agonist × 3 doses over 60–90 min
$O_2$ to maintain saturation ≥95%
If no wheezing and PEFR or $FEV_1$ >70% baseline, discharge with follow-up

IF OXIMETRY <90%, $FEV_1$ <1.0 L, or PEFR <100 L/min ON PRESENTATION:
Continue nebulized albuterol
Start intravenous corticosteroids
Consider intravenous aminophylline
Obtain arterial blood gases
Admit to intensive care unit
Consider intubation

IF PEFR OR $FEV_1$ >40% BUT <70% BASELINE AFTER $\beta_2$-AGONIST:
Obtain arterial blood gases
Continue inhaled $\beta_2$-agonist every 1–4 hr
Start intravenous corticosteroids in most cases
Consider intravenous aminophylline
Admit most cases to hospital

$FEV_1$ = forced expiratory volume in the first second; PEFR = peak expiratory flow rate.

## Labor and Delivery Management

Asthma medications should not be discontinued during labor and delivery. Although asthma is usually quiescent during labor, consideration should be given to assessing PEFRs when the patient is admitted and at 12-hour intervals. The patient should be kept hydrated and should receive adequate analgesia to decrease the risk of bronchospasm. If systemic corticosteroids have been used in the previous 4 weeks, hydrocortisone (100 mg every 8 hours, intravenously) should be administered during labor and for the 24-hour period after delivery to prevent adrenal crisis.

Patients who have well-controlled mild asthma at term do not need intensive fetal monitoring during labor. Other patients should have continuous electronic fetal monitoring at presumed fetal viability. With few exceptions, delivery should follow spontaneous labor, or induction of labor should be for obstetric indications. It is rarely necessary to deliver a fetus via cesarean section for an acute asthma exacerbation. Usually, maternal and fetal distress can be managed by aggressive medical management. Occasionally, delivery may improve the respiratory status of a patient who has unstable asthma and who fetus is mature.

Cervical ripening can be accomplished with either laminaria tents or prostaglandin PGE$_2$ gel. Oxytocin is indicated for labor induction or augmentation. Either oxytocin or PGE$_2$ is indicated for the management of spontaneous or induced abortions or for postpartum hemorrhage; 15-methyl PGF$_2\alpha$ and methylergonovine can cause bronchospasm. If the patient is receiving a systemic β-mimetic drug for asthma control, a non-β-mimetic tocolytic should be used. Magnesium sulfate, which is a bronchodilator, is a safe choice for treating preterm labor or preeclampsia. Indomethacin, a potent tocolytic, can induce bronchospasm in the aspirin-sensitive patient. There are no reports of the use of calcium channel blockers for tocolysis among patients with asthma.

Lumbar anesthesia can reduce oxygen consumption and minute ventilation during labor. Fentanyl may be a better analgesic than meperidine, which causes histamine release. However, meperidine is rarely associated with the onset of bronchospasm during labor. Regional anesthesia is appropriate for nonemergent cesarean delivery, although a 2% incidence of bronchospasm has been reported. Ketamine is useful for induction of general anesthesia because it can prevent bronchospasm.

Communication among obstetric, anesthetic, and pediatric caregivers is important for optimal care. An analysis of maternal and fetal status and potential complications caused by either asthma per se or asthma pharmacologic therapy should be communicated.

## Breast Feeding

In general, only small amounts of asthma medications enter breast milk. The use of prednisone, theophylline, antihistamines, beclomethasone, β-agonists, or cromolyn is not considered a contraindication for breast feeding. However, among sensitive individuals, theophylline may cause toxic effects in the neonate, including vomiting, feeding difficulties, jitteriness, and cardiac arrhythmias.

### REFERENCES

American Academy of Pediatrics Committee on Drugs: Transfer of drugs and other chemicals into human milk. Pediatrics 84:924–936, 1989.

Arwood LL, Dasta JF, Friedman C: Placental transfer of theophylline: Two case reports. Pediatrics 63:844–846, 1979.

Bailey K, Herrod H, Younger R, et al: Functional aspects of T-lymphocyte subsets in pregnancy. Obstet Gynecol 66:211–215, 1985.

Briggs GG, Freeman RK, Yaffe SJ: In Drugs in Pregnancy and Lactation, 3rd ed. Baltimore, Williams & Wilkins, 1990, pp 237–238, 520–521.

Brogden RN, Sorkin EM: Nedocromil sodium: An updated review of its pharmacological properties and therapeutic efficacy in asthma. Drugs 45:693–715, 1993.

Cockcroft DW, Murdock KY: Comparative effects of inhaled salbutamol, sodium cromoglycate, and beclomethasone dipropionate on allergen-induced early asthmatic responses, last asthmatic responses, and increased bronchial responsiveness to histamine. J Allergy Clin Immunol 79:734–740, 1987.

Dombrowski MP, Bottoms SF, Boike GM, et al: Incidence of preeclampsia among asthmatic patients lower with theophylline. Am J Obstet Gynecol 155:265–267, 1986.

Dombrowski MP, Brown CL, Berry SM: Preliminary experience with triamcinolone acetonide during pregnancy. J Matern Fetal Med 5:310–313, 1996.

Doull IJM, Freezer JN, Holgate ST: Growth of prepubertal children with mild asthma treated with inhaled beclomethasone dipropionate. Am J Respir Crit Care Med 151:1715–1719, 1995.

Dutoit JI, Salome CM, Woolcock AJ: Inhaled corticosteroids reduce the severity of bronchial hyperresponsiveness in asthma but oral theophylline does not. Am Rev Respir Dis 136:1174–1178, 1987.

Ernst P, Spetzer WO, Suissa S, et al: Risk of fatal and near-fatal asthma in relation to inhaled coriticosteroid use. JAMA 268:3462–3464, 1992.

Evans DJ, Taylor DA, Zetterstrom O, Chung KF, et al: A comparison of low-dose inhaled budesonide plus theophylline and high-dose inhaled budesonide for moderate asthma. N Engl J Med 337:1412–1428, 1997.

Fanta CH, Rossing TH, McFadden ER: Treatment of acute asthma: Is combination therapy with sympathomimetics and methylxanthines indicated? Am J Med 80:5–10, 1986.

Fitzsimons R, Greenberger PA, Patterson R: Outcome of pregnancy in women requiring corticosteroids for severe asthma. J Allergy Clin Immunol 78:349–353, 1986.

Fung DL: Emergency anesthesia for asthma patients. Clin Rev Allergy 3:127–141, 1985.

Geddes DM: Inhaled corticosteroids: Benefits and risks. Thorax 47:404–407, 1992.

Greenberger PA, Patterson R: Beclomethasone dipropionate for severe asthma during pregnancy. Ann Intern Med 98:478–480, 1983.

Greenberger PA, Patterson R: The outcome of pregnancy complicated by severe asthma. Allergy Proc 9:539–543, 1988.

Groot CAR, Lammers J-WJ, Molema J, et al: Effect of inhaled beclomethasone and nedocromil sodium on bronchial hyperresponsiveness to histamine and distilled water. Eur Respir J 5:1075–1082, 1992.

Haahtela T, Jarvinen M, Kava T, et al: Comparison of β$_2$-agonist, terbutalline, with an inhaled corticosteroid, budesonide, in newly detected asthma. N Engl J Med 325:338–392, 1991.

Hägerdal M, Morgan CW, Sumner AE, et al: Minute ventilation and oxygen consumption during labor with epidural analgesia. Anesthesiology 59:425–427, 1983.

Hendeles L, Jenkins J, Temple R: Revised FDA labeling guideline for theophylline oral dosage forms. Pharmacotherapy 15:409–427, 1995.

Hirshman CA, Downes H, Farbood A, et al: Ketamine block of bronchospasm in experimental canine asthma. Br J Anaesth 51:713–718, 1979.

Joad JP, Ahrens RC, Lindgren SD, et al: Relative efficacy of maintenance therapy with theophylline, inhaled albuterol, and the combination for chronic asthma. J Allergy Clin Immunol 79:78–85, 1987.

Kerrebijn KF: Use of topical corticosteroids in the treatment of childhood asthma. Am Rev Respir Dis 141:S77–S81, 1990.

Knorr B, Matz J, Bernstein JA, et al: Montelukast for chronic asthma in 6 to 14 year old children. JAMA 279:1181–1186, 1998.

Kraan J, Koeter GH, Van Der Mark THW, et al: Dosage and time effects of inhaled budesonide on bronchial hyperactivity. Am Rev Respir Dis 137:44–48, 1988.

Lipworth BJ: Airway and systemic effects of inhaled corticosteroids in asthma: Dose response relationship. Pulm Pharmacol Ther 9:19–27, 1996.

Lowhagen O, Rak S: Modification of bronchial hyperreactivity after treatment with sodium cromoglycate during pollen season. J Allergy Clin Immunol 75:460–467, 1985.

Mabie WC, Barton JR, Wasserstrum N, et al: Clinical observations on asthma in pregnancy. J Matern Fetal Med 1:45–50, 1992.

National Asthma Education Program, Guidelines for the Diagnosis and Management of Asthma, Expert Panel Report, August 1991, NIH Publication No. 91-3042.

National Asthma Education Program, Management of Asthma During Pregnancy, Report of the Working Group on Asthma and Pregnancy, September 1993, NIH Publications No 93-3279.

Nelson HS, Spector SL, Whitsett TL, et al: The bronchodilator response to inhalation of increasing doses of aerosolized albuterol. J Allergy Clin Immunol 72:371–375, 1983.

Nolten W, Rueckert P: Elevated free cortisol index in pregnancy: possible regulatory mechanisms. Am J Obstet Gynecol 139:492–498, 1981.

Packe GE, Douglas JG, McDonald AF, et al: Bone density in asthmatic patients taking high dose inhaled beclomethasone dipropionate and intermittent systemic corticosteroids. Thorax 47:414–417, 1992.

Pauwels R, Van Renterghem D, Van Der Straeten M, et al: The effect of theophylline and enprofylline on allergen-induced bronchoconstriction. J Allergy Clin Immunol 76:583–590, 1985.

Perlow JH, Montgomery D, Morgan MA, et al: Severity of asthma and perinatal outcome. Am J Obstet Gynecol 167:963–967, 1992.

Pirson Y, Van Lierde M, Ghysen J, et al: Retardation of fetal growth in patients receiving immunosuppressive therapy [letter]. N Engl J Med 313:328, 1985.

Puolijoki H, Liippo K, Herrala J, et al: Inhaled beclomethasone decreases serum osteocalcin in postmenopausal asthmatic women. Bone 13:285–288, 1992.

Reid DM, Nicoll JJ, Smith MA, et al: Corticosteroids and bone mass in asthma: Comparisons with rheumatoid arthritis and polymyalgia rheumatica. BMJ 293:1463–1465, 1986.

Reinisch JM, Simon NG, Karow WG, et al: Prenatal exposure to prednisone in humans and animals retards intrauterine growth. Science 202:436–439, 1978.

Rossing TH, Fanta CH, McFadden ER: Medical House Staff of the Peter Bent Brigham Hospital: A controlled trial of the use of single versus combined drug therapy in the treatment of acute episodes of asthma. Am Rev Respir Dis 123:190–194, 1982.

Salmeron S, Guerin JC, Godard P, et al: High doses of inhaled corticosteroids in unstable chronic asthma: A multicenter, double-blind, placebo-controlled study. Am Rev Respir Dis 140:167–171, 1989.

Schatz M, Zeiger RS, Harden KM, et al: The safety of inhaled β-agonist bronchodilators during pregnancy. J Allergy Clin Immunol 82:686–695, 1988.

Schatz M, Zeiger RS, Hoffman CP: Intrauterine growth is related to gestational pulmonary function in pregnant asthmatic women. Kaiser-Permanente Asthma and Pregnancy Study Group. Chest 98:389–392, 1990.

Schatz M, Zeiger R, Hoffman C, et al: Perinatal outcomes in the pregnancies of asthmatic women: A prospective controlled analysis. Am J Respir Crti Care Med 151:1170–1174, 1995.

Sears MR, Taylor DR, Print CG, et al: Regular inhaled β-agonist treatment in bronchial asthma. Lancet 336:1391–1396, 1990.

Shapiro GG, Konig P: Cromolyn sodium: A review. Pharmacotherapy 5:156–170, 1985.

Spitzer WO, Suissa S, Ernst P, et al: The use of β-agonists and the risk of death and near death from asthma. N Engl J Med 326:501–506, 1992.

Stenius-Aarniala BS, Teramo PK: Asthma and pregnancy: A prospective study of 198 pregnancies. Thorax 43:12–18, 1988.

Svendsen UG, Frolund L, Madsen F, et al: A comparison of the effects of sodium cromoglycate and beclomethasone dipropionate on pulmonary function and bronchial hyperreactivity in subjects with asthma. J Allergy Clin Immunol 80:68–74, 1987.

Tabachnik E, Zadik Z: Clinical and laboratory observations: Diurnal cortisol secretion during therapy with inhaled beclomethasone dipropionate in children with asthma. J Pediatr 118:294–297, 1991.

Thomas BC, Stanhope R, Grant DB: Impaired growth in children with asthma during treatment with conventional doses of inhaled corticosteroids. Acta Paediatr 83:196–199; 1994.

Tinkelman DG, Reed CE, Nelson HS, et al: Aerosol beclomethasone dipropionate compared with theophylline as primary treatment of chronic, mild to moderately severe asthma in children. Pediatrics 92:64–77, 1993.

Twentyman OP, Finnerty JP, Holgate ST: The inhibitory effect of nebulized albuterol on the early and late asthmatic reactions and increase in airway responsiveness provoked by inhaled allergen in asthma. Am Rev Respir Dis 144:782–787, 1991.

Wendel PJ, Ramin SM, Barnett-Hamm C, et al: Asthma treatment in pregnancy: A randomized controlled study. Am J Obstet Gynecol 175:150–154; 1996.

Wenzel SE: New approaches to anti-inflammatory therapy for asthma. Am J Med 104:287–300, 1998.

Woolcock AJ, Yan K, Salome CM: Effects of therapy on bronchial hyper-responsiveness in the long-term management of asthma. Clin Allergy 18:165–176, 1988.

Woolcock AJ, Jenkins C: Corticosteroids in the modulation of bronchial hyperresponsiveness. Immunol Allergy Clin North Am 10:543–557, 1990.

Yeh TF, Pildes RS: Transplacental aminophylline toxicity in a neonate [letter]. Lancet 1(8017):910, 1977.

Zaborny, BA, Lukacsko P, Barinov-Colligaon I, Ziemniak JA: Inhaled corticosteroids in asthma: A dose-proportionality study with triamcinolone acetonide aerosol. J Clin Pharmacol 32:463–469, 1992.

# 37

# Hypertensive Disorders in Pregnancy

DOREL ABRAMOVICI
FARID MATTAR
BAHA M. SIBAI

Hypertensive disorders are common medical complications of pregnancy. High blood pressure complicates 5 to 10% of all pregnancies and is the second leading cause of maternal death in the United States and a leading cause of perinatal mortality and morbidity worldwide.

Hypertension is the hallmark for the diagnosis of these disorders. Although the clinical manifestations may be similar, the underlying etiologies may differ (chronic hypertension, renal disease, preeclampsia) (Table 37–1).

## Classification of Hypertensive Disorders

The terminology and definitions used to describe the hypertensive disorders of pregnancy have been confusing and inconsistent. The American College of Obstetricians and Gynecologists (ACOG) describes two distinct entities in the pregnant woman: chronic hypertension and pregnancy-induced hypertension (PIH). PIH is defined as a multiorgan disease process that may involve more than just elevated blood pressure. We believe the term PIH is vague and broad and can be confused with gestational hypertension. As such, the ACOG definition and classification scheme has pitfalls regarding clinical diagnosis and management.

In this chapter, hypertensive disorders are divided into three major categories: chronic hypertension, gestational hypertension, and preeclampsia. The subcategories of preeclampsia (eclampsia, HELLP [hemolysis, elevated liver enzymes, and low platelet count] syndrome, and superimposed preeclampsia) are also discussed.

## Chronic Hypertension

Chronic hypertension complicates 1 to 5% of pregnancies. Essential hypertension is by far the most common cause of chronic hypertension during pregnancy. This diagnosis can be reached only after excluding potentially correctable underlying causes, such as renovascular disease, coarctation of the aorta, pheochromocytoma, and Cushing's syndrome.

Table 37–1  Hypertensive Disorders of Pregnancy

| Clinical Findings | Chronic Hypertension | Gestational Hypertension* | Preeclampsia |
|---|---|---|---|
| Time of onset of hypertension | <20 wk of gestation | Usually in third trimester | ≥20 wk of gestation |
| Degree of hypertension | Mild or severe | Mild | Mild or severe |
| Proteinuria* | Absent | Absent | Usually present |
| Serum urate (>5.5 mg/dl) (0.33 mmol/L) | Rare | Absent | Present in almost all cases |
| Hemoconcentration | Absent | Absent | Present in severe disease |
| Thrombocytopenia | Absent | Absent | Present in severe disease |
| Hepatic dysfunction | Absent | Absent | Present in severe disease |

*Defined as ≥1+ by dipstick testing on two occasions or ≥300 mg in a 24-hour urine collection.
From Sibai BM: Treatment of hypertension in pregnant women. N Engl J Med 335:257–265, 1996.

## DIAGNOSIS AND CLASSIFICATION OF CHRONIC HYPERTENSION

The diagnosis of chronic hypertension during pregnancy is usually based on either a history of hypertension before pregnancy or a blood pressure of at least 140/90 mm Hg before 20 weeks of gestation. This diagnosis is made more difficult because during normal pregnancy, blood pressure decreases gradually to a nadir between 14 and 24 weeks of gestation, and then increases to prepregnancy values in the third trimester.

In pregnancy, chronic hypertension is classified into mild (systolic blood pressures between 140 and 159 mm Hg, diastolic blood pressures between 90 and 109 mm Hg or both) and severe (systolic blood pressures of at least 160 mm Hg, diastolic blood pressures of at least 110 mm Hg, or both).

## MATERNAL AND FETAL RISKS OF CHRONIC HYPERTENSION

Pregnancies complicated by chronic hypertension are associated with increased maternal and perinatal risks, such as superimposed preeclampsia (10 to 50%), abruptio placentae (0.5% to 10%), fetal growth restriction, and preterm birth. The frequency of these complications increases in women who have long-standing severe hypertension and in those who have pre-existing cardiovascular or renal disease.

## MANAGEMENT OF CHRONIC HYPERTENSION

Management depends on the severity of maternal disease. Patients are classified as having low-risk hypertension (essential hypertension without associated medical disorders or target organ involvement) or high-risk hypertension (patients who have severe hypertension and those who have target organ damage or associated medical disorders).

The majority of patients who have this disorder have low-risk chronic hypertension and thus have a favorable maternal and perinatal prognosis without the use of antihypertensive drugs. Our experience indicates that there is no benefit to be derived from the use of antihypertensive drugs in the management of these pregnancies. Antihypertensive drugs are discontinued (or not initiated) at the time of the first prenatal visit. In the low-risk group, only 15% of women subsequently require drug therapy because of exacerbated severe hypertension. Fetal testing should include weekly nonstress tests starting at 34 weeks of gestation and serial ultrasound examinations for fetal growth every 4 weeks starting at 28 weeks of gestation.

On the other hand, fetal and maternal morbidity are increased in pregnant women who have high-risk chronic hypertension. The use of antihypertensive drugs is continued or initiated in these women and in those whose diastolic blood pressure at time of first prenatal visit is at least 105 mm Hg. Additionally, these patients require more frequent antenatal visits and may need recurrent hospitalization for stabilization of blood pressure and treatment of associated medical disorders. Fetal evaluation includes a nonstress test, a biophysical profile twice weekly, or both (starting at 32 weeks of gestation), as well as serial ultrasonographic examinations for fetal growth every 4 weeks (beginning at 26 weeks of gestation). In both low- and high-risk chronic hypertensive patients who have normal fetal testing, pregnancy may continue until 41 weeks of gestation. Labor may be induced after 37 weeks of gestation if the cervix is favorable (Bishop's score ≥6).

The medications commonly used to control maternal blood pressure are described in Table 37–2.

# Gestational Hypertension

Gestational hypertension is the development of elevated blood pressure (without other symptoms of pre-

**Table 37-2** Antihypertensive Drugs in Pregnancy

### Common Drugs for Chronic Therapy of Hypertension

| Class | Drug | Starting Dose | Maximum Dose |
|---|---|---|---|
| Central $\alpha_2$-antagonist | Methyldopa | 250 mg tid | 4 g/d |
| Calcium channel blocker | Nifedipine | 10 mg qid | 120 mg/d |
| $\alpha/\beta$ blocker | Labetalol | 150 mg | 2400 mg/d |

### Common Drugs for Acute Therapy of Severe Hypertension

| Class | Drug | Dose |
|---|---|---|
| Arteriolar dilator | Hydralazine | 5–10 mg IV q 15–30 min |
| Calcium channel blocker | Nifedipine | 10–20 mg PO q 30 min |
| $\alpha/\beta$ blocker | Labetalol | 20–40–80 mg IV every 20 min (up to 300 mg) |
| Arterial/venous dilator | Nitroprusside | 0.2–0.5 µ/kg min |

*tid = three times daily; qid = four times daily; bid = two times daily; IV = intravenously; PO = orally.
From Witlin AG, Sibai BM: Hypertension in pregnancy: Current concepts of preeclampsia. Annu Rev Med 48:115–127, 1997.

---

eclampsia) after 20 weeks of gestation in a previously normotensive woman. Gestational hypertension may be an early manifestation of preeclampsia (20%) or unrecognized chronic hypertension. A diagnosis of gestational hypertension is made if blood pressure is elevated to 140/90 mm Hg on at least two separate occasions more than 4 hours apart. The diagnosis may be made antepartum, during labor, or postpartum, but most patients are diagnosed late in the third trimester. Usually, pregnancy outcome is favorable without drug therapy. In these patients, management includes outpatient follow-up with relative rest and twice weekly evaluation of blood pressure and urine protein levels in a physician's office. Clinical fetal evaluation and nonstress testing begin at the time of diagnosis and are performed at least once a week. Ultrasonography to evaluate fetal growth is performed every 3 to 4 weeks. Induction of labor is initiated at ≥38 weeks of gestation if the cervix is ripe (Bishop's score ≥ 6). Pregnancy can be continued until 41 weeks of gestation.

## Preeclampsia

Preeclampsia is defined as the occurrence of hypertension, edema, and proteinuria after 20 weeks of gestation in a previously normotensive woman. Hypertension is defined as a sustained blood pressure elevation to 140/90 mm Hg. The current ACOG technical bulletin disputes earlier reports that suggested the diagnosis of preeclampsia if there is an increase of 30 mm Hg systolic or 15 mm Hg diastolic from baseline second trimester values. Proteinuria is defined as a concentration of ≥.1 g/L in at least two random urine specimens (collected 6 hours or more apart) or ≥.3 g in 24-hour collection.

Preeclampsia is classified as mild or severe primarily on the basis of the degree of blood pressure elevation, degree of proteinuria, or involvement of other organ systems (Table 37–3).

Eclampsia is the occurrence of seizures or coma (not attributed to any other cause) in a woman who has preeclampsia.

## MILD PREECLAMPSIA

All patients who are diagnosed as having mild preeclampsia should be evaluated and observed closely for early detection of worsening of the disease process. All women are questioned about symptoms of headache, visual disturbances, and epigastric pain and are instructed to report any signs of labor, abdominal pain, or vaginal bleeding.

Laboratory tests (hematocrit, platelet count, and liver enzymes) are performed twice a week. This evaluation is important because the patient may develop thrombocytopenia and abnormal liver enzymes even with mild blood pressure levels. Fetal evaluation

**Table 37-3** Criteria for Severe Preeclampsia

Blood pressure >160 mm Hg systolic or >110 mm Hg diastolic
Acute onset renal failure
Oliguria <500 ml/24 hr
Grand mal seizures (eclampsia)
Pulmonary edema
HELLP syndrome (hemolysis, elevated liver enzymes, low platelets)
Thrombocytopenia (<100,000/µl)
Symptoms suggesting significant end-organ involvement: headache, visual disturbances, or epigastric or right-upper quadrant pain

Data from Witlin AG, Sibai BM: Hypertension in pregnancy: Current concepts of preeclampsia. Annu Rev Med 48:115–127, 1997.

should include serial ultrasonography for growth and amniotic fluid volume, daily fetal movement count (kick count), and nonstress testing (or biophysical profile) twice a week. The optimal management of mild preeclampsia remote from term is controversial, and either outpatient management or hospitalization is considered appropriate. Ideally, all patients are initially evaluated in the hospital. Candidates for outpatient management are those in whom good compliance is expected, symptoms of severe preeclampsia are absent, hypertension is mild, proteinuria is <1 g/24 hr, and fetal testing is reassuring.

Patients are instructed to follow a regular diet with no salt restriction and maintain relative bed rest. Diuretics, antihypertensive drugs, and sedatives are not used. These agents do not improve pregnancy outcome and may increase the incidence of fetal growth retardation. Any evidence of disease progression (symptoms or laboratory abnormalities) or acute severe hypertension is an indication for prompt hospitalization.

Conservative management is inappropriate if there are signs of progression to severe preeclampsia at ≥34 weeks of gestational age or if fetal monitoring test results are abnormal (Table 37–4). Because uteroplacental blood flow may be suboptimal in patients who have preeclampsia, conservative management of mild disease beyond term is not beneficial. Therefore, after 37 weeks of gestation, labor should be induced as soon as the cervix is favorable or at the completion of 40 weeks of gestation.

## SEVERE PREECLAMPSIA

The clinical course of severe preeclampsia may be characterized by progressive deterioration in both maternal and fetal conditions. Once the diagnosis of preeclampsia has been made, definitive therapy in the form of delivery is the desired goal, because it is the only cure for the disease.

**Table 37–4** Indications for Delivery in Mild Preeclampsia

Gestational age ≥40 wk
Gestational age ≥37 wk
    Bishop score ≥6
    Fetal weight ≤10th percentile
    Nonreactive nonstress test
Gestational age >34 weeks
    Labor
    Rupture of membranes
    Vaginal bleeding
    Persistent headaches or visual symptoms
    Epigastric pain, nausea, vomiting
Abnormal biophysical profile
Criteria for severe preeclampsia

The ultimate goals of therapy must always be safety of the mother first and then delivery of a live, mature newborn who will not require intensive and prolonged neonatal care.

The choice between expectant management and immediate delivery usually depends on one or more of the following factors:
1. Presence of labor
2. Fetal gestational age
3. Maternal condition
4. Fetal condition

Traditionally, preeclamptic women who meet established criteria for severe disease are delivered expeditiously. Although delivery is always appropriate therapy for the mother, it may not be appropriate for the fetus remote from term. There is universal agreement to deliver all patients who are at >34 weeks of gestation or if there is evidence of maternal or fetal distress before that time.

These patients receive magnesium sulfate ($MgSO_4$) intravenously to prevent convulsions and antihypertensive medications as needed to control maternal blood pressure within a safe range (diastolic <110 mmHg), followed by induction of labor. If delivery of a preterm infant (<35 weeks of gestation) is anticipated at a level I or II hospital, the mother should be transferred to a tertiary care center. The current conservative management protocol for patients who have severe preeclampsia was summarized by Sibai in 1991.

Conservative management should be considered only at a tertiary care center, where intensive maternal and neonatal care facilities are available (Fig. 37–1). The patient should be admitted to the labor and delivery area for close observation of the maternal and fetal conditions. Intravenous $MgSO_4$ should be administered and blood pressure controlled (diastolic blood pressure <110 mm Hg) with bolus injections of hydralazine (5 mg IV every 20 minutes up to cumulative total of 20 mg), intravenous (IV) labetalol (20 mg, up to cumulative total of 300 mg), or oral nifedipine (10 mg, up to cumulative total of 120 mg).

Women displaying persistent severe hypertension or other signs of maternal or fetal deterioration during the observational period are usually delivered within 24 hours, regardless of gestational age or fetal lung maturity. Some of these women have marked improvement in blood pressure and symptoms after hospitalization. If diastolic blood pressure remains <110 mm Hg after 24 hours of observation in labor and delivery, $MgSO_4$ should be discontinued and the patient followed closely in the hospital. Maternal and fetal status is then monitored daily. Maternal evaluation includes monitoring of blood pressure, uterine activity, abdominal pain, vaginal bleeding, and symptoms reflecting cerebral status. Laboratory evaluation includes daily platelet count and liver enzymes. Fetal

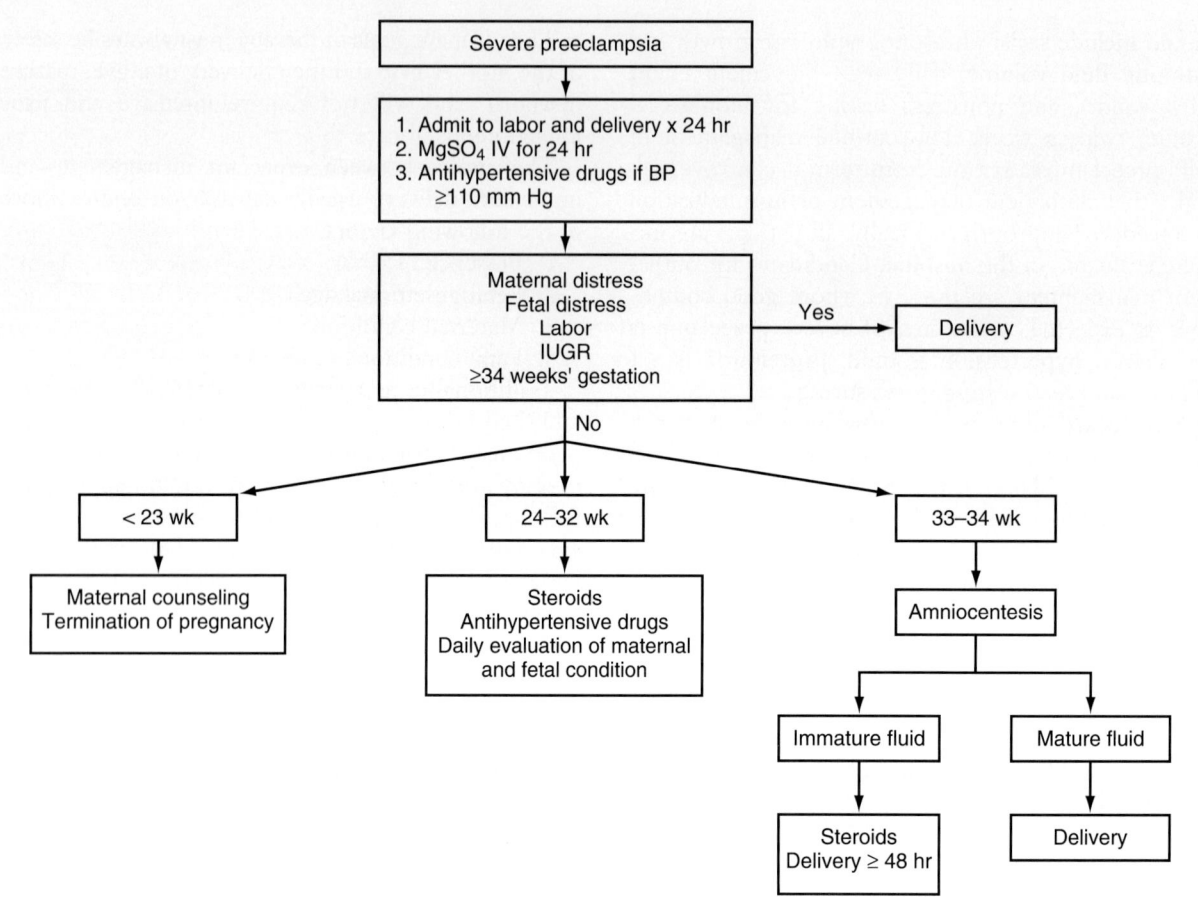

```
┌─────────────────────────┐
│   Severe preeclampsia   │
└───────────┬─────────────┘
            ▼
┌─────────────────────────────────┐
│ 1. Admit to labor and delivery  │
│    × 24 hr                      │
│ 2. MgSO₄ IV for 24 hr           │
│ 3. Antihypertensive drugs if BP │
│    ≥110 mm Hg                   │
└───────────┬─────────────────────┘
            ▼
┌─────────────────────────┐   Yes    ┌──────────┐
│   Maternal distress     │─────────▶│ Delivery │
│   Fetal distress        │          └──────────┘
│   Labor                 │
│   IUGR                  │
│   ≥34 weeks' gestation  │
└───────────┬─────────────┘
            │ No
   ┌────────┼────────┐
   ▼        ▼        ▼
 <23 wk  24–32 wk  33–34 wk
```

Figure 37–1  Management of severe preeclampsia. Conservative management should be performed only at a tertiary care center, where intensive maternal and neonatal care facilities are available. IUGR = intrauterine growth rate; MgSO₄ = magnesium sulfate.

well-being is monitored with nonstress tests, biophysical profile, and ultrasonographic assessment for fetal growth. All these patients receive steroids to accelerate fetal lung maturity.

Occasionally, a patient may develop severe preeclampsia at <28 weeks of gestation. These pregnancies are associated with high maternal and perinatal mortality and morbidity. If gestation is ≤22 weeks, we offer the patient the choice of pregnancy termination with prostaglandin $E_2$ ($PGE_2$) vaginal suppositories. These patients receive IV MgSO₄, and hypertension is controlled with either bolus injections of hydralazine or IV labetalol, as needed.

All other patients with gestation beyond 22 weeks are offered the option for conservative management. The pregnancy may then continue until either maternal or fetal jeopardy develops, or until the patient reaches 34 weeks of gestation, at which time labor is induced.

The diagnosis of superimposed preeclampsia is made if there is an exacerbation in hypertension accompanied by the acute onset of proteinuria (at least 1 g/24 hr). In cases of underlying renal disease, proteinuria and hyperuricemia may already be present, and the diagnosis should be based on signs of severe preeclampsia such as thrombocytopenia, or symptoms such as headache, visual disturbances, or epigastric pain. Patients who have superimposed preeclampsia are treated the same as patients who have preeclampsia.

## HELLP SYNDROME

The most frequently encountered disorder of microangiopathic destruction of red blood cells and platelets during pregnancy is a variant of severe preeclampsia known as HELLP syndrome. The term *HELLP syndrome* was first coined by Weinstein in 1982 and is an acronym for hemolysis (H), elevated liver enzymes (EL), and low platelets (LP). The reported incidence of this syndrome ranges from 2 to 12%, but its presence is associated with high maternal and perinatal mortality and morbidity. Our criteria for the diagnosis of HELLP syndrome are summarized in Table 37–5.

The typical patient who has HELLP syndrome is Caucasian, multiparous, and ≥25 years of age; she

**Table 37–5** Criteria for HELLP Syndrome

HEMOLYSIS
  Abnormal peripheral smear
  Total bilirubin >1.2 mg/dl
  Lactic dehydrogenase (LDH) >600 U/L

ELEVATED LIVER FUNCTIONS
  Serum aspartate aminotransferase (AST) >70 U/L
  Lactic dehydrogenase (LDH) >600 U/L

LOW PLATELETS
  Platelet count <100,000/mm³

HELLP = hemolysis, elevated liver enzymes, low platelets.
Courtesy of University of Tennessee, Memphis.

---

usually develops the disorder remote from term. The majority (80%) manifest this disorder at <36 weeks of gestation.

Patients who have HELLP syndrome may have various signs and symptoms. A total of 70% of patients complain of epigastric or right upper quadrant pain, and 40% have nausea or vomiting. A total of 90% have nonspecific viral-like symptoms with malaise for several days before the disorder is apparent. These patients usually demonstrate significant weight gain and generalized edema. Ten to 15% of patients have a diastolic blood pressure <90 mmHg. Proteinuria depends on the disease duration; however, it can be absent in 6% of patients. The nonspecific nature of these symptoms commonly results in misdiagnosis of this life-threatening disease (Table 37–6).

Complications associated with HELLP syndrome include placental abruption, renal failure, ascites, and rupture of a liver hematoma. A rare complication of HELLP syndrome is transient nephrogenic diabetes insipidus, which is caused by elevated circulatory levels of vasopressinase. Most of the perinatal deaths are related to placental abruption, intrauterine hypoxia, and extreme prematurity. As many as 30% of infants born to mothers who have HELLP syndrome are growth retarded.

Patients who are not near term should be referred to a tertiary care center, and initial management should be the same as that for severe preeclampsia (Table 37–7). The first priority is to assess and stabilize maternal condition, particularly coagulation abnormalities, and then evaluate fetal well-being. Then, a decision must be made as to whether immediate delivery is indicated. Amniocentesis for fetal lung maturity may be performed in these patients as indicated without an increased risk of bleeding complications. Steroid use to accelerate fetal lung maturation is indicated, but the health of the mother or the fetus should not be jeopardized by delaying delivery for this reason alone.

All patients with true HELLP syndrome, irrespective of gestational age, should be delivered within 48 hours. The presence of this syndrome is not an indication for immediate delivery by cesarean section. Labor may be initiated with oxytocin infusions, exactly as for routine induction. In a patient with an unripe cervix and a gestational age of <30 weeks, the use of either a ripening agent or elective cesarean section is appropriate. After 30 weeks of gestation, labor is induced regardless of cervical Bishop score.

If maternal analgesia is necessary, intermittent 25- to 50-mg IV doses of meperidine hydrochloride may be used. The use of pudendal block or epidural anesthesia is contraindicated in HELLP syndrome patients because of the risk of bleeding into these areas. General anesthesia should be used for cesarean section.

---

**Table 37–6** Medical and Surgical Disorders Confused With HELLP Syndrome

Acute fatty liver of pregnancy
Appendicitis
Diabetes insipidus
Gallbladder disease
Gastroenteritis
Glomerulonephritis
Hemolytic uremic syndrome
Hepatic encephalopathy
Hyperemesis gravidarum
Idiopathic thrombocytopenia
Kidney stones
Peptic ulcer
Pyelonephritis
Systemic lupus erythematosus
Thrombotic thrombocytopenic purpura
Viral hepatitis

HELLP = hemolysis, elevated liver enzymes, low platelets.

---

**Table 37–7** Management Outline of Antepartum HELLP Syndrome

ASSESS AND STABILIZE MATERNAL CONDITION:
- If disseminated intravascular coagulopathy present, correct coagulopathy
- Antiseizure prophylaxis with magnesium sulfate
- Treatment of severe hypertension
- Transfer to tertiary care center if appropriate
- Computed tomography or ultrasound of the abdomen if subcapsular hematoma of the liver is suspected

EVALUATE FETAL WELL-BEING:
- Nonstress testing
- Biophysical profile
- Ultrasonographic biometry

EVALUATE FETAL LUNG MATURITY IF <35 WEEKS OF GESTATION:
- If mature → delivery
- If immature → steroids → delivery

HELLP = hemolysis, elevated liver enzymes, low platelets.

Platelet transfusions are indicated before or after delivery if the platelet count is <10,000/mm³. However, repeated platelet transfusions are not recommended, as consumption occurs rapidly and the effect is transient. Correction of thrombocytopenia is particularly important before cesarean section. Our policy is to transfuse 6 to 10 units of platelets in all patients with a count of <50,000/mm³ before we intubate for cesarean section.

Generalized oozing from the operative site is common. To minimize the risk of hematoma formation, we recommend placement of a subfascial drain, with the bladder flap left open. The wound should also be left open and should be closed primarily within 72 hours. If these recommendations are not followed, a 20% incidence of hematoma formation will result.

After delivery, the patient should be monitored in the recovery room for at least 24 hours, including hourly evaluation, maternal vital signs, and intake and output. Thirty percent of HELLP syndrome cases occur in the puerperium; thus, vigilance is mandatory. Most patients show evidence of resolution of the disease process within 72 hours after delivery; however, some may require several days. In such patients, MgSO₄ therapy may have to be continued for more than 24 hours. Such patients are at risk for development of pulmonary edema from fluid overload, fluid mobilization, and compromised renal function.

## ECLAMPSIA

Eclampsia is defined as the development of convulsions, coma, or both unrelated to other cerebral conditions during pregnancy and the postpartum period in patients with signs and symptoms of preeclampsia. Eclampsia complicates approximately 1 per 1000 to 1500 deliveries and is present in 3.5% of twin pregnancies. It is primarily a disease of young primigravidas, with an increased incidence seen among indigent women. Other risk factors include molar pregnancies, chronic hypertension or renal disease, previous preeclampsia or eclampsia, and nonimmune hydrops fetalis. Eclamptic convulsions are a life-threatening emergency for both mother and fetus. Seventy-five percent of eclamptic cases develop before delivery, and 25% occur postpartum. Although hypertension is the hallmark for the diagnosis of eclampsia, it does not necessarily have to exist in the severe range (≥160/110 mmHg). Moreover, 20% of all eclamptic patients do not have proteinuria. Symptoms preceding an eclamptic convulsion vary, but headache (83%) and visual disturbances (49%) are the most common.

Eclampsia is an obstetric emergency that requires prompt treatment. The following are principles of treatment:

1. Support of cardiorespiratory function
2. Control of convulsions and prevention of recurrent convulsions
3. Correction of maternal hypoxemia and acidosis
4. Control of severe hypertension
5. Initiation of the delivery process

The most urgent aspect of therapy is to ensure maternal oxygenation and minimize the risk of aspiration, rather than to stop the convulsive episode (most eclamptic convulsions resolve spontaneously in 60 to 90 seconds). Drugs to shorten or abolish the initial convulsion should not be given, but MgSO₄ should be given to prevent further seizures.

After controlling the maternal convulsions, oxygen saturation should be monitored continuously to ensure the presence of normal tissue oxygenation. Maternal hypoxemia or acidemia may result from aspiration, repeated convulsions, respiratory depression resulting from the use of multiple anticonvulsive agents, or all of these combined. To avoid toxic side effects, it is necessary to correct hypoxemia and acidemia before administering anesthetic drugs.

Uterine hyperactivity, consisting of increased frequency and tone, and fetal heart rate changes usually appear during and after an eclamptic convulsion (Table 37–8). These changes are commonly transient, 3 to 15 minutes in duration, and most resolve spontaneously after the convulsions conclude, or after correction of maternal hypoxemia and acidosis. An emergency cesarean section should not be performed based on these findings, as this approach might prove detrimental to both the mother and newborn. If changes persist despite corrective measures, placental abruption, fetal distress, or both, should be suspected, especially in the preterm or growth-retarded fetus.

The primary treatment of eclampsia is delivery of the fetus and placenta. After convulsions and severe hypertension are well controlled and the patient has been stabilized, preparation for delivery should be initiated. Fetal heart rate and uterine activity must be monitored continuously during labor. If labor is not well established and fetal distress is not noted, it is possible to use IV oxytocin to induce labor in all

**Table 37–8** Transitory Changes Associated With Eclamptic Convulsions

| UTERINE HYPERACTIVITY |
| --- |
| Increased frequency of contractions |
| Increased tone |

| FETAL HEART RATE CHANGES |
| --- |
| Bradycardia |
| Compensatory tachycardia |
| Decreased beat-to-beat |
| Late decelerations |

patients at 30 weeks of gestation or beyond, irrespective of the extent of cervical dilatation or effacement.

A similar approach is appropriate for patients at <30 weeks of gestation if the cervix is favorable for induction. For an unfavorable cervix, cesarean section is recommended. Our previous experience of a high incidence of intrapartum complications, such as placental abruption and nonreassuring fetal heart rate in women developing eclampsia before 30 weeks, justifies the use of this method.

Convulsions occurring 48 hours after delivery are commonly referred to as late postpartum eclampsia. They require a careful search for underlying disease such as epilepsy, space-occupying lesion of the central nervous system, pheochromocytoma, hypertensive encephalopathy, intracerebral hemorrhage, or metabolic diseases. $MgSO_4$ remains the drug of choice for prevention and treatment of those seizures. Therapy should continue until diuresis is noted and blood pressure is stabilized, and for at least 24 hours after the last convulsion.

## PREVENTION AND CONTROL OF CONVULSIONS

Parenteral $MgSO_4$ ($MgSO_4 \cdot 7H_2O$ USP) is the drug of choice for treatment and prevention of eclamptic convulsions. It has been the standard treatment for the last 30 years and is associated with reduction in maternal and neonatal morbidity related to eclampsia. Major advantages include its relative safety when used properly. All women diagnosed as having preeclampsia, particularly those with severe disease, should be given $MgSO_4$ both during labor and postpartum.

Table 37–9 describes the common regimens of administering $MgSO_4$. Patellar reflexes, urine output, and respiratory rate of all patients receiving $MgSO_4$ therapy should be checked hourly. Loss of patellar reflexes is the first sign of magnesium toxicity and is an indication for discontinuation of $MgSO_4$ infusion. Signs and symptoms of $MgSO_4$ toxicity are a direct result of smooth muscle weakness and include respiratory depression and lethargy (Table 37–10). Magnesium toxicity can be reversed by slow IV administration of 1 g of 10% calcium gluconate.

For the rare case of seizures unresponsive to $MgSO_4$, sodium amobarbital, 250 m/g IV, can be given by slow push over 3 minutes.

## THERAPY OF SEVERE HYPERTENSION

The objective of treating severe hypertension in pregnancy is to prevent multiorgan failure, cerebrovascular accidents, and congestive heart failure without compromising uteroplacental blood flow.

**Table 37–9** Specific Recommended Regimens for Treating Eclamptic Convulsions

PRITCHARD'S IM REGIMEN

Loading dose: 4 g IV (20% solution obtained by mixing 8 ml of 50% $MgSO_4$ and 12 ml of sterile water) over 3–5 min + 10 g IM (20 ml of 50% $MgSO_4$, ½ dose in each buttock)
Maintenance dose: 5 g IM (20% solution) q4h

ZUSPAN'S IV REGIMEN

Loading dose: 4 g IV over 5–10 min
Maintenance dose: 1–2 g IV per hr

SIBAI'S IV REGIMEN

Loading dose: 6 g IV over 20–30 min (6 g of 50% solution diluted in 150 ml $D_5W$)
Additional 2 g over 5–10 min (1–2 times) can be given with persistent convulsions
If convulsions persist (2% of cases), 250 mg sodium amobarbital over 3 min given IV
In status eclampticus: intubation and muscular paralysis
Maintenance dose: 2–3 g $MgSO_4$ IV per hr (40 g $MgSO_4$ in 1 L $D_5$/LR at 50 ml/hr)

$D_5W$ = 5% dextrose in water; IM = intramuscularly; IV = intravenously; $MgSO_4$ = magnesium sulfate.

Antihypertensive treatment is initiated when systolic blood pressure is >180 mm Hg or diastolic pressure is ≥110 mm Hg. The goal is to slowly reduce the diastolic blood pressure to 90 to 105 mm Hg. Antihypertensive agents of choice have a rapid onset and a relatively short duration of action, the latter proving beneficial in the event of overtitration. Hydralazine hydrochloride (Apresoline) is safe and effective for managing severe hypertension during pregnancy. It can be administered in increments of 5-to 10-mg IV bolus every 20 minutes. This regimen requires monitoring blood pressure every 5 minutes for at least 30 minutes after IV administration. Another alternative is labetalol, which can be adminis-

**Table 37–10** Magnesium Toxicity

| MANIFESTATIONS |
|---|
| Loss of patellar reflex (8–12 mg/dl) |
| Feeling of warmth, flushing (9–12 mg/dl) |
| Somnolence (10–12 mg/dl) |
| Slurred speech (10–12 mg/dl) |
| Muscular paralysis (15–17 mg/dl) |
| Respiratory difficulty (15–17 mg/dl) |
| Cardiac arrest (30–35 mg/dl) |

| MANAGEMENT |
|---|
| Discontinue $MgSO_4$ |
| Obtain Mg level |
| If Mg level ≥ 15 mg/dl: |
|     Give 1 g calcium gluconate IV |
|     Intubate |
|     Assist ventilation |

IV = intravenously; Mg = magnesium; $MgSO_4$ = magnesium sulfate.

tered IV in doses of 20 to 80 mg every 20 minutes up to 300 mg. Unlike hydralazine, labetalol does not cause maternal tachycardia, flushing, or headaches.

Nifedipine, a calcium channel blocker, is used as an oral alternative. Neither adverse fetal effects nor changes in uteroplacental flow have been reported after short- or long-term therapy with this agent. The maximum daily dose is 120 mg. Common side effects include headache, flushing, tachycardia, and fatigue. Other hypertensive drugs are rarely needed for the management of these patients, and diuretics should be used only in the presence of pulmonary edema.

## INTRAPARTUM AND POSTPARTUM MANAGEMENT OF PREECLAMPSIA

Objectives of intrapartum management of patients with preeclampsia are the following:
1. Control of hypertension
2. Prevention of seizures using $MgSO_4$
3. Effecting delivery
4. Prevention of fluid overload/pulmonary edema

The presence of preeclampsia is not an indication for cesarean section. Labor can be initiated with oxytocin in the same manner as for routine induction in all patients with a gestational age of >30 weeks and in all those who have a favorable Bishop's score ($\geq$6). Cervical ripening agents such as prostaglandin $E_2$ ($PGE_2$) gel or misoprostol ($PGE_1$ analog) may be used. In patients with an unfavorable cervix and gestational age of <30 weeks, it is appropriate to consider the use of either cervical ripening agents or elective cesarean section. After delivery, the patient must be monitored closely for least 12 hours. Most women show resolution of the disease process within 48 to 72 hours after delivery. Those who recover more slowly or deteriorate are at risk for development of pulmonary edema from transfusion of blood products, fluid mobilization, and compromised renal function.

## PREDICTION AND PREVENTION OF PREECLAMPSIA

Prevention of preeclampsia requires knowledge of its etiology and availability of methods for prediction of those at risk. The etiology and underlying pathophysiology of preeclampsia remain unknown. No clinical, biophysical, or biochemical test has been reliable for use as a screening test to predict or identify women at risk for preeclampsia.

Clinical trials using salt restriction, diuretic drugs, and antihypertensive drugs failed to demonstrate a reduction in the incidence of hypertensive disorders in pregnancy.

Low-dose aspirin was reported to reduce the incidence and severity of preeclampsia. However, the results of recent randomized trials in nulliparous women and women at risk for preeclampsia did not support the use of aspirin in pregnancy.

Investigators examining the relationship between calcium intake and the incidence of eclampsia in different countries have identified an inverse relationship between calcium intake and the incidence of preeclampsia. Recently, a large, prospective, multi-center study assigned low-risk women to either 2 g/day of calcium or placebo from 21 weeks of gestation until delivery. This study concluded that there was no reduction in the incidence of preeclampsia within the calcium group. Currently, there is no method to prevent preeclampsia.

## REFERENCES

American College of Obstetricians and Gynecologists: Hypertension in pregnancy. ACOG Tech Bull no. 219, January 1996.

Barton JR, Sibai BM: Care of the pregnancy complicated by HELLP syndrome. Obstet Gynecol Clin North Am 18:165–79, 1991.

Belizan JM, Villar J: The relationship between calcium intake and edema, proteinuria, and hypertension-gestosis: An hypothesis. Am J Clin Nutr 33:2202, 1980.

Caritis SN, Sibai B, Hauth J, et al, for the National Institute of Child Health and Human Development Network of Maternal-Fetal Medicine Units: Low-dose aspirin to prevent preeclampsia in women at high risk. N Engl J Med 338:701–705, 1998.

CLASP (Collaborative Low Dose Aspirin Study in Pregnancy) Collaborative Group: A randomized trial of low-dose aspirin for the prevention and treatment of preeclampsia among 9364 pregnant women. Lancet 343:619–629, 1994.

Davey DA, MacGillivray I: The classification and definition of the hypertensive disorders of pregnancy. Am J Obstet Gynecol 158:892–898, 1988.

Levine RJ, Hauth JC, Curet LB, et al: Trial of calcium to prevent preeclampsia. N Engl J Med 337:69–76, 1997.

Long PA, Oats JN: Preeclampsia in twin pregnancy, severity and pathogenesis. Aust N Z J Obstet Gynecol 27:1, 1987.

Lubarsky SL, Barton JR, Friedman SA, et al: Late postpartum eclampsia revisited. Obstet Gynecol 83:502–505, 1994.

National High Blood Pressure Education Program Working Group Report on High Blood Pressure in Pregnancy. Am J Obstet Gynecol 163:1689–1712, 1990.

Rubin PC: Beta-blockers in pregnancy. N Engl J Med 305:1323, 1981.

Sibai BM: Magnesium sulfate is the ideal anticonvulsant in preeclampsia-eclampsia. Am J Obstet Gynecol 162:1141–1145, 1990.

Sibai BM: Diagnosis and management of chronic hypertension in pregnancy. Obstet Gynecol 78:451–461, 1991.

Sibai BM: Management of preeclampsia. Clin Perinatol 18:793–808, 1991.

Sibai BM: Treatment of hypertension in pregnant women. N Engl J Med 335:257–265, 1996.

Sibai BM, Barton JR, Akl S, et al: A randomized prospective comparison of nifedipine and bed rest versus bed rest alone in the management of preeclampsia remote from term. Am J Obstet Gynecol 167:879–884, 1992.

Sibai BM, Gonzalez AR, Mabie WC, Moretti M: A comparison of labetalol plus hospitalization versus hospitalization alone in the management of preeclampsia remote from term. Obstet Gynecol 70:323–327, 1987.

Sibai BM, Mabie WC, Shamsa F, et al: A comparison of no

medication versus methyldopa or labetalol in chronic hypertension during pregnancy. Am J Obstet Gynecol 162:960–967, 1990.

Sibai BM, Ramadan MK, Usta I, et al: Maternal morbidity and mortality in 442 pregnancies with hemolysis, elevated liver enzymes, and low platelets (HELLP syndrome). Am J Obstet Gynecol 169:1000–1006, 1993.

Sibai BM, Taslimi M, Abdella TN, et al: Maternal and perinatal outcome of conservative management of severe preeclampsia in midtrimester. Am J Obstet Gynecol 152:32–37, 1985.

Sibai BM, Taslimi MM, El-Nazer A, et al: Maternal-perinatal outcome associated with the syndrome of hemolysis, elevated liver enzymes, and low platelets in severe preeclampsia. Am J Obstet Gynecol 155:501–509, 1986.

Steegers EA, van Lakwijk HP, Jougsma HW, et al: Physiological implications of chronic dietary sodium restriction during pregnancy: A longitudinal prospective randomized study. Br J Obstet Gynaecol 98:980–987, 1991.

Witlin AG, Sibai BM: Hypertension in pregnancy: Current concepts of preeclampsia. Annu Rev Med 48:115–127, 1997.

# 38

# Illicit Substance Abuse During Pregnancy

VIRGINIA DELANEY-BLACK
CHANDICE Y. COVINGTON
SUDIPTA DHAR
ROBERT J. SOKOL

Women who abuse substances during pregnancy may be understandably reluctant to acknowledge abuse, particularly within the punitive social and legal environment that exists in the United States. In some states, for example, a history of substance abuse by a mother, especially of cocaine, may result in foster care placement of her children or at least a social services referral. It is likely that fear of identification of substance abuse may also lead to lack of prenatal care for some women. Studies that rely primarily on historical information are likely to underidentify the exposed group. This underidentification or misclassification of exposure may lead to type II errors: failure to identify abnormalities in outcome associated with prenatal cocaine exposure. Additional difficulties may be encountered in interpreting outcomes because of variation in the extent or timing of exposure. Urine testing, for example, identifies only recent exposure. Positive results are dependent on both the amount of drug used and the assay used. For example, radioimmunoassay and mass spectrography are more sensitive than thin-layer chromatography. Meconium testing, on the other hand, may not identify first-trimester exposure. Even if a woman reports her drug use honestly, substances purchased on the street are neither produced nor sold under rigorous conditions. It is also quite likely that contaminants (with potentially toxic effects) are included in her purchase. Estimating frequency of drug use and the cost of the purchased supply may provide crude estimates of the amount of drug exposure.

Human studies are also hampered by the inability to exercise control over other important variables. Failure to sufficiently account for critical extraneous factors (e.g., influences of the home, neighborhood, community, maternal characteristics) have significantly restricted the ability of research designs to identify effects of prenatal cocaine exposure. Moreover, drug abuse studies are frequently limited to women from low socioeconomic groups, and other covariants may be extremely important. We have observed that inadequate nutrition, poor prenatal care, older age, and previous pregnancies are characteristically associated with maternal cocaine use even when the comparison sample is selected from subjects of the same socioeconomic background. Furthermore, the home environment and subsequent child development may be negatively affected by continued drug abuse. Repeated changes in custody, foster care placement, or informal family arrangements may be necessitated by the unavailability of a suitable home environment. Unfortunately, alternative homes may also lack an environment conducive to development of a healthy child. These limitations must be acknowledged in identifying the effects of prenatal substance abuse.

## Prenatal Cocaine Exposure

### COCAINE: PROPERTIES AND METABOLISM IN PREGNANCY

Cocaine, or benzoylmethylecgonine, is an alkaloid that can be snorted, injected, ingested, or—in its freebase form—smoked. It is one of several alkaloids found in the leaves of the coca shrub indigenous to South America. The first extraction product, coca paste, contains about 80% cocaine. After conversion to a salt, it is diluted with a variety of adulterants (including arsenic) to a concentration of 40 to 50%. Dissolving the salt in an alkaline solution and recrystallizing produces a highly purified version, known as crack, which can be smoked.

Cocaine inhibits presynaptic reuptake of catecholamine and blocks the reuptake of dopamine and serotonin in the central nervous system. Thus, the concentration of the neurotransmitter remains elevated in the synapse, resulting in cocaine's characteristic euphoric effect. Cocaine is highly addictive. Repetitive use is associated with compulsive behavior despite potential negative consequences of drug use. Koob reports that the mesoaccumbens dopamine pathway from the midbrain ventral tegmental area to the nucleus accumbens is the site of its reinforcing effects.

Once absorbed, cocaine is metabolized by plasma and liver cholinesterase to water-soluble metabolites excreted by the kidney. Blood levels usually peak quickly. In the central nervous system (CNS), the levels are 20-fold higher. Depending on the laboratory technique, metabolites may be present in adult urine for 3 to 6 days after exposure. Its half-life depends on route of absorption and plasma cholinesterase activity. Cholinesterase activity is decreased in the pregnant woman and fetus, thus increasing the plasma half-life and enhancing physiologic effects. Placental cholinesterase in the term placenta may partially protect the fetus as evidenced by placental microsomes obtained from 12 placentas of women who were not drug abusers. However, cholinesterase activity in the less mature placenta has not been studied. Furthermore, low or absent cholinesterase activity occurs in 1 to 13% of normal adults. This enzymatic deficiency may account for some of the reported variability in cocaine toxicity. Additionally, a combination of alcohol and cocaine may result in the production of cocaethylene, which in adults has been associated with a longer half-life (2 hours for cocaethylene vs. 38 minutes for cocaine) and a greater risk for sudden death in adult users.

### PREVALENCE OF COCAINE ABUSE

Cocaine use, particularly in the form of crack, increased significantly in the United States in the 1980s, reaching across both racial and socioeconomic lines. The reported incidence of maternal admission of at least one-time use of cocaine during pregnancy is 10 to 11% in pregnant women. When urine drug screening was added, conservative estimates of cocaine use during pregnancy rose to 13 to 17%. In our own delivery rooms during the late 1980s, a 31% prevalence was reported by Ostrea and associates who used newborn meconium, a sensitive drug screen for prenatal cocaine exposure. Among women who had no prenatal care, Spence and associates reported a 62% prevalence of cocaine use. More recent evidence suggests that prenatal cocaine use has decreased. By using intrapartum urine samples in a Southern urban setting, Miller and associates documented a prevalence of less than 10%, and in a mixed urban and suburban sample, only 3.4% of infants had positive meconium samples.

### COCAINE EFFECTS ON PREGNANCY

In animals, cocaine has been shown to decrease placental blood flow, increase maternal blood pressure and fetal heart rate, decrease fetal partial pressure of oxygen, increase spontaneous abortions, increase maternal mortality, reduce maternal weight gain, decrease litter size and weight, and increase postnatal mortality. Human studies of cocaine exposure during pregnancy have reported an increase in spontaneous abortions, fetal deaths, premature labor, and premature rupture of the membranes. Other pregnancy complications, such as meconium staining of the amniotic fluid and fetal distress, have been associated with cocaine use in some but not all studies. Among the inconsistent findings is abruptio placentae, which has been reported to be increased among cocaine users in several studies. This lack of conformity is likely to relate to the timing of cocaine exposure as well as other obstetric factors, including cigarette smoking.

### COCAINE EFFECTS ON THE NEWBORN

Unlike heroin, cocaine is not associated with a specific withdrawal syndrome. Even in pregnancies complicated by multiple drug use, infants born to cocaine-abusing women had lower abstinence scores than those exposed to heroin and methadone. Although necrotizing enterocolitis, cardiovascular abnormalities (arrhythmias and hypertension), and sudden infant death syndrome (SIDS) have all been reported in children exposed prenatally to cocaine, the primary areas for concern have more recently focused on intrauterine growth, duration of pregnancy, and neurobehavioral outcome.

### Fetal Growth and Gestational Age

Multiple studies have reported a decrease in infant weight associated with cocaine use during pregnancy. These results were attenuated when exposure was limited to early pregnancy. A large controlled study by Pettiti and Coleman demonstrated a significant reduction in weight even after adjusting for covariants. More recently, by using historical reports of drug use during pregnancy, the investigators in a large study were able to demonstrate a dose-response relationship between prenatal cocaine exposure and birth weight. In both a homogeneous sample and a large controlled study, a negative correlation was found between gestational age and cocaine exposure.

### Fetal Head Growth

Several authors have described a reduction in fetal head growth related to prenatal cocaine exposure, including the recent report of a dose-response relationship when cocaine exposure was documented by hair analysis. Sokol and associates demonstrated a reduction in neonatal head circumference after prenatal cocaine exposure, which persisted after adjustment for both prematurity and birth weight. These findings suggest that cocaine may have a specific effect on fetal brain growth. Decreased head growth has been associated with developmental delay in a number of perinatal and developmental studies.

### Neurologic Outcomes

Cerebral infarction, neonatal seizures, and abnormal electroencephalogram (EEG) have all been described after prenatal cocaine exposure. The initial case reports do not describe the base population or other maternal risk factors. In other studies, assessments were not blinded. However, data from the day of birth indicate that cocaine exposure was associated with higher peak systolic and diastolic neonatal blood pressure and mean cerebral blood flow velocity.

Assessments of cocaine-exposed infants using the Brazelton Neonatal Behavioral Assessment Scale (BNBAS) have reported numerous and conflicting results, perhaps related to factors such as variation in sample size and selection, amount and timing of exposure, control for polysubstance abuse, gestational age at birth, and age at testing. Despite the inconsistent findings, studies demonstrate a dose-response relationship between cocaine exposure and neonatal behavior. Tronick and associates characterized exposure by historical report and found alterations in reflexes, state regulation, autonomic stability, and excitability. Delaney-Black and associates used meconium testing for their quantitative estimate of exposure and found poorer scores for motor and regulation of state.

## EARLY CHILDHOOD OUTCOME OF PRENATAL COCAINE EXPOSURE

Evaluation of outcomes for preschool and school-aged children has been limited. Preliminary studies from several authors have failed to identify a significant, direct effect of prenatal cocaine exposure on cognitive outcome. One study reported an intelligence quotient (IQ) difference, but failed to account for important covariants. Childhood behavior after prenatal exposure continues to be controversial. Howard and colleagues noted that children exposed to several different drugs performed within normal limits on structured instruments, namely pediatric assessments that provided examiner-guided structure to an activity; however, these same children showed striking deficits when assessed in unstructured free play. Other investigators have reported immature play strategies, more irritability, and more emotional and behavioral problems. Griffith and associates and Hawley and associates reported differences in parent reports of child behavior. Griffith's group identified anxiety, depression, and withdrawal, whereas Hawley's group reported more aggression and delinquent behavior. In contrast, Richardson and associates reported that the cocaine-exposed group had significantly fewer behavioral problems at the age of 6 years than the control group.

The social, medical, and psychological comorbidities associated with cocaine abuse often predispose the caregiver to parenting failure. Compared with control mothers, cocaine-abusing mothers are more likely to have a history of abuse and exposure to violence, to have experienced more negative life events, to be polydrug users, and to be malnourished. In addition, cocaine-exposed mothers are more likely to have signs of depression, personality disorders, and affective disorders, which compromise the mother's ability to read and respond appropriately to the child's communicative signals. Thus, neither the parent nor the child is able to regulate personal behavior, or respond to the other's behavior successfully. When there is a dyadic problem, the child is susceptible to neglect and abuse. Less maternal attention to the infant and higher rates of neglect and abuse have been related to cocaine dependence, making assessments of the role of prenatal exposure difficult.

# Heroin Abuse in Pregnancy and Its Postnatal Outcome

## BACKGROUND

3,6-Diacetylmorphine, better known as heroin, is a narcotic that became a popular drug of abuse in the 1960s. It is estimated that one quarter of a million women are intravenous drug abusers and that 90% of them are in the childbearing age group. Consequently, 9000 women addicted to narcotics give birth each year. Heroin, like other narcotics, is known to cross the placental barrier. The specific risk factors for infants born to narcotic-addicted women can be divided into three interrelated categories: prenatal exposure to hard drugs, which can influence the growth and development of the fetus; abstinence (withdrawal) symptoms after birth, when the infant is no longer supplied with the addictive substance the mother used; and the specific social circumstances that result from the addiction to illegal substances, which can affect the development of the children. Researchers have focused their studies on all three categories of risk factors and produced interesting results. Studies on laboratory animals and in vitro studies of human cells have shown effects of prenatal heroin exposure on growth parameters, neurobehavior, and development.

## OBSTETRIC COMPLICATIONS

Many drug-abusing women neglect their health; therefore, they are predisposed to various problems that affect the morbidity and mortality of their infants. Weight gain in pregnancy is poor, and obstetric complications associated with heroin addiction include abortion, abruptio placentae, amnionitis, and chorioamnionitis. Placental insufficiency, intrauterine growth retardation, preeclampsia and eclampsia, antepartum hemorrhage, meconium-stained amniotic fluid, preterm delivery, and precipitous labor and delivery are more common among heroin-addicted women. Lam and associates reported that heroin users had significantly shorter second-stage labor, and that the ratio of placental weight to birth weight was also significantly higher. Some studies have shown 200 to 400% increases in the incidence of premature rupture of membranes in heroin users. Naeye and associates reported an increased incidence of acute infection in mothers who abused heroin, most of whom delivered prematurely. The incidence of hepatitis B, human immunodeficiency virus (HIV) infection, and syphilis is also higher among heroin addicts. Maternal discontinuance of heroin during pregnancy can result in fetal withdrawal. Fetal withdrawal is associated with increased fetal movements and potential hypoxia in both animals and humans. Wong and Lao suggested that Doppler assessment of umbilical artery flow velocity waveform may be useful in detecting withdrawal in narcotic users.

## NEONATAL OUTCOME

A number of controlled and uncontrolled studies have attempted to evaluate the impact of prenatal heroin use on neonates. Increased risk of fetal anomalies, ranging from 4 to 14%, has been reported in several uncontrolled studies. Most researchers agree, however, that no definite pattern or syndrome has been detected.

Fricker and Segal noted an impressive incidence of neonatal hypoglycemia in infants exposed to prenatal heroin, which may be related to prematurity and intrauterine growth retardation, because these findings have not been confirmed. Additionally, a decreased incidence of respiratory distress syndrome in 33 premature infants born to heroin addicts has been reported, suggesting that heroin may act as an enzyme inducer. Nevertheless, respiratory distress syndrome certainly does occur in premature infants born to heroin users.

## MORTALITY

A high incidence of stillbirths has been observed among heroin addicts. Several uncontrolled studies have reported a 6 to 8% stillbirth rate in women using heroin, although other studies have not confirmed these results. The perinatal mortality rate of 5 to 11% has been reported from among the offspring of heroin addicts. The incidence of SIDS in infants of heroin-addicted mothers has been reported to be greater than that of nonuser control groups.

## NEONATAL ABSTINENCE SYNDROME

A major concern in infants exposed to narcotics such as heroin is withdrawal symptoms or neonatal abstinence syndrome (NAS). NAS is a generalized disorder characterized by signs and symptoms of CNS hyperirritability, gastrointestinal dysfunction, respiratory distress, and vague autonomic symptoms, including yawning, sneezing, mottling, and diarrhea. The disorder is explained by postnatal overstimulation of central $\alpha_2$-adrenergic receptors, whose numbers increase as a result of fetal heroin exposure. Fetuses of chronic heroin users become physically dependent on heroin because it crosses the placenta. The onset of withdrawal symptoms may be from a few minutes after birth up to 2 weeks of age and last for 6 to 8 weeks. However, symptoms of irritability may persist for more than 3 months. The Finnegan scoring system has been used frequently to quantitate the presence and degree of withdrawal. Wilson and associates reported severe NAS in 68% of offspring of heroin addicts. Similar results were found in two other studies. Stimmel and associates found that 45% of these infants exhibited severe withdrawal symptoms.

Providing adequate nutrition to infants who have NAS is a problem because the sucking response may be uncoordinated and ineffectual. Kron and associates demonstrated that heroin-exposed infants were significantly depressed with respect to sucking rate and nutrient consumption. Much of the morbidity associated with NAS can be eliminated by appropriate assessment of symptoms and expeditious initiation of treatment. Paregoric and phenobarbital are commonly used to treat NAS. Wilson and associates described a phase of subacute withdrawal after hospital discharge. This phase, consisting primarily of hyperphagia and hyperacusis, rarely persisted after 6 months of age.

## INFECTIONS

The infants of heroin addicts are subjected to higher risk of infection because of high rates of transmission from mothers in utero, during delivery, or in the postpartum period. Moreover, Lam and associates found an increased incidence of clinically overt neonatal sepsis in their study on heroin-addicted mothers. The total infection rate of 43.5% was reported among infants of heroin addicts who were asymptomatic carriers of hepatitis B virus. However, this prevalence is likely to vary from site to site. In infants born to mothers with first- or second-trimester hepatitis B, only 1 in 10 were infected, but if acute maternal infection occurred during the third trimester or within 2 months of delivery, 76% of infants were infected. An Italian multicenter study reported that 32.6% of infants born to heroin-addicted, HIV-positive mothers were infected with the virus, and 21% of them died at a median age of 10.2 months. Additionally, screening for hepatitis, HIV infection, and other sexually transmitted diseases is essential in this high-risk group.

## GROWTH PARAMETERS

The most consistent perinatal effect of heroin was seen in fetal growth. Several controlled studies showed that offspring of heroin-addicted mothers had as much as a 340 g weight reduction compared with the weight of infants of drug-free control groups. The limitations in these studies were that the drug-free control subjects were not matched for confounding variables, and statistical control subjects were not enrolled. Some studies report that birth weight was lower in infants born to heroin-addicted mothers compared with infants of methadone-addicted mothers. In contrast to heroin, methadone use during pregnancy has been associated with improved weight and less intrauterine growth retardation. However, caution must be used in interpreting these results because of the lack of statistical control; data from other uncontrolled studies showed virtually no difference in birth weights between heroin and methadone groups.

## NEONATAL NEUROBEHAVIOR

As previously described, tremulousness and hyperirritability are common signs of NAS in newborns. A shrill, high-pitched cry and sleep disturbances are also common. The normal sucking response of the newborn may become uncoordinated and ineffectual in prenatally heroin-exposed neonates. In a controlled study performed at Hutzel Hospital in Detroit, the investigators reported increased irritability, tremulousness, and jerkiness of motor and hand-mouth movements. Addicted infants were less cuddly, particularly at 24 hours of age, and showed a deficit in habituation, poor response to visual stimuli, and decreased orientation to auditory stimulus. Several of these differences in neurobehavior between addicted and nonaddicted groups were related to the severity of withdrawal. Kaplan reported alertness to be within normal limits by 28 days, although tremulousness remained. Strauss and associates reported similar findings. Dinges and associates reported abnormal sleep patterns with an increase in rapid eye movement sleep and decrease in quiet sleep in infants of heroin addicts. A significantly greater proportion of addicted infants woke during EEG sleep recordings, suggesting that wakefulness is increased during opiate withdrawal.

## LONG-TERM CONSEQUENCES

Several longitudinal studies were conducted to assess long-term consequences of prenatal exposure to heroin on children. These studies are difficult to interpret, however, because of problems superimposed by the addicts' lifestyles and limitations of study designs, especially lack of appropriate control groups. There is a general agreement that heroin produces intrauterine growth retardation; however, longitudinal investigations have reported variable outcome for later growth. Head growth may be impaired. In general, mental and psychomotor development in prenatally heroin-exposed infants were not affected at the end of the first year. Developmental delay and behavioral problems have been reported in later childhood and associated with prenatal heroin or methadone exposure.

Behaviorally, the problems of the heroin-exposed children were related to impulsiveness, aggressiveness, and peer relations. These behavioral problems were thought to be manifestations of impaired attention and organizational abilities. The heroin-exposed group was rated more active than the other groups during physical examination. Ornoy and associates in 1993 reported that a high proportion of children born to heroin-dependent mothers exhibited inattention, hyperactivity, and a variety of behavioral abnormalities suggestive of attention deficit hyperactive disorder (ADHD). Similarly, Davis and Templer, Wilson and associates, and Hickey and associates identified inattentive behavior related to prenatal exposure. When distracters were added to the task, the heroin group failed to suppress vagal tone compared with control subjects. However, the heroin-exposed group made fewer correct responses in the task than the control subjects, suggesting that the normal physiologic responses to increased attentional demand may be impaired in the heroin group.

# Marijuana Use in Pregnancy and Postnatal Outcome

## BACKGROUND AND METABOLISM

Marijuana is derived from the plant *Cannabis sativa* and can contain any of the plant material, including seeds and flowers. There are 60 compounds unique to cannabis. Marijuana is one of the most commonly used illicit drugs among pregnant women. A total of 21% of women between the ages of 18 and 25 years reported using the drug at least once during the year preceding the interview and 9% during the preceding month. Overall, the lifetime prevalence of marijuana use is higher in white women than in black or Hispanic women, but the black women were more likely to report current use. A number of research studies have evaluated the postnatal consequences of marijuana use in pregnancy, because delta-9-tetrahydrocannabinol, the principal psychoactive component of marijuana, is known to cross the human-placental barrier and, therefore, has potential teratogenic effects on fetal organogenesis.

## MARIJUANA USE DURING PREGNANCY

Prevalence rates of marijuana use during pregnancy vary with method and time of assessment. In the Maternal Health Practice and Child Development Project phase 1 (MHPCD-1) study, researchers reported that 31% of women used marijuana in the first trimester and 42% used it at least once in the year before conception. Marijuana users had a lower socioeconomic status and a median age of 22 years (range 18 to 42 years). Only 60% had graduated from high school. A study of a low-income sample from Denver found that 32% of the women used marijuana in the first trimester of pregnancy. Similarly, a prevalence rate of 23% by interview and 16% by urinalysis was identified in a low-income, inner-city sample in Boston. In a middle-class sample, the prevalence rate was 13% during the first and 10% during the third trimester. Most women decreased their use of the drug by the end of the first trimester. This decrease in use occurs especially after confirmation of pregnancy.

## NEONATAL EFFECTS

Several studies have evaluated the effects of prenatal marijuana use on the neonate. An increase in birth complications, fetal distress, and meconium staining has been reported.

## INTRAUTERINE GROWTH

Continued controversy exists regarding the impact of marijuana on intrauterine growth. A prospective study of 1226 women recruited and interviewed at the Prenatal Clinics of Boston City Hospital reported reductions of 79 g in birth weight and 0.5 cm in length after controlling for confounding variables. A dose-response decrement in birth weight has also been reported. Other investigators have found only an alteration in birth length. In the Ottawa Prenatal Prospective Study of middle-class volunteers, after adjustment for covariants, the investigators reported no significant effects of first- or third-trimester marijuana use on any of the growth parameters. Lester and Dreher studied ganja (a form of marijuana that is three to four times more potent than that used in the United States) in Jamaica. Infants born to mothers using ganja weighed more than infants of mothers in the control group. Although both groups were matched for social status, the environment of the ganja users was more stimulating and had more resources available than that of the control families, perhaps accounting for this finding.

## IMPACT ON THE LENGTH OF GESTATION

Conflicting data on the effects of marijuana on duration of pregnancy have been reported. Length of gestation and prematurity were not significantly affected by prenatal marijuana exposure in studies conducted by Day and associates, Hatch and Brack, and Quazi and Mriano. However, another study reported a statistically significant reduction in gestational length by less than 1 week in offspring of women who smoked marijuana six or more times a week compared with abstainees. Furthermore, although Gibson and Baghurst found that 25% of their heaviest users had premature infants, other studies showed no difference in duration of gestation.

## IMPACT ON MORPHOLOGY

In general, researchers have not found any significant relationship between prenatal marijuana use and morphologic abnormalities in neonates, although sporadic case reports have been published. A case report by Quazi and Mriano showed facial anomalies that were reminiscent of those reported in fetal alcohol syndrome in offspring of marijuana users in pregnancy.

## IMPACT ON NEONATAL NEUROBEHAVIOR

An equivocal relationship has been found between prenatal marijuana use and neurobehavioral outcome of the offspring. In the Ottawa Prenatal Prospective Study, the investigators found that the exposed neonates had altered visual responsiveness and increased tremors and startles on the BNBAS. In contrast, infants of Jamaican women using ganja had a better state of control, were less irritable, and had fewer tremors than nonexposed infants on the BNBAS. Richardson and associates and Hayes and associates could not identify any effect of prenatal marijuana exposure on neonatal behavior.

## CHILDHOOD OUTCOME

The few follow-up studies evaluating long-term consequences of prenatal marijuana exposure have not shown any long-term negative effects on growth. Researchers generally report no effect of prenatal marijuana use on infant development.

## Treatment Protocols for the Pregnant Addict

Effective treatment is not possible without identification of substance abuse. Hence, the first step in treatment must be the consistent inclusion of nonjudgmental questions regarding the use of drugs of abuse in the prenatal history. When incorporated into the medical history with other habits, including cigarette and alcohol use, important confidential information may be shared. Work by Chasnoff and associates, using anonymous drug testing, has identified that medical suspicion of drug use is highly inaccurate and may be attributed to other unrelated factors, including poverty. When prenatal care is combined with treatment of drug abuse, pregnancy outcome is improved. Because of the effects of the illicit drugs per se and the associated effects of poor nutrition, suboptimal prenatal care, and use of legal substances, such as cigarettes and tobacco, these pregnancies should be considered to be high risk. Therefore, all pregnancies complicated by illicit drug use should have ultrasonographic assessment of fetal growth (see Chapters 23 and 31). Antenatal fetal assessment by nonstress testing or biophysical profile (see Chapter 21) should be started in most cases by 32 weeks of gestation or earlier, depending on clinical assessment of the case.

Drug treatment of the drug addict must focus on two areas: pharmacologic interventions, when available, to assist with the physiologic effects of withdrawal, and behavioral interventions to alter the psychological factors that contribute to drug addiction. When possible, pharmacologic modalities should provide agonist substitution for both the initial detoxification period and the chronic maintenance program. Antagonists that block the effect of the drug of abuse may also play an important role in treatment. When necessary, symptomatic treatment, although not directly related to the effect of the abused drug, may also be effective in reducing symptoms. For the pregnant addict, drug therapy must be chosen carefully to avoid deleterious effects on the fetus. Behavioral modification has focused on individual and group psychotherapy, contingency management to identify consequences of continued drug abuse, provision of a therapeutic community, skill development, and support groups, such as Narcotics Anonymous.

Few data are available regarding pharmacologic interventions for cocaine exposure. Newer experimental drugs for cocaine addiction have not been tested during pregnancy. Psychological interventions may be appropriate for this population. Concern for the welfare of her unborn baby is a powerful motivating factor in reducing drug use during pregnancy, providing a "window of opportunity" for patient commitment to sobriety. A reduction in both cigarette and alcohol use is common in the second and third trimesters after confirmation of the pregnancy. Similarly, efforts to reduce illicit drug abuse may also be more successful.

## MANAGEMENT OF THE PREGNANT HEROIN ADDICT

Substantial data are available to provide guidance in the care of the pregnant heroin addict. Although earlier work suggested that the pregnant heroin addict undergo drug withdrawal before delivery, current recommendations acknowledge that for many women achieving a drug-free state during pregnancy is neither possible nor advisable. Rapid withdrawal from heroin has been shown to affect the fetus adversely and has been associated with both fetal distress and seizures. Hence, current recommendations advocate methadone maintenance. This therapy, in conjunction with behavioral modification, removes the woman from the drug-seeking culture, reduces fluctuation of the drugs to the fetus, and can be associated with improved prenatal care, including nutrition. It also offers the addicted woman an opportunity to restructure her life and continue stabilization after pregnancy.

Substantial data that became available over the last three decades have identified the therapeutic effects of methadone maintenance programs. Reductions in obstetric risk factors, pregnancy complications, and fetal loss have all been reported. Neonatal withdrawal, however, is a well-known complication and must be treated appropriately. Methadone may be given orally and has a half-life of 24 hours, hence, once-a-day dosing is appropriate. There is no euphoria or opiate abstinence symptoms in the appropriately maintained methadone patient. Methadone dosage schedules must be determined individually to reduce maternal symptoms and continue fetal well-being. In the nonpregnant patient, doses may range from 60 to 100 mg day. High doses in early pregnancy have been associated with normal fetal growth. However, these high doses are associated with significant neonatal abstinence symptoms. Additionally, plasma levels of methadone show marked intrapatient and interpatient variability and are usually lower in pregnancy, likely related to the changes in fluid compartments during pregnancy. Hence, lower dose methadone treatments in pregnancy may result in onset of withdrawal symptoms. Further reduction of methadone late in pregnancy reduces neonatal abstinence.

Monitoring of ongoing heroin use can be evaluated by urine drug testing three times a week. Less frequent testing may miss persistent heroin use.

Additional treatment protocols have been recommended, but safety of these protocols for the pregnant heroin addict is often inadequate or not available. Among these alternative protocols are the nonopioid, longer acting, methadone-like agents, as well as opioid antagonists. One of the newer nonopioid alternatives is clonidine, an $\alpha_2$-adrenergic agonist. Clonidine does not reduce anxiety, potentially reducing its effectiveness. An early study has reported less sedation associated with a related agent, lofexidine. Alternatively, longer acting methadone-like agents have been approved by the Food and Drug Administration. Kreek has reviewed newer experimental approaches to the treatment of patients with heroin addiction.

Additional monitoring of the heroin addict in pregnancy is mandated by the increase in pregnancy complications, including intrauterine growth retardation and stillbirths. Furthermore, the heroin abuser is at higher risk for sexually transmitted diseases, including syphilis, gonorrhea, herpes, and HIV infection. Early HIV and serology testing are warranted, as is rescreening for syphilis late in pregnancy.

## MANAGEMENT OF THE PREGNANT COCAINE ADDICT

Unfortunately, clinical care of the cocaine addict has been hampered both by underreporting and lack of available treatment centers for pregnant women. Although data obtained from birth certificates in New York reported peak prevalence of cocaine exposure at less than 3%, national data from the same area reported prevalence rates of more than 20%. In one study, almost one third of the cocaine-exposed mothers received no prenatal care. The same authors reported that in their New York hospital more than 50% of low-income women who received no prenatal care were cocaine exposed. Yet a survey conducted at the peak of the cocaine epidemic in New York revealed that more than half of the programs excluded pregnant women, two thirds excluded Medicaid recipients, and 97% excluded crack-addicted patients.

Comprehensive reviews of the general treatment of cocaine dependency are available, as well as reviews specifically addressing pregnancy. In the 1997 monograph from the National Institute on Drug Abuse, McCance suggested that the 2- to 10- week withdrawal period associated with cocaine abstinence is ideal for trials of new pharmacotherapies because of the high risk of drug relapse. Combined with behavioral modification, this two-tiered approach has the potential to reduce drug use. The use of a cocaine agonist is particularly relevant during the period of cocaine craving. Although randomized control trials have been performed with antidepressants and dopaminergic agents (antagonists: haloperidol and flupenthixol; agonists: bromocriptine and amantadine), substantive effects have yet to be confirmed. Potential new treatments have focused on both cocaine antagonists, which attenuate the effects of cocaine, and agonists, which share some but not all of cocaine's associated symptoms. McCance outlined many of these preclinical treatment trials. Additionally, anticocaine antibodies have been recommended to reduce the reinforcing behavior of cocaine. However, these treatment protocols have not been shown to be safe for the pregnant cocaine addict.

Additional drugs of abuse are likely to be used by the cocaine addict. Although methadone has been recommended for opioid addiction, heroin addicts who also abuse cocaine frequently eliminate or reduce cocaine while on methadone maintenance. Hence, further study of the efficacy of methadone for cocaine addiction may be warranted. Current treatment of the pregnant cocaine addict includes initial daily doses of 20 to 40 mg of methadone to relieve symptoms of abstinence. This dose can be adjusted as needed. Additionally, alcohol treatment should also parallel treatment for cocaine. Women should be monitored carefully for fetal well-being (see Chapter 21), as well as drug use across the pregnancy. Regular urine screening during pregnancy is recommended for the detection of metabolites of cocaine. It must be remembered, however, that even negative urine tests cannot be equated with abstinence. As previously noted, sporadic urine testing severely underestimates drug use. Many factors affect the duration of cocaine metabolites in urine, including the sensitivity of the screening test, the dose used, and the time since last exposure. The duration of time during which drug detection occurs is not linearly related to the drug dose. Instead, a log-linear relationship exists. Hence, small doses may go undetected. Even once-a-week testing leaves close to 80% "safe" time.

Alternatives to maternal urine drug testing include analyses of maternal hair and neonatal meconium. Maternal hair has the advantages of providing data across pregnancy. Washing the sample should eliminate second-hand drug use. However, the effects of hair care products have not been adequately evaluated. Furthermore, many women are reluctant to provide hair, although only 100 mg of samples are necessary. Neonatal meconium is easily obtained and has good sensitivity and specificity. Ostrea identified little cross-reactivity with other compounds. However, because meconium accumulates in the second and third trimesters, first-trimester drug exposure is unlikely with this technique.

Treatment protocols for the cocaine addict often include individual or group psychotherapy, sometimes in the context of the therapeutic community. Although originally designed for male addicts, these programs have gained some financial support for pregnant women in some communities. Inclusion of prepartum women and the ability of women to retain custody of their children (often within the therapeutic community) have been attributes of some of the more successful programs.

To be effective, treatment for the pregnant opioid or cocaine addict requires evaluation of the associated factors that contribute to the drug addiction. Drug therapy to reduce withdrawal and drug craving, behavioral interventions, and personalized prenatal care should help to reduce drug use and to optimize pregnancy outcome. For the addict, a single treatment admission is unlikely to eliminate drug use. Rehospitalization or outpatient treatment may need to be repeated. Community supports, including home visitation programs, may be effective in establishing ongoing care for both mother and child.

## REFERENCES

Abel EL: Prenatal exposure to cannabis: A critical review of effects on growth, development, and behavior. Behav Neurol Biol 29:137, 1980.

Abrams CAL: Cytogenic risks to the offspring of pregnant addicts. J Addict Dis 2:63, 1975.

Acker, D, Sachs BP, Tracey KS, et al: Abruptio placentae associated with cocaine use. Am J Obstet Gynecol 146:220, 1983.

Ambre J: The urinary excretion of cocaine and metabolites in humans: A kinetic analysis of published data. J Anal Toxicol 9:241, 1985.

Astley SJ, Claren SK, Little RE, et al: Analysis of facial shape in children gestationally exposed to marijuana, alcohol, and/or cocaine. Pediatrics 89:67, 1992.

Ball SA, Mayes LC, DeTeso, JA, Schottenfeld RS: Maternal attentiveness of cocaine abusers during child-based assessments. Am J Addict 6:135, 1997.

Barabach LM, Glazer G, Norris SC: Maternal perception and parent-infant interaction of vulnerable cocaine-exposed couplets. J Perinat Neonatol Nurs 6:76, 1992.

Barr HM, Streissguth AP, Martin DC, et al: Infant size at 8 months of age: Relationship to maternal use of alcohol, nicotine and caffeine during pregnancy. Pediatrics 74:336, 1984.

Beckwith L, Rodning C, Norris D, et al: Spontaneous play in two-year-olds born to substance-abusing mothers. Infant Ment Health J 12:189, 1994.

Beeghly M, Tronick EZ: Effects of prenatal exposure to cocaine in early infancy: Toxic effects on the process of mutual regulation. Infant Ment Health J 15:158, 1994.

Berenson AB, Wilkinson GS, Lopez LA: Effects of prenatal care on neonates born to drug-using women. Substance Use Misuse 31:1063, 1996.

Blackard C, Tennes K: Human placenta transfer of cannabinoids. N Engl J Med 311:797, 1984.

Blinick G, Jerez E, Wallach RC: Methadone maintenance, pregnancy and progeny. JAMA 225:477, 1973.

Blinick G, Wallach RC, Jerez E: Pregnancy in narcotic addicts treated by medical withdrawal. Am J Obstet Gynecol 105:997, 1969.

Burkett G, Yasin S, Palon D: Perinatal implications of cocaine exposure. J Reprod Med 35, 35, 1990.

Carzoli RP, Murphy SP, Hammer-Knisely J, et al: Evaluation of auditory brain stem response in full-term infant of cocaine-abusing mothers. Am J Dis Child 145:1013, 1991.

Chaney NE, Franke J, Wadlington WB: Cocaine convulsions in a breast-feeding baby. J Pediatr 108:134, 1988.

Chasnoff IJ: Drug use and women: Establishing a standard of care. Ann NY Acad Sci 562:208, 1989.

Chasnoff IJ, Burns KA, Burns WJ, Schnoll SH: Prenatal drug exposure: Effects on neonatal and infant growth and development. Neurobehav Toxicol Teratol 8:357, 1986.

Chasnoff IJ, Burns WJ, Schnoll SH, Burns KA: Cocaine use in pregnancy. N Engl J Med 313:666, 1985.

Chasnoff IJ, Bussey ME, Savidh R, et al: Perinatal cerebral infarction and maternal cocaine use. J Pediatr 108: 456, 1986.

Chasnoff IJ, Griffith DR, MacGregor S, et al: Temporal patterns of cocaine use in pregnancy: Prenatal outcome. JAMA 261:1741, 1989.

Chasnoff I, Landress HJ, Barrett ME: Prevalence of illicit-drug or alcohol use during pregnancy and discrepancies in mandatory reporting in Pinellas County, Florida. N Engl J Med 322:1202,1990.

Chavez CJ, Ostrea EM Jr, Stryker JC, et al: SIDS among infants of drug dependent mothers. J Pediatr 95:407, 1975.

Chazotte C, Youchah J, Freda MC: Cocaine use during pregnancy and low birth weight: The impact of prenatal and drug treatment. Semin Perinatol 19:293, 1995.

Cherukuri R, Minkoff H, Feldman J, et al: A cohort study of alkaloid cocaine ("crack") in pregnancy. J Obstet Gynecol 72:147, 1988.

Choteau M, Brickner-Namerow P, Leppert P: The effect of cocaine abuse on birth weight and gestational age. J Obstet Gynecol 72:351, 1988.

Church MW, Overbeck GW, Andrzejczak AL: Prenatal cocaine exposure in the Long-Evans rat: I. Dose-dependent effects on gestation, mortality and postnatal maturation. Neurotox Teratol 12:327, 1989.

Cone EJ, Dickerson SL: Efficacy of urinalysis in monitoring heroin and cocaine abuse patterns: Implications in clinical trials for treatment of drug dependence. NIDA Res Monogr 128:46, 1992.

Cone EJ, Menchen SL, Paul BD, et al: Validity testing of commercial urine cocaine metabolite assays: Assay detection times, individual excretion patterns, and kinetics after cocaine administration to humans. J Forens Sci 34:15, 1989.

Connaughton JF, Reeser D, Schut J, et al: Perinatal addiction: Outcome and management. Am J Obstet Gynecol 129:679, 1977.

Cozens DD, Clark R, Palmer AK, et al: The effect of crude marihuana extract on embryonic and fetal development of the rabbit. *In* Nahas GG, Paton WD (eds): Marijuana: Biologic Effects. Oxford, Pergamon Press, 1979, pp 469–479.

Cregler LL, Mark H: Cardiovascular dangers of cocaine abuse. Am J Cardiol 57:1185, 1986.

Critchley HOD, Woods SM, Barson AJ, et al: Fetal death in utero and cocaine abuse. Br J Obstet Gynecol 95:195, 1988.

Cuthill JD, Beroniade V, Salvatori VA, et al: Evaluation of clonidine suppression of opiate withdrawal reactions: A multidisciplinary approach. Can J Psychiatry 35:377, 1990.

Dahl RE, Scher MS, Williamson DE, et al: A longitudinal study of prenatal marijuana use: Effects on sleep and arousal at age 3 years. Pediatr Adolesc Med 149:145, 1995.

Davis DD, Templer DI: Neurobehavioral functioning in children exposed to narcotics in utero. Addict Behav 13:275, 1988.

Day NL, Cottreau CM, Richardson GA: The epidemiology of alcohol, marijuana and cocaine use among women of childbearing age and pregnant women. Clin Obstet Gynecol 36:232, 1993.

Day NL, Richardson GA: Prenatal marijuana use, epidemiology, methodologic issues, infant outcome. Clin Perinatol 18:77, 1990.

Day NL, Richardson GA, Goldschmidt L, et al: Effect of prenatal marijuana exposure on the cognitive development of offspring at age three. Neurotoxicol Teratol 11:49, 1990.

Day NL, Sambamoorthi U, Taylor P, et al: Prenatal marijuana use and neonatal outcome. Neurotoxicol Teratol 13:329, 1991.

Delaney-Black V, Covington C, Ostrea E Jr, et al: Prenatal cocaine and neonatal outcome: Evaluation of dose-response relationship. Pediatrics 98:735, 1996.

Dewey WL: Cannibinoid pharmacology. Pharmacol Rev 38:151, 1986.

Dinges DF, Davis MM, Glass P: Fetal exposure to narcotics: Neonatal sleep as a measure of nervous system disturbances. Science 209:619, 1980.

Dobercznk TM, Shanzer S, Seine RJ, et al: Neonatal neruologic and electroencephalographic effects of intrauterine cocaine exposure. J Pediatr 113:354, 1988.

Dole VP, Kreek MJ: Methadone plasma level: Sustained by a reservoir of drug in tissue. Proc Natl Acad Sci USA 70:10, 1973.

Egelko S, Galanter M, Edwards H, Marinelli K: Treatment of perinatal cocaine addiction: Use of the modified therapeutic community. Am J Drug Alcohol Abuse 22:185, 1996.

Elk R, Mangus LG, LaSoya RJ, et al: Behavioral interventions: Effective and adaptable for the treatment of pregnant cocaine-dependent women. J Drug Issues 27:625, 1997.

Ellenhorn M, Barceloux D: Medical Toxicology. New York, Elsevier Science, 1988, pp 644–661.

Fantel AG, Macphail BJ: The teratogenicity of cocaine. Teratology 26:17, 1982.

Farkas KJ, Parran TV: Treatment of cocaine addiction during pregnancy. Clin Perinatol 20:29, 1993.

Farrar HC, Kearns GL: Cocaine: Clinical pharmacology and toxicology. J Pediatr 115:665–675, 1989.

Finnegan LP et al: Neonatal abstinence syndrome: Assessment and pharmacotherapy. *In* Rubaltelli FF, Garnati B (eds): National Therapy: An Update. New York, Excerpta Medica, 1986.

Finnegan LP, Kandall SR: Maternal and neonatal effects of alcohol and drugs. *In* Lowinson JH, Ruiz P, Millman RB, et al (eds): Substance Abuse: A Comprehensive Textbook. Baltimore, Williams & Wilkins, 1992, pp 628–656.

Finnegan LP, Hagan T, Kaltenbach KL: Scientific foundation of clinic practice: Opiate use in pregnant women. Bull N Y Acad Med 67:223, 1991.

Finnegan P: Effects of maternal opiate abuse on the newborn. Symposium, Drug Toxicity in the Newborn. April 5, 1984.

Frank DA, Zuckerman BS, Amaro H, et al: Cocaine use during pregnancy: Prevalence and correlates. Pediatrics 82:888, 1988.

Fricker HS, Segal S: Narcotic addiction, pregnancy and newborn. Am J Dis Child 132:360, 1978.

Fried PA, Mankin JE: Neontal behavioral correlates of prenatal exposure to marijuana, cigarettes, and alcohol in a low-risk population. Neurotoxicol Teratol 9:1, 1987.

Fried PA, O'Connell CM: A comparison of the effects of prenatal exposure to tobacco, alcohol, cannabis and caffeine on birth size and subsequent growth. Neurotoxicol Teratol 9:79, 1987.

Fried PA, Watkinson B: 12- and 24-month neurobehavioral follow-up of children prenatally exposed to marijuana, cigarettes and alcohol. Neurotoxicol Teratol 10:305, 1988.

Fried PA, Watkinson B: 36- and 48-month neurobehavioral follow-up of children prenatally exposed to marijuana, cigarettes, and alcohol. Neurotoxicol Teratol 11:49, 1990.

Fried PA, Watkinson B, Grant A, et al: Changing patterns of soft drug use prior to and during pregnancy: A prospective study. Drug Alcohol Dependence 6:323, 1980.

Fried PA, Watkinson B, William A: Marijuana use during pregnancy and length of gestation. Am J Obstet Gynecol 150:23, 1984.

Friedler G, Cochin J: Growth retardation in offspring of female rats treated with morphine prior to conception. Science 175:654, 1972.

Fulroth R, Phillips B, Durand DJ: Perinatal outcome of infants exposed to cocaine and or heroin in utero. Am J Dis Child 143:905, 1989.

Gibson GT, Baghurst PA: Maternal alcohol, tobacco and cannabis consumption and outcome of pregnancy. Aust N Z J Obstet Gynecol 23:15, 1983.

Gillogley KM, Evans AT, Hansen RL, et al: The perinatal impact of cocaine, amphetamine and opiate use detected by universal intrapartum screening. Am J Obstet Gynecol 163:1535, 1990.

Glass L, Evans EE: Physiological effects of intrauterine exposure to narcotics. *In* Rementeria JL (ed): Drug Abuse in Pregnancy and Neonatal Effects. St. Louis, CV Mosby, 1997, pp 108–115.

Glass L, Rajegowda BK, Evans HF: Absence of respiratory distress syndrome in premature infants of heroin-addicted mothers. Lancet 2:685, 1971.

Glass L, Rajegowda BK, Mukherjee TK, et al: Effects of heroin on corticosteroid production in pregnant addicts and their fetuses. Am J Obstet Gynecol 117:416, 1973.

Gold MS, Pottash ALC, Extein I: Clonidine in acute opiate withdrawal. N Engl J Med 302:1421, 1980.
Griffith DR, Azuma SD, Chasnoff IJ: Three-year outcome of children exposed prenatally to drugs. J Am Acad Child Adolesc Psychiatry 33:20, 1994.
Hack M, Breslau N, Weissman B, et al: Effect of very low birth weight and subnormal head size on cognitive abilities at school age. N Engl J Med 325:231, 1991.
Hadeed AJ, Siegel SR: Maternal cocaine use during pregnancy: Effect on the newborn infant. Pediatrics 84:205, 1989.
Hamburg M, Tallman JF: Chronic morphine administration increases the apparent number of alpha-2-adrenergic receptors in rat brain. Nature 291:493, 1981.
Handler A, Kistin N, Davis F, et al: Cocaine use during pregnancy. Perinatal outcomes. Am J Epidemiol 133:818, 1991.
Harper RG, Solish GI, Puow HM, et al: The effect of methadone treatment program upon heroin addicts and their newborn infants. Pediatrics 54:300, 1974.
Hatch EE, Brack MB: Effect of marijuana use in pregnancy on fetal growth. Am J Epidemiol 124:986, 1986.
Hawley TL, Halle TG, Drasin, RE, et al: Children of addicted mothers: Effect of the 'crack epidemic' on the caregiving environment and the development of preschoolers. Am J Orthopsychiatry 65:364, 1995.
Hayes JS, Dreher M: Newborn outcome with maternal marijuana use in Jamaican women. Pediatr Nurs 14:107, 1988.
Hayes JS, Lampert R, Dreher MC, et al: Five-year follow-up of rural Jamaican children whose mothers used marijuana during pregnancy. West Ind Med J 40:120, 1991.
Heier LA, Carpanzano CR, Mast J, et al: Maternal cocaine abuse: The spectrum of radiologic abnormalities in the neonatal CNS. Am J Neuroradiol 12:951, 1991.
Hickey JE, Suess PW, Newlin DB, et al: Vagal tone regulation during sustained attention in boys exposed to opiates in utero. Addict Behav 2:43, 1995.
Hill RM, Tennyson LM: Maternal drug therapy: Effect on fetal and neonatal growth and neurobehavior. Neurotoxicology 7:121, 1986.
Hingson R, Alpert JJ, Day N, et al: Effects of maternal drinking and marijuana use on fetal growth and development. Pediatrics 70:539, 1982.
Hoegerman G, Schnoll S: Narcotic use in pregnancy. Clin Perinatol 18:51, 1991.
Howard J, Beckwith L, Espinosa M, Tyler R: Development of infants born to cocaine-abusing women: Biologic/maternal influences. Neurotoxicol Teratol 17:403, 1995.
Howard J, Beckwith L, Rodning C, et al: The development of young children of substance-abusing parents: Insights from seven years of intervention and research. Subst Abuse Fam 9:1564, 1989.
Hutchings DE: Methadone and heroin during pregnancy: A review of behavioral effects in human and animal offspring. Neurobehav Toxicol Teratol 4:429, 1982.
The impact of acquired immunodeficiency syndrome on drug abuse treatment. Drug Abuse and Drug Abuse Research. The Third Triennial Report to Congress from the Secretary, Department of Health and Human Services, pp 48–60.
Italian Multicenter Study: Epidemiology, clinical features, and prognostic factors of pediatric HIV infection. Lancet 2:1043, 1988.
Jasinski DR, Johnson RE, Kocher TE: Clonidine in morphine withdrawal: Differential effects on signs and symptoms. Archiv Gen Psychiatry 42:1063, 1985.
Johnson LH, Diano, A, Rosen TS: 24-month neurobehavioral follow-up of children of methadone maintained mothers. Infant Behav Dev 7:115, 1984.
Jones RT: The pharmacology of cocaine. NIDA Res Monogr 50:34, 1984.
Limitations of neurologic and behavioral assessments in the newborn infant. In Gluck L (ed): Intrauterine Asphyxia and the Developing Fetal Brain. Chicago, 1978, pp 431–432.
Kaltenbach K, Graziani LJ, Finnegan LP: Pediatr Res 12:372, 1978.
Kaltenbach K, Graziani LJ, Finnegan LP: Methadone exposure in utero: Developmental status at one and two years of age. Pharmacol Biochem Behav 11(suppl):15, 1979.

Kandall SR, Albin S, Lowinson J, et al: Differential effects of maternal heroin and methadone use on birth weight. Pediatrics 58:681, 1976.
Kron RE, Finnegan LP, Kaplan SL: The assessment of behavioral change in infants undergoing narcotic withdrawal: Comparative data from clinical and objective methods. Addict Dis 2:257, 1975.
Kendall SR, Gartner LM: Late presentation of drug withdrawal symptoms in newborn. Am J Dis Child 127:58, 1974.
Kendall SR, Gaines J, Habel L, et al: Relationship of maternal substance abuse to subsequent SIDS in offspring. J Pediatr 23:120, 1993.
Kitchen WH, Doyle LW, Ford GW, et al: Very low birth weight and growth to age 8 years. II: Head dimension and intelligence. Am J Dis Child 146:46, 1992.
Kleber HD: Approaches in the treatment of cocaine abusers. Cocaine: A symposium. Sponsored by the Wisconsin Institute on Drug Abuse, 1990, pp 54–58.
Koob, GF: Drug addiction: The yin and yang of hedonic homeostasis. Neuron, 16:893, 1996.
Kramer LD, Locke GE, Ogunyemi A, et al: Neonatal cocaine-related seizures. J Child Neurol 5:60, 1990.
Kreek MJ: Goals and rationale for pharmacotherapeutic approach in treating cocaine dependence: Insights from basic and clinical research. NIDA Research Monograph. 175:5, 1997.
Kron RE, Litt M, Phoenix MD, Finnegan LP: Neonatal narcotic abstinence: Effects of pharmacotherapeutic agents and maternal drug usage on nutritive sucking behavior. J Pediatr 88:637, 1976.
Lam SK, To WK, Duthie SJ, Ma HK: Narcotic addiction in pregnancy with adverse maternal and perinatal outcome. Aust N Z J Obstet Gynecol 32:216, 1992.
Landry DW, Yang GX: Anti-cocaine catalytic antibodies: A novel approach to the problem of addiction. Addiction 91:1699, 1996.
Lester, BM, Corwin MJ, Sepkoski C, et al: Neurobehavioral syndromes in cocaine-exposed newborn infants. Child Dev 62:694, 1991.
Lester BM, Dreher M: Effects of marijuana use during pregnancy on newborn cry. Child Dev 60:765, 1989.
Lifschitz MH, Wilson GS, Smith EO, et al: Fetal and postnatal growth of children born to narcotic dependent women. J Pediatr 102:686, 1983.
Lipsitz PJ, Blatman S:Newborn infants of mothers on methadonic maintenance. NY State J Med 74:994, 1974.
Ling W, Klett CJ, Gillis RP: A cooperative study on methadryl acetate. Arch Gen Psychiatry 35:345, 1978.
Little BB, Snell LM, Palmore MK, et al: Cocaine use in pregnant women in a large public hospital. Am J Perinatol 5:206, 1988.
Lodge A, Marcus MM, Ramer CM: Part II. Behavioral and electrophysiological characteristics of the addicted neonate. Addict Dis 2:235, 1975.
Macgregor SN, Keith LG, Chasnoff IJ, et al: Cocaine use during pregnancy: Adverse perinatal outcome. Am J Obstet Gynecol 157:686, 1987.
Madden JD: Problems pertaining to care of newborn infants of drug addicted women. J Reprod Med 20:303, 1978.
Martin JC, Barr HM, Martin DC, et al: Neonatal neurobehavioral outcome following prenatal exposure to cocaine. Neurotoxicol Teratol 18:617, 1996.
McCance EF: Overview of potential treatment medications for cocaine dependence. NIDA Res Monogr 175:36, 1997.
McCartney JS, Fried PA: Prenatal cigarette exposure and central auditory processing abilities in 6 to 11-year-old children. Teratology 47:456, 1993.
Metosky P, Vondra J: Prenatal drug exposure and play and coping in toddlers: A comparison study. Infant Behav Dev 18:15, 1995.
Miller JM, Boudreaux MC, Regan FA: A case-control study of cocaine use in pregnancy. Am J Obstet Gynecol 172:180, 1995.
Mitchell JL, Consensus Panel Chair: Pregnant, Substance Abusing Women. Rockville, MD, US Department of Health and Human Services (Center for Substance Abuse Treatment), 1993.
Mofenson HC, Caraccio TR: Cocaine. Pediatr Ann 17:864, 1987.
Moore T, Sorg J, Miller L, et al: Hemodynamic effects of intravenous cocaine on the pregnant ewe and fetus. Am J Obstet Gynecol 155:883–888, 1986.
Naeye RL, Blanc W, Leblanc W, et al: Fetal complications of maternal heroin addiction, abnormal growth, infections, and episodes of stress. J Pediatr 83:1055, 1973.

Newman RG, Bashkow S, Calko D:Results of 313 consecutive live births of infants delivered to patients in New York City methadone maintenance treatment program. Am J Obstet Gynecol 121:233, 1975.

O'Brien WB, Devlin CJ: In Lowinson JH, Ruiz P, Millman RB (eds): Substance Abuse: A Comprehensive Textbook, 3rd ed. Baltimore, Williams & Wilkins, 1997, pp 400–429.

O'Connell CM, Fried PA: An investigation of prenatal cannabis exposure and minor physical anomalies in the low-risk population. Neurobehav Toxicol Teratol 6:345, 1984.

ORLAAM Product Labeling. Roxane Laboratories, Inc. Columbus, Ohio.

Ornoy A, Michaelevkaya V, Lukashov I, et al: The developmental outcome of children born to heroin-dependent mothers, raised at home or adopted. Child Abuse Neglect 10:385, 1996.

Oro AS, Dixon SD: Perinatal cocaine and methamphetamine exposure: Maternal and neonatal correlates. J Pediatr 111:571, 1987.

Ostrea EM: Meconium drug analysis in mothers' babies and cocaine. In Lewis M, Bendarsky M (eds): The Role of Toxins in Development. Hillsdale, NJ, Erlbaum Associates, 1995.

Ostrea EM Jr, Brady M, Gause S, et al: Drug screening of newborns by meconium analysis: A large-scale, prospective, epidemiologic study. Pediatrics 89:107, 1992.

Ostrea EM, Chavez CJ: Perinatal problems (excluding neonatal withdrawal) in maternal drug addiction: A study of 830 cases. J Pediatr 94:292, 1979.

Paluzzi PA, Emerling J, Leiva P, et al: Impact of enhanced model of prenatal care for substance abusers in a comprehensive treatment program. In Harris LS (ed): Problems of Drug Dependence, 1994: Proceedings of the 56th Annual Scientific Meeting, The College on Problems of Drug Dependence, Inc., vol. 2: Abstracts 181. Washington, DC, NIDA Research Monograph, 1995.

Payte JT, Khure ET: Principles of methadone dose determination. In State Methadone Treatment Guidelines, vol 1. Rockville, MD, Center for Substance Abuse Treatment, Treatment Improvement Protocol Services, 1993, pp 45–58.

Pelosi MA, Frattarola H, Apuzzio J, et al: Pregnancy complicated by heroin addiction. Obstet Gynecol 45:512, 1975.

Perlmutter JF: Drug addiction in pregnant women. Obstet Gynecol 99:569, 1967.

Pettiti, D, Coleman, C: Cocaine and the risk of low birth weight. Am J Public Health 80:25, 1990.

Pond SM, Kreek MJ, Tong TG: Altered methadone pharmacokinetics in methadone maintained pregnant women. J Pharmacol Exp Ther 233:1, 1985.

Quazi QH, Mriano E: Abnormalities in offspring associated with prenatal marijuana exposure. Dev Pharmacol Ther, 8:141, 1985.

Rajegowda BA, Glass L, Evans HE, et al: Methadone withdrawal in newborn infants. J Pediatr 81:532, 1972.

Randall P: Cocaine and alcohol mix in body to form even longer lasting, more lethal drug. JAMA 267:1043, 1992.

Reddy AM, Harper RG, Stern G: Observations on heroin and methadone withdrawal in newborns. Pediatrics 48:353, 1971.

Rementeria JL, Janakammal S, Hollander M: Multiple births in drug-addicted women. Am J Obstet Gynecol 122:958, 1975.

Rementeria JL, Nunag NN: Narcotic withdrawal in pregnancy: Stillbirth incidence with a case report. Am J Obstet Gynecol 116:1152, 1973.

Richardson GA, Conroy ML, Day, NL: Prenatal cocaine exposure: Effects on the development of school-age children. Neurotoxicol Teratol 18:627, 1996.

Richardson GA, Day NL, Taylor PM: The effect of prenatal alcohol, marijuana and tobacco exposure on neonatal behavior. Infant Behav Dev 12:199, 1989.

Roe DA, Little BB, Bawdon RE, Gilstrap LC: Metabolism of cocaine by human placentas: Implications for fetal exposure. Am J Obstet Gynecol 163:715, 1990.

Rosenberg K, Bateman DM, Des Jarlais DC: Underestimating cocaine use during pregnancy. Am J Public Health 87:687, 1997.

Rosner MA, Keith L, Chasanoff I: The Northwestern University Drug Dependence Program: The impact of intensive prenatal care on labor and delivery outcome. Am J Obstet Gynecol 144:23, 1982.

Ryan L, Ehrlich S, Finnegan L: Cocaine abuse in pregnancy: Effects on the fetus and newborn. Neurotoxicol Teratol 9:295, 1987.

Salerno LJ: Prenatal care: In Rementeria JL (ed): Drug Abuse in Pregnancy and Neonatal Effects. St Louis, CV Mosby, 1977, p 19.

Sallee FR, Katikaneni LP, McArthur PD, et al: Head growth in cocaine-exposed infants: Relationship to neonate hair level. Dev Behav Pediatr 16:77, 1995.

Sardemann H, Madsen KS, Friis-Hansan B: Follow-up of children of drug-addicted mothers. Arch Dis Child 51:131, 1976.

Schweitzer IL, Dunn AE, Peter RL, et al: Viral hepatitis B in neonates and infants. Am J Med 55:762, 1973.

Shih L, Cone-Wesson B, Reddix B: Effects of maternal cocaine abuse on the neonatal auditory system. Int J Pediatr Otorhinolaryngol 15:245, 1988.

Shiraki K, Yoshihara N, Kawana T, et al: Hepatitis B surface antigen and chronic hepatitis in infants born to asymptomatic carrier mothers. Am J Dis Child 131:644, 1977.

Sofia RD, Strasbaugh JE, Banerjee BN: Teratologic evaluation of synthetic Δ9-THC in rabbits. Teratology 19:361, 1979.

Sokol RJ, Martier S, Ager J, et al: Evidence of lack of brain-sparing associated with prenatal cocaine exposure. Presented SGI, San Antonio, Texas, March, 1991.

Spence MR, Williams R, Di Gregorio GJ, et al: The relationships between recent cocaine use and pregnancy outcome. Obstet Gynecol 78:326, 1991.

Stern R: The pregnant addict. Am J Obstet Gynecol 94:253, 1966.

Stewart DJ, Inaba T, Lucassen M, Kalow W: Cocaine metabolism: Cocaine and norcocaine hydrolysis by liver and serum esterase. Clin Pharmacol Ther 25:464, 1979.

Stewart Woods NS, Eyler FD, Behnke M, Conlon M: Cocaine use during pregnancy: Maternal depressive symptoms and infant neurobehavior over the first month. Infant Behav Dev 16:83, 1993.

Stimmel B, Goldberg J, Reaiman A, et al: Fetal outcome in narcotic-dependent women: The importance of the type of maternal narcotic used. Am J Drug Alcohol Abuse 9:383, 1983.

Stone ML, Salerno LJ, Green M, et al: Narcotic addiction in pregnancy. Am J Obstet Gynecol 109:716, 1971.

Strauss ME, Andresko MA, Stryker JC, et al: Methadone maintenance during pregnancy: Pregnancy, birth and neonate characteristics. Am J Obstet Gynecol 120:895, 1974.

Strauss ME, Lessen-Firestone JK, Chavez CJ, et al: Children of methadone-treated women at 5 years of age. Pharmacol Biochem Behav 11(suppl):3, 1979.

Strauss ME, Starr RH, Ostrea EM, et al: Behavioral concomitants of prenatal addiction to narcotics. J Pediatr 89:842, 1976.

Streissguth AP, Barr HM, Sampson PD, et al: IQ at age 4 in relation to maternal alcohol use and smoking during pregnancy. Dev Psychol 25:3, 1989.

Tennes K, Avitable N, Blackard C, et al: Marijuana prenatal and postnatal exposure in the human. NIDA Research Monograph 59:1400, 1985.

Treatment lacking for pregnant addicts (Editorial). Science 247:285, 1990.

Treatment of morphine-type dependency by withdrawal methods (Editorial). JAMA 219:1161, 1972.

Tronick EZ, Frank DA, Cabral H, et al: Late dose-response effects of prenatal cocaine exposure on newborn neurobehavioral performance. Pediatrics 98:76, 1996.

Umans JG, Szeto HH: Precipitated opiate abstinence in utero. Am J Obstet Gynecol 151:441, 1985.

van de Bor M, Walther, FJ, Sims ME: Brain-stem transmission time in infants exposed to cocaine in utero. J Pediatr 85:733, 1990.

Vining E, Kosten TR, Kleber HD: Clinical reliability of rapid clonidine-naltrexone detoxification for opioid abusers. Br J Addict 83:567, 1988.

Warner EA, Kosten TR, O'Connor PG: Pharmacotherapy for opioid and cocaine abuse. Pharmacol Biochem Behav 57:551, 1997.

Washton AM, Gold MS, Pottash AC, et al: Adolescent abusers. Lancet 2:764, 1984.

Washton AM, Resnick RB, Geyer G: Opiate withdrawal using

lofexidine, a clonidine analog with fewer side effects. J Clin Psychiatr 44:335, 1983.

Wasserman DR, Leventhal JM: Maltreatment of children born to cocaine-dependent mothers. Am J Dis Child 147:1324, 1993.

Wilson GS: Clinical studies of infants and children exposed prenatally to heroin. Ann NY Acad Sci 562:183, 1989.

Wilson GS, Desmond MM, Verniaud WM: Early development of infants of heroin addicted mothers. Am J Dis Child 126:45, 1973.

Wilson GS, Desmond M, Wait RB: Follow-up of methadone-treated and untreated narcotic-dependent women and their infants: Health, developmental, and social implications. J Pediatr 98:716, 1981.

Wilson GS, McCreary R, Kean J, et al: The development of preschool children of heroin addicted mothers: A controlled study. Pediatrics 63:135, 1979.

Wong WM, Lao TT: Abnormal unbilical artery flow velocity waveform: A sign of fetal narcotic withdrawal? Aust N Z J Obstet Gynecol 37:358, 1997.

Woods JR, Pressinger MA: Pregnancy increases cardiovascular toxicity to cocaine. Am J Obstet Gynecol 162:529, 1990.

Zelson C, Rubio E, Wasserman E: Neonatal narcotic addiction: Ten year observation. Pediatrics 48:178–189, 1971.

Zelson C, Sook JL, Casalino M: Neonatal narcotic addiction. N Engl J Med 289:1216, 1973.

Zuckerman B, Amoro H, Cabral H: The validity of self-report of marijuana and cocaine use among pregnant adolescents. J Pediatr 115:812, 1989.

Zuckerman B, Frank DA, Hingson R, et al: Effects of maternal marijuana and cocaine use on fetal growth. N Engl J Med 320:762, 1989.

# 39

# Infections in Pregnancy

TRACY COWLES
BERNARD GONIK

Infection of the female urogenital tract is not an uncommon complication of pregnancy. Responsible organisms include a vast array of viruses, bacteria, and parasites. As in most gynecologic infections, organisms complicating pregnancy tend to be polymicrobial.

Infectious complications during pregnancy lead to an increase in morbidity and mortality for both patients—the fetus and the mother. Premature rupture of the membranes (PROM), premature labor (PTL), and preterm birth (PTB) can be the result of infection. Pyelonephritis, endometritis, and sepsis are common examples of maternal morbidity. Neonatal infection, occurring when the immature immunologic system is less protective, may predispose to meningitis, pneumonia, sepsis, or death.

Early diagnosis and aggressive treatment of infection during pregnancy may substantially lower the associated morbidity and mortality. This chapter discusses common clinical disorders and specific infectious organisms that occur during pregnancy.

## Clinical Disorders

### URINARY TRACT INFECTION

Urinary tract infections (UTIs) are the most common medical complication of pregnancy. They may be classified as asymptomatic bacteriuria (ASB), cystitis, or pyelonephritis. ASB, defined as greater than 100,000 organisms in the urine of a patient who lacks symptoms, is present in approximately 5 to 10% of the pregnant population. The prevalence of bacteriuria is related to lower socioeconomic status, sickle cell trait or disease, and diabetes mellitus. *Escherichia coli* is by far the predominating organism (80 to 90%). *Proteus mirabilis, Klebsiella pneumoniae*, and group B β-hemolytic streptococci (GBS) are also commonly identified pathogens.

If untreated, 20 to 30% of women who have ASB will develop pyelonephritis. ASB is also associated with an increased risk of preterm birth and delivery of low birth weight infants. Appropriate screening for and treatment of ASB lower these risks significantly. The goal of antibiotic treatment for pregnant women with ASB is sterile urine for the remainder of the pregnancy. This is usually accomplished with a short course of sulfisoxazole, cephalexin, or nitrofurantoin and monthly culture surveillance. Recurrences are common (approximately one third of patients) and suppressive therapy with macrodantin is instituted after the culture is again cleared with a short course of antibiotic therapy.

Acute cystitis occurs in 1.3% of pregnancies and seems to be a separate clinical entity from ASB and acute pyelonephritis. Cystitis, unlike the other two, does not tend to be preceded by bacteriuria in the initial screening cultures, does not recur as frequently, and is not the result of upper tract involvement. The most common pathogen is *E. coli*, and antibiotic treatment with cephalexin, sulfonamides, or nitrofurantoin is appropriate.

The incidence of acute pyelonephritis during pregnancy is 1 to 2.5%, with an estimated recurrence rate of 10 to 18% during the same pregnancy. Clinical manifestations include fever, costovertebral angle tenderness, nausea, vomiting, and symptoms of lower UTI such as frequency, dysuria, and urgency. The pregnant patient may become quite ill with severe dehydration, transient renal dysfunction, respiratory distress, and septicemia.

The microbiology of pyelonephritis is similar to that described for lower tract disease in pregnancy. Initial antibiotic therapy includes the use of an aminoglycoside or an advanced generation penicillin or cephalosporin. Therapy can be tailored to the results of the urine culture when this information becomes available. Clinical response is usually rapid; 85% of patients show a decrease in temperature elevation within 48 hours. Recurrence of the pyelonephritis may be as high as 60% if suppressive antimicrobial therapy is not maintained throughout the duration of the pregnancy. Renal calculi and anatomic obstruction can be responsible for a failure to respond to otherwise effective antibiotic treatment. Sonography, limited exposure intravenous pyelography, or magnetic resonance imaging may be used to evaluate a patient who continues with fever or worsening symptoms.

# Preterm Labor and Premature Rupture of the Membranes

Prematurity complicates 7 to 10% of all births and is responsible for a disproportionately large fraction of perinatal morbidity and mortality. Although the mechanisms underlying PROM and PTL are imperfectly understood, it appears that infection and inflammation may cause 20 to 40% of preterm births. A variety of evidence supports these findings:

1. Histologic chorioamnionitis is more common in PTB
2. Clinical infection is increased in both infant and mother in cases of PTB
3. Several specific organisms are associated with PTB
4. Amniotic fluid cultures are positive in 10 to 15% of women who have PTI
5. Bacteria and bacterial products induce PTB in animal models
6. Antibiotics lower PTB in some studies

Antibiotics have been used in certain clinical situations to prevent PTB. It is fairly clear from the literature that appropriate treatment of *Neisseria gonorrhoeae*, *Chlamydia trachomatis*, ASB, and bacterial vaginosis improves pregnancy outcome. It is less clear that treating group B streptococcus (GBs), *Trichomonas vaginalis*, or genital mycoplasmas decreases the risk of PTL or preterm PROM (PPROM).

Antibiotics have also been used in women with PTL, PROM, or both to attempt to prolong the pregnancy and to decrease maternal and neonatal morbidity and mortality. In the setting of PTL with intact membranes, antibiotic therapy does not consistently prolong the time until delivery, decrease maternal chorioamnionitis or endometritis, or decrease neonatal infectious morbidity. However, prophylaxis against neonatal GBS infection is indicated. If bacterial vaginosis or *T. vaginalis* is present, these should be treated appropriately.

Antibiotic therapy may be more useful in the patient with PPROM. Antibiotic prophylaxis to prevent neonatal GBS sepsis is indicated. There is now evidence that broader spectrum antibiotics may prolong the time from rupture of membranes until delivery. In addition, a decrease in chorioamnionitis and an improvement in neonatal outcomes, such as sepsis and intraventricular hemorrhage, may result. Protocols using ampicillin-amoxicillin plus erythromycin or ampicillin sulbactam followed by amoxicillin clavulanate have been studied.

# Intra-Amniotic Infection

Clinically evident intrauterine infection complicates 1 to 10% of pregnancies, leading to an increase in maternal morbidity and perinatal morbidity and mortality. The clinical diagnosis of intra-amniotic infection (IAI) is made on the basis of maternal fever, foul odor of the amniotic fluid, and leukocytosis. Ruptured membranes are invariably present and, along with fever and leukocytosis, are the most common findings. Uterine tenderness and foul-smelling amniotic fluid are more specific but are present in only a minority of cases.

Laboratory criteria likewise tend to be nonspecific. Peripheral blood leukocytosis commonly occurs in normal labor. Maternal bacteremia occurs in only 10% of patients. Positive Gram's stains and colony counts higher than $10^2$/ml of amniotic fluid are associated with clinical infection. However, in unselected patients who have ruptured membranes, bacteria are often demonstrated in the amniotic fluid despite a lack of clinical evidence of infection.

Before the rupture of membranes and labor, the amniotic cavity is almost always sterile. Instrumentation, such as amniocentesis, percutaneous umbilical sampling, and intrauterine transfusion can introduce bacteria into the previously sterile environment. Viral infection most commonly infects the fetus and amniotic fluid via hematogenous spread through the placenta and umbilical cord. *Listeria monocytogenes* may cause fulminant IAI by this route. The most likely route of infection associated with IAI, however, is the ascending route.

Recent studies have demonstrated that IAI is a polymicrobial infection, involving aerobic and anaerobic bacteria. Organisms include *Bacteroides* species, group B streptococcus, other streptococci, *Gardnerella vaginalis*, *E. coli*, and other gram-negative rods. *Chlamydia* does not seem to contribute to the incidence of IAI, although this possibility remains controversial.

Antibiotic therapy should be initiated after establishing the diagnosis of IAI. Broad-spectrum intravenous (IV) antibiotics, frequently ampicillin and an aminoglycoside, are given to limit maternal sepsis and initiate fetal therapy. Cesarean section, although more frequently performed in the presence of IAI, is undertaken only for obstetric indications. If cesarean section is undertaken, clindamycin or other agents with anaerobic coverage are added to the therapeutic regimen to reduce the risk of antibiotic failure during the postoperative period. Complications of maternal infection are more frequent after a cesarean section than after vaginal delivery and may include endometritis (up to 30%), wound infection (3 to 5%), sepsis (2 to 4%), pelvic abscess formation, and septic pelvic thrombophlebitis.

# Bacterial Vaginosis

Bacterial vaginosis (BV) is a common disorder in which there is a shift from the normal lactobacilli of the vagina to a high concentration of organisms, including *G. vaginalis*, a wide range of anaerobic organisms, and genital mycoplasmas. The classic clinical findings are present in Table 39–1. The prevalence of BV is approximately 10 to 30% in pregnant women, the majority of whom are asymptomatic. BV has been linked to adverse outcomes of pregnancy, including PTL, PROM, and chorioamnionitis. Evidence suggests that treatment of BV in pregnancies at risk for

**Table 39–1** Clinical Characteristics of Bacterial Vaginosis

- Gray-white homogeneous discharge
- Elevated pH of vaginal discharge >4.5
- Fishy amine odor on mixing discharge with 10% potassium hydroxide
- Clue cells on wet preparation

preterm birth improves pregnancy outcome. It is less clear that treatment in nonsymptomatic, low-risk pregnancies is helpful.

Metronidazole (500 mg twice a day for 7 days) is extremely effective in the treatment of nonpregnant women. Because of reported carcinogenicity in rodents and mutagenicity in bacteria, clinicians have been reluctant to use this drug during pregnancy, particularly during the first trimester. Intravaginal clindamycin cream and metronidazole gel have been efficacious. Treatment of the male partner does not alter the course of the disease or prevent recurrence.

# Viral Pathogens

## VARICELLA-ZOSTER

The varicella-zoster virus (VZV) is a member of the herpesvirus group. Exposure in childhood results in chickenpox, and 85 to 95% of young adults have developed an immunity to the virus. A total of 10 to 20% of adults experience a reactivation of the virus, developing the painful skin lesions of herpes zoster along one or two adjacent dermatomes, commonly called shingles.

VZV is a highly contagious virus, with an inoculation period of 13 to 17 days. Children usually experience a 2- to 3-day period in which pruritic vesicles cover the head, neck, and trunk. Adults compose only 2% of chickenpox cases but frequently have a more severe illness. They account for 25% of the mortality, which is primarily due to varicella pneumonia. Pregnant women may be at particularly high risk of death when they develop this complication and may benefit from the administration of acyclovir. A live attenuated varicella vaccine has been developed, but it is not currently recommended for use in pregnancy.

The incidence of varicella in pregnancy has been estimated at 5:10,000. Even when pregnant women give a negative or uncertain history of childhood varicella infection, serologic testing reveals that approximately 80% of them are immune to VZV.

Varicella-zoster immune globulin (VZIG) has been used in pregnant women who do not have antibody to VZV to prevent or modify the course of the disease. Administration within 96 hours after exposure is necessary. The ability of VZIG to block vertical transmission is unknown.

A congenital VZV syndrome has been described in infants born to mothers who were infected with the virus in the first trimester. The physical stigmas of the syndrome include scarred, dermatomal skin lesions with ipsilateral limb deformities and central nervous system (CNS) abnormalities, including intracranial calcifications, cortical and optic atrophy, and chorioretinitis. The frequency of defects consistent with congenital VZV syndrome after infection in the first trimester has been reported to range from 0 to 9%. There is no evidence that occurrence of this syndrome follows second- or third-trimester infection of varicella-zoster.

Congenital infection can occur without structural abnormalities. Fetuses exposed to varicella infection during the second half of pregnancy up to 21 days before delivery may develop zoster in infancy. Fetuses who were exposed between 6 and 20 days before delivery may benefit from transplacental passage of the maternal antibody and may display minimal evidence of chickenpox at birth. Infants delivered to mothers who develop varicella less than 5 days before or up to 2 days after delivery are at much higher risk. Lacking passively acquired maternal antibody, these infants have a 15 to 30% chance of manifesting congenital varicella infection. Immediate administration of ZVIG and acyclovir to these infants may lower their mortality rate to less than 10%.

## Rubella

Before the introduction of the vaccination in 1969, rubella was a common childhood infection, with 85% of young adults demonstrating immunity. Epidemics occurred at 6- to 9-year intervals, with major pandemics every 10 to 30 years. Maternal rubella infection early in pregnancy frequently results in fetal malformations consistent with the congenital rubella syndrome (CRS). The epidemiology of this infection has changed with the licensure of the vaccine; cases of both rubella and CRS have decreased dramatically.

The rubella infection is subclinical in 30% of adults. Symptomatic disease occurs 14 to 21 days after infection. A mild course of fever and malaise accompanied by rash and lymphadenopathy is typically present. Diagnosis on clinical grounds is difficult; serologic confirmation of a fourfold increase in antibody titer is required.

Fetal infection can occur after an instance of maternal rubella viremia at any stage of pregnancy. Prospective studies of women who have confirmed rubella during pregnancy show that the risk of congenital infection varies from 80% in the first 12 weeks to 30% with exposure at 23 to 30 weeks and 100% if exposed during the last month of pregnancy. Multiple defects occur after very early exposure; almost every fetus exposed during the first month of pregnancy develops abnormally. Full-blown CRS includes sensorineural hearing loss, mental retardation, cardiac malformations, and ocular defects. Delayed manifestations of CRS can occur, including insulin-dependent diabetes mellitus, thyroid disease, and encephalopathy. Deafness and eye abnormalities not evident at birth can develop.

Despite recommendations for universal immunization, it is estimated that as many as 20% of women of reproductive age in the United States are seronegative for rubella. The live attenuated vaccine should not be administered for 3 months before conception or during pregnancy because of theoretical fetal risks. No vaccine-related cases of CRS have been reported, although there is a small risk of congenital infection (0 to 2%).

Because of the high percentage of pregnancies affected after exposure to rubella infection, counseling regarding the termination of pregnancy should be offered. Congenital infection can be demonstrated by reverse transcription-nested polymerase chain reaction (PCR) or detection of fetal serum immunoglobulin (IgG) after 22 to 24 weeks of gestation.

## Herpes Simplex Virus

Herpes simplex virus (HSV) infections are common and can be grouped into two serologic subtypes, HSV-1 and HSV-2. The most common clinical manifestations of HSV-1 are orolabial lesions, although this virus may be responsible for 15 to 20% of genital infections. The most common infection caused by HSV-2 is genital herpes.

It is estimated that more than 500,000 new cases occur annually, contributing to a pool of more than 30 million cases. Seroepidemiologic studies of obstetric populations show that antibody to HSV-2 is present in 17 to 46% of patients, depending on the population source.

The clinical manifestations of genital HSV infection may occur as one of three syndromes. Primary infection is usually associated with multiple painful genital vesicles, which proceed to an ulcerative stage frequently accompanied by inguinal adenopathy. Systemic symptoms include fever, malaise, myalgias, headache, and nausea. A first-episode, nonprimary infection occurs when the first clinical episode of HSV appears in a patient who has existing antibodies to HSV-1 or HSV-2. The clinical course is similar to that of recurrent disease. Recurrent disease can occur more frequently after HSV-2 infections. Mild local lesions occur and last about half as long as initial lesions. Systemic manifestations are absent. Asymptomatic shedding of the virus is not uncommon.

Transplacental infection is rarely reported. Primary HSV infections during the first trimester seem to increase the frequency of spontaneous abortions, stillbirths, and prematurity. The major risk of infection for the neonate is intrapartum exposure to an infected birth canal. This risk is particularly increased in women who acquire the infection shortly before delivery. Approximately 40% of infants delivered in this situation become infected, resulting in high rates of mortality and neurologic sequelae. Of infants delivered vaginally, approximately 5% in the presence of overt lesions and less than 1% exposed to asymptomatic shedding are infected. A cesarean section, performed as soon as possible after rupture of membranes, has been recommended to minimize viral exposure during an active HSV infection. However, cesarean delivery decreases the risk of neonatal infection even when it has been hours or days since rupture of membranes. In the absence of prodromal symptomatology or genital lesions (with careful inspection), vaginal delivery should be allowed.

Studies of the use of acyclovir to suppress HSV recurrence at term, thus decreasing the rate of cesarean section, have been undertaken. Using acyclovir in this manner may be particularly helpful in patients whose pregnancies are complicated by primary herpes infection. The Centers for Disease Control (CDC) does not currently recommend acyclovir therapy for this indication; therefore, individual patients should be counseled regarding potential risks and benefits. A registry has been established by the manufacturer, and no increase in the rate of birth defects has been found in women receiving the drug during pregnancy.

## Cytomegalovirus

Cytomegalovirus (CMV) is a ubiquitous virus that infects most people in their lifetime. In adults, primary infection is usually asymptomatic. Reactivation of latent infection can occur with viral shedding. The virus can be transmitted to the fetus after primary or recurrent infection.

CMV acquisition rates vary inversely with socioeconomic status. Seroepidemiologic studies in the United States indicate that 50 to 60% of pregnant middle-class women have antibodies to CMV, compared with 70 to 85% of those from lower socio-economic groups. Approximately 2 to 2.5% of susceptible women acquire CMV infection during pregnancy.

Seroconversion is the best demonstration of primary infection. Demonstration of IgM indicates primary infection within the previous 60 days. A single positive IgG antibody titer does not necessarily indicate primary infection. Even rising titers do not readily distinguish primary from recurrent infection because antibody titers can transiently rise in these circumstances.

Vertical transmission can occur after either primary or recurrent CMV infection. A total of 1 to 2% of all infants born in the United States have documented congenital infection. Congenital CMV infection occurs in 30 to 40% of infants born to mothers experiencing primary CMV infection during pregnancy. The rate of transmission after recurrent infection is probably similar to that of primary disease, although the percentage of infants who are symptomatic at birth or who develop serious sequelae is much lower.

Of infants born with CMV infection, 10% are symptomatic at birth. Infant mortality in this group is 20 to 30%, and most suffer long-term serious sequelae. Hepatosplenomegaly, microcephaly, optic abnormalities, intellectual impairment, and sensorineural hearing loss occur. Most infants (>90%) identified at birth as being infected are asymptomatic. Approximately 15 to 25% of these infants may suffer late sequelae, including neurologic abnormalities, sensorineural hearing loss, and mental retardation.

Prenatal diagnosis can be made on the basis of abnormal ultrasonographic findings and PCR or culture evidence of CMV in amniotic fluid samples. Specific treatment is not available and routine screening is not indicated.

## Hepatitis

Hepatitis A virus (HAV) is an RNA virus that is responsible for approximately 30 to 35% of cases of acute hepatitis. Infection produces a mild, self-limiting illness that does not result in a chronic carrier state. Transmission is by an oral-fecal route; parenteral transmission is rare. Infection with HAV does not seem to increase the risk of adverse pregnancy outcome. Although perinatal transmission has not been documented, administration of immunoglobulin to neonates born within 2 weeks of maternal illness is recommended.

Hepatitis C virus (HCV) is responsible for 20 to 40% of all hepatitis and accounts for up to 90% of posttransfusion hepatitis. Infection is asymptomatic in 65 to 75% of patients; 25% of patients are icteric and 10% become quite ill. Chronic hepatitis develops in 70%, with 35% progressing to cirrhosis and 20 to 25% developing hepatocellular carcinoma over 20 to 30 years. Vertical transmission occurs, with rates of 0 to 18% reported in HIV-negative and 6 to 36% in HIV-positive pregnant women. The majority of children thus infected develop chronic hepatitis. Postexposure immunoglobulin seems to offer little protection to newborns; an effective HCV vaccine has not been developed. α-Interferon-2b has been shown to clear the virus in 40 to 50% of infected patients.

Hepatitis E (HEV) is responsible for outbreaks of enterally acquired hepatitis in developing countries. Although many cases remain subclinical, the case fatality rate is higher (1 to 2%) than that seen with

HAV (1 to 2:1000). A chronic carrier state and perinatal transmission do not appear to occur.

Hepatitis B virus (HBV) accounts for 40 to 50% of hepatitis cases in the United States. Acute infection occurs in 1 to 2:1000 pregnancies and chronic infection complicates 0.5 to 1.5% of pregnancies. The incubation period for acute HBV varies from 45 to 150 days. At least 50% of healthy adults and children are asymptomatic. Symptoms can include anorexia, malaise, weakness, and abdominal pain. Clinical signs include jaundice, icterus, hepatic tenderness, and weight loss. The acute course usually runs 3 to 4 weeks, but symptoms may persist up to 6 months.

The diagnosis of HBV is based on serologic markers. Surface antigen (HBsAg) is the first marker to appear in acute infection and is present before the onset of clinical symptoms. At about the same time, e antigen (HBeAg) appears. This antigen disappears before clinical symptoms resolve and is usually followed by the antibody (anti-HBe). Antibody to the surface antigen (anti-HBs) appears during the convalescent period, and high titers are an indication of immunity. The core antigen (HBcAg) is not present in serum in sufficient quantities to be clinically useful. The antibody to HBcAg is typically present in the window between detectable HBsAg and anti-HBs.

Approximately 10% of patients with acute HBV infection become chronic carriers. These patients fail to develop anti-HBs and the HBsAg persists. In chronic active infection, HBeAg may persist for years, followed by the gradual seroconversion to anti-HBe. Asymptomatic carriers are characterized by the presence of HBsAg and anti-HBc; liver function tests are normal.

The transmission rate of HBV from mother to infant varies with the clinical setting. Most evidence suggests that the neonate is infected at the time of delivery as a consequence of exposure to contaminated blood and genital tract secretions. Infants who are seronegative at birth convert after an incubation period of 2 to 4 months. Women who are infected in the third trimester have an increased chance (up to 75%) of passing the virus to their infants. The most predictive marker for vertical transmission is the HBeAg; when this antigen is present, the transmission rate reaches 80 to 90%. In chronic carriers, the additional presence of anti-HBe drops the transmission rate to 10 to 20%.

Most hepatitis infections in infants are asymptomatic. Most infants who are infected at birth become chronic carriers of HBsAg. Many develop adverse sequelae, including cirrhosis, chronic active hepatitis, and primary hepatocellular carcinoma.

The CDC and the American College of Obstetrics and Gynecology advocate routine screening of all patients at their first antepartum visit and perhaps repeat screening during the third trimester of those in especially high-risk situations. The prevention of neonatal hepatitis depends on the prompt administration of immunoglobulin and hepatitis B vaccination. The CDC now recommends immunization of all infants. Pregnancy is not a contraindication to vaccination or administration of hepatitis B immunoglobulin in those at risk of infection.

## Bacterial Pathogens

### GONORRHEA

*N. gonorrhoeae*, a gram-negative diplococcus, is most commonly found in the urogenital tract but can infect the pharynx and conjunctiva and, when disseminated, causes sepsis and arthritis. It is a common disease of women of reproductive age, and is especially prevalent in the 15- to -19-year-old age group.

Gonococcal infections in pregnant women tend to be asymptomatic. Most common symptoms when noted are vaginal discharge and dysuria. Cervical cultures are recommended at the first prenatal visit and repeat cultures in the high-risk patient in the third trimester would be appropriate. The CDC recommendation for treatment reflects the increasing identification of penicillinase-producing *N. gonorrhoeae* species. A single dose of ceftriaxone, 125 mg intramuscularly, or cefixime, 400 mg orally, and then erythromycin base, 250 mg four times a day for 7 days, has been recommended. This antibiotic regimen also treats the frequently (40 to 60%) concomitant chlamydial infections.

Untreated maternal endocervical gonococcal infection has been associated with perinatal complications, such as prematurity, PROM, and IUGR. These associations are controversial; gonorrheal infection may simply be a marker for other confounding variables associated with poor pregnancy outcome. Neonatal conjunctivitis and postpartum endometritis can be caused by gonorrhea.

## Group B Streptococcal Infection

GBS is an important cause of maternal and neonatal infection. Asymptomatic vaginal colonization with GBS occurs in 15 to 40% of pregnant women. Colonization can be transient, making vaginal culture in the midtrimester an imperfect predictor of culture status at delivery.

Although approximately two thirds of infants born to colonized mothers become asymptomatic colonized carriers themselves, only one symptomatic GBS infection occurs for every 100 colonized infants. Symptomatic infection is divided into early onset, with symptoms present at birth or shortly thereafter (incidence 1.3 to 3:1000 live births), and late onset, with symptoms appearing more than 7 days after delivery (incidence 1 to 1.7:1000 live births). Early-onset disease is characterized by sepsis and overwhelming pneumonia. Mortality in term infants is 10 to 20%; the preterm mortality rate is three to four times higher. Late-onset disease begins more insidiously between 1 and 12 weeks of life. The majority of these infants develop meningitis, and half may suffer long-term sequelae.

Three factors play a particularly important role in symptomatic GBS in the newborn: prematurity, PROM, and intrapartum fever. There is an approximately 10- to 15-fold increase in the risk of early-onset GBS infection in preterm infants.

Intrapartum maternal fever is indicative of IAI, which is frequently associated with GBS infection. Postpartum endometritis, characterized by high fever, tachycardia, and tender uterine fundus, occurs in 15 to 25% of women following PROM and is even higher after cesarean section. Wound infection and sepsis may follow GBS infection. The diagnosis of intrapartum IAI or postpartum infection mandates broad-spectrum antibiotic coverage for suspected polymicrobial infection. Ampicillin is the most frequently used drug to combat GBS; the first- and second-generation cephalosporins, erythromycin, and clindamycin also provide adequate coverage.

Major efforts have gone into attempting to block vertical transmission by the administration of prophylactic antibiotics. Until recently, however, little agreement had been reached as to the most appropriate protocol for prevention of newborn disease. In 1996, the CDC published prevention guidelines in conjunction with representatives from the American College of Pediatrics. Based on epidemiologic assumptions and an array of clinical trials, two prevention strategies were recommended. In the first, intrapartum antibiotic prophylaxis was suggested for women identified as GBS carriers by prenatal cultures collected at 35 to 37 weeks of gestation, and for those with premature labor or rupture of membranes earlier than 37 weeks of gestation (Fig. 39–1). The second strategy was based solely on the use of intrapartum antibiotic prophylaxis in women who had the previously discussed risk factors for vertical transmission. Intravenous penicillin G was recommended for prophylaxis; either clindamycin or erythromycin was substituted for patients with known allergy (Fig. 39–2).

New avenues of prevention of neonatal GBS infections are being actively explored. The use of a maternal vaccination may allow placental transfer of antibodies that could reduce or eliminate neonatal infection. Other research is directed at the use of hyperimmune and monoclonal intravenous immuno-

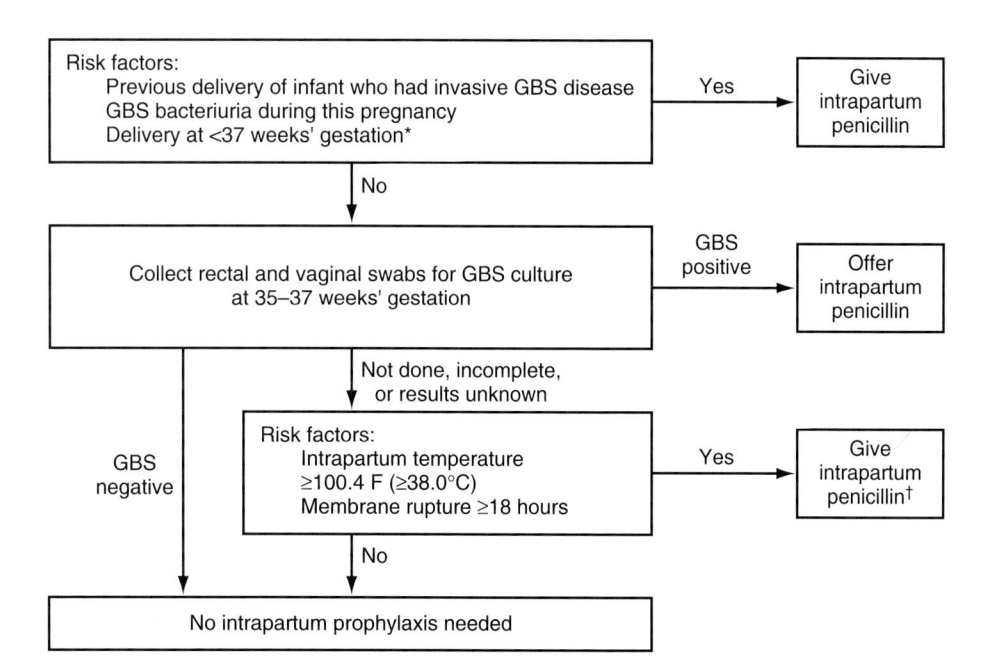

**Figure 39–1** Algorithm for prevention of early-onset group B streptococcal (GBS) disease in neonates, using prenatal screening at 35–37 weeks' gestation. *If membranes rupture at <37 weeks' gestation and the mother has not begun labor, collect GBS culture and either (1) administer antibiotics until cultures are completed and the results are negative, or (2) begin antibiotics only when positive cultures are available. No prophylaxis is needed if culture obtained at 35–37 weeks' gestation was negative. †Broader spectrum antibiotics may be considered at the physician's discretion, based on clinical indications. (From Centers for Disease Control: Prevention of perinatal group B streptococcal disease: A public health perspective. MMWR 45:1–24, 1996.)

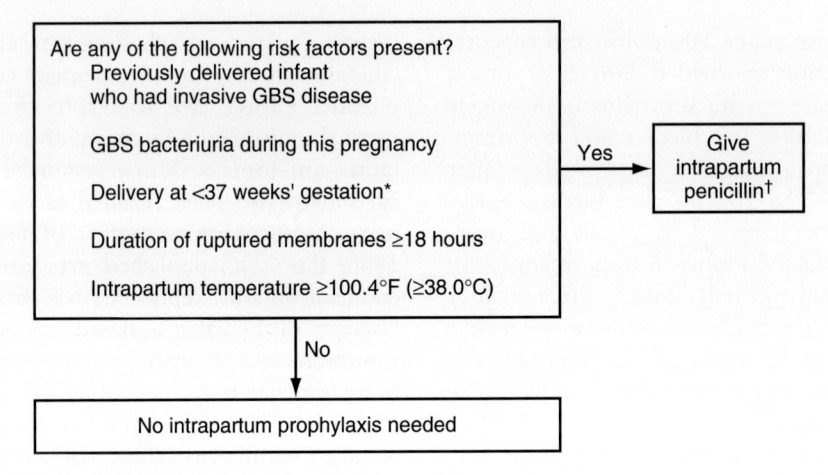

Figure 39–2  Algorithm for prevention of early-onset group B streptococcal (GBS) disease in neonates, using risk factors. *If membranes ruptured at <37 weeks' gestation, and the mother has not begun labor, collect group B streptococcal culture and either (1) administer antibiotics until cultures are completed and the results are negative, or (2) begin antibiotics only when positive cultures are available. †Broader spectrum antibiotics may be considered at the physician's discretion, based on clinical indications. (From Centers for Disease Control: Prevention of perinatal group B streptococcal disease: A public health perspective. MMWR 45:1–24, 1996.)

globulin as adjuvant therapy or prophylaxis for the very preterm neonate.

## Syphilis

Syphilis is found more frequently in poor, urban, and minority populations. A dramatic increase in the number of syphilis cases in young women was reported in the late 1980s and early 1990s, with a concomitant resurgence in neonatal cases. This rise is blamed on the increase in exchanging illegal drugs (primarily crack cocaine) for sex and a broader surveillance definition for congenital syphilis.

After an incubation period of 10 to 90 days from exposure to *Treponema pallidum*, the painless, hard chancre of primary (P) syphilis appears. Although this chancre is readily apparent in males, it is frequently located in the vagina or on the cervix of females and passes unnoticed by the patient. During the second (S) stage 6 weeks to 6 months after primary inoculation, there is involvement of all major organ systems. The patient may present with a maculopapular rash of the palms and soles, condyloma latum, and generalized lymphadenopathy. The findings clear spontaneously as the patient enters the latent stage. If they are untreated, approximately one third of patients develop tertiary syphilis, with involvement of the CNS, cardiovascular system, and gumma formation.

Clinical diagnosis, especially in pregnant patients, of "the great imitator" may be difficult. Antepartum diagnosis relies on serologic screening with the use of nontreponemal tests such as the Venereal Disease Research Laboratory test or the rapid plasma reagin test. False-positive results occur in 1 to 2% of tests and may be caused by recent febrile illness, subclinical autoimmune disease, or laboratory error. Reactive nontreponemal tests are confirmed by specific antibody tests, such as the microhemagglutination assay for antibodies to *T. pallidum* or the fluorescent treponemal antibody absorption test.

Treponemes appear capable of crossing the placenta at any point in pregnancy, and infection can cause preterm delivery, stillbirth, and congenital infection, neonatal death, or both. Congenital syphilis causes fetal or perinatal death in 40 to 50% of affected infants. Spontaneous abortion and stillbirth may be the result of overwhelming infection of the placenta and resultant nonimmune hydrops. Older literature suggests that transmission occurs in virtually all of the infants born to mothers with P and S syphilis, although only half of the infants may be symptomatic. The rate of transmission drops to 40% with early latent stages (<2 years) and 6 to 14% with late latent stages. Even with appropriate antepartum diagnosis and antibiotic treatment of the mother, 11% of infants may demonstrate CNS involvement.

Clinical manifestations may appear as early (first 2 years of life) or late congenital syphilis. Early disease is associated with hemolytic anemia, hepatosplenomegaly, and cutaneous bullous eruptions. Periostitis, osteochondritis, and meningitis are common findings. Late stigmata include periostitis, abnormal deviation, saddle nose, saber shins, eighth nerve deafness, and CNS abnormalities.

Prevention of congenital syphilis requires prenatal care, antepartum screening, and appropriate antibiotic therapy. The CDC recommendations state that regardless of gestational age, infected pregnant

Table 39–2  Syphilis Treatment During Pregnancy

| Type | Treatment |
| --- | --- |
| Primary or secondary | BPG 2.4 million units IM × 1 |
| Latent | |
| Early (<1 yr) | BPG 2.4 million units IM × 1 |
| Late (>1 yr) | BPG 2.4 million units IM × 3 (weekly) |
| Tertiary | BPG 2.4 million units IM × 3 (weekly) |
| Neurosyphilis | Aqueous penicillin G 18–24 million units/d IV × 10–14 d; or procaine penicillin 2.4 million units/d IM and probenecid 500 mg qid PO × 10–14 d |

BPG, benzathine penicillin G; IV = intravenously; IM = intramuscularly; PO = orally; qid = four times a day. If patient is allergic to penicillin, desensitize and treat. Do not use tetracycline or erythromycin. There are insufficient data pertaining to azithromycin or ceftriaxone to allow recommendations to be made.
Modified from 1998 guidelines for treatment of sexually transmitted diseases. MMWR 47(R-1):1–111, 1998.

women should be treated immediately with penicillin appropriate for the stage of syphilis as recommended for nonpregnant patients (Table 39–2). Patients who have a history of penicillin allergy may be treated with penicillin after negative skin testing or penicillin desensitization. Tetracycline is not recommended during pregnancy because of adverse fetal effects. Although erythromycin may be acceptable treatment in adults, it does not cross the placenta readily and may not treat the fetus as well as penicillin. Maternal follow-up includes monthly nontreponemal serologic testing. A rise in titers or lack of a fourfold drop in titers over 3 months indicates a need for retreatment. All patients should be offered counseling and testing for HIV antibody due to the frequent associations of the two infections.

As in nonpregnant patients, treatment of the early stages of syphilis may precipitate the Jarisch-Herxheimer reaction. This syndrome consists of fever, myalgias, and headaches beginning several hours after therapy. In addition, uterine contractions and decreased fetal movement can occur. Transient late decelerations and perinatal deaths have been described.

At birth, the placenta and cord should be examined by dark-field microscopy for treponemes. Neonatal serum should be examined for IgM. Cerebrospinal fluid evaluation and long-bone radiography may be indicated. Both mother and infant require close follow-up to ensure disease eradication.

## Chlamydia

*C. trachomatis* is the most common sexually transmitted organism, and more than 4 million infections occur annually. It is generally believed that 5 to 10% of sexually active women in the United States carry chlamydia in their cervix. A total of 40 to 60% of women who have positive gonorrhea cultures have a concomitant chlamydial infection. The anatomic site in the female genital tract most frequently infected with *C. trachomatis* is the cervix. The ensuing endocervicitis may be asymptomatic or more commonly associated with a hypertrophic cervical erosion and copious mucopurulent discharge containing a high number of polymorphonuclear leukocytes. *C. trachomatis* is a common cause of tubal infertility.

Cell culture has long been the "gold standard" for diagnosis of chlamydial infection. Recently, rapid nonculture detection kits that rely on conjugated monoclonal antibodies or enzyme immunoassay have been promoted. The performance of only a few of these tests has been adequately tested in large-scale clinical trials. The treatment of choice in chlamydial infections has been doxycycline and azithromycin in nonpregnant women. Erythromycin base or succinate (or ampicillin if gastrointestinal intolerance develops) is used for treatment during pregnancy.

*C. trachomatis* infection may be associated with such adverse pregnancy outcomes as prematurity, PROM, IUGR, and postpartum endometritis. Antepartum treatment of chlamydia during pregnancy appears to improve pregnancy outcome. Screening at the first prenatal visit with rescreening in high-risk groups in the third trimester is recommended. Treatment may lower the incidence of neonatal conjunctivitis and pneumonia.

## Toxoplasmosis

*Toxoplasmosis gondii* is a parasite of felines, although other mammals and some avian species may be infected. Human infestation is usually the result of eating undercooked contaminated meat or contact with the feces of an infected cat.

The prevalence of seropositivity in the United States is approximately 20%, depending on geography, lifestyle, and keeping of pets. The chance for seroconversion during pregnancy is less than 0.1%. Acute infection is subclinical in the vast majority of adults. Diagnosis relies on detection of IgM, IgA, and IgE in conjunction with rising, high, or both titers of IgG. Serology and its interpretation can be difficult; the diagnosis of acute infection should be confirmed by a reference laboratory.

A variety of tests have been used to make the diagnosis of fetal infection in utero. Ultrasonographic evaluation may detect ventriculomegaly, ascites, hepatomegaly, or intracranial calcifications. Polymerase chain reaction (PCR) testing of amniotic fluid samples has replaced cordocentesis for diagnosis of fetal infection.

Intrauterine infection is possible only during primary infection or reactivation of an immunocompromised host. Latent infection may be reactivated, causing fetal infection, in transplant recipients or patients who have acquired immunodeficiency syndrome (AIDS); it is unlikely to adversely affect pregnancy outcome in healthy women. The transmission rate increases from 20 to 54 to 65% in the first, second, and third trimesters, respectively. The severity of fetal disease is inversely related to the gestational age at the time of infection. Most (up to 90%) infected infants are asymptomatic at birth. However, abnormalities in the infected infant include chorioretinitis, hydrocephaly, microcephaly, mental retardation, hepatosplenomegaly, jaundice, and lymphadenopathy.

Antibiotics administered to pregnant women who have acute infection may reduce vertical transmission and lessen the severity of newborn disease. Spiramycin, used in Europe, is available through the Food and Drug Administration to decrease vertical transmission. Azithromycin has been used to treat *T. gondii* in AIDS patients and may be an effective alternative to spiramycin. If fetal infection is demonstrated, pyrimethamine and sulfadiazine should be added to reduce severity of the congenital infection.

## REFERENCES

Alger LS: Toxoplasmosis and parvo virus B19. Infect Dis Clin North Am 11:55–75, 1997.
Barron SD, Pass RF: Infectious causes of hydrops fetalis. Semin Perinatol 19:493–501, 1995.
Boyer KM, Gotoff AP: Antimicrobial prophylaxis of neonatal group B streptococcal sepsis. Clin Perinatol 15:831–850, 1988.
Brown ZA, Selke S, Zeh J, et al: The acquisition of herpes simplex virus during pregnancy. N Engl J Med 337:509–515, 1997.
Centers for Disease Control: Hepatitis B virus: A comprehensive strategy for eliminating transmission in the United States through universal vaccination: Recommendations of the Immunization Practices Advisory Committee (ACIP). MMWR 40(RR-13):1–25, 1991.
Centers for Disease Control: Recommendation for the prevention and management of *Chlamydia trachomatis* infections, 1993. MMWR 42:1–37, 1993.
Centers for Disease Control: 1993 Sexually transmitted disease treatment guidelines. MMWR 42(RR-14):1–102, 1993.
Centers for Disease Control: Prevention of perinatal group B streptococcal disease: A public health perspective. MMWR 45:1–24, 1996.
Centers for Disease Control. Prevention of varicella: Recommendations of the Advisory Committee on Immunization Practices. MMWR 45(RR-11):1–36, 1996.
Christmas JT, Wendel GD, Bawdon RE, et al: Concomitant infection with *Neisseria gonorrhoeae* and *Chlamydia trachomatis* in pregnancy. Obstet Gynecol 74:295–298, 1989.
Daffos F, Forestier F, Capella-Pavlovsky M: Prenatal management of 746 pregnancies at risk for congenital toxoplasmosis. N Engl J Med 318:271–275, 1988.
Dinsmoor MJ: Hepatitis in the obstetric patient. Infect Dis Clin North Am 11:77–91, 1997.
Gibbs RS, Eschenbach DA: Use of antibiotic to prevent preterm birth. Am J Gynecol Obstet 177:375–380, 1997.
Haddad J, Langer B, Astruc D, et al: Oral acyclovir and recurrent genital herpes during late pregnancy. Obstet Gynecol 82:102–104, 1993.
Hunt CM, Carson KL, Sharara AI: Hepatitis C in pregnancy. Obstet Gynecol 89:883–890, 1997.
Joesoef MR, Schmid GP: Bacterial vaginosis: Review of treatment options and potential clinical indications for therapy. Clin Infect Dis 20:S72–S79, 1995.
Lewis R, Mercer BM: Adjunctive care of preterm labor and the use of antibiotics. Clin Obstet Gynecol 38:755–770, 1995.
McGregor JA: Chlamydial infection in women. Obstet Gynecol Clin North Am 16:565–592, 1989.
McGregor JA, French JI, Seo K: Premature rupture of membranes and bacterial vaginosis. Am J Obstet Gynecol 169:463–466, 1993.
McCoy MC, Katz VL, et al: Bacterial vaginosis in pregnancy: An approach for the 1990s. Obstet Gynecol Surv 50:482–488, 1995.
Mellinger AK, Cragan JD, Atkinson WL, et al: High incidence of congenital rubella syndrome after a rubella outbreak. Pediatr Infect Dis J 14:573–578, 1995.
Mercer BM, Arheart KL: Antimicrobial therapy in expectant management of preterm premature rupture of the membranes. Lancet 346:1271–1279, 1995.
Millar LK, Cox SM: Urinary tract infections complicating pregnancy. Infect Dis Clin North Am 11:13–26, 1997.
Miller E, Craddock-Watson JE, Pollak TM: Consequence of confirmed maternal rubella at successive stage of pregnancy. Lancet 2:781–784, 1982.
Nelson CT, Demmler GJ: Cytomegalovirus infection in the pregnant mother, fetus and newborn infant. Clin Perinatol 24:151–166, 1997.
Power RD: New directions in the diagnosis and therapy of urinary tract infections. Am J Obstet Gynecol 164:1387–1389, 1991.
Romero R, Oyarzun E, Mazor M, et al: Meta-analysis of the relationship of asymptomatic bacteriuria and preterm delivery/low birth weight infant. Obstet Gynecol 73:576–582, 1989.
Ryan GM, Abdella TN, McNeeley SG, et al: *Chlamydia trachomatis* infection in pregnancy and effect of treatment on outcome. Am J Obstet Gynecol 162:34–39, 1990.
Sanchez PJ, Wendel GD: Syphilis in pregnancy. Clin Perinatol 24:71–90, 1997.
Scott LL, Hollier LM, Dias K: Perinatal herpesvirus infections: Herpes simplex, varicella and cytomegalovirus. Infect Dis Clin North Am 11:27–53, 1997.
Strauss SE, Ostrove JM, Inchauspe G, et al: NIH conference. Varicella-zoster infections: Virology, natural history, treatment and prevention. Ann Intern Med 108:221–237, 1988.
Tanemura M, Suzumori K, Yagami Y, et al: Diagnosis of fetal rubella infection with reverse transcription and nested polymerase chain reaction: A study of 34 cases diagnosed in fetuses. Am J Obstet Gynecol 174:578–582, 1996.
Wendel GD: Sexually transmitted diseases in pregnancy. Semin Perinatol 14:171–178, 1990.

# 40

# Human Immunodeficiency Virus Infection in Pregnancy

THEODORE JONES

In less than two decades, human immunodeficiency virus (HIV) has taken center stage in the world's battle against infectious disease. HIV is an incurable infection that leads to a terminable disease, acquired immunodeficiency syndrome (AIDS), and approximately 30 million adults and 1.4 children are infected worldwide. In addition, the number of cases of AIDS is over 8.7 million. It is estimated that nearly 10,000 new HIV infections are contracted every day.

In the United States, approximately 440,000 cases of AIDS have been reported to the Centers for Disease Control and Prevention (CDC) and it is estimated that over 1 million US citizens are HIV-1 affected but remain asymptomatic. Nearly 82% of infected patients are men and 18% are women. This differs slightly from the world demographics, where 24 to 30% of infected people are women. Additionally, close to 90% of patients are 20 to 49 years of age, prime reproductive years for women. Currently, women account for 14% of the cumulative cases of AIDS reported in the United States. In 1996, 20% of the new cases of AIDS among adults and adolescents reported to the CDC were women. In fact, women and adolescents as demographic groups represent two of the fastest growing segments of the population contracting the infection. The transmission of HIV from mother to infant may occur during pregnancy, labor, and delivery and postpartum via breast feeding. When considering the most likely time of transmission, the period at or around delivery may contribute approximately 64 to 70% of infected babies. In contrast, a smaller percentage of infants are infected in utero or through breastfeeding. Estimates in recent years indicate approximately 7000 HIV-infected women have given birth annually in the United States. When one assumes a 14 to 30% perinatal transmission rate, an estimated 1000 to 2000 HIV-infected children are born each year in the United States. These children with perinatally acquired HIV infection account for over 90% of the pediatric AIDS cases in the United States.

## Virology

HIV-1 is one of several RNA retroviruses possessing the enzyme reverse transcriptase. This unusual enzyme permits genomic RNA to be transcribed into double-stranded DNA. Another enzyme, integrase, facilitates the incorporation of viral DNA into the host cell genome. Cell-mediated immunity is affected by the virus's tendency to attach itself to subpopulations of T lymphocytes known as CD4+ cells (also known as T4 or T-helper lymphocytes). These cells coordinate the action of the immune system to combat viruses, bacteria, and certain malignancies. HIV leads to a slow and progressive destruction of T cells.

Once incorporated into the genome of the host, the virus uses the cellular machinery of its host to make multiple new copies of itself. The process of viral propagation will eventually lead to host cell damage. In the case of HIV infection, there is a gradual depletion of CD4+ cells. This is accompanied by an inability of B lymphocytes to produce effective antibody to HIV or other microorganisms; depression of cytotoxic response; decreased secretion of interleukin-2, which then inhibits clonal expansion of mature CD4+ cells; and an inability of surviving CD4+ cells to perform antigen recognition function. These events lead to progressive deterioration of the host immune system with progression toward AIDS for most infected individuals.

## Adult Pathogenesis

The incubation period of HIV is approximately 1 to 3 weeks, during which time there is a veritable explosion of viral replication. Symptoms during this time are similar to those of a viral or flu-like syndrome—headache, muscle aches, fever, malaise, fatigue—and may last for 2 to 3 weeks. After the peak viral load is achieved, there is a gradual fall in viral load until a steady state concentration of virus is reached, known as the *set point*. The set point is, in effect, a balance between the virus's ability to replicate and the host's ability to protect itself by the neutralization and removal of virus. New viral particles are produced at an average rate of $10^{10}$ per day, and most are produced by replication in CD4+ lymphocytes. Because only 2% of CD4+ cells are circulating at any given time, the rest of the cells are in the lymphoid tissue found throughout the body. The host possesses the ability of clearing large amounts of virus on a daily basis, although the degree of success achieved by the host depends on its level of immunologic control and other cellular factors (genetic). The concept of a set point is an important one. It becomes the principal determinant of the rate of progress of disease and may be the major determinant of the long-term response to antiretroviral therapy (ART). When the viral load set point is high, there is more viral replication and more rapid destruction of host CD4+ cells. This will frequently lead to a more rapid appearance of opportunistic infections and cancers. In addition, higher viral activity allows for the occurrence of more viral genomic mutations, affording additional chances for the development of viral resistance to ART therapy.

A new and intriguing finding is the chemokine-receptor gene mutation on the *CCR4* receptor. Some individuals have been noted to be homozygous or heterozygous for a mutation in the *CCR4* gene characterized by a 32-nucleotide deletion ($\Delta 32$). In homozygous individuals, the receptor is absent on the surface of the host cells, whereas individuals who are heterozygous possess reduced amounts. Persons who have been exposed to HIV on multiple occasions but did not acquire the infection seem to be homozygous for the gene deletion. When an HIV-seropositive person is heterozygous for the *CCR4* $\Delta 32$ mutation, some protection against the acquisition of the virus and prolonged AIDS-free survival are noted.

## Routes of Transmission

The principle mechanisms for dissemination of the virus include exposure to genital body fluids during sexual activity (generally repeated exposure); receiving virus-contaminated blood, blood products, or drug injection using needles and syringes previously used by an infected person; and vertical transmission from infected mothers to their newborns. Transmission of virus by sexual contact with infected secretions has become the most important, accounting for most cases encountered worldwide. Multiple sexual partners is a principal risk factor for both heterosexual and homosexual transmission, although the latter appears to be of questionable significance to women. Male-to-female transmission is approximately twice as frequent as female-to-male transmission. Host infectiousness appears to increase as the concentration of virus in the genital tract increases. Viral concentration is higher in individuals with primary infection or with advanced disease. It would appear that women are infected more easily when in contact with the infected secretions of men than vice versa. There also appears to be a direct relationship between the number of encounters an individual has with an infected person and their risk of acquiring the disease. However, this does not preclude the possibility of a person having sex with an infected person once and becoming infected. In addition, other factors have been implicated that would make the risk of acquiring the disease a much more complex issue. Rectal intercourse appears to be more dangerous than vaginal intercourse due to a predisposition for mucosal tears. Additionally, the rectal mucosa is a preferred site for viral replication. The predisposition of substance abusers to engage in risky sexual activity within and outside their community places them in added jeopardy.

Transmission of the virus by the parenteral route appears to be the most potent means of acquiring HIV. Early in the epidemic, the inability of the blood banking community to effectively screen potential donors allowed many unsuspecting recipients of infected blood or blood products to receive large inocula of virus intravascularly, producing infection and more rapid progression to AIDS. This was especially true for individuals with hemophilia who often received many transfusions of factor VIII concentrate from pooled donors per year. In 1984, 70% of persons with hemophilia A and 34% of those with hemophilia B were found to be HIV seropositive. The sharing of needles and hypodermic syringes by drug-injecting substance users is an important cause of the epidemic's spread throughout the United States and Europe.

Vertical transmission of HIV accounts for well over 90% of the incidence of HIV infection in children. It is discussed in detail later in the chapter.

## Diagnosis

A thorough history in women seeking health care should always involve some assessment of their risk for contracting HIV infection. Risk factors for HIV infection are well-known and are listed in Table 40–1. A simple way of incorporating a question about HIV infection into the interview is to ask every woman who is sexually active "What do you do to keep from getting infected with the AIDS virus (or with HIV)?" Every sexually active women who has ever had exposure to male sexual secretions without using a barrier method should be thought of as at risk for acquiring the infection. Additional signs and symptoms include fatigue, history of recent tuberculosis disease, and recurrent episodes of diseases, such as pneumonia, vaginal candidiasis, pelvic inflammatory disease, or intractable diarrhea. Physical evaluation should focus on evidence of immunosuppression, such as lymphadenopathy, oral thrush, or abnormal pulmonary findings on auscultation and percussion.

Most new infections of HIV are diagnosed by serologic testing, because the majority of patients are asymptomatic (even patients with primary infection frequently have no symptoms or do not have symptoms severe enough to lead to medical evaluation). The average time for seroconversion to occur after infection with HIV is 44 days. Laboratory evaluation for the detection of antibodies in plasma or serum uses an enzyme immunoassay (EIA). The discovery of antibodies yields a reactive test that is automatically repeated to confirm its results. Commercially pro-

**Table 40–1** Risky Behavior that Increases Chance of Acquiring HIV Infection

High-risk sexual practices
    Receptive anal/vaginal intercourse with ejaculation and without a condom
    Receptive vaginal intercourse with spermicidal foam but without a condom
    Receptive anal intercourse with withdrawal before ejaculation
Multiple sexual partners
Sharing nonsterile needles during drug injection
Sexual practice with some risk of HIV transmission
    Oral sex with men with or without ejaculation
    Oral sex with women
Drugs that reduce inhibition to engaging in high-risk behaviors
    Alcohol
    Mood-altering drugs
Partner bisexuality may be hidden risk

duced EIA kits have sensitivities greater than 97% and specificities greater than 99.4%. This is then confirmed with a Western blot test for specific antibodies. Patients should not be informed of their screening test status until confirmatory testing is completed. Direct tests for HIV are indicated when a primary HIV infection is suspected; to determine the HIV status of a newborn infant born to a seropositive mother; or indeterminate results from serologic testing are obtained. Testing options include viral culture, p24 antigen detection, and detection of HIV-1 proviral DNA with polymerase chain reaction (PCR). The latter test is the most widely available and sensitive: it detects HIV DNA, which has been integrated into the genome of CD4+ lymphocytes and is the test of choice for all three indications (Fig. 40–1).

## Perinatal Transmission of Human Immunodeficiency Virus

### Modes of Transmission

Mother-to-child transmission of HIV has a risk that ranges from about 14 to 34%. The risk varies geographically, with lower rates reported in European centers than the rates documented in African nations. There are three distinct time periods during pregnancy during which an HIV-infected woman may transmit the virus to her fetus or neonate: intrauterine, intrapartum, and postpartum. Virus found in the products of conception from spontaneous and therapeutic abortions suggests that *intrauterine transmission* may occur as early as 8 to 14 weeks of gestation. It has also been postulated that the virus may contribute

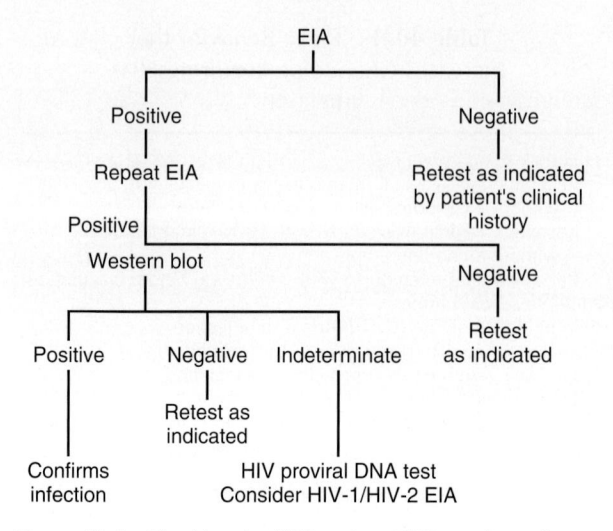

**Figure 40–1** Algorithm for HIV testing. DNA = deoxyribonucleic acid; EIA = enzyme immunoassay; HIV = human immunodeficiency virus.

to the early pregnancy wastage seen in first- and early second-trimester losses and that some infected gestations successfully progress to viability and delivery. The incidence of perinatal transmission to the fetus by the intrauterine route ranges between 20 and 40%. Most transmission is thought to occur during the last trimester of pregnancy, possibly in the last few weeks of gestation.

Several factors make *intrapartum transmission* the putative route of vertical transmission of HIV in the majority of fetuses. Infected newborns frequently show the appearance of virus after the first week of life rather than during their initial week of life. Similarly, first-born twins have nearly three times the rate of vertical transmission as their second-born sibling. Currently, 40 to 80% of cases of vertical transmission are attributed to the intrapartum period. Laboratory evaluation is notable for an absence of virus in the neonatal peripheral blood at birth followed by the appearance of virus on viral culture and on HIV-PCR testing. A clinical course similar to that of HIV-infected adults is seen. *Postpartum transmission* is an infrequent cause of vertical transmission. Current estimates indicate a risk for infection through breastfeeding of 14%.

## Mechanisms of Transmission

The mechanism for intrauterine transmission remains unclear, although fetal or fetal cell contact with free virus in the maternal blood or amniotic fluid and cell-to-cell transmission at the level of the placenta are the most probable causes. Similarly, an association of vertical HIV transmission with the first-born twin and with increasing duration of ruptured membranes implicates contact with the virus in the maternal genital tract as a probable mechanism of infection for intrapartum transmission. Additionally, there appears to be a relationship between clinical chorioamnionitis and vertical transmission. There is a suggestion of intrapartum transmission occurring with contact between fetal cells and HIV-infected maternal white blood cells present in the placenta. Transmission may also occur by infection of the fetal/neonatal gastrointestinal mucosa by HIV-infected maternal cells or free virus present in the amniotic fluid. HIV has been found in both colostrum and breast milk; the relationship between the specific timing and the length of breast feeding to risk for transmission is not clear. There is evidence of transmission by breast-feeding as late as 30 months of life.

## Risks for Vertical Transmission

There are many factors associated with vertical transmission, creating an interactive tapestry that is multifactorial and under continuing revision. *Maternal immune status* reveals an increasing risk of vertical HIV transmission with decreasing maternal CD4 cell count and CD4%. Transmission risk for the lowest quartile maternal CD4% is three times that for the CD4% in the highest quartile maternal CD4%. There is also an increase in risk for transmission as CD8% increases.

*Maternal viral load* is directly correlated with vertical transmission. Measurements of maternal viral load by quantitative HIV RNA-PCR during pregnancy and at delivery reveal that vertical HIV transmission increases as maternal viral burden rises. Earlier reports failed to identify a threshold level for quantitative culture or for RNA-PCR above which transmission always occurred. Likewise, there does not appear to be an RNA-PCR level below which transmission never occurs. However, a more recent study found 0 of 22 and 0 of 34 infants infected among women who were both zidovudine (ZDV) users and nonusers, respectively, with viral loads below 1000 HIV RNA copies/ml. This transmission rate was contrasted with a transmission rate of 7 of 34 and 19 of 30 infants born to women who were ZDV users and nonusers, respectively, with a viral load above 100,000 HIV RNA copies/ml. Decreasing the viral load during gestation is associated with a decrease in perinatal transmission, although the magnitude of the effect remains unclear. Table 40–2 describes the relationship between vertical transmission risk and immune status.

Obstetric risks contribute to intrapartum transmission and are of primary importance to the development of effective prevention interventions. Prolonged duration of ruptured membranes, defined as longer than 4 hours, increases the risk for vertical transmis-

Table 40–2  Maternal Immune Status and Viral Load: Risk for Transmission

| Risk | Immune Status |
|---|---|
| High | Low CD4 count with high viral load |
| Intermediate | Low CD4 count with low viral load |
| | or |
| | High CD4 count with high viral load |
| | or |
| | Intermediate CD4 count with intermediate viral load |
| Low | High CD4 count with low viral load |

sion almost twofold. Factors such as bleeding during pregnancy, placental abruption, amniocentesis, and episiotomy have been identified as potential factors in transmission but have not been clarified in previous studies. A few studies have suggested that placental and/or clinical chorioamnionitis may increase the risk for vertical HIV transmission by the intrapartum but not the intrauterine route.

Maternal cofactors have also been identified as causally related to the risk of vertical transmission. Maternal drug use during pregnancy is associated with a twofold increased risk for vertical transmission. Secondary factors of substance abuse, such as altered immune function, viral variations, changes in nutrition, systemic coinfections, and sexually transmitted diseases, all influence transmission. Syphilis, ulcerative genital diseases, cervicitis, and bacterial vaginosis increase the risk of heterosexual transmission and may also increase the risk for vertical HIV transmission. In addition, coinfection with hepatitis C confers a twofold increase on vertical HIV transmission.

## Prevention of Vertical Transmission

### Drug Therapy

The Pediatric AIDS Clinical Trials Group (PACTG) reported in February 1994 that Protocol 076 demonstrated that a three-part regimen of ZDV reduced the risk of vertical HIV transmission by nearly 70%. Included in the regimen was oral ZDV begun between 14 and 34 weeks gestation and continued throughout pregnancy, followed by intravenous ZDV during labor and oral administration of ZDV to the infant for 6 weeks after delivery (Table 40–3).

Recommendations were made later that year by the US Public Health Service (USPHS) for the use of ZDV for reduction of perinatal HIV-1 transmission and then the following year for universal prenatal HIV-1 counseling and HIV-1 testing with consent for all pregnant women in the United States. The use of ZDV has increased dramatically in various reports since the advocacy of its use.

Although ZDV therapy is still an important component of perinatal transmission reduction, a more enlightened understanding of the importance of viral load reduction has led to a reconsideration of the USPHS recommendations. ZDV monotherapy for medical care has been demonstrated to be less effective than combination antiretroviral therapies. Combination therapies have been tested clinically and found to produce maximal and sustained suppression of viral replication. The goal of antiretroviral therapy is to achieve the lowest possible viral load (preferably below the levels of detection of sensitive plasma HIV RNA assays limits) for as long as possible. Potent combination antiretroviral therapy utilizing drugs not previously used by the patient accomplishes this goal more efficiently and limits the potential for selection of antiretroviral-resistant HIV variants. Table 40–4 contains information about available antiretroviral agents.

Clinical trials have yet to demonstrate that antiretroviral drugs other than ZDV are effective in reducing perinatal transmission. However, potent combination antiretroviral regimens that substantially suppress viral replication and improve clinical status in infected adults are available and are being used with regularity in men and nonpregnant women. Expert panels that previously recommended only ZDV for vertical transmission prophylaxis are now advocating the consideration of combination antiretroviral therapy for pregnant women as well. Pregnant women should have a thorough understanding of the benefits and risks associated with the use of combination therapy (Table 40–5). Prophylaxis should be started as early as possible in pregnancy after 14 weeks. Emphasis should be placed on adherence throughout pregnancy, because it is unclear which of the three components of ZDV therapy is most important.

## Minimizing Obstetric Risks

Several risk factors for vertical transmission have been noted near the time of delivery. Long duration of ruptured membranes leads to nearly twice the risk of

Table 40–3  Currently Recommended Regimen of Zidovudine for Fetal Protection

Zidovudine, 100 mg 5 times a day or 200 mg tid, administered antenatally to the time of labor
Zidovudine, 2 mg/kg loading dose followed by 1 mg/kg per hr intrapartum or administered for 4 hr before scheduled cesarean section
Zidovudine, 2 mg/kg per dose qid to the neonate from birth through 6 wk of life

## Table 40–4  Antiretroviral Agents

| Antiretroviral Drug | Dosing | Elimination | Major Toxicity |
|---|---|---|---|
| **NUCLEOSIDE REVERSE TRANSCRIPTASE INHIBITORS** | | | |
| Zidovudine (AZT, ZDV, Retrovir) | 200 mg tid or 300 mg bid | Liver then renal | Bone marrow suppression; GI Sx, headache, insomnia |
| Didanosine (ddI, Videx) | >60 kg–200 mg bid<br><60 kg–125 mg bid | Renal | Pancreatitis, peripheral neuropathy, nausea, diarrhea |
| Zalcitabine (ddC, Hivid) | 0.75 mg q8h | Renal | Peripheral neuropathy, stomatitis |
| Stavudine (d4T, Zerit) | >60 kg–40 mg bid<br><60 kg–30 mg bid | Renal | Peripheral neuropathy |
| Lamivudine (3TC, Epivir) | 150 mg bid | Renal | Minimal |
| **NON-NUCLEOSIDE REVERSE TRANSCRIPTASE INHIBITORS** | | | |
| Nevirapine (Viramune) | 200 mg daily × 14 d, >90% then 200 mg bid | Liver then renal | Rash, induces cytochrome P-450 enzymes |
| Delavirdine (Rescriptor) | 400 mg tid | Liver then renal | Rash, induces cytochrome P-450 |
| **PROTEASE INHIBITORS** | | | |
| Indinavir (Crixivan) | 800 mg q8h, 30% empty stomach | Biliary, cytochrome P-450s | Nephrolithiasis, GI intolerance, headache, dizziness, rash, thrombocytopenia |
| Ritonavir (Norvir) | 600 mg q12h, with food | Biliary, cytochrome P-450s | GI symptoms, paresthesias, asthenias, ↑ triglycerides, transaminases |
| Nelfinavir (Viracept) | 750 mg q8h, with food | Biliary, cytochrome P-450s | Diarrhea |
| Saquinavir (Invirase) | 600 mg q8h, with high-fat meal | Biliary, cytochrome P-450s | GI symptoms, headache, ↑ transaminases |

GI = gastrointestinal; Sx = symptoms.

vertical HIV transmission. Theoretical risks include exposure to maternal blood due to obstetric events such as placental abruption or episiotomy. These risks, along with invasive procedures such as scalp electrode placement, amniocentesis, and cordocentesis, have yet to be confirmed but remain a subject of concern. Similarly, the route of delivery as a mitigating factor for vertical transmission remains unclear. In previous evaluations, the European Collaborative Study Group demonstrated a 35% reduction in infection in infants delivered by both elective and nonelective cesarean section when compared with infants delivered vaginally (11.7 vs. 17.6%). Although many potential confounding factors were controlled, indications for cesarean section varied between centers, and few patients used antiretroviral therapy. It remains unclear whether the protective effect of cesarean section will persist with routine use of antiretroviral therapy, especially highly active antiretroviral therapy (HAART).

Considering current data and accepted theories of intrapartum transmission, prudent obstetric management would include the following:

1. Application of scalp electrode and fetal scalp puncture for pH determination should be avoided.
2. Avoidance of artificial rupture of membranes is recommended to decrease risk of exposure.
3. Expeditious delivery after rupture of membranes is advised.

## Obstetric Management

### IDENTIFICATION OF PREGNANT WOMEN WITH HUMAN IMMUNODEFICIENCY VIRUS INFECTION

The USPHS strategy for the reduction of vertical transmission depends on offering women with known HIV seropositivity ZDV prophylaxis. Critical to this plan is a woman's knowledge of her HIV serostatus. Reliance solely on a patient's perception of risk or a health-care worker's assumptions about risk on review of history leads to missed diagnoses in women who are infected but without obvious risk factors. Indeed, selective screening of presumed "high-risk" patients failed to identify 40 to 70% of HIV-seropositive women in various series in the literature.

All obstetric care providers should discuss the risk of perinatal HIV transmission with their patients. In addition, health-care providers should routinely offer and recommend HIV antibody testing for all pregnant women and all women considering pregnancy.

**Table 40–5** Preclinical and Clinical Data Relevant to Use of Antiretrovirals in Pregnancy

| Antiretroviral Drug | FDA Pregnancy Category* | Placental Passage (Newborn/Maternal Drug Ratio) | Long-Term Animal Carcinogenicity Studies | Effects on Reproduction | Concerns Specific to Pregnancy |
|---|---|---|---|---|---|
| **NUCLEOSIDE ANALOGUE REVERSE TRANSCRIPTASE INHIBITORS** | | | | | |
| Zidovudine (ZDV, AZT) | C | Yes (human, 0.85) | Positive (rodent, vaginal tumors high doses) | Increased resorption in rats and rabbits. No teratogenicity in rats, rabbits at usual dose. Increased malformations at near lethal dose in rats | None identified |
| Zalcitabine (ddC) | C | Yes (rhesus, 0.30–0.50) | Positive (rodent, thymic lymphomas, (1000× human dose) | Hydrocephalus in rats at >2000× human dose; decreased birth weight at >1000× human dose | None identified |
| Didanosine (ddI) | B | Yes (human, 0.5) | Negative (no tumors, lifetime rodent study) | No impaired fertility or teratogenicity noted in rats, rabbits | Pregnancy may complicate diagnosis if pancreatitis |
| Stavudine (d4T) | C | Yes (rhesus, 0.76) | Not completed | Increased resorption at >200× human doses, decreased sternal ossification at >400× human doses | None identified |
| Lamivudine | C | Yes (human, ≈1.0) | Negative (no tumors, lifetime rodent study) | Increased resorption in rabbits but not rats. No increase in malformations | None identified |
| **NON-NUCLEOSIDE REVERSE TRANSCRIPTASE INHIBITORS** | | | | | |
| Nevirapine | C | Yes (human, 1.0) | Not completed | Impaired fertility in rats at clinically used doses. No increase in malformation in rats, rabbits. Decreased fetal weight in rats at clinically used doses | None identified |
| Delavirdine | C | Unknown | Not completed | Increased resorptions, fetal deaths in rats, rabbits at high doses. Increased ASD/VSD in rats at high doses | None identified |
| **PROTEASE INHIBITORS** | | | | | |
| Saquinavir | B | Unknown | Not completed | No embryolethality or teratogenicity in rats or rabbits at 4–5× human dose | None identified |
| Indinavir | C | Crosses in rats but not rabbits | Not completed | Fertility not affected in rats, rabbits. Normal fetal weights. Increase in supernumerary ribs in rats, no teratogenicity in rabbits | Concern for hyperbilirubinemia, kernicterus in newborn. Must ensure adequate hydration in newborn |
| Ritonavir | B | 1.0 in rats | Not completed | No teratogenicity in rats, rabbits. Increased resorptions, decreased fetal weight in rabbits | None identified |
| Nelfinavir | B | Unknown | Not completed | No effect on fertility, malformations in rats, rabbits | |

ASD = atrial septal defect; VSD = ventricular septal defect.

*FDA pregnancy categories: A, adequate and well-controlled studies of pregnant women fail to demonstrate a risk to the fetus during the first trimester of pregnancy (and there is no evidence of risk during later trimesters); B, animal reproduction studies fail to demonstrate a risk to the fetus and adequate and well-controlled studies of pregnant women have not been conducted; C, safety in human pregnancy has not been determined, animal studies are either positive for fetal risk or have not been conducted, and the drug should not be used unless the potential benefit outweighs the potential risk to the fetus; D, positive evidence of human fetal risk based on adverse reaction data from investigational or marketing experiences, but the potential benefits from the use of the drug in pregnant women may be acceptable despite its potential risks; X, Studies in animals or reports of adverse reactions have indicated that the risk associated with the use of the drug for pregnant women clearly outweigh any possible benefit. Information included in these guidelines may not represent FDA approval or approved labeling for the particular product or indications in question. Specifically, the terms "safe" and "effective" may not be synonymous with the FDA-defined legal standards for product approval (Data from MMWR 47:RR-2–RR-5).

At admission for labor and delivery, routine history taking should include determination of HIV serostatus, including prior HIV testing, test results, and risk history. This is particularly important in women who have not received prenatal care, because prevalence of HIV among them may be higher.

On occasion, women will refuse testing after HIV counseling is given. Critical to success in counseling is ensuring that sufficient information about HIV and the test has been given; that it was provided in an understandable, believable, and supportive way; and that no confusion was created about her options and the risks and benefits of antiretroviral therapy. Ideally, this information should be communicated as routine obstetric care to aid patients in making an informed decision about HIV testing.

## EVALUATION OF PREGNANT HUMAN IMMUNODEFICIENCY VIRUS-INFECTED WOMEN

Care for pregnant HIV-infected women should begin with a thorough discussion of her disease, both pregnancy and nonpregnancy issues. It is important to emphasize to patients that pregnancy does not appear to accelerate the course of HIV infection. The obstetric course, on the other hand, may be adversely affected by the presence of HIV. The frequency of preterm delivery, intrauterine growth retardation, stillbirth, neonatal mortality, and puerperal endometritis are all increased.

Physical examination should look for evidence of immunocompromise, such as the presence of lymphadenopathy, oral thrush, or auscultatory abnormalities. Health-care providers should be alert for the symptoms and signs of acute retroviral syndrome, which is characterized by fever, malaise, lymphadenopathy, and skin rash. This syndrome frequently occurs in the first few weeks after HIV infection before antibody test results become positive. Recent data indicate that initiation of antiretroviral therapy during this period can delay the onset of HIV-related complications and might influence prognosis.

Evaluation should include screening for potentially harmful infectious disease exposure. Screening for tuberculosis with PPD (skin) testing no longer needs to be accompanied by placement of skin controls to screen for anergy. However, a positive PPD test is obtained with skin induration of at least 5 mm rather than the 10-mm cutoff used in HIV-seronegative individuals. If a patient is immunocompromised (i.e., low CD4 cell count), serology for exposure to *Toxoplasmosis gondii* and Cytomegalovirus should be obtained. Assessment of the patient should also include the status of immunizations. Indicated immunoprophylaxis includes vaccinations for hepatitis A, hepatitis B, influenza, and pneumococcus. A word of caution is necessary: a booster dose of pneumococcal vaccine is given 5 years after the first dose. Different response rates have been noted in patients who have received vaccine therapy (Table 40-6).

The higher prevalence of cervical dysplasia in HIV-seropositive patients makes careful evaluation of the cervix with cytology important. Evaluation should be performed more frequently than in HIV-seronegative woman, with Pap smears twice a year as the generally accepted frequency. Less is known about the impact of HIV infection on the natural history and response to therapy of sexually transmitted diseases (STDs). The natural history of many STDs may be modified by HIV infection. An association between HIV and syphilis has been reported: there appears to be a higher incidence of HIV infection among women with reactive syphilis serology. In addition, syphilis may follow a more fulminant course among HIV-seropositive individuals along with increased difficulties with false-negative and false-positive reaction on laboratory testing. Indeed, central nervous system syphilitic infection has been documented with primary syphilis rather than the usual years of latency seen in noninfected individuals.

The combination of two laboratory results, the absolute (or percentage) CD4+ lymphocyte count and the quantitative measure of plasma HIV RNA (often called the "viral load"), provides much more prognostic information than either alone. A patient's level of plasma HIV RNA strongly indicates the expected rate of progression of their HIV disease; higher RNA levels correlate with more rapid progression. Quantitative plasma HIV RNA can be measured using one of three tests (reverse transcriptase [RT]-PCR known as Amplicor by Roche, bDNA by Chiron, and NASBA by Organin Technika), but results should not be compared across methods. Further, because of variability in all of these tests, baseline values before treatment are best obtained by averaging two separate assays on two separate specimens drawn on different days. Because acute illnesses and vaccinations can transiently raise viral load, HIV RNA testing should be postponed several weeks after an illness or vaccination. A patient's CD4+ lymphocyte count indicates how far immune destruction has

**Table 40-6** Patient Response Rates to Vaccination in Asymptomatic HIV Infection

| Vaccine | Response (%) |
| --- | --- |
| Hepatitis B | 25-60 |
| Influenza | 50-90 |
| Pneumococcal | 88 |

progressed. A patient with a low viral load (<3000 copies by RT-PCR) and high CD4+ count (>750 cells) has nearly a zero probability of progressing to AIDS within 3 years, whereas a patient with a high viral load (>110,000 copies by RT-PCR) and low CD4+ count (<200 cells) has an 86% chance of developing AIDS within the next 3 years.

## COUNSELING

Patients should be given an overview of HIV infection and its pathogenesis and clinical course. The importance of ongoing medical care should be highlighted and vigorously encouraged. The risk for vertical transmission should be discussed and the results of PACTG Protocol 076 should be described in sufficient detail to help the patient understand its pivotal role in decreasing the risk of vertical transmission. The immunologic and virologic testing results of the patient should be used as clinical markers for the discussion. A useful illustration for the patient with asymptomatic HIV infection to aid her and her family in understanding where they are in their clinical course at the time of counseling is that of a train (HIV disease) on a railroad track heading for a precipice (AIDS). Where she is on the track correlates with her CD4+ absolute cell count: the higher the count, the further away from the cliff she is at that moment. Low counts find the patient closer to the precipice. The speed at which the train is traveling is analogous to the viral load: patients with high viral loads are traveling quickly and are destined to arrive at the diagnosis of AIDS more quickly than those with low or undetectable viral loads.

Counseling should include information about the availability of ZDV therapy and other antiretroviral therapy options. Recommendations for therapy should consider the patient's need for medical therapy using combination antiretroviral therapy. Such a determination is made using the same criteria to evaluate nonpregnant women: physical examination, immunologic and virologic status, and past retroviral therapy experience. Information concerning the safety of drugs in pregnancy is derived from animal toxicity data, anecdotal reports, registry data, and clinical trials. At this time, little information is available regarding the pharmacokinetics and safety of antiretrovirals during pregnancy with the exception of ZDV. With this consideration, drug therapy choices should be focused on the individual after discussion with the woman about the available data from preclinical and clinical testing of the individual drugs. Table 40–5 contains information that may be used during counseling. Interestingly, two recent studies in mice raise the concern that ZDV may have a transplacental carcinogenic effect. An independent panel of the National Institutes of Health reviewed the data from the two studies and was unanimous in concluding that "the known benefits of AZT in preventing perinatal transmission appear to far outweigh the hypothetical concerns of transplacental carcinogenesis." The panel strongly emphasized the need for active and thorough discussion of the information with all HIV-infected pregnant women.

# Special Considerations

## ACQUIRED IMMUNODEFICIENCY SYNDROME

Advanced HIV disease or AIDS results from the unrelenting viral replication and the gradual loss of immune system mechanisms for viral control, resulting in large amounts of virus in the circulation and declining CD4 cell counts (<200 cells/μl). This may be manifested as loss of lean body mass or as a wasting syndrome. Eventually, there is an increased risk for opportunistic infections and neoplastic processes.

The most common opportunistic infection is the pneumonia caused by the protozoan *Pneumocystis carinii*. Other significant infections include toxoplasmic encephalitis, pulmonary and extrapulmonary tuberculosis, disseminated infection with *Mycobacterium avium complex*, and cryptococcosis. Table 40–7 contains appropriate prophylaxis for these selected opportunistic infections.

Once the need for prophylaxis is reached, with the rapid changes now encountered in the treatment of HIV/AIDS and the rapidly growing knowledge base necessary to care competently for infected patients, joint management of the patient with an infectious disease specialist is strongly encouraged.

## OCCUPATIONAL RISK FOR HEALTH-CARE WORKERS

There is an ever-present risk for health-care workers contracting the virus in their care of HIV-infected patients. The estimated risk for infection after parental or mucous membrane exposure is 0.36%. Sharp injury with a hollow needle presents the greatest threat for critical exposure that could lead to seroconversion. Risk of HIV exposure is minimized by adhering to the following:
1. Avoidance of needle-stick injuries
2. Use of gloves, gowns, caps, masks, and eye coverings to avoid exposure to contaminated blood or body fluids

**Table 40–7** Prophylaxis for Selected Opportunistic Infections

| Condition | Indication for Prophylaxis | Antibiotic Regimen |
| --- | --- | --- |
| *Pneumocystis carinii* pneumonia | Previous infection or CD4 < 200/mm$^3$ | TMP-SMZ-1 ds tablet qd indefinitely |
| Toxoplasmosis | CD4 < 100/mm$^3$ + serology | TMP-SMZ-1 ds tablet qd indefinitely |
| Tuberculosis | +PPD > 5 mm; no active disease on chest radiograph | INH; 300 mg qd, plus pyridoxine, 50 mg qd, ×12 mo |
| Disseminated infection with *Mycobacterium avium* complex | CD4 < 50/mm$^3$ | Azithromycin 1200 mg/wk |
| Cryptococcosis | CD4 < 50/mm$^3$ | Routine prophylaxis not recommended. Patients who have been treated for an acute cryptic infection should receive fluconazole, 200 mg qd, indefinitely |

TMP-SMZ = trimethoprim and sulfamethoxazole; ds = double strength.

3. Covering exudative skin lesions
4. Mechanical suction for resuscitation with mouthpiece
5. Appropriate sterilization and disinfection of instruments and lines

Postexposure prophylaxis with ZDV is now known to be effective, decreasing the risk of seroconversion by 79%. With consideration of this success, the value of perinatal transmission prophylaxis and the value of combination antiretroviral therapy, the CDC now recommends triple therapy for postexposure prophylaxis (ZDV + lamivudine + indinavir).

## REFERENCES

Barlett JG: Medical Management of HIV Infection. Baltimore, Port City Press, 1998, pp 41–60.

Centers for Disease Control and Prevention: National HIV Serosurveillance Summary: Results Through 1991. Vol 3. Atlanta, US Department of Health and Human Services, Public Health Service, 1994.

Centers for Disease Control and Prevention: 1997 USPHS/IDSA guidelines for the prevention of opportunistic infections in persons infected with human immunodeficiency virus. MMWR 46:1–46, 1997.

Cohen CR, Duerr A, Pruithithada N, et al: Bacterial vaginosis and HIV seroprevalence among female commercial sex workers in Chiang Mai, Thailand. AIDS 9:1093–1097, 1995.

Connor EM, Sperling RS, Gelber R, et al: Reduction of maternal-infant transmission of human immunodeficiency virus type 1 with zidovudine treatment. N Engl J Med 331:1173–1180, 1994.

Datta P, Embree JE, Kreiss JK: Resumption of breast-feeding in later childhood: A risk factor for mother to child human immunodeficiency virus Type I transmission. Pediatr Infect Dis J 11:974–976, 1992.

Davis SF, Byers RH, Lindegren ML, et al: Prevalence and incidence of vertically acquired HIV infection in the United States. JAMA 247:952–955, 1995.

Dickover R, Garratty EM, Herman SA, et al: Identification of levels of maternal HIV-1 RNA associated with risk of perinatal transmission. Effect of maternal zidovudine treatment on viral load. JAMA 275:599–605, 1996.

Dunn DT, Newell ML, Ades HE, et al: Risk of human immunodeficiency virus type 1 transmission through breast-feeding. Lancet 340:585–588, 1992.

Ecker JL: The cost effectiveness of human immunodeficiency virus screening in pregnancy. Am J Obstet Gynecol 174:716–721, 1996.

Garcia PM, Kalish L, Pih J, et al: Maternal human immunodeficiency viris (HIV) RNA level correlates with the risk but does not predict the timing of perinatal transmission [Abstract]. Am J Obstet Gynecol 178:52, 1998.

Goedert JJ, Duliege A-M, Amos CI, et al: International Registry of HIV-exposed twins: High risk of HIV infection for first born twins. Lancet 338:1471–1475, 1991.

Gurtler L: Difficulties and strategies of HIV diagnosis. Lancet 348:176–179, 1996.

Haulir DV, Richman DD: Viral dynamics of HIV: Implications for drug development and therapeutic strategies. Ann Intern Med 124:984–994, 1996.

Hershow RC, Riester KA, Lew J, et al: Increased vertical transmission of human immunodeficiency virus from hepatitis C virus–coinfected mothers. J Infect Dis 176:414–420, 1997.

Holtom PD, Larsen RA, Leal ME, et al: Prevalence of neurosyphilis in HIV infected patients with latent syphilis. Am J Med 93:9–12, 1992.

Hughes MD, Johnson VA, Hirsch MS, et al: Monitoring plasma HIV-I RNA levels in addition to CD4+ lymphocyte count improves assessment of antiretroviral therapeutic response. Ann Intern Med 126:929–938, 1997.

Kroner BL, Rosenberg PS, Aledort LM, et al: HIV-1 infection incidence among persons with hemophilia in the United States and western Europe, 1978–1990. Multicenter Hemophilia Cohort Study. AIDS 7:279–286, 1994.

Laga M, Manoka A, Kivuvu M, et al: Non-ulcerative sexually transmitted diseases as risk factors for HIV-1 transmission in women: Results from a cohort study. AIDS 7:95–102, 1993.

Landesman SH, Kalish LA, Burns DN, et al: Obstetrical factors and the transmission of human immunodeficiency virus type 1 from mother to child. The Women and Infants Transmission Study. N Engl J Med 334:1617–1623, 1996.

Lindsay MK: A protocol for routine voluntary antepartum human immunodeficiency virus antibody screening. Obstet Gynecol 168:476–479, 1993.

Mann J, Tarantola D (eds.): AIDS in the World. Global AIDS Policy Coalition. Vol 11. London, Oxford University Press, 1996.

Mano H, Sherman JC: Fetal human immunodeficiency virus Type 1 infection in different organs in the second trimester. AIDS Res Hum Retrovir 7:83–88, 1991.

Matheson PB, Abrams EJ, Thomas PA, et al: Efficacy of antenatal zidovudine in reducing perinatal transmission of human immunodeficiency virus type 1. The New York City Perinatal HIV Transmission Collaborative Study Group. J Infect Dis 172:353–358, 1995.

Mellors JW, Rinaldo CR Jr, Gupta P, et al: Prognosis in HIV-1 infection predicted by the quantity of virus in plasma. Science 272:1167–1170, 1996.

Minkoff H, Augenbraun M: Antiretroviral therapy for pregnant women. Am J Obstet Gynecol 176:478–489, 1997.

Mofenson L: Epidemiology and determinants of vertical HIV transmission. Semin Pediatr Infect Dis 5:252–265, 1994.

Moodley J, Moodley D, Pillay K, et al: Antiviral effect of lamivudine alone and in combination with zidovudine in HIV-infected pregnant women. Proceedings of the Fourth Conference on Retroviruses and Opportunistic Infections, Washington DC, January 22–26, 1997, Abstract 607, p 176.

National Institute of Allergy and Infectious Diseases: Summary of the meeting of a panel to review studies of transplacental toxicity of AZT. National Institutes of Health, January 14, 1997.

Newell ML, Dunn D, Peckham CS, et al: Caesarean section and risk of vertical transmission of HIV-1 infection: European Collaborative Study. Lancet 343:1464–1467, 1994.

Panel on Clinical Practices for Treatment of HIV Infection: Guidelines for the use of Antiretroviral Agents in HIV-Infected Adults and Adolescents. Washington DC, US Public Health Service, 1997.

Peckham C: Mother to child transmission of the human immunodeficiency virus. N Engl J Med 333:298–302, 1995.

Public Health Service: Guidelines for the management of healthcare worker exposures to HIV and recommendations for post exposure prophylaxis. MMWR 47(RR-7):1–28, 1998.

Public Health Service Task Force: Recommendations for the use of antiviral drugs in pregnant women infected with HIV-1 for maternal health and for reducing perinatal HIV-1 transmission in the United States. MMWR 47:1–30, 1998.

Rodriguez EM, Mofenson LM, Chang BH, et al: Association of maternal drug use during pregnancy with maternal HIV culture positivity and perinatal HIV transmission. AIDS 10:273–282, 1996.

Royce RA, Sena A, Cates W, et al: Sexual transmission of HIV. N Engl J Med 336:1072–1078, 1997.

Saag MS: Use of HIV viral load in clinical practice: Back to the future. Ann Intern Med 126:983–985, 1997.

Sperling RS, Shapiro DE, Coombs RW, et al: Maternal viral load, zidovudine treatment, and the risk of transmission of human immunodeficiency virus type 1 from mother to infant. Pediatric AIDS Clinical Trials Group Protocol 076 Study Group. N Engl J Med 335:1621–1629, 1996.

Wright TC, Ellerbrock TV, Chaisson MA, et al: Cervical intraepithelial neoplasia in women with human immunodeficiency virus: Prevalence, risk factors, and validity of Papanicolaou smears. Obstet Gynecol 84:591–597, 1994.

# 41

# Drug Therapy in Pregnancy

IVANA M. VETTRAINO
ROBERT A. WELCH

The average woman ingests three to four prescription and nonprescription medications during pregnancy. Few birth defects have been specifically linked to these medications. Despite this fact, there remains a public and professional distrust of anything consumed that may be perceived as a potential harm to the developing offspring. The pharmaceutical industry has been unable to provide assistance in this area because of justified concerns over liability. Benefits of a medication in pregnancy must be weighed against the potential risks before prescribing. The US Food and Drug Administration (FDA) has established categories of drugs that assess these risks (Table 41–1). Only a handful of medications are known human teratogens (Table 41–2).

The purpose of this chapter is to provide a comfort level for the clinician prescribing drugs for pregnant patients. It is presented in two sections. The first gives an overview of frequently prescribed classes of drugs in pregnancy. This portion takes a *drugs to use, drugs to avoid* approach. The second section suggests preferred drugs for specific medical conditions often encountered in pregnancy. It makes recommendations of which drugs are considered current best selections. Both themes merge in Box 41–1, an extensive appendix summarizing preferred drugs for specific medical conditions in pregnancy.

Drug use in pregnancy is a rapidly changing area and there may be some drugs that are released from the time of this writing to ultimate publication. There are also developing combinations of drugs for a variety of diseases that appear to have great promise but have not been tested in pregnancy. Before embarking on these newer combinations, the reader is cautioned to consider some of the basic principles of drug metabolism contained in the following pages.

## Special Considerations

### TERATOLOGY

Teratology is the study of abnormal development. Initially limited to structural malformations, teratology has now been expanded to include developmental aberrations such as intrauterine growth restriction, abortion, stillbirth, and other functional deficits. A teratogen is any substance, organism, physical agent, or deficiency state present during embryonic or fetal life capable of inducing abnormal structure or function. Approximately 3 to 5% of congenital malformations have been attributed to prenatal drug exposure.

Table 41-1  FDA Fetal Risk Categories

| Category | Definitions |
|---|---|
| A | Controlled studies in humans have failed to demonstrate a fetal risk. |
| B | Reproduction studies in animals have failed to demonstrate a fetal risk, but controlled studies in humans do not exist or reproduction studies in animals have shown an adverse effect, but controlled studies in humans *have not confirmed* the adverse effect. |
| C | Reproduction studies in animals have shown adverse fetal effects, but controlled studies in humans do not exist or studies in animals and humans do not exist. |
| D | There is positive evidence in humans of teratogenicity or adverse fetal effects. Benefits of maternal use of the drug may outweigh the potential risk. |
| X | Studies in animals and humans show fetal abnormalities and adverse fetal outcomes. Fetal risk outweighs benefits of use. The drug should be considered contraindicated for use in women who are or who may become pregnant. |

Data from FDA published definitions U.S. Food and Drug Administration. Pregnancy labeling. Washington, DC, FDA Drug Bull 9:23–24, 1979.

Table 41-2  Medications Categorized as Category X

| | |
|---|---|
| Aminopterin | Leuprolide |
| ACE inhibitors | Lovastatin |
| Coumarin derivatives | Methotrexate |
| Chenodiol | Mifepristone/misoprostol |
| Danazol | Phencyclidine |
| Diethylstilbestrol | Quinine |
| Ethanol | Radioactive iodine |
| Etretinate | Ribavirin |
| Flurazepam | Temazepam |
| Iodinated glycerol | Trimethadione |
| Isotretinoin | |

ACE = angiotensin-converting enzyme.

The greatest susceptibility to a teratogenic agent is during the embryonic period, from the second to eighth weeks postconception (days 18 to 55). This is the epic of critical fetal organ formation (Table 41-3). It is classically believed that before this time, exposure to a teratogen will either cause abortion or the embryo will survive unscathed (the "all-or-none" effect). Teratogens can have variable impact on the developing offspring. Important influences in the ultimate effects include amount of drug or metabolite reaching the fetus, gestational age at time of exposure, duration of exposure, genotypes of the mother and offspring, and interactions between multiple medications.

Teratogenic effects can also be species specific. One example is the increased frequency of orofacial clefting in rat pups resulting from administered corticosteroids, yet this effect is not seen in humans.

## PHYSIOLOGIC CHANGES IN PREGNANCY

Maternal physiologic changes may influence drug metabolism and circulating levels of active drug. The pulmonary changes of increased tidal volume and minute ventilation can enhance the metabolism of inhalation anesthetics and other inhaled drugs. Increased circulating progesterone causes smooth muscle relaxation that decreases gastrointestinal transit time, although absorption of drug from the gastrointestinal tract has not been shown to change significantly between pregnant and nonpregnant states. Drug distribution is affected by increases in plasma volume and body fat and decreases in plasma albumin concentration. These effects influence availability of drugs and metabolites that are polar, fat soluble, and highly protein bound, respectively.

Hepatic enzyme systems can become more easily induced, resulting in increased drug metabolism. This effect is most concerning for some of the anticonvulsant medications. Those depending on renal clearance generally are cleared at an increased rate because of dramatic elevations in renal blood flow and glomerular filtration rate.

## PLACENTAL TRANSFER OF DRUGS

Most drugs cross the placenta by simple diffusion, making the term *placental barrier* somewhat of an outdated misnomer. The rate of drug transfer is governed by Fick's principle (a substance will seek to diffuse equally throughout a space). In general, the rate of transfer is determined by the drug's molecular weight, concentration of the free drug, lipid permeability, placental surface area, and uteroplacental blood flow. Drugs with a molecular weight above 1000 Da do not cross the placenta. However, most drugs and their metabolites are approximately 500 Da and thus readily cross.

Table 41-3  Critical Periods in Embryonic Development

| Days From Conception | Developmental Event |
|---|---|
| 1 | — |
| 5–7 | Implantation/blastula |
| 24–25 | Anterior neuropore closes |
| 26–27 | Posterior neuropore closes |
| 27–28 | Upper limb buds form |
| 29–30 | Lower limb buds form |
| 46–47 | Heart septation occurs |
| 56–58 | Palate closes |
| 84 | Second trimester begins |

Data from Moore KL: The Developing Human: Clinically Oriented Embryology, 4th ed. Philadelphia, WB Saunders, 1988.

## BOX 41–1  PREFERRED DRUGS FOR SPECIFIC MEDICAL CONDITIONS IN PREGNANCY

| Situation | Preferred Drug(s) | Optional Drug(s) | Remarks |
|---|---|---|---|
| • Acne | Topical agents | Oral erythromycin<br>Topical retinoic acid | Isotretinoin (Accutane) is contraindicated. |
| • Allergic rhinitis | Pseudoephedrine, intranasal saline drops/spray, intranasal corticosteroids, cetirizine hydrochloride, loratadine | Cromolyn sodium<br>Fexofenadine | For unresponsive patients, a trial amoxicillin (3-wk course), erythromycin (3-wk course), or azithromycin can be prescribed. |
| • Antiretrovirals | Zidovudine | Didanosine (ddI)<br>Lamivudine (3TC)<br>Stavudine (d4T)<br>Zalcitabine (ddC) | Protease inhibitors should only be used in study protocols. |
| • Analgesics | Oral: acetaminophen<br>Intravenous (IV)/intramuscular (IM): Demerol, morphine | Oral: acetaminophen with codeine<br>Intranasal: butorphanol tartrate | Oral propoxyphene/acetaminophen can be used if a codeine allergy exists.<br>Salicylates and NSAIDs should be avoided. |
| • Anemia<br>Iron,<br>folate,<br>vitamin B$_{12}$ | Ferrous sulfate, ferrous gluconate<br>Folic acid supplementation<br>IM: vitamin B$_{12}$ | | Folic acid supplementation is recommended for all women contemplating pregnancy and during the first trimester of pregnancy.<br>For severe anemia, blood transfusions may be required. |
| • Anesthetics (local) | Lidocaine, tetracaine, procaine, chloroprocaine | Bupivicaine | |
| • Antibiotics | Penicillins, cephalosporins, clindamycin, gentamicin, macrolides (erythromycin, azithromycin, etc.), miconazole, nitrofurantoin | Monobactams (aztreonam), carbapenam, vancomycin; fluoroquinolones (for resistant infections only) | Metronidazole can be used after the first trimester. Tetracycline, chloramphenicol, chloroquine should not be used. Trimethoprim and sulfonamides should be used only in the second trimester because of theoretical risks with use in the first and late third trimester. |
| • Anticoagulation | Heparin (conventional), Heparin (low molecular weight) | Dipyridamole, urokinase, streptokinase | Coumarin derivatives are contraindicated. |
| • Antifungals | OTC topical preparations, nystatin, miconazole, clotrimazole, terconazole | Fluconazole, itraconazole, amphotericin B | Griseofulvin is contraindicated.<br>Experience in human pregnancy with butoconazole is lacking. |
| • Asthma | Albuterol, metaproterenol, theophylline, prednisone, inhaled corticosteroids | Terbutaline, cromolyn sodium | β-Adrenergic receptor blocking agents should be avoided in patients who have asthma. |
| • Anxiety disorders | Lorazepam | Alprazolam | Diazepam should be avoided if possible. |

| BOX 41-1 | PREFERRED DRUGS FOR SPECIFIC MEDICAL CONDITIONS IN PREGNANCY *Continued* | | |
|---|---|---|---|
| *Situation* | *Preferred Drug(s)* | *Optional Drug(s)* | *Remarks* |
| • Cardiac arrythmias | Adenosine, atropine, digoxin, propanolol, labetolol, lidocaine | Procainamide, verapamil, quinidine, esmolol, flecainide, diltiazem | Amiodarone has been associated with adverse effects on neonatal thyroid function. Digoxin is contraindicated in the patient with Wolff-Parkinson-White syndrome. In emergency situations, treat as if the patient *were not* pregnant. |
| • Cold sores | Over-the-counter (OTC) topical ointment creams | Oral, acyclovir/valacylovir | |
| • Constipation | Docusate sodium, magnesium hydroxide (milk of magnesia), Metamucil | Magnesium citrate, senna preparations | Enemas should only be used under the guidance of an obstetric caregiver. |
| • Cough | Diphenhydramine, dextromethorphan | Codeine | |
| • Depression | Tricyclic antidepressants (desipramine, nortriptyline); fluoxetine | | Patients who have psychiatric disorders should be comanaged with their psychiatric caregiver. |
| • Dermatitis | 1% hydrocortisone cream, oral corticosteroids, diphenhydramine, calamine lotion | Hydroxyzine hydrochloride (Atarax), Astemizole (Hismanal) | |
| • Diabetes | Insulin (recombinant) | Insulin (beef or pork) | Oral hypoglycemics should be avoided. |
| • Diarrhea | Kaopectate, loperamide | Diphenoxylate hydrochloride, codeine | Bismuth subsalicylate should be avoided because it contains salicylate. |
| • Diuretics | Lasix | | In general, should be avoided during pregnancy. Acetazolamide and spironolactone should not be used. |
| • Fever | Acetaminophen | | Salicylates and nonsteroidal anti-inflammatory drugs (NSAIDs) should be avoided. |
| • Gastroesophageal reflux/peptic ulcer disease | Antacids, ranitidine, famotidine | Sucralfate, cimetidine | There is no experience with omeprazole in pregnancy. Nizatidine is category C. Endoscopy if symptoms are unrelenting. |
| • Headache | See analgesics | | |
| • Hypertension | Methyldopa, labetolol, hydralazine | Atenolol, propanolol, nifedipine | ACE inhibitors are contraindicated. In general, a patient who has chronic hypertension and who is well controlled should not have her antihypertensive changed unless the medication is contraindicated. |

*Box continued on following page*

### BOX 41–1 PREFERRED DRUGS FOR SPECIFIC MEDICAL CONDITIONS IN PREGNANCY Continued

| Situation | Preferred Drug(s) | Optional Drug(s) | Remarks |
| --- | --- | --- | --- |
| Hyperthyroidism | Propylthiouracil (PTU) | Methimazole; β-adrenergic blockers for symptoms | Radioactive iodine is contraindicated. Surgery may be necessary. |
| Hypothyroidism | L-Thyroxine | | |
| Inflammatory bowel disease | Corticosteroids (prednisone); sulfasalazine | Olsalazine, azathioprine | Folic acid supplementation is particularly important for those receiving sulfasalazine. |
| Lice/scabies | Nix creme rinse; crotamiton (10%) lotion or cream | | Lindane should be reserved for resistant infections. Contacts should be treated. |
| Mania (bipolar disease) | Lithium | Chlorpromazine; haloperidol | Fetal echocardiogram should be performed in those patients exposed to lithium. |
| Myasthenia gravis (MG) | Pyridostigmine, steroids | Azathioprine | Plasmapharesis may be used in emergency situations. Any drug with curare-like effects is contraindicated, including magnesium sulfate, aminoglycosides, muscle relaxants. *Before use*, a drug should be investigated for possible side effects in MG. |
| Nausea/vomiting | Trimethobenzamide, promethazine, prochlorperazine, vitamin B_6, meclizine | Metoclopramide, ondansetron hydrochloride | |
| Pinworms/parasites | Mebendazole | Thiabendazole, pyrantel pamoate | Contacts also need to be treated. |
| Pruritis | Topical agents: camphor, phenol, calamine; corticosteroid creams. Systemic agents: antihistamines, diphenhydramine, hydroxyzine | Cetirizine hydrochloride, loratadine | |
| Psoriasis | Topical corticosteroid creams and ointments | | |
| Raynaud's disease | Calcium channel blocking agents (nifedipine) | Prazosin, phenoxybenzamine | |
| Rheumatoid arthritis | Glucocorticoids | Azathioprine, sulfasalazine, cyclosporine | Hydroxychloroquine, NSAIDs, and salicylates should be avoided. Gold salts and penicillamine are contraindicated. |
| Sedatives/hypnotics | Diphenhydramine, promethazine | Zolpidem, droperidol, secobarbital, morphine | Triazolam, pentobarbital, and flurazepam are contraindicated. |
| Seizures | | | The medication that best controls the patient's seizure disorder should be used. Polytherapy should be avoided if possible (see text). |

| BOX 41-1 | PREFERRED DRUGS FOR SPECIFIC MEDICAL CONDITIONS IN PREGNANCY Continued |||| 
|---|---|---|---|
| Situation | Preferred Drug(s) | Optional Drug(s) | Remarks |
| • Smoking cessation | Nicotine gum or patches | | Bupropion hydrochloride should not be used. |
| • Systemic lupus erythematosus | Prednisone (glucocorticoids) | | Azathioprine, cyclosporine for steroid-unresponsive disease. Hydroxychloroquine should be avoided. NSAIDs should be avoided. |
| • Vaccinations | Polio, tetanus toxoid, rabies, influenza, hepatitis B, diphtheria pneumococcus, cholera, plague, immunoglobulins | | Exposure to rubella, mumps, measles, pertussis, smallpox, varicella, typhoid, and yellow fever should be avoided. |

The rate of drug transfer across the placenta appears to increase in late pregnancy. The extent to which the placenta and fetus are able to metabolize drugs probably plays an important role in determining the extent of adverse effects. These mechanisms are, in part, genetically regulated and there is still much to be learned about them.

## Selected Classes of Drugs

### ANALGESICS

Acetaminophen in regular or extra strength is commonly used during pregnancy and has not been associated with adverse fetal or neonatal effects. Maternal liver damage is a potential risk with overdose or with excessive use in patients who have prior liver disease. Conversely, regular-strength aspirin (325 mg) should be avoided during pregnancy. In the mother it can result in postpartum hemorrhage, prolonged gestation, and prolonged labor. It readily crosses the placenta and can alter fetal and neonatal platelet function. Because it is a prostaglandin synthetase inhibitor, it has the hypothetic risk of premature closure or constriction of the ductus arteriosus. Newborn pulmonary hypertension may result from aspirin and chronic use during pregnancy may also be associated with oligohydramnios.

"Low-dose aspirin" (≤81 mg/d) has not been associated with the adverse effects seen with regular-strength aspirin. Speculation of an increased risk for abruptio placentae associated with low-dose aspirin use has not been substantiated in subsequent studies. Both acetaminophen and aspirin are common ingredients in a wide variety of combination medications and care should be taken to examine the individual ingredients in combination products (e.g., cough and cold remedies).

Nonsteroidal anti-inflammatory drugs (NSAIDs) have not been associated with congenital malformations. However, prolonged usage during pregnancy can result in oligohydramnios. Use after 32 to 34 weeks' gestation may induce constriction of the fetal ductus arteriosus with resulting pulmonary hypertension in the newborn. Some case reports suggest that fetal exposure in the 24 to 48 hours preceding birth may increase the risk of newborn intraventricular hemorrhage, oliguria, and necrotizing enterocolitis. Of course, prematurity alone may account for these same morbidities without the use of these drugs.

### ANTIASTHMATICS

Asthma can be life threatening and often deserves aggressive treatment. The National Institutes of Health have published a consensus statement addressing treatment of asthma in pregnancy. Generally, exacerbations of asthma in pregnancy are treated similarly to those occurring in the nonpregnant state. Medications typically used for this treatment are acceptable for use in all trimesters of pregnancy. See the chapter on asthma for an in-depth discussion of the pharmacologic therapy during pregnancy (Chapter 36).

### ANTICOAGULANTS

Approximately 1 of every 2500 pregnancies is complicated by deep vein thrombosis (DVT) and/or pulmonary embolism (PE). Thromboembolic disorders are a leading cause of maternal morbidity and mortality. Patients also may be found to have congenital antithrombus deficiency disorders (e.g., proteins C and S, antithrombin III) that require prophylaxis during pregnancy. Heparin remains the drug of choice for the treatment or prophylaxis of DVT or PE. Because heparin consists of a group of large charged molecules, it does not cross the placenta. Thus, it has not been shown to be teratogenic. It can be administered intravenously or subcutaneously. Maternal side effects can occur with prolonged high-dose use and include thrombocytopenia, osteopenia, osteoporosis, alopecia, and excessive postpartum bleeding. Heparin allergy in pregnancy is rare. The anticoagulant effect of heparin can be reversed with protamine sulfate (0.5 mg for every 100 units of heparin, up to 50 mg).

Low-molecular-weight heparin (LMWH) has been recently introduced and is gaining popularity in pregnancy. With a molecular weight of 4000 to 6000 Da, it does not cross the placenta, and no teratogenic effects have been reported. Route of administration is subcutaneous, but it is associated with fewer side effects than regular heparin and no greater bleeding tendency. Dosing is once daily, based on maternal weight, and does not require frequent monitoring with serial activated prothrombin time (aPTT) levels. The ease of administration, simple follow-up, and decreased risk of adverse effects are a clear advantage for long-term use. Unfortunately, LMWH remains more expensive than regular heparin. In addition, a recent FDA advisory cautions the use of regional analgesia and anesthesia in patients who are receiving treatment with LMWH due to reports of epidural and spinal hematomas with resulting neurologic injury. The use of regional analgesia/anesthesia is contraindicated in any patient who is fully anticoagulated regardless of anticoagulant.

Coumarin derivatives (e.g., warfarin sulfate) are known teratogens and contraindicated in pregnancy. Their anticoagulant activity is produced through depression of the vitamin K–dependent clotting factors (II, VII, IX, and X). Coumarins are small molecules that readily cross the placenta and cause bleeding diathesis in the developing embryo/fetus. Between 15 and 25% of offspring exposed to coumarins in the first trimester will show effects known as the fetal warfarin syndrome (Table 41–4).

Thrombolytic agents are rarely indicated during pregnancy. Streptokinase, alteplase, and urokinase have not been directly associated with teratogenesis. The common side effect of high fever during their use presents a hypothetic risk to the fetus. Bleeding complications associated with thrombolytics also limit their use in patients who are postpartum. Postepisiotomy, lacerations and extensions, or postcesarean birth may be particularly susceptible to this complication. Thrombolytic use in pregnancy should be limited to life-threatening circumstances when other medications or devices (i.e., Greenfield filter) are not sufficiently effective.

**Table 41–4** Teratogenic Fetal Effects of Coumarin Derivatives

Nasal hypoplasia
Stippled epiphyses
Optic atrophy
Central nervous system abnormalities
Microcephaly
Deafness
Fetal growth restriction
Mental retardation

Data from Hall JG, Pauli RM, Wilson KM: Maternal and fetal sequelae of anticoagulation during pregnancy. Am J Med 68:122–140, 1980.

## ANTICONVULSANTS

Approximately one million women of reproductive age have a seizure disorder. Women taking anticonvulsant drugs are two to three times more likely to have a child with a congenital malformation. Consensus guidelines have been published to provide guidance in counseling patients with a seizure disorder in pregnancy. One anticonvulsant drug is no longer believed to be less teratogenic than another. Thus, the most efficacious drug for the patient should be used.

Polytherapy with anticonvulsants should be avoided, if possible. The lowest serum drug level that is effective in controlling seizures should be maintained throughout pregnancy. Combinations of phenobarbital, valproic acid, and carbamazepine should be avoided because combinations of these drugs have been associated with increased rates of fetal malformations. Maternal serum alpha-fetoprotein levels, a targeted ultrasonography study at 18 to 20 weeks of gestation, and fetal echocardiography should be offered to patients taking anticonvulsants. Folic acid supplementation in a dose of 4 mg/d is also recommended. It is important that these patients understand that the adverse effects from grand mal seizures outweigh the potential teratogenic risks of anticonvulsant drugs.

The most frequently prescribed anticonvulsants in pregnancy are phenobarbital, phenytoin, valproic acid, and carbamazepine. Secondary to changes in the volume of distribution and induction of hepatic enzyme systems, drug levels should be monitored on a regular basis during pregnancy and in the postpartum period. With the exception of valproic acid, anticonvulsant drugs can decrease fetal vitamin K–dependent coagulation factors that increase the risk for neonatal hemorrhage. Some authorities suggest maternal supplementation with oral vitamin K in doses of 10 to 20 mg/d during the last month of pregnancy. Most importantly, the neonate should receive intramuscular vitamin K (1 mg neonatal concentration) shortly after birth.

## ANTIEMETICS

Hyperemesis gravidarum is experienced by many pregnant women. Nausea and vomiting can also occur throughout pregnancy for a variety of reasons (e.g., gastroenteritis). The phenothiazines and piperazines are frequently prescribed to ameliorate these symptoms. It appears that they can generally be used in all trimesters to help alleviate these conditions with little risk to the fetus. Moderate to high-dose vitamin $B_6$ appears to be safe and effective for early pregnancy vomiting. Metoclopramide has also been used for the treatment of nausea and as an enhancer of gastric motility without reported teratogenic effects.

## ANTIHYPERTENSIVES

Chronic hypertension is among the most prevalent medical complications of pregnancy. In general, if a patient has hypertension before pregnancy that has been difficult to control, she should not be changed from the effective drug unless there is a known fetal risk. Angiotensin-converting enzyme (ACE) inhibitors are contraindicated in pregnancy and have been associated with adverse outcomes, especially when used in the second and third trimesters. Exposure to this class of drugs has been associated with fetal hypocalvaria, renal anomalies, oligohydramnios, pulmonary hypoplasia, and stillbirth. ACE inhibitors should not be prescribed for gravidas or women contemplating pregnancy unless absolutely no other alternative exists.

Methyldopa remains the most commonly prescribed antihypertensive for women contemplating pregnancy or for those already pregnant. Years of use in the general population have demonstrated safety in pregnancy. Adrenergic blockers continue to grow in popularity in this country. Most experience with their use in pregnancy comes from the United Kingdom where there have not been reports of teratogenic effects or adverse newborn outcomes. Caution should be exercised when considering prescribing this group of drugs to women with diabetes mellitus or asthma because they can cause exacerbation of these entities.

Calcium channel blocking agents have varied effects on human gestation. Nifedipine is now frequently used as a tocolytic, and no adverse fetal effects have been documented. Verapamil may decrease uterine blood flow, and exposure in pregnancy may increase the risk for fetal malformations. This drug should be used cautiously in pregnancy. There is little reported experience with the use of cardiazem and nicardipine in pregnancy.

Diuretic use in pregnancy remains controversial. Although there does not appear to be an increased risk for adverse fetal effects, their use may limit the increase in plasma volume considered necessary in normal gestation. Additionally, the use of thiazide diuretics in the third trimester may cause neonatal thrombocytopenia. Acetazolamide and spironolactone should be avoided because of potential teratogenic effects.

## ANTIMICROBIALS

### Antibiotics

Antibiotics are among the most commonly prescribed medications in pregnancy. In general, the penicillins and cephalosporins have not been associated with any pregnancy-associated risks. For those with allergies to penicillin, the macrolide antibiotics (erythromycin and azithromycin), appear to be safe alternatives. Extensive use of these medications during pregnancy has shown no increase in adverse fetal or neonatal effects. Erythromycin estolate, however, is contraindicated in pregnancy because of an association with maternal cholestatic hepatitis.

The tetracyclines were one of the first classes of drugs noted to be teratogenic to the developing offspring. They are associated with abnormal development of teeth and bone, congenital defects, and maternal liver toxicity. Their use should be avoided in pregnancy. Trimethoprim is a folic acid antagonist and poses a theoretical risk to the fetus, although studies have not shown an increase in fetal or neonatal complications associated with this drug. Sulfonamides do not appear to be teratogenic to humans. They do compete with bilirubin binding to plasma albumin and have a risk of causing severe jaundice and associated kernicterus in the newborn. It is generally considered unwise to use sulfonamide antibiotics in the late third trimester of pregnancy. Along with nitrofurantoin, sulfonamides have been associated with hemolytic anemia in patients with glucose-6-phosphate dehydrogenase deficiency.

Metronidazole has been reported to decrease the risk of premature birth because of its utility in treating bacterial vaginosis. Case reports describe congenital malformations in newborns exposed in the first trimester of pregnancy. Because this has created some controversy, prescribing this drug in the first trimester should be done only if the perceived benefits far exceed the potential risks. This medication appears to be safe when prescribed in pregnancy after the first trimester.

## Antifungals

Topical antifungals such as clotrimazole, miconazole, and nystatin have not been associated with an increase in congenital anomalies. It appears that the systemic antifungals, fluconazole and amphotericin B, can also be used where indicated. Griseofulvin is contraindicated during pregnancy because of increased risk for central nervous system and skeletal abnormalities in laboratory animals.

## Antivirals

Experience with antivirals in pregnancy has been driven by a need for their use in sexually transmitted diseases. Acyclovir and valcyclovir are commonly prescribed for the treatment of herpes simplex virus (HSV). Their mechanism of action is specific for viral DNA, and this allows their use for HSV outbreaks during pregnancy. Recent studies have demonstrated a role for acyclovir in suppression of HSV recurrences in the last trimester of pregnancy.

Zidovudine is indicated for the management of human immunodeficiency virus infection during pregnancy and especially intrapartum (Table 41–5). The Zidovudine in Pregnancy Registry has not shown an increase in congenital malformations in exposed offspring. Drugs that inhibit viral replication, zalcitabine and stavudine, can apparently be used as needed. There is currently no information available for the use of protease inhibitors in pregnancy. See Chapter 40 for a comprehensive discussion.

## IMMUNOSUPPRESSANTS

Immunosuppressant drugs are predominantly used in the management of autoimmune disorders and of transplant rejection. These agents and their metabolites cross the placenta. In general, their benefits outweigh potential risks. Experience with azathioprine, prednisone, cyclosporine, and tacrolimas has shown little risk to the fetus. Unfortunately, azathioprine can cause neonatal hematologic abnormalities, including pancytopenia. Further, the safety of monoclonal antibody use in pregnancy is unknown. Gold salts should be avoided during pregnancy and for the first few months before pregnancy. These agents accumulate in the fetal liver and kidney, resulting in newborns with renal and hematologic complications.

**Table 41–5** Recommendations for Zidovudine Use in Pregnancy

Antepartum: Zidovudine (ZDV)—100 mg orally five times a day or 200 mg three times a day starting at 14 to 34 wk gestation and continuing for the duration of pregnancy.
Intrapartum: A loading dose of 2 mg/kg intravenously over an hour followed by a continuous intravenous infusion of 1 mg/kg per hr until delivery.
Newborn therapy: ZDV syrup—2 mg/kg every 6 hr starting within 8 to 12 hr of life and continuing for 6 wk.

Data from Centers for Disease Control and Prevention: Recommendations of the U.S. Task Force on the use of zidovudine to reduce perinatal transmission of human immunodeficiency virus. MMWR 42:1, 1994.

## LOCAL ANESTHETICS

Physicians are often consulted by dentists regarding the risks of these drugs in pregnancy. Local anesthetics are not associated with teratogenic effects.

## PSYCHOTROPICS

### Antidepressants

The selective serotonin reuptake inhibitors (fluoxetine, sertraline, and paroxetine) have become the most frequently prescribed antidepressant drugs. They are easy to take and have fewer side effects than other classes of antidepressants. Compliance is high and rates of discontinuation are low. Fluoxetine is the most commonly prescribed antidepressant in the United States. Experience with its use has shown no increase in congenital malformations in those children exposed in utero. Studies have suggested that infants exposed in the third trimester had increased rates of preterm birth, low birth weight, and poor neonatal transition. These outcomes remain controversial, and further studies are needed.

Tricyclic antidepressants are the oldest prescribed members of this class of medications (Table 41–6). They have noted maternal side effects consisting of constipation, sedation, lightheadedness, and tachycardia. Tricyclic antidepressant use during the third trimester of pregnancy has been associated with newborn tachyarrhythmias, urinary retention, and withdrawal-like symptoms.

Monoamine oxidase inhibitors are rarely used during pregnancy. They are associated with a significant

**Table 41–6** Tricyclic Antidepressants

| | | |
|---|---|---|
| Amitriptyline | Desipramine* | Imipramine |
| Amoxapine | Doxepin | Nortriptyline* |
| Clomipramine | | |

*Recommended because of fewer side effects.

risk of hypertensive crisis if a low-tyrosine diet is not followed with its use.

## Antipsychotics

Most drugs in this category are dopamine antagonists. Maternal side effects include sedation, orthostatic hypotension, dry mouth, constipation, and extrapyramidal effects. Neonates exposed to these drugs can exhibit extrapyramidal effects. Teratogenesis has not been specifically found with this group of drugs. It should be noted that for unexplained reasons psychotic women have an increased rate of offspring with congenital malformations.

Lithium is the drug of choice for treatment of bipolar disorder. Its use in the first trimester has been linked to an increased incidence of fetal cardiac malformations. The most notable of these is Ebstein's anomaly (inferior displacement of the tricuspid valve). Pregnant patients who have taken lithium in the first trimester should undergo fetal echocardiography.

## Anxiolytics

The drugs in this class are also known as tranquilizers. Benzodiazepines constitute the majority prescribed. They are not associated with congenital malformations but have substantial newborn effects. Diazepam can cause newborn depression and withdrawal symptoms. Alprazolam and lorazepam may result in neonatal hypotonia ("floppy baby" syndrome) when used in the third trimester. Avoidance of these drugs in pregnancy is recommended.

## OVER-THE-COUNTER DRUGS

Over-the-counter (OTC) drugs are often not considered "drugs" by many patients. Increasingly, medications previously available only by prescription are now available OTC. The safety of these drugs in pregnancy is often erroneously assumed by pregnant women because of their OTC status. The contents should be reviewed carefully by the health-care provider. Many of the cough and cold remedies contain alcohol.

"Alternative medicine" has been accompanied by "alternative drugs." Our populace now spends more money on these approaches to health than traditional medicine. These herbal medications should be used with caution. They have escaped FDA review, and the list of ingredients can be incomplete or cryptic. Some herbal teas prescribed by alternative medicine practitioners should be avoided in pregnancy because of their stimulant properties. Finally, too much of a given drug may be contained in these preparations. As an example, more than 10,000 IU of vitamin A is known to be teratogenic. Patients should be asked regularly about medications or supplements they are ingesting.

# Conclusions

It appears that a number of drugs can be safely prescribed during pregnancy. Only a limited number are known or suspected human teratogens. The most important principle to follow when considering the use of a drug periconceptionally or during pregnancy is the identification and assessment of benefits and risks to the patient and her conceptus. Yet, undiscovered risks warrant the approach of minimized drug consumption whenever possible during pregnancy.

### REFERENCES

Allen LD, Desai G, Tynan MJ: Prenatal echocardiographic screening for Ebstein's anomaly for mothers on lithium therapy. Lancet 2:875, 1982.

American College of Obstetricians and Gynecologists: Seizure disorders in pregnancy. ACOG Educational Bulletin 231. Washington, DC, ACOG, 1996.

American College of Obstetricians and Gynecologists: Human immunodeficiency virus infections in pregnancy. ACOG Educational Bulletin 232. Washington, DC, ACOG, 1997.

American College of Obstetricians and Gynecologists: Teratology. ACOG Educational Bulletin 236. Washington, DC, ACOG, 1997.

Andrews EB, Yankaskas BC, Cordero JF, et al: Acyclovir in pregnancy registry: Six years experience. Obstet Gynecol 79:7, 1992.

Aselton P, Jick H, Milunsky A, et al: First trimester drug use and congenital disorders. Obstet Gynecol 65:451, 1985.

Barbour LA: Current concepts of anticoagulant therapy in pregnancy. Obstet Gynecol Clin North Am 24:499, 1997.

Bergman U, Rosa FW, Baum C, et al: Effects of fetal exposure to benzodiazepines during fetal life. Lancet 340:694, 1992.

Bracken MB, Holford TR: Exposure to prescribed drugs in pregnancy and association with congenital malformations. Obstet Gynecol 58:336, 1981.

Briggs GG, Freeman RK, Yaffe SJ: Drugs in Pregnancy and Lactation, 4th ed. Baltimore, Williams & Wilkins, 1994.

Brumfitt W, Pursell R: Trimethoprim/sulfamethoxazole in the treatment of bacteriuria in women. J Infect Dis 128:657, 1973.

Burtin P, Taddio A, Arburunu O, et al: Safety of metronidazole in pregnancy: A meta-analysis. Am J Obstet Gynecol 172:525, 1995.

Butters L, Kennedy S, Rubin PC: Atenolol in essential hypertension during pregnancy. Br Med J 301:587, 1990.

Centers for Disease Control and Prevention: Recommendations for the use of folic acid to reduce the number of cases of spina bifida and other neural tube defects. MMWR 41:1, 1992.

Centers for Disease Control and Prevention: Birth outcomes following zidovudine therapy in pregnant women. MMWR 43:409, 1994.

Chambers CD, Johnson KA, Dick LM, et al: Birth outcomes in pregnant women taking fluoxetine. N Engl J Med 335:1010, 1996.

Chez RA, Jonas WB: Complementary and alternative medicine. Part I. Clinical studies in obstetrics. Obstet Gynecol Surv 52:704, 1997.

Chez RA, Jonas WB: The challenges of complementary and alternative medicine. Am J Obstet Gynecol 177:1156, 1997.

Childress CH, Katz VL: Nifedipine and its indications in obstetrics and gynecology. Obstet Gynecol 8:616, 1994.
CLASP Collaborative Group: Low dose aspirin in pregnancy and early childhood development: Follow up of the collaborative low dose aspirin study in pregnancy. Br J Obstet Gynaecol 102:861, 1995.
Cohen DL, Orzel J, Taylor A: Infant of mothers receiving gold therapy. Arthritis Rheum 24:104, 1981.
Cohen LS, Friedman JM, Jefferson JW, et al: A re-evaluation of risk of in utero exposure to lithium. JAMA 271:146, 1994.
Corby DG: Aspirin in pregnancy: maternal and fetal effects. Pediatrics 62(suppl):930, 1978.
Cornelissen M, Steegers-Theunissen R, Kolle L, et al: Supplementation of vitamin K in pregnant women receiving anticonvulsant therapy prevents neonatal vitamin K deficiency. Am J Obstet Gynecol 168:884, 1993.
Dahlman TC: Osteoporotic fractures and recurrence of thromboembolism during pregnancy and the puerperium in 184 women undergoing thromboprophylaxis with heparin. Am J Obstet Gynecol 168:1265, 1993.
Dean JL, Wolf JE, Ranzini AC, et al: Use of amphotericin B during pregnancy: Case reports and review. Clin Infect Dis 18:364, 1994.
Delgado-Escueta AV, Janz D: Consensus guidelines: Preconception counseling, management, and care of the pregnant woman with epilepsy. Neurology 42(suppl):149, 1992.
Dulitzki M, Pauzner R, Langevitz P, et al: Low-molecular weight heparin during pregnancy and delivery: Preliminary experience with 41 pregnancies. Obstet Gynecol 87:380, 1996.
Elia J, Katz IR, Simpson GM: Teratogenicity of psychotherapeutic medications. Psychopharmacol Bull 28:531, 1987.
Friedman JM: Teratogen update: Anesthetic agents. Teratology 37:69, 1988.
Ginsberg JS, Kowalchuk G, Hirsh J, et al: Heparin therapy during pregnancy: Risks to the mother and fetus. Arch Intern Med 149:2233, 1989.
Goldbar KG: Psychotropics. Semin Perinatol 21:154, 1997.
Goldstein DJ, Corbin LA, Sundell KL: Effects of first trimester fluoxetine exposure on the newborn. Obstet Gynecol 89:713, 1997.
Gordon MC, Samuels P: Indomethacin. Clin Obstet Gynecol 38:697, 1995.
Greenberg F: Possible metronidazole teratogenicity and clefting. Am J Med Genet 22:825, 1985.
Harman K: "Floppy-infant" and maternal diazepam. Lancet 2:612, 1977.
Hill LM, Kleinberg F: Effects of drugs and chemicals on the fetus and newborn. Part 1. Mayo Clin Proc 59:707, 1984.
Jelovsek FR, Mattison DR, Chen JJ: Prediction of risks for human developmental toxicity: How important are animal studies for hazard identification? Obstet Gynecol 74:624, 1989.
Koren G, Bologa M, Long D, et al: Perception of teratogenic risk by pregnant women exposed to drugs and chemicals during the first trimester. Am J Obstet Gynecol 160:1190, 1989.
Koren G, Pastuszak A, Ito S: Drugs in pregnancy. N Engl J Med 338:1128, 1998.
Kutscher AH, Zegarelli EV, Tovell HM, et al: Discoloration of the deciduous teeth induced by the administration of tetracycline antepartum. Am J Obstet Gynecol 96:291, 1966.
Lee P: Anti-inflammatory therapy during pregnancy and lactation. Clin Invest Med 8:328, 1985.
Lindhout D, Hoppener RJ, Meinardi H: Teratogenicity of antiepileptic drug combinations with special emphasis on epoxidation (carbamazepine). Epilepsia 25:77, 1984.
Lip GY, Beavers M, Churchill D, et al: Effect of atenolol on birth weight. Am J Cardiol 79:1436, 1997.
Little BB: Immunosuppressive drugs and pregnancy. Semin Perinatol 21:143, 1997.
Lumpkin MM. FDA Public Health Advisory—Reports of epidural or spinal hematomas with the concurrent use of low molecular weight heparin and spinal/epidural anesthesia or spinal puncture. Washington, DC, FDA Talk Paper, Dec. 15, 1997.
Macones GA, Robinson CA: Is there justification for using indomethacin in preterm labor? An analysis of neonatal risks and benefits. Am J Obstet Gynecol 177:819, 1997.
Magee LA, Conover B, Schick B, et al: Exposure to calcium channel blockers in human pregnancy: A prospective controlled multicentre cohort study. Teratology 49:372A, 1994.
Malone FD, D'Alton ME: Drugs in pregnancy: Anticonvulsants. Semin Perinatol 21:114, 1997.
Mastrobattista JM: Angiotensin converting enzyme inhibitors in pregnancy. Semin Perinatol 21:124, 1997.
Maternal adaptations to pregnancy. In Cunningham FG, MacDonald PC, Gant NF, et al (eds): Williams Obstetrics, 20th ed. Stamford, CT, Appleton & Lange, 1997, pp 158, 191.
Mattison DR: Minimizing toxic hazards to fetal health. Contemp Obstet Gynecol 37:81, 1982.
McCormick WM, George H, Donner A, et al: Hepatotoxicity of erythromycin estolate during pregnancy. Antimicrob Agents Chemother 12:630, 1977.
McEwen LM: Trimethoprim/sulfamethoxazole mixture in pregnancy. Br Med J 4:490, 1971.
Merlob P, Litwin A, Mor N: Possible association of acetazolamide administration during pregnancy and metabolic disorders in the newborn. Eur J Obstet Gynaecol Reprod Biol 35:85, 1990.
Messina M, Biffignandi P, Ghiga E, et al: Possible contraindications to spironolactone during pregnancy. J Endocrinol Invest 2:222, 1979.
Metneki J, Czeizel A: Griseofulvin teratology. Lancet 1:1042, 1987.
Miller LJ: Psychopharmacology during pregnancy. Prim Care Update Obstet Gynecol 3:79, 1996.
Moore KL: The Developing Human: Clinically Oriented Embryology, 4th ed. Philadelphia, WB Saunders, 1988, p 131.
Murphy PA: Alternative therapies for nausea and vomiting of pregnancy. Obstet Gynecol 91:149, 1998.
Murray L, Seger D: Drug therapy during pregnancy and lactation. Emerg Med Clin North Am 12:129, 1994.
National Asthma Education Program: Report of the Working Group on Asthma and Pregnancy: Executive summary: Management of asthma during pregnancy. National Heart, Lung and Blood Institute. Bethesda, MD, NIH Publication 93-3279A, March 1993.
National High Blood Pressure Education Program Working Group: Report on high blood pressure in pregnancy. Am J Obstet Gynecol 163:1691, 1990.
Norton ME, Merrill J, Cooper BAB, et al: Neonatal complications after the administration of indomethacin for preterm labor. N Engl J Med 329:1602, 1993.
Nulman I, Rovert J, Stewart DE, et al: Neurodevelopment of children exposed in utero to antidepressant drugs. N Engl J Med 336:258, 1997.
Parisi VM, Salinas J, Stockmar KJ: Fetal vascular responses to maternal nicardipine administration in the hypertensive ewe. Am J Obstet Gynecol 161:1035, 1989.
Pastuszak A, Schick-Boschetto B, Zuber C, et al: Pregnancy outcomes following first trimester exposure to fluoxetine (Prozac). JAMA 269:2246, 1993.
Piper JM, Mitchel EF, Ray WA: Prenatal use of metronidazole and birth defects: No association. Obstet Gynecol 82:348, 1993.
Polak JF, Wilkinson DL: Ultrasonographic diagnosis of symptomatic deep venous thrombosis in pregnancy. Am J Obstet Gynecol 165:625, 1991.
Powell RD, DeGowin RL, Alving AS: Nitrofurantoin induced hemolysis. J Lab Clin Med 62:1002, 1963.
Ramsey-Goldman R, Schilling E: Immunosuppressive drug use during pregnancy. Rheum Clin North Am 23:149, 1997.
Rasanen J, Jouppila P: Fetal cardiac function and ductus arteriosus during indomethacin and sulindac therapy for threatened preterm labor: A randomized study. Am J Obstet Gynecol 175:20, 1995.
Read MD, Wellby DE: The use of calcium antagonist (nifedipine) to suppress preterm labor. Br J Obstet Gynaecol 93:933, 1986.
Rementaria JL, Bhatt K: Withdrawal symptoms in neonates from intrauterine exposure to diazepam. J Pediatr 90:123, 1977.
Rosa FW, Baum C, Shaw M: Pregnancy outcomes after first trimester vaginitis drug therapy. Obstet Gynecol 69:751, 1987.
Rossoff LJ: Diagnosis, treatment, and prevention of venous thromboembolism in women. Prim Care Update 1:108, 1994.
Rothman KJ, Moore LL, Singer MR, et al: Teratogenicity of high vitamin A intake. N Engl J Med 333:1369, 1995.
Rubin CP, Craig GF, Gavin K, et al: Prospective survey of use of therapeutic drugs, alcohol, and cigarettes during pregnancy. Br Med J 292:81, 1986.

Sahakian V, Rouse D, Sipes S, et al: Vitamin $B_6$ is effective therapy for nausea and vomiting of pregnancy: A randomized, double-blind placebo-controlled study. Obstet Gynecol 78:33, 1991.

Scialli AR: Safe medications during pregnancy. Contemp Obstet Gynecol 27:40, 1983.

Scott LL, Sanchez PJ, Jackson L, et al: Acyclovir suppression to prevent cesarean delivery after first-episode genital herpes. Obstet Gynecol 87:69, 1996.

Sexson WR, Barak Y: Withdrawal emergent syndrome in an infant associated with maternal haloperidol therapy. J Perinatol 9:170, 1989.

Shepard TH: Human teratogenicity. Adv Pediatr 33:225, 1986.

Shepard TH: Catalog of Teratogenic Agents, 8th ed. Baltimore, Johns Hopkins University Press, 1995.

Sibai BM, Caritis SN, Thom E, et al: Prevention of preeclampsia with low-dose aspirin in healthy, nulliparous pregnant women. The National Institute of Child Health and Human Development Network of Maternal-Fetal Medicine Units. N Engl J Med 329:1213, 1993.

Sibai BM, Caritis SN, Thom E, et al: Low-dose aspirin in nulliparous women: Safety of continuous epidural block and correlation between bleeding time and maternal-neonatal bleeding complications. National Institute of Child Health and Human Development Maternal-Fetal Medicine Network. Am J Obstet Gynecol 172:1553, 1995.

Sibai BM, Grossman RA, Grossman HG: Effects of diuretics on plasma volume in pregnancies complicated with long term hypertension. Am J Obstet Gynecol 150:831, 1984.

Simone C, Derewlany LO, Koren G: Drug transfer across the placenta: Considerations for treatment and research. Clin Perinatol 21:463, 1994.

Slone D, Siskind V, Heinonen OP, et al: Antenatal exposure to phenothiazines in relation to congenital malformations, perinatal mortality rate, birth weight, and intelligence quotient score. Am J Obstet Gynecol 128:486, 1977.

Stevenson RE, Burton M, Ferlauto GJ, et al: Hazards of oral anticoagulants during pregnancy. JAMA 243:1549, 1980.

Stiffman MN, Adam P: Acyclovir in pregnancy for prevention of neonatal herpes. J Family Pract 44:29, 1997.

Sturridge F, de Sewiet M, Letsky E: The use of low-molecular weight heparin for thromboprophylaxis in pregnancy. Br J Obstet Gynaecol 101:69, 1994.

Toglia MR, Weg JG: Venous thromboembolism during pregnancy. N Engl J Med 335:305, 1996.

Turrentine MA, Braems G, Ramirez MM: Use of thrombolytics for the treatment of thromboembolic disease during pregnancy. Obstet Gynecol Surv 50:534, 1995.

Ulmsten U, Anderson KE, Wingerup L: Treatment of preterm labor with calcium antagonist nifedipine. Arch Gynecol 229:1, 1980.

Vermilion ST, Scardo JA, Lashus AG, et al: The effect of indomethacin tocolysis on fetal ductus arteriosus constriction with advancing gestational age. Am J Obstet Gynecol 177:256, 1997.

Vuckovic N, Nichter M: Changing pattern of pharmaceutical practice in the United States. Soc Sci Med 44:1285, 1997.

Walker BE: Induction of cleft palate in rats with anti-inflammatory drugs. Teratology 4:39, 1971.

Walley PJ, Adams RH, Combes B: Tetracycline toxicity in pregnancy. JAMA 189:357, 1964.

Warkany J: Teratogen update: Lithium. Teratology 38:593, 1988.

Weinstein MR, Goldfield MD: Cardiovascular malformations with lithium use during pregnancy. Am J Psychiatry 132:529, 1975.

Weisberg M: Treatment of vaginal candidiasis in pregnant women. Clin Ther 8:563, 1986.

Yerby MS: Pregnancy, teratogenesis, and epilepsy. Neurol Clin 12:749, 1994.

# GYNECOLOGIC ONCOLOGY

# 42

# Premalignant Disorders of the Lower Genital Tract

MICHELE FOLLEN MITCHELL

## Definition

The concept that invasive cancer develops from intraepithelial precursor lesions was proposed in the early 1900s by clinicians who studied the cervix. They recognized that intraepithelial lesions that are histologically similar to invasive cervical cancer frequently occur adjacent to invasive cancers; these lesions were found to have a high capacity to progress to invasive cancer if left untreated. These lesions were referred to as carcinoma in situ (CIS). Later, other types of intraepithelial lesions of the cervix were identified; these lesions are histologically less severe than CIS but can also progress to invasive cervical cancer if left untreated. These lesions were referred to as dysplasia and were classified in degree from mild to severe. Observations of abnormalities similar to those of the squamous epithelium in the cervix were also made in the squamous epithelial layer of the vulva and vagina.

In the 1960s, based on the results of follow-up studies in patients and supporting evidence derived from electron microscopy, clonality studies, and tissue culture studies, Richart proposed that these dysplastic precursor lesions in the cervix formed a biologic continuum that he termed cervical intraepithelial neoplasia, or CIN. The terminology was so easily accepted that it was quickly applied to the vulva (vulvar intraepithelial neoplasia, or VIN) and the vagina (vaginal intraepithelial neoplasia, or VAIN). The CIN continuum concept was based on the premises that precursor lesions share a similar etiology and biology and that they eventually advance to invasive cancer. Since that time, it has become clear that untreated higher grade cervical lesions are more likely to progress to invasive cancer and that many lower grade cervical lesions regress. The natural history of untreated VIN and VAIN appears similar.

Cervical, vulvar, and vaginal intraepithelial neoplasias were classified in three grades: grade 1 (mild dysplasia) is characterized by undifferentiated cells that extend up to one third of the distance from the basement membrane to the surface epithelium; grade 2 (moderate dysplasia), characterized by extension from one third to two thirds of this distance; and grade 3 (severe dysplasia and CIS), characterized by extension over more than two thirds of this distance. The pathologic diagnosis of intraepithelial neoplasia is based on seven morphologic criteria: increased nuclear size, altered nuclear shape, increased nuclear stain uptake, nuclear pleomorphism, increased mitosis, abnormal mitosis, and disordered or absent maturation. The term invasive cancer is used to describe lesions in which the malignant cells penetrate the underlying basement membrane and infiltrate the stroma. As the pathobiology of these precursors increasingly focused on the role of human papillomavirus (HPV), its hallmark, koilocytotic atypia, also called condyloma, became a recognized part of the spectrum, preceding intraepithelial neoplasia.

Squamous intraepithelial lesions (SIL) is the term now used to describe intraepithelial neoplasia of the lower genital tract. With the goal of increasing agreement among observers and taking into account the role HPV may play in the pathobiologic continuum, a new classification system for reporting cervical smears, the Bethesda system, was introduced in 1988. In this system, noninvasive squamous lesions are classified as atypical squamous cells of undetermined significance (ASCUS), including lesions with cells that have abnormal nuclear characteristics but without changes suggestive of koilocytotic atypia, or CIN 1; atypical glandular cells of uncertain significance (AGCUS); low-grade SIL (LGSIL), including koilocytotic lesions and CIN 1; and high-grade SIL (HGSIL), including CIN 2, CIN 3, and CIS. This cytologic classification is now used to describe histopathologic lesions. In the cervix, the histopathologic correlates for ASCUS and AGCUS are atypias and inflammation. The role of atypias and inflammation in the pathologic continuum is unknown. Parallel to the application of CIN terminology to the vulva and vagina, some pathologists report vulvar and vaginal histopathology using the LGSIL and HGSIL classifications. The three evolving terminologies for describing the premalignant disorders are summarized in Figure 42–1.

## Diagnostic Considerations and Strategies

### HISTORY

Epidemiologic studies have long suggested a sexually transmitted etiology for cervical neoplasia. The risk for cervical neoplasia is higher among women who have multiple sexual partners, women who have their first sexual intercourse at an early age, and women whose sexual partners are promiscuous. In addition, socioeconomic status, reproductive history, smoking habits, oral and barrier contraceptive use, dietary factors, characteristics of the sexual partner (e.g., smoking habits), immunosuppression, and frequency of Papanicolaou smears have been implicated as risk factors for cervical neoplasia. The etiologic role of several sexually transmitted agents has been studied; these agents include herpes simplex virus type 2, *Chlamydia trachomatis*, *Trichomonas vaginalis*, cytomegalovirus, *Neisseria gonorrhoeae*, and *Treponema pallidum*.

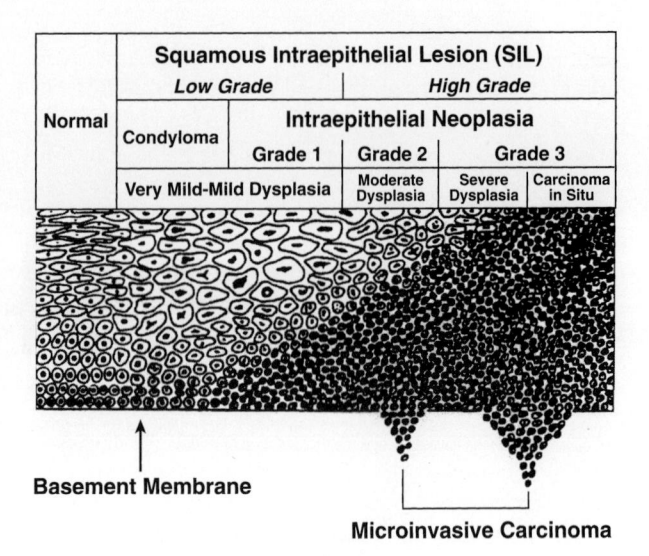

**Figure 42–1** Pathologic continuum of intraepithelial neoplasias. Three different terminologies have been used to refer to these lesions. At top is the current terminology, the Bethesda system. (From Wright TC, Kurman RJ, Ferenczy A: Precancerous lesions of the cervix. *In* Kurman RJ (ed): Blaustein's Pathology of the Female Genital Tract, 4th ed New York, Springer-Verlag, 1994, p 246.)

Since the mid-1970s, substantial evidence has accumulated to support the role of some types of HPV in the etiology of cervical neoplasia. Current epidemiologic data support a strong and central role for HPV in the etiology of cervical neoplasia in women worldwide. Furthermore, the involvement of HPV appears to explain many of the established risk factors for cervical neoplasia, including sexual behavior and cigarette smoking, which are risk factors for HPV infection as well. The association between HPV infection and neoplasia is particularly strong with specific high-risk HPV types, with increasing viral load, and with coinfection of patients with different HPV types. This association has been independent of the HPV assay method used and epidemiologic study design. However, although HPV is the most important risk factor for intraepithelial neoplasia of the lower genital tract, the presence of other cofactors seems to be necessary for the development of disease. The difference between the high prevalence of HPV infection in young healthy women and the low incidence of cervical, vaginal, and vulvar neoplasia, as well as the low rate of progression of untreated intraepithelial lesions, supports the hypothesis that HPV may be a necessary but not sufficient factor for intraepithelial neoplasia. The introduction of more accurate and effective methods for detection of HPV infection has improved the opportunity of conducting larger epidemiologic studies to reassess the independent or joint effect of previously established risk factors and HPV. In addition, the role of HPV persistence in the progression of intraepithelial neoplasia and the determinants of HPV persistence need further evaluation.

Both vulvar and vaginal SILs are believed to have risk factors similar to those of cervical SILs, and HPV is the most important. Thus, a good medical risk factor history for a patient suspected to have intraepithelial neoplasia of the lower genital tract would include age, race, educational or socioeconomic level, smoking status, history of exposure to HPV, history of genital warts, history of other sexually transmitted diseases, immunosuppressive medical illnesses, immunosuppressive medication use, age at first sexual intercourse of patient and partner, number of sexual partners of patient and partner, barrier and nonbarrier contraceptive use, reproductive history, frequency of screening exams and Papanicolaou smears, dietary history (focusing on low vitamin A intake), family history of cancer, personal history of cancer and exposure to radiation, and history of vulvar dystrophy. The medical history should concentrate on these risk factors and on previous treatments in the history of present illness and should also include past medical history, family medical history, and review of systems.

## PHYSICAL EXAMINATION AND EVALUATION

The physical examination should be comprehensive and should include a gynecologic examination. During the gynecologic examination, the following tests should be performed: a Papanicolaou smear, cervical cultures for gonorrhea and chlamydia, a wet drop of any vaginal discharge, a culture of any vesicular lesion to rule out herpes, and, finally, pancolposcopy of the vulva, perineum, vagina, and cervix. Diagrams or photographs of vulvar, vaginal, and cervical condylomas and intraepithelial lesions should be made, noting location, appearance, and presence or type of vascular atypia (Fig. 42–2). Colposcopically directed biopsies should be performed on any suspicious areas of the vulva, vagina, and cervix.

Colposcopists agree on the terminology for the classification of vascular atypia: fine punctation, coarse punctation, mosaiform atypia, mosaicism, and atypical vessels. Atypical vessels are suggestive of malignant lesions. Coarse punctation is more often associated with higher grade lesions than is fine punctation. Similarly, mosaicism is more often associated with higher grade lesions than is mosaiform atypia.

### Vulva

Generally, vulvar condylomas present as raised hyperkeratotic papules, which are often pigmented. Vulvar

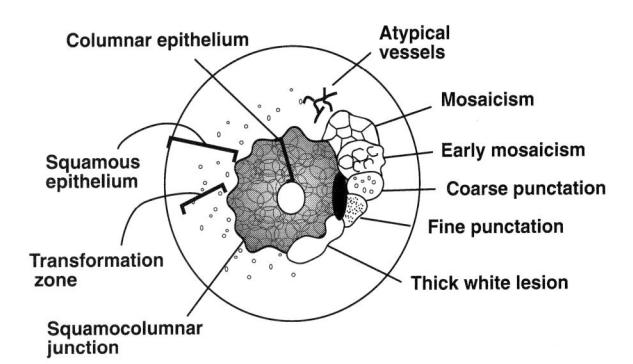

**Figure 42–2** Diagram of the vascular atypia of the vulva, the vagina, and the cervix. (From Mitchell MF, Tortolero-Luna GT, Wright T, et al: Cervical human papillomavirus infection and intraepithelial neoplasia: A review. Monogr Natl Cancer Inst 21:17, 1996.)

intraepithelial lesions appear as discrete erythematous, pigmented, or thick white lesions and may involve either non–hair- or hair-bearing areas of the labia majora or labia minora. Perianal lesions may be particularly difficult to visualize. Thus, careful inspection of the vulva and perianum with white light is mandatory. This should be followed by covering the entire vulva and perianum with acetic acid-soaked gauze, leaving it in place for a minimum of 5 minutes, and then carefully inspecting with the colposcope with both white and green light. If vascular atypia is present on the vulva, it usually appears as punctation. If hair growth is particularly dense, the area can be shaved to aid inspection.

Punch biopsies of representative abnormal-appearing areas of the vulva and perianum are performed after application of local anesthesia. Dermal punches measuring 3 to 5 mm provide adequate samples. Hemostasis after biopsy is achieved with nitrate sticks.

### Vagina

Vaginal condylomas appear as raised hyperkeratotic papules. Vaginal intraepithelial lesions appear as discrete erythematous, or thick and thin white lesions. Generally, 2 full minutes exposure to acetic acid applied with several soaked cotton balls is sufficient for visualization of these lesions. Careful inspection with the colposcope using both white and green light should ensue. Care must be taken to visualize the entire vagina. Because the speculum hides the anterior and posterior vault, it should either be removed and placed sideways in the vault or slowly removed so that the vault can be visualized as it collapses. I prefer using the speculum to visualize the lateral vault in the anterior and posterior dimension and then moving the speculum laterally to visualize the anterior and posterior vault. Colposcopically directed biopsies of representative abnormal-appearing areas should be taken with sharp biopsy forceps, such as the mini-Townsend forceps. Hemostasis is achieved with Monsel's paste, a combination of ferrous subsulfate and benzoin solution.

### Cervix

Cervical condylomas and intraepithelial lesions manifest as erythematous or, more often, white epithelium with or without the presence of vascular atypia. After exposure to acetic acid for 2 minutes, careful inspection with the colposcope should be performed using both white and green light. The colposcopic diagram of the cervix should include the location of the os, the squamocolumnar junction, the transformation zone, the location and size of the lesion or lesions, and the presence or absence of vascular atypia. Colposcopically directed biopsies should be taken of representative abnormal-appearing areas using a sharp biopsy forceps, such as the mini-Townsend. An endocervical curettage using an endocervical curette with a basket is mandatory unless the patient is pregnant. Hemostasis is achieved with Monsel's paste.

### LABORATORY EVALUATION

All lesions should be biopsied. Assumptions should not be made about the diagnosis from visualization alone. Many a patient who has had an invasive cancer of the vulva, vagina, or cervix has been treated for months as a patient who had a condyloma by an unsuspecting clinician. No treatment plan can be generated without a biopsy.

All patients should have any referral cytology and pathology specimens reviewed by the pathologist, who works closely with the clinician. The importance of reviewing this material cannot be overemphasized.

Interrater agreement between cytologists and pathologists is excellent for high-grade lesions and poor for low-grade lesions and ASCUS and AGCUS lesions of vulva, vagina, and cervix. Atypical metaplasia and inflammation of the cervix, vaginal atrophy, and vulvar inflammation can be sources of confusion to cytologists, histopathologists, and colposcopists. Careful coordination of effort to come to a consensus diagnosis rewards both the patient and the clinician. This can only be achieved by careful review of previous and current specimens and by the colposcopic exam.

Some clinicians perform HPV testing of the cervix using the Virapap or Hybrid Capture assay (Digene Diagnostics, Inc., Silverspring, MD), although its utility has not been proved. Serum human immunodeficiency virus (HIV) testing should be performed after appropriate counseling. Additional preventive medicine guidelines should be followed, depending on the current health status of the patient and whether the obstetrician/gynecologist is also the primary care physician.

## DIFFERENTIAL DIAGNOSIS

The differential diagnosis for lesions of the vulva includes invasive cancer, VIN or vulvar SIL, vulvar dystrophy, atrophy, benign nevi, and inflammation. The differential diagnosis for lesions of the vagina includes invasive cancer, VAIN or vaginal SIL, atrophy, and inflammation. The differential diagnosis for lesions of the cervix includes invasive cancer, CIN or SIL, HPV infection, and acute or chronic inflammation. The crucial goal in diagnosis of premalignant disorders of the lower genital tract is excluding invasive cancer.

## Treatment

### TREATMENT OF CONDYLOMAS

#### Vulvar Condylomas

Vulvar condylomas cause discomfort, and patients often request treatment. Therapy is appropriate in any case to control the disease. Treatments have included surgical excision, ablation, and experimental vaccines. Surgical excision has been carried out in the past with the scalpel and electrocautery and is carried out in the present with loop excision electrocautery (wire cautery). Ablation has been carried out using devices (including cryotherapy and $CO_2$ laser ablation) and chemicals (including podophyllin, trichloroacetic acid, idoxuridine, and fluorouracil [5-FU]). A vaccine trial using vaccines produced from the patient's own warts was reported in 1972. This approach is still being investigated in a more sophisticated form that stimulates both the humoral immune response and the cell-mediated immune response. Overall cure rates for all therapies together range from 15 to 20% for short periods of follow-up. Long-term failure rates range from 40 to 60%.

New classes of medications that are becoming available include antiviral and immunomodulatory agents. An example of an antiviral agent is cidofovir, a nucleotide analog that acts by inhibiting DNA polymerase. It is active against a number of DNA viruses, such as herpes virus and HPV. Unlike the antiviral agents acyclovir and ganciclovir, which require activation by a viral protein kinase, cidofovir is active independent of the presence of viral infection. Cidofovir is currently under study as a treatment for genital warts in HIV-infected patients. A topical immunomodulatory agent that is being studied is imiquimod, a heterocyclic amine. It stimulates monocytes, macrophages, and keratinocytes to produce interferon and other cytokines. In clinical trials of the treatment of anogenital warts, there was a 50% response rate to imiquimod (5%) applied three times weekly for 16 weeks. In a second trial, daily treatment with the 5% imiquimod dose led to a 70% response rate. In the long term, HPV vaccine trials will eventually be of great interest.

### Vaginal Condylomas

Vaginal condylomas are rarely symptomatic and patients are usually treated when they receive concomitant therapy for vulvar condylomas or SIL of the cervix. Vaginal condylomas can be removed by surgical excision or ablation. Vaginal condylomas have been excised surgically in the past with the scalpel and electrocautery. Now, the latter procedure is performed with loop excision electrocautery. Ablation has been carried out using cryotherapy and carbon dioxide ($CO_2$) laser ablation as well as podophyllin, trichloroacetic acid, and 5-FU. Cure rates range from 10 to 12% for short periods of follow-up. Long-term failure rates range from 60 to 80%. Therapies such as cidofovir and imiquimod will eventually be of interest for this population. Over the long term, a vaccine directed at treatment will be of much interest.

### Cervical Condylomas

Cervical condylomas may represent subclinical or latent cervical HPV infections. In these cases, the infection may cause only atypia of the cervix. If the atypia is caused by HPV and affects only the cervical epithelium, patients are evaluated and treated as if they had LGSIL. Because many LGSIL lesions regress, many clinicians simply monitor these patients with cytology and colposcopy at regular intervals, reserving treatment for higher grade lesions. HPV testing would be clinically useful if it helped in deciding which patients with LGSIL need to treated or followed more aggressively.

## TREATMENT OF PREMALIGNANT DISORDERS

### Vulvar Intraepithelial Lesions

Intraepithelial lesions of the vulva have been treated in the past by vulvectomy, wide local excision, 5-FU cream, laser ablation, cryotherapy, and radiation. Vulvectomy and wide local excision have similar success rates, and because wide local excision is less deforming, it has become the standard of surgical care for most patients who have these lesions. Laser ablation has a higher cure rate than 5-FU, cryotherapy, or radiation and is now used more frequently than these other ablative therapies.

VIN or vulvar SIL can be well-treated by wide local excision or laser ablation. The cure rates for both are similar, ranging from 80 to 90%. If the vulva has been adequately sampled and the pathology carefully reviewed, the diagnosis should be known to the surgeon before the planned procedure. In patients younger than 45 to 50 years of age, laser ablation, which does not produce a specimen, has a role if invasive cancer has been ruled out. Because patients who are older than 50 years are more likely to harbor invasive or microinvasive cancer, wide local excision is preferable because it yields a specimen.

For labial lesions that are smaller than 2 cm in size, wide local excision can be performed with local anesthesia in a clinic, using a scalpel or the electrosurgical excision procedure. Larger lesions should be excised with the patient under general anesthesia and with the scalpel following the skin lines. Clitoral lesions should always be excised with the patient under general anesthesia because of the pain associated with this highly innervated area. Closure should be achieved with durable suture material, preferably using a mattress technique. Patients may be instructed to use sitz baths and a hair dryer on the vulva one to two times daily. The incisions heal in 4 to 6 weeks, leaving a scar.

For small labial lesions, laser ablation can be performed with the patient under local anesthesia in an outpatient clinic. Again, patients who have larger labial or any size clitoral lesions should be treated with use of general anesthesia. The technique using laser treatment for patients who have VIN or vulvar SIL is well described by Reid and involves penetrating well into the reticular dermis. Patients may be instructed to use sitz baths and an antibacterial cream on the vulva three to four times per day. Healing occurs over 4 to 8 weeks, and often there is very little scarring.

### Vaginal Intraepithelial Lesions

Vaginal intraepithelial lesions have been treated in the past with radiation, vaginectomy, 5-FU, laser, and electrocautery. The most successful techniques are vaginectomy, 5-FU, and laser.

Lesions of the vagina should be carefully reviewed to exclude the diagnosis of atrophy, a common source of atypia in postmenopausal and other estrogen-deficient patients. The treatment for patients who have atrophy is an estrogen vaginal cream. Colposcopically visualized lesions and abnormal smears resulting from atrophy disappear after 1 to 2 months of daily use of estrogen cream. Careful consideration of atrophy as a cause of abnormalities cannot be overemphasized. Again, however, the most important lesion to exclude is invasive cancer of the vagina.

For vaginal lesions that are suggestive in any way of invasion or that are found in patients older than 50 years in whom atrophy has been excluded, vaginectomy should be performed. Vaginectomy, partial or total, is difficult and should be performed by a surgeon who has experience in these procedures. The involved area of the vagina must be incised, which is a challenging procedure because the anterior vagina overlies the bladder, the ureters, or the urethra, and the posterior vagina overlies the rectum. Because the blood supply of the vagina runs in the lateral walls, lesions in these areas are no less difficult to remove. Total vaginectomies are usually accompanied by skin-grafting procedures to create neovaginas. The cure rate following excision is 90%.

Lesions that are not thought to be suggestive of invasion, especially in women younger than 45 to 50 years old, can be treated with 5-FU cream or laser ablation. Neither procedure yields a specimen, and thus both are inadequate in the patient in whom invasion is suspected. 5-FU cream can be applied in a variety of regimens; the most common is vaginal application for 5 nights per month for 1 to 6 months with colposcopic follow-up. Many groups treat the patient for 3 months and then reevaluate. 5-FU causes sloughing of the vaginal mucosa and is best used in patients who have large lesions and those who are not currently sexually active. The cure rate following 5-FU treatment is 85%.

Laser ablation is well suited to patients who have small lesions (1 to 1.5 cm) or who desire early resumption of sexual activity. The treatment can be tailored to the size of the lesion and can be accomplished in one visit. Generally, laser ablation of the vagina is best performed with the patient under general anesthesia. A microscope is used to help visualize the area of interest. After the procedure, sitz baths and application of an antibacterial vaginal cream are recommended twice daily. Estrogen should be added if the patient is hypoestrogenic. The cure rate following laser ablation is 80%.

## Cervical Intraepithelial Neoplasia or Squamous Intraepithelial Lesions

In patients who have biopsy-proven SIL of the cervix and negative findings on endocervical curettage, a satisfactory colposcopy result and congruent Papanicolaou smear and biopsy results (specifically, the Papanicolaou smear results must not indicate higher grade disease than the biopsy), ablation of the transformation zone has been the standard of care for several decades. However, ablation is not sufficient if there is a possibility of invasive cancer in patients who have biopsy-proven SIL of the cervix and positive findings on endocervical curettage; an unsatisfactory colposcopy result; a Papanicolaou smear result worse than the biopsy result; suspicion of invasion based on the Papanicolaou smear, colposcopy, or biopsy; suspicion of adenocarcinoma in situ or adenocarcinoma; or a history of noncompliance with follow-up. In such cases, cone biopsy has been the standard of care for several decades. The triage scheme for making this decision is illustrated in Figure 42–3.

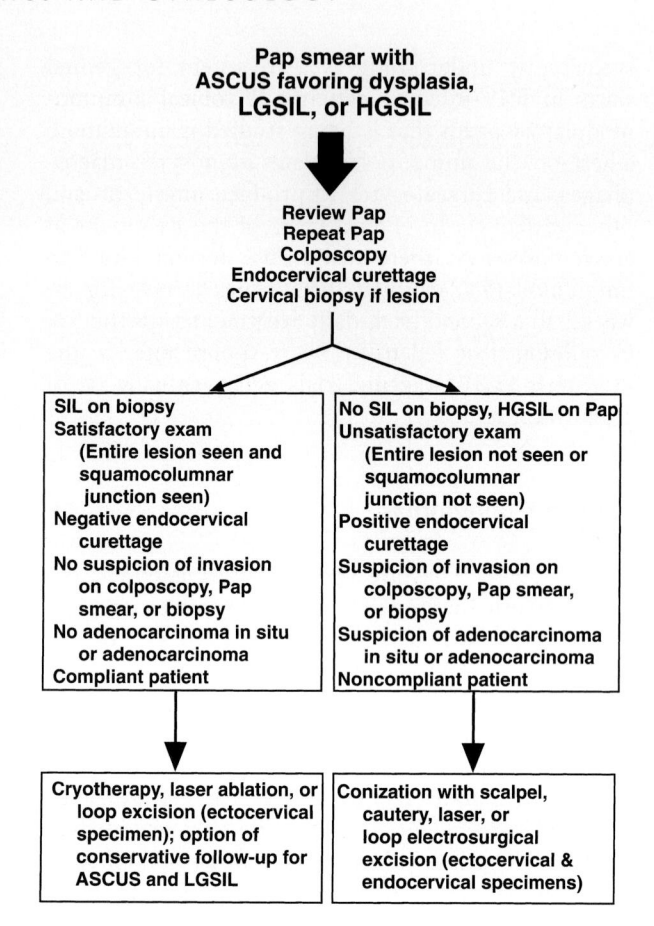

**Figure 42–3** Triage of patients who have abnormal Papanicolaou smears. (From Mitchell MF, Tortolero-Luna GT, Wright T, et al: Cervical human papillomavirus infection and intraepithelial neoplasia: A review. Monogr Natl Cancer Inst 21:17, 1996.)

## Ablative Techniques

Several techniques for ablation are available: cryotherapy, laser ablation, loop excision of the transformation zone or the loop electrosurgical excision procedure, electrocautery, Semm cold coagulation, electrocoagulation diathermy, and interferon therapy. Cryotherapy, laser ablation, and the loop electrosurgical excision procedure are most commonly used (Fig. 42–4).

Cryotherapy involves the application to the cervix of a metal probe through which compressed gases with boiling points in the cryogenic range are passed. The drop in temperature of the probe causes an ice ball to form in the tissue, leading to tissue dehydration and destruction. To perform cryotherapy, a large Graves' speculum is placed in the vagina, and a nipple-tipped probe of a size appropriate to cover the lesion and transformation zone is selected. K-Y jelly (Johnson & Johnson Medical, Inc., Arlington, TX) can be applied to the probe before applying the probe to the cervix. Tongue blades are used along the vaginal walls for protection. The patient's cervix is treated for 3 minutes, thawed, and treated again for 3 minutes so that an ice ball extends 5 mm beyond the lesion and transformation zone. Cryotherapy remains a trusted tool because of its reliability, ease of use, and low cost. Its disadvantages include the lack of ability to tailor the treatment to the size of the lesion and the lack of a tissue specimen.

Laser vaporization, introduced in 1977, uses a $CO_2$ laser attached to a colposcope to create a monochromatic, coherent, and collimated light that destroys tissue by evaporation. To perform laser ablation, a $CO_2$ laser colposcopy unit (Leisegang Medical, Inc., Boca Raton, FL) is used. The procedure includes the placement of a large ebonized Graves' speculum with suction attachment. The laser is set at 20 watts on continuous mode, and the spot size is 1 mm. Small dots are made around the lesion and the transformation zone, and the laser is then used to ablate an area 8 mm deep around the canal and 6 mm deep at the edge. Rulers can be used to check the depth, and the procedure is continued until the appropriate depth is achieved. Hemostasis is achieved by increasing the spot size and defocusing the beam. Ferric subsulfate solution (Monsel's solution) is applied at the end of the procedure. The laser has the advantage of being easily tailored to the size of the lesion; the disadvantage is that the laser is an expensive piece of equipment, requires a moderate amount of training to be used properly, and produces toxic effects (e.g., burns, eye injuries). Also, no specimen is obtained with this technique.

The loop electrical excision procedure, introduced in 1989, uses a bipolar electric current through a thin wire to excise a portion of the cervix. For the loop electrocautery excision procedure (LEEP), machines are available from several companies, including Cooper Medical Gynemed Division, Leisegang Medical Corp., Valleylab, Inc., and Cabot Medical Corp. The procedure includes placement of a large plastic Graves' speculum and a plastic vaginal retractor. The 20- by 8-mm loop is used to remove the lesion and the entire transformation zone. The area of interest is removed in one piece if it is 4 cm or smaller in diameter. If the area is larger than 4 cm, it is removed in two sections. The bed is coagulated with the ball electrode, and ferric subsulfate solution is placed in the bed. This technique is reasonably reliable and easy to use, can be tailored to the size of the lesion, and produces a tissue specimen. The disadvantages of the technique are increased risk of bleeding, infection, and increased cost. Bleeding rates in the literature vary from 2 to 7%. The potential advantage of a specimen is underscored by the fact that unsuspected adenocarcinoma in situ or microinvasive squamous carcinoma is found in 2 to 3% of specimens.

In nonrandomized studies, cryotherapy and laser ablation have similar cure rates (80 to 90%), and the LEEP performs slightly better (90 to 95%). In nonrandomized studies, three types of lesions have been associated with persistent or recurrent disease: the higher grade lesion, the lesion with endocervical gland involvement, and the larger lesion, which occupies more than two thirds of the surface area of the cervix.

Cryotherapy and laser ablation were subjected to a randomized clinical trial by Berget and associates. These investigators showed initial cure rates of 90% for 103 patients treated by laser ablation and 91% for 101 patients treated by cryotherapy; longer term follow-up put the cure rates at 91% for patients treated with laser and 96% for those treated with cryotherapy. My colleagues and I performed a randomized clinical trial of all three therapies. Patients were stratified by important prognostic variables

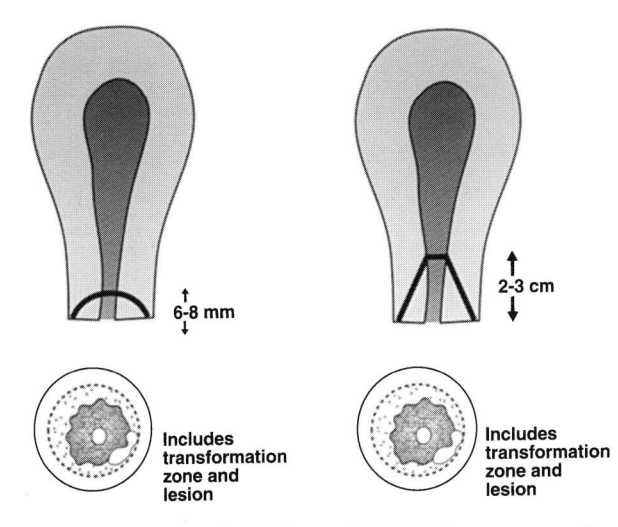

Figure 42–4 Cervical cone biopsy for cervical squamous epithelial lesions (SIL). (From Mitchell MF, Tortolero-Luna GT, Wright T, et al: Cervical human papillomavirus infection and intraepithelial neoplasia: A review. Monogr Natl Cancer Inst 21:17, 1996.)

(grade of lesion, endocervical involvement, and size of lesion) before randomization. Recurrence and persistence rates were 20% for all three therapies with 2 years of follow-up. We concluded that the three treatments performed equally well and that a cost-effectiveness analysis was needed.

### Cone Biopsy

Several techniques of cone biopsy are available: scalpel (cold knife), cautery (hot knife), laser, and loop excision.

Cone biopsies remove the endocervical canal, and specimens range in size from 2 to 3 cm in height around the canal and include the transformation zone of the ectocervix. Because the endocervical canal is included, they are diagnostic as well as therapeutic treatments (Figure 42–4).

The scalpel, cautery, and laser remove the cervix in one conical piece and are performed with the patient under general anesthesia. The scalpel and cautery are used similarly by outlining the transformation zone and lesion and removing a conical piece of tissue 3 cm in height. Hemostasis is achieved with cautery and suture ligation. Cure rates approach 95 to 98%.

The loop cone removes the cervix in 2 to 3 specimens. The advantage of loop cone cauterization is that it can be performed in the clinic in less than 5 minutes using local anesthesia. One randomized study showed many uninterpretable specimens using LEEP, but other studies showed comparable complication rates and specimens using LEEP. We showed a lower cure rate in patients who underwent a LEEP cone in a randomized study comparing LEEP with cold knife and laser conization. The major reason for the lower cure rate was considered to be that the height of the LEEP cones, which was 2 cm rather than the 3 cm obtained with the scalpel and laser cones. LEEP cones can be made to extend higher by taking an additional sample with the endocervical loop. The first ectocervical specimen is 8 to 10 mm deep. Two endocervical specimens can then be obtained with the 10- by 10-mm loop; the margin of the higher specimen should be marked to facilitate pathologic analysis.

## Controversies and New Developments

Advances in understanding the role of HPV in carcinogenesis and immunobiology of HPV infection may be exploitable in developing new treatment strategies. Several new diagnostic and screening approaches and chemoprevention strategies may change the way SILs are detected and treated in the future.

### BIOLOGY

The high-risk oncogenic HPV viruses produce two oncoproteins from the early region open reading frames: E6 and E7 (Fig. 42–5). These oncoproteins interact with endogenous cell cycle regulatory proteins: E6 with p53 and E7 with RB, p107, and cyclin A. The interaction of virally derived proteins with cell cycle regulatory proteins leads to deregulation of cell cycle progression and appears to be a critical step in cervical squamous carcinogenesis. Other HPV early region open reading frames produce E2, E4, and E5 proteins. Integration of HPV DNA into the host genome frequently disrupts the open reading frame for E2 protein, which controls transcription; this results in further overexpression of E6 and E7. E5 protein has weak transforming activity, whereas E4 is involved in maturation and viral replication. The capsid proteins are produced by late region open reading frames: L1 is the major capsid protein and L2 the minor.

Although HPV plays a critical role in the process of cervical carcinogenesis, interactions with other oncogenes, such as ras and myc, and alterations of chromosome 3 may be important for the final transition to cancer. Current investigators are trying to identify useful biomarkers to help prognosticate which high-grade lesions are likely to progress to cancer and which low-grade lesions are likely to progress to high-grade lesions.

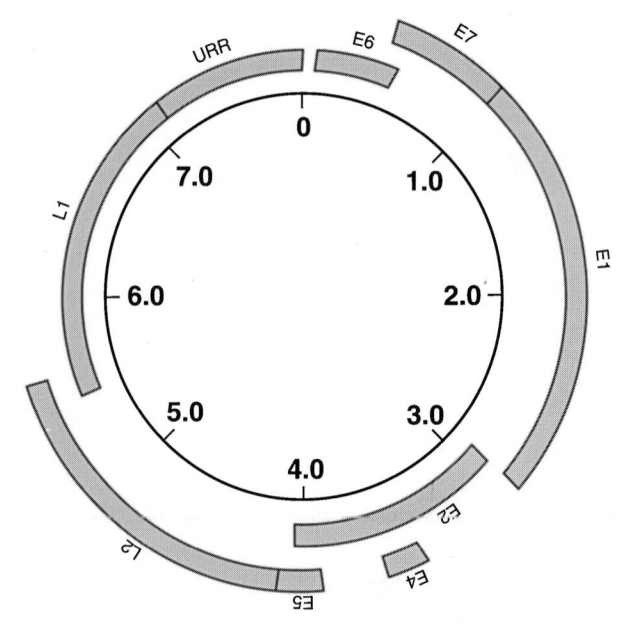

**Figure 42–5** The HPV genome.

## IMMUNOBIOLOGY

Studies of cytomorphologically normal Papanicolaou smears demonstrate that HPV prevalence is age-dependent, with the peak number of infections occurring in women aged 20 to 24 years. Clinically, if the Papanicolaou smear is normal and no lesion is visualized colposcopically, these infections are referred to as latent or subclinical. Once a lesion is evident cytologically and colposcopically, HPV infection is assumed to be productive; HPV DNA may be episomal (outside the host cell DNA) or integrated (incorporated into the host cell DNA). These infections are believed to last for 10 to 20 years; after this period of time, some regress, some persist, and some progress.

Many groups have investigated the humoral or serum antibody response to these infections. There is substantial evidence suggesting that both spontaneous regression and persistence of cutaneous HPV-associated warts are related to immunologic responses in the individual. In general, in the majority of viral infections, evidence of immunity is based on demonstrating the presence of virus-specific antibodies. In the past, the serologic analysis of HPV-associated mucocutaneous infections—clinical (visible to the naked eye), subclinical (visible using the colposcope), and latent (not visible by colposcope or naked eye, but HPV-positive by molecular biologic detection)—in patients was hampered by lack of a suitable antigen as a target and also by inability to propagate the virus. However, with the advent of recombinant DNA technology and other immunologic methodologies, we are now better able to study the immune response to HPV infection, and a vaccine that stimulates the humoral immune system may soon be available.

For efficient immunoprevention and immunotherapy of HPV infection, it will be important to understand the role of T-cell responses directed against various HPV proteins. The T-cell system makes up the cell-mediated immune response. Viral proteins, which appear on the infected cell surface in the form of peptides in the context of major histocompatibility complex (MHC) molecules, activate autologous T cells (both helper T cells and cytotoxic T cells [CTL]), expressing appropriate receptors. The E6 and E7 oncoproteins of HPV found in cervical biopsies are, therefore, considered attractive candidates for immune intervention strategies. Using both in vitro and in vivo approaches, investigators have identified several peptides from the E6 and E7 oncoproteins that are capable of inducing HPV-specific T-cell responses in both animal and human models.

These results suggest that initial cervical infections might be prevented by a humoral vaccine aimed at the capsid proteins L1 and L2, possibly administered before the onset of sexual activity in population-based vaccination programs. Once persistent infection is in place or a lesion is present, efforts might be better aimed at cell-mediated immunity using cocktails of peptides from the HPV E6 and E7 oncoproteins, with the intention of causing regression of disease; these vaccines would be therapeutic and would be used in a well-defined group of women who would have the disease.

## OTHER SCREENING AND DIAGNOSTIC TECHNIQUES

Several approaches have been considered to improve the performance of screening cytology or to better diagnose high-grade lesions at the time of the initial visit. These approaches include targeted rescreening, colposcopic screening, cervicography (review of a picture of the cervix after acetic acid exposure), HPV DNA testing (differentiating low-risk and high-risk viral types), speculoscopy (viewing the cervix under chemiluminescence), digital-imaging colposcopy, fluorescence spectroscopy (viewing the excitation and emission wavelengths of light reflected from the cervix), and computer-assisted automated image analysis of Papanicolaou smear readings. Further studies are needed to determine the clinical benefits and cost-effectiveness of these tests.

## NEW TREATMENT APPROACHES

Several chemoprevention trials that use micronutrients or pharmaceuticals to try to prevent or delay development of cancer in healthy populations have been carried out in the cervix. None of the micronutrient studies have demonstrated statistically significant regression of CIN lesions in randomized trials. Topical transretinoic acid caused significant regression of CIN 2 but not CIN 3 in the trial of Meyskens and associates. We showed a 50% regression rate for CIN 3 in a phase I, dose-finding study of difluoromethylornithine, a polyamine synthesis inhibitor. Because chemopreventives affect the patient systemically, they may be particularly advantageous in the patient who has multifocal disease or who is immunodepressed. No trials of chemopreventives have yet been carried out in vulvar or vaginal intraepithelial lesions.

## REFERENCES

Baker GE, Tyring SK: Therapeutic approaches to papillomavirus infections. Dermatol Clin 15:331, 1997.
Becker TM, Wheeler CM, McGough NS, et al: Contraceptive and reproductive risk factors for cervical dysplasia in Southwestern

Hispanic and non-Hispanic white women. Int J Epidemiol 23:913, 1994.

Bellina JH: The use of the carbon dioxide laser in the management of condyloma acuminatum with eight-year follow-up. Am J Obstet Gynecol 147:375, 1984.

Berget A, Andreasson B, Bock JE, et al: Outpatient treatment of cervical intraepithelial neoplasia: The CO2 laser versus cryotherapy, a randomized trial. Acta Obstet Gynecol Scand 66:531, 1987.

Beutner KR, Ferenczy A: Therapeutic approaches to genital warts. Am J Med 102:28, 1997.

Boone CW, Kelloff GJ, Steele VE: Natural history of intraepithelial neoplasia in humans with implications for cancer chemoprevention strategy. Cancer Res 52:1651, 1992.

Bosch FX, Muñoz N, de Sanjose S, et al: Human papillomavirus and cervical intraepithelial neoplasia grade III/carcinoma in situ: A case-control study in Spain and Colombia. Cancer Epidemiol Biomarkers Prev 2:415, 1993.

Brinton LA: Epidemiology of cervical cancer—Overview. IARC Sci Publ No. 119, 3, 1992.

Brinton LA, Nasca PC, Mallin K, et al: Case-control study of cancer of the vulva. Obstet Gynecol 18:71, 1990.

Brinton LA, Nasca PC, Mallin K, et al: Case-control study of in situ and invasive cancer of the vagina. Gynecol Oncol 38:49, 1990.

Dillner J: Antibody responses to defined HPV epitopes in cervical neoplasia: Review. Papillomavirus Report 5:35, 1994.

Dillner J: Immunobiology of papillomavirus. Prospects for vaccination. Cancer 5:181, 1992.

Edwards CL, Tortolero-Luna G, Linares AC, et al: Vulvar intraepithelial neoplasia and vulvar cancer. Obstet Gynecol Clin North Am 23:295, 1996.

Fahey MT, Irwig L, Macaskill P: Meta-analysis of Pap test accuracy. Am J Epidemiol 141:680, 1995.

Koss LG: Cervical (Pap) smear: New directions. Cancer 71:1406, 1993.

Koss LG: The Papanicolaou test for cervical cancer detection: A triumph and a tragedy. JAMA 261:737, 1989.

Koss LG, Stewart FW, Foote FW, et al: Some histological aspects of behavior of epidermoid carcinoma in situ and related lesions of the uterine cervix. Cancer 16:1160, 1963.

Koutsky L: Role of epidemiology in defining events that influence transmission and natural history of anogenital papillomavirus infection. JNCI 83:978, 1991.

Koutsky LA, Holmes KK, Critchlow CW, et al: A cohort study of the risk for cervical intraepithelial neoplasia grade 2 or 3 in relation to papillomavirus infection. N Engl J Med 327:1272, 1992.

Linares AC, Storment J, Rhodes-Morris H, et al: A comparison of three cone biopsy techniques for evaluation and treatment of squamous intraepithelial lesions. J Gynecol Tech 3:151, 1997.

Meyskens FL, Surwit EA, Moon TE, et al: Enhancement of regression of cervical intraepithelial neoplasia II (moderate dysplasia) with topically applied all-trans-retinoic acid: A randomized trial. JNCI 86:539, 1994.

Mitchell MF, Hittelman WK, Lotan R, et al: Chemoprevention trials and surrogate endpoint biomarkers in the cervix. Cancer 76:1956, 1995.

Mitchell MF, Tortolero-Luna G, Lee JJ, et al: Phase I dose de-escalation trial of alpha-difluoromethylornithine in patients with cervical intraepithelial neoplasia grade 3. Clin Cancer Res 4:310, 1998.

Mitchell MF, Tortolero-Luna G, Wright T, et al: Cervical human papillomavirus infection and intraepithelial neoplasia: A review. J Natl Cancer Inst Monogr 21:17, 1996.

Mitchell MF, Tortolero-Luna G, Cook E, et al: A randomized clinical trial of cryotherapy, laser vaporization, and loop electrosurgical excision procedure for treatment of squamous intraepithelial lesions of the cervix. Obstet Gynecol 92:737, 1998.

Mitchell MF: The natural history of CIN and management of the abnormal Pap smear. In Rubin SC, Hoskins WJ (eds): Cervical Cancer and Preinvasive Neoplasia. Philadelphia, Lippincott-Raven Publishers, 1996, p 103.

Mitchell MF: Preinvasive diseases of the female lower genital tract. In Gershenson DM, DeCherney AH, Curry SL (eds): Operative Gynecology. New York, WB Saunders, 1993, p 231.

Morrison EB, Ho GF, Vermund SH, et al: Human papillomavirus infection and other risk factors for cervical neoplasia: A case-control study. Int J Cancer 49:6, 1991.

Munoz N, Bosch FX: Epidemiology of cervical cancer. IARC Sci Publ 94:9, 1989.

Munoz N, Bosch FX: HPV and cervical cancer: Review of case-control and cohort studies. IARC Sci Publ 119:251, 1992.

Munoz N, Bosch FX, de Sanjose S, et al: Risk factors for cervical intraepithelial neoplasia grade III/carcinoma in situ in Spain and Colombia. Cancer Epidemiol Biomarkers Prev 2:423, 1993.

National Cancer Institute Workshop: The 1988 Bethesda system for reporting cervical/vaginal cytologic diagnoses. JAMA 262:931, 1989.

Olsen AO, Gjoen K, Sauer T, et al: Human papillomavirus and cervical intraepithelial neoplasia grade II-III: A population-based case-control study. Int J Cancer 61:312, 1995.

Oster AG: Natural history of cervical intraepithelial neoplasia: A critical review. Int J Gynecol Pathol 12:186, 1993.

Powell LC: Condyloma acuminatum: Recent advances in development, carcinogenesis, and treatment. Clin Obstet Gynecol 21:1061, 1972.

Regan JW, Fu YS: The uterine cervix. In Silverberg SG (ed): Principles and Practice of Surgical Pathology, vol 2. New York, Wiley, 1983, p 124.

Reid R: Superficial laser vulvectomy. I. The efficacy of extended superficial ablation for refractory and very extensive condyloma. Am J Obstet Gynecol 151:1047, 1985.

Reid R: Superficial laser vulvectomy. III. A new surgical technique for appendage-conserving ablation of refractory condylomas and vulvar intraepithelial neoplasia. Am J Obstet Gynecol 152:504, 1985.

Reid R, Elfont EA, Zirkin RM, et al: Superficial laser vulvectomy. II. The anatomic and biophysical principles permitting accurate control over the depth of dermal destruction with the carbon dioxide laser. Am J Obstet Gynecol 152:261, 1985.

Richart RM: Cervical intraepithelial neoplasia: A review. In Sommers SC (ed): Pathology Annual. East Norwalk, CT, Appleton-Century-Crofts, 1973, p 301.

Schiffman MH, Bauer HM, Hoover RN, et al: Epidemiology evidence showing that human papillomavirus infection causes most cervical intraepithelial neoplasia. JNCI 85:958, 1993.

Schottenfeld D, Mitchell MF, Hong WK: Screening and chemoprevention of gynecologic tumors. Obstet Gynecol Clin North Am 23:285, 1996.

# 43

# Vulvar and Vaginal Cancers

JUDITH K. WOLF
THOMAS W. BURKE

Malignant tumors of the lower female genital tract are uncommon. Annually, fewer than 5000 women in the entire United States are diagnosed with cancer of the vulva or vagina. Consequently, few physicians have extensive clinical experience in diagnosis and treatment of women who have these malignancies. Because many of these tumors develop after a preinvasive phase, arise in a readily accessible site, and produce recognizable symptoms, early diagnosis is possible in most cases. By adhering to careful diagnostic guidelines, the general gynecologist should be able to provide an accurate diagnosis for all women who have symptoms or examination abnormalities. Moreover, treatment of women who have early-stage disease produces excellent results. This chapter provides a straightforward framework for the diagnosis, evaluation, and treatment of women who have these cancers.

## Vulvar Cancer

### DEFINITION

Vulvar malignancies comprise a series of rare cancers that arise from the skin or skin appendages of the vulva. Consequently, their histology mimics that of tumors found in other cutaneous sites, with squamous cell tumors accounting for about 85% of vulvar cancers, malignant melanoma accounting for about 10%, and adenocarcinomas originating in skin glands or Bartholin's glands accounting for approximately 5%.

### HISTORY

Two clinically distinct subsets of vulvar cancer patients have been identified. The classical picture is one of gradual development of a solitary ulcerated cancer, frequently arising in an area of chronic vulvar dystrophy in an elderly woman. A more recently described example is that of a younger woman with multifocal lesions arising in a background of squamous dysplasia and human papillomavirus (HPV) changes.

Potential risk factors for development of squamous cell carcinoma and carcinoma in situ of the vulva are listed in Table 43–1. Many of these factors represent observed associations reported over a period of years, without conclusive scientific evidence of a direct association. Those for which there is more significant documentation of an association include HPV infection (especially type 16), previous abnormal Papani-

**Table 43–1** Possible Risk Factors for the Development of Vulvar Carcinoma and Carcinoma In Situ

Sexually transmitted infections
    Chronic granulomatous lesions
    Syphilis
    Herpes simplex virus
    Human papillomavirus*
Chronic vulvar conditions
    Lichen sclerosus
    Hypertrophic dystrophy
Lifestyle factors
    Previous abnormal Papanicolaou smear*
    Multiple sexual partners*
    Cigarette smoking*
Systemic medical conditions
    Hypertension
    Diabetes mellitus
    Obesity
    Immunosuppression

*Indicates strong evidence of an association.

colaou smear, cigarette smoking, and exposure to multiple sexual partners.

**Physical Examination.** Because vulvar cancers develop on an exposed skin surface, a visually identifiable lesion is always present and readily accessible for biopsy. Unfortunately, diagnostic delays are common. Although many women who have vulvar cancer may detect a pruritic and palpable mass, they often do not seek a gynecologic evaluation immediately because they are embarrassed or attempt to self-medicate a presumed benign condition. Equally disconcerting is that many women who report for examination receive empiric topical treatment without a histologic diagnosis. Consequently, the key to the diagnosis of vulvar malignancies is careful inspection and biopsy of any identified abnormality.

Most vulvar cancers occur laterally on the labia majora, but 20 to 30% originate in midline sites at the perineal body or clitoris. Systematic inspection of the entire vulvar surface should be a part of every gynecologic examination. Application of dilute acetic acid and colposcopic magnification may be useful in selecting sites for biopsy in women who have extensive or multifocal disease.

The lymphatic drainage of the vulvar skin tends to proceed stepwise to the ipsilateral superficial inguinal nodes, the deep inguinal nodes, and, finally, the pelvic nodes (Fig. 43–1). Although variations in this pattern can be seen, aberrant drainage routes that result in unexpected lymphatic metastases are uncommon. Palpation of the left and right sides of the groin for lymphadenopathy is an important component of the examination of the woman who has a vulvar lesion. Firm, enlarged, or matted nodes should be carefully noted. Nevertheless, lymph node metastases are known to occur in the absence of palpable adenopathy in about 15% of early cancers. All patients who have malignancy require a complete physical examination. Because vulvar cancers rarely appear with distant metastases, this portion of the examination should be directed toward the detection of other concomitant medical problems.

## DIAGNOSTIC CONSIDERATIONS AND DIFFERENTIAL DIAGNOSIS

Any vulvar lesion requires biopsy for histologic diagnosis. This is particularly important because chronic inflammatory lesions (hypertrophic dystrophy and lichen sclerosus), HPV-induced changes (flat condylomas and genital warts), dysplasias (primarily carcinoma in situ), and cancer (all histologic types) may have similar features of irritation, surface irregularity, abnormal pigmentation, and ulceration. In addition, it is not unusual for more than one such lesion to coexist with another. When extensive involvement of the vulva is present, multiple biopsies may be required to arrive at the correct diagnosis.

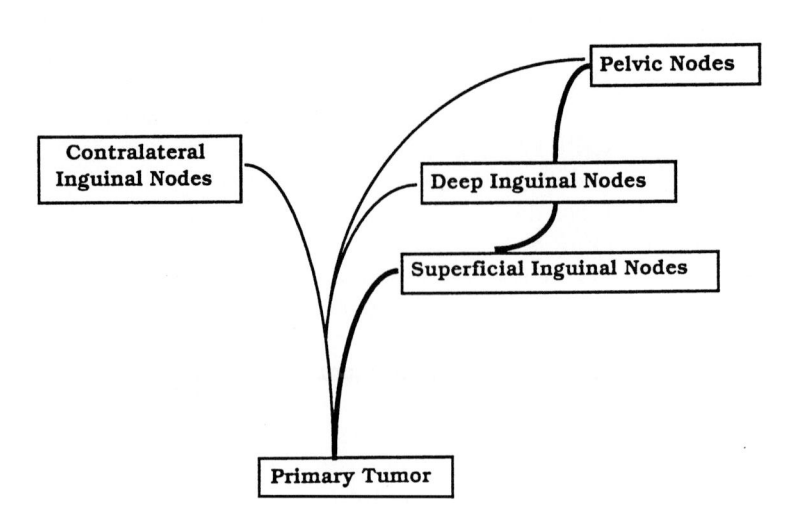

**Figure 43–1** Vulvar lymphatic drainage routes. The lymphatic drainage of the vulvar skin tends to proceed stepwise. Initial drainage is to the 5 to 8 ipsilateral lymph nodes that comprise the superficial inguinal group. Subsequently, lymph drains to the deep inguinal nodes and then the retroperitoneal pelvic nodes. In some cases, lymphatic drainage may bypass the superficial group and drain directly to the deep inguinal or pelvic nodes, or to nodes on the opposite side of the groin. Although uncommon, such aberrant lymphatic patterns may explain the small percentage of women who develop unexpected lymph node failure.

## Table 43–2  FIGO Staging for Vulvar Carcinoma (1995)

| STAGE 0 | Carcinoma in situ |
|---|---|
| STAGE I | Tumor confined to vulva or perineum and measuring ≤2 cm; no lymph node metastases<br>Stage IA  Maximum stromal invasion <1 mm<br>Stage IB  Stromal invasion >1 mm |
| STAGE II | Tumor confined to the vulva or perineum and measuring >2 cm in greatest dimension; no lymph node metastases |
| STAGE III | Tumor of any size that has spread to the vagina, urethra, or anus; any tumor with unilateral inguinal node metastases |
| STAGE IV | Advanced local or distant disease<br>Stage IVA  Tumor that has invaded the bladder or rectal mucosa, upper urethra, or pelvic bone; any tumor with bilateral inguinal node metastases<br>Stage IVB  Tumor with distant metastases |

Once the target site for biopsy has been determined, infiltrate the vulva with 1 to 2% plain lidocaine from a dental cartridge syringe through a 31-gauge needle. A 3- to 5-mm disposable Keyes punch biopsy instrument is then used to obtain a full-thickness sample from the selected site.

## LABORATORY AND DIAGNOSTIC EVALUATION

Pretreatment staging for women who have vulvar cancer combines a detailed evaluation of the primary tumor for size and local extension with histologic assessment of the inguinal lymph nodes (Table 43–2). The local extent of most primary vulvar cancers can be readily and accurately determined by physical examination. When large tumors are encountered, additional diagnostic studies may be necessary to provide a more objective evaluation of deep tissue spread. The workup for a given patient should be tailored to the examination findings. Cystoscopy can be used to detect invasion of the upper urethra or bladder mucosa. Similarly, proctoscopy should be employed to detect involvement of the rectum. Computerized tomography (CT) or magnetic resonance imaging (MRI) may be helpful in identifying retroperitoneal lymphadenopathy above the groin or invasion of the bony structure of the pelvis. Patients who have symptoms or examination findings that suggest the possibility of distant metastases should have further diagnostic studies directed at those sites.

Because groin palpation is associated with a significant failure rate in the detection of lymph node spread to this site, the current modification of the staging system requires histologic evaluation of the inguinal lymph nodes for staging purposes. However, the extent of the sampling procedure is not specified in the staging rules. In practice, lymph node dissection is tailored to the size and location of the primary tumor in situations in which surgical therapy is the primary treatment modality. Limited lymph node biopsy or fine-needle aspiration cytology may be used to assess the groin node status of advanced lesions or those with palpable lymphadenopathy.

Routine pretreatment evaluation should also include a complete blood count, serum hepatic function tests, blood urea nitrogen (BUN) plus creatinine tests, and chest radiography. Further assessment of baseline organ functions should be considered in women who have significant comorbid conditions.

## TREATMENT

Surgical resection is the major treatment modality for women who have invasive vulvar cancer. The extent of the resection depends upon the size and location of the tumor, the depth of stromal invasion, and the biases of the treating physician. Because carcinoma in situ lesions are more likely to occur in younger women and have a strong potential for recurrence, $CO_2$ ablation may be the best option for women who have intraepithelial disease. This procedure preserves tissue and function in a patient who may require multiple episodes of treatment over her lifetime. However, if microinvasion is suspected or documented by outpatient punch biopsy, excisional biopsy should be considered for both diagnosis and treatment. Excision of stage IA lesions along with a 1-cm gross margin is adequate. Groin dissection is not routinely performed in these cases because the risk of lymphatic spread is negligible. For women who have either intraepithelial or early stromal invasive lesions, careful and regular follow-up is mandatory. A substantial percentage of women in these categories develop new or recurrent vulvar disease (Fig. 43–2).

More extensive operative approaches are necessary for women who have gross lesions. En bloc resection of the entire vulva with simultaneous dissection of the superficial and deep inguinal lymph nodes is the classic approach to the treatment of stages I and II vulvar cancers. This therapy results in 80 to 90% rates of long-term disease-free survival. Many recent reviews have shown that similarly excellent outcomes can be achieved with more conservative surgical resections. These approaches typically combine radical wide excision of the primary tumor along with at least a 2-cm tissue margin, with groin dissection tailored to the tumor location and the operative findings. Dissection of ipsilateral superficial inguinal nodes is performed for lateral lesions, whereas bilateral superficial dissection is performed for midline tumors of

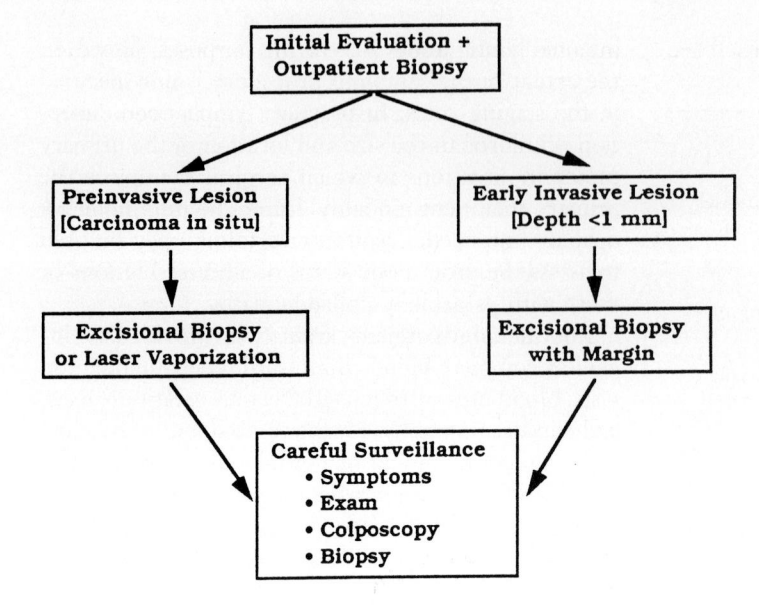

**Figure 43-2** Treatment algorithm for early lesions. Very early vulvar cancers are those that demonstrate a depth of stromal invasion of less than 1 mm. The risk of lymphatic metastases in this setting is exceedingly small; hence, groin dissection is not required. Such early invasive lesions should be distinguished from intraepithelial disease (carcinoma in situ) by an appropriate biopsy. For either type of lesion, excision with a margin of normal tissue is adequate therapy. Careful post-treatment surveillance is important because the risk of recurrent or new disease is significant.

the clitoris or perineal body (Fig. 43-3). If clinically positive nodes are encountered, an attempt should be made to resect all gross disease. More conservative resections provide an equivalent opportunity for cure, preserve body image and sexual function to a greater degree, and significantly reduce surgical morbidity and late lymphatic complications compared with outcomes of radical vulvectomy. Postoperative irradiation of the vulva, both sides of the groin, and the pelvis should be considered in women who have lymph node spread.

In rare cases, patients neglect obvious vulvar cancer for an extended time and do not seek treatment until they have massive disease that is not amenable to surgical resection short of exenteration. However, treatment with external beam irradiation, with or without concomitant systemic chemotherapy, may produce impressive clinical responses, even in women who have advanced lesions. Such therapy can be preceded or followed by limited resection of the gross tumor. Survival rates of 30 to 40% have been achieved when distant spread has not yet occurred, but clinical experience with these combined modality approaches is limited.

Patients who do not respond to local treatment of the vulva can often be successfully salvaged by repeat surgical excision. However, treatment failure in the groin or at any distant site is usually fatal. Experience with systemic chemotherapy has been disappointing. Responses tend to be unusual and brief when they occur.

The preceding discussion applies primarily to the treatment of women who have squamous cell carcinomas. Because of the rarity of malignant melanoma on the vulva, less information regarding its clinical behavior is available. Older reports have tended to recommend radical resection. However, more recent experiences suggest that similar outcomes can be ob-

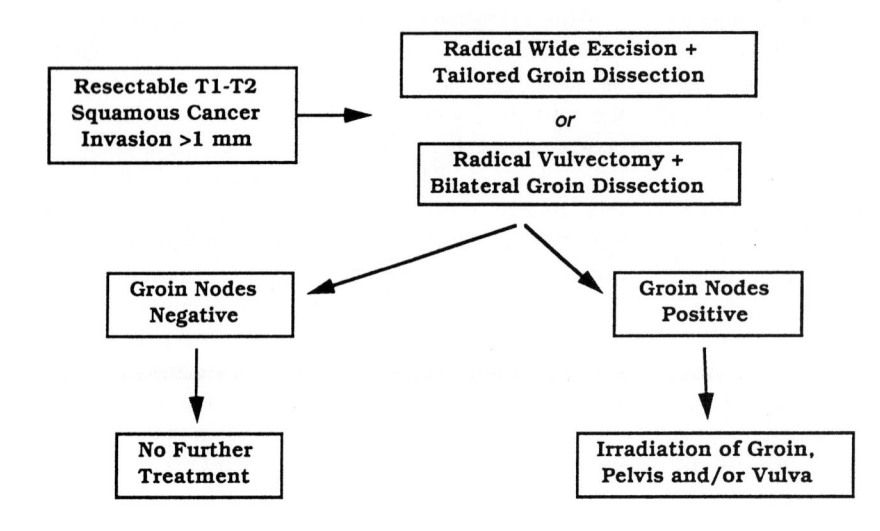

**Figure 43-3** Treatment algorithm for resectable cancers. Grossly identifiable tumors can be resected by classical radical vulvectomy and bilateral en bloc groin dissection or by radical wide excision and selective groin dissection. The current trend is toward more conservative surgical approaches. Postoperative irradiation is recommended for women who have positive lymph nodes. Treatment fields should include the vulva, both sides of the groin, and the lower pelvic nodes.

tained with the more conservative concept discussed for squamous tumors. The presence of nodal metastases is generally considered to indicate the presence of systemic disease. Patients who have such disease are ideal candidates for clinical trials. Irradiation may enhance local and regional control in patients who have vulvar melanoma, and some have used it for high-risk and node-positive patients. This experience is largely anecdotal and not universally accepted.

## CONTROVERSIES

A number of minor controversies continue to surround the treatment of women who have early vulvar cancers. Although most gynecologic oncologists would probably support a more conservative approach than radical vulvectomy with groin dissection, there is considerable variation in the recommendations of how conservatively a resection should be performed. Some have suggested that resection of the primary tumor along with a 2-cm margin is adequate; others would argue for an even less radical 1-cm margin, and still others for a more aggressive resection by hemivulvectomy. We have used the concept that the ipsilateral superficial inguinal nodes accurately predict true lymph node status and have used unilateral superficial dissection as our standard approach for treatment of patients who have lateral tumors. Others would argue that bilateral dissections should always be performed, or that deep inguinal nodes should be included in all groin dissections. Further experience and more extensive data will be needed to resolve these issues. However, it is important to recognize that these represent areas of refinement in the surgical management of vulvar cancer rather than major divergent concepts.

There is also considerable variation in approaches to the management of women who have very advanced vulvar cancers. Because of the clinical rarity of such cases, no standard approach has yet been defined. Multimodal therapy using some combination of surgery and radiotherapy, with or without concomitant chemotherapy, is used in most centers. The precise timing and sequence of each mode of treatment and the specific details of delivery vary widely.

# Vaginal Cancer

## DEFINITION

Vaginal malignancies are the least common gynecologic cancers in the United States, accounting for less than 2% of all tumors. Most vaginal cancers are squamous carcinomas (90%), with other less common cell types (melanoma, adenocarcinoma, sarcoma, endodermal sinus tumor) comprising the remaining 10%. Both squamous carcinoma and melanoma occur most commonly in the seventh and eighth decades of life, whereas leiomyosarcoma is most common during the later reproductive years. Endodermal sinus tumors and some rare sarcomas are cancers of infants and children. Clear cell adenocarcinomas occur mostly in adolescents and young adults.

## HISTORY

Squamous vaginal carcinomas may be preceded by a premalignant intraepithelial phase known as vaginal intraepithelial neoplasia (VAIN). Lenehan and Benedet report an approximate 5% incidence of progression from carcinoma in situ to invasive cancer, even with treatment. VAIN is diagnosed in 1 to 3% of patients who have cervical intraepithelial neoplasia (CIN). Many women who have VAIN, however, have had previous CIN or cervical cancer. HPV infection is thought to be a major etiologic factor in the development of VAIN. Previous irradiation and chronic immunosuppression are also risk factors. In approximately 80% of cases, VAIN occurs in the upper vagina.

Most asymptomatic patients who have invasive vaginal carcinoma have stage I disease. About 60% of women who have vaginal cancer have had a previous hysterectomy. Consequently, Papanicolaou smear screening of the vagina remains an important issue even after hysterectomy. As many as one third of patients who have vaginal cancer have had cervical cancer treated 5 or more years earlier. Previous irradiation of the vagina may be a risk factor for development of vaginal cancer. The most common symptom associated with cancer is vaginal bleeding. Patients may also complain of a watery, malodorous discharge. More than 75% of patients who have such symptoms have an advanced stage of the disease.

## PHYSICAL EXAMINATION

Squamous carcinoma arises within the vaginal mucosa and spreads locally by invading the underlying tissues. Examination of a patient who has known or presumed vaginal cancer includes careful exploration of the entire vaginal, vulvar, and pelvic areas. Careful visual inspection of the entire vagina can be achieved by rotating the speculum to visualize all the walls, first with the naked eye and then with colposcopy and acetic acid. This type of examination is especially important for women who have VAIN and early lesions. The relationship of the tumor to both cervix and vulva should be assessed. Rectovaginal examination can aid in evaluating involvement of submucosa, paravaginal tissue, rectum, and pelvic wall.

Vaginal cancers usually have an exophytic growth pattern and project into the vaginal canal. Forty percent occur in the upper vagina, where involvement of the cervix may obscure the actual site of origin. By convention, tumors that involve the cervix are classified as cervical carcinomas. Fifteen percent of cancers originate in the distal vagina, where they may be difficult to distinguish from lesions arising in the vulva or urethra. About one third of tumors are advanced at diagnosis and involve the entire length of the vagina. Tumor involvement of the anterior, posterior, and lateral vaginal walls is about equal. Deeply invasive vaginal cancers can spread directly into the bladder or rectum.

Lymphatic spread is a common metastatic route. The pattern of lymphatic spread depends on the location of the tumor. Tumors of the lower third of the vagina spread to the inguinal lymph nodes as do vulvar cancers. Tumors of the upper two thirds of the vagina spread, as does cervical cancer, to pelvic and then para-aortic lymph nodes (Fig. 43–4). Careful palpation of the inguinal and supraclavicular nodes is essential when examining the patient who has vaginal cancer.

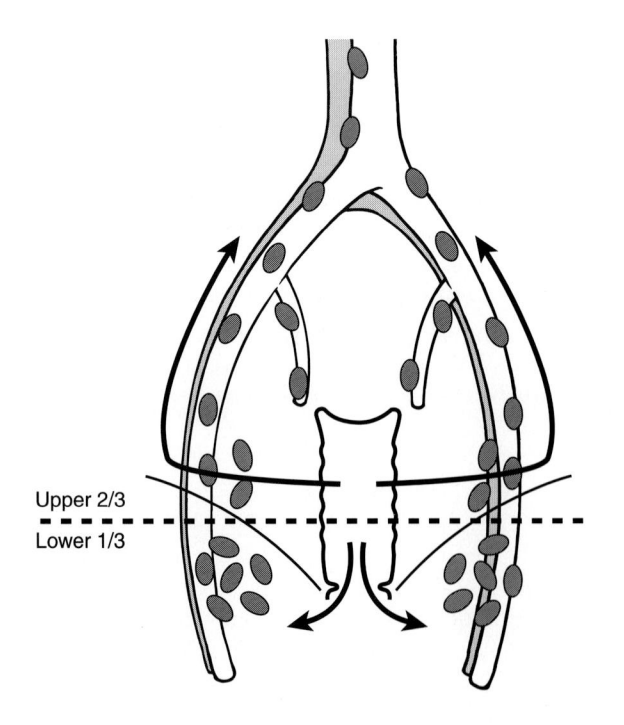

**Figure 43–4** Vaginal lymphatic drainage routes. Lesions arising in the upper two thirds of the vagina drain to retroperitoneal lymph nodes along the pelvic wall in a pattern similar to that seen in cervical cancer. Tumors originating in the lower third of the vaginal canal drain primarily to the superficial inguinal nodes as seen in vulvar cancers.

## DIAGNOSTIC CONSIDERATIONS AND DIFFERENTIAL DIAGNOSIS

The differential diagnosis of vaginal cancer includes benign growths, infectious processes, premalignant changes (VAIN), and metastatic malignancies from other organs. As with incidence of cancer, benign vaginal tumors are rare. Most are cystic lesions that are small, single, and asymptomatic. Epidermoid inclusion cysts occur in the distal vagina after trauma (e.g., delivery of a baby) and are 1 to 2 cm in diameter. Cysts can also arise within müllerian remnants located in the anterolateral vagina near the fornices. These average 3 cm in diameter and are lined by mucinous epithelium. The Gartner duct cyst, or mesonephric duct cyst, is usually small, asymptomatic, and anterolateral. Any large or symptomatic cyst should be removed.

Vaginal polyps are usually small, are occasionally multiple, and occur in adult women. They typically consist of fibrovascular stroma covered by squamous epithelium. Benign rhabdomyomas can be of two types: the cardiac type, or hamartoma, which is associated with tuberous sclerosis, and the fetal type. These muscle tumors occur in the vagina, cervix, or vulva of middle-aged women and are usually small, soft, and asymptomatic. Vaginal leiomyomas occur in the anterior vaginal wall of women between the fourth and fifth decades. The lesions are usually less than 5 cm in diameter and can cause dyspareunia.

Ulcerative vaginal lesions may be benign or malignant. They may be infectious, as in herpes simplex virus outbreaks; autoimmune, as in Behçet's syndrome; or traumatic, as in lesions caused by tampon use. They may also be a manifestation of a dermatosis, such as lichen planus or pemphigoid. History, culture, biopsy, and detection of other skin or mucosal lesions usually lead to the appropriate diagnosis.

Interestingly, metastatic involvement of the vagina by other cancers is more frequent than development of primary cancer. Tumors that metastasize to the vagina are most commonly other pelvic malignancies, particularly cervical cancers. Adenocarcinoma from the upper genital tract (i.e., endometrium, ovary) or from other sites (i.e., kidney, breast, colon, pancreas) can spread to the vagina.

The most common nonsquamous primary tumor of the vagina is vaginal adenocarcinoma. It can arise from müllerian remnants, vaginal adenosis, or endometriosis; from the Gartner duct epithelium; or as a result of intrauterine exposure to diethylstilbestrol (DES).

The next most common primary malignancy is malignant melanoma. The average age when diagnosis is made in patients who have such disease is 55 years. Most patients complain of vaginal bleeding, usually of less than 3 months' duration, and often accompanied by a foul discharge. Though melanoma can occur anywhere in the vagina, 45% of cases occur in the anterior vagina and 58% in the distal third. Melanoma of the vagina is a highly malignant disease, with a reported 5-year survival rate of 15 to 20%.

## LABORATORY AND DIAGNOSTIC EVALUATION

Diagnostic measures used to evaluate a woman who has newly diagnosed or suspected vaginal cancer begin with a history and a physical examination. Efforts should be made to elicit historical risk factors, such as previous VAIN, CIN, or cancer; HPV infection; immunosuppression; or previous pelvic irradiation. Physical examination should include careful examination of all pelvic organs and lymph nodes. For small lesions, colposcopy of the vagina using 3% acetic acid may be helpful in identifying abnormal areas. Biopsy of any suspicious lesion should confirm the diagnosis of cancer and exclude preinvasive or benign conditions. Diagnostic imaging studies recommended for International Federation of Gynecology and Obstetrics (FIGO) staging include a chest radiograph and intravenous pyelogram. Depending upon the size and location of the lesion, cystoscopy, sigmoidoscopy, or both may be needed to evaluate bladder or rectal involvement (Table 43–3). Assessment of pelvic lymph nodes by CT, MRI, or lymphangiography may be useful, especially for lesions of the upper vagina or bulky tumors.

The staging rules for vaginal cancer are shown in Table 43–4. Stage at diagnosis is the most important prognostic factor for squamous carcinoma. Distribution rates of stages at diagnosis are approximately 25% at stage I, 33% at stage II, 25% at stage III, and 16% at stage IV. The reported 5-year survival rate for stage I is 70%; stage II, 45%; stage III, 30%; and stage IV, 18%. Five-year survival rate for all stages is approximately 42%. Chu and Beechinor report a slightly worse prognosis for women who have large, poorly differentiated tumors, and a slightly better outcome for lesions arising in the upper vagina than for those in the lower vagina. Perez and colleagues reported 100% survival rate for patients with stage I lesions with less than 2.5 mm of invasion. Primary adenocarcinomas of the vagina may have a slightly worse overall prognosis than that of squamous tumors.

**Table 43–3** Diagnostic and Laboratory Evaluation of Women Who Have Vaginal Cancer

Physical examination
    Visualization and palpation of vulva and vagina
    Bimanual and rectovaginal pelvic examination
    Evaluation of inguinal and supraclavicular lymph nodes
Colposcopy (using dilute acetic acid)
Biopsy
Chest radiograph
Intravenous pyelography
Lymphangiogram
Additional studies as indicated
    Cystoscopy
    Flexible sigmoidoscopy
    CT of abdomen and pelvis
    MRI of abdomen and pelvis

CT = Computed tomography; MRI = magnetic resonance imaging.

**Table 43–4** International Federation of Gynecology and Obstetrics Staging for Vaginal Cancer

| | |
|---|---|
| STAGE I | Carcinoma is limited to the vaginal wall. |
| STAGE II | Carcinoma involves the subvaginal tissue, but has not extended to the pelvic sidewall. |
| STAGE III | Carcinoma extends to the pelvic sidewall. |
| STAGE IV | Carcinoma extends beyond the true pelvis or has involved the mucosa of the bladder or rectum. Stage IVA Tumor has spread to adjacent organs. Stage IVB Tumor has spread to distant organs. |

## TREATMENT

Treatment of vaginal cancer needs to be individualized and must take into account stage, size, and location of the lesion; the presence or absence of the uterus; and whether the patient has been previously irradiated. Both surgery and irradiation appear to be equally effective for early lesions. A basic treatment algorithm is outlined in Figure 43–5.

Surgery may be particularly suited for patients who have lesions in the posterior fornix that are located away from the bladder and rectum. Surgery also should be considered in the younger patient who has a small cancer or any patient for whom preservation of vaginal function for coitus is important or feasible. Even for lesions extending over a large part of the vagina, vaginectomy, with or without a radical hysterectomy, can be combined with reconstruction.

Although surgery may be considered in selected cases, radiation is the treatment of choice for most patients who have vaginal cancers. Treatment should include the pelvic lymph nodes, parametrium, vaginal tube, and paravaginal tissues and structures to a level 2 cm below the lowest extent of the lesion. If the lesion is in the lower vagina, treatment should also incorporate the inguinal lymph nodes. Standard radiation treatment includes 40 to 50 Gy external beam plus brachytherapy, given either through an interstitial implant or by intracavitary treatment.

There is no consensus as to the best treatment for advanced tumors. Therefore, therapy must be

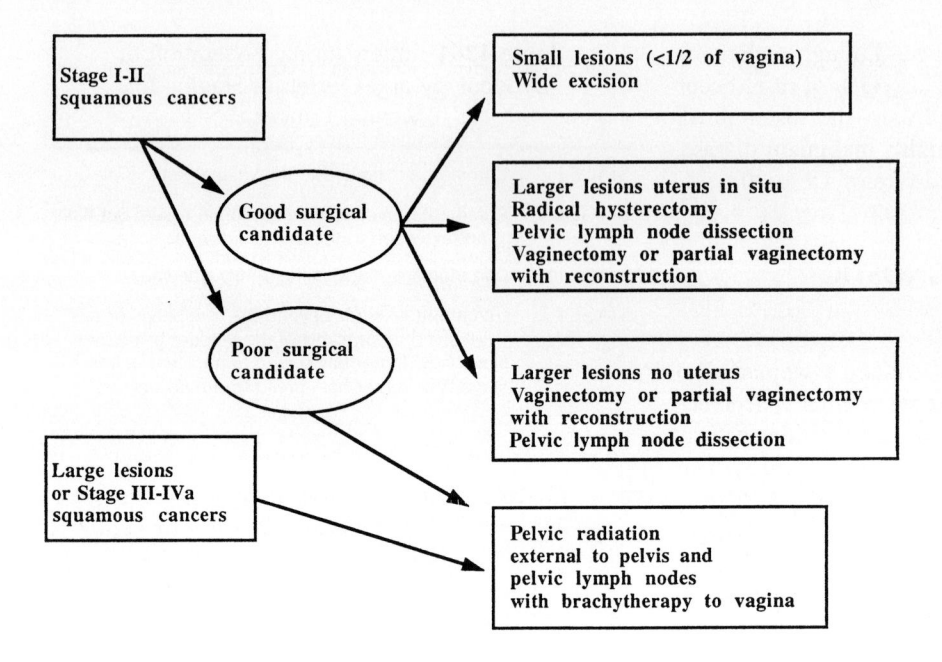

**Figure 43-5** Treatment algorithm for vaginal cancer. Surgery is a major treatment modality for preinvasive and small tumors, particularly those originating in the upper vagina. Radiotherapy, usually given as a combination of external beam and brachytherapy, is an appropriate treatment for tumors of all sizes. Irradiation should be considered the primary treatment modality for women who are poor operative candidates or who have large cancers.

designed for the individual patient. With radiation alone, local failure rates are as high as 50% and complication rates as high as 25%. Consequently, combined modality treatment (e.g., exenteration after external beam radiation, or chemotherapy in combination with radiation) is often employed.

Treatment options for vaginal melanoma include conservative local excision, radical surgery (including exenteration), radiation, or a combination of limited surgery and radiation. Distant failure is common, and, unfortunately, there is no active systemic treatment available.

Rare vaginal tumors include sarcoma botryoides and endodermal sinus tumor, which occur in infants or small children. These tumors appear with vaginal bleeding and may extend into the bladder or rectum. They spread through both the lymphatic and the blood systems. Currently, excellent cure rates are obtained with chemotherapy, usually employing a regimen containing vincristine, actinomycin D, and cyclophosphamide (VAC) and doxorubicin combined with limited surgical resection.

Treatment of patients who have soft tissue sarcomas is generally by resection with wide local excision. The addition of radiation has no known benefit. The behavior of such tumors is predicted by mitotic count and the degree of cellular atypia.

## CONTROVERSIES

Because of the rarity of vaginal cancer and its similarities to cervical cancer (upper vaginal lesions) and vulvar cancer (lower vaginal lesions), treatment has generally paralleled the standard treatment recommendations for patients who have these two cancers.

Areas of investigation for both cervical and vulvar cancer include combining chemotherapy with radiation therapy for large unresectable tumors. If chemoradiation becomes the standard of care for clinical subsets of patients who have either cervical or vulvar cancer, it may also eventually become the preferred treatment for similar vaginal lesions.

## REFERENCES

Al-Kurdi M, Monaghan JM: Thirty years experience in the management of primary tumors of the vagina. Br J Obstet Gynaecol 88:1145–1150, 1981.

Anderson WA, Sabio H, Durso N, et al: Endodermal sinus tumor of the vagina: The role of primary chemotherapy. Cancer 56:1025–1027, 1985.

Ansink AC, Krul MRL, DeWeger RA, et al: Human papillomavirus, lichen sclerosus, and squamous cell carcinoma of the vulva: Detection and prognostic significance. Gynecol Oncol 52:180–184, 1994.

Ball HG, Berman ML: Management of primary vaginal carcinoma. Gynecol Oncol 14:154–163, 1982.

Ballon SC, Lagasse LD, Chang NH, et al: Primary adenocarcinoma of the vagina. Surg Gynecol Obstet 149:233–237, 1979.

Bell J, Sevin BU, Averette H, et al: Vaginal cancer after hysterectomy for benign disease: Value of cytologic screening. Obstet Gynecol 64:699–702, 1984.

Benedet JL, Saunders BH: Carcinoma in situ of the vagina. Am J Obstet Gynecol 148:695–700, 1984.

Benedet JL, Murphy KJ, Fairey RN, et al: Primary invasive carcinoma of the vagina. Obstet Gynecol 62:715–719, 1983.

Berek JS, Heaps JM, Fu YS, et al: Concurrent cisplatin and 5-fluorouracil chemotherapy and radiation therapy for advanced-stage squamous carcinoma of the vulva. Gynecol Oncol 42:197–201, 1991.

Berman ML, Soper JT, Creasman WT, et al: Conservative surgical management of superficially invasive stage I vulvar carcinoma. Gynecol Oncol 35:352–357, 1989.

Binder SW, Huang I, Fu YS, et al: Risk factors for the development of lymph node metastasis in vulvar squamous carcinoma. Gynecol Oncol 37:9–16, 1990.

Boronow RC: Combined therapy as an alternative to exenteration for locally advanced vulvo-vaginal cancer: Rationale and results. Cancer 49:1085–1091, 1982.

Brinton LA, Nasca PC, Mallin K, et al: Case-control study of cancer of the vulva. Obstet Gynecol 75:859–866, 1990.

Burke TW, Stringer CA, Gershenson DM, et al: Radical wide excision and selective inguinal node dissection for squamous cell carcinoma of the vulva. Gynecol Oncol 38:328–332, 1990.

Burke TW, Levenback C, Coleman RC, et al: Surgical therapy of T1 and T2 vulvar carcinoma: Further experience with radical wide excision and selective inguinal lymphadenectomy. Gynecol Oncol 57:215–220, 1995.

Choo YC, Anderson DG: Neoplasms of the vagina following cervical carcinoma. Gynecol Oncol 14:125–132, 1982.

Chu AM, Beechinor R: Survival and recurrence patterns in the radiation treatment of carcinoma of the vagina. Gynecol Oncol 19:298–307, 1989.

Chung AF, Woodruff JM, Lewis JL Jr: Malignant melanoma of the vulva: A report of 44 cases. Obstet Gynecol 45:638–646, 1975.

Chung AF, Casey MJ, Flannery JT, et al: Malignant melanoma of the vagina: A report of 19 cases. Obstet Gynecol 55:720–727, 1980.

Copeland LJ, Gershenson DM, Saul PB, et al: Sarcoma botryoides of the female genital tract. Obstet Gynecol 66:262–266, 1985.

Creasman WT: New gynecologic cancer staging. Obstet Gynecol 58:157, 158, 1995.

Curry SL, Wharton JT, Rutledge F: Positive lymph nodes in vulvar squamous carcinoma. Gynecol Oncol 9:63–67, 1980.

DiSaia PJ, Creasman WT, Rich WM: An alternative approach to early cancer of the vulva. Am J Obstet Gynecol 133:825–830, 1979.

Downey GO, Okagaki T, Ostrow RS, et al: Condylomatous carcinoma of the vulva with special reference to human papillomavirus DNA. Obstet Gynecol 72:68–73, 1988.

Eddy GL, Singh KL, Gangler TS: Superficially invasive carcinoma of the vagina following treatment for cervical cancer: A report of 6 cases. Gynecol Oncol 136:376–379, 1990.

Franklin EW, Rutledge FD: Epidemiology of epidermoid carcinoma of the vulva. Obstet Gynecol 39:165–172, 1972.

Frick HC, Jacox HW, Taylor HC: Primary carcinoma of the vagina. Am J Obstet Gynecol 101:695–703, 1968.

Hacker NF, Van der Velden J: Conservative management of early vulvar cancer. Cancer 71:1673–1677, 1993.

Hacker NF, Berek JS, Julliard GJF, et al: Preoperative radiation therapy for locally advanced vulvar cancer. Cancer 54:2056–2061, 1984.

Heaps JM, Fu YS, Montz FJ, et al: Surgical-pathologic variables predictive of local recurrence in squamous cell carcinoma of the vulva. Gynecol Oncol 38:309–314, 1990.

Hopkins MP, Reid GC, Morley GW: The surgical management of recurrent squamous cell carcinoma of the vulva. Obstet Gynecol 75:1001–1005, 1990.

Houghton CRS, Iversen T: Squamous cell carcinoma of the vagina: A clinical study of the location of the tumor. Gynecol Oncol 13:365–372, 1982.

Kalra JK, Grossman AM, Krumholz BA, et al: Preoperative chemoradiotherapy for carcinoma of the vulva. Gynecol Oncol 12:256–260, 1981.

Kaufman RH, Friedrich EG Jr, Gardner NL: Benign Disease of the Vulva and Vagina, 3rd ed. Chicago, Year Book Medical Publishers, 1989.

Kelley JL III, Burke TW, Tornos C, et al: Minimally invasive vulvar carcinoma: An indication for conservative surgical therapy. Gynecol Oncol 144:240–244, 1991.

Kucera H, Vavra N: Radiation management of primary carcinoma of the vagina: Clinical and histopathological variables associated with survival. Gynecol Oncol 40:12–16, 1991.

Lenahan PM, Meffe F, Lickrish GM: Vaginal intraepithelial neoplasia: Biologic aspects and management. Obstet Gynecol 68:333–337, 1986.

Manetta A, Pinto JL, Larson JE, et al: Primary invasive carcinoma of the vagina. Obstet Gynecol 72:77–81, 1989.

Morley GW: Infiltrative carcinoma of the vulva: Results of surgical treatment. Am J Obstet Gynecol 124:874–888, 1976.

Morrow CP, Rutledge FN: Melanoma of the vulva. Obstet Gynecol 39:745–752, 1972.

Norris JH, Taylor HB: Polyps of the vagina. Cancer 22:227–232, 1966.

Parry-Jones E: Lymphatics of the vulva. J Obstet Gynaecol Br Empire 70:751–765, 1963.

Perez CA, Arneson AN, Dehner LP, et al: Radiation therapy in carcinoma of the vagina. Obstet Gynecol 44:862–872, 1972.

Peters WA III, Kumar NB, Morley GW: Carcinoma of the vagina: Factors influencing treatment outcome. Cancer 55:892–897, 1985.

Phillips GL, Bundy BN, Okagaki T, et al: Malignant melanoma of the vulva treated by radical hemivulvectomy: A prospective study of the Gynecology Oncology Group. Cancer 73:2626–2632, 1994.

Podratz KC, Symmonds RE, Taylor WF: Carcinoma of the vulva: Analysis of treatment failures. Am J Obstet Gynecol 143:340–351, 1982.

Pradhan S, Tobon H: Vaginal cysts: A clinicopathologic study of 41 cases. Int J Gynecol Pathol 5:35–46, 1986.

Pride GL, Buchler DA: Carcinoma of the vagina ten or more years following pelvic irradiation therapy. Am J Obstet Gynecol 127:513–517, 1977.

Rhatigan RM, Mojaddi Q: Adenosquamous carcinomas of the vulva and vagina. Am J Clin Pathol 60:208–217, 1973.

Rubin SC, Young J, Mikuta JJ: Squamous carcinoma of the vagina: Treatment complication and long-term follow-up. Gynecol Oncol 20:346–353, 1985.

Rutledge FN, Mitchell MF, Munsell MF, et al: Prognostic indicators for invasive carcinoma of the vulva. Gynecol Oncol 42:239–244, 1991.

Rutledge F, Smith JP, Franklin EW: Carcinoma of the vulva. Am J Obstet Gynecol 106:1117–1130, 1970.

Stehman FB, Bundy BN, Dvoretsky PM, et al: Early stage I carcinoma of the vulva treated with ipsilateral superficial inguinal lymphadenectomy and modified radical hemivulvectomy: A prospective study of the Gynecologic Oncology Group. Obstet Gynecol 79:490–497, 1992.

Thomas G, Dembo A, DePetrillo A, et al. Concurrent radiation and chemotherapy in vulvar carcinoma. Gynecol Oncol 34:263–267, 1989.

Weed JC, Cozier C, Daniel SJ: Human papilloma virus in multifocal invasive female genital tract malignancy. Obstet Gynecol 62(Suppl):83S–87S, 1983.

# 44

# Cervical Cancer

ROBERT E. BRISTOW
FREDRICK J. MONTZ

Carcinoma of the uterine cervix continues to be a leading cause of cancer-related death among women worldwide, with approximately 500,000 cases diagnosed annually. The age-standardized incidence rates of cervical cancer show significant geographic variation, ranging from 4 cases per 100,000 women in Israel to 83.2 cases per 100,000 women in Brazil, where cervical cancer is the most common female malignancy. Among women in the United States, cancer of the uterine cervix is the sixth most common solid malignant neoplasm, being surpassed in frequency only by cancer of the breast, lung, colorectum, endometrium, and ovary. The American Cancer Society has estimated that in 1998 there were 13,700 new cases of invasive cervical cancer and 4900 deaths from the disease in the United States. The average age at which cervical cancer is diagnosed is 52.2 years; the distribution is bimodal, however, with peaks at 35 to 39 years and 60 to 64 years.

## Definitions

*Human papillomavirus* (HPV) is a family of double-stranded DNA viruses with a predilection for the human anogenital tract, thought to be a key etiologic agent in the development of cervical neoplasia.

*Cervical intraepithelial neoplasia* (CIN) is a preinvasive lesion of the cervical epithelium characterized by hyperproliferation and cellular abnormalities; subsequent risk of invasive cervical cancer is determined by the degree of neoplasia: CIN 1, CIN 2, CIN 3, carcinoma in situ.

*Papanicolaou smear* is a screening method for detecting cervical cancer and its precursors through cytologic evaluation of cells obtained from the cervix and vagina.

*Conization* is a surgical procedure in which a conically shaped section of cervix is excised, usually for diagnostic purposes.

*Radical hysterectomy* is a surgical treatment method for early stage cervical cancer involving removal of the cervix and uterus along with portions of the vagina, uterosacral and cardinal ligaments, parametria, and regional lymph nodes.

*External beam therapy* is a radiation treatment method in which the radiation source is outside the patient; it is used to treat the regional lymph nodes and soft tissues and shrink the primary cervical tumor.

*Brachytherapy* is an intracavitary radiation treatment method used to deliver a high dose of radiation to the central tumor mass.

## Diagnostic Considerations

### RISK FACTORS

Several reproductive and sexual characteristics have emerged as important risk factors for cervical cancer

**Table 44–1** Risk Factors for Invasive Cervical Cancer

| Factors Influencing Risk | Estimated Relative Risk* |
|---|---|
| Older ages | 2 |
| Residency in Latin America, Asia, Africa† | 2–6 |
| Lower levels of education or income | 2–3 |
| African American, Hispanic, Native American | 2 |
| Multiparity | 2–4 |
| Early age at first sexual intercourse | 2–4 |
| Multiple sexual partners | 2–5 |
| Presence of detectable HPV | 4–40 |
| Previous STDs (especially genital warts, HSV) | 2–10 |
| Long-term smoking | 2–4 |
| Long-term oral contraceptive use | 1.5–2 |
| No prior regular Pap smear screening | 2–6 |
| Diet low in carotene, vitamin C | 2–3 |

*Relative risks depend on the study and referent groups used.
†Certain parts of Latin America, Asia, and Africa.
STD = sexually transmitted disease; HSV = herpes simplex virus.
Adapted from Brinton LA, Hoover RN: Epidemiology of gynecologic cancers. In Hoskins WJ, Perez CA, Young RC (eds): Principles and Practice of Gynecologic Oncology, 2nd ed. Philadelphia, Lippincott-Raven, 1997, p 3.

(Table 44–1). This has lead to the hypothesis that the primary etiologic agent (or agents) of cervical cancer is sexually transmitted. During the past decade, epidemiologic evidence has accumulated implicating HPV infection as the most likely causative agent of squamous cell carcinoma of the cervix and its precursors. HPV is known to colonize mucosal or cutaneous epithelium, initially resulting in formation of warts at the site of infection. Based on differences in DNA sequencing, over 70 different types of HPV have been identified, more than 20 of which infect the anogenital tract. HPV types 6 and 11 are associated with preinvasive cervical lesions (CINs). Conversely, HPV types 16, 18, 31, 45, and 56 are associated with invasive carcinoma. HPV DNA has been isolated in virtually all cases (93%) of cervical cancer and its precursor lesions. Case-control studies have shown that the presence of HPV infection increases the relative risk of developing cervical cancer from approximately 4- to 40-fold. Although HPV infection is thought to be a necessary component of cervical neoplastic transformation, it is unlikely to be entirely sufficient because other environmental cofactors (low socioeconomic status, race, long-term smoking) also appear to be important (Table 44–1).

*Cervical cytology* has proven to be the most efficacious and cost-effective method for cervical cancer screening. By increasing the detection of preinvasive and early invasive disease, the Papanicolaou smear has decreased both the incidence and mortality from cervical cancer in those populations with cervical cancer screening programs. A single negative Papanicolaou smear may decrease the risk of developing cervical cancer by 45%, and nine negative smears during a lifetime decrease the risk by as much as 99%. Eddy, using a mathematical model, indicated that in women aged 35 to 64 years, screening intervals of 10, 5, and 3 years would reduce the incidence of invasive cervical cancer by 64, 84, and 91%, respectively. One half of women with newly diagnosed invasive cervical carcinoma have never had a Pap smear, and another 10% have not had a smear in the 5 years preceding diagnosis. Underscreened populations include older women, the uninsured, ethnic minorities, and women of lower socioeconomic status, particularly those in rural areas.

The American College of Obstetrics and Gynecology and the American Cancer Society currently recommend that pelvic examination and Pap smear screening begin annually at age 18 years or at the onset of sexual activity. After three consecutive satisfactory normal examinations, Pap smears may be performed at up to 3-year intervals in low-risk women at the discretion of the physician; annual screening is prudent for women with one or more risk factors for cervical cancer or its precursor lesions. Screening should be continued for women over the age of 65 years because 25% of all cases of cervical cancer and 41% of deaths from the disease occur in women in this age group.

It is estimated that over one million women in the United States are diagnosed annually with CIN by means of the Pap smear. It is now recognized that most early CIN lesions will regress spontaneously if untreated; nevertheless, CIN refers to a lesion that may progress to invasive carcinoma. In a comprehensive review of the literature spanning over 40 years, Oster compiled data from multiple studies showing that for CIN 1 lesions the approximate likelihood of spontaneous regression is 60%, the likelihood of persistence is 30%, that of progression to CIN 3 is 10%, and the risk of progression to invasive carcinoma is 1% (Table 44–2). Approximately one third of high-grade lesions (CIN 2 or 3) will spontaneously regress, whereas most of these lesions will persist or progress. The risk of CIN 3 progressing to invasive carcinoma was found to be at least 12%. The duration of follow-up ranged from 4 months to 20 years.

**Table 44–2** Natural History of Cervical Intraepithelial Neoplasia

| | Regression | Persistence | Progression to CIS | Progression to ICC |
|---|---|---|---|---|
| CIN 1 | 57% | 32% | 11% | 1% |
| CIN 2 | 43% | 35% | 22% | 5% |
| CIN 3 | 32% | 56% | — | 12% |

CIS = carcinoma in situ; ICC = invasive cervical carcinoma.
From Oster AG: Natural history of cervical intraepithelial neoplasia: A critical review. Int J Gynecol Pathol 12:186–192, 1993.

## HISTORY

The most common presenting symptom of cervical cancer is abnormal vaginal bleeding or discharge. Abnormal bleeding may take the form of postcoital spotting, intermenstrual bleeding, menorrhagia, or postmenopausal spotting. If cervical bleeding has been chronic, the patient may complain of fatigue or other symptoms related to anemia. A serosanguineous or yellowish vaginal discharge frequently accompanies cervical cancer. If the lesion is advanced or necrotic, the discharge may be associated with a foul odor. Locally advanced disease or tumor necrosis may result in pelvic pain. Similarly, tumor extension to the pelvic sidewall may cause sciatic or back pain associated with hydronephrosis. Advanced stage cervical carcinoma with bladder or rectal involvement can present with hematuria or hematochezia, respectively.

## PHYSICAL EXAMINATION

Patients with invasive cervical cancer may have a normal general physical examination; however, a visible lesion on the cervix can usually be appreciated on pelvic examination. Early lesions may be focally indurated, ulcerated, or present as a slightly elevated and granular area that bleeds readily on contact. Larger lesions have two major types of gross appearance: exophytic or endophytic. Exophytic tumors characteristically have a polypoid or papillary appearance and may involve the upper vagina. Endophytic tumors can be hidden from view in the endocervical canal but can be appreciated on bimanual examination. Particular attention should be directed at examination of the inguinal and supraclavicular fossa lymphatic-bearing regions to rule out distant metastatic disease.

## DIFFERENTIAL DIAGNOSIS

The differential diagnosis for cervical cancer is broad and includes both benign and malignant conditions. Besides cervical cancer, another gynecologic malignancy that may present with abnormal vaginal bleeding is endometrial carcinoma. Endometrial carcinoma may extend into the cervical stroma and give the impression of a barrel-shaped, endophytic, cervical carcinoma arising in the endocervical canal. The incidence of endometrial carcinoma increases with age, so that this is a less likely diagnostic possibility in a young premenopausal patient. A cervical leiomyoma is a benign tumor that is sometimes mistaken for invasive cervical cancer. Severe erosive cervicitis may cause abnormal gynecologic bleeding and may have the appearance of a malignant lesion. In patients of reproductive age, complications of pregnancy must always be considered in the differential diagnosis of abnormal bleeding. Rarely, a cervical ectopic pregnancy may present as a bleeding cervical mass and may be mistaken for an invasive carcinoma.

# Diagnostic Evaluation and Staging

## DIAGNOSTIC EVALUATION

The diagnostic assessment of cervical carcinoma is based largely on clinical evaluation. Determination of the clinical stage depends on careful inspection and palpation of the cervix, vagina, and pelvis. Frequently, this is best accomplished at the time of examination under anesthesia. A histologic diagnosis of invasive cervical cancer is obtained by colposcopic examination with endocervical curettage and directed cervical biopsies, by cervical conization, or by biopsy of grossly visible lesions.

Cervical conization, a procedure in which a conically shaped section of cervix is surgically excised, is particularly useful for evaluating the presence or absence of early invasive carcinoma. Diagnostic indications for conization include an unsatisfactory colposcopy, a positive endocervical curettage, and a lack of correlation among cervical cytology, colposcopy, and biopsy (Table 44–3). When a cervical punch biopsy shows microinvasive carcinoma, conization is indicated to rule out frankly invasive disease because treatment recommendations hinge on the depth of invasion and the associated risk of lymphatic metastases. If cervical biopsy or endocervical curettage indicates the presence of cervical adenocarcinoma in situ, conization should also be performed to exclude the presence of a coexisting invasive adenocarcinoma.

An intravenous pyelogram and flat plate radiographic examination of the chest are additional staging procedures that are usually performed to assess ureteral obstruction or distantly metastatic disease,

**Table 44–3** Indications for Conization of the Cervix

1. Abnormal cytology with unsatisfactory colposcopy (squamocolumnar junction not seen).
2. Limits of the cervical lesion cannot be visualized colposcopically.
3. Positive endocervical curettage.
4. Lack of correlation between cytology, biopsy, and colposcopic findings.
5. Microinvasive carcinoma on biopsy or colposcopy suspicious for carcinoma.
6. Adenocarcinoma in situ on biopsy or endocervical curettage.

### Table 44–4  Staging Procedures for Cervical Carcinoma

| | |
|---|---|
| Physical examination | Examination under anesthesia recommended |
| Radiologic studies | Chest x-ray |
| | Intravenous pyelogram |
| | Barium enema |
| | Skeletal x-ray |
| Procedures | Colposcopy |
| | Cervical biopsy |
| | Conization |
| | Endocervical curettage |
| | Cystoscopy |
| | Proctoscopy |
| Optional studies* | Computed tomography |
| | Lymphangiography |
| | Ultrasonography |
| | Magnetic resonance imaging |
| | Radionucleotide scanning |
| | Laparoscopy/laparotomy |

*Not allowed by FIGO.

respectively. Skeletal x-rays may also be performed for those patients with symptoms suggestive of bony metastasis. Lymphangiography, arteriography, computed tomography (CT), magnetic resonance imaging, and laparoscopy or laparotomy findings may be helpful in planning treatment strategy; however, the results of these tests cannot be used to assign the clinical stage. Staging procedures allowed by International Federation of Gynecology and Obstetrics (FIGO) convention are shown in Table 44–4.

### STAGING

In 1995, FIGO revised the clinical staging system of cervical carcinoma (Table 44–5). Stage I neoplasms are those that are clinically confined to the cervix. In the current staging classification, stage IA1 (microinvasive carcinoma) is defined as a tumor with cervical stromal invasion no greater than 3.0 mm in depth beneath the basement membrane and no wider than 7.0 mm. The stage IA2 definition is applied to those lesions with 3.1 to 5.0 mm of invasion and a breadth of no greater than 7.0 mm. This distinction reflects data indicating that patients with less than 3 mm of invasion are at very low risk of metastatic disease and may be treated more conservatively. Larger lesions confined to the cervix are also subclassified into stage IB1 (no greater than 4 cm in maximal diameter) and stage IB2 (greater than 4 cm in maximal diameter), reflecting the prognostic importance of tumor volume. Careful palpation of the pelvic soft tissue may reveal tumor extension to the upper two thirds (stage IIA) or lower one third of the vagina (stage IIIA). Tumor extension into the parametrial tissue (stage IIB) or to the pelvic side wall (stage IIIB) is best appreciated on rectovaginal examination. The distribution of patients by clinical stage is stage I 38%, stage II 32%, stage III 26%, and stage IV 4%.

## Spread of Disease

Lymphatic spread of cervical carcinoma follows an orderly and reasonably predictable pattern (Fig. 44–1). The primary lymph node groups most frequently involved are the obturator, external iliac, and internal iliac. Secondary nodal involvement (common iliac, para-aortic) rarely occurs in the absence of primary nodal disease. Tumor cells commonly spread through

### Table 44–5  FIGO Staging of Cervical Carcinoma

| | |
|---|---|
| Stage 0 | Carcinoma in situ, intraepithelial carcinoma |
| Stage I | The carcinoma is strictly confined to the cervix |
| Stage IA | Invasive cancer identified only microscopically. All gross lesions even with superficial invasion are stage IB cancers. Invasion is limited to measured stromal invasion with maximum depth of 5 mm and no wider than 7 mm. |
| Stage IA1 | Measured invasion of stroma no greater than 3 mm in depth and no wider than 7 mm |
| Stage IA2 | Measured invasion of stroma greater than 3 mm but no greater than 5 mm in depth and no wider than 7 mm |
| Stage IB | Clinical lesions confined to the cervix or preclinical lesions greater than stage IA |
| Stage IB1 | Clinical lesions no greater than 4 cm in size |
| Stage IB2 | Clinical lesions greater than 4 cm in size |
| Stage II | The carcinoma extends beyond the cervix but has not extended to the pelvic wall. The carcinoma involves the vagina but not as far as the lower third. |
| Stage IIA | No obvious parametrial involvement |
| Stage IIB | Obvious parametrial involvement |
| Stage III | The carcinoma has extended to the pelvic wall. On rectal examination, there is no cancer-free space between the tumor and the pelvic wall. The tumor involves the lower third of the vagina. All cases of hydronephrosis or nonfunctioning kidney are included unless known to be due to another cause. |
| Stage IIIA | No extension to the pelvic wall |
| Stage IIIB | Extension to the pelvic wall, hydronephrosis, or nonfunctioning kidney |
| Stage IV | The carcinoma has extended beyond the true pelvis or has clinically involved the mucosa of the bladder or rectum. Bullous edema does *not* permit a case to be allocated to stage IV. |
| Stage IVA | Spread of growth to adjacent organs |
| Stage IVB | Spread to distant organs |

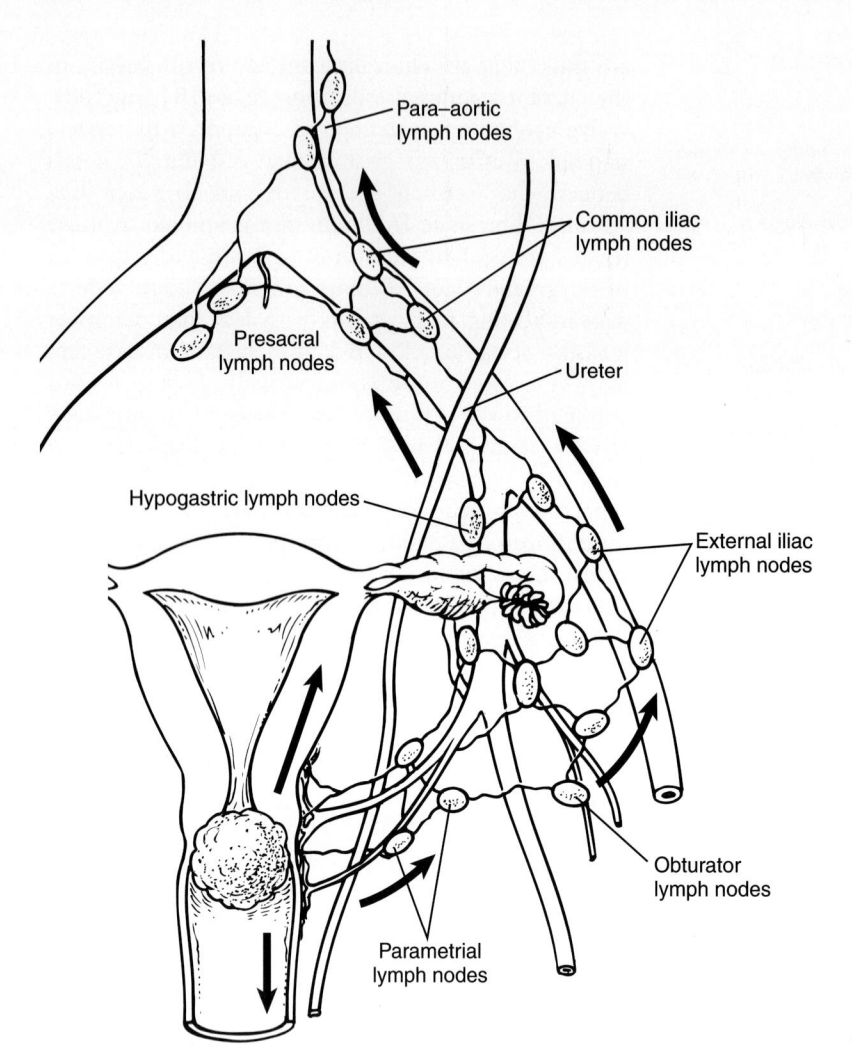

**Figure 44–1** Anatomic pathways for spread of cervical cancer.

the parametrial lymphatic vessels, expanding and replacing the parametrial lymph nodes. These individual tumor masses enlarge and become confluent, eventually replacing the normal parametrial tissue.

The endometrium is involved in 2 to 10% of cervical cancer cases treated with surgery, although the overall incidence (including nonsurgical cases) is unknown. Ovarian metastases are present in less than 1% of patients with squamous carcinoma and slightly more than 1% of patients with adenocarcinoma undergoing surgical treatment. When the primary tumor has extended beyond the confines of the cervix, the upper vagina is involved in 50% of cases.

## Pathology

Squamous cell carcinoma accounts for 75 to 90% of cervical cancers and is classified into three different histologic grades. Well-differentiated tumors constitute about 5% of squamous cell carcinomas, whereas most (85%) squamous tumors are moderately differentiated. Poorly differentiated tumors have a rapid growth rate and may be difficult to recognize as having originated in squamous cells.

Adenocarcinoma of the cervix accounts for approximately 10 to 15% of invasive cervical neoplasms. Although cervical adenocarcinomas have been reported to have a worse prognosis than similar stage squamous carcinomas, this difference is due, at least in part, to the tendency of adenocarcinomas to grow endophytically and establish a large tumor volume before clinical detection. When cervical adenocarcinomas and squamous carcinomas are matched by patient age, clinical stage, tumor volume, and treatment method, survival outcomes are not significantly different.

Small cell carcinoma of the cervix is fortunately uncommon, because these tumors behave in a clinically aggressive fashion and demonstrate a marked propensity to metastasize to local and distant sites. Other less common histologic subtypes of cervical cancer include glassy cell carcinoma, adenosquamous carcinoma, adenoid cystic carcinoma, and leiomyosarcoma.

# Prognostic Factors

Clinical stage at the time of presentation is the most important determinant of subsequent survival. Approximate 5-year survival rates are 97% for stage IA, 85% for stage IB, 60% for stage II, 45% for stage III, and 18% for stage IV disease. Among surgically treated patients, survival is directly related to the number and location of lymph node metastasis, and the frequency of positive lymph nodes increases with the stage of disease (Table 44–6). For all stages of disease, the 5-year survival rate is 75.2% when both pelvic and para-aortic lymph nodes are negative. Survival decreases to 45.6% with positive pelvic nodes and drops to 15.4% when para-aortic nodes are involved. Larger tumor volume and increasing depth of invasion are associated with a worse prognosis. Histologic differentiation is also of prognostic importance, because the 5-year survival rate decreases from 74.5% for patients with well-differentiated tumors to 63.7% for those with moderately differentiated tumors and 51.4% for those with poorly differentiated tumors.

# Treatment

## SURGERY

There are three distinct variations or types of hysterectomy commonly used in the treatment of cervical cancer. A *type I* hysterectomy, or standard extrafascial total abdominal hysterectomy, ensures complete removal of the cervix with minimal disruption to surrounding structures and is appropriate treatment for stage IA1 disease. A *type II* hysterectomy is also referred to as a modified radical hysterectomy. This procedure involves dissection of the ureters from the parametrial and paracervical tissues down to the ureterovesicular junction (Fig. 44–2). This permits removal of all parametrial tissue medial to the ureters and the medial half of the uterosacral ligament and proximal 1 to 2 cm of vagina. In a *type III* or radical abdominal hysterectomy, the ureters are completely dissected from within the paracervical tunnel and the bladder and rectum are extensively mobilized. This operation involves removal of all the parametrial tissue out to the pelvic side wall, complete resection of the uterosacral ligaments, and excision of the upper one third to one half of vagina. Pelvic lymphadenectomy is typically performed with both the type II and type III operations.

Urinary dysfunction resulting from partial denervation of the detrusor muscle during excision of the paracervical and paravaginal tissues is the most common complication observed after radical hysterectomy. Ureterovaginal and vesicovaginal fistulas occur in 2 and 0.9% of patients, respectively.

## RADIATION THERAPY

The two primary modalities of irradiation used to treat cervical cancer are external beam and brachytherapy. *External beam irradiation* is used to treat the whole pelvis and the lateral parametria, including the common iliac and para-aortic lymph nodes. External therapy also serves to decrease central tumor volume, reducing the anatomic distortion produced by larger tumor masses and allowing optimization of subsequent intracavitary therapy.

After external therapy, *brachytherapy* is used to treat the central disease, including the cervix, vagina, and medial parametria. Depending on the volume of disease to be treated, a variety of intracavitary techniques can be used in the treatment of cervical cancer. The intrauterine tandem with vaginal colpostats is the standard application device; however, unusual vaginal or tumor anatomy may be more effectively treated with interstitial needle implants or a vaginal cylinder.

The optimal dose for invasive carcinoma of the cervix is delivered with a combination of whole pelvis and intracavitary therapy. Two reference points in the pelvis are used to describe the total prescribed radiation dose. *Point A* is 2 cm lateral and 2 cm superior to the external cervical os. *Point B* is 3 cm lateral to point A and corresponds to the pelvic side wall. The combined dose of brachytherapy and teletherapy believed to be adequate for central control is between 7500 and 8500 cGy to point A. Depending on the bulk of parametrial and side wall disease, the dose to point B is usually 4500 to 6500 cGy.

Radiation therapy is associated with both acute and chronic complications. Proctosigmoiditis and hemorrhagic cystitis occur in up to 8 and 3% of patients

Table 44–6 Incidence of Pelvic and Para-Aortic Lymph Node Metastasis by FIGO Stage of Cervical Carcinoma

| Stage | n | Positive Pelvic Nodes (%) | Positive Para-Aortic Nodes (%) |
|---|---|---|---|
| IA1 | 179 | 0.5 | 0 |
| IA2 | 178 | 6.2 | <1 |
| IB | 1926 | 15.9 | 2.2 |
| IIA | 110 | 24.5 | 11 |
| IIB | 324 | 31.4 | 19 |
| III | 125 | 44.8 | 30 |
| IVA | 23 | 55 | 40 |

Modified from Hatch KD: Cervical cancer. *In* Berek JS (ed): Practical Gynecologic Oncology, 2nd ed. Baltimore, Williams & Wilkins, 1994, p 243.

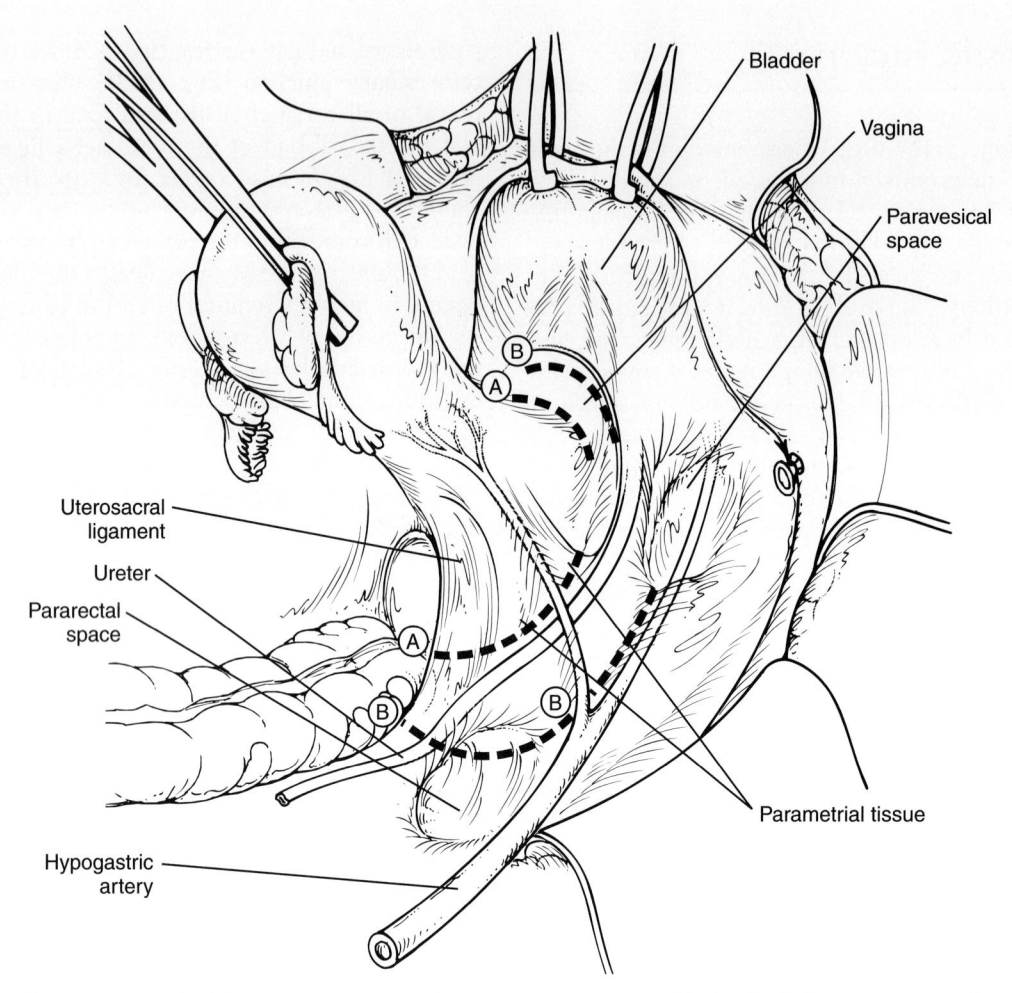

**Figure 44–2** Radical hysterectomy. *Incision lines A,* A type II, or modified radical, hysterectomy involves removal of all parametrial tissue medial to the ureters, the medial half of the uterosacral ligament, and the proximal 1 to 2 cm of the vagina. *Incision lines B,* In a type III, or radical hysterectomy, all parametrial tissue (including the cardinal ligament) out to the pelvic side wall is removed, the uterosacral ligaments are completely resected, and the upper third to half of the vagina is excised.

undergoing radiation therapy for cervical cancer, respectively. Vaginal stenosis is the most common chronic complication of radiation therapy for cervical cancer and is seen in up to 70% of cases. Rectovaginal and vesicovaginal fistulas each occur in approximately 1% of cervical cancer patients treated with irradiation. Two percent of patients experience small bowel obstruction as a consequence of radiation therapy, more commonly in those patients with vascular disease or a history of previous abdominal surgery.

## GENERAL MANAGEMENT BY STAGE

### Stage IA1

Extrafascial hysterectomy is adequate treatment for this group of patients. Conization may be used selectively if preservation of fertility is desired, provided the surgical margins are free of disease (Fig. 44–3). In the absence of lymph–vascular space invasion (LVSI), the incidence of pelvic lymph node metastasis is about 0.3% and lymphadenectomy is not indicated. When LVSI is present, the risk of pelvic node metastasis increases to 2.6%. In these cases we recommend conization with pelvic lymphadenectomy that may be performed by either the laparoscopic or extraperitoneal approach.* In medically inoperable patients, stage IA1 cervical carcinoma can be treated with intracavitary therapy only (point A dose 6000 cGy in one insertion or 7500 cGy in two insertions).

### Stage IA2

Microinvasive cervical carcinoma with stromal invasion of 3.1 to 5.0 mm is associated with positive pelvic lymph nodes in 6.2% of cases. The preferred

---

*Some gynecologic oncologists, however, believe that conization with lymphadenectomy is not sufficient treatment in the presence of LVSI; they recommend hysterectomy and lymphadenectomy. Further studies are needed to answer this question.

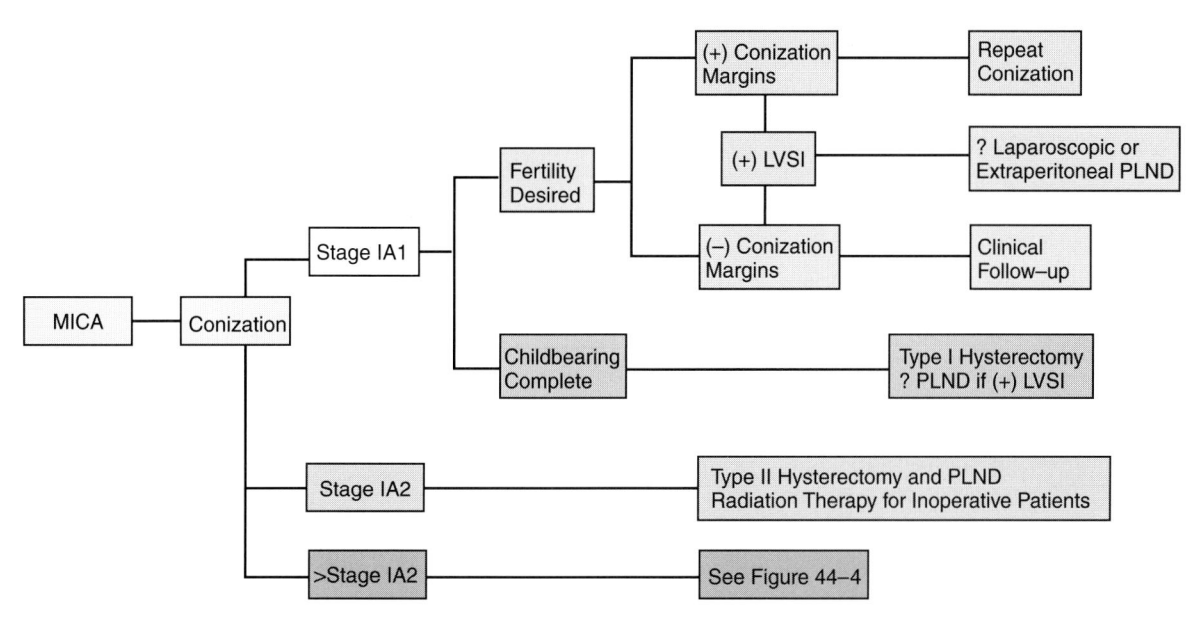

**Figure 44–3** Management algorithm for microinvasive carcinoma of the cervix. LVSI = lymph vascular space invasion; MICA = microinvasive carcinoma on colposcopically directed cervical biopsy; PLND = pelvic lymph node dissection.

treatment for these lesions is modified radical (type II) hysterectomy with pelvic lymphadenectomy.

## Stages IB1, IB2, and IIA

Both radical abdominal hysterectomy (type III) with pelvic lymphadenectomy or radiation therapy are equally effective in treating stages IB and IIA carcinoma of the cervix. Numerous uncontrolled studies support the merits of each modality, with no significant differences in pelvic tumor control or overall survival. The choice of treatment modality should be individualized, although surgery is generally the preferred method because it permits assessment of central tumor volume and the retroperitoneal lymph nodes (Fig. 44–4). Patients can then be offered an individualized treatment plan based on their precise disease status. Surgery also permits conservation of the ovaries, which is desirable in younger patients. Surgical treatment may not be advisable in the presence of significant coexistent medical problems, however. Radiation therapy can be used for most patients regardless of age, body habitus, or coexistent medical

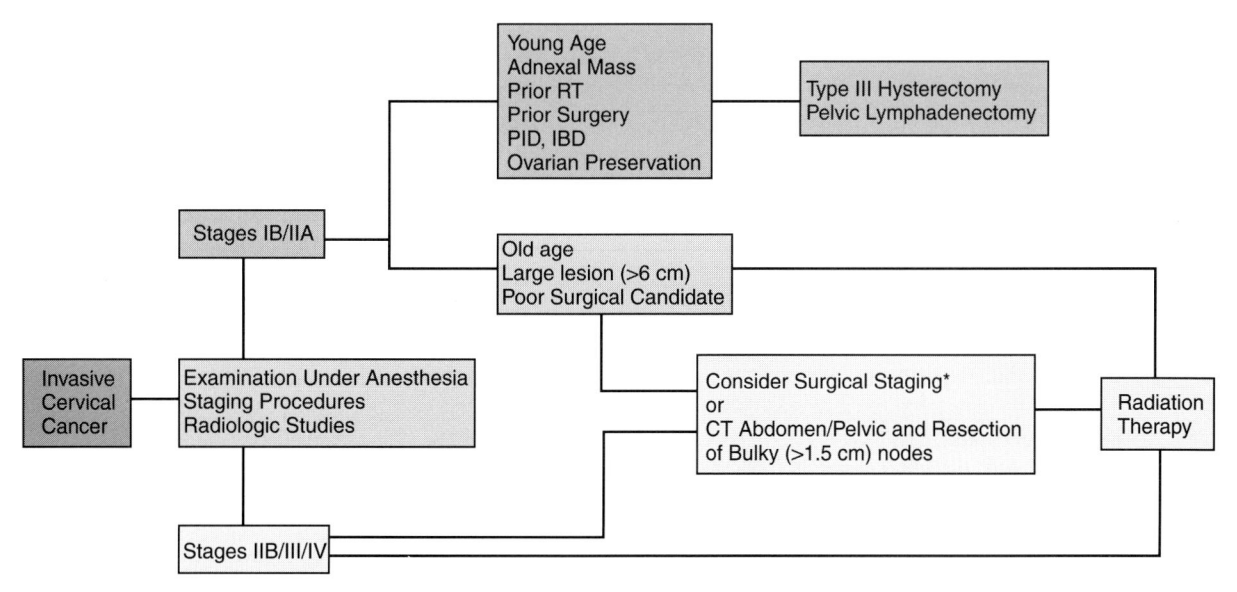

**Figure 44–4** Management algorithm for invasive cervical carcinoma. IBD = inflammatory bowel disease; PID = pelvic inflammatory disease; RT = radiation therapy.

conditions. Stage IB or IIA disease can be effectively treated with a total irradiation dose (whole pelvis and intracavitary) to point A of 7000 to 8500 cGy. Relative contraindications to radiation therapy include prior abdominal surgery, previous pelvic radiation, inflammatory bowel disease, pelvic inflammatory disease, or a coexistent adnexal neoplasm.

Treatment should be individualized for patients with bulky stage I (IB2) tumors. Although some clinicians limit the use of radical hysterectomy to patients with small cervical lesions (<4 cm), acceptable survival rates can be obtained from primary surgical treatment in patients with bulky disease confined to the cervix. Five-year survival rates range from 73 to 82% after radical hysterectomy and pelvic lymphadenectomy for cervical lesions larger than 4 cm. Survival decreases to 66% for lesions larger than 6 cm. When radiation treatment is chosen, tumor expansion of the endocervix and lower uterine segment can distort cervical anatomy and lead to suboptimal application of intracavitary radiation. The central failure rate is 17% in patients with lesions greater than 6 cm treated with radiation alone. In such situations, a "completion" extrafascial hysterectomy is usually performed after radiation therapy.

**Stages IIB, III, and IV**

Radiation therapy, given as a combination of external and intracavitary treatments, is the treatment of choice for patients with stage IIB and more advanced disease. The average total dose of irradiation required to control disease within the treated area in 90% of cases ranges from 5000 cGy for lesions less than 2 cm to over 8000 cGy for tumor volumes exceeding 6 cm. The maximum tolerated dose to point A is 9500 cGy. Patients with stage IVB disease are usually treated with chemotherapy alone or in combination with local irradiation. These patients have a uniformly poor prognosis regardless of treatment modality.

## Surgical Staging

Discrepancies between clinical staging of cervical cancer and surgicopathologic findings occur in 17 to 38% of patients with clinical stage I disease and in as many as 44% of patients with stage III disease. Although not permitted by FIGO for assignment of clinical stage, the disparity between clinical and surgical findings has led some to emphasize surgical staging of cervical carcinoma to identify occult tumor spread so that appropriate, directed adjunctive or extended field radiation therapy may be offered. Surgical staging of cervical carcinoma involves pelvic and para-aortic lymph node dissection and may include evaluation of the parametria with multiple biopsies to delineate side wall extension. Both transperitoneal and extraperitoneal surgical approaches have been advocated; the extraperitoneal route is generally associated with fewer complications and does not delay institution of radiation therapy.

An additional benefit of surgical staging is that it provides an opportunity for surgical resection of grossly enlarged lymph nodes. Potish and associates reported that in women with advanced cervical cancer who underwent surgical excision of grossly enlarged pelvic lymph nodes before definitive radiation therapy, the 5-year survival rate was comparable (56%) with that of women with only microscopically positive pelvic nodes (57%). Alternatively, CT of the abdomen and pelvis can be used to evaluate the retroperitoneal lymph nodes before initiating radiation therapy in patients with locally advanced cervical cancer. Surgical exploration is then reserved for those patients with grossly enlarged lymph nodes (>1.5 cm) on CT (Fig. 44-4).

## Chemotherapy

Chemotherapy is indicated for those patients with extrapelvic metastases and those patients with recurrent disease who are not candidates for radiation or surgical treatment. Cisplatin has been the most extensively studied agent and has demonstrated the most significant clinical response rates. In patients with recurrent or metastatic disease, complete clinical responses to cisplatin have been observed in approximately 24% of cases, with an additional 16% of patients demonstrating a partial response. Other agents demonstrating at least partial activity against cervical cancer include carboplatin, ifosfamide, doxorubicin, etoposide, vinblastine, vincristine, 5-fluorouracil, mitomycin-C, vinorelbine, and methotrexate. In general, response rates are less favorable in those patients who have previously received radiation therapy.

The administration of chemotherapeutic agents before radical hysterectomy has been termed *neoadjuvant chemotherapy*. Cisplatin, bleomycin, and vinblastine have been the most extensively used combination. When chemotherapy is administered before surgery, complete clinical response rates range from 17 to 44%, with overall response rates of 80 to 90%. In addition to increasing surgical resectability, preoperative chemotherapy also decreases the number of positive pelvic lymph nodes and, in some studies, has improved 2- and 3-year survival rates.

Chemotherapy given concurrently with radiation therapy for advanced cervical cancer is referred to as chemoradiation. The rationale for this approach is based on the sensitization of cervical cancer cells to irradiation by some chemotherapeutic agents and the potential to eliminate microscopic systemic metastasis. The most commonly used agents are 5-fluorouracil, hydroxyurea, and cisplatin.

## Posttreatment Surveillance

Among patients who fail primary treatment for cervical cancer, recurrence is detected within 1 year in 50% of cases and within 2 years in more than 80% of patients. Pelvic examination and lymph node evaluation, including supraclavicular nodes, should be performed every 3 months for 2 years and then every 6 months for additional 3 years. Of patients with locally recurrent cervical cancer, over 70% will have abnormal cervical or vaginal cytology; therefore, appropriate cytologic smears should be obtained at the time of each routine examination. Any palpable mass should be evaluated by CT with fine-needle aspiration cytology if indicated. A chest x-ray should be obtained annually to detect pulmonary metastases.

## Treatment of Recurrent Cervical Cancer

Cervical cancer detected within the first 6 months after completion of primary therapy is often termed *persistent cancer*, whereas that diagnosed later is referred to as *recurrent disease*. Appropriate treatment of recurrent cervical cancer is dictated by both the site of recurrence and the method of primary therapy. In general, those patients developing recurrent disease after primary surgical therapy should be considered for radiation therapy. Conversely, surgical treatment should be considered for those patients with recurrent disease after initially receiving irradiation. Distantly metastatic recurrent tumor is not amenable to either modality alone and is an indication for palliative chemotherapy and possibly radiation therapy for local control and alleviation of symptoms.

Only when recurrent cervical cancer is confined to the central pelvis are patients candidates for curative surgical intervention. Total hysterectomy is inadequate treatment for centrally recurrent cervical cancer. Additionally, when radical hysterectomy is performed after therapeutic doses of irradiation, 20 to 50% of patients experience ureteral strictures, urinary fistulas, or other serious complications. Therefore, pelvic exenteration is usually the procedure of choice for centrally recurrent cervical cancer. Before exenterative surgery, a thorough evaluation should be performed to rule out extrapelvic metastases. The clinical triad of unilateral leg edema, sciatic pain, and ureteral obstruction is strongly suggestive of tumor extension to the pelvic side wall and is a contraindication to surgery. Approximately 25% of patients with recurrent cervical cancer are deemed satisfactory candidates for exenterative surgery.

Anterior exenteration combines radical cystectomy with radical hysterectomy and vaginectomy and is indicated for recurrent cervical carcinoma limited to the cervix, anterior vagina, and/or bladder. Posterior exenteration is indicated for lesions confined to the posterior fornix and rectovaginal septum and combines radical hysterectomy and vaginectomy with resection of the rectum. Total pelvic exenteration is the procedure most often required for recurrent cervical cancer and involves the en bloc resection of the bladder, uterus, vagina, and rectum. With proper patient selection and sound surgical judgment, 5-year survival rates after pelvic exenteration range from 45 to 61%.

## Controversies and Special Problems

### ADJUVANT RADIATION THERAPY AFTER SURGERY

Data are limited concerning the efficacy of postoperative pelvic irradiation in patients at high risk of recurrence after radical hysterectomy and pelvic lymphadenectomy. High-risk prognostic factors include microscopic parametrial invasion, pelvic lymph node metastases, deep cervical invasion, and positive or close surgical margins. No survival benefit has been demonstrated for patients with one or two positive lymph nodes receiving postoperative radiation therapy when compared with surgery alone. Although there are no controlled studies, retrospective data suggest that postoperative irradiation after radical hysterectomy may provide a modest gain in survival in patients with three or more positive pelvic lymph nodes. Combined surgical and radiation therapy results in increased morbidity, however, because lymphedema has been reported in up to 23.4% of patients receiving combined therapy.

### POSITIVE LYMPH NODES ENCOUNTERED AT RADICAL HYSTERECTOMY

The management of patients with grossly positive lymph nodes encountered at the time of radical hysterectomy has been controversial. Radiation therapy is clearly indicated in such circumstances. In the interest of minimizing postoperative radiation-related complications and preservation of cervical anatomy for intracavitary radiation placement, some clinicians advocate aborting the surgical procedure once metastatic disease is confirmed on histologic frozen section. Conversely, there are limited data indicating that acceptable survival rates can be obtained with surgical resection of grossly involved nodes in conjunction with radical hysterectomy. Hacker and associates reported that even in patients with grossly positive para-aortic lymph nodes, the 5-year survival rate was 48% after radical hysterectomy, resection of all macroscopic nodal disease, and adjunctive radiation therapy. Serious morbidity occurred in 18% of patients in this series.

## INCIDENTAL CERVICAL CANCER FOUND AT SIMPLE HYSTERECTOMY

Invasive cervical cancer may be incidentally discovered in the surgical specimen after extrafascial hysterectomy. For disease more advanced than stage IA1 (without LVSI), simple hysterectomy is inadequate treatment because the parametria, vaginal cuff, and pelvic lymph nodes may harbor residual tumor. Additional treatment is dictated by the volume of disease and the surgical margins of resection.

Radical surgery after simple hysterectomy for invasive cervical cancer includes radical parametrectomy, resection of the cardinal ligaments, excision of the vaginal cuff, and pelvic lymphadenectomy. Radiation therapy alone can be used for older patients or those who are poor surgical candidates. Five-year survival is 95 to 100% for patients with microscopic disease only in the hysterectomy specimen, whereas 82 to 84% of those with macroscopic disease and negative surgical margins survive 5 years. If the surgical margins of resection are microscopically involved with carcinoma, 5-year survival ranges from 38 to 87%; survival drops to 20 to 47% for patients with gross residual tumor.

The use of postoperative radiation therapy is dictated by the surgical and pathologic findings. Tumor at the surgical margins of resection or gross residual disease is an absolute indication for adjunctive radiation therapy.

## REFERENCES

Alvarez RD, Gelder MS, Gore H, et al: Radical hysterectomy in the treatment of patients with bulky early stage carcinoma of the cervix uteri. Surg Gynecol Obstet 176:539–542, 1993.
American College of Obstetrics and Gynecology: Committee opinion: Recommendations on frequency of Pap test screening. Int J Gynaecol Obstet 49:210–211, 1995.
Anderson GH, Boyes DA, Benedet JL, et al: Organisation and results of the cervical cytology screening programme in British Columbia, 1955–85. Br Med J 296:975–978, 1988.
Boyce J, Fruchter R, Nicastri A: Prognostic factors in stage I carcinoma of the cervix. Gynecol Oncol 12:154–165, 1981.
Brinton LA, Hoover RN: Epidemiology of gynecologic cancers. In Hoskins WJ, Perez CA, Young RC (eds): Principles and Practice of Gynecologic Oncology, 2nd ed. Philadelphia, Lippincott-Raven, 1997, pp 3–29.
Buckley SL, Tritz DM, Van Le L, et al: Lymph node metastases and prognosis in patients with stage IA2 cervical cancer. Gynecol Oncol 63:4–9, 1996.
Cervical cancer. Consensus Statement. Bethesda 14:1–38, 1996.
Chung CK, Nahhas WA, Zaino R, et al: Histologic grade and lymph node metastasis in squamous cell carcinoma of the cervix. Gynecol Oncol 12:348–354, 1981.
Creasman WT: New gynecologic cancer staging. Gynecol Oncol 58:157–158, 1995.
Creasman WT, Soper JT, Clarke-Pearson D: Radical hysterectomy as therapy for early carcinoma of the cervix. Am J Obstet Gynecol 155:964–969, 1986.
Delgado G, Bundy BN, Fowler WC, et al: A prospective surgical pathological study of stage I squamous carcinoma of the cervix: A Gynecologic Oncology Group Study. Gynecol Oncol 35:314–320, 1989.
Eddy DM: Screening for cervical cancer. Ann Intern Med 113:214–226, 1990.
Eluf-Neto J, Booth M, Munoz N, et al: Human papillomavirus and invasive cancer in Brazil. Br J Cancer 69:114–119, 1994.
Hacker NF, Wain GV, Nicklin JL: Resection of bulky positive lymph nodes in patients with cervical carcinoma. Int J Gynecol Cancer 5:250–256, 1995.
Hatch KD: Cervical cancer. In Berek JS (ed): Practical Strategies in Gynecologic Oncology, 2nd ed. Baltimore, Williams & Wilkins, 1994, pp 243–283.
Hreshchyshyn MM, Aron BS, Boronow RC, et al: Hydroxyurea or placebo combined with radiation to treat stage IIIb and IV cervical cancer confined to the pelvis. Int J Radiat Oncol Biol Phys 5:317–322, 1979.
Kilgore LC, Soong S-J, Gore H, et al: Analysis of prognostic factors in adenocarcinoma of the cervix. Gynecol Oncol 31:137–153, 1988.
Kim DS, Moon H, Kim KT, et al: Two-year survival: Preoperative adjuvant chemotherapy in the treatment of cervical cancer stages Ib and II with bulky tumor. Gynecol Oncol 33:225–230, 1989.
Kosary CL: FIGO stage, histology, histologic grade, age and race as prognostic factors in determining survival for cancers of the female gynecologic system: An analysis of 1973–87 SEER cases of cancers of the endometrium, cervix, ovary, vulva, and vagina. Semin Surg Oncol 10:31–46, 1994.
Krebs HB, Helmkamp BF, Sevin B-U, et al: Recurrent cancer of the cervix following radical hysterectomy and pelvic node dissection. Obstet Gynecol 59:422–427, 1982.
Lagasse LD, Creasman WT, Shingleton HM, et al: Results and complications of operative staging in cervical cancer: Experience of the gynecologic oncology group. Gynecol Oncol 9:90–98, 1980.
Morrow CP, Shingleton HM, Averette HE, et al: Is pelvic irradiation beneficial in the postoperative management of stage Ib squamous cell carcinoma of the cervix with pelvic lymph node metastases treated by radical hysterectomy and pelvic lymphadenectomy? A report from the Presidential Panel at the 1979 Annual Meeting of the Society of Gynecologic Oncologists. Gynecol Oncol 10:105–110, 1980.
Munoz N, Bosch FX, de Sanjose S, et al: The causal link between human papillomavirus and invasive cancer: A population-based case-control study in Columbia and Spain. Int J Cancer 52:743–749, 1992.
Omura GA: Chemotherapy for stage IVB or recurrent cancer of the uterine cervix. J Natl Inst Monogr 21:123–126, 1996.
Oster AG: Natural history of cervical intraepithelial neoplasia: A critical review. Int J Gynecol Pathol 12:186–192, 1993.
Parker SL, Tong T, Bolden S, et al: Cancer statistics, 1997. CA Cancer J Clin 47:5–27, 1997.
Perez CA, Camel HM, Kuske RR, et al: Radiation therapy alone

in the treatment of carcinoma of the uterine cervix: A 20-year experience. Gynecol Oncol 23:127–140, 1986.

Peterson F: Annual report on the results of treatment of gynecologic cancer. Radiumhemmet, Stockholm, Sweden, International Federation of Gynecology and Obstetrics (F.I.G.O.). Oxford, Isis Medical Media, 1994, p 132.

Piver MS, Rutledge F, Smith JP: Five classes of extended hysterectomy for women with cervical cancer. Obstet Gynecol 44:265–272, 1974.

Plentl AA, Friedman EA: Lymphatic System of the Female Genitalia: The Morphologic Basis of Oncologic Diagnosis and Therapy. Vol II: Clinical Significance of Cervical Lymphatics. Philadelphia, WB Saunders, 1971, pp 85–115.

Potish RA, Downey GO, Adcock LL, et al: The role of surgical debulking in cancer of the uterine cervix. Int J Radiat Oncol Biol Phys 17:979–984, 1989.

Rabin S, Browde S, Nissenbaum M, et al: Radiotherapy and surgery in the management of stage IB and IIA carcinoma of the cervix. S Afr Med J 65:374–377, 1984.

Reeves WC, Brinton LA, Garcia M, et al: Human papillomavirus (HPV) infection and cervical cancer in Latin America. N Engl J Med 320:1437–1441, 1989.

Sardi J, Sananes C, Giaroli A, et al: Neoadjuvant chemotherapy in locally advanced carcinoma of the cervix uteri. Gynecol Oncol 38:486–493, 1990.

Shingleton HM, Orr JW: Recurrent cancer: Exenterative surgery. *In* Shingleton HM, Orr JW: Cancer of the Cervix. Philadelphia, JB Lippincott, 1995.

Simon NL, Gore H, Shingleton HM, et al: Study of superficially invasive carcinoma of the cervix. Obstet Gynecol 68:19–24, 1986.

Thomas G, Dembo A, Beale F: Concurrent radiation, mitomycin-C and 5-fluorouracil in poor prognosis carcinoma of the cervix: Preliminary results of a Phase I-II study. Int J Radiat Oncol Biol Phys 10:1785–1790, 1984.

Zander J, Baltzer J, Lohe KJ, et al: Carcinoma of the cervix: An attempt to individualize treatment; results of a 20 year cooperative study. Am J Obstet Gynecol 139:752–759, 1981.

… 45 …

# Uterine Cancers

GUNTER DEPPE
ADNAN R. MUNKARAH

## Endometrial Cancer

Endometrial cancer is the most common female genital cancer in the United States. The American Cancer Society estimated that in 1997, 34,900 new cases were diagnosed, and 6000 women died of the disease. The death rate is relatively low compared with the incidence rate because the vast majority of patients are diagnosed when the disease is in its early stages and confined to the uterus. In fact, the most common presenting manifestation, abnormal uterine bleeding in the perimenopausal or postmenopausal woman, leads the patient to seek medical attention early in the course of the disease.

Endometrial cancer is a disease primarily of postmenopausal women; median patient age is 61 years. However, up to 25% of cases occur in perimenopausal women; 5% of patients are younger than 40 years old at the time of diagnosis.

### RISK FACTORS

Most risk factors associated with an increased incidence of endometrial cancer seem to be related to a hyperestrogenic state. (Table 45–1) Patients with endometrial cancer can be divided into two distinct groups based on their epidemiologic and histologic characteristics. The first group includes women with a history of exposure to high levels of estrogen. The endometrial cancers they develop most likely begin as endometrial hyperplasia and progress to carcinoma. The tumors are usually well to moderately differentiated and appear at an early stage with only superficial myometrial invasion and infrequent lymph node metastases. The second group of patients tends to be older than women in the first group and usually are without evidence of prolonged estrogen exposure. Their neoplasms often are high-grade lesions with more undifferentiated cell types and are associated with lymph node metastases and poor prognosis.

Tamoxifen is a nonsteroidal antiestrogen that is

**Table 45–1** Estimated Risk Ratios for Endometrial Cancer According to Selected Risk Factors

| Risk Factor | Risk Ratio |
|---|---|
| Overweight | |
|   20–50 lb | 3.0 |
|   >50 lb | 10.0 |
| No children vs. 1 child | 2.0 |
| No children vs. 5 children | 5.0 |
| Late menopause (≥ age 52 yr vs. <49 yr) | 2.4 |
| Diabetes mellitus | 2.7 |
| Unopposed estrogen therapy | 6.0 |

Data from Rose PG: Endometrial carcinoma. N Engl J Med 335:640, 1998.

frequently used as an adjuvant treatment in women with breast cancer. Reports in the literature suggest an association between tamoxifen use and the development of endometrial cancer. In the National Surgical Adjuvant Breast and Bowel Project (NSABP) trial, Fisher found a sevenfold increased risk of endometrial cancer after 5 years of tamoxifen therapy. However, the expected benefit of reducing breast cancer recurrence in this patient population outweighs this potential risk of endometrial cancer. Women treated with tamoxifen should have a yearly pelvic examination and Papanicolaou smear. An endometrial biopsy should be performed if vaginal bleeding occurs. In the absence of any symptoms, the present data do not support the routine use of endometrial biopsy or transvaginal sonography as screening tools in women on tamoxifen.

## DIAGNOSIS

### History

A complete medical history should be obtained, with special focus on the patient's age, onset of menopause, and use of steroid contraceptives or hormone replacement therapy.

Any personal or family history of other malignancies including breast, gastrointestinal, and ovarian cancers should be noted. Postmenopausal bleeding is defined as vaginal bleeding that occurs 12 months after the last normal menstrual period. It is the presenting sign of endometrial cancer in about 90% of patients. Premenopausal patients may present with increased menstrual flow, decreased menstrual interval, or intermenstrual bleeding. Other rare manifestations associated with advanced stage disease include dyspnea secondary to pulmonary involvement and severe pain secondary to bone metastases.

### Physical Examination

In addition to a complete physical examination, a pelvic examination should include careful visual inspection of vulva, vagina, cervix, and palpation of the pelvic organs. Most women with endometrial cancer do not have significant abnormalities on physical examination. An enlarged uterus is the most common finding but is nonspecific. Adnexal masses may be detected in patients with simultaneous ovarian endometrioid adenocarcinoma or ovarian granulosa cell tumor. Cervical or vaginal metastases may be noted and reflect more advanced stages of the disease. During the physical examination, the gastrointestinal and urinary tract should be ruled out as the possible source of postmenopausal bleeding.

### Diagnostic Procedures

If no gross lesions are noted in the lower genital tract during the physical examination, a Papanicolaou smear and endometrial biopsy should be performed. It is worth noting that the Papanicolaou smear is done to exclude cervical pathology and is abnormal in only 50% of patients with endometrial cancer. Several endometrial biopsy devices are available for office use. They consist of plastic or stainless steel, with suction generated either electrically with a suction pump or mechanically by an attached syringe (i.e., Novak curette, Vabra aspirator, Pipelle). If office endometrial biopsy is negative, then dilatation and curettage (D&C) is indicated in most patients. The diagnostic accuracy of a D&C for detecting endometrial hyperplasia or cancer exceeds 90%. Hysteroscopy has been used by some in the evaluation of postmenopausal bleeding. Although hysteroscopy is helpful in selected cases, we do not recommend its routine use in all patients. In fact, a recent study showed that hysteroscopy did not improve the sensitivity of D&C in the detection of endometrial hyperplasia or cancer. Transvaginal ultrasonography (TVS) has been used to visualize the endometrial stripe and aid in the diagnosis of endometrial pathology. In one study, all women with an endometrial stripe thickness exceeding 8 mm had histologic evidence of hyperplasia or polyps. Present studies are focusing on the ability of TVS to detect endometrial cancer and determine the presence of myometrial invasion. Serum cancer antigen 125 (CA 125), a tumor marker helpful in the management of women with ovarian cancer, is elevated in most patients with advanced or metastatic endometrial cancer. Some investigators have used serial serum levels to determine response to therapy in patients with metastatic disease.

## DIFFERENTIAL DIAGNOSIS

Endometrial hyperplasias and malignancies account for 20 to 30% of cases of postmenopausal bleeding. Other possible etiologies are listed in Table 45–2. Because colonic tumors are common in the age group of women diagnosed with endometrial cancer, we recommend routine rectal examination and guaiac testing on the stools. We follow the American Cancer Society recommendations for lower gastrointestinal endoscopy.

## PATHOLOGY OF ENDOMETRIAL CANCER

### Endometrial Hyperplasia

The classification of hyperplasia by the International Society of Gynecological Pathologists has been help-

| Table 45–2 Causes of Postmenopausal Bleeding | |
|---|---|
| Uterine | Ovarian |
|   Atrophic endometrium |   Functioning stromal tumors |
|   Exogenous estrogen |   Epithelial tumors |
|   Hyperplasia | Tubal |
|   Polyps |   Carcinoma |
|   Adenocarcinoma | Extragenital |
|   Sarcoma |   Gastrointestinal |
| Vulvar |     Hemorrhoids |
|   Carcinoma |     Fissures |
|   Trauma |     Adenomas, polyps, carcinoma |
|   Intraepithelial neoplasia |   Urinary tract |
| Vaginal |     Caruncle |
|   Carcinoma |     Urethral prolapse |
|   Vaginal atrophy |     Infections |
|   Trauma | |
| Cervical | |
|   Carcinoma | |
|   Polyps | |

ful in standardizing nomenclature and defining therapy options and outcome (Table 45–3). Complex hyperplasia is distinguished from simple hyperplasia by increased glandular complexity and crowding. Only lesions with nuclear atypia are designated atypical. Progression from hyperplasia to carcinoma occurs in less than 3% of patients with lesions without cytologic atypia, whereas 8% of patients with simple atypical hyperplasia and 23% of patients with complex atypical hyperplasia develop carcinoma. Patient age, presence of an estrogen-secreting ovarian tumor, and exogenous hormone administration may also influence the risk of progression. Endometrial hyperplasia with atypia requires a thorough evaluation. If this diagnosis is made by office endometrial biopsy, coexistent cancer should be excluded by D&C.

## Endometrial Cancers

Endometroid adenocarcinoma is the most common histologic subtype of all uterine cancers and accounts for about 60% of all corpus malignancies. Other recognized subtypes are listed in Table 45–4. Of these, papillary serous (~5%) and clear cell carcinoma (~6%) are particularly virulent, with a high tendency for lymph node involvement and abdominal spread.

Table 45–3 Classification of Endometrial Hyperplasia

1. Endometrial hyperplasia without atypia
    Simplex
    Complex
2. Atypical endometrial hyperplasia
    Simplex
    Complex

Table 45–4 Classification of Endometrial Carcinoma

Endometrioid adenocarcinoma
  Adenocarcinoma
    Secretory
    Ciliated cell
    Adenocarcinoma with squamous differentiation
Papillary serous adenocarcinoma
Clear cell adenocarcinoma
Mucinous adenocarcinoma
Squamous cell carcinoma
Mixed carcinoma
Undifferentiated carcinoma

The prognosis of patients with either tumor is usually poor. Christopherson and associates estimated a 5-year survival rate of 80% for stage I endometroid adenocarcinomas compared with 68% for papillary serous carcinomas and 44% for clear cell carcinomas. Adenocanthoma was a common term used for lesions that had benign-appearing squamous elements in addition to the malignant glandular component. Adenosquamous carcinoma was a term reserved for adenocarcinomas that also had malignant squamous features. In the last few years, it has been proposed that the term *adenocarcinoma with squamous differentiation* be used, without concern for the degree of differentiation of the squamous elements. The behavior of these tumors appears to be related to the architectural and nuclear grade of the glandular component.

## TREATMENT

### Endometrial Hyperplasia

The presence or absence of cytologic atypia should be one of the main factors used to plan therapy. For women with endometrial hyperplasia and no atypia, first-line treatment should consist of periodic progestins. A repeat biopsy should be performed in about 4 months to exclude persistent hyperplasia. In younger women with infertility owing to anovulation, induction of ovulation may be the therapy of choice. In cases of atypical hyperplasia, treatment is dictated by patient's age and desire for future fertility. In the young woman who has not completed her family, continuous progestational therapy with megestrol acetate (40 to 160 mg/day) or medroxyprogesterone acetate (40 to 100 mg/day) is recommended for at least a few months with follow-up endometrial sampling. In the older patient population, hysterectomy is the treatment of choice (Fig. 45–1).

### Endometrial Cancer

An accurate understanding of the natural progression of endometrial cancer aids in treatment planning and

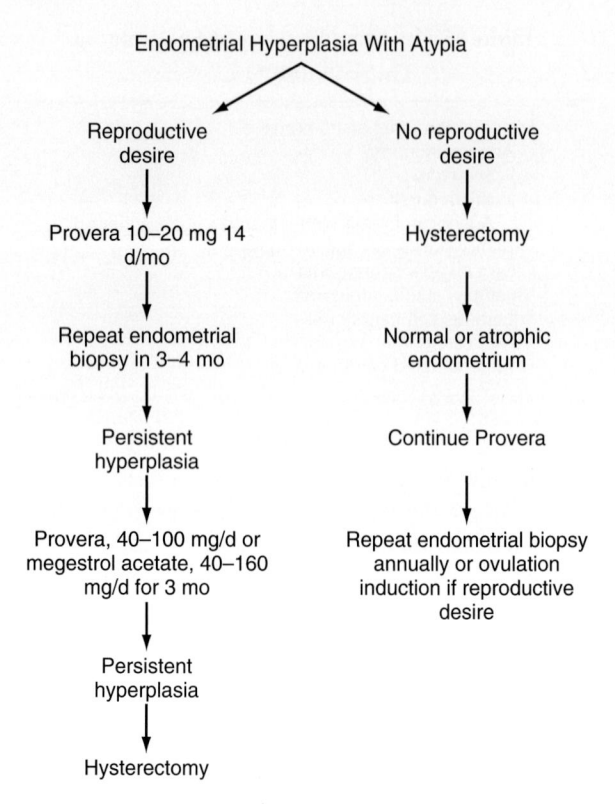

Figure 45–1  Management of endometrial hyperplasia.

**Table 45–5** Preoperative Evaluation for Early Stage Endometrial Cancer

| | |
|---|---|
| History | Liver function studies |
| Physical examination | Serum glucose |
| Complete blood count | Urinalysis |
| Serum creatinine | Electrocardiogram |
| Electrolytes | Chest radiograph study |

these studies as an adjunct to the planned surgical procedure. We reserve the use of CT and MRI to cases with highly suspected distant metastatic disease and to the few patients with significant medical illnesses who are not candidates for primary surgical therapy.

## Surgery

The primary therapy for most patients with endometrial cancer is surgical and consists of exploratory laparotomy, peritoneal washings, hysterectomy, and

patient counseling. One of the main routes of endometrial cancer spreads is by direct extension through the myometrium, cervix, parametrium, vagina, and fallopian tubes. The development of intra-abdominal metastases and malignant peritoneal cytology may occur as a result of deep invasion through the myometrial wall or by retrograde flow of the malignant cells through the fallopian tubes. Involvement of pelvic and aortic lymph nodes occurs through lymphatic dissemination. Hematogenous spread may lead to lung, liver, brain, and bone metastases. More than 70% of patients with endometrial cancer have disease localized to the pelvis at the time of diagnosis. In most patients, the first step in the treatment is surgical exploration for hysterectomy, salpingo-oophorectomy, and possible staging.

## Preoperative Evaluation

Routine preoperative investigation for early stage endometrial cancer is shown in Table 45–5. A chest radiograph film is usually ordered to rule out pulmonary metastases. Cystoscopy, sigmoidoscopy, colonoscopy, or barium enema can be used if bladder or rectal involvement or a concomitant colon cancer is suspected. A pelvic and abdominal computed tomography (CT) or magnetic resonance imaging (MRI) may be helpful in determining the extent of metastatic disease. However, there are no data to support a cost-benefit effect of the routine use of any of

**Table 45–6** FIGO Staging for Endometrial Carcinoma

| Stage | Description |
|---|---|
| IA G 1,2,3 | Tumor limited to endometrium |
| IB G, 1,2,3 | Invasion of less than half of the myometrium |
| IC G 1,2,3 | Invasion of more than half of the myometrium |
| IIA G 1,2,3 | Endocervical glandular involvement only |
| IIB G, 1,2,3 | Cervical stromal invasion |
| IIIA G 1,2,3 | Tumor invades serosa +/or adnexa +/or positive peritoneal cytology |
| IIIB G 1,2,3 | Vaginal metastases |
| IIIC G 1,2,3 | Metastases to pelvic +/or para-aortic lymph nodes |
| IVA G 1,2,3 | Tumor invasion of bladder +/or bowel mucosa |
| IVB G 1,2,3 | Distant metastases including intra-abdominal and/or inguinal lymph nodes |

Histopathology—degree of differentiation. Cases of carcinoma of the corpus should be graded according to the degree of histologic differentiation as follows:
  Grade 1 = 5% or less of a nonsquamous or nonmorular solid growth pattern
  Grade 2 = 6–50% of a nonsquamous or nonmorular solid growth pattern
  Grade 3 = More than 50% of a nonsquamous or nonmorular solid growth pattern

Notes on Pathologic Grading
1. Notable nuclear atypia inappropriate for the architectural grade, raises the grade of a Grade 1 or Grade 2 by 1.
2. In serous adenocarcinomas, clear-cell adenocarcinomas, and squamous cell carcinomas, nuclear grading takes precedence.
3. Adenocarcinomas with benign squamous differentiation are graded according to the nuclear grade of the glandular component.

Rules Related to Staging
1. Because corpus cancer is now staged surgically, procedures previously used for determination of stages are no longer applicable (e.g., findings from functional dilatation and curettage to differentiate between stage I and stage II).
2. There may be a small number of patients with corpus cancer who will be treated primarily with radiation therapy. If that is the case, the clinical staging, adopted by FIGO in 1971, still would apply, but designation of that staging system would be noted.
3. Ideally, width of the myometrium should be measured along with the width of tumor invasion.

FIGO = International Federation of Gynecology and Obstetrics.

### Table 45–7  Surgical Staging for Endometrial Cancer

Abdominal hysterectomy and bilateral salpingo-oophorectomy
Peritoneal cytology
Inspection and palpation of abdominal and pelvic organs including diaphragm, liver, omentum, peritoneum, retroperitoneal nodes
Omental biopsy or subcolic omentectomy*
Selective biopsy of retroperitoneal nodes†

*Patients with papillary serous and clear-cell cancers
†Frozen section of uterus is used by some to select patients for lymphadenectomy
Data from Chen SS, Spiegel G: Stage I endometrial carcinoma. Role of omental biopsy and omentectomy. J Reprod Med 36:627–629, 1991; Malviya VK, Deppe G, Malone JM, et al: Reliability of frozen section examination in identifying poor prognostic indicators in stage I endometrial adenocarcinoma. Gynecol Oncol 34:299–304, 1989.

bilateral salpingo-oophorectomy. Unlike the previous clinical staging system, the revised International Federation of Gynecology and Obstetrics (FIGO) staging system for endometrial cancer is based on the surgicopathologic findings (Table 45–6). Thus, for a complete surgical staging, selective pelvic and periaortic lymph node biopsies are required (Table 45–7). However, the therapeutic benefit of complete surgical staging for all patients has been debated. Clinical judgment and adequate knowledge of the disease process should be the basis of deciding on the extent of the operation. Factors that increase the risk of lymphatic spread include high-grade lesions, papillary serous and clear cell histology, deep myometrial invasion, and isthmus and cervical involvement. Most gynecologic oncologists use these criteria to determine whether to proceed with lymph node sampling (Table 45–8).

In morbidly obese patients diagnosed with a well-differentiated carcinoma, an abdominal surgery may carry a significant morbidity. In these selected cases, vaginal hysterectomy with bilateral salpingo-oophorectomy is recommended. Prospective studies are currently evaluating the use of laparoscopic assisted hysterectomy with bilateral salpingo-oophorectomy and pelvic and periaortic lymph node sampling in endometrial cancer patients. The goal of such an approach is to achieve shorter hospitalizations, reduced care costs, and faster recuperation.

Advanced metastatic disease presents a significant management dilemma to the gynecologic oncologist.

### Table 45–8  Endometrial Cancer Indications for Retroperitoneal Lymph Node Sampling

Enlarged pelvic or aortic nodes
Grade 2 or 3 lesions
Clear-cell or serous histology
Isthmus-cervix extension
Myometrial invasion >50%

### Table 45–9  Prognostic Factors in Endometrial Cancers

| | |
|---|---|
| Stage | Adnexal involvement |
| Age | Intraperitoneal spread |
| Histologic grade | Peritoneal cytology |
| Histologic type | DNA-ploidy |
| Myometrial invasion | Overexpression of p53 |
| Isthmus-cervix extension | Hormone receptor status |
| Vascular space invasion | |

Prognosis for these patients is very poor, and survival is limited. In patients whose metastases are limited to the peritoneal cavity, recent retrospective studies have suggested possible benefit for optimal tumor debulking, a concept adopted from the management of ovarian cancer. The value of this approach needs further investigation.

## Postoperative Therapy

The postoperative management of patients with endometrial cancer is dictated by many considerations including the patient's age and medical condition, tumor histology, and surgical stage. In patients with early stage disease, multiple prognostic factors have been investigated to determine the risk of recurrence and the benefits of adjuvant therapy (Table 45–9). For patients with stage I tumors, deep myometrial invasion and presence of extensive vascular invasion are used by some as indications for adjuvant pelvic radiation.

In patients with extrauterine spread, surgery is not sufficient treatment. A variety of additional therapies have been used depending on the site of metastasis and the philosophy and experience of the treating centers. These therapies have included pelvic radiation, pelvic radiation with extended field, whole abdominal radiation, and chemotherapy (Table 45–10). Current randomized studies are comparing radiation

### Table 45–10  Treatment for Endometrial Cancer According to Surgical Stage

| Stage | Postoperative Treatment |
|---|---|
| IA G12 | None |
| IA G3<br>1B G123 | None or vaginal cuff radiation |
| 1C<br>IIA<br>IIB<br>IIIA | All grades — Pelvic radiation |
| IIIB*<br>IVA<br>IVB* | All grades — Pelvic and aortic radiation<br>Pelvic and abdominal radiation<br>Individualize |

*Consider cytotoxic or hormonal therapy.

to combination chemotherapy in selected groups with advanced tumors. Patients with clinical stage II who have gross cervical involvement are occasionally treated with preoperative radiation followed by surgery. Another acceptable approach is to perform a radical (modified) hysterectomy and then proceed with radiotherapy. For women with advanced or recurrent endometrial cancer, who have well-differentiated and receptor-positive disease, a therapy preferred by some authors is progestins. For patients who fail hormonal therapy, combination chemotherapeutic regimens with doxorubicin, platinum, or paclitaxel-based combinations are recommended.

### Nonsurgical Treatment

Progestational therapy has been described as a treatment option for young patients with well-differentiated carcinomas who desire to preserve their fertility. Good success rates have been described; however, available data regarding this therapy are quite limited, and patients need adequate counseling about possible risks and failure rates. In women at high surgical risk, pelvic radiation has been used as primary treatment for endometrial cancer, and acceptable levels of complications and tumor control rates have been reported. The risk of treatment failure is definitely higher with pelvic radiation alone compared with surgical treatment.

## ENDOMETRIAL PAPILLARY SEROUS CARCINOMA

In 1982, Hendrickson and colleagues introduced the term *uterine papillary serous carcinoma* for a highly malignant form of endometrial adenocarcinoma that histologically resembles the common papillary serous cancers of the ovary. It spreads primarily through lymphatics and by peritoneal metastases. Postmenopausal bleeding, abdominal or pelvic mass, and abdominal bloating are the most common presenting symptoms. It is not strongly associated with obesity, hypertension, or the hyperestrogenic states. Because this tumor simulates the behavior of ovarian cancer, surgical staging and cytoreductive surgery should be based on principles for ovarian cancer treatment. For patients whose tumors have been adequately staged and optimally debulked, postoperative therapies being evaluated include whole abdominal radiation and paclitaxel (Taxol)-based combination chemotherapy.

# Uterine Sarcomas

Uterine sarcomas are much less common than endometrial carcinoma. They can arise from either the endometrium or the myometrium. They can generally be divided into four major groups: (1) malignant mixed müllerian tumors (MMMT), (2) leiomyosarcomas, (3) endometrial stromal sarcomas (ESS), and (4) adenosarcomas. ESS are further subdivided into high-grade sarcomas and low-grade sarcomas; the latter is also referred to as endolymphatic stromal myosis. MMMT are the most common and account for 50% of uterine sarcomas, followed by leiomyosarcomas (40%) and ESS approximately 6 to 8%.

## DIAGNOSIS

The different subtypes of uterine sarcomas affect women of different ages. MMMT and high-grade ESS tend to occur later in life. The average age at diagnosis of MMMT is usually in the seventh decade. Leiomyosarcomas occur at a younger age, with an average age of 53 years at the time of diagnosis. Low-grade stromal sarcoma is usually diagnosed in the premenopausal years.

Abnormal vaginal bleeding is the presenting complaint in 75 to 95% of patients with uterine sarcoma. Other signs and symptoms include pelvic pain (30%), pelvic mass (20 to 50%), and purulent vaginal discharge. Abnormal physical examination findings include an enlarged uterus, pelvic mass, or a polypoid tumor protruding through the cervical os. Laboratory evaluation is similar to that described for endometrial cancer. Because of the high incidence of extrauterine spread, radiologic testing (CT scan, MRI) to rule out metastases is more frequently used.

## PATHOLOGY

MMMT, also known as carcinosarcomas, are composed of malignant epithelial and malignant connective tissues. The epithelial element is usually a high-grade adenocarcinoma. The malignant connective tissue element can be homologous (stromal sarcoma) or heterologous (rhabdomyosarcoma, chondrosarcoma, osteosarcoma to uterine tissues). Stage for stage, the prognosis of patients with heterologous and homologous MMMT is similar. In leiomyosarcomas, the malignant cells usually arise from the myometrial smooth muscle. The criteria for diagnosis of malignancy in a uterine smooth muscle tumor are based on mitotic count and cellular atypia. The tumors are considered frankly malignant if they exhibit (1) more than 10 mitoses per 10 high-powered fields (HPF), based on counts of 40 or more consecutive HPF, or (2) 5 to 10 mitoses per 10 HPF with cellular atypia.

## TREATMENT

### Malignant Mixed Müllerian Tumors

The initial step in the treatment of these tumors is exploratory laparotomy, hysterectomy, bilateral salpingo-oophorectomy, selective pelvic and periaortic lymph node dissection, lymph and omental sampling. Clinical staging in these tumors is quite unreliable; 15 to 40% of clinical stages I/II are understaged according to surgicopathologic findings. If the disease is confined to the pelvis, the use of postoperative adjuvant pelvic radiation reduces the incidence of local recurrence. Unfortunately, it does not improve overall survival because distant recurrences continue to be a significant problem contributing to the death of these patients. In cases with diffuse metastases, combination chemotherapy is usually given postoperatively. Active drugs include cisplatin, doxorubicin (Adriamycin), and ifosfamide.

### Leiomyosarcomas

These tumors are frequently diagnosed at the time of surgery for symptomatic enlarging fibroids or pelvic mass. The surgery should include total hysterectomy and bilateral salpingo-oophorectomy. All patients with lymph node metastases seem to have clinical evidence of extrauterine spread; therefore, some authors do not recommend routine sampling of clinically normal lymph nodes in the absence of other signs of metastases. Leiomyosarcomas are aggressive tumors; up to 70% of patients with early stage disease have a recurrence within 2 years of diagnosis. Radiation therapy does not seem to be effective with these tumors. Active chemotherapy agents include Adriamycin and dimethyl triazeno imidazole carboxamide (DTIC). In some patients with a solitary pulmonary recurrence, cures have been achieved with local resections.

## ENDOMETRIAL STROMAL SARCOMAS

### Low-Grade Sarcomas

Treatment of these tumors is usually surgical with hysterectomy. Bilateral salpingo-oophorectomy is usually recommended because there is high risk of recurrence in the retained ovaries, and these tumors are hormonally responsive. Late relapses are seen even in patients with early stage disease. Recurrent tumors are slow growing and often amenable to surgical resection. In patients with recurrent or advanced disease, progestins are usually prescribed with good tumor response. Long-term survival is expected with these lesions.

### High-Grade Sarcomas

As for the other uterine sarcomas, total abdominal hysterectomy, bilateral salpingo-oophorectomy, and surgical staging should be performed first. Adjuvant pelvic radiation improves local control in patients with disease confined to the pelvis. For women with more advanced disease, chemotherapy is usually recommended. Unfortunately, high-grade uterine sarcomas are aggressive tumors and cure rates are low.

## REFERENCES

Barter JF, Smith EB, Sapak CA, et al: Leiomyosarcoma of the uterus: A clinicopathologic study of 21 cases. Gynecol Oncol 21:220–227, 1985.

Ben-Yehuda OM, Kim YB, Leuchter RS: Does hysteroscopy improve upon the sensitivity of dilatation and curettage in the diagnosis of endometrial hyperplasia or carcinoma? Gynecol Oncol 68:4–7, 1998.

Berchuck A, Rubin SC, Hoskins WJ, et al: Treatment of uterine leiomyosarcoma. Obstet Gynecol 71:845–850, 1988.

Cacciatore B, Lehtovirta P, Wahlstrom T, Ylostalo P: Preoperative sonographic evaluation of endometrial cancer. Am J Obstet Gynecol 160:133–137, 1989.

Chen SS: Propensity of retroperitoneal lymph node metastasis in patients with stage I sarcoma of the uterus. Gynecol Oncol 1989;32:215–217, 1989.

Chen SS, Spiegel G: Stage I endometrial carcinoma. Role of omental biopsy and omentectomy. J Reprod Med 36:627–629, 1991.

Christopherson WM, Connelly PJ, Alberhasky RC: Carcinoma of the endometrium. V. An analysis of these prognosticators in patients with favorable subtypes and stage I disease. Cancer 51:1705–1709, 1983.

Creasman WT, Morrow CP, Bundy BN: Surgical pathologic spread patterns of endometrial cancer. A Gynecologic Oncology Group study. Cancer 60:2035–2041, 1987.

DeFusco PA, Gaffey TA, Malkasian GD, et al: Endometrial stromal sarcoma: Review of Mayo clinical experience 1945–1980. Gynecol Oncol 35:8–14, 1989.

Fisher B, Costatino JP, Redmond CK, et al: Endometrial cancer in tamoxifen-treated breast cancer patients: Findings from the National Surgical Adjuvant Breast and Bowel Project (NSABP) B-14. J Natl Cancer Inst 86:527–537, 1994.

Gitsch G, Friedlander ML, Wain GV, Hacker NF: Uterine papillary serous carcinoma. Cancer 75:2239–2243, 1995.

Goff BA, Rice LW, Fleischhacker D, et al: Uterine leiomyosarcoma and endometrial stromal sarcoma: lymph node metastases and sites of recurrence. Gynecol Oncol 50:105–109, 1993.

Harlow BL, Weiss NS, Lofton S: The epidemiology of sarcomas of the uterus. J Natl Cancer Inst 76:399–402, 1986.

Harouny VR, Sutton GP, Clark SA, et al: The importance of peritoneal cytology in endometrial carcinoma. Obstet Gynecol 72:394–398, 1988.

Hendrickson M, Ross J, Martinez A, et al: Uterine papillary serous carcinoma: a highly malignant form of endometrial adenocarcinoma. Am J Surg Pathol 6:93–108, 1982.

Kedar RP, Bourne TH, Powles TJ, et al: Effects of tamoxifen on uterus and ovaries of postmenopausal women in a randomized breast cancer prevention trial. Lancet 343:1318–1321, 1994.

Kilgore LC, Partridge EE, Alvarez RD, et al: Adenocarcinoma of the endometrium: survival comparisons of patients with or without pelvic node sampling. Gynecol Oncol 56:29–33, 1995.

Kurman RJ, Kaminski PF, Norris HJ: The behavior of endometrial hyperplasia: a long-term study of "untreated" hyperplasia in 170 patients. Cancer 56:403–412, 1985.

Larson B, Silfversward C, Nilsson B, Pettersson F: Mixed müllerian tumors of the uterus—prognostic factors: A clinical and histopathologic study of 147 cases. Radiother Oncol 17:123–132, 1990.

Levenback C, Rubin SC, McCormack PM, et al: Resection of pulmonary metastases from uterine sarcomas. Gynecol Oncol 45:202–205, 1992.

Malviya VK, Deppe G, Malone JM, et al: Reliability of frozen section examination in identifying poor prognostic indicators in stage I endometrial adenocarcinoma. Gynecol Oncol 34:299–304, 1989.

Morrow CP, Bundy N, Kurman RJ, et al: Relationship between surgical-pathological risk factors and outcome in clinical stage I and II carcinoma of the endometrium: A Gynecologic Oncology Group study. Gynecol Oncol 40:55–65, 1991.

Olt G, Berchuck A, Bast RC Jr: The role of tumor markers in gynecologic oncology. Obstet Gynecol Surv 45:570–577, 1990.

Omura GA, Major FJ, Blessing JA, et al: A randomized study of adriamycin with and without dimethyl triazeno imidazole carboxamide in advanced uterine sarcomas. Cancer 52:626–632, 1983.

Orr JW, Holiman JL, Orr PF: Surgical stage I corpus cancer. Is teletherapy necessary? Proceedings of the American Gynecological and Obstetrical Society. Asheville, North Carolina, September 1, 5–7, 1995, pp 34–35.

Orr JW, Orr PF, Taylor PT: Surgical staging endometrial cancer. Clin Obstet Gynecol 39:656–668, 1996.

Parker SL, Tony T, Bolden S, et al: Cancer statistics, 1997. CA Cancer J Clin 47:5–27, 1997.

Peters WA III, Andersen WA, Thornton N Jr, et al: The selective use of vaginal hysterectomy in the management of adenocarcinoma of the endometrium. Am J Obstet Gynecol 146:285–289, 1983.

Piver MS, Rutledge FN, Copeland L, et al: Uterine endolymphatic stroma myosis: A collaborative study. Obstet Gynecol 64:173–178, 1995.

Rose PG, Piver MS, Tsukada Y, Lau T: Patterns of metastasis in uterine sarcoma. Cancer 63:935–938, 1989.

Rose PG. Endometrial carcinoma. N Engl J Med 335:640–649, 1996.

Rose PG, Sommers RM, Reale FR, et al: Serial serum CA-125 measurements for evaluation of recurrence in patients with endometrial carcinoma. Obstet Gynecol 84:12–16, 1994.

Rutquist LE, Johansson H, Signomklav T, et al: Adjuvant tamoxifen therapy for early stage breast cancer and second primary malignancies. J Natl Cancer Inst 87:645–651, 1995.

Silva EG, Tornos CS, Follen-Mitchell M: Malignant neoplasms of the uterine corpus in patients treated for breast carcinoma: the effects of tamoxifen. Int J Gynecol Pathol 13:248–258, 1994.

Sutton GP, Stehman FB, Michael H, et al: Estrogen and progesterone receptors in uterine sarcomas. Obstet Gynecol 68:709–719, 1986.

Wolfson AH, Wolfson DJ, Sittler SY, et al: A multivariate analysis of clinicopathologic factors for predicting outcome in uterine sarcomas. Gynecol Oncol 52:56–62, 1994.

Zaino RJ, Kurman RJ: Squamous differentiation in carcinoma of the endometrium: A critical appraisal of adenoacanthoma and adenosquamous carcinoma. Semin Diagn Pathol 5:154–171, 1998.

Zaino RJ, Kurman RJ, Herbald D, et al: The significance of squamous differentiation in endometrial carcinoma: Data from a Gynecologic Oncology Group Study. Cancer 68:2293–2302, 1991.

# 46

# Epithelial Ovarian Carcinoma

ANNETTE BICHER

## Epidemiology

Epithelial ovarian cancer is the leading cause of death from gynecologic malignancy in the United States. There was an estimated 25,400 new cases and 14,500 deaths related to ovarian cancer in 1998. It is the fifth leading cancer site following breast, lung, colorectum, and endometrium. It is also the fifth leading cause of cancer death following lung, breast, colorectal, and pancreatic carcinoma. Approximately 1 in 70 women will develop the disease, and 1 in 100 will die of disease. The median age of diagnosis is 63. The incidence of ovarian cancer is relatively high in North America and Northern Europe relative to Japan. In addition, whites have an increased risk relative to African Americans; however, this difference may be narrowing.

Epithelial ovarian tumors account for three fifths of all ovarian lesions including benign neoplasms. Malignant epithelial tumors (including borderline malignancies) account for 90% of all ovarian cancers. Two thirds of these are frankly malignant; one third are borderline.

## Risk Factors

Parity is an important risk factor for epithelial ovarian cancer. Women who have been pregnant have a 30 to 60% decreased risk relative to women who are nulliparous. Multiple pregnancies increase this protective effect. A history of breast-feeding has also been shown to decrease the risk, although the duration of lactation is not a factor (Table 46–1).

Several small case-cohort studies suggest that the use of the ovulation-inducing drug clomiphene citrate for a prolonged period of time (12 or more ovulatory cycles) may have a lifetime risk of 5 to 6%. The patients studied primarily developed borderline malignancies and the cohorts are small, thus making these results preliminary in nature. The use of oral contraceptives has repeatedly been shown to be protective, leading to a 30 to 60% decreased risk of developing ovarian cancer relative to women who have not used oral contraceptives. A study by the World Health Organization (WHO) compared 368

**Table 46–1** Risk Factors for Epithelial Ovarian Cancer

| Risk Factors | Protective Factors |
| --- | --- |
| Nulligravity | Pregnancy |
| Family history of ovarian cancer | Oral contraceptives |
| Personal history of breast cancer | Breast-feeding |
| BRCA1 mutation carrier | History of hysterectomy |
| History of infertility | |
| Ovulation induction drug (?) | |

women with ovarian cancer and 2397 matched controls. A decreased relative risk of 0.75 was noted in women who had ever used oral contraceptives. In addition, increasing duration of use provided a further decrease in risk.

Women with a prior history of breast cancer have a fourfold increased risk of ovarian cancer. In addition, women with a personal history of ovarian cancer have a twofold to fourfold increased risk of breast cancer. These findings further suggest an important role for altered hormonal balance in the etiology of ovarian carcinoma. However, exogenous hormone replacement therapy has not been associated with an increased risk of ovarian cancer.

## Genetic Factors

It is important to distinguish familial and hereditary ovarian cancer. In familial disease, a woman with a single family member with ovarian cancer has a lifetime risk of 4 to 5% relative to a lifetime risk of 1.6% for the general population. The risk increases to 7% if two relatives (not both first-degree) are affected. The average age of onset of this entity is similar to sporadic disease. Hereditary ovarian cancer syndromes, on the other hand, are defined as women with at least two first-degree relatives with ovarian cancer. These patients may have a lifetime probability of up to 50%, and the average age of diagnosis is 48. Approximately 1 to 5% of ovarian carcinomas can be attributed to hereditary disease. Three distinct genotypes of hereditary ovarian cancer have been identified:

1. Breast and ovarian cancer syndrome accounts for 65 to 75% of all hereditary ovarian cancer cases. The majority are linked to BRCA1 or BRCA2.
2. Hereditary ovarian cancer syndrome accounts for 10 to 15% of all hereditary cases. Most of these families are linked to BRCA1. The question has arisen whether these patients represent breast-ovarian cancer syndrome families where breast cancer has not yet appeared.
3. Lynch II syndrome with associated hereditary nonpolyposis colon cancer (autosomal dominant). These patients have three or more first-degree relatives with colon or endometrial cancer, at least two of whom are diagnosed with colon cancer at less than 50 years of age. These patients have a 3.5-fold increased risk of ovarian cancer and compose 10 to 15% of hereditary ovarian cancer cases.

## Pathology

Epithelial tumors arise from the ovarian serosa. The celomic cavity forms during embryonic life and is lined by mesothelium, which is of mesodermal origin. Portions of the mesothelium form the serosal epithelium, which covers the gonadal ridge. During ovarian development, the surface epithelium extends into the ovarian stroma and forms inclusion glands and cysts. When malignant transformation occurs, a variety of müllerian differentiations can be exhibited. These include serous, mucinous, endometrioid, clear cell, transitional cell, and mixed epithelial lesion. These cell types can lead to benign, borderline, and frankly malignant lesions. The incidence of each by cell type is listed in Table 46–2.

Benign epithelial tumors are most commonly serous or mucinous. They are often large, frequently between 15 and 30 cm in diameter. Benign serous tumors are more commonly bilateral. Borderline tumors or tumors of low malignant potential (LMP) contain some histologic features suggestive of cancer. This differentiation is frequently made on an architectural basis rather than on a cytologic evaluation alone. The tumors share an excellent prognosis even when they have spread. Even advanced stage disease has a 5-year survival or approximately 80%. However, these lesions are notorious for late recurrence with associated morbidity and mortality. Malignant ovarian tumors frequently present as complex solid and cystic masses with areas of necrosis and hemorrhage. Destructive growth helps distinguish these lesions from borderline tumors.

Almost half of all common epithelial tumors are serous neoplasms. Of these approximately half are benign, one sixth are borderline, and one third are malignant. Patients tend to present with benign and borderline lesions at a younger age; the mean ages of

**Table 46–2** Approximate Frequencies of Epithelial Tumors

| Histology | Benign (%) | Borderline (%) | Invasive (%) | Total (%) |
|---|---|---|---|---|
| Serous | 23 | 7 | 16 | 46 |
| Mucinous | 29.5 | 5 | 2 | 36.5 |
| Endometrioid | Rare | 1.5 | 6 | 7.5 |
| Mesenchymal and mixed | Rare | Rare | 0.7 | 0.7 |
| Clear cell | Rare | Rare | 3 | 3 |
| Transitional and Brenner | 2 | Rare | Rare | 2 |
| Squamous | Rare | Rare | Rare | Rare |
| Mixed epithelial | 1.5 | 0.5 | 0.5 | 2.5 |
| Undifferentiated | — | — | 1.5 | 1.5 |
| Unclassified | Rare | Rare | 0.3 | 0.3 |
| Total | 56 | 14 | 30 | 100 |

Adapted from Russel P: Surface epithelial-stromal tumors of the ovary. In Kurman RJ (ed): Blaustein's Pathology of the Female Genital Tract. New York, Springer Verlag, 1995, p 706.

diagnosis are 45 and 48, respectively. Microscopically, the characteristic epithelium of serous tumors resembles that of the fallopian tube.

Approximately one third (36%) of epithelial ovarian tumors are mucinous; 81% of these are benign and approximately one sixth are borderline. Only 5% of mucinous epithelial neoplasms are malignant. Pseudomyxoma peritonei is most often associated with borderline lesions. This phenomenon is characterized by copious mucin and clusters of well-differentiated mucinous cells throughout the peritoneal cavity. Current data suggest that this tumor may originate in the appendix with metastasis to the ovary, or there may be concomitant primary tumors, accounting for lesions in both organs. For these reasons, when mucinous histology is found in either a borderline or malignant ovarian tumor, an appendectomy should be performed as part of the original surgical procedure.

Microscopically, mucinous tumors are lined by cells that resemble either the mucinous cells of the endocervix or those forming the lining of the colon. Pseudomyxoma peritonei or ovarii is most often associated with the intestinal cell type.

Endometrioid tumors compose approximately 8% of all epithelial neoplasms. Benign endometrioid tumors are rare. The majority of these tumors are malignant, and one fifth are borderline. Histologically, these tumors resemble adenocarcinomas of the endometrium. Almost 25% of endometrioid ovarian tumors are associated with concomitant endometrial cancers. An additional 10% of cases are associated with endometriosis.

Clear cell tumors are uncommon and make up only 3% of epithelial tumors. They are almost all malignant, and approximately 50% of cases are associated with endometriosis. Histologically, the tumor is characterized by "hobnail cells" and clear cells. It has been suggested that these tumors are more aggressive than the other histologic subtypes; however, this remains controversial.

Transitional-cell tumors are the least common of the epithelial neoplasms (2%). They are of urothelial differentiation and thought to arise from transitional cell metaplasia. Brenner tumors are primarily benign, although rarely they can present with borderline or frankly malignant features. The transitional-cell carcinoma is considered a separate entity that lacks any demonstrable antecedent. This is different from a malignant Brenner tumor, which arises from demonstrable preexisting benign or proliferative Brenner tumor. Transitional cell carcinomas tend to be more aggressive than malignant Brenner tumors and more frequently present with advanced stage disease. Relative to other epithelial variants, however, these tumors tend to have a better response to chemotherapy.

## Patterns of Spread

There are two primary modes of spread of epithelial ovarian cancers. One involves exfoliation and implantation. Once the tumor penetrates through the ovarian capsule the malignant cells exfoliate into the peritoneal cavity. Frequently they follow the normal circulation of the peritoneal cavity in clockwise fashion and implant themselves in the right paracolic gutter and the right hemidiaphragm; however, all intra-abdominal peritoneal surfaces are at risk.

The second mode of metastasis is via the retroperitoneal lymphatics that drain the ovary. These follow the ovarian blood supply in the infundibulopelvic ligament to the nodes that lie in the para-aortic chain up to the level of the vena cava. In addition, some lymphatics pass through the broad ligament and the parametria, which terminate in the pelvic nodes. Included in this mode are the external iliac, hypogastric, and obturator lymph node chains. Spread to the inguinal lymphatics can occur through the course of the round ligament, although this is less common.

## History and Physical Examination

The majority (75 to 85%) of patients with ovarian cancer present with nonspecific symptoms attributable to advanced disease. These include diffuse abdominal pain and abdominal distention or a bloating sensation. Other symptoms include back pain, alterations in bowel or bladder habits, gastroesophageal reflux, and dyspareunia. Unfortunately, these nonspecific complaints are often attributed to other disease processes such as gastritis, irritable bowel syndrome, colitis, or endometriosis. They are often caused by malignant ascites and/or a large intra-abdominal mass.

Early stage disease, however, is often asymptomatic and is frequently diagnosed as an incidental finding on routine pelvic examination. The majority of palpable adnexal masses are benign, and in premenopausal women, ovarian cancer represents less than 5% of ovarian neoplasms. The majority of these lesions are physiologic and regress in one to three menstrual cycles.

A complete physical examination can reveal findings indicative of the degree of disease. Because of the incidence of pleural effusion, ascites, and a large abdominal mass in advanced disease, it is imperative to include a detailed examination. A careful lymph node survey is also important, especially in advanced stage disease where supraclavicular, inguinal, and periumbilical (Sister Mary Joseph's) nodes can be involved. In addition, breast and colon cancer are more common than primary ovarian tumors and should be adequately evaluated as part of the examination.

The pelvic examination can often be quite revealing, especially the rectovaginal examination. Here, it is possible to assess the posterior uterine surface, the uterosacral ligaments, the pouch of Douglas, and the parametria. The majority of ovarian tumors lie posterior to the uterus or, owing to their size, may ascend to the upper abdomen. The rectovaginal examination allows detection of cul-de-sac nodularity, neoplastic disease involving the rectovaginal septum, and posterior tumors that would not be appreciated otherwise.

## Diagnostic Testing

The standard workup for the patient with an uncharacterized pelvic mass should include ultrasonography or an abdominopelvic computed tomography (CT) scan (if clinically indicated) after a thorough physical examination. Ultrasonographic findings more frequently associated with malignancy include irregular borders of the ovarian mass, multiple dense septations, papillary projections, the presence of solid elements, bilateral lesions, and ascites. Color flow Doppler allows potential differentiation of benign from malignant lesions. Malignant tumors often have neovascularity with vessel walls that have little smooth muscle support. These vessels have a characteristic wave form with a low resistivity index (RI = peak systolic–end diastolic Doppler shift/peak systolic Doppler shift). There is controversy over which RI value to use as a cutoff point between malignant and benign. However, most experts agree that it should lie between 0.4 and 0.5. The CT scan is helpful in defining liver and spleen metastases, pleural nodules, and omental disease in patients who are strongly suspected of having advanced disease. A chest x-ray film should be obtained preoperatively to rule out a pleural effusion. Colonoscopy or a barium enema is not routinely recommended, although in specific clinical settings they may be of value.

In addition, appropriate laboratory studies including an assessment of renal and liver status, as well as cancer antigen 125 (CA 125) level, should be obtained. CA 125 is a glycoprotein that is detectable by immunoradiometric assay. Elevated serum levels are detected in 80 to 85% of patients with epithelial ovarian cancer. Serous histology is most closely associated with an elevated level, whereas mucinous lesions have a low incidence of abnormal serum levels. Elevations of the CA 125 are nonspecific and can indicate many other conditions, especially in premenopausal patients. These include endometriosis, fibroids, conditions leading to peritonitis (e.g., pelvic inflammatory disease, diverticulitis, pancreatitis), or pregnancy. In addition, CA 125 levels can be elevated in other malignancies including gastrointestinal primary tumors and breast cancer with metastases to the peritoneal cavity. In postmenopausal women with an asymptomatic pelvic mass, however, an elevated serum CA 125 (>65 U/ml) had a sensitivity of 97% and a specificity of 76% for ovarian cancer. Thus, in postmenopausal patients, an elevated CA 125 and a complex pelvic mass indicate the need for prompt surgical exploration.

## Screening

Currently there are no good screening tests for epithelial ovarian carcinoma recommended for the general population. Multiple international studies have been conducted but have not found adequate sensitivity, specificity, or positive predictive value of generalized testing for ovarian cancer. Screening with regular physical examinations, CA 125 testing, and pelvic ultrasonography is recommended, however, for the segment of the population with a family history consistent with hereditary ovarian cancer.

## Differential Diagnosis

Ovarian cancer is frequently asymptomatic in its early stages. On the other hand, patients with advanced stage disease commonly present with ascites and an abdominal/pelvic mass. Advanced colon cancer, primary peritoneal cancer, and metastatic lesions to the ovary from either the gastrointestinal tract or the breast should all be considered in the patient's evaluation. In patients who present with adnexal masses and no other evident pathology on either physical examination or radiologic studies, the differential diagnosis mainly includes benign ovarian lesions (especially endometriosis in the younger population), germ cell tumors of the ovary, and sex cord–stromal ovarian lesions. Factors such as the patient's age, physical examination, CA 125 results, and ultrasonographic findings clearly alter the differential diagnosis.

## Surgical Staging

Primary therapy for ovarian cancer involves a combined modality approach. An initial staging laparotomy followed by systemic chemotherapy is indicated in most cases. The natural history and early patterns of spread form the basis of the current surgical stag-

#### Table 46–3  Staging System for Ovarian Cancer—FIGO (1986)

Stage I: Growth limited to the ovaries
IA  Growth limited to one ovary; no ascites; no tumor on the external surfaces, capsule intact.
IB  Growth limited to both ovaries; no ascites; no tumor on the external surfaces, capsule intact.
IC  Tumor limited to one or both ovaries with any of the following: capsule ruptured, tumor on ovarian surface, malignant cells in ascites, or peritoneal washings.

Stage II: Tumor involves one or both ovaries with pelvic extension
IIA  Extension and/or implants on uterus and/or tube(s). No malignant cells in ascites or peritoneal washings.
IIB  Extension to other pelvic tissues. No malignant cells in ascites or peritoneal washings.
IIC  Pelvic extension (IIA or IIB) with malignant cells in ascites or peritoneal washings.

Stage III: Tumor involves one or both ovaries with microscopically confirmed peritoneal metastasis outside the pelvis and/or regional lymph node metastasis
IIIA  Microscopic peritoneal metastasis beyond the pelvis
IIIB  Macroscopic peritoneal metastasis beyond the pelvis 2 cm or less in greatest dimension
IIIC  Peritoneal metastasis beyond the pelvis more than 2 cm in greatest dimension and/or regional lymph node metastasis.

Stage IV: Distant metastasis (excludes peritoneal metastasis, for example, liver parenchyma, pleural space)

---

ing system. The International Federation of Gynecology and Obstetrics (FIGO) staging system (Table 46–3), most recently revised in 1986, reflects our current understanding of the disease. Unfortunately, more than 60% of women with epithelial ovarian cancer have advanced stage disease at the time of diagnosis.

The staging procedure entails an exploratory laparotomy, total abdominal hysterectomy, bilateral salpingo-oophorectomy (TAH-BSO), bilateral pelvic and para-aortic lymph node sampling, an omentectomy, and biopsy or removal of any suspicious lesions, as well as random peritoneal biopsies including the pelvic side walls, cul-de-sac, paracolic gutters, and the hemidiaphragms (Table 46–4). Upon entering the peritoneal cavity, ascites should be aspirated or a peritoneal lavage performed for evaluation by cytopathology. If the tumor is encapsulated, it should be removed intact if possible because the spillage of malignant cells increases the patient's stage and may adversely affect her prognosis.

#### Table 46–4  Surgical Staging Laparotomy

Peritoneal washings
Salpingo-oophorectomy ± hysterectomy
Omentectomy
Multiple peritoneal biopsies
Diaphragmatic sampling (cytologic smears or biopsies)
Retroperitoneal lymph node sampling

---

Conservative surgery with preservation of the uterus and possibly one ovary should be considered in selected cases. These include young women who desire future fertility and whose tumor appears confined to either one or both ovaries and exhibits a low grade histology. In the case of unilateral disease, the patient can have a unilateral salpingo-oophorectomy with the previously mentioned staging biopsies and be advised to undergo hysterectomy and removal of the remaining ovary after she has completed childbearing. In the case of bilateral disease, the patient has the option of bilateral salpingo-oophorectomy with full staging biopsies and preservation of the uterus. This would allow her to pursue pregnancy with donor egg–assisted reproductive technology in the future.

However, if the disease is advanced at the time of diagnosis, the procedure of choice is a TAH-BSO accompanied by a maximal cytoreductive effort, regardless of the patient's age. Lymph node dissection is usually performed in this setting if it would alter the patient's stage, or if their removal would affect the cytoreductive effort. With advanced stage or bulky disease, an attempt should be made to remove as much tumor as possible.

Controversy exists with regard to management of patients with incompletely staged apparent stage IA or IB grade 1 tumors. Four treatment options have been considered: relaparotomy (or laparoscopy), chemotherapy followed by relaparotomy, chemotherapy alone assuming the patient has higher-stage or grade of tumor, or observation alone and treating only at the time of recurrence. Patients with suspected stage IA or IB grade 2 or 3 tumors or suspected IC, II, III, or IV disease who have been incompletely staged pose less controversy regarding management. In patients with suspected residual disease, relaparotomy or laparoscopy is recommended. In those with no suspected residual disease, chemotherapy with subsequent relaparotomy or laparoscopy is generally accepted. In patients with bulky stage II and IV disease who are not surgical candidates, neoadjuvant chemotherapy should also be considered. However, pathologic diagnosis should be confirmed by fine-needle aspiration or paracentesis in this cohort. If a significant response to chemotherapy is noted and the patient's overall condition has improved, an interval cytoreductive effort may be indicated.

## Prognostic Factors

Multiple clinicopathologic variables are significant prognostically (Table 46–5). The most important is tumor stage. In patients with stage I disease who have undergone a comprehensive staging laparotomy, the

**Table 46–5** Prognostic Factors

| | |
|---|---|
| Stage | Tumor grade |
| Preoperative disease volume | Histologic subtype |
| Residual disease volume | Patient performance status |

5-year survival is 90%. Similarly, patients with stage II disease (only 10 to 15% of ovarian cancer patients) have a 5-year survival of 80%. The 5-year survival of those with stages III and IV disease drops dramatically to 15% and 5%, respectively. Residual disease volume has been directly correlated with survival in patients with advanced disease. Multiple studies have been performed with variable definitions of optimal cytoreduction, ranging from <1 to <3 cm of residual disease. Hoskins and colleagues summarized this information, and noted a median survival of 36.7 months in 388 patients who were optimally cytoreduced vs. 16.6 months in 537 patients with suboptimal residual disease. A Gynecologic Oncology Group (GOG) study revealed that survival for patients with advanced ovarian cancer progressively decreases as the maximal residual increases. There was no survival benefit after the residual tumor volume exceeded 2 cm. The currently accepted standard within the GOG is ≤1 cm residual disease. Within this optimal group of patients, there is a survival difference between patients with microscopic residual and those with any macroscopic disease <1 cm. Thus, the best survival is seen in those patients with no gross evidence of disease after debulking. However, tumor biology must be considered as well. Given an equal size of residual disease, patients with larger-volume initial metastatic disease have shorter long-term survival.

Histologic subtype has less prognostic significance than do other factors such as stage, volume of disease, and grade. Although it has been suggested that mucinous ovarian adenocarcinomas may have a better overall survival, this is thought to reflect the fact that the majority of mucinous lesions are grade 1 or 2. Transitional cell carcinomas are also thought to have a better overall prognosis. On the other hand, it has been suggested that clear cell carcinoma of the ovary is more aggressive than other epithelial ovarian malignancies. This possibility remains controversial; studies for the other common epithelial histologies reveal similar survival rates once they are stratified for stage and cell type.

The preoperative CA 125 level has been shown, on univariate analysis, to have prognostic significance. On multivariate analysis, however, it is not an independent prognostic factor, probably because of the association of the CA 125 level with disease volume. However, postoperative CA 125 levels were of prognostic significance.

Many molecular factors are currently under investigation as possible prognostic factors, including cytologic factors such as ploidy as well as genetic factors. Some of the genes currently being evaluated include *p53* (a tumor suppressor gene), *ERB-B2* (codes for a protein that is similar in structure to EGFR, the epidermal growth factor receptor), *mdr* (the multidrug resistance gene), and possibly *ERCC1* (a DNA repair gene).

## Chemotherapy

Chemotherapy after surgical debulking plays an essential role in the treatment of advanced stage disease (Fig. 46–1). This is well established in both retrospective and prospective randomized trials. During the last 25 years, there has been significant improvement in both the response rates and median survival rates of ovarian cancer patients treated with surgery and chemotherapy; however, the overall 5-year survival has not changed significantly.

Early studies in the 1970s with the use of a single-agent alkylating drugs showed a response rate in the 20% range. The concept of combination therapy was next introduced with the addition of doxorubicin, which led to response rates of approximately 35%. In the early 1980s, cisplatinum was found to have significant activity in epithelial ovarian carcinoma. With the advent of cisplatinum and the use of combination chemotherapy, further improvement in survival was noted. Combination chemotherapy with

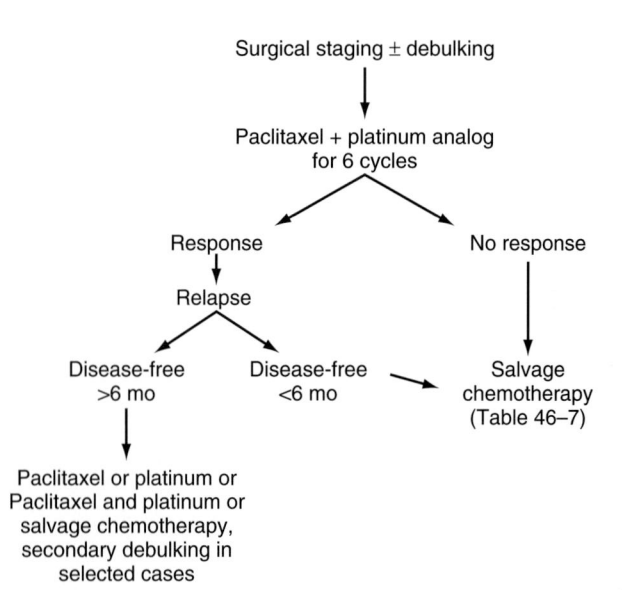

**Figure 46–1** Advanced stages of disease (stages III & IV). (Adapted from Sharpless NE, Seiden MV: Advanced ovarian cancer: Recent progress and current challenges. Contemp Ob Gyn 43:123, 1998.)

**Table 46–6** Definitions of Disease Response

Clinical Complete Response: Resolution of all disease by physical examination radiographs and CA 125
Partial Clinical Response: >50% reduction in the sum of the products of the bidirectional measurements of tumor masses lasting at least 4 weeks
Progressive Disease: Development of pathologically documented new lesions and/or >25% increase in the sum of the products of the bidirectional measurements of tumor masses
Pathologic Complete Responses: No evidence of tumor at second-look surgical evaluation

platinum and an alkylating agent as first-line treatment led to complete and overall response rates of 30 to 40% and 60 to 70%, respectively (Table 46–6). By using these combinations, the median progression-free survival durations were 13 to 15 months, with the median survival of 17 to 25 months. Until 1996, a regimen of cyclophosphamide and cisplatinum was considered the treatment of choice for epithelial ovarian cancer. Two randomized trials reported in 1992 found that carboplatin in combination with cyclophosphamide was equally effective and less toxic than cisplatinum and cyclophosphamide. Carboplatin is a platinum analog that is less neurotoxic and nephrotoxic but more myelosuppressive than cisplatinum.

Paclitaxel was introduced in phase I and II trials in the late 1980s and early 1990s. It is derived from the Pacific yew tree (*Taxus brevifolia*) and has novel mechanisms of action that are synergistic with platinum agents. Paclitaxel was initially found to have significant activity in ovarian cancer when it was tested in patients with disease refractory to platinum-based therapy.

Thus, paclitaxel was a novel agent with significant activity in epithelial ovarian cancer without cross-resistance with platinum compounds. The GOG conducted a randomized phase III trial comparing cyclophosphamide and cisplatinum with paclitaxel and cisplatinum in women with stage III and IV ovarian cancer. The combination of paclitaxel and cisplatinum yielded a higher complete (51% vs. 31%) and overall tumor response (73% vs. 60%) compared with cyclophosphamide and cisplatinum ($P = .01$). The progression-free (18 vs. 13 months) and median survival (38 vs. 24 months) were significantly longer ($P < .001$) in the paclitaxel combination group. These results are especially impressive given that the patients with stage III disease were all suboptimally debulked (>1 cm residual disease), and the remainder of the patients had stage IV disease. The paclitaxel combination had managable associated toxicity, more patients were able to complete six cycles of this regimen than the cisplatinum/cyclophosphamide combination. Thus, paclitaxel in combination with a platinum is currently considered standard initial treatment after cytoreductive surgery for patients with advanced disease.

Because carboplatin has shown similar efficacy in advanced epithelial ovarian cancer with a decreased incidence of nonhematologic toxicity, studies were undertaken to evaluate the combination of paclitaxel infused over 3 hours with carboplatin. This combination allowed for improved patient tolerance and complete outpatient administration. Currently three large randomized trials are comparing paclitaxel and carboplatin with paclitaxel and cisplatinum in patients with previously untreated advanced epithelial ovarian cancer.

## Early Stage Disease

In well-staged ovarian cancer, if early stage disease is discovered, treatment with chemotherapy depends on the exact stage and grade of the tumor (Fig. 46–2). The basic recommendations made by both the National Comprehensive Cancer Network (NCCN) and the National Institutes of Health (NIH) consensus conference on ovarian cancer are similar. Patients with stage IA grade 1 and stage IB grade 1 tumors do not require adjuvant therapy. All patients with grade 3 tumors require adjuvant therapy, as do all patients with clear cell histology. Patients with Stage IC grade 1, 2, or 3 require postoperative chemotherapy with the exception of some grade 1 tumors, in which observation may be indicated. All stage II patients, regardless of grade, should receive chemotherapy. Currently recommended regimens in this setting are paclitaxel and either cisplatin or carboplatin for a total of three to six cycles. The GOG is exploring the combination of paclitaxel and carboplatin in the treatment of patients with early stage disease who have poor prognostic factors. The most effective ad-

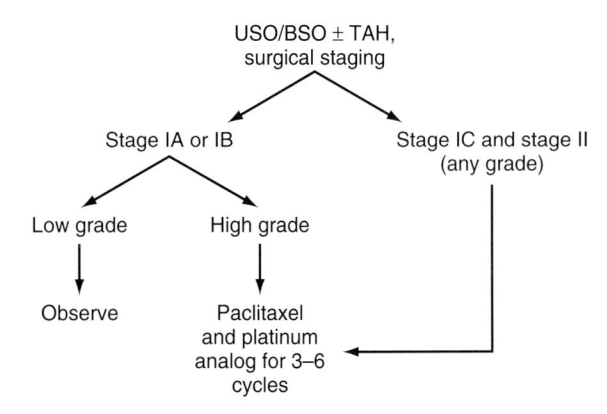

**Figure 46–2** Early stages of disease. BSO = bilateral salpingo-oophorectomy; TAH = total abdominal hysterectomy; USO = unilateral salpingo-oophorectomy.

juvant therapy in early stage disease has not been established. Thus, patients with high-risk stage I cancers should ideally be enrolled in clinical trials to identify optimal adjuvant therapy to improve survival.

## Management of Low Malignant Potential Disease

The main treatment for tumors of LMP is surgical. The surgical approach for these patients is the same as that for patients with invasive epithelial ovarian cancer (see previous discussion). In patients with early stage disease, there is no role for adjuvant chemotherapy. Five-year survival rates have ranged from 90 to 100%.

In contrast to invasive epithelial ovarian cancer, only 20% of patients with LMP disease tumors present with advanced stage disease. The postoperative management of women with stage III and IV LMP tumors is not well established. Gershenson and Silva surgically determined the response to chemotherapy in 20 patients with metastatic serous ovarian tumors of low malignant potential who had macroscopic residual disease after initial surgery. The overall response rate was 80% (40% complete response [CR] and 40% partial response [PR]).

The 5-year survival rates for patients with advanced-stage LMP ovarian tumors have ranged from 64 to 96%. There is a steady decline in survival after 5 years, suggesting the indolent clinical course of this disease. This is likely due to a low growth fraction, which may also explain their refractoriness to chemotherapy. There appears to be a subset of lesions that behave aggressively with rapid disease recurrence after surgery. Kaern and colleagues used cellular DNA content to identify patients with an unfavorable prognosis who may benefit from chemotherapy. Aneuploid lesions appear to have a significantly worse 15-year survival (20%) relative to diploid lesions (75%). A prospective study evaluating the benefit of chemotherapy for these tumors has not been reported.

## Management After Initial Therapy

In advanced ovarian cancer, the optimal management following induction chemotherapy is being investigated. Overall, approximately 50% of patients obtain a clinical complete response (no evidence of disease on radiographic studies or physical examination after initial therapy). However, only 30% of all patients with ovarian cancer have a complete pathologic response at second-look surgery after platinum-based therapy. The most important prognostic factor for complete pathologic response is tumor volume at the completion of initial cytoreduction before the initiation of chemotherapy. Of those patients who do achieve a surgical complete response, up to 50% subsequently develop a recurrence.

The use of second-look surgery to assess disease response to chemotherapy is currently a matter of debate. The term *second-look laparotomy* specifically refers to a systematic surgical re-exploration with multiple biopsies in patients without any clinical evidence of disease. Retrospective studies compare the survival of patients who have undergone a second-look laparotomy vs. those who have shown no difference in survival. Because of these findings and the inherent morbidity of a second laparotomy, the use of this procedure is accepted only in patients who are on a specific protocol that incorporates it. Laparoscopy has also been used in this setting. However, in the face of a negative laparoscopy, residual disease has been documented in 55% of patients at laparotomy. Because of this high false-negative rate, a laparotomy should be performed on those patients with a negative laparoscopy to confirm pathologic complete response in protocol patients.

The benefit of secondary cytoreductive operations in ovarian cancer, either at the time of second-look operation or otherwise, has not been clearly demonstrated. The use of secondary cytoreduction at the time of recurrence after initial platinum-based chemotherapy has also been evaluated. In patients whose tumors remain sensitive to chemotherapy, cytoreduction to an optimal residual tumor appears to be of benefit. The current NCCN guidelines recommend that patients with a low-grade or focal recurrence after a long disease-free interval be considered for secondary cytoreductive surgery followed by chemotherapy. Occasionally, when the disease is focal in this setting, radiation therapy has also been used.

In patients who achieve a surgically confirmed complete response, there is presently no evidence that further therapy will decrease the relapse rate. However, several ongoing prospective trials are evaluating the role of consolidation therapy. Different treatment options include intraperitoneal (IP) chemotherapy, IP radioisotopes, high-dose chemotherapy, and systemic chemotherapy with non–cross-resistant agents.

Currently, most patients with a clinical and/or pathologic complete response of disease are followed closely with interval CA 125 levels, physical examinations, and abdominal CT and chest x-ray studies. Elevations of the CA 125 level can indicate tumor progression many months before any clinical evidence of disease. At this point, there is no evidence that initiating chemotherapy for a rising CA 125 level improves survival.

## Recurrent Disease

Long-term survival in epithelial ovarian cancer patients is primarily affected by the initial chemotherapy regimen. In patients who experience relapse after first-line platinum-based chemotherapy, the response to salvage treatment depends mainly on the disease-free interval after their initial treatment. Patients who develop recurrence within 6 months of completion of initial platinum-based chemotherapy are considered to have platinum-resistant disease. Their response to retreatment with platinum-based therapy is less than 10%. Patients who respond to their initial platinum-based regimen with a greater than 6-month disease-free interval are considered to have platinum-sensitive disease. It has been suggested that longer intervals without treatment may allow either for the regrowth of platinum sensitive cells or for platinum-resistant cells to lose their drug resistance.

In patients with platinum-sensitive disease who develop recurrence of disease, current recommendations for therapy include retreatment with platinum-based combination therapy, single-agent platinum, or single-agent paclitaxel. Retreatment of these patients with a second platinum-based regimen results in overall response rates of 26 to 77% depending on the treatment-free interval. Patients with an interval >24 months achieved a significantly greater overall response rate than those with an interval <24 months.

## Second-Line Chemotherapy Options

Patients with platinum-resistant disease have a poor response (<10%) to retreatment with platinum-based therapy. There are numerous alternatives for salvage therapy (Table 46–7); however, response rates to these agents are predominantly <25%. Because of this overall response rate, the choice of therapy should be based on multiple factors. These should include quality of life, toxicity profile, nature of prior drug toxicity, patient preference, and ease of administration.

## Future Directions

Based on the data from the GOG trial using paclitaxel and cisplatinum as up-front therapy it is not yet possi-

**Table 46–7** Chemotherapy for Recurrent Disease

| Drug | Response Rate (%) | Main Toxicities |
|---|---|---|
| Oral etoposide | 27–34 | Hematologic |
| Topotecan | 13–23 | Hematologic |
| Weekly Taxol | 29–31 | Hematologic |
| Doxil | 20–31 | Stomatis and hand/foot syndrome |
| Gemcitabine | 29 | Nausea and vomiting |
| Altretamine | 18–39 | Nausea and vomiting |
| Ifosfamide | 14 | Hematologic, nephrotoxic, neurologic |
| Vinorelbine | 15 | Neutropenia, anemia, worsening neuropathy |
| Tamoxifen | 13 | |

Response rate includes clinical complete response and clinical partial response.

ble to answer questions regarding long-term survival. However, after 3 years of follow-up, disease recurrence or progression has been seen in 70% of patients. Thus, it is unlikely that this treatment will have a significant impact on the cure rate of this disease. Several efforts regarding chemotherapy dosing schedules, new agents, and new approaches are under investigation to improve the actual cure rate of this disease.

IP chemotherapy has been under investigation in different clinical settings for many years. A recent study by Alberts and colleagues demonstrated decreased toxicity and increased efficacy of IP vs. intravenous cisplatinum in optimally debulked stage III ovarian cancer patients. However, patients in the control arm of this study did not receive the current standard of care. Thus, it is unclear whether the benefit of IP cisplatinum as part of a paclitaxel-containing regimen would merit the inconvenience and expense.

Issues related to the dose, schedule, and duration of infusion of paclitaxel are all being investigated. In addition, it is possible that higher doses of paclitaxel with growth factor support would be more effective.

The concept of dose intensity has been taken one step further with the treatment of poor-prognosis patients with very high dose chemotherapy and subsequent autologous peripheral blood stem cell transplant (PBSCT). This technique has been studied in women with recurring ovarian cancer. A review of 100 patients with recurrent tumor that could be debulked with surgery or salvage chemotherapy to a minimal residual state was recently reported. These patients subsequently received high-dose chemotherapy with PBSCT rescue, and a median survival of 30 months was demonstrated. A subset of patients may experience prolonged palliation with this approach. Clinical trials have recently begun with high-dose chemotherapy with PBSCT in selected patients with untreated ovarian cancer or as a consolidation treatment after induction therapy with standard doses of drugs. This therapy should be used only in an investigational setting.

Other novel approaches such as phototherapy, gene therapy, hyperthermia, and immunotherapy are under investigation. Current ongoing phase I genetic trials include use of a Her2/neu peptide based vaccine, p53 vaccine in conjunction with chemotherapeutic agents, as well as trials incorporating EGFR modulators. Additional studies with selective antibodies, as well as hyperthmic peritoneal perfusion with carboplatin, are ongoing. Antiangiogenic agents such as CAI are also under investigation, either alone or in combination with chemotherapeutic agents (paclitaxel).

## Summary

Epithelial ovarian carcinoma is a lethal malignancy. Adequate surgical staging and cytoreduction should be performed in all patients who are surgical candidates. The current recommended primary chemotherapy includes intravenous paclitaxel and a platinum analog. Promising new agents and new regimens, including dose intensification with or without stem cell support, are under investigation. Although progress has been made in extending disease-free survival, most women with epithelial ovarian cancer will die of their disease. New approaches to this disease are needed both to aid in the diagnosis of early stage disease (given that 75% of cases are stage III/IV at diagnosis) and to augment or replace current treatment to improve the cure rate of epithelial ovarian cancer.

### REFERENCES

Abu-Rustum NR, Aghajanian C, Barakat RR, et al: Salvage weekly paclitaxel (Taxol) for recurrent ovarian cancer. Semin Oncol 24:515–567, 1997.

Abu-Rustum NR, Barakat RR, Siegel PL, et al: Second-look operation for epithelial ovarian cancer: laparoscopy or laparotomy? Obstet Gynecol 88:549–553, 1996.

Alberts DS, Green S, Hannigan EV, et al: Improved therapeutic index of carboplatin plus cyclophosphamide versus cisplatin plus cyclophosphamide: Final report by the Southwest Oncology Group of a phase III randomized trial in stages III and IV ovarian cancer. J Clin Oncol 10:706–717, 1992.

Alberts DS, Liu PY, Hannigan EV, et al: Intraperitoneal cisplatin plus intravenous cyclophosphamide versus intravenous cisplatin plus intravenous cyclophosphamide for stage III ovarian cancer. N Engl J Med 335:1950–1955, 1996.

Boyd J, Rubin SC: Hereditary ovarian cancer: Molecular genetics and clinical implications. Gynecol Oncol 64:196–206, 1997.

Burke W, Daly M, Garber J: Recommendations for follow-up care of individuals with an inherited predisposition to cancer. II. JAMA 277:997–1003, 1997.

Carlson JF, Skates SJ, Singer DE: Screening for ovarian cancer. Ann Intern Med 121:124–132, 1994.

Chambers JT: Borderline ovarian tumors: A review of treatment. Yale J Biol Med 62:351–365, 1989.

Claus EB Schildkraut JM, Thompson WD, et al: The genetic attributable risk of breast and ovarian cancer. Cancer 77:2318–2324, 1996.

Connelly E, Markman M, Kennedy A, et al: Paclitaxel delivered as 3 hr infusion with cisplatin in patients with gynecologic cancers: Unexpected incidence of neurotoxicity. Gynecol Oncol 62:166–168, 1996.

du Bois A, Nitz U, Schroder W, et al: Cisplatin/paclitaxel versus carboplatin/paclitaxel as first-line chemotherapy in ovarian cancer: interim analysis of an AGO Study Group trial (Abstract 1272). Proc Am Soc Clin Oncol 16:357, 1997.

Easton DF, Ford D, Bishop DT: Breast and ovarian cancer incidence in BRCA1-mutation carriers. Breast Cancer Linkage Consortium. Am J Hum Genet 56:265–271, 1995.

Einhorn N, Sjovall K, Knapp RC, et al: Prospective evaluation of serum CA 125 levels for early detection of ovarian cancer. Obstet Gynecol 80:17–18, 1992.

Gershenson DM, Silva EG: Serous ovarian tumors of low malignant potential with peritoneal implants. Cancer 65:578, 1990.

Gordon A, Bookman M, Malmstrom H, et al: Efficacy of topotecan in advanced epithelial ovarian cancer after failure of platinum and paclitaxel: International Topotecan Study Group trial (Abstract 763). Proc Am Soc Clin Oncol 15:282, 1996.

Gruppo Interregionale Cooperativo Oncologico Ginecologia: Long-term results of a randomized trial comparing cisplatin with cisplatin and cyclophosphmide with cisplatin, cyclophosphamide, and adriamycin in advanced ovarian cancer. Gynecol Oncol 45:115–117, 1992.

Ho AF, Beller U, Speyer JL, et al: A reassessment of the role of second-look laparotomy in advanced ovarian cancer. J Clin Oncol 5:1316–1321, 1987.

Hoskins WJ, Bundy BN, Thigpen JT, et al: The influence of cytoreductive surgery on recurrence-free interval and survival in small volume stage III epithelial ovarian cancer: a Gynecologic Oncology Group study. Gynecol Oncol 47:159–166, 1992.

Hoskins WJ, McGuire WP, Brady MF, et al: The effect of diameter of largest residual disease on survival after primary cytoreductive surgery in patients with suboptimal residual epithelial ovarian cancer. Am J Obstet Gynecol 170:974–980, 1994.

Jenison EL, Montag AG, Griffiths CT, et al: Clear cell adenocarcinoma of the ovary: A clinical analysis and comparison with serous carcinoma. Gynecol Oncol 32:65–71, 1989.

Kaern J, Trope C, Kjorstad KE, et al: Cellular DNA content as a new prognostic tool in patients with borderline tumors of the ovary. Gynecol Oncol 38:452–457, 1990.

Kaufman DW, Kelly JP, Welch WR, et al: Noncontraceptive estrogen use and epithelial ovarian cancer. Am J Epidemiol 130:1142–1151, 1989.

Kaufmann M, Bauknecht T, Jonat W, et al: Gemcitiabine (GEM) in cisplatin-resistant ovarian cancer. (Abstract 758). Proc Am Soc Clin Oncol 14:272, 1995.

Kavanagh K, Tresukosol D, Edwards C, et al: Carboplatin reinduction after taxane in patients with platinum-refractory epithelial ovarian cancer. J Clin Oncol 13:1584–1588, 1995.

Kennedy AW, Biscotti CV, Hart WR, et al: Histologic correlates of progression-free interval and survival in ovarian clear cell adenocarcinoma. Gynecol Oncol 50:334–338, 1993.

Klaasen U, Wilke H, Strumberg D, et al: Phase I study with a weekly 1 h infusion of paclitaxel in heavily pretreated patients with metastatic breast and ovarian cancer. Eur J Cancer 32A:547–549, 1996.

Kohn EC, Sarosy GA, Davis P, et al: A phase I/II trial of dose intense paclitaxel with cisplatin and cyclophosphamide as initial therapy of poor-prognosis advanced stage epithelial ovarian cancer. Gynecol Oncol 62:181–191, 1996.

Kurjak A, Predanic M: New scoring system for prediction of ovarian malignancy based on trasvaginal color Doppler sonography. J Ultrasound Med 11:631–638, 1992.

Landis SH, Murray T, Bolden S, et al: Cancer Statistics, 1998. CA Cancer J Clin 48:6–29, 1998.

Makar A, Kristensen GB, Kaern J, et al: Prognostic value of pre- and postoperative serum CA 125 levels in ovarian cancer: New aspects and multivariate analysis. Obstet Gynecol 79:1002–1010, 1992.

Malkasian GD Jr, Knapp RC, Lavin DJ, et al: Preoperative evaluation of serum CA-125 levels in premenopausal and postmenopausal patients with pelvic masses: discrimination of benign form malignant disease. Am J Obstet Gynecol 159:341–346, 1988.

Markman M, Rothman R, Hakes T, et al: Second-line platinum therapy in patients with ovarian cancer previously treated with cisplatin. J Clin Oncol 9:389–393, 1991.

McGuire WP, Hoskins WJ, Brady MF, et al: Cyclophosphamide and cisplatin compared with paclitaxel and cisplatin in patients with stage III and stage IV ovarian cancer. N Engl J Med 334:1–6, 1996.

Michael H, Roth LM, Koxylo PK: Recent developments in the pathology of ovarian epithelial tumors of low malignant potential and related neoplasms. Pathol Annu 28:1–22, 1993.

National Institutes of Health Consensus Conference: Ovarian cancer: screening, treatment, and follow-up. JAMA 273:491–497, 1995.

National Institutes of Health Consensus Development Conference Statement: Ovarian cancer: Screening, treatment, and follow-up. April 5–7. Gynecol Oncol 55:S4–S14, 1994.

Neijt JP, Hansen M, Hansen SW, et al: Randomized phase III study in previously untreated epithelial ovarian cancer FIGO stage IIB, IIC, III, IV, comparing paclitaxel-cisplatin and paclitaxel-carboplatin (Abstract 1259). Proc Am Soc Clin Oncol 352a, 1997.

Omura G, Bundy B, Berek J, et al: Randomized trial of cyclophosphamide plus cisplatin with or without doxorubicin in ovarian carcinoma: a Gynecologic Oncology Group study. J Clin Oncol 7:457–465, 1989.

Ozols RF: Gynecologic Oncology Group trials in ovarian carcinoma. Semin Oncol 24(suppl2):S2-10–S2-12, 1997.

Ozols RF: Update of the NCCN Ovarian Cancer practice guidelines. Oncology 11:95–105, 1997.

Ozols RF: Treatment of recurrent ovarian cancer: Increasing options "recurrent" results (Editorial). J Clin Oncol 15:2177–2180, 1997.

Ozols RF, Vermorken JB: Chemotherapy of advanced ovarian cancer: Current status and future directions. Semin Oncol 24(suppl2):S2-1–S2-9, 1997.

Reed E: The chemotherapy of ovarian cancer. Principles and Practice of Oncology Updates 10:1–12, 1996.

Robboy SJ, Bentlew RC, Krigman H, et al: Synoptic reports in gynecologic pathology. Int J Gynecol Pathol 13:161–174, 1994.

Rose PG, Blessing JA, Mayer AR, et al: Prolonged oral etoposide as second line therapy for platinum resistant (PLATR) and platinum sensitive (PLATS) ovarian carcinoma: A Gynecologic Oncology Group study (Abstract 762). Proc Am Soc Clin Oncol 15:282, 1996.

Rossing MA, Daling JR, Weiss NS, et al: Ovarian tumors in a cohort of infertile women. N Engl J Med 331:771–776, 1994.

Rowinsky EK, Donehower RC: Paclitaxel (Taxol). New Engl J Med 332:1004–1014, 1995.

Rubin S, Hoskins W, Saigo P, et al: Prognostic factors for recurrence following negative second-look surgery in ovarian cancer patients treated with platinum-based chemotherapy. Gynecol Oncol 42:137–141, 1991.

Safra T, Jeffers S, Groshen S, et al: Doxil(D) in platinum-refractory epithelial ovarian cancer (EOC): results from three consecutive phase I/II studies (Abstract 1248). Proc Am Soc Clin Oncol 16:349a, 1997.

Segna RA, Dottino PR, Mandeli JP, et al: Secondary cytoreduction for ovarian cancer following cisplatin therapy. J Clin Oncol 11:434–439, 1993.

Sharpless NE, Seiden MV: Advanced ovarian cancer: recent progress and current challenges. Contemp Ob Gyn 43:123–137, 1998.

Staging Announcement: FIGO Cancer Committee. Gynecol Oncol 25:383, 1986.

Stiff PJ, Bayer R, Kerger C, et al: High-dose chemotherapy with autologous transplantation for persistent relapsed ovarian cancer: A multivariate analysis of survival for 100 consecutively treated patients. J Clin Oncol 15:1309–1317, 1997.

Swenerton K, Jeffrey J, Stuart G, et al: Cisplatin-cyclophosphamide versus carboplatin-cyclophosphamide in advanced ovarian cancer: A randomized phase III study of the National Cancer Institute of Canada Clinical Trials Group. J Clin Oncol 10:718–726, 1992.

Taylor KJ, Schwartz PE: Screening for early ovarian cancer. Radiology 192:1–10, 1994.

ten Bokkel Huinink W, Gore M, Carmichael J, et al: Topotecan versus paclitaxel for the treatment of recurrent epithelial ovarian cancer. J Clin Oncol 15:2183–2193, 1997.

Tidy J, Mason WP: Endometrioid carcinoma of the ovary: A retrospective study. Fr J Obstet Gynecol 95:1165–1169, 1988.

Whittemore AS: Characteristics relating to ovarian cancer risk: Implications for prevention and detection. Gynecol Oncol 55:S15–S19, 1994.

Whittemore AS: The risk of ovarian cancer after treatment for infertility. N Engl J Med 331:805–806, 1994.

Whittemore AS, Gong G, Itnyre J: Prevalence and contribution of BRCA1 mutations in breast cancer and ovarian cancer: Results from three US population-based case-control studies of ovarian cancer. Am J Hum Genet 60:496–504, 1997.

The WHO collaborative study of neoplasia and steroid contraceptives. Epithelial ovarian cancer and combined oral contraceptives. Int J Epidemiol 18:538, 1989.

Yancik R: Ovarian cancer. Age contrasts in incidence, histology, disease stage at diagnosis, and mortality. Cancer 71:517–523, 1993.

Young RC, Walton LA, Ellenberg SS, et al: Adjuvant therapy in Stage I and II epithelial ovarian cancer. Results of two prospective randomized trials. N Engl J Med 322:1021–1027, 1990.

# — 47 —

# Germ Cell and Stromal Ovarian Tumors

ROBERT T. MORRIS
ADNAN R. MUNKARAH

Neoplasms may develop from any of the three main histologic components of the ovary: surface epithelium, primordial germ cells, or stroma. Tumors arising from these tissues are clinically distinct and therefore require separate discussions. Epithelial ovarian neoplasms constitute approximately two thirds of all ovarian neoplasms (see Chapter 46). The nonepithelial ovarian neoplasms (germ cell tumors and sex cord stromal tumors) are less common than epithelial neoplasms. Nearly 95% of all germ cell tumors are benign; malignant germ cell tumors account for less than 5% of all ovarian cancers. They typically occur in girls and young women, are highly malignant, and grow rapidly. Only during the last two decades have we defined their pathologic criteria, clarified their terminology, and developed solid treatment principles. By contrast, sex cord stromal tumors of the ovary, which account for less than 10% of ovarian cancers, may occur at any age, although the peak age of incidence is during the postmenopausal years. Because of their extreme rarity, the multiplicity of histologic patterns with associated confusing terminology, and their typical indolent behavior, malignant stromal tumors represent a therapeutic challenge. This chapter focuses on the diagnosis and management of the nonepithelial tumors.

Ovarian germ cell tumors (OGCT) represent approximately 25% of all ovarian neoplasms, and 5 to 10% of all ovarian malignancies. In the first two decades of life, nearly 75% of ovarian tumors are of germ cell origin, and one third of these will be malignant. OGCTs are almost exclusively found in adolescence and early adult life. They are occasionally diagnosed in premenarchal girls and rarely in postmenopausal women. The median age for malignant OGCT is 16 to 20 years in contrast to 56 years for epithelial ovarian cancer. Because of the involved age group, a significant proportion (15 to 20%) of malignant germ cell tumors are diagnosed during pregnancy or in the puerperium. Whereas the majority of epithelial cancers are diagnosed at an advanced stage, 60 to 70% of malignant OGCT are stage I at diagnosis.

Before 1973, the multiplicity of histologic patterns and lack of a standardized nomenclature precluded significant progress in management. The institution of the current classification system by the World Health Organization (WHO) in 1973 represented a major advance in standardizing the nomenclature and histologic criteria (Table 47–1). Because of the rarity and complex histologic appearance of these lesions, consultation with an experienced gynecologic pathologist should be obtained when a malignant germ cell tumor is encountered.

In adults, the great majority of OGCT are benign

**Table 47–1** World Health Organization Classification of Germ Cell Tumors

>    Dysgerminoma
>    Endodermal sinus tumor
>    Embryonal carcinoma
>    Polyembryoma
>    Choriocarcinoma
>    Teratomas
>        Immature
>        Mature (dermoid cyst)
>        Monodermal (struma ovarii, carcinoid)
>        Mixed forms
>    Gonadoblastoma

(95%) and consist of mature cystic teratoma (dermoid cyst). These are composed of mature ectoderm, mesoderm, and endoderm. Teeth, hair, and sebaceous material are prominent in most; however, some may be composed entirely of thyroid tissue (struma ovarii). Unlike the malignant germ cell tumors, the mature cystic teratomas are frequently bilateral. Bilateral involvement is observed in approximately 15% of patients.

Dysgerminoma is the most common ovarian germ cell malignancy, representing nearly 50% of all germ cell malignancies and 2% of all ovarian malignancies. In young women, it is the most common ovarian cancer. It is the only malignant germ cell tumor with a significant incidence of bilateral ovarian involvement (10 to 15%). Dysgerminoma is also notable for its increased frequency in dysgenetic gonads.

In contrast to the benign mature cystic teratoma, immature teratomas are highly malignant. Immature teratoma is graded by its relative content of primitive embryonic elements, which are predominantly neuroectodermal. Accurate grading is essential because treatment and prognosis correlate with tumor grade. Patients with stage I grade 1 tumors are adequately treated with surgery alone, whereas nearly 70% of patients with grade 3 tumors develop recurrence if no adjuvant chemotherapy is given.

Yolk sac tumors (endodermal sinus tumors), like immature teratomas, account for 20% of ovarian germ cell cancers. These aggressive tumors recapitulate primitive gut and almost always stain positively for alpha-fetoprotein (A-FP). Embryonal carcinoma and nongestational ovarian choriocarcinoma are exceptionally rare lesions that are often associated with elevated serum tumor markers.

# Germ Cell Tumors

## HISTORY AND PHYSICAL EXAMINATION

Most benign OGCT are discovered as an incidental finding on physical examination, radiologic examination, or intraoperatively. When symptoms exist they are most frequently pain, pelvic pressure, or abdominal distention. Malignant OGCT are associated with abdominal pain and a palpable mass in approximately 85% of patients. Rupture, hemorrhage, or torsion of these malignancies may occur and present with acute abdominal pain in 10% of patients. Because of the young affected age group, acute abdominal pain is often misdiagnosed as appendicitis. Less common presenting symptoms include abdominal distention, vaginal bleeding, and fever. In contrast to epithelial ovarian cancer, gastrointestinal symptoms and abdominal bloating resulting from ascites are rarely encountered and herald advanced disease (Table 47–2).

A thorough physical examination is mandatory; however, a pelvic mass is most frequently the only abnormality. Benign mature cystic teratomas tend to be smaller than malignant germ cell tumors. Most mature cystic teratomas are usually less than 15 cm in diameter, whereas the malignant OGCT have a median size of 16 cm. Careful attention should be directed to the detection of abdominal masses, ascites, and pleural effusions.

## DIAGNOSTIC CONSIDERATIONS

A comprehensive discussion of the evaluation of an adnexal mass is beyond the scope of this chapter. Cystic masses less than 8 cm in postmenarchal women are most often functional ovarian cysts and appropriately managed with ovarian suppression and re-examination after 8 weeks. However, prompt evaluation and treatment of an adnexal mass is required if it is solid, large (>10 cm), diagnosed in the premenarchal years, or associated with ascites or peritonitis. The differential diagnosis in these patients most significantly includes ovarian neoplasm, as well as pregnancy-related events, infectious etiologies, and less likely functional cysts. With the exception of the few patients who present with acute abdominal findings, these patients require a methodic and thorough evaluation.

**Table 47–2** Clinical Presentation of Ovarian Germ Cell Tumors

| Symptoms | (%) |
| --- | --- |
| Palpable mass | >80 |
| Abdominal pain | >80 |
| Tumor rupture | 20 |
| Ascites | 20 |
| Acute abdomen | 10 |
| Other | |
|     Fever | |
|     Bleeding | |
|     Isosexual precocity | |

## LABORATORY AND DIAGNOSTIC EVALUATION

Benign OGCT (mature cystic teratoma) have no reliable serum tumor marker. However, the production of serum tumor markers by many of the malignant OGCT aids in their diagnosis. More important, tumor markers may be used in monitoring the response to treatment and in surveillance after completion of therapy. Table 47–3 illustrates the typical findings in the sera of patients with the various histologic types. Yolk sac tumor (endodermal sinus tumor) and choriocarcinoma are the prototypical tumors producing A-FP and human chorionic gonadotropin (hCG), respectively. Immature teratoma will occasionally have elevated AFP levels. Dysgerminoma, the most common malignant OGCT, has been traditionally considered devoid of tumor markers. Therefore, normal A-FP and hCG levels are not sufficient to exclude the diagnosis of malignant OGCT. Recently, lactic dehydrogenase isoenzymes and neuron-specific enolase have been studied as potential markers for dysgerminoma.

Malignant OGCT, particularly dysgerminoma, may arise from dysgenetic gonads. In premenarchal patients with an adnexal mass, the evaluation must include a karyotype. The karyotype will be useful in determining surgical management; bilateral gonadectomy is usually recommended in patients with dysgenetic gonads.

Radiologic imaging techniques are frequently used in evaluating patients with adnexal masses. The sonographic appearance of mature cystic teratomas is usually heterogeneous owing to the sebaceous material and frequent calcifications. These calcifications are also frequently identified on abdominal x-rays studies. Malignant OGCT characteristically contain a large solid component, as well as complex architecture on pelvic sonography. In patients suspected of having malignant OGCT, the metastatic evaluation should include a chest x-ray film to assess for mediastinal disease, as well as pulmonary metastases. Because of the propensity for lymphatic metastasis, computed tomography (CT) of the abdomen and pelvis may be useful in assessing retroperitoneal disease and possible liver metastases.

## TREATMENT

### Surgery

The initial treatment approach for patients suspected of having an OGCT is surgery, for both diagnosis and therapy. After an adequate vertical midline incision is made, the extent of disease should be determined by inspection and palpation. If the disease seems to be confined to one or both ovaries, it is important to perform proper staging biopsies. An ovarian cystectomy may be performed initially if the mass is not obviously malignant. Intraperitoneal spillage of cyst content should be avoided at the time of resection. Preliminary intraoperative pathologic diagnosis using frozen sections should direct the surgical management. If a mature cystic teratoma is found, unilateral cystectomy with close inspection of the contralateral ovary is curative. If a malignant OGCT is encountered, staging is mandatory. Adequate staging consists of taking one or more peritoneal cytologic specimens (and ascitic fluid, if present), random biopsies of tissue from the omentum, abdominal and pelvic peritoneum, and retroperitoneal lymph nodes. Although OGCT may metastasize by exfoliation into the peritoneal cavity or by contiguous extension to other abdominopelvic structures, an important distinction from epithelial ovarian cancers is that OGCT have an increased tendency for lymphatic metastasis. This necessitates close inspection and biopsy of pelvic and periaortic lymph nodes during surgical staging. The International Federation of Gynecology and Obstetrics (FIGO) surgical staging system used for epithelial ovarian cancer is also applied to malignant germ cell and stromal tumors.

Preservation of reproductive potential is a critical issue in the treatment of malignant OGCT because of the young age of most patients. Because most tumors are stage I and few are bilateral, unilateral oophorectomy with thorough staging is sufficient for most patients. A large series reported in the 1970s and early 1980s demonstrated that 5 to 10% of patients with malignant germ cell tumors will also have contralateral benign cystic teratomas. Ovarian cystectomy with preservation of the contralateral normal ovarian tissue is recommended in that setting. In patients with dysgenetic gonads or bilateral ovarian involvement, bilateral oophorectomy should be performed; however, the uterus can often be preserved. Normal intrauterine pregnancy may be achieved with modern reproductive technology and donor (or banked) oocytes.

Most patients who undergo surgery for malignant

**Table 47–3** Serum Tumor Markers in Malignant Germ Cell Tumors of the Ovary

| Histology | Alpha-Fetoprotein | Human Chorionic Gonadotropin |
|---|---|---|
| Dysgerminoma | − | ± |
| Endodermal sinus tumor | + | − |
| Immature teratoma | ± | − |
| Mixed germ cell tumor | ± | ± |
| Choriocarcinoma | − | + |
| Embryonal carcinoma | ± | + |
| Polyembryoma | ± | + |

OGCT do so outside major centers, and for most of them, the staging information available upon referral is inadequate. The lack of adequate information may subsequently lead to a compromise in the chemotherapeutic management of the patient in terms of type of regimen, dose intensity, or duration of chemotherapy. In patients without bulky residual disease after the initial surgery, it is probably inadvisable to delay chemotherapy with surgical re-exploration for the sole purpose of gaining more precise staging information. On the other hand, in patients who may potentially avoid toxic chemotherapy by confirming stage I disease, re-exploration with formal staging should be considered. This group of patients includes those with probable stage IA dysgerminoma or stage IA grade 1 immature teratoma.

In patients with bulky metastatic disease, recent evidence suggests that tumor debulking with smaller residual disease improves prognosis. In fact, in a study of the Gynecologic Oncology Group (GOG), 68% of patients with incompletely resected disease did not respond to a combination of vincristine, dactinomycin, and cyclophosphamide (VAC) compared with 28% of patients with completely resected disease treated with the same regimen. In a subsequent GOG study in which patients were treated with the combination of vinblastine, bleomycin, and cisplatin (VBP), those with clinically nonmeasurable disease had a greater likelihood of remaining progression free than those with measurable disease (65% vs. 34%). It remains uncertain whether these differences are attributable to surgical skill and aggressiveness or to differences in tumor biology. Most agree that debulking is warranted if the risk of major morbidity is low.

## Chemotherapy

Until the advent of combination chemotherapy in the mid-1960s, the prognosis for most patients with malignant ovarian germ cell tumors was dismal; virtually all patients with advanced disease died. Even in stage I disease, only 5 to 20% of patients survived after treatment with surgery alone. In the entire series from the M.D. Anderson Cancer Center (MDACC) 30 of 33 patients treated with surgery alone had recurrent disease. Equally dismal survival rates resulted from postoperative treatment with radioisotopes, external radiation therapy, or single-alkylating agent chemotherapy. Currently, the only patients with malignant OGCT who should be considered for treatment with surgery alone are those with well-documented stage IA, grade 1 pure immature teratoma or stage IA pure dysgerminoma.

Beginning in approximately 1970, VAC began to be used for patients with nondysgerminomatous tumors. Studies by Gershenson and by the GOG demonstrated 72 to 86% progression-free survival rates in patients with completely resected early stage disease treated with VAC. In patients with established metastatic disease, sustained remission was achieved in only 33 to 44% of patients. Although the VAC regimen is still used in many large centers worldwide, it began to lose popularity in the late 1970s with the introduction of cisplatin into clinical trials. VBP was superior to the VAC regimen. In a prospective trial of the GOG, 53% of patients with advanced stage or recurrent disease treated with VBP remained disease free at a median follow-up of 52 months. However, toxicity was high, with nearly 50% requiring dose modification and 5% treatment-related deaths.

Over the last two decades, the combination of bleomycin, etoposide, and cisplatin (BEP) has become the standard regimen for malignant ovarian germ cell tumors. In prospective randomized trials, BEP showed equal if not superior efficacy and less toxicity than VBP in patients with testicular cancer (the male analog of malignant ovarian germ cell tumors). Recent experience with the BEP regimen in malignant ovarian germ cell tumors has been favorable; sustained remission rates in the range of 95% have been reported (Table 47–4).

The optimal duration of treatment is somewhat unclear. For patients with stage I or completely resected metastatic tumors, three to four cycles appear to be adequate, but for patients with bulky residual tumor, five to six cycles may be indicated. For patients with positive tumor marker findings, it seems adequate to administer two cycles after normalization of the serum levels. For patients without measurable disease or without elevated serum tumor marker lev-

**Table 47–4** Combination Chemotherapy Regimens for Malignant Germ Cell Tumors of the Ovary

| Regimen | Dosage |
| --- | --- |
| VAC | |
|   Vincristine | 1–1.5 mg/m² IV on d 1 |
|   Actinomycin D | 0.5 mg/d IV for 5 d |
|   Cyclophosphamide | 150 mg/m² for 1 d IV for 5 d |
|   Repeat cycles at 4-wk intervals | |
| VBP | |
|   Vinblastine | 0.3 mg/kg IV in divided doses on d 1 and 2 |
|   Bleomycin | 15 mg/day for 5 d by continuous infusion |
|   Cisplatin | 100 mg/m² IV on d 1 |
|   Repeat cycles at 3 to 4 wk intervals | |
| BEP | |
|   Bleomycin | 20–30 U IV on d 1 |
|   Etoposide | 75 mg/m² for 1 d IV for 5 d |
|   Cisplatin | 20 mg/m² for 1 d IV for 5 d |
|   Repeat cycles at 3 to 4 wk intervals | |

els, it is more difficult to determine the precise duration of treatment.

All patients with dysgerminoma require adjuvant therapy, with the possible exception of completely staged stage IA pure dysgerminoma. Radiation therapy has been the traditional postoperative treatment for patients with metastatic dysgerminoma. Although dysgerminoma is exquisitely radiosensitive and survival rates with such treatment have been excellent, fertility is almost always destroyed. Because of the high antitumor activity, acceptable toxicity profile, and the preservation of reproductive potential, chemotherapy has replaced radiation therapy as the standard postoperative therapy. Surveying the entire experience of the treatment of dysgerminoma with BEP, it appears that three to four cycles are adequate therapy, even for patients with bulky residual disease. This holds true for the majority of patients who will have stage I disease, as well as for patients with advanced disease. Radiation therapy, therefore, should be reserved for salvage therapy or unusual circumstances such as severe concurrent medical conditions.

In summary, all patients with malignant ovarian germ cell tumors require chemotherapy after initial surgical resection and staging, with the possible exception of stage IA grade 1 immature teratoma and stage IA pure dysgerminoma. Three to four courses of the BEP combination have evolved as the standard regimen for adjuvant treatment; however, the duration of therapy requires individualization according to stage, residual disease, and tumor marker status.

## Post-Therapy Surveillance

Since the advent of successful combination chemotherapy for malignant OGCT, clinical management for patients with these lesions has been similar to that for epithelial ovarian cancer. Namely, patients who were clinically disease free at the completion of a planned number of chemotherapy cycles routinely underwent second-look laparotomy (SLL). However, during the last two decades, the role of SLL in OGCT has diminished. Although SLL has been used routinely, data from the late 1980s and early 1990s indicate that it is rarely useful after non-platinum-based combination therapy for malignant OGCT. Studies by Gershenson and by Williams demonstrate that few patients benefit from SLL and support the philosophy of limiting the use of SLL in this population as much as possible. For patients whose initially positive tumor markers have normalized, especially those with early stage disease, the procedure is not recommended. Some patients with initially negative tumor markers, advanced stage disease, or a teratoma component may benefit from SLL. Nevertheless, as better therapies are developed and refined, SLL inevitably will become obsolete, except in unusual circumstances.

After completing chemotherapy, patients are examined at monthly intervals for the first year and less frequently thereafter. If serum tumor markers are initially positive, patients are monitored at monthly intervals during the first 2 years (the most likely time frame for recurrence). Imaging studies are performed as indicated and are used more commonly in patients with initially negative tumor markers.

## Salvage Chemotherapy

Information is sparse regarding salvage therapy for patients with malignant OGCT who have persistent, progressive, or recurrent disease after initial chemotherapy. Patients who were not treated initially with a platinum-based regimen are best treated with cisplatin at the time of recurrence. Almost all patients currently receive cisplatin-containing combination regimens as first-line treatment; the salvageability of these patients is much more germane. For the purpose of prognosis and appropriate therapy selection, it is important to distinguish between platinum-resistant and platinum-sensitive tumors. Patients with the former have progressive disease during therapy or within 4 to 6 weeks of stopping therapy; those with the latter have relapses more than 4 to 6 weeks after discontinuing treatment. For platinum-sensitive patients, the combination of cisplatin and ifosfamide with etoposide or vinblastine has been used with limited response rates. For patients with platinum-resistant tumors, treatment options are limited and include either high-dose chemotherapy or phase II drugs.

## Late Sequelae

Most patients with ovarian germ cell tumors require chemotherapy, and fortunately most will survive. With the marked improvement in prognosis over the last two decades, long-term sequelae of surgery and chemotherapy have become a focus of attention. The most notable issues are ovarian function and development of secondary malignancies.

Preservation of reproductive function is a primary concern in these young and highly curable patients. Gershenson studied reproductive function in 40 successfully treated female patients with OGCT. Most received the VAC regimen; the median number of chemotherapy cycles was 16. During chemotherapy 19 of 33 (67%) experienced regular menses and 11 (33%) had amenorrhea or oligomenorrhea. After chemotherapy 36 of 39 (92%) postmenarchal patients had no serious or persistent menstrual dysfunction.

Nine (23%) experienced transient menstrual irregularities, which resolved within 9 months after completion of therapy. Eleven of 16 (69%) patients attempting to become pregnant were successful and delivered 22 healthy infants. Four patients reported infertility; however, only one of these sought medical consultation. These favorable results are in contrast to those for men in which impaired gametogenesis after treatment of testicular germ cell tumors is well documented.

The risk of secondary malignancies is a recognized late effect of chemotherapy for germ cell tumors. Most of the available data are from the treatment of testicular germ cell tumors; however, Williams and colleagues reported one case of leukemia after BEP for OGCT. The use of etoposide has been associated with the development of acute monocytic or myelomonocytic leukemia. Review of several large retrospective studies demonstrates that 0.09% to 0.8% of patients developed leukemia after treatment with standard-dose etoposide-containing regimens. In addition, etoposide-induced leukemias appear sooner after chemotherapy than does alkylating agent-induced leukemia.

## PROGNOSIS

Malignant ovarian germ cell tumors represent one of the true success stories in oncology. Whereas the prognosis was almost uniformly grave regardless of disease stage, modern oncologic management now is curative for almost all patients. In patients with early stage completely resected disease, survival rates are 90 to 100% after adjuvant chemotherapy. In the minority of patients with advanced stage or bulky residual disease, 50 to 80% survive without recurrence. The most important prognostic factors are histologic type, stage, and residual disease. Yolk sac tumors and immature teratomas tend to be more aggressive lesions, whereas dysgerminoma is the least aggressive.

# Sex Cord Stromal Tumors of the Ovary

## DEFINITION

Sex cord stromal tumors constitute approximately 8% of ovarian tumors and 7% of ovarian malignancies. These solid tumors are derived from the mesenchyme of the embryonic gonad. Such neoplasms may contain any element of the sex cord: granulosa cells, thecal cells, Sertoli cells, Leydig cells, or stromal cells. Table 47–5 shows the WHO classification for sex cord stromal tumors of the ovary. Because of the normal endocrinologic function of this ovarian compartment, the majority of hormonally active gynecologic neoplasms fall under this category. The relative rarity of this group of tumors precludes any definitive statements regarding optimal treatment of the malignant variants.

**Table 47–5** World Health Organization Classification of Sex Cord Stromal Tumors

Granulosa stromal cell
   Granulosa cell
   Thecoma-fibroma
Androblastomas; Sertoli-Leydig cell tumors
   Well-differentiated (Pick's adenoma, Sertoli cell tumor)
   Intermediate differentiation
   Poorly differentiated
   With heterologous elements
Lipid cell tumors
Gynandroblastoma
Unclassified

Ovarian fibromas account for nearly half of the stromal tumors. They may occur at any age; the average age is 48 years. They range in size from microscopic to massive and are almost always benign. Meigs' syndrome (ovarian fibroma, ascites, and pleural effusion) is a dramatic syndrome associated with approximately 1% of ovarian fibromas. Most patients with a solid ovarian tumor, ascites, and a pleural effusion have an epithelial ovarian carcinoma rather than Meigs' syndrome.

Granulosa cell tumors are divided into adult and juvenile types. Together they account for 70% of malignant sex cord tumors. The average age for the adult type is 52, whereas 90% of the juvenile type occurs in prepubertal girls. Estrogen production is common; two thirds of patients experience irregular vaginal bleeding. In patients with granulosa cell tumors, endometrial hyperplasia is detected in approximately half, and adenocarcinoma in approximately 10%. Isosexual precocious pseudopuberty may be seen in premenarchal girls. The average tumor diameter is 12 cm; the tumors are predominantly cystic with solid components. Similar to germ cell malignancies, most (90%) granulosa cell tumors are stage I at diagnosis. For granulosa cell tumors, stage appears to be the strongest prognostic factor. Other factors that have been studied for their influence on survival include age, tumor size, tumor size, tumor rupture, mitotic index, cellular atypia, capsular invasion, and lymphatic invasion; but none has been shown to have a consistent effect. Flow cytometric DNA ploidy correlates with the clinical course of granulosa cell tumors in some studies.

Sertoli-Leydig cell tumors are a rare ovarian malignancy, accounting for approximately 0.5% of ovarian cancers. One third are hormonally active and present with signs of virilization. The average age at diagnosis in one large series was 25 years. Almost all are unilateral and stage I at diagnosis. For Sertoli-Leydig cell tumors, the only definite prognostic factors appear to be stage and tumor differentiation. The presence of heterologous elements also seems to be unfavorable.

## HISTORY AND PHYSICAL EXAMINATION

Diagnosis of sex cord stromal tumors is rarely made before surgical exploration. As with germ cell tumors, many of these tumors are detected at the time of routine examination. Frequently, these lesions are large and may present with pain, pelvic pressure, or abdominal distention. Symptoms of hormonal imbalance such as irregular bleeding, precocious puberty, or virilization in the clinical setting of a predominantly solid adnexal mass should raise the question of a sex cord stromal tumor. Evaluation and diagnostic considerations for the stromal cell tumors are the same as for germ cell tumors, with the exception of tumor markers. Although sex cord stromal tumors do not consistently produce serum tumor markers as do certain germ cell tumors, several produce markers that can be monitored both during and after therapy. Serial serum levels of estradiol or testosterone may be followed in patients having estrogenic or androgenic tumors, respectively. In addition, granulosa cell tumors may produce serum inhibin, and Sertoli-Leydig cell tumors may produce serum AFP.

## TREATMENT

### Surgery

Adequate surgical management of sex cord stromal tumors of the ovary consists of an exploratory laparotomy through an adequate vertical midline incision. Suspicious lesions should be assessed intraoperatively by using frozen sections. Benign lesions such as fibromas or thecomas are treated as other benign ovarian neoplasms. Oophorectomy should be curative. If the tumor is malignant and seems to be confined to one ovary in a young patient, unilateral salpingo-oophorectomy and complete staging biopsies are appropriate. If the malignancy is bilateral or if the patient is postmenopausal, bilateral salpingo-oophorectomy with or without hysterectomy is indicated. If the tumor is obviously metastatic, an effort at aggressive cytoreductive surgery should be made, although no scientific evidence of the benefits of such surgical management exists. If conservative surgery without hysterectomy is contemplated in a patient with a granulosa cell tumor, a uterine curettage should be performed at the time of laparotomy to exclude the possibility of a concurrent endometrial cancer.

### Chemotherapy

Based on available information, surgery alone appears to be optimal therapy for patients with benign tumors, as well as most nonmetastatic sex cord stromal malignancies: juvenile granulosa cell tumors, Leydig cell tumors, and well-differentiated Sertoli-Leydig cell tumors. For patients with metastatic disease of any type (primary, advanced, or recurrent) or those with poorly differentiated Sertoli-Leydig cell tumors of any stage, postoperative therapy is necessary. For patients with stage IA adult type granulosa cell tumors, the decision concerning the need for postoperative therapy is more difficult. No histologic criteria provide definite information to guide the clinician. If the tumor is unruptured, no further therapy seems indicated. For patients with ruptured tumors, management is more controversial. Some experts suggest that tumor rupture worsens the prognosis, although others doubt such an association.

Information regarding the chemotherapeutic treatment of these tumors has been limited primarily to small series or case reports. Single agent therapy appears to have limited activity, and more effort has been directed at combination chemotherapy. Most recent regimens include cisplatin and have been similar to those used for germ cell tumors (VBP and BEP). Overall response rates of 60 to 80% have been reported in small series, including a recent study by the Gynecologic Oncology Group.

There may also be a role for hormonal therapy in metastatic granulosa cell tumors. Few case reports have described arrest of tumor growth and stabilization of disease with progesterone, tamoxifen, or a long-acting gonadotropin-releasing hormone agonist analog.

## PROGNOSIS

Overall, the malignant stromal ovarian tumors tend to be indolent lesions, with the vast majority being diagnosed as stage I. In patients with early stage disease, 80 to 90% experience progression-free survival. Patients with extraovarian or advanced stage disease have 5-year survival rates of 20 to 50%. Prognostic factors include histologic type, stage, rupture of tumor, and tumor size.

# Unresolved Issues and Future Directions

Now that the histologic classification and terminology have been standardized and biologic behavior of these rare tumors have been clarified, the principal challenges for the future include the refinement of selection criteria for adjuvant therapy and clarification of the relative roles of available modalities. The continued search for optimal therapy includes new phase II chemotherapy trials and expanded experience with a variety of hormonal agents. However, progress in this area will continue to be hampered by the rarity of these tumors and their indolent behavior.

## REFERENCES

Boshoff C, Begent RH, Oliver RT, et al: Secondary tumours following etoposide containing therapy for germ cell cancer. Ann Oncol 6:35–40, 1995.

Bower M, Fife K, Holden L, et al: Chemotherapy for ovarian germ cell tumours. Eur J Cancer 32:593–597, 1996.

Culine S, Kattan J, Lhomme C, et al: A phase II study of high-dose cisplatin, vinblastine, bleomycin, and etoposide (PVeBV regimen) in malignant nondysgerminomatous germ-cell tumors of the ovary. Gynecol Oncol 54:47–53, 1994.

DePalo G, Pilotti S, Kenda R, et al: Natural history of dysgerminoma. Am J Obstet Gynecol 143:799–807, 1982.

Gershenson DM: Menstrual and reproductive function after treatment with combination chemotherapy for malignant ovarian germ cell tumors. J Clin Oncol 6:270–275, 1988.

Gershenson DM, Copeland LJ, Del Junco G, et al: Second-look laparotomy in the management of malignant germ cell tumors of the ovary. Obstet Gynecol 67:789–793, 1986.

Gershenson DM, Copeland LJ, Kavanagh JJ, et al: Treatment of malignant nondysgerminomatous germ cell tumors of the ovary with vincristine, actinomycin-D, and cyclophosphamide. Cancer 56:2756–2761, 1985.

Gershenson DM, Kavanagh JJ, Copeland LJ, et al: Treatment of malignant nondysgerminomatous germ cell tumors of the ovary with vinblastine, bleomycin and cisplatin. Cancer 57:1731–1737, 1986.

Gershenson DM, Morris M, Burke TW, et al: Treatment of poor-prognosis sex cord-stromal tumors of the ovary with the combination of bleomycin, etoposide, and cisplatin. Obstet Gynecol 87:527–531, 1996.

Gershenson DM, Morris M, Cangir A, et al: Treatment of malignant germ cell tumors of the ovary with belomycin, etoposide, and cisplatin (BEP). J Clin Oncol 8:715–720, 1990.

Gershenson DM, Wharton JT: Malignant germ cell tumors of the ovary. In Alberts DS, Surwit EA (eds): Ovarian Cancer. Boston: Martinus Nijhoff, 1985, pp 227–269.

Homesley HD, Bundy BN, Hurteau JA, et al: Bleomycin, etoposide, and cisplatin combination therapy of ovarian granulosa cell tumors and other stromal malignancies: A Gynecologic Oncology Group Study. Gynecol Oncol 72:131–137, 1999.

Jacobs AJ, Harris M, Deppe G, et al: Treatment of recurrent germ cell tumors with cisplatin, vinblastine, and belomycin. Obstet Gynecol 59:129–132, 1982.

Jimerson GK, Woodruff JD: Ovarian extraembryonal teratoma. Am J Obstet Gynecol 127:302–305, 1977.

Jimerson GK, Woodruff JD: Ovarian extraembryonal teratoma. II. Endodermal sinus tumor mixed with other germ cell tumors. Am J Obstet Gynecol 127:302–305, 1977.

Klemi PK, Joensuu H, Salmi T: Prognostic value of flow cytometric DNA content analysis in granulosa cell tumor of the ovary. Cancer 65:1189–1193, 1990.

Kurman RJ, Norris HJ: Endodermal sinus tumor of ovary. A clinical and pathological analysis of 71 cases. Cancer 38:2404–2419, 1976.

Kurman RJ, Norris HJ: Malignant mixed germ cell tumors of the ovary. Obstet Gynecol 48:579–589, 1976.

Malkasian GD, Webb MJ, Jorgensen EO: Observations on chemotherapy of granulosa cell carcinomas and malignant ovarian teratomas. Obstet Gynecol 44:885–888, 1974.

Martikainen H, Penttinen J, Huhtaniemi I, et al: Gonadotropin-releasing hormone agonist analog therapy effective in ovarian granulosa cell malignancy. Gynecol Oncol 35:406–408, 1989.

McCaffrey JA, Mazumdar M, Bajorin DF, et al: Ifosfamide and cisplatin-containing chemotherapy as first-line salvage therapy in germ cell tumors: response and survival. J Clin Oncol 15:2559–2563, 1997.

Motzer RJ, Mazmdar M, Bosl GJ, et al: High-dose carboplatin, etoposide, and cyclophosphamide for patients with refractory germ cell tumors: Treatment results and prognostic factors for survival and toxicity. J Clin Oncol 14:1098–1105, 1996.

Norris HJ, Zirkin HJ, Benson WL: Immature malignant teratoma of the ovary. Cancer 37:2359–2372, 1976.

Schwartz PE, MacLusky N, Sakamoto H, et al: Steroid-receptor proteins in nonepithelial malignancies of the ovary. Gynecol Oncol 15:305–315, 1983.

Serov SF, Sully RE, Sobin LJ: Histological typing of ovarian tumors. I. World Health Organization. International Histological Classifications of Tumors. Geneva, World Health Organization, 1973.

Slayton RE, Park RC, Silverberg SG, et al: Vincristine, dactinomycin, and cyclophosphamide in the treatment of malignant germ cell tumors of the ovary: A Gynecologic Oncology Group study (a final report). Cancer 56:243–248, 1985.

Smith JP, Rutledge FN: Advances in chemotherapy for gynecologic cancer. Cancer 36:669–674, 1975.

Stephenson WT, Poirier SM, Rubin L, et al: Evaluation of reproductive capacity in germ cell tumor patients following treatment with cisplatin, etoposide, and bleomycin. J Clin Oncol 13:2278–2280, 1995.

Williams SD, Birch R, Einhorn LH, et al: Treatment of disseminated germ-cell tumors with cisplatin, bleomycin, and either vinblastine or etoposide. N Engl J Med 316:1435–1440, 1987.

Williams SD, Blessing JA, DiSaia PJ, et al: Second-look laparotomy in ovarian germ cell tumors: The Gynecologic Oncology Group experience. Gynecol Oncol 52:287–291, 1994.

Williams SD, Blessing JA, Hatch KD, et al: Chemotherapy of advanced dysgerminoma: Trials of the Gynecologic Oncology Group. J Clin Oncol 9:1950–1955, 1991.

Williams SD, Blessing JA, Moore DH, et al: Cisplatin, vinblastine, and bleomycin in advanced and recurrent ovarian germ cell tumors. Ann Intern Med 111:22–27, 1989.

Williams SD, Liao SY, Ball H, et al: Adjuvant therapy of ovarian germ cell tumors with cisplatin, etoposide and bleomycin: A trial of the Gynecologic Oncology Group. J Clin Oncol 12:701–706, 1994.

Young RH, Scully RE: Ovarian Sertoli-Leydig cell tumors: A clinicopathological analysis of 207 cases. Am J Surg Pathol 9:543–569, 1985.

Zambetti M, Escobedo A, Pilotti S, et al: Cisplatinum/vinblastine/bleomycin combination chemotherapy in advanced or recurrent granulosa cell tumors of the ovary. Gynecol Oncol 36:317–320, 1990.

# 48

# Surgical Complications

CHARLES LEVENBACK

Complications are an inevitable aspect of medical practice. The risk of complications must be balanced against the ancient admonition to the physician: "First, do no harm." Fear of complications should not prevent decisive action when delay will only escalate the risks. On the other hand, overly aggressive management can lead to disaster for the patient. This balancing act is at the core of the art of medicine.

Surgical complications are morbid events that occur during or after the operation and that are not an essential part of the disease or procedure. Complications may be divided into categories by organ system involved, by the presenting symptoms, or by the timing of the complication in relation to the procedure; but all of these categories are arbitrary and can obscure how complications can be interrelated.

The most disastrous clinical situations involve a cascade of events that, each considered alone, may be manageable. For example, a major vessel laceration repaired promptly may have only minor consequences; but if blood loss is excessive, hypotension, shock, coagulopathy, adult respiratory distress syndrome (ARDS), and multiorgan system failure can follow. Physicians tend to view complications as solely their responsibility; however, this is rarely the situation. In the example of intraoperative hemorrhage, the effect of the bleeding can be reduced if the anesthesiologist has large bore intravenous access prepared, nurses react promptly and efficiently to requests for additional instruments and sutures, the blood bank has the correct units available quickly, and a critical care specialist and well-staffed intensive-care unit (ICU) are available. Understanding the specific health care delivery system as a whole and its limitations is another important part of preventing complications.

An outstanding clinician always strives to anticipate and prevent complications. When complications do occur, their management can be a true test of an individual's judgment and skill as a surgical subspecialist. The goal of this chapter is to assist the clinician in first preventing surgical complications and then, when complications do occur, recognizing and managing them appropriately to reduce adverse consequences. A full description of all potential complications of gynecologic surgery is not possible here. Instead, common intraoperative and postoperative complications are reviewed, with emphasis on practical clinical management.

The first part of the chapter reviews prevention of complications through careful preoperative planning. The second section deals with management of three common intraoperative complications: hemorrhage, genitourinary tract injury, and gastrointestinal tract injury. The final section reviews the management of the frequent postoperative complications of fever, oliguria, and shortness of breath.

# Preoperative Evaluation

## HISTORY AND PHYSICAL EXAMINATION

A major aspect of preoperative preparation is risk assessment and complication prevention. The operating surgeon has an ethical obligation to perform personally (or through a responsible designee) a complete history and physical examination on patients undergoing elective procedures. Most operating rooms have medical staff guidelines for timeliness of history and physical examination, and these should be observed for the benefit of both patient and physician.

The elements of a complete history and physical examination are listed in Table 48–1. Medication use for cardiac, pulmonary, or endocrine disorders should be fully investigated. Regular use of over-the-counter medications such as aspirin may require postponement of major elective surgery. If the patient has undergone radiation therapy, the radiation field and dose should be known.

Physical examination should be complete and include pelvic and rectal examinations. The history of each surgical scar, particularly on the abdomen or pelvis, should be known. Reoperation on patients with a history of abdominal or pelvic malignancy can be especially hazardous and the operative notes, if available, should be reviewed.

## RISK ASSESSMENT

Several risk assessment scoring systems have been developed to assist in estimating the risk of mortality or morbidity from major surgery. The American Society of Anesthesiologists categories correlate with complication risk; however, the usefulness of this system (Table 48–2) for clinicians is limited, as the classes are broadly defined.

Goldman and colleagues developed a multifactorial index of cardiac risk in noncardiac surgical procedures (Table 48–3). Patients with heavily weighted risks, such as those with myocardial infarction within the last 6 months, abnormal cardiac rhythm, jugular venous distention, or an extra heart sound, should be evaluated by a cardiologist to reverse correctable abnormalities and to assist in postoperative management. Advice to the anesthesiologist such as "avoid hypotension" is not helpful and is a sign of an inexperienced consultant. Although there are flaws in the Goldman classification, this index remains a useful tool for cardiac risk assessment.

Increasing age, body cavity surgery, smoking, and obesity are the primary risk factors for pulmonary complications. Pulmonary function tests remain the mainstay for quantifying risks. In general a 1-second forced expiratory volume of less than 65% of predicted value (usually less than 1000 ml) indicates high risk, and a value of less than 70% of predicted value

**Table 48–1** Elements of a Preoperative History and Physical Examination

Chief problem or introductory statement
History of present illness
Review of systems
Obstetric/gynecologic history
Family history
Social history
Medication use (including over-the-counter drugs)
Allergies to medications
Physical examination including vital signs
Review of laboratory, pathology, medical record, and imaging data
Assessment
Plan, including alternatives

**Table 48–2** American Society of Anesthesiologists (ASA) Physical Status Classification

| Class | Description |
|---|---|
| I | Healthy |
| II | Mild systemic disease—no functional limitation |
| III | Severe systemic disease—definite functional limitation |
| IV | Severe systemic disease that is a constant threat to life |
| V | Moribund patient unlikely to survive 24 hours with or without operation |

Adapted from Wolters U, Wolf T, Stützer H, et al: ASA classification and perioperative variables as predictors of postoperative outcome. Br J Anaesth 77:217–222, 1996.

**Table 48–3** Goldman Multifactorial Preoperative Index Score to Estimate Cardiac Risk

| Preoperative Finding | Points |
|---|---|
| $S_3$ gallop or jugular venous distention | 11 |
| Myocardial infarct within 6 months | 10 |
| Premature ventricular beats (>5/min) | 7 |
| Rhythm other than sinus or premature atrial contractions | 7 |
| Age >70 years | 5 |
| Emergency surgery | 4 |
| Intraperitoneal surgery | 3 |
| Valvular stenosis | 3 |
| Poor medical condition | 3 |
|   K < 3.0 mEq/L | |
|   $HCO_3$ < 20 mEq/L | |
|   BUN > 50 mg/dl | |
|   Creatinine > 3.0 mg/dl | |
|   $Po_2$ < 60 mm Hg | |
|   $Pco_2$ > 50 mm Hg | |
|   Chronic liver disease | |
|   Bedridden | |

BUN = blood urea nitrogen.

**Table 48–4** Factors That Increase Surgical Risk in Patients with Liver Cirrhosis

Ascites
Total bilirubin > 3.5 mg/dl
Alkaline phosphatase > 70 U/dl
PT/PTT increased > 2 seconds over control
Serum albumin < 3.0 g/dl
Emergency surgery

PT = prothrombin time; PTT = partial thromboplastin time.

(usually between 1000 and 2000 ml) indicates medium to high risk.

Cessation of smoking even 48 hours before surgery can reduce carboxyhemoglobin levels. It requires 2 to 6 weeks of abstention from smoking to improve mucociliary function and reduce sputum production. If surgery can be postponed this long and the patient will commit to smoking cessation, surgical risk can be reduced.

The surgical risk factors associated with cirrhosis of the liver are shown in Table 48–4. In one study, the mortality rates were 20% for patients with two or three of these factors and 33% for patients with four or five risk factors. Suture line failure, peritonitis, and sepsis were common complications in another study in which the mortality rate was 21% for all patients with nonbleeding cirrhosis. Clinical experience indicates that patients commonly underestimate alcohol intake. A detailed drinking history, therefore, should include questions regarding the type and volume of intake and the frequency of binge drinking.

Diabetes mellitus increases the risk of hyperglycemia and hypoglycemia, impaired wound healing, and infection. Blood glucose concentrations should be stabilized at less than 250 mg/dl before surgery. There is controversy regarding how tightly glucose concentrations need to be controlled and the best way of achieving this, especially in the postoperative period when patient caloric intake is reduced. The most common technique is to obtain glucose values every 6 to 8 hours and prescribe insulin as needed until oral intake resumes.

Assessment of bleeding tendency begins with a detailed history as outlined in Table 48–5. Many patients do not consider aspirin and nonsteroidal anti-inflammatory drugs (NSAIDs) in the same category of importance as their prescription medications; therefore, specific questions regarding the use of NSAIDs must be asked. Patients who take aspirin regularly should discontinue its use 7 to 10 days before surgery.

Numerous factors can increase the risk of deep vein thrombosis (DVT) and pulmonary embolism (Table 48–6). Virtually all patients undergoing surgery for known or suspected gynecologic malignancy are at increased risk for DVT and should receive prophylaxis.

## PREOPERATIVE LABORATORY TESTING

There has been a recent emphasis on limiting preoperative testing after years of unnecessary universal testing, which included chest x-ray studies, coagulation studies, and urinalysis on all patients, even though these studies rarely altered the management plan. Furthermore, chemistry and hematology surveys have been "unbundled" so that specific studies must be selected individually. The minimum laboratory evaluation of a healthy patient less than 40 years of age undergoing major abdominal surgery is a complete blood count and blood typing and screening for antibodies. An electrocardiogram is routine in patients 40 years or older. Other indicated tests include pulmonary function tests and arterial blood gases in patients with chronic obstructive pulmonary disease (COPD), measurement of glucose concentrations in

**Table 48–5** Information to Obtain During Preoperative Assessment of Hemostatic Function

Personal medical history
  Abnormal bleeding after minor surgery
  Reoperation for bleeding
  Hematoma requiring drainage
  Blood transfusion
  Gingival bleeding
  Bruising without trauma
Family history
  Same as above
Associated illnesses
  Hepatic
  Renal
  Hematologic
  Nutrition
Drug intake within the last 10 days
  Aspirin
  Anti–vitamin K drugs
  NSAIDs
  Antibiotics

NSAIDs = nonsteroidal anti-inflammatory drugs.

**Table 48–6** Risk Factors for Deep Vein Thrombosis (DVT)

| Strong risk factors | Equivocal risk factors |
| --- | --- |
| Age >50 years | Obesity |
| Immobilization | Varicose veins |
| Previous DVT | Oral contraceptive use |
| General anesthesia | Hormone replacement therapy |
| Major abdominal surgery | Thrombocytosis |
| Pregnancy | |
| Malignant disease | |
| Hypercoagulable state | |
| Tissue trauma | |

patients with diabetes, thyroid function tests in patients receiving thyroid hormone replacement therapy, and liver function tests in patients with a history of excessive alcohol use. Patients with gastrointestinal symptoms such as vomiting and diarrhea should be evaluated for electrolyte abnormalities. These studies can be of great value in understanding baseline organ function and in optimizing a patient for the stress of surgery. They also serve as a baseline reference point if complications arise postoperatively.

## PREOPERATIVE IMAGING STUDIES

Imaging studies may be performed as part of the preoperative evaluation for screening, staging, or diagnostic purposes. Screening chest radiography is commonly performed in patients over the age of 60 years. A chest x-ray film and intravenous pyleogram (IVP) are part of the staging evaluation for patients undergoing radical hysterectomy for cervical cancer. Pelvic ultrasonography and chest radiography are appropriate in a patient with a suspicious pelvic mass. For patients with cancer, additional imaging studies that evaluate the extent of disease, such as computed tomography, may influence the decision to operate and the planned procedure. Routine IVP and barium enema x-ray study in all patients undergoing hysterectomy are not indicated.

Preoperative evaluation is an opportunity to bring patients up to date with screening tests for both gynecologic and nongynecologic cancers. American Cancer Society screening recommendations are shown in Table 48–7. Procedures such as breast biopsy, mastectomy, and colon resection can be combined with gynecologic procedures with little additional risk, given proper perioperative evaluation and preparation.

## CONSULTATIONS

Consultation should be obtained when appropriate. For a patient at risk for cardiopulmonary complications, consultation with an internist, cardiologist, pulmonologist, anesthesiologist, or critical-care specialist may be appropriate, depending on the practice situation. If the diagnosis is in doubt, such as the etiology of a pelvic mass, then consultation from another surgical specialist should be sought. For procedures that overlap specialties and subspecialties, such as incontinence procedures and certain cancer procedures, "turf" issues should never be a factor in deciding on the best treatment plan for a patient. Rather than proceeding, the clinician must find trustworthy colleagues with whom to work and must treat them with respect by consulting them preoperatively, rather than only in the operating room or postoperatively, for assistance in managing predictable or preventable complications. If the consultant informs the surgeon that the patient is not ready for elective surgery and that further testing is recommended, it must be remembered that this is for the benefit of the clinician as well as for the patient.

## PREVENTIVE MEASURES

Mechanical bowel preparation reduces contamination of the peritoneal cavity in the event of spillage and can aid in visualization of the pelvis by reducing gas and stool, particularly in laparoscopic procedures. Antibiotic preparation in combination with mechanical bowel preparation reduces coliform bacterial counts even further and is recommended for colon resection or if there is a high risk of enterotomy. A variety of regimens are described in the literature, including cathartics, enemas, and lavage solutions. Table 48–8 describes one common bowel preparation

Table 48–7  American Cancer Society Screening Recommendations for the Early Detection of Cancer

| Type of Cancer | Test | Age (Years) | Frequency |
|---|---|---|---|
| Breast | Self-examination | 20+ | Monthly |
|  | Clinical examination | 20–40 | Every 3 years |
|  |  | over 40 | Yearly |
|  | Mammography | 40+ | Every Year |
| Cervix | Pap test and pelvic examination | 18+ or at start of sexual activity | Yearly |
|  |  |  | May decrease frequency if 3 consecutive Pap tests are normal |
| Endometrium | Endometrial biopsy | High-risk patients | Physician discretion |
| Colon/rectum | Fecal occult blood | 50+ | Yearly |
|  | Digital rectal exam (DRE) and flexible sigmoidoscopy | 50+ | Every 5 years |
|  | DRE and colonoscopy | 50+ | Every 10 years |
|  | DRE and double-study contrast barium enema | 50+ | Every 5–10 years |

**Table 48–8** Bowel Preparation Regimen for Major Surgery with Possible Large Bowel Resection

| Timing on Day Before Surgery | Step to Take |
| --- | --- |
| Up till 1:00 PM | Regular diet |
| After 1:00 PM | Clear liquids |
| 1:00–5:00 PM | 4 polyethylene glycol electrolyte solution |
| 6:00 PM | Neomycin, 2 tablets orally |
|  | Metronidazole, 2 tablets orally |
| 10:00 PM | Repeat oral antibiotics |
| Midnight forward | Nothing by mouth |

regimen. Randomized studies indicate that most patients may receive bowel preparation safely as outpatients. Inpatient bowel preparation can be justified for elderly patients or those with cardiac instability or pre-existing dehydration.

Intravenous prophylactic antibiotics clearly reduce the incidence of infection after vaginal hysterectomy and most likely have the same beneficial effect for patients undergoing abdominal hysterectomy. The most likely pathogens for gynecologic procedures are enteric gram-negative bacilli, anaerobes, group B streptococci, and enterococci. The chosen drug should be safe, offer good pelvic coverage, be inexpensive, and not be one used for treatment of major postoperative infections. For most patients, a cephalosporin such as cefazolin or cefoxitin will suffice. Ampicillin and gentamicin are recommended for endocarditis prophylaxis in high-risk patients, with vancomycin as a substitute for patients with penicillin allergy.

Perioperative subcutaneous heparin, various types of compression boots, and several of the newer once-a-day low-molecular-weight heparin compounds have been shown to reduce the risk of DVT and pulmonary embolism in a variety of patient populations. In general, the risk of bleeding complications with heparin compounds is about 2%, and these complications are usually minor. Heparin-induced thrombocytopenia is quite rare. Use of compression boots avoids these complications; however, these boots are contraindicated in patients with arterial insufficiency, can impede postoperative ambulation, and may not fit obese patients.

Shaving body hair is not mandatory and should be done in the operating room, if at all. Preoperative showers have not been found to be cost-effective.

These preventive measures offer a good opportunity to exploit the benefits of clinical pathways. Standardization of preoperative testing and preparation helps maintain quality and good outcomes, reduces costs, and improves efficiency.

## CONSENT

Potential complications should be identified and discussed with the patient as part of the process of informed consent. Informed consent always involves a discussion of the indications for the procedure, risks, benefits, and alternatives. Consent can be a relatively straightforward process or a complex one, and it cannot be rushed. The complexity of the consent process is not necessarily related to the risk of the procedure. Although consent can be obtained by a physician-in-training, the operating surgeon should personally review the salient aspects of the consent process with the patient.

# Intraoperative Complications

## HEMORRHAGE

The blood supply to the pelvis is rich, and the extensive collateral circulation in the pelvis can make control of hemorrhage difficult. Gynecologists should know the vascular anatomy of the pelvis and how to open the retroperitoneal space to locate the hypogastric (internal iliac) and uterine arteries. Pelvic surgeons should also know the blood supply of the major pelvic organs, bladder, rectum, and reproductive organs as well as the blood supply of the ureter.

Many of the severe sequelae of hemorrhage can be avoided by planning a quick response. If there is a risk of hemorrhage, such as in complex gynecologic oncology surgery, blood should be typed and screened for antibodies before surgery, and the availability of matched units should be confirmed. The surgeon and anesthesiologist should discuss venous access and place a central line when appropriate. If major vessel injury occurs, the surgeon must make a series of quick and crucial decisions. Ideally, the bleeding is controlled with pressure, packing, or clamps while blood is ordered, a second suction set up, additional venous access is placed, the incision is extended, vascular clamps and sutures are opened, and (if necessary) consultants are called. If hypotension can be avoided, coagulopathy, shock, and end-organ damage may also be prevented. Common sites of hemorrhage include the vaginal cuff angles during hysterectomy, pelvic side wall vessels (in particular hypogastric and obturator veins) during tumor reduction, and the inferior vena cava during lymph node dissection. Arterial bleeding is usually quickly identified and easily controlled with a single well-placed clamp or clip.

Diffuse venous bleeding can be much more difficult to manage because multiple sites may be involved and the more fragile veins can be injured before they are fully exposed making identification difficult. Smaller vessels can be grasped with a vascular pick up and a hemoclip or fine clamp placed. Small venous lacerations can be controlled by precision placement of a series of clips. Larger venous lacerations require suturing with 5-0 or 6-0 vascular suture material such as silk or Prolene. Vessel loops or vascular clamps may be required to obtain control of the bleeding.

If these measures fail and blood loss continues, then hypogastric artery litigation should be considered. This procedure is performed by passing a 0 silk suture around the hypogastric artery a minimum of 2 cm distal to the origin from the common iliac artery. Bilateral hypogastric artery ligation results in an 85% decrease in the pulse pressure distal to the ligation. However, in one obstetric series of 18 patients with postpartum bleeding, just over half the patients still required hysterectomy to control the bleeding. Hypogastric artery ligation is not effective in the special situation of hemorrhage during sacrospinous ligament fixation, as the inferior gluteal artery is the most likely source of bleeding. Clips, packing, or embolization is recommended in this situation.

Unfortunately, bleeding from multiple sites can continue even after bilateral hypogastric artery ligation. Attempts to ligate each bleeder individually will slow down the progress of the operation and increase blood loss. Bleeding of this nature usually occurs only after the surgeon is past the point of retreat. The surgeon must remain calm, get the specimen out, and pack the area for at least 5 minutes. When the packs are removed, the bleeding is inevitably less, and individual sites are more easily seen. In addition, hemostatic materials such as Gelfoam, Surgicel, and thrombin spray will be much more effective.

In extreme situations, the pack cannot be removed. In this situation, several rolls of packing material tied together are left in the pelvis and exit through the vagina or abdominal stab wounds. This pack can then be removed 24 to 48 hours later in the ICU or in the operating room. Although this procedure can be complicated by nerve injury, bowel obstruction, and "empty pelvis syndrome," it is effective in most patients.

## GENITOURINARY TRACT COMPLICATIONS

Cystostomy is a relatively common complication of gynecologic surgery owing to the proximity of the bladder to the cervix and vagina. Cystostomy is usually identified by the presence of urine or the Foley catheter balloon in the pelvis. A small leak can be confirmed by filling the bladder with saline mixed with methylene blue through the Foley catheter. With the bladder opened, urine should be seen ejecting from the ureteral orifices. Intravenous injection of indigo carmine may help in this process. If the injury does not involve the trigone of the bladder, a simple double layer repair with absorbable suture material can be performed. Failure to identify cystostomy or a more subtle form of injury, such as passing vaginal cuff sutures through the bladder base, may result in a vesicovaginal fistula manifested by leakage of urine from the vagina 3 days to 2 weeks after surgery. After repair of a cystostomy, the Foley catheter is left in place for 5 to 7 days. A cystogram can be performed before removal of the catheter to confirm the security of the repair. Laparoscopic cystostomy can be repaired laparoscopically with intracorporeal or extracorporeal knot-tying techniques.

Intraoperative ureteral trauma may be more difficult to identify and manage. The common sites of injury are at the infundibulopelvic ligament, the tunnel under the uterine artery, and the ureterovesical junction. Possible various injuries to the ureter include transection, crush injury, suture ligation, resection of a segment, and ureterovaginal fistula, particularly of the distal ureters during radical hysterectomy (Fig. 48–1). If the ureter is clamped or tied and this is recognized before transection, the clamp or suture should be removed. If the ureter appears viable, with good vascularization and peristalsis, no further action is necessary. If revascularization is tentative, a ureteral stent may be placed for 7 to 10 days. This can be performed by cystostomy or cystoscopy.

If the ureter is actually transected or even a portion resected, the location of the injury will determine the type of repair. Any reanastomosis should be tension free and stented. The bladder and even the kidney can be mobilized to ensure a tension-free anastomosis. A psoas hitch or Boari flap can be used to extend the bladder and compensate for lost ureteral length. If the injury involves the distal ureter, reimplantation should be performed. This technique requires tunneling of the ureter through the bladder wall and suturing the bladder mucosa to the ureteral mucosa (Fig. 48–2).

Ureteroureterostomy is performed when the transection is above the pelvic brim. The reanastomosis is performed with full-thickness 4-0 absorbable sutures over a Silastic stent. Transureteroureterostomy is a rarely performed variation whereby one ureter is anastomosed to the contralateral side because of the loss of a large section of one ureter. This procedure places both renal units at risk for stenosis or infection. An alternative is interposing a segment of ileum between the bladder and ureter. In urgent situations in which time under anesthesia is critical, the cut ureter may be tied off and nephrostomy performed intraoperatively or postoperatively.

Several authors have recently emphasized a cautious approach to ureteral trauma recognized postoperatively. Management with percutaneous nephros-

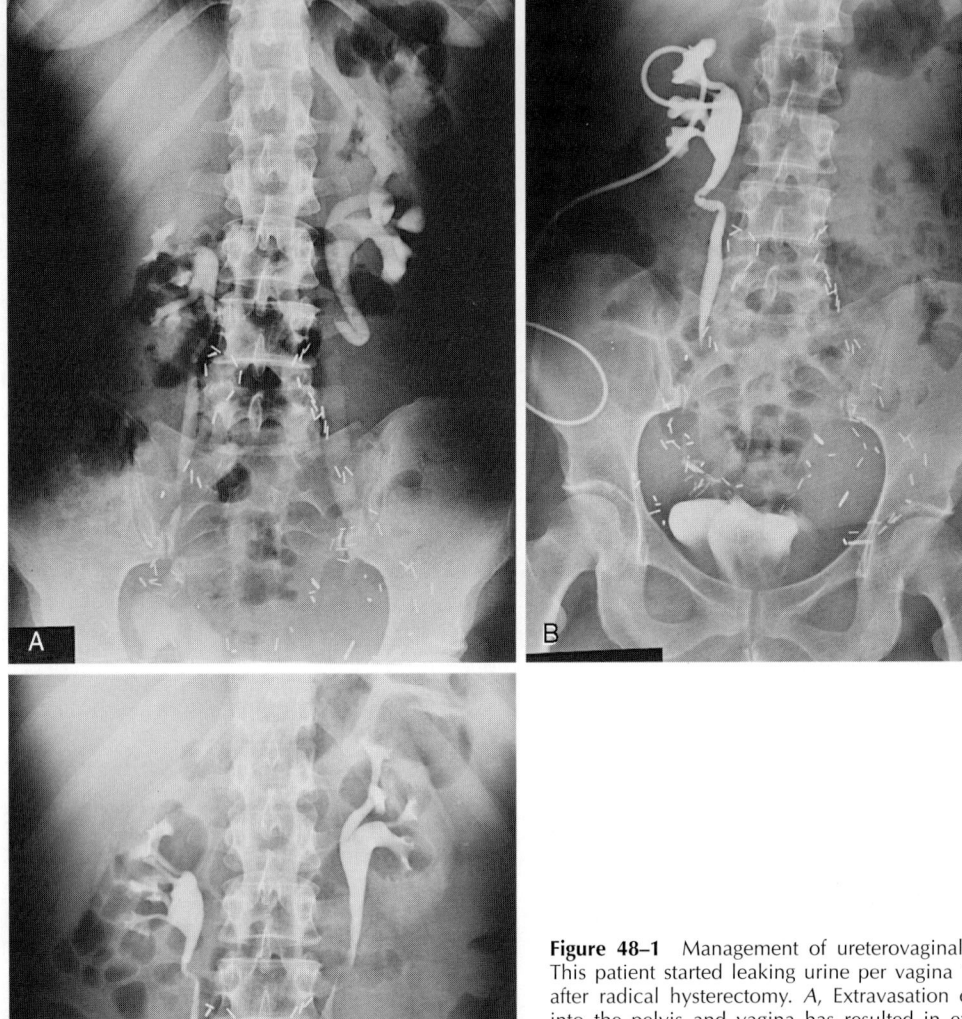

**Figure 48–1** Management of ureterovaginal fistula. This patient started leaking urine per vagina 10 days after radical hysterectomy. *A*, Extravasation of urine into the pelvis and vagina has resulted in extensive soft tissue inflammation and induration. *B*, A nephrostogram several weeks later shows leakage directly to the vagina. *C*, An intravenous pyelogram was performed after ureteroneocystostomy and a psoas hitch was performed 4 months after identification of the fistula.

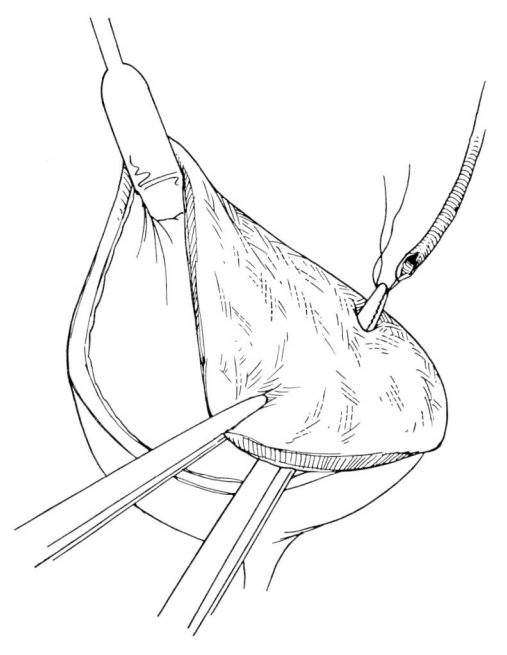

**Figure 48–2** Technique for ureteroneocystostomy. The anastomosis must be tension-free and water-tight. (From Morris M, Burke TW: Surgery of the genitourinary tract in relation to gynecology. *In* Gershenson DM, DeCherney AH, Curry SL (eds): Operative Gynecology. Philadelphia, WB Saunders, 1993, p. 436.)

tomy tubes and retrograde or antegrade stents appears to reduce the need for reoperation, as some leaks may heal with rest and diversion. If reoperation is necessary, the morbidity is reduced compared with immediate attempts at reconstruction as the intense inflammatory reaction to urine in the pelvis subsides.

## GASTROINTESTINAL TRACT COMPLICATIONS

Intraoperative bowel complications are rare in patients undergoing surgery for benign gynecologic indications. When injuries do occur, they are usually related to adhesions from previous surgery, intraabdominal infection, or anatomy distorted by pelvic disease. Under these conditions, the bowel may become fixed in place and vulnerable to traction injuries. When the abdomen is entered through a previous scar, fixation of the bowel to the scar may be encountered. Vigorous traction to separate the fascial edges can tear small bowel loops adhering to the scar. After the abdomen is opened, intraloop adhesions should be taken down to the extent necessary to reach the site of the pelvic disease. Loops of terminal ileum or sigmoid colon fixed in the pelvis can be especially challenging. Gentle traction, countertraction, identification of structures, and, above all, patience are required in these situations.

Serosal injuries to the bowel are common during difficult dissections. Not all serosal tears require oversewing; however, if the mucosa is visible, serosal repair with 3-0 absorbable sutures should be performed. If an enterotomy occurs, the loop of bowel should be fully identified before repair. A single-layer closure of interrupted 3-0 delayed absorbable sutures placed 3 mm apart and perpendicular to the path of the bowel contents is adequate (Fig. 48–3). The small bowel lumen should be about the diameter of a nickel after repair, and the closure should be water-tight.

In the event of colonic injury in a patient who has not undergone bowel preparation, the question of whether a colostomy is needed is frequently raised. The decision is based on the extent of the injury, the volume of fecal spillage, and the general condition of the pelvis. In the event of an extensive injury in the presence of a pelvic tumor or abscess, diversion will reduce the risk of postoperative perforation or fistula. Under more favorable conditions, primary closure with a broadening of the antibiotic coverage is acceptable.

## Postoperative Complications

### FEVER

Fever is a common postoperative finding. A physical examination should be performed that, at a minimum, includes review of all vital signs, mental status assessment, auscultation and percussion of the chest, and inspection of the incision and lower extremities. A pelvic or rectal examination should be performed if there is any suspicion of a surgical site infection or hematoma in the pelvis. The primary goal of this assessment is to separate a fever owing to infection from that owing to other causes such as atelectasis or drug reaction. Fever associated with atelectasis usually

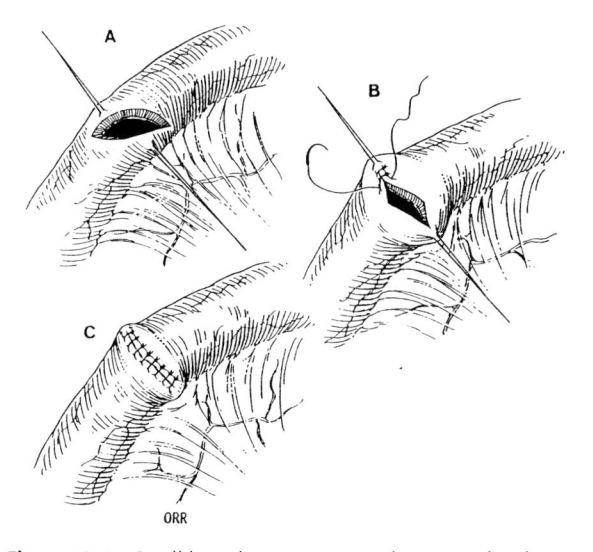

**Figure 48–3** Small bowel enterotomy can be repaired with interrupted 3-0 sutures perpendicular to the direction of the fecal flow to preserve the diameter of the lumen. (From Orr JW Jr, Shingleton HM (eds): Complications in Gynecologic Surgery. Philadelphia, JB Lippincott, 1994, p. 117.)

occurs in the first 24 to 48 hours and is low grade and not associated with other signs of infection. A chest x-ray film usually cannot distinguish between atelectasis and pneumonia in this early postoperative period; however, the study is indicated and can be of great assistance in the evaluation of evolving findings in a high-risk patient. If the clinical diagnosis is atelectasis, the treatment is mobilization, incentive spirometry, and occasionally nebulizers. There is no need for antibiotic therapy at this point.

Conversely, in some situations antibiotic therapy is indicated solely on clinical grounds. Patients with a high fever and shaking chills should be assumed to be bacteremic, and there is no need to wait for culture reports or blood count results before starting antibiotics in this situation.

Fevers that occur 72 to 96 hours after surgery are frequently surgical site infections. "Pelvic cellulitis" is a diagnosis of exclusion. The fever workup will have excluded pulmonary or urinary sources, and there is usually a mild leukocytosis. In this situation, blood cultures are usually negative, and vaginal cuff cultures do not help with antibiotic selection. Patients usually respond promptly to any one of a number of antibiotic therapies. The "gold standard" in this situation is clindamycin and gentamicin as this regimen is inexpensive, is safe in patients with normal renal function, and has broad gram-negative and anaerobic coverage. There are numerous alternatives, such as the newer cephalosporins, ticarcillin and clavulanic acid, sulbactam and ampicillin, and the carbapenems. Clinicians should always be alert to allergic reactions to antibiotics, particularly to penicillins. Vancomycin is the treatment of choice for gram-positive coverage in patients with penicillin allergies.

The pelvis is particularly vulnerable to fluid collections because of gravity and poor drainage. If a patient does not respond to antibiotics, an abscess or infected hematoma should be considered. A bedside digital rectal examination can frequently give a quick answer. Pelvic ultrasonography may also be of use; however, computed tomography of the abdomen and pelvis is the best diagnostic procedure in most situations. A collection with air-fluid levels should be drained; however, infected hematomas usually respond to antibiotics only without drainage. Drainage can usually be achieved with percutaneous placement of a drain by an interventional radiologist, although reoperation is necessary in rare cases.

The treatment of wound infection deserves special note. At times it can be difficult to determine if a patient has a wound cellulitis, which will respond to antibiotics alone, or a true wound infection, which requires drainage and debridement. If cellulitis is the correct diagnosis, improvement should be seen within 24 to 48 hours after beginning antibiotic therapy. If the wound is weeping, fluctuant, or foul smelling, it should be opened, drained, and debrided without delay. Antibiotics may be given, depending on the severity of the infection. The fascia should be carefully inspected. A probe such as a cotton-tipped applicator is insufficient for this purpose; digital probing is required to identify fascial defects. If necrotic fascia is found, it should also be debrided, even when this requires removal of some of the suture material in the wound. Necrotic tissue leads to continued contamination of the wound and inhibition of granulation tissue formation. As long as the peritoneal cavity is not exposed and the wound is clean, it will granulate; even loops of bowel sealing the base of the wound will granulate. A true evisceration is rare with current antibiotic prophylaxis and closure techniques. When it occurs, however, a prompt return to the operating room is needed.

## OLIGURIA

Major abdominal surgery results in numerous changes in the fluid and electrolyte balance of the body. It is difficult to accurately measure fluid losses, including blood loss. Renal blood flow may be altered by hypotension or reduced cardiac function, intrinsic renal function may be altered by any one of a number of pharmacologic agents, and the physiologic response to surgery is fluid retention mediated by an increase in aldosterone and antidiuretic hormone. These factors all help reduce urine output.

Oliguria is usually defined as less than 400 ml urine/day, although another definition for severely ill patients is 0.5 ml/kg/hr. A urine output in the postoperative period of at least 30 ml/hr or at least 120 ml in a 4-hour period is desirable. The causes for oliguria are usually divided into prerenal and postrenal causes and intrinsic renal disease. Prerenal azotemia occurs when renal blood flow is not adequate to excrete the obligatory solute load; the most common cause is intravascular volume depletion. Renal vein thrombosis and renal artery stenosis are much less common causes of prerenal azotemia. Postoperative postrenal obstruction is usually iatrogenic such as bilateral ureteral trauma.

The differential diagnosis of azotemia caused by intrinsic renal disease is quite daunting. In the immediate postoperative period, acute tubular necrosis (ATN) is the most common explanation for oliguria or azotemia in the absence of obvious prerenal causes. In the vast majority of patients, postoperative ATN is caused by hypotension or a nephrotoxic drug; aminoglycosides, NSAIDs, and radiographic contrast material are the most common nephrotoxins. In one study of the causes of ATN, about half the patients had more than one acute insult contributing to the renal injury.

Evaluation of a patient with postoperative oliguria begins with a review of the medical history, preoperative laboratory data, anesthesia record, and medication record. Any pre-existing renal or cardiac dysfunction should be identified and baseline blood urea nitrogen (BUN) and creatinine values reviewed. Possible sources of preoperative dehydration such as outpatient bowel preparation, diarrhea, and vomiting should be reviewed. Complete input and output for the intraoperative and postoperative periods, including losses resulting from ascites or nasogastric suction, should be calculated. The graphic anesthesia record can be quickly scanned for periods of hypotension. Finally, the correct dosing of all drugs should be confirmed and nephrotoxins identified. If there is a central venous catheter in place, the central venous pressure should be measured.

Appropriate laboratory assessment includes hemoglobin (to exclude anemia), BUN, and creatinine. A chest x-ray film may be helpful in documenting fluid overload. Urinary electrolytes can help distinguish the causes of oliguria.

After the medical record and physical examination, are reviewed, the appropriateness of a fluid challenge can usually be determined. Contraindications to a fluid challenge include suspected pulmonary edema or congestive heart failure. The volume of the fluid challenge depends on the patient: a 250-ml bolus may be all that an elderly patient with underlying cardiac dysfunction can tolerate, whereas a youthful patient with adequate organ function reserve can tolerate a 1000-ml fluid challenge. In most situations, a 500-ml challenge of normal saline is acceptable. If a patient is anemic, blood is the best replacement for depleted fluid.

If the patient has signs of fluid overload or has failed to respond to a generous fluid challenge, diuresis should be induced using furosemide; again, the dose depends on the clinical situation. The initial dose of furosemide is usually between 10 and 40 mg, and the vast majority of patients will respond to this dose. Patients who do not respond may require escalating doses. If a patient does not respond, ATN is a strong possibility, and consultation with a renal specialist is appropriate.

Another useful therapeutic intervention is the use of renal doses of dopamine by continuous infusion in the range of 2 µg/kg/min. This results in selective renal vessel vasodilatation and improved renal blood flow and urine output. It is especially useful for patients who have underlying renal disease or other medical problems and who cannot tolerate the large shifts in fluid volume associated with hydration or diuretics.

## SHORTNESS OF BREATH

General anesthesia leads to impaired gas exchange in several ways. Chest wall and diaphragmatic mechanics are compromised, leading to decreased lung volumes and forced expiratory volume. Reduced clearance of mucus and bacteria increases dead space and collapse of the alveolar spaces. The gag reflex is compromised, increasing the risk of aspiration.

Knowledge of preoperative pulmonary function and of the baseline physical examination findings is vital when a patient with shortness of breath is evaluated. A history of heavy smoking, COPD, and obesity increases the risk of pulmonary complications. The results of any preoperative testing should be reviewed. The anesthesia record can help alert the clinician to difficulties with intubation, oxygenation, or compliance during the procedure. The duration of the procedure is also a significant risk factor. A preoperative chest x-ray film is valuable in a patient with postoperative respiratory distress.

Careful physical examination may be of help but is frequently difficult. Ventilatory rate is an important vital sign and the only one not commonly measured with a mechanical device. Astute clinicians frequently measure ventilatory rate themselves and find significant differences from the commonly reported 20 breaths per minute. An assistant may be needed to help turn a patient for auscultation of the complete lung field.

Atelectasis is commonly found in the first 24 to 48 hours and is almost always associated with a fever. The dyspnea and tachypnea associated with atelectasis are usually mild. Bedside pulse oxymetry may show a reduction in oxygen saturation, which will respond rapidly to coughing and incentive spirometry. If atelectasis is suspected, a chest x-ray film is not required before initiating treatment. A symptomatic response and reduction in fever should be seen within 24 to 48 hours after the onset of fever. A chest x-ray film is mandatory if the patient does not respond to first-line therapy.

Initially it can be difficult to distinguish atelectasis from pneumonia on clinical and radiographic grounds. Pneumonia usually occurs after atelectasis. Pneumonia should be suspected in high-risk patients (elderly patients, smokers, patients with a history of COPD, those who underwent long surgery, and obese patients) or when treatment for atelectasis does not control fever. Over half of hospital-acquired pneumonias are caused by gram-negative bacilli such as *Escherichia coli*, *Pseudomonas aeruginosa*, and *Klebsiella pneumoniae*. Sputum cultures should be obtained before starting antibiotics, although they will be useful only if results are positive and the patient does not respond to first-line antibiotic therapy. Third-generation cephalosporins, ticarcillin/clavulanic acid, or imipenem with or without aminoglycosides are all choices for the treatment of hospital-acquired pneumonia.

A small proportion of postoperative patients experience progressive dyspnea, tachypnea, and hypoxemia between 24 and 72 hours after surgery despite treatment for atelectasis, administration of antibiotics and/or oxygen, and careful fluid management. Although pneumonia and pulmonary edema are still in the differential diagnosis, ARDS should be suspected. Once ARDS is part of the differential diagnosis, the patient should be transferred to ICU because (1) close nursing observation is required, (2) respiratory failure and intubation are probable, (3) invasive hemodynamic monitoring is necessary, and (4) the contribution of an intensivist will be crucial to the patient's care. The chest x-ray findings in ARDS and pulmonary edema are the same, and each can be complicated by pneumonia (Fig. 48-4). The primary distinguishing factor is pulmonary capillary wedge pressure (PCWP) measured with a pulmonary artery catheter. The PCWP is elevated in patients with pulmonary edema, which is treated with diuresis and treatment of any cardiac or renal disease. The PCWP is low or normal in patients with ARDS, which is treated with fluid restriction, positive pressure ventilation, and treatment of any identifiable underlying causes such as sepsis. Unfortunately, precipitating causes such as massive transfusion or aspiration of gastric contents cannot be reversed. The mortality rate for patients with ARDS is in the 50% range. This patient population is currently the subject of clinical trials, in particular with various immunotherapies targeted at cytokines such as tumor necrosis factor and interleukins, which mediate endothelial injury in the lung.

In most clinical situations, dyspnea is progressive. However, some patients have truly acute shortness of breath. In this situation, pulmonary embolism should be considered. The classic symptoms of pulmonary embolism include chest pain, hemoptysis, tachycardia, dyspnea, and tachypnea; however, any of these may be the only symptom. The workup in this situation includes an electrocardiogram, blood gas analysis, and chest x-ray study. Hypoxemia in the presence of a normal chest x-ray film increases the suspicion of a pulmonary embolism, and a ventilation perfusion scan should be performed. Unfortunately, ventilation perfusion scans are frequently "indeterminate," and often cannot be obtained on nights and weekends. If a pulmonary embolism is detected, clinicians must decide whether to administer anticoagulants, with the associated risks of bleeding and thrombocytopenia. Massive pulmonary embolism is usually fatal.

## REFERENCES

Alberti KGMM, Thomas DJB: The management of diabetes during surgery. Br J Anaesth 51:693-710, 1979.

Antimicrobial prophylaxis in surgery. *In* Abramowicz M, Rizack MA (eds): Med Lett 34:5-8, 1992.

Barksdale PA, Elkins TE, Sanders CK, et al: An anatomic approach to pelvic hemorrhage during sacrospinous ligament fixation of the vaginal vault. Obstet Gynecol 91:715-718, 1998.

Beck DE, Fazio VW: Current preoperative bowel cleansing methods. Results of a survey. Dis Colon Rectum 33:12-15, 1990.

Burchell RC: Physiology of internal iliac artery litigation. J Obstet Gynaecol Br Commonw 75:642-651, 1968.

Burke TW, Levenback C: Gastrointestinal tract. *In* Orr JW, Shingleton HM (eds): Complications of Gynecologic Surgery: Prevention, Recognition and Management. Philadelphia, JB Lippincott, 1994, p 116.

Caprini JA, Arcelus JI, Hasty JH, et al: Clinical assessment of venous thromboembolic risk in surgical patients. Semin Thromb Hemost 17:304-312, 1991.

The choice of antibacterial drugs. *In* Abramowicz M, Rizack MA (eds). Med Lett 40:33-41, 1998.

Dajani AS, Taubert KA, Wilson W, et al: Prevention of bacteria endocarditis. Recommendatons by the American Heart Association. JAMA 277:1794-1801, 1997.

Doberneck RC, Sterling WA, Allison DC: Morbidity and mortality after operation in nonbleeding cirrhotic patients. Am J Surg 146:306-309, 1983.

Evans S, McShane P: The efficacy of internal iliac artery litigation in obstetric hemorrhage. Surg Gynecol Obstet 160:250-253, 1985.

Finan MA, Fiorica JV, Hoffman MS, et al: Massive pelvic hemorrhage during gynecologic cancer surgery: "pack and go back." Gynecol Oncol 62:390-395, 1996.

Frazee RC, Roberts J, Symmonds R, et al: Prospective, randomized trial of inpatient *vs.* outpatient bowel preparation for elective colorectal surgery. Dis Colon Rectum 35:223-226, 1992.

Gallup DG, Talledo OE, King LA: Primary mass closure of midline incisions with a continuous running monofilament suture in gynecologic patients. Obstet Gynecol 73:675-677, 1989.

Gass GD, Olsen GN: Preoperative pulmonary function testing to predict postoperative morbidity and mortality. Chest 89:127-135, 1986.

Goldman L: Cardiac risks and complications of noncardiac surgery. Ann Intern Med 98:504-513, 1983.

Goldman L, Caldera D, Nussbaum S, et al: Multifactorial index of cardiac risk in noncardiac surgical procedures. N Engl J Med 297:845-850, 1977.

Grossman RA: Oliguria and acute renal failure. Med Clin North Am 65:413-427, 1981.

Hemsell DL: Prophylactic antibiotics in gynecologic and obstetric surgery. Rev Infect Dis 13(suppl 10):S821-S841, 1991.

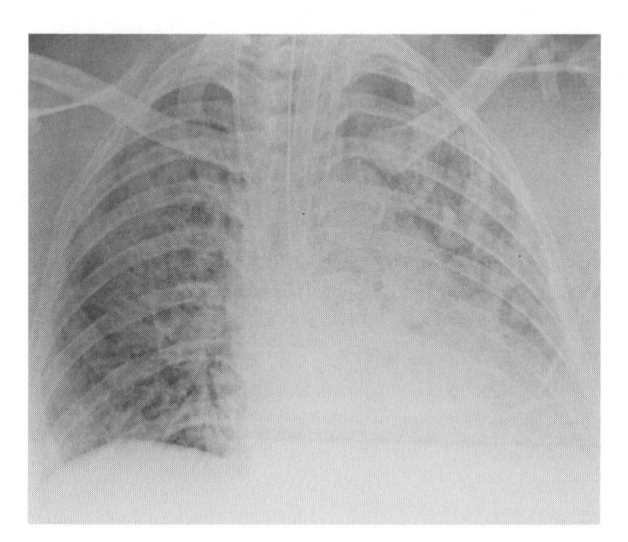

**Figure 48-4** Bilateral fluffy pulmonary infiltrates characteristic of adult respiratory distress syndrome (ARDS) and pulmonary edema.

Jakab F, Ráth Z, Sugár I, et al: Complications following major abdominal surgery in cirrhotic patients. Hepatogastroenterology 40:176–179, 1993.

Klopfenstein CE: Preoperative clinical assessment of hemostatic function in patients scheduled for a cardiac operation. Ann Thorac Surg 62:1918–1920, 1996.

Lask D, Abarbanel J, Luttwak Z, et al: Changing trends in the management of iatrogenic ureteral injuries. J Urol 154:1693–1695, 1995.

Lynch W, Davey PG, Malek M, et al: Cost-effectiveness analysis of the use of chlorhexidine detergent in preoperative whole-body disinfection in wound infection prophylaxis. J Hosp Infect 21:179–191, 1992.

Meirow D, Moriel EZ, Zilberman M, et al: Evaluation and treatment of iatrogenic ureteral injuries during obstetric and gynecologic operations for nonmalignant conditions. J Am Coll Surg 178:144–148, 1994.

Morris M, Levenback C, Burke TW, et al: An outcomes management program in gynecologic oncology. Obstet Gynecol 89:485–492, 1997.

Nezhat CH, Seidman DS, Nezhat F, et al: Laparoscopic management of intentional and unitentional cystotomy. J Urol 156:1400–1402, 1996.

Orr JW, Holloway RW, Orr PJ: Pulmonary complications. *In* Orr JW, Shingleton HM (eds): Complications in Gynecologic Surgery: Prevention, Recognition, and Management. Philadelphia, JB Lippincott, 1994, p 70.

Pearce AC, Jones RM: Smoking and anesthesia: perioperative abstinence and perioperative morbidity. Anesthesiology 61:576–584, 1984.

Prough DS, Zaloga GP: Management of acute oliguria in the elderly patient. Int Anesthesiol Clin 26:112–118, 1988.

Rasmussen HH, Ibels LS: Acute renal failure. Multivariate analysis of causes and risk factors. Am J Med 73:211–218, 1982.

Tisi GM: Preoperative evaluation of pulmonary function. Validity, indications, and benefits. Am Rev Respir Dis 119:293–310, 1979.

Weinmann EE, Salzman EW: Deep-vein thrombosis. N Engl J Med 331:1630–1641, 1994.

Wolters U, Wolf T, Stützer H, et al: ASA classification and perioperative variables as predictors of postoperative outcome. Br J Anaesth 77:217–222, 1996.

# 49

# Gestational Trophoblastic Disease

DONALD PETER GOLDSTEIN
ROSS STUART BERKOWITZ

## Definition

Gestational trophoblastic disease (GTD) originates from placental tissue and comprises a group of interrelated tumors that are classified histologically as complete and partial mole, invasive mole, choriocarcinoma, and placental site trophoblastic tumor (PSTT). PSTT is an uncommon variant of choriocarcinoma composed almost entirely of mononuclear intermediate trophoblasts without chorionic villi. It is well recognized that these conditions have varying propensities for local invasion and dissemination. Even in the presence of widespread metastases, however, they are among the rare human tumors that can be cured with chemotherapy. When persistent GTD develops after evacuation of an hydatidiform mole, the resulting tumor is either an invasive mole, choriocarcinoma, or, on rare occasion, PSTT. The tumor that develops after a term pregnancy or miscarriage histologically is choriocarcinoma or PSTT.

The worldwide incidence of GTD is difficult to determine precisely because of the wide disparity that exists in reporting statistics. Table 49–1 summarizes the incidence of molar pregnancy and persistent GTD after various antecedent pregnancies in the United States.

## Diagnostic Considerations and Strategies

### MOLAR PREGNANCY

Hydatidiform mole may be categorized as either complete or partial on the basis of karyotype, gross morphology, and histopathology (Table 49–2).

### Clinical Presentation

The clinical presentation of complete mole has changed significantly over the past 2 decades. The widespread use of ultrasound and the availability of quantitative human chorionic gonadotropin (hCG) testing are responsible for the shift in the diagnosis of complete mole from the second to the first trimester. Although vaginal bleeding remains the most common presenting symptom, currently patients are diagnosed routinely before the other classical signs and symptoms develop (Table 49–3). Patients with partial mole usually do not present with the dramatic clinical features that in the past were characteristic of complete mole. Most commonly, they present with the signs

**Table 49-1** Incidence of Molar Pregnancy and Persistent Gestational Trophoblastic Disease (GTD) After Various Antecedent Pregnancies

| Antecedent Pregnancy (Incidence : Pregnancy) | Persistent GTD Nonmetastatic (%) | Metastatic (%) |
|---|---|---|
| Complete mole (1 : 1250) | 15 | 5 |
| Partial mole (1 : 750) | 3 | Rare |
| Post-term CCA (1 : 150,000) | 20 | 80 |
| Post-term PSTT (rare) | 90 | 10 |
| Ectopic CCA (1 : 50,000) | 80 | 20 |
| Ectopic mole (rare) | 90 | 10 |
| Postabortal CCA (1 : 5000) | 50 | 50 |
| Postabortal PSTT (rare) | 90 | 10 |

CCA, choriocarcinomas; PSTT, placental site trophoblastic tumor.

**Table 49-3** Classical Signs and Symptom of Complete Molar Pregnancy*

- Uterus >dates
- hCG >100,000 mIU/ml
- Theca lutein ovarian cysts >6 cm
- Preeclampsia
- Hyperthyroidism
- Hyperemesis
- Trophoblastic embolism

*Patients with one or more of these signs and symptoms are at increased risk of development of persistent gestational trophoblastic disease (so-called *high-risk mole*).

and symptoms of incomplete or missed abortion, and the diagnosis is made by the pathologist. However, the current practice of very early uterine evacuation has made the accurate morphologic diagnosis of complete mole more difficult to distinguish from partial mole or nonmolar spontaneous abortion. A delay in the diagnosis of molar pregnancy, either partial or complete, can occur when a viable fetus is present. On rare occasions, a complete mole develops with a coexisting normal pregnancy or partial mole. When the diagnosis is delayed into the second trimester, excessive uterine enlargement, preeclampsia, hyperthyroidism, hyperemesis, and theca lutein ovarian cysts frequently occur in association with very high levels of hCG, often exceeding 1,000,000 mIU/ml.

## Diagnosis

Ultrasound has been a reliable and sensitive technique for the diagnosis of complete mole. Classically, most complete moles produce a characteristic vesicular pattern because the chorionic villi are diffusely hydropic. However, in the first trimester, the sonographer may be unable to differentiate the small molar villi from the degenerating chorionic villi of the hydropic abortus. When there is sonographic ambiguity, the clinician can use the hCG level, which generally increases more rapidly when molar trophoblast is present. Ultrasonography also may facilitate the diagnosis of partial mole by demonstrating focal cystic spaces in the placenta and an increase in the transverse diameter of the gestational sac. Rarely, the sonogram exhibits the classical picture of partial mole by the presence of a fetus with multiple congenital anomalies associated with a focally hydropic placenta.

## PERSISTENT GESTATIONAL TROPHOBLASTIC DISEASE

Persistent GTD is diagnosed when there is clinical, radiologic, pathologic, and/or hormonal evidence of persistent trophoblastic tissue. Although persistent GTD most commonly develops after a complete or partial molar pregnancy, it may occur after any type of gestation. Rarely, the type of antecedent pregnancy cannot be documented.

## Clinical Presentation

Locally invasive or nonmetastatic GTD can develop after any pregnancy but most commonly occurs after molar evacuation in 15% of cases. It is characterized by a plateau or re-elevation of the hCG level and abnormal uterine bleeding. Histologically, the tumor usually consists of invading molar villi, but also can be characterized by choriocarcinoma, or PSTT. Because PSTT secretes very small amounts of hCG, a large tumor burden may be present before hCG levels are detectable.

In approximately 5% of patients with complete mole, metastatic disease develops, which may consist histologically of either invasive mole or choriocarcinoma. Patients in whom GTD develops after nonmolar gestations have a higher incidence of metastases because the histology is that of choriocarcinoma, which has a propensity to invade blood vessels and

**Table 49-2** Comparison of Morphologic and Genetic Features of Complete and Partial Molar Pregnancy

| Features | Complete Mole | Partial Mole |
|---|---|---|
| Fetal or embryonic tissue | Absent | Present |
| Hydropic swelling | Diffuse | Focal |
| Trophoblast hyperplasia | Diffuse | Focal |
| Scalloping of villi | Absent | Present |
| Stromal inclusions | Absent | Present |
| Karyotype | 46XX (90%) | Triploid (90%) |
|  | 46XY (10%) | Diploid (10%) |

disseminate hematogenously early in the course of the disease. The most common metastatic sites are the lung (80%), the vagina (30%), the brain (10%) and the liver (10%). Brain and liver metastases usually develop only when choriocarcinoma is present and generally are considered to be late manifestations of the disease. Because trophoblastic tumors are highly vascular, metastases often present with signs and symptoms of hemorrhage, such as hemoptysis, acute abdominal pain, melena, hematuria, or acute neurologic symptoms.

## Diagnosis and Staging

The optimal management of GTD requires a thorough evaluation to determine the extent of disease before treatment. All patients with persistent GTD should undergo a thorough evaluation, including a complete history and physical examination, baseline hCG levels, complete blood count (CBC) and urinalysis, hepatic, renal and thyroid tests, pelvic sonography, and chest radiography. Because 40% of patients in whom persistent GTD develops after molar evacuation have been shown to have pulmonary micrometastases, a chest computed tomography (CT) scan also may be obtained when readily available. Additional imaging should depend on the clinical presentation. Asymptomatic patients with a normal pelvic examination and chest radiograph are unlikely to have liver or brain metastases.

The International Federation of Gynecology and Obstetrics (FIGO) has recommended an anatomic staging system to standardize data collection and to serve as a guide to proper management (Table 49–4). Stage I includes all patients with persistently elevated

**Table 49–4** International Federation of Gynecology and Obstetrics (FIGO) Staging System for Gestational Trophoblastic Disease

STAGE
 I—Disease confined to the uterus
 II—Disease extending outside the uterus but limited to the genital structures (adnexa, vagina, broad ligament)
 III—Disease extending to the lungs, with or without known genital tract involvement
 IV—Disease at other metastastic sites

SUBSTAGE
 A—No risk factors
 B—One risk factor
 C—Two risk factors

RISK FACTORS
 Human chorionic gonadotropin (hCG) >100,000 mIU/ml
 Duration from termination of the antecedent pregnancy to diagnosis >6 mo

**Table 49–5** World Health Organization Prognostic Scoring System for Gestational Trophoblastic Disease

| Parameter | Score 0 | 1 | 2 | 4 |
|---|---|---|---|---|
| Age (yrs) | <39 | >39 | | |
| Antecedent pregnancy | Mole | Abortion | Term | |
| Interval (mo)† | <4 | 4–6 | 7–12 | >12 |
| Pretreatment hCG (log) | <3 | <4 | <5 | >5 |
| Largest tumor (cm) | | 3–5 | >5 | |
| Site of metastases | | Spleen Kidney | GI Liver | Brain |
| No. of metastases identified | | 1–4 | 5–8 | >8 |
| Previously failed chemotherapy (no. of agents) | | | Single | >2 |

hCG, human chorionic gonadotropin; GI, gastrointestinal.
*The total score for a patient is obtained by adding the individual scores for each prognostic factor. Total score <5 = low risk, 5–7 = medium risk, 8 = high risk.
†"Interval" is the time (mos) between the end of the antecedent pregnancy and the start of chemotherapy.

hCG levels with no evidence of disease outside the uterus. Stage II includes all patients with tumor outside the uterus but confined to the vagina and/or pelvis. Stage III patients have pulmonary metastases. Stage IV includes patients with far-advanced disease involving the brain, liver, kidneys, gastrointestinal tract, and/or other distant foci. The histologic diagnosis in these patients is usually choriocarcinoma, and the antecedent pregnancy is most commonly term. Fatal drug-resistant GTD is encountered almost exclusively in stage IV.

In addition to anatomic staging, a prognostic scoring system has been proposed by the World Health Organization (WHO) to predict the likelihood of drug resistance and assist in the selection of appropriate chemotherapeutic protocols (Table 49–5). When the prognostic score is 8 or higher, the patient is considered to be at high risk for drug resistance, and intensive combination chemotherapy is considered mandatory to achieve optimal results. In general, patients with stage I disease have low risk scores and patients with stage IV disease have high risk scores. The prognostic scoring system appears to be most valuable in those patients with stage II and III disease, for whom the proper selection of the initial chemotherapeutic regimen may be crucial.

There is a strong sentiment among clinicians who deal with these tumors on a regular basis to combine the staging and prognostic scoring systems to more accurately assess the patient's risk of drug resistance and to assist the clinician in formulating a rational treatment regimen. Table 49–6 is an algorithm for the diagnosis and staging of persistent GTD using both the FIGO and prognostic scoring systems.

**Table 49-6** Algorithm for the Staging and Management of Gestational Trophoblastic Disease

```
                    Persistent hCG Elevation
                              ↓
        ┌───── Chest radiograph and/or CT; Vaginal examination ─────┐
        │                     │                                     │
  Chest negative       Chest negative                        Chest positive
  Vagina negative      Vagina positive                    Vagina positive or negative
        │                     │                                     │
        │                     └──────────────┬──────────────────────┘
        │                                    │
        │                              Head/Liver CT
        │                                    │
        │                          ┌─────────┴─────────┐
        │                       Positive             Negative
        │                          │                   │
        ↓                          │                   ↓
    Stage I                   Stage II             Stage III
    Initial-SA                Initial-SA           Initial: LR-SA
    Salvage-Triple            Salvage-Triple               HR-Combination
                                   ↓                 Salvage: Experimental
                              Stage IV
                              Initial: Combination
                              Salvage: Experimental: ? Stem cell transplant
```

hCG, human chorionic gonadotropin; CT, computed tomography; SA, single agent; LR, low risk; HR, high risk.

# Treatment

## MOLAR PREGNANCY

### Surgical Evacuation

When a presumptive diagnosis of molar pregnancy has been made, the patient should be evaluated carefully to identify potential medical complications such as pre-eclampsia; electrolyte imbalance due to hyperemesis; hyperthyroidism, which could lead to anesthetic complications such as thyroid storm; anemia caused by persistent vaginal bleeding; and theca lutein ovarian cysts. Once a patient's medical status has been stabilized, the decision regarding the most appropriate means of evacuation must be made. As aforementioned, this is less of a problem because currently diagnosis of complete molar pregnancy is made earlier, during the first rather than the second trimester, which has led to a marked reduction in the incidence of medical complications. The evacuation of a partial molar pregnancy is usually not a problem because the diagnosis usually is made postfacto by the pathologist after termination of what was thought to be a missed or incomplete abortion. The two situations that still may be associated with a high incidence of medical complications are the second trimester partial mole and a complete mole with coexisting fetus.

Suction evacuation is the preferred method of evacuation, regardless of uterine size, in patients who desire to preserve fertility. When a second-trimester fetus is present, the technique is similar to that used for a late dilatation and evacuation, including preoperative placement of laminaria when feasible. As the cervix is being dilated, the surgeon may encounter brisk uterine bleeding due to the passage of retained blood. Shortly after commencing suction evacuation, uterine bleeding usually is well controlled and the uterus rapidly involutes. If the uterus is larger than 14 weeks' size, it is advisable to massage the fundus during the procedure. An oxytocin drip should be started at the onset of cervical dilatation. The diameter of the cannula used should coincide with the uterine size. It is advisable to explore the uterine cavity with a sharp curette after suctioning to ensure complete removal of chorionic tissue. Excessively vigorous curettement should be avoided, however, because of the risk of endometrial damage, which can result in uterine synechia. Rh-D–negative patients should receive Rh immune globulin.

Acute respiratory distress due to massive trophoblastic pulmonary embolization is a rare but potentially life-threatening complication that can develop within minutes or hours after evacuation of large moles. This usually is a self-limiting condition that clears spontaneously in 72 to 96 hours. Pulmonary embolization and congestive heart failure due to excessive fluid load should be ruled out or treated empirically. In most instances, however, careful monitoring of oxygen saturation is all that is required. The use of a ventilator may be necessary when spontaneous resolution is delayed.

If the patient no longer desires to preserve fertility, a gravid hysterectomy may be the optimal method of evacuation, particularly in patients older than 40 years of age who are at increased risk of developing persistent GTD. Decompression of large theca lutein cysts can be carried out at the time of surgery. Trophoblastic embolization also has been encountered in patients who undergo hysterectomy for large complete moles and invasive moles. When hysterectomy is contemplated, counsel the patient that although removal of the uterus eliminates the risk of invasive disease, it does not prevent metastases that may have occurred before surgery.

### Natural History of Molar Pregnancy

Uterine invasion and metastases occur in 16% and 6% of patients, respectively, after evacuation of complete mole. The risk of persistent GTD is much higher in patients who manifest signs of marked trophoblastic growth, including hCG levels greater than 100,000 mIU/ml, uterine size larger than expected for date of gestation, and theca lutein cysts larger than 6 cm. An increased risk of postmolar GTD, also has been observed in women older than 40 years of age. The incidence of postmolar tumor has not been affected by earlier diagnosis. In contrast, the risk of locally invasive disease developing in a patient with partial mole is only 3%, and metastases are quite rare.

### Prophylactic Chemotherapy

The use of chemotherapy at the time of evacuation of complete mole to reduce the incidence of persistent GTD remains controversial. Both methotrexate and actinomycin D have been shown to reduce the risk of postmolar GTD in patients who present with high-risk complete moles characterized by a larger-than-dates uterus, theca lutein ovarian cysts, and markedly elevated hCG levels. Chemotherapy also has been used prophylactically in women older than 40 years of age in whom postmolar tumor is more likely to develop. The greater awareness by clinicians of the importance of hCG testing has reduced the necessity for the use of chemoprophylaxis.

### Hormonal Follow-Up

After molar evacuation, all patients should be observed with weekly hCG measurements until they are normal for 3 consecutive weeks and then monthly for at least 3 months. Follow-up for longer than 3 months may not be essential because persistent GTD can be detected within that period of time in virtually all instances. Patients are encouraged to use effective contraception during the entire interval of follow-up. In this regard, birth control pills or medroxy progesterone acetate (Depo-Provera) injections may be safely prescribed immediately, but intrauterine devices should not be inserted before the hCG level becomes undetectable because of the risk of uterine perforation or bleeding if tumor is present. Any plateau in the hCG level for 3 or more weeks, or re-elevation, is sufficient evidence on which to base a diagnosis of persistent GTD and initiate treatment.

Pregnancy may be undertaken after the hCG level has been undetectable for at least 3 months. After treatment for either a partial or complete mole, patients can anticipate normal reproductive function except for a 1% risk of another mole developing. For this reason, we recommend that an ultrasound be performed in the first trimester of any subsequent pregnancy to confirm the presence of a healthy fetus. We also recommend that an hCG test be performed at the time of the 6-week postpregnancy check-up to exclude occult GTD.

## PERSISTENT GESTATIONAL TROPHOBLASTIC DISEASE

### Stage I (Nonmetastatic)

Single-agent chemotherapy is the preferred treatment in patients with stage I disease who want to preserve fertility (Table 49–7). Primary single-agent chemotherapy with either methotrexate or actinomycin D (or both used sequentially) induced complete remission in more than 90% of patients at the New England Trophoblastic Disease Center (NETDC) (Table 49–8). The remaining resistant patients subsequently achieved remission with either combination chemotherapy or surgical intervention with either local resection or hysterectomy. Patients with locally invasive tumor who are resistant to either single-agent or combination chemotherapy and want to preserve fertility are candidates for local resection. When local resection is contemplated, magnetic resonance imaging (MRI) scanning of the uterus may be used to determine the precise size and location of the tumor.

Courses of chemotherapy in most centers are administered at set intervals of 1 to 3 weeks on the basis of the protocol selected until the hCG level becomes undetectable. An alternative method, which we have found to be equally effective, consists of administering a course of chemotherapy and then monitoring the hCG levels weekly. Further therapy is withheld

**Table 49–7** Protocols for the Management of Stage I Gestational Trophoblastic Disease

INITIAL THERAPY

Methotrexate with folinic acid rescue as follows:

Methotrexate, 1 mg/kg, IM or IV on d 1, 3, 5, 7, and folinic acid, 0.1 mg/kg, PO on d 2, 4, 6, 8

or

Methotrexate, 100 mg/m² in 250 ml normal saline IV followed immediately by a 12-hr IV infusion of 200 mg/m² with folinic acid rescue; folinic acid rescue is administered as 15 mg PO q12hr × 4 doses to start 24-hr after commencement of methotrexate administration

SEQUENTIAL THERAPY (OR AS PRIMARY THERAPY IF HEPATOTOXICITY IS PRESENT)

Dactinomycin 12 μg/kg IV bolus qd × 5

SALVAGE THERAPY

Triple therapy as follows:
- Methotrexate with folinic acid rescue (as above)
- Dactinomycin D 12 μg/kg IV bolus qd × 5
- Cyclophosphamide 3 mg/kg IV bolus qd × 5

---

as long as the hCG level continues to decrease. We consider a one log (10-fold) decrease in the hCG level as indicative of tumor sensitivity to the chemotherapy agent. If the response is inadequate, then drug resistance is assumed and another agent is substituted. Complete remission is defined as three consecutive weekly undetectable hCG levels. At this point, no further therapy is administered and the patient is observed with monthly hCG tests for 1 year before pregnancy is permitted. We encourage the use of oral contraceptives during this time. We do not use consolidation therapy in postmole patients but do administer at least two additional courses of chemotherapy after the first normal hCG value in patients with nonmolar disease (i.e., choriocarcinoma) in whom the risk of relapse is increased.

**Table 49–8** Results of Treatment of Stage I Gestational Trophoblastic Disease—New England Trophoblastic Disease Center (7/65–12/96)

| Remission Therapy | % | (No. of Patients) |
|---|---|---|
| **Initial** | 93.5 | (441) |
| Sequential single agent | 91.6 | (404) |
| Hysterectomy | 6.6 | (29) |
| Other | 1.8 | (8) |
| | 100 | (441) |
| **Salvage** | 6.5 | (35) |
| Triple therapy | 85.7 | (30) |
| Hysterectomy/local resection | 11.4 | (4) |
| Other | 2.9 | (1) |
| | 100 | (35) |

Patients who no longer wish to preserve fertility may be treated with hysterectomy and adjuvant single-agent chemotherapy. Adjuvant therapy is recommended in this situation for three reasons: (1) to reduce the likelihood of disseminating viable tumor cells at surgery, (2) to maintain a cytotoxic level of chemotherapy in the blood stream and tissues in case viable tumor cells are disseminated at surgery, and (3) to treat any occult metastases that already may be present. Chemotherapy has not been shown to increase postoperative complications.

## Stages II and III

The NETDC protocols for the management of stage II and III patients are summarized in Tables 49–9 and 49–10. In general, single-agent chemotherapy induced complete remission in more than 80% of patients with low-risk disease (WHO prognostic score <8). Conversely, high-risk patients require combination chemotherapy to achieve similar results. Patients resistant to the primary agents used in most instances respond to the salvage therapy.

Vaginal metastases may bleed profusely, and there-

**Table 49–9** Protocols for the Management of Stages II and III Gestational Trophoblastic Disease—New England Trophoblastic Disease Center (7/65–12/96)

LOW RISK (WHO SCORE <8)

| | |
|---|---|
| Initial therapy | Sequential single agent |
| Salvage therapy | Triple therapy as follows: |
| | MAC = methotrexate, dactinomycin, cyclophosphamide, or |
| | EMA = methotrexate 100 mg/m² IV on d 1 followed immediately by a 12-hr IV infusion of 200 mg/m² with folinic acid rescue on d 2 and 3, dactinomycin 12 μg/kg IV bolus on d 1 and 2, and etoposide 100 mg/m² IV infusion on d 1 and 2. Folinic acid rescue is administered as 30 mg PO or IM q12hr × 6 doses starting 32 hr after commencement of methotrexate. |

HIGH RISK (WHO SCORE = OR >8)

| | |
|---|---|
| Initial therapy | Combination chemotherapy—EMA/CO or EMA/EP |
| | EMA/CO = EMA on d 1 and 2 and then vincristine 1 mg/m² IV and cyclophosphamide 600 mg/m² IV on d 8. Each cycle is repeated every 14 d. |
| | EMA/EP = EMA on d 1 and 2 and then etoposide 100 mg/m² and cisplatin 60 mg/m² on d 8. Each cycle is repeated every 14 d. |
| Salvage therapy | Experimental protocols |
| | Possible stem cell rescue |

WHO, World Health Organization.

fore, biopsy should be avoided. Bleeding can be controlled by packing or wide local excision using mattress sutures. Angiographic embolization also can be used when bleeding persists.

Thoracotomy has a limited role in the management of stage III tumors because lung metastases are usually multifocal. If a patient has a solitary pulmonary nodule that persists despite adequate therapy, its removal may obviate the need for more intensive treatment. Before undertaking pulmonary resection, however, a thorough metastatic workup should be instituted. Persistent solitary nodules in a patient with normal hCG levels usually consist of fibrosis and do not require removal.

Hysterectomy sometimes is required in patients with metastatic disease to control bleeding, debulk tumor, or treat sepsis.

## Stage IV

Tables 49–11 and 49–12 summarize the current management of stage IV disease at the NETDC. These patients are at high risk for the development of rapidly progressive disease despite intensive therapy. For that reason, these patients should be referred either to a trophoblastic disease center or to a clinician who has substantial experience with treating GTD. All patients with stage IV disease are high risk for developing drug resistance and should be treated intensively with combination chemotherapy and the selective use of radiation therapy and surgery. Aggressive management in this manner has improved survival from 30% before 1975 to greater than 70% currently.

The management of hepatic metastases is particularly difficult and challenging. Local resection may be required to control bleeding or to excise resistant tumor. Angiographic embolization has shown promise in the management of other types of hepatic metastases tumors and may be applicable here as well.

Cerebral metastases should be treated promptly with either radiation or intrathecal methotrexate in addition to intensive combination chemotherapy. Brain irradiation appears to decrease tumor vascularity and thus reduce the risk of life-threatening hemorrhage. Craniotomy should be performed to manage acute bleeding or to provide acute decompression.

Splenic, renal, gastrointestinal and other metastatic sites may require surgical intervention if patients are symptomatic and/or resistant to drug therapy. High-

**Table 49–11** Protocols for the Management of Stage IV Gestational Trophoblastic Disease—New England Trophoblastic Disease Center (7/65–12/96)

**INITIAL THERAPY**

- Combination chemotherapy (EMA/CO or EMA/EP)
- Brain metastases should be treated with whole head irradiation (3000 cGy)
- Craniotomy may be required to manage complications
- Liver metastases may require resection to manage complications
- Hysterectomy is indicated for bulk disease, infection, and hemorrhage

**SALVAGE THERAPY**

High-dose combination chemotherapy with stem cell rescue

EMA/CO, etoposide, methotrexate, dactinomycin, and leucovorin; EMA/EP, etoposide, methotrexate, dactinomycin, and cisplatin.

**Table 49–10** Results of Treatment of Stages II and III Gestational Trophoblastic Disease—New England Trophoblastic Disease Center

| Remission Therapy | % | (No. of Patients) |
|---|---|---|
| **Low risk** (WHO score <8) | 66.5 | (107) |
| Initial | | |
|   Sequential single-agent therapy | 81.2 | (87) |
| Salvage | | |
|   Triple therapy | 19.8 | (20) |
| | 100 | (107) |
| **High risk** (WHO score >8) | 32.5 | (54) |
| Initial | | |
|   Sequential single-agent therapy | 27.7 | (15) |
|   Triple therapy | 55.6 | (30) |
| Salvage | | |
|   Combination chemotherapy | 16.6 | (9) |
| | 100 | (54) |

WHO, World Health Organization.

**Table 49–12** Results of Treatment of Stages IV Gestational Trophoblastic Disease—New England Trophoblastic Disease Center (7/65–12/96)

| Remission Therapy | % | (No. of Patients) |
|---|---|---|
| <1975 | | (20) |
| Initial | | |
|   Sequential single-agent therapy | 83 | (5) |
| Salvage | | |
|   Triple therapy (MAC) | 17 | (1) |
| | 6 | (30%) |
| >1975 | | (18) |
| Initial | | |
|   Sequential single-agent chemotherapy | 2 | |
|   Triple or combination chemotherapy | 2 | |
| Salvage | | |
|   High-dose sequential single-agent chemotherapy | 4 | |
|   Triple or combination chemotherapy | 8 | |
| | 16/18 | (88.8%) |

**Table 49–13** Subsequent Pregnancy Outcome in Patients Treated with Chemotherapy for Gestational Trophoblastic Disease (New England Trophoblastic Disease Center, 1965–1997)

| Total Pregnancies | Live Births | Term Deliveries | Premature Deliveries | Stillbirths | Spontaneous Abortions |
|---|---|---|---|---|---|
| 504 | 375 (74%) | 348 (69%) | 27 (5%) | 8 (1.5%) | 10 (2%) |

dose therapy with either stem cell or bone marrow transplant may be an appropriate salvage therapy in selected patients.

## Follow-Up

All patients with stages I, II, and III GTD should be observed with weekly hCG level tests until they are normal for 3 consecutive weeks and then monthly for 12 months. Pregnancy may be undertaken after 12 months of normal hCG levels. In patients with stages II and III disease, in whom the risk of late relapse is increased, hCG testing should be continued at 6-month intervals for 5 years. If pregnancy ensues in the interim, follow-up is resumed at the 6-week post-pregnancy checkup.

Patients with stage IV disease should be observed at monthly intervals for 24 months before pregnancy is permitted because of the increased risk of late recurrence. Follow-up should be continued at 6-month intervals for 5 years as in stages II and III disease.

## Subsequent Pregnancy

Patients treated successfully for GTD also can expect normal reproductive function subsequent to completion of their follow-up (Tables 49–12 and 49–13). It is particularly reassuring that the frequency of congenital malformations is not increased because chemotherapy is potentially mutagenic and teratogenic.

## REFERENCES

Berkowitz RS, Goldstein DP: Chorionic tumors. N Engl J Med 335:1740–1748, 1996.

Berkowitz RS, Im SS, Bernstein MR, et al: Gestational trophoblastic disease: Subsequent pregnancy outcome, including repeat molar pregnancy. J Reprod Med 43:81–86, 1998.

Berkowitz RS, Goldstein DP: Presentation and management of molar pregnancy. In Hancock BW, Newlands ES, Berkowitz RS (eds): Gestational Trophoblastic Disease. London, Chapman and Hall, 1997, pp 127–142.

Bracken MD: Incidence and etiology of hydatidiform mole. Br J Obstet Gynaecol 94:1123–1135, 1987.

Fine C, Bundy AL, Berkowitz RS, et al: Sonographic diagnosis of partial molar pregnancy. Obstet Gynecol 71:854–857, 1989.

Goldstein DP, Berkowitz, RS: Gestational trophoblastic neoplasms: Clinical principles of diagnosis and management. Philadelphia, WB Saunders, 1982, pp 1–301.

Goldstein DP, Berkowitz RS: Current management of complete and partial molar pregnancy. J Reprod Med 39:139–146, 1994.

Kohorn EA: Staging and assessing trophoblastic tumors: A possible solution to an intractable problem. J Reprod Med 43:33–36, 1998.

Leopold GR: Diagnostic ultrasound in the detection of molar pregnancy. Radiology 98:171–176, 1971.

Mosher R, Goldstein DP, Berkowitz RS, et al: Complete hydatidiform mole: Comparison of clinicopathologic features, current and past. J Reprod Med 43:21–27, 1998.

Mutch DG, Soper JT, Baker ME, et al: Role of computed axial tomography of the chest in staging patients with non-metastatic gestational trophoblastic tumors. Obstet Gynecol 68:348–352, 1986.

Newlands ES, Bagshawe KD, Begent RHJ, et al: Results with the EMA/CO (etoposide, methotrexate, actinomycin D, cyclophosphamide, vicristine) regimen in high risk gestational trophoblastic tumors, 1979 to 1989. Br J Obstet Gynaecol 98:530–557, 1991.

Rice LW, Berkowitz RS, Lage JM, et al: Persistent gestational trophoblastic disease after partial hydatidiform mole. Gynecol Oncol 36:358–362, 1990.

Soto-Wright V, Bernstein MR, Goldstein DP, et al: The changing clinical presentation of complete molar pregnancy. Obstet Gynecol 86:775–779, 1995.

Steller MA, Genest DR, Bernstein MR, et al: Clinical feature of multiple conception with partial or complete molar pregnancy and co-existing fetuses. J Reprod Med 39:147–154, 1994.

World Health Organization Scientific Group on Gestational Trophoblastic Tumors: Technical Report Series No. 692. Geneva, WHO, 1983.

# 50

# Cancer in Pregnancy

WENDY R. BREWSTER

PHILIP J. DiSAIA

The coexistence of pregnancy with malignant disease occurs in approximately 1000 live births and therefore is a relatively rare occurrence. Over the past 30 years, breast and gynecologic cancers have been the most commonly diagnosed cancers during pregnancy. The recent trend of delaying childbearing to the latter portion of the reproductive years will undoubtedly result in an increased frequency of cancer diagnosis in older parturients. It is difficult to conceive of a set of circumstances more stressful for a patient and her physician than the discovery of a malignancy during pregnancy. Such situations give rise to many questions and concerns: Is immediate termination of the pregnancy necessary to ensure a favorable outcome to the mother? Can therapy be safely deferred until fetal viability is attained? Will treatment of the malignancy be detrimental to the developing fetus? Is there a possibility of metastases to the conceptus?

In theory, the hormonal, metabolic, hemodynamic, and immunologic changes that occur during pregnancy may impose many possible adverse effects in the pregnant woman afflicted with cancer. The theoretical concerns are greatest for tumors arising in tissues and organs that are under hormonal control or that respond to hormonal stimulation. The increased vascularity of the breasts and pelvic organs, the enhanced lymphatic drainage of these organs, and the state of immunologic tolerance that characterizes pregnancy could contribute to early dissemination of the malignant process. This hypothetical reasoning has not been substantiated in most instances by clinical data; however, it has often led to erroneous conclusions resulting in a recommendation for therapeutic abortion.

## Pelvic Malignancies in Pregnancy

### CERVICAL CANCER

Cervical cancer is the most frequently diagnosed invasive neoplasm in pregnancy and comprises approximately 25% of all malignancies in pregnant women. It occurs in approximately 1 per 2000 to 2500 pregnancies. On the other hand, nearly 3% of all cervical cancers are found during pregnancy. These statistics underscore the need for careful evaluation of all pregnant women for cervical cancer and its precursor lesions.

As part of every first prenatal visit, the physician should obtain a Papanicolaou smear from both the cervix and lower endocervical canal. Occult malignancies in the endocervix often are not detected if this area is not evaluated with either a cotton-tipped applicator or an endocervical aspirator. A wire brush sampling device should be avoided in pregnancy because of the small risk of rupturing the fetal membranes and the ease with which bleeding can be induced.

Although invasive cervical cancer is an uncommon cause of bleeding in pregnancy, a high index of suspicion will avoid unnecessary delays in the diagnosis of the occasional case. Thus, a careful speculum examination of the lower genital tract to rule out the existence of a friable exophytic lesion is essential to evaluate this complaint. This will also facilitate the diagnosis of other nonobstetric causes of bleeding, such as a cervical polyp and vaginal laceration.

The methods used for diagnosis and treatment of cervical cancer and its precursors in either pregnant or postpartum patients are the same as those used in the nonpregnant patient (Table 50–1). Although the Pap smear is a sensitive screening tool, one should not rely on it to rule out invasive disease in the presence of a suspicious cervical lesion, because up to 30% of invasive cancers can be associated with negative cytology. Thus, a small office punch biopsy of any suspicious lesion should be done even in the presence of a normal Pap smear. The moderate bleeding that ensues can be controlled by the application of Monsel's solution or silver nitrate.

The general philosophy for diagnosis and treatment of intraepithelial neoplasia of the cervix detected during pregnancy is one of careful diagnosis and expectant therapy. The pregnant patient who has an abnormal Pap smear must be colposcopically evaluated. Depending on the experience of the colposcopist, areas of abnormality that clearly are not invasive, such as those with minimal white epithelium without underlying atypical vascular changes, may be observed without biopsy until the postpartum period. Patients with intraepithelial neoplasia of the cervix may deliver vaginally with subsequent reassessment in the postpartum period. Interestingly, many of these patients do not demonstrate persistent intraepithelial neoplasia when re-evaluated 6 weeks' postpartum. Although an explanation for these changes is obscure, it probably results from either spontaneous regression or traumatic loss of the epithelium during the birth process.

When a suspicion of invasion exists during pregnancy based on clinical or cytologic assessment, a carefully directed biopsy of sufficient depth to permit an accurate diagnosis should be carried out. A diagnosis of suspected microinvasion on biopsy must be followed as soon as possible by a cone biopsy to rule out frankly invasive disease. This is the only absolute indication for conization during pregnancy. The performance of a cone biopsy in the pregnant patient is a formidable undertaking with an increased risk of hemorrhage and spontaneous abortion. In reviewing the scientific literature, Hannigan compiled data that showed a 12 to 13% risk of bleeding complications associated with this procedure. To reduce this potentially serious adverse effect, we recommend using six hemostatic sutures evenly distributed around the portio of the cervix close to the vaginal reflection. These sutures effectively reduce blood flow to the cone bed, evert the squamocolumnar junction, and facilitate performance of a shallow cone biopsy with little interruption of the endocervical canal. Because pregnancy itself causes the squamocolumnar junction to be everted, the need for sampling tissue high in the endocervix is limited. The surgical procedure described for pregnancy might be envisioned as excising a "coin" rather than a cone of tissue. The loop electrocautery excision procedure (LEEP) procedure is especially well adapted to excision of a shallow cone of sufficient breadth and depth to permit treatment decisions while ruling out a more extensive invasive process. In the pregnant patient, such a procedure should be done in the operating room rather than in the office setting because of the increased potential for bleeding.

Cervical conization will identify patients with microinvasion whose pregnancy can proceed to term without appreciable maternal risk from those with frank invasion in whom consideration must be given to early interruption of the pregnancy. The Society of Gynecologic Oncologists defines microinvasion or early stromal invasion of the cervix as an invasive cancer that does not penetrate the stroma more than 3 mm below the basement membrane of the epithelium from which the invasive lesion arises, does not manifest vascular or lymphatic invasion, is free of confluent tongues of tumor, and does not extend to the margins of the surgical specimen. By International Federation of Gynecology and Obstetrics (FIGO) staging criteria, these lesions must be less than 7 mm in diameter to qualify as stage IA1. When these histologic criteria for stage IA1 have been met,

**Table 50–1** Recommendations for Management of the Pregnant Patient with Abnormal Cytologic Findings

| Results of Colposcopically Directed Biopsy | Management |
| --- | --- |
| CIN I–III (cytology consistent with CIN) | Deter further diagnostic and therapeutic procedures until 6 wk post partum |
| CIN I–III (cytology consistent with invasive cancer) | Cone biopsy* |
| Microinvasive tumor | Cone biopsy* |
| Invasive cancer | Radical hysterectomy or radiotherapy |

*Proceed to radical hysterectomy or radiotherapy if invasive cancer is present.
CIN = cervical intraepithelial neoplasia.
Modified from DiSaia PJ, Creasman WT: Clinical Gynecologic Oncology. St. Louis, CV Mosby, 1997.

the patient is advised that pregnancy may continue safely to term. Cesarean section is not necessary for this group of patients, and the route of delivery should be determined by obstetric indications. A recommendation for postpartum hysterectomy is not essential in these patients with early stromal invasion if they desire to bear more children and are good candidates for subsequent periodic monitoring.

A second category of microinvasive cancer includes the lesions in which the depth of invasion is between 3.1 to 5.0 mm and the lesion is less than 7 mm in diameter (i.e., FIGO stage IA2). An expectant approach to definitive management may be considered in such patients; however, definitive treatment by modified radical hysterectomy with pelvic lymphadenectomy should be considered after delivery.

The therapy for invasive cervical cancer in pregnancy depends on the stage of disease, the duration of pregnancy, and the patient's desire and religious convictions (Table 50–2). Although many early reports suggested that pregnancy might accelerate the growth of carcinoma of the cervix, more recent studies show that pregnancy has little effect on tumor growth. When pregnant and nonpregnant cervical cancer patients are matched by age, pregnancy is found to have little adverse effect on the overall survival for this disease. In addition, patients with diethyl stilbestrol (DES)–associated clear cell carcinoma of the cervix and vagina diagnosed during pregnancy have a 5- and 10-year survival rate that is not significantly different from that which is reported for nonpregnant women with this diagnosis.

Generally, patients in the first half of pregnancy are advised to undergo definitive therapy immediately, and thus interruption of the pregnancy usually is advised. The exceptions to this philosophy in patients with "early stromal invasion" (stages IA1 and IA2) have already been discussed. Recent studies suggest that treatment delays in patients diagnosed with stage IB cervical cancer even before the 20th week of gestation might not result in a significant reduction in survival. The quality of these studies is limited by the small number of patients and the variability of gestational ages at the time of diagnosis of cervical cancer.

For patients who have passed the 20th week of gestation, therapy may be delayed until fetal viability is reached, unless hemorrhage forces early intervention. Timing of delivery by cesarean section is usually determined by the status of fetal lung maturity. One option of treatment for patients with stages IB and IIA disease is to perform a radical hysterectomy with bilateral pelvic lymphadenectomy at the time of cesarean delivery. Cesarean radical hysterectomy around the 34th week of gestation will usually ensure fetal viability while delaying definitive therapy a maximum of 14 weeks for patients diagnosed during the second half of pregnancy. If studies of fetal lung maturity at that time suggest that respiratory distress syndrome is likely, surgery may be postponed until lung maturity is ensured, with repeat tests done on a weekly basis. Such an approach necessitates careful coordination of efforts between the gynecologic oncologist and the perinatologist to ensure the best possible outcome for both mother and fetus. Implicit in this concept is the need for a neonatal intensive care unit for care of the preterm newborn.

Another option of treatment for patients with frankly invasive cancer is radiation therapy. Whole-pelvis external irradiation must be initiated immediately after the abdominal incision of the cesarean section has healed. Intracavitary radiation can follow, thus allowing time for complete uterine involution and adequate placement of the brachytherapy devices. The basic radiotherapeutic plan used for cancer of the cervix in the nonpregnant patient generally can

**Table 50–2** Suggested Therapy for Cervical Cancer in Pregnancy

| Length of Pregnancy | Stage of Cancer | |
|---|---|---|
| | I–IIA | IIB–IIIB |
| Up to 20 wk | 4500 WP: If spontaneous abortion, 6000 mg/hr brachytherapy or equivalent<br>If no abortion, modified radical hysterectomy<br>*or*<br>Radical hysterectomy with bilateral pelvic lymphadenectomy | 5000 WP: If spontaneous abortion, 5000 mg/hr brachytherapy or equivalent<br>If no spontaneous abortion, type II radical hysterectomy, no lymphadenectomy, and 5000 mg/hr brachytherapy |
| Beyond 20 wk | Cesarean section when fetus viable followed by 5000 WP and 5000 mg/hr brachytherapy or equivalent<br>*or*<br>Cesarean radical hysterectomy with bilateral pelvic lymphadenectomy | Cesarean section when fetus viable followed by 5000–6000 WP and 4000–5000 mg/hr brachytherapy or equivalent |

WP = whole-pelvis irradiation, with number indicating cGy.
Modified from DiSaia PJ, Creasman WT: Clinical Gynecologic Oncology. St. Louis, CV Mosby, 1997.

be used for patients in whom only cesarean section has been performed after uterine involution is completed.

Patients with stages IB and IIA disease can be treated with either surgery or radiation. The question of which is preferable remains the subject of endless debate. There is a lack of conclusive evidence that supports a survival advantage for either of the modalities. The modified radical or Wertheim-type radical hysterectomy at the time of cesarean section carries some advantages in the young parturient. It allows the patient to return home with her infant without needing further therapy, permits preservation of ovarian function, and is associated with less frequent sexual dysfunction than radiotherapy. One of the most common adverse effects of radical hysterectomy is bladder dysfunction. Because some patients might require adjuvant radiotherapy after surgery, bilateral ovarian transposition out of the pelvis is recommended to avoid their ablation. The complication rate of radical hysterectomy with bilateral pelvic lymphadenectomy should not exceed that for nonpregnant patients. Although vascular supply to the pelvis is increased, normal tissue planes are very distinct and facilitate easier pelvic dissection.

Radiation therapy is the treatment of choice for the more advanced stages of cervical cancer. If therapy is begun in the first trimester, spontaneous abortion will generally occur within the first 5 weeks of radiotherapy. Spontaneous abortion usually occurs within 7 weeks of the initiation of therapy if begun in the second trimester. Treatment then is completed with intracavitary or interstitial brachytherapy. If spontaneous abortion does not occur by completion of the external beam therapy, we usually prefer to proceed with a modified radical hysterectomy without pelvic lymphadenectomy to excise the residual central neoplasm. We believe this approach is preferable to completion of therapy with brachytherapy because the gravid uterus is not suitable for intracavitary radium or cesium. This strategy delivers potentially curative doses of radiation to the pelvic lymph nodes, followed by surgical resection of the remaining central tumor. An alternative approach in the patient who has not aborted is to evacuate the uterus by means of a hysterotomy followed by conventional intracavitary irradiation delivered within 1 to 2 weeks.

The prognosis of patients with cervical cancer is a function of stage, tumor volume, and histologic type. The prognosis in patients with either small cell cancer, undifferentiated cancers of neuroendocrine type, or poorly differentiated adenosquamous cancers is dismal.

## OVARIAN CANCER

With respect to malignancies arising from within the pelvis, ovarian cancers are second in frequency to cervical cancer but occur in only 1 in 20,000 to 30,000 pregnancies. The diagnosis of ovarian masses during pregnancy is complicated by their shifting location as the gravid uterus moves out of the pelvis and the difficulty in distinguishing between the consistency of a gravid uterus and an ovarian neoplasm. Additionally, the routine use of ultrasonography to assess fetal development increases the likelihood of finding unexpected ovarian masses and creates the clinical dilemma of identifying subclinical masses that rarely prove to be malignant. In addition to ovarian tumors, the differential diagnosis of a pelvic mass in pregnancy includes a retroverted pregnant uterus, a pedunculated uterine leiomyoma, carcinoma of the rectosigmoid colon, a pelvic kidney, a retroperitoneal mass, and a uterine congenital anomaly such as an accessory uterine horn.

During pregnancy, the complications associated with ovarian masses include pelvic impaction, obstructed labor, torsion, hemorrhage or rupture of the cyst, and, rarely, malignancy. Although malignancy is relatively uncommon in pregnancy, it should always be foremost in the clinician's mind. Torsion of an ovarian neoplasm is particularly common in pregnancy, with a reported incidence of 10 to 15%. Most cases of ovarian torsion occur either when the uterus is growing at a rapid rate between the 8 and 16th weeks of gestation or when the uterus is involuting rapidly during the puerperium. About 60% of the cases of torsion occur in the first half of pregnancy and most of the remaining cases in the puerperium. The presenting symptoms are usually sudden lower abdominal pain, nausea with vomiting, and, in some instances, a shock-like syndrome; the abdomen is often tense and tender. If the ovarian mass obstructs the birth canal during labor, exploratory laparotomy is indicated for both delivery of the infant and management of the ovarian neoplasm. Obstruction of the birth canal during labor by a neoplasm can result in rupture of the ovarian mass followed by hemorrhage, peritonitis, tumor dissemination, or shock. Even if an ovarian cyst does not rupture, the trauma of labor can cause hemorrhage into the tumor followed by necrosis and suppuration.

Most ovarian masses found in early pregnancy are corpus luteum cysts and usually are no more than 5 cm in diameter. With expectant management, more than 90% of these functional cysts disappear as pregnancy progresses and are undetectable by the 14th week of gestation. Guidelines for the management of an ovarian mass during pregnancy are similar to those generally recommended in the nonpregnant premenopausal woman. If a cyst remains unchanged or increases in size during a 6- to 8-week observation period, the patient should undergo abdominal exploration. For solid ovarian masses of any size or cystic enlargement more than 8 cm in diameter, an observation period is not required before surgical intervention because such masses usually are neoplastic. Experience has showed that fetal wastage can be minimized with laparotomy performed between 18 and 20 weeks of gestation.

In the asymptomatic patient with a pelvic mass who on the basis of ultrasonography findings and physical examination is presumed to be at low risk for a malignancy, it is prudent to delay operative intervention until the second trimester. This approach permits the spontaneous resolution of a probable functional cyst and minimizes the risk of interfering with the pregnancy. We have advocated the "no touch technique" at laparotomy where there is a concerted effort made to avoid contact with the uterus. This seems to decrease uterine irritability in the postoperative period. Some authors have reported up to a fivefold increase of second trimester pregnancy loss associated with operative intervention for a pelvic mass. We have not experienced this adverse effect of operative intervention when surgery is performed between 18 and 22 weeks and believe that the benefits of earlier cancer diagnosis and prevention of subsequent complications outweigh the risks of operative intervention.

In the patient with a mass that is suspicious for malignancy, diagnostic studies, an ultrasonography of the abdomen and pelvis, and/or magnetic resonance imaging should be performed to look for ascites or metastases. If clinically indicated, a limited barium enema can be done to rule out colonic cancer; if possible this radiologic study should be avoided, especially during the first trimester of pregnancy, to prevent the potential mutagenic effects of ionizing radiation to the developing fetus during organogenesis. Abdominal examination is unreliable even when ascites is present because of the large uterus.

Epithelial ovarian cancers (serous, mucinous, endometrioid, and clear cell adenocarcinomas) account for nearly half of malignant ovarian neoplasms diagnosed in pregnancy. Characteristically, these tumors are of early stage and low grade; indeed, many epithelial cancers of the ovary during pregnancy prove to be tumors of low malignant potential (LMP). If the surgeon finds an ovarian malignancy in pregnancy, treatment should be appropriate for the stage of disease. The first priority is to stage the patient's disease properly (refer to Chapter 11). The exploration should be performed through a midline or paramedian incision extending above the umbilicus. The operative procedure should include collection of peritoneal fluid or washings for cytologic evaluation, visualization of the liver and diaphragm, biopsy of the omentum and peritoneum in the pelvis and pericolic areas, and careful evaluation of the pelvic and periaortic lymph nodes.

Patients with stage IA epithelial ovarian cancers may be treated conservatively with a unilateral salpingo-oophorectomy, provided a thorough staging and exploration of the abdominal cavity has been carried out. More advanced epithelial lesions should not be treated conservatively unless they are LMP tumors, in which case definitive surgical therapy can be deferred until fetal viability is achieved. The decision regarding the degree of surgical intervention, which might include hysterectomy while the fetus is still immature, ultimately rests with the patient and her desire to continue the pregnancy. It is extremely important that thorough preoperative counseling of the patient concerning all possible findings is completed by the surgeon.

Germ cell tumors are common ovarian neoplasms in pregnancy; these include dysgerminoma, embryonal carcinomas, immature teratomas, endodermal sinus tumors, and mixed germ cell tumor. Dysgerminomas are the most commonly reported of all malignant germ cell tumors, and mature teratomas are the most common benign neoplasms found in pregnancy. Malignant germ cell neoplasms usually present as stage IA and can be managed with a unilateral salpingo-oophorectomy and staging biopsies. However, most patients would require postoperative combination chemotherapy (except for stage I dysgerminomas and stage I grade 1 and 2 immature teratomas). In addition, these tumors are very chemosensitive, and cure rates are high with such therapy. Therefore, when a malignant ovarian germ cell tumor is diagnosed during the first or second trimester, the patient and her physician are faced with difficult treatment choices, including interrupting the pregnancy and initiating chemotherapy immediately, preserving the pregnancy and beginning chemotherapy with the fetus in situ, or preserving the pregnancy and delaying chemotherapy until the fetus is either more mature or is delivered. The third of these options is the least acceptable; it is well known that these tumors are very aggressive and progress rapidly if left untreated. Therefore, a delay in therapy might endanger the patient's life.

The option of preserving the pregnancy and giving chemotherapy is complicated by the fact that very limited data are available regarding the effects of chemotherapy on the fetus. Although retrospective studies have not shown a significant increased incidence of congenital anomalies in patients treated in the second and third trimesters, many of the newer agents have not been used extensively in pregnancy.

Because of the uncertain effects of chemotherapy in the second and third trimester of pregnancy and the risk of early recurrence of cancer in the patient for whom adjuvant chemotherapy is delayed for several months, the patient and her family must be counseled carefully concerning the risks vs. benefits of all treatment options. The best available data suggest that the fetal risk of antineoplastic agents when initiated after the first trimester is small, and continuation of the pregnancy probably will not result in congenital malformations. Nevertheless, many patients and their families are unwilling to face the uncertainties associated with a continued pregnancy.

Patients with stage I ovarian dysgerminoma have an excellent prognosis after surgery alone. Because of the risk of lymphatic spread, surgery should consist of unilateral adnexectomy and optimal staging, including both pelvic and periaortic lymph node sampling. Emergency surgical intervention and obstetric complications are commonly reported in patients with dysgerminomas. Karlen and associates reviewed 27 cases of dysgerminoma associated with pregnancy. Obstetric complications occurred in almost 50% and fetal demise in 25%. Torsion and incarceration were found commonly in this group of patients whose neoplasms averaged 25 cm in diameter.

When granulosa-theca cell tumors and Sertoli-Leydig cell tumors are found in pregnancy, it is recommended that these are managed conservatively as in the young nonpregnant patient because these usually are neoplasms with low malignant potential and typically present as stage I disease.

In summary, diagnosing and treating a pregnant woman with an ovarian tumor is a complex matter for the clinician, the solution of which often is not clearcut. The difficulty arises when both patient and physician resist an abdominal exploration during pregnancy because of the fear of precipitating fetal loss. We believe that the potential danger to the mother of a delay in diagnosis and treatment exceeds the risk to the fetus. Most dangers seen with ovarian tumors are those created by acts of omission rather than of commission. The possibility of ovarian cancer must be kept foremost in the minds of physicians caring for pregnant patients, and any adnexal mass in pregnancy persisting after the 18th week of gestation, excluding thin-walled unilocular cysts, should be surgically removed.

## BLADDER CANCER

Carcinoma of the bladder is seen most frequently after the childbearing years but occasionally is diagnosed in pregnancy. Ninety-five percent of cases are transitional cell carcinomas, starting in the region of the trigone and spreading by direct extension via the lymphatic system or by hematogenous route to regional and distant sites. The prognosis is directly related to the extent of disease and grade of tumor. Well-differentiated superficial lesions can be managed by either local fulguration, intravesical chemotherapy, or BCG. The more advanced or aggressive cancers require partial or total urinary bladder removal with lymphadenectomy to facilitate a cure. Radiation therapy also has been used with curative intent, but a gravid uterus can complicate this situation markedly. Neither bladder removal nor pelvic irradiation is appropriate during pregnancy if the patient wishes to ensure fetal viability. Scattered attempts at surgical extirpation with preservation of the pregnancy have resulted in high rates of fetal wastage. The mode of delivery of the fetus must be individualized according to the length of gestation and patient and physician preference.

## COLORECTAL CANCER

Colon cancer is a rare complication in pregnancy, with a reported frequency of 1 in 50,000 to 100,000 pregnancies. Sixty percent of all colorectal cancers are found in the distal colon and rectum. This distribution is not affected by the age of the patient or her pregnancy status. A delay in diagnosis can occur because rectal bleeding, which often provides the first clue, is commonly ascribed to hemorrhoids, a frequent complaint during pregnancy.

When colorectal cancer is diagnosed in the first trimester of pregnancy, it generally should be treated as in nonpregnant patients. Radical surgery at this stage frequently is followed by abortion, and simultaneous hysterotomy should be considered seriously. The fallopian tubes, ovaries, and uterus should be resected if metastases or tumor fixation to these areas is found. Oophorectomy is recommended for all low-lying colonic tumors because of the high incidence of metastatic disease to the ovaries; at times, occult metastases are found even in the normal-appearing ovary. In 1968, Barber and Brunschwig advocated routine hysterectomy between 10 and 20 weeks of gestation to provide better exposure for adequate margins in resection. The treatment of colorectal cancer during the third trimester remains controversial. Some surgeons believe that with adequate exposure the cancer can be removed without disturbing the uterus and its contents. Others hold that resection should be carried out 2 weeks after cesarean section, at which time the patient has regained her strength and the uterus and pelvic vasculature are less troublesome to the surgeon. The principles of en bloc dissection of the tumor and its lymph nodes and wide margins of tumor-free tissue are as necessary during pregnancy as in the nonpregnant state.

Unfortunately, the gravid uterus presents technical problems of exposure deep in the pelvis that can necessitate modifying the usual operative approach. Occasionally, hysterotomy or hysterectomy must be performed to facilitate exposure. Colon cancer in young patients has a poor survival rate compared with postmenopausal women. The young pregnant patient has equivalent prognoses, stage for stage, as nonpregnant patients.

## Extrapelvic Malignancies in Pregnancy

### MELANOMA

Melanomas account for 8% of cancers in pregnancy. It has been speculated that malignant melanoma may be one of the few malignancies that pregnancy adversely affects. In fact, pregnancy is associated with increased adrenocorticotropic hormone (ACTH) production, resulting in heightened intrinsic melanocyte-stimulating hormone (MSH) activity. In addition, MSH secretion by the pituitary gland increases after the second month of pregnancy. As a result, increased skin pigmentation is characteristic of pregnancy and is observed in the nipple, vulva, linea nigra, and, on occasion, in pre-existing nevi. Despite these physiologic changes, retrospective studies have not shown any therapeutic benefit of abortion or oophorectomy in the management of the pregnant patient diagnosed with melanoma.

All melanomas masquerade as nevi before their diagnosis. Pigmented lesions with irregular borders or surface contour and those that have undergone enlargement or a color change must be excised to rule out the presence of a melanoma. Variations in the color of a lesion should lead the clinician to be suspicious. Shades of red or pink suggest inflammation, whereas a bluish hue may result from pigmented cells within the dermis, both conditions suggesting a malignant diagnosis. A policy of waiting and watching a suspicious pigmented lesion may be detrimental, because early excision of a melanoma often is lifesaving.

There are conflicting data regarding the biologic behavior of melanomas diagnosed during pregnancy. There are some reports in the literature that suggest that malignant melanomas are thicker in pregnant vs. nonpregnant women, which is a poor prognostic factor in itself. This finding might be explained by longer delays in diagnosis of malignant melanoma during pregnancy compared with the nonpregnant state because of the hyperpigmentation commonly associated with pregnancy. White and associates reported a study of 71 women between 15 and 30 years old with melanomas, 30 of whom were pregnant. The 5-year survival rate in the pregnant patients was 73%, whereas that in the nonpregnant patients was 53%. The authors concluded that differences in survival were not significant between the two groups. George and associates compared the outcome of 115 pregnant women with melanoma in pregnancy with 330 nonpregnant patients. They reported that spread to regional nodes might be more rapid in the pregnant patient, but stage for stage, there was no significant difference in the outcomes between the two groups. Grin and associates reviewed five well-controlled case studies comprising 427 women diagnosed with malignant melanoma, most of whom had stage I disease. All five studies showed no adverse effect of pregnancy on overall survival; however, among women who recurred there was a reduced disease-free survival in the pregnant women reported in three studies.

The frequent recommendation that women delay conception for 2 years after treatment for malignant melanoma is based mainly on the time during which recurrences are most likely to be identified. Two case-controlled studies by Reintgen and associates and MacKie and associates failed to identify any difference in the disease-free survival or overall survival in women with stage I melanoma who became pregnant within 5 years of diagnosis of their cancer.

Metastasis of maternal cancers to products of conception is rare despite the significant number of pregnancies that are at risk. This is partly due to an unexplained resistance of the placenta to invasion by maternal malignancies as shown in many animal models. In a comprehensive review of the subject by Dildy and associates, only 53 cases of malignancy metastatic to the products of conception were reported between 1966 and 1987, including 12 that metastasized to the fetus. Although melanoma accounts for only 8% of cancers associated with pregnancy, they are responsible for 30% of all tumors metastasizing to the placenta and more than half of metastasizing tumors to the fetus.

### BREAST CANCER

Breast cancer complicates 1 of 3500 to 10,000 pregnancies. It is estimated that 1 to 2% of patients with breast cancer are pregnant when diagnosed, constituting a difficult challenge in counseling and treatment. Pregnant patients tend to present with a larger primary tumor and a higher incidence of positive nodes than nonpregnant patients and thus tend to have a poorer prognosis. Conversely, patients with negative nodes in pregnancy have a prognosis similar to that of nonpregnant patients with early-stage disease. The more advanced stage of disease in most pregnant patients has been attributed to multiple factors. The breast engorgement typical in pregnancy can delay the diagnosis by obscuring a mass for many months. Additionally, there is increased vascularity and lymphatic drainage from the breast in pregnancy, which potentially might assist the metastatic disease process. The major factor influencing the tendency for advanced disease at presentation in pregnancy has been conclusively attributed to the young age of the patient population. Breast cancer is a more aggressive disease in the young, and pregnant patients are usually young.

Obstetricians more than any other physicians have the opportunity to detect breast cancer early in pregnancy through regular examinations and indirectly by educating patients in self-examination. Needle aspiration of masses or ultrasonography will distinguish a cyst or galactocele from a solid tumor. If bloody fluid is obtained, it should be examined cytologically. For solid masses, the sensitivity of fine-needle aspiration (FNA) cytology during pregnancy ranges between 50 and 95%. Core needle biopsy with stereotactic guidance or excision biopsy should be done on masses from which fluid cannot be aspirated and on suspicious masses in which FNA cytology is nondiagnostic.

Pregnancy does not appear to augment the rate of growth or spread of breast cancer, and abortion does not improve the prognosis. Initial treatment usually is surgical if the pregnancy is allowed to continue and can consist of radical, modified radical, or simple mastectomy, depending on the extent of disease and the histologic type of tumor. Lumpectomy and quadrantectomy rarely are used because the lesions usually are large with less well-defined clinical margins than in the nonpregnant patient. The more extensive operations are tolerated well during pregnancy, and the results of treatment are much the same, stage for stage, as in the nonpregnant state.

Despite the trend toward limited surgery combined with radiotherapy for breast conservation, this approach should not be used in pregnancy because the dose to the fetus from radiation scatter would be unacceptably high. Even in early pregnancy, when the distance between the breast and uterus is the greatest, radiation scatter to the fetus might be 10 to 20 rad for the total treatment course. This dose is unacceptable in early pregnancy during organogenesis. Later in pregnancy, when the fundus approaches the xiphoid process, 100 rad or more might be delivered to the fetus.

Optimal treatment of breast cancer during pregnancy is confusing because of a lack of controlled studies evaluating survival of comparable patients in different treatment groups. Most authorities recommend a radical or modified radical mastectomy without delay in patients with stage I or II and some stage III disease. The extent of surgery in treating advanced breast cancer remains a subject of extensive debate throughout the world. The reported overall survival rate for women diagnosed with breast cancer during pregnancy is poor, reflecting advanced stage of disease at diagnosis in most. Holleb and Farrow reported a series of 283 patients with breast carcinoma in pregnancy; 73 had inoperable disease and 210 received surgery with or without postoperative radiation. Ninety-three percent of patients with inoperable disease died within 2 years of the diagnosis, including all 7 who had undergone interruption of pregnancy. Continuation of pregnancy did not seem to affect survival adversely, with 33% 5-year survival in the group who carried to term vs. 17% in those who underwent abortion. For the small subgroups of patients, these survival differences were not significant. Anderson and associates reported the experience at the Memorial Sloan-Kettering Cancer Center with breast cancer in women younger than 30 years. Two hundred twenty-seven cases were identified, of whom 22 had pregnancy-associated breast cancer. The authors confirmed that pregnancy-associated breast cancers were usually larger and present in more advanced stages at diagnosis than in young women who were not pregnant. The survival probability for women with early-stage disease was independent of the pregnancy status.

Although many clinicians believe that localized breast cancer in the first trimester of pregnancy is a valid reason to recommend pregnancy termination, therapeutic abortion has not been found to increase survival, and the presence of a fetus does not compromise proper surgical management. Thus, we do not believe that pregnancy termination is an essential component of effective treatment of early disease despite the theoretic advantage of removing the source of massive estrogen production. On the other hand, therapeutic abortion is usually necessary for effective palliation in patients with advanced estrogen receptor-positive breast cancers. In the first trimester of pregnancy, this can be accomplished by suction curettage of the uterus; later in pregnancy, termination is accomplished by prostaglandin vaginal suppositories, hysterotomy, or hysterectomy. When the pregnancy enters the third trimester, the decision for premature delivery depends heavily on the patient's wishes and the urgency for treatment. A short wait until the fetus is viable might not be accompanied by significant progress of the neoplasm. Continued gestation represents no threat to the fetus because the risk that cancer will traverse the placenta and metastasize to the fetus is negligible.

Nugent and O'Connell found that only 30% of breast cancers in pregnancy were estrogen receptor positive. It is unclear whether this observation reflects true hormone receptor negativity or whether the high levels of circulating estrogen occupy all available estrogen receptor binding sites, resulting in false-negative receptor assays. The relatively infrequent responsiveness to oophorectomy in patients who develop cancers while pregnant suggests that these tumors frequently are receptor negative. In this situation the pregnant patient with advanced disease might elect to undergo primary chemotherapy without hormonal ablation by abortion plus castration. After the first trimester of pregnancy, the apparent risks of chemotherapy to the fetus are small and pregnancy can be allowed to proceed.

Chemotherapy has been used after the first trimester to palliate advanced disease. Alkylating agents, 5-fluorouracil, and vincristine are relatively safe and have been used while the fetus is still in utero. Methotrexate should be avoided if possible, particularly in the first trimester. The possible role for adjuvant chemotherapy is still uncertain; however, recent reports suggest that combination chemotherapy can significantly improve survival in premenopausal patients when used in an adjuvant setting. The National Institutes of Health currently recommends adjuvant systemic chemotherapy for selected patients, including premenopausal women with axillary node metastases, a category into which most pregnant breast cancer patients fall. These women are most likely to benefit from cyclophosphamide and 5-fluorouracil with either doxorubicin or methotrexate.

As many as 7% of premenopausal women have one or more pregnancies after mastectomy for breast cancer, 70% of which can be expected within the first 5 years after treatment. How should the physician advise the patient who has had a mastectomy for breast cancer about future pregnancies? Should they be avoided? Should they be terminated if they occur? The recommendations should be influenced by two major considerations: whether pregnancy promotes recurrence of cancer and the probability of having achieved a cure. It is generally observed that women who become pregnant after mastectomy survive surprisingly well, far better than those whose pregnancy coexisted with the primary tumor and often better than mastectomy patients overall. This phenomenon of a favorable outcome for patients who became pregnant after treatment for breast cancer might be a function of selection, because most women will wait at least 2 years after treatment, during which many tumors destined to recur will do so. In addition, only women with a good prognosis are likely to achieve counsel recommending subsequent pregnancies. Finally, even though hormonal stimulation by a pregnancy might accelerate a recurrence in a patient with cancer, it is probable that in the pregnant patient whose cancer recurs, the cancer would have recurred eventually even had she not become pregnant. Thus, the issue becomes one of disease-free interval and duration of survival in these patients rather than probability of cure. Although it may be presumptuous to conclude on the basis of retrospective studies that pregnancy protects against recurrence after mastectomy, it is reasonably safe to conclude that it does not increase the risk of recurrence. Consequently, if a pregnancy occurs, there appears to be no justification for recommending its termination in patients without evidence of recurrence. Finally, patients must be cautioned that an uneventful pregnancy after a cancer diagnosis in no way guarantees against subsequent recurrence. Indeed, there are cases on record in which multiple pregnancies eventually have been followed by recurrence. We usually recommend that women with favorable tumors without regional or distant spread wait at least 3 years before attempting pregnancy. All such patients should undergo extensive evaluation before conception, including bone and liver scans, chest x-rays, and mammography of the opposite breast, and all must be followed closely during pregnancy. Follow-ups at 10 and 15 years are always necessary in breast cancer because late recurrences occur frequently.

There is no uniform agreement about the role of breastfeeding in the postpartum patient with breast cancer. Because many data implicate a viral etiology for breast cancer in laboratory animals, there is concern that a virus might cause human breast cancer as well. Therefore, the possibility exists that the contralateral breast is contaminated with the etiologic agent, which might even be passed on to the fetus. This theory has never been borne out in fact, but most surgeons recommend artificial feeding in such cases to avoid vascular enrichment in the opposite breast, which also might contain a neoplasm. This approach is especially important if systemic cytotoxic therapy is planned, because antineoplastic agents are detectable in breast milk and might cause neonatal bone marrow suppression. There are, however, no convincing data that nursing affects the prognosis of breast cancer patients adversely.

## BONE TUMORS

Both benign and primary or metastatic malignant bone tumors can be found in pregnant women and can pose problems in diagnosis and treatment. The diagnosis frequently can be suspected from the characteristic radiographic findings in a patient with bony asymmetry or pain. When the diagnosis is uncertain and malignancy is suspected, a biopsy must be done. Benign bone tumors rarely are a problem in pregnancy; however, two benign tumors that can affect pregnancy and delivery are endochondromas and benign exostosis, both of which can develop at the pelvic brim. These neoplasms may interfere with progression of labor and engagement of the fetal head by causing mechanical obstruction at the pelvic inlet, necessitating cesarean section.

Primary malignant bone tumors are rarely associated with pregnancy. The most common primary malignant tumors seen in the childbearing years are Ewing's sarcoma, osteogenic sarcoma, and osteocystoma. These tumors usually involve the clavicle, sternum, spine, humerus, or femur and are associated with local pain, mass, and disability. Signs and symptoms of myelitis with radiating pain, paresthesias, and weakness can be produced by primary sarcoma of the spine.

Primary bone cancer is aggressive, frequently metastasizing by the hematogenous route at the time of diagnosis. It is treated initially with surgical excision, usually without regard for the pregnancy. In the past, radiation therapy and chemotherapy were delayed until delivery if the tumor had not metastasized at the time of diagnosis. Because pregnancy does not affect the growth of bone cancers and because these tumors do not affect the pregnancy, indications for pregnancy termination did not exist. Unfortunately, survival in the group of patients for whom chemotherapy was delayed was uniformly poor, with most patients dying of disseminated cancer within 24 months. Within the past 20 years, the treatment of osteogenic sarcomas has become much more successful, combining adjuvant chemotherapy often with more limited surgery than advocated previously. Aggressive chemotherapy administered soon after amputation or resection is crucial to prevent the development of clinically detectable metastases in patients with these tumors. Therefore, it is appropriate to recommend early termination of pregnancy for patients whose cancers are discovered in the first or early second trimester. If the diagnosis is made later in pregnancy, early delivery of the infant should be effected, and intensive multiple-agent chemotherapy with doxorubicin, methotrexate, and cisplatin should be instituted. Alternatively, because the risk of fetal malformations induced by chemotherapy during the second half of the pregnancy is low, continuation of pregnancy despite administration of a methotrexate-containing multiple-drug regimen can be considered. The rarity of these tumors in pregnancy precludes concrete treatment recommendations based on extensive clinical experience. Because most recurrences from bone malignancy appear within the first 3 years of initial therapy, recommendations for future pregnancies should be deferred until that interval has passed.

In women of childbearing age, the most common malignancies that metastasize to bone are those of breast, cervix, thyroid, and kidney. Metastases occur most frequently in the skull, ribs, spine, and long bones, except for those from the cervix, which can extend directly to involve the pelvis. Patients can present with pain, a pathologic fracture, or paralysis, but some asymptomatic patients are identified by routine chest x-ray during pregnancy. This finding necessitates careful evaluation for a primary site, with definitive therapy dictated by the source of tumor and the duration of pregnancy at the time of diagnosis.

## THYROID CANCER

Both benign diseases and cancers of the thyroid gland occur more commonly in women than in men. Approximately 65% of all patients with carcinoma of the thyroid are women. Although most patients with thyroid carcinoma are in their 50s and 60s, about 15% are below age 30. Some younger patients with thyroid cancer have an antecedent history of thymic radiation during infancy or facial skin radiation in the treatment of adolescent acne.

The identification of a thyroid nodule is usually by physical examination. Physical examination is not sufficient to ensure that the palpated mass is solitary. Thyroid nodules can be present in approximately 1% of women of childbearing age. Seventy-five percent of thyroid nodules discovered and evaluated during pregnancy are benign colloid nodules. Because approximately 15% of solitary thyroid nodules are malignant, prompt investigation of these nodules is warranted. Because thyroid scanning in pregnancy is contraindicated, evaluation should consist of measuring serum-free $T_4$ and $T_3$ to rule out a benign toxic adenoma and ultrasonography to rule out a cystic mass, which is rarely (<2%) malignant. The approach to the evaluation of thyroid nodules in pregnancy should be similar to that for nonpregnant patients. If a solitary solid cold nodule is found, FNA or percutaneous needle biopsy is warranted. Pregnancy does not affect the reliability of this procedure.

The diagnosis of carcinoma of the thyroid during pregnancy is not an absolute indication to terminate the pregnancy; neither is pregnancy a contraindication to necessary surgery. Thyroidectomy should be performed for malignant lesions of the papillary type even during pregnancy because they tend to be quite aggressive. Definitive treatment of follicular carcinomas can be delayed until the postpartum period because they are much more indolent than papillary tumors. Radioactive iodine therapy when indicated must be withheld until after delivery. The recurrence rate is not influenced by subsequent pregnancies but is related to many other factors such as tumor size, histologic type, and grade. Anaplastic cancers are associated with a dismal outlook. Younger patients with thyroid cancer have been reported to have a better prognosis than older ones.

## REFERENCES

Anderson BO, Petrek JZ, Byrd DR, et al: Pregnancy influences breast cancer stage at diagnosis in women 30 years of age and younger. Ann Surg Oncol 2:204, 1996.

Barber HRK, Brunschwig A: Gynecologic cancer complicating pregnancy. Am J Obstet Gynecol 85:156, 1963.

Bottles K, Taylor R: Diagnosis of breast masses in pregnant and lactating women by aspiration cytology. Obstet Gynecol 66:765, 1985.

Brodsky JB, Cohen EN, Brown BW, et al: Surgery during pregnancy and fetal outcome. Am J Obstet Gynecol 138:1165, 1980.

Creasman WT, Rutledge F, Fletcher G: Carcinoma of the cervix associated with pregnancy. Obstet Gynecol 36:495, 1970.

Dildy GA, Moise KJ, Carpenter RJ, et al: Maternal malignancy metastatic to the products of conception: A review. Obstet Gynecol Surv 44:535, 1989.

Duggan B, Muderspach LI, Roman LD, et al: Cervical cancer in pregnancy: Reporting on planned delay in therapy. Obstet Gynecol 82:596, 1993.

George PA, Fortner JG, Pack GT: Melanoma with pregnancy: Report of 115 cases. Cancer 13:854, 1960.

Gharib H: Fine needle aspiration biopsy of thyroid nodules: Advantages, limitations and effect. Mayo Clin Proc 69:44, 1994.

Grin CM, Driscoll MS, Grant-Kels JM: Pregnancy and prognosis of malignant melanoma. Semin Oncol 23:734, 1996.

Hannigan EV: Cervical cancer in pregnancy. Clin Obstet Gynecol 33:837, 1990.

Holleb AI, Farrow JH: The relation of carcinoma of the breast and pregnancy in 283 patients. Surg Gynecol Obstet 115:65, 1962.

Karlen JR, Akbari A, Cook WA: Dysgerminoma associated with pregnancy. Obstet Gynecol 53:330, 1979.

MacKie RM, Bufalino R, Morabito A, et al: Lack of effect of pregnancy on outcome of melanoma. Lancet 337:653, 1991.

Nugent P, O'Connell T: Breast cancer and pregnancy. Arch Surg 120:1221, 1985.

Reintgen DS, McCarty KS, Vollmer RT, et al: Malignant melanoma and pregnancy. Cancer 55:1340, 1985.

Sivanesaratnam V, Jayalaksmi P, Loo C: Surgical management of early invasive cancer of the cervix associated with pregnancy. Gynecol Oncol 48:68, 1992.

Sorosky JI, Squatrito R, Ndubisi BU, et al: Stage I squamous cell carcinoma in pregnancy: Planned delay in therapy awaiting fetal maturity. Gynecol Oncol 59:207, 1995.

van der Vange N, Weverling GJ, Ketting BW, et al: The prognosis of cervical cancer associated with pregnancy: A matched cohort study. Obstet Gynecol 85:1022, 1995.

White LP, Linden G, Breslow L, et al: Studies on melanoma. The effect of pregnancy on survival in human melanoma. JAMA 117:235, 1961.

Wiebe VJ, Sipila PE: Pharmacology of antineoplastic agents in pregnancy. Crit Rev Oncol Hematol 16:75, 1994.

# PRODUCTIVE ENDOCRINOLOGY AND INFERTILITY

# 51

# Spontaneous Abortion

SANDRA A. CARSON

Questions regarding spontaneous abortion come up daily in clinical practice. This is not surprising, because 2 of 15 pregnancies result in miscarriage. Furthermore, in the United States, 3 to 4% of married women of reproductive age experience more than two spontaneous abortions. Patients want to know what to do, what to avoid, and what went wrong.

Most spontaneous abortions occur because of karyotypic abnormalities in the fetus. Almost 70% of first trimester abortuses are karyotypically abnormal; 30% of second trimester abortuses and 3% of stillbirths are karyotypically abnormal. The remaining nongenetic causes include anatomic, infectious, hormonal, immune, and environmental factors. Therapy begins with education and takes patience, understanding, and time.

## Background

For decades, obstetricians believed in the concept of habitual abortion. With each spontaneous abortion, the risk of pregnancy losses was believed to escalate, so that after three spontaneous abortions a patient was believed to have an 80 to 90% risk of subsequent pregnancy loss. Studies led by Warburton in the 1960s documented the risks of women who experienced pregnancy losses, refuted the concept of habitual abortion, and provided accurate statistics from real patients (Table 51–1). Before these studies were available, the incorrect figures were used as controls in clinical trials evaluating pregnancy loss and various therapeutic regimens. This practice led to unwarranted acceptance of interventions, such as treatment with diethylstilbestrol (DES). Today, we have the task of educating women on the true risk of pregnancy loss, which rises from 15% in the first pregnancy to 35% after one spontaneous abortion but does not increase thereafter. If the woman has at least one liveborn child, the risk of her first spontaneous abortion is 15%, and after one spontaneous abortion it rises to between 25 and 30% with no subsequent increase.

Maternal age, not gravidity per se, increases the

Table 51–1 Recurrence Risk Figures Useful for Counseling Women Who Have Repeated Spontaneous Abortions

|  | Previous Abortions | % Risk |
|---|---|---|
| Women with liveborn infants | 0 | 12 |
|  | 1 | 24 |
|  | 2 | 26 |
|  | 3 | 32 |
|  | 4 | 26 |
| Women without liveborn infants | 2 or more | 40–45 |

Data from Warburton D, Fraser FC: Spontaneous abortion risks in man: Data from reproductive histories collected in a medical genetics unit. Am J Hum Gen 16:1, 1964.

risk of spontaneous abortion: Twice as many pregnancies are lost at age 40 as at age 20. Although one might suspect that the reason for this increase is the known increase in aneuploid conception with increasing maternal age, this does not wholly account for the rapid rise in spontaneous abortion. Indeed, increasing numbers of euploid pregnancies are lost with increasing maternal age. This suggests that some unknown uterine factor—perhaps decreased uterine blood supply, chronic infections, or diminished luteal response—changes with age. The diagnostic and therapeutic approaches to these patients begin with education provided with patience and understanding. The next step is to conduct a thorough laboratory examination to rule out all known causes and implement directed therapy.

Patients who experience recurrent pregnancy loss would benefit by undergoing the battery of tests that are outlined in Table 51–2. In general, these tests are performed after three spontaneous abortions or, in a woman older than 35 years of age, after two spontaneous abortions. Although there is no greater likelihood of finding an abnormal test after three spontaneous abortions than after one, cost-effectiveness, as well as practical considerations regarding the ability of the laboratories to process all specimens, supports this rule of thumb. In the event of an abnormal test at the initiation of treatment, the test should be repeated after treatment has ensued. In addition, patients should be instructed to avoid smoking cigarettes and drinking alcohol and to minimize their exposure to environmental chemicals that are known to increase the risk of spontaneous abortion, as mentioned later in this chapter.

## Medical History and Physical Examination

The patient's medical history should begin with her obstetric history. A previous stillbirth, a child with an anomaly, or a karyotypically abnormal pregnancy loss heightens the suspicion of a genetic etiology for pregnancy loss. Fetal losses in the second trimester may suggest a uterine anatomic abnormality. Similarly, a family history of pregnancy loss or abnormal newborns may suggest a chromosomal abnormality. Patients who are exposed to environmental and occupational chemicals may identify potential toxins. The patient's use of toxins, such as nicotine and alcohol, should be elicited. Finally, past medical illness, chronic disease, and current medication may reveal factors associated with spontaneous abortion.

Physical examination occasionally elicits evidence of a chronic disease in patients who experience pregnancy loss. However, except for the presence of uterine leiomyomas and the occasional palpable bicornuate uterus, there are no physical findings that suggest the etiology of spontaneous abortion.

## Genetics

Patients who have a karyotypically abnormal abortus are more likely to have another abortus that is abnormal. Most abnormalities stem from the process of gamete formation or occur after fertilization takes place. In 2 to 5% of couples, a chromosomal abnormality exists in the parents that results in abnormal gametes. Most often, this is a chromosomal translocation.

Translocations, inversions, and deletions may be found in patients who experience recurrent spontaneous abortions. The rate of abnormality is increased if the couple has a history of a stillbirth or a child with anomalies. Also, parents who have siblings who have been delivered of stillbirths or anomalous children have a 10% risk of carrying a chromosomal abnormality. In this regard, obstetric history and family history are exceedingly important in advising the couple who have recurrent spontaneous abortions.

## Anatomic Abnormalities

**Müllerian Fusions Defects.** Müllerian defects of all types are associated with a higher incidence of pregnancy loss, presumably caused by a less vascular implantation site. Among these the septate uterus is the most common anatomic abnormality, carrying a 70% risk of spontaneous abortion. Patients who have surgical resection of the uterine septum before attempting another pregnancy have a higher term pregnancy rate than those who do not. The surgery carries relatively little morbidity when performed through the hysteroscope. Conversely, metroplasty for bicor-

**Table 51–2** Evaluation of Couples Who Have Recurrent Spontaneous Abortions

Karyotype in both parents
Karyotype in any subsequent abortus
Endometrial biopsy
- Histologic dating
- *Ureaplasma Urealyticum* culture

Hysterosalpingogram or hysteroscopy
Lupus erythematosus screen
Antiphospholipid levels
- Lupus anticoagulant
- Anticardiolipin

nuate uterus may be associated with mechanical infertility.

**Intrauterine Synechiae.** Adhesions may develop after overzealous curettage of the uterus during the postpartum period, after intrauterine surgery (e.g., myomectomy) or after endometritis. Dense, avascular intrauterine adhesions (Asherman's syndrome) may interfere with placentation and usually are a result of multiple previous uterine curettages. Treatment consists of hysteroscopic lysis of adhesions and the procedure entails little risk in the hands of a skilled surgeon. No randomized study data exist to confirm the efficacy of hysteroscopic lysis of adhesions in preventing subsequent spontaneous abortion; however, in one series, 89.6% of patients conceived after lysis of adhesions with the spontaneous abortion rate ranging from 5.9 to 21.4%.

**Leiomyomas.** Location rather than size of leiomyomas is probably most important. Submucosal leiomyomas may result in fetal loss through several theoretical mechanisms:

1. Endometrial thinning over the surface of the myoma that may impair decidualization and implantation.
2. Necrosis within the myoma (red degeneration) caused by hormonally stimulated growth may exceed the blood supply and lead to uterine contractions and fetal expulsion.
3. The myoma may encroach on the space required by the developing fetus and lead to fetal expulsion in the second trimester.

Therapeutic efficacy of myomectomy has not been documented in controlled trials but only suggested by surgical cohorts with increased postoperative term pregnancy rates of approximately 40 to 50%. As in incomplete müllerian fusion, careful patient selection is important, and the increased risk of mechanical infertility resulting from postoperative adhesions must be considered.

## Endocrine Abnormalities

**Diabetes Mellitus.** Poorly controlled insulin-dependent diabetes mellitus may increase the risk of spontaneous abortion. However, euglycemic patients who have diabetes mellitus do not have an increased risk of pregnancy loss. Therefore, unless indicated by history, there is no reason to screen routinely for diabetes mellitus in patients who have recurrent spontaneous abortions.

**Luteal Phase Defect.** The luteal phase defect results when the endometrium fails to develop appropriately for implantation and placentation cannot be supported adequately. The condition results from either deficient progesterone secretion or poor endometrial response to adequate progesterone stimulation. Endometrial histologic dating lagging at least 3 days behind the actual postovulatory date in two menstrual cycles is diagnostic of luteal phase defect. Because of the pulsatile nature of progesterone secretion, serum progesterone levels are of poor diagnostic value.

Of over 100 studies published since 1965 regarding luteal phase defect, none used a concomitant randomized control group. The data most suggestive that luteal phase defect is a valid entity are derived from a study of 33 infertile women whose luteal phase defect was documented by two out-of-phase biopsies. Although the study involved women who had infertility rather than recurrent abortions, no abortions occurred in the 14 women who conceived after progesterone treatment. Of the 16 women whose luteal phase defect was not corrected, there were 4 pregnancies, all of which ended in spontaneous abortion. The study suggests a role for luteal phase defect in infertility but even more hints that luteal phase defect indeed may lead to spontaneous abortion.

The current belief is that luteal inadequacy is a result of inadequate follicular development and, ultimately, leads to spontaneous abortion in women who conceive. Therefore, clomiphene citrate therapy to improve follicular development may be superior to progesterone therapy. Clomiphene citrate may be administered in doses of 50 mg for 5 days beginning between day 3 and day 5 of the menstrual cycle. To ensure that luteal phase difficulty is corrected with these therapies, an endometrial biopsy should be performed during the treatment cycle.

More current investigations are pursuing the role of molecules such as $\beta_3$ integrins, which may be important in implantation. Factors affecting the concentration of these hormones in the endometrium may reflect a novel way of diagnosing what histologically has become known as the luteal phase defect.

## Infection

Few prospective studies exist that compare a cohort of patients who have spontaneous abortions with a fertile population in terms of the prevalence of any organism. The only organism for which such data exist is *Ureaplasma urealyticum*. Women who have *Ureaplasma urealyticum* endometritis have a higher prevalence of spontaneous abortion. Furthermore, women who have positive endometrial cultures for *Ureaplasma urealyticum* should be treated along with their partners with doxycycline, 100 mg twice a day, for 2 to 3 weeks. Such treatment has been shown to increase resultant term pregnancies. Therefore, couples who have recurrent spontaneous abortions should be screened for *T-Mycoplasma* organism. Cultures for other organisms are not necessary.

## Immunologic Disorders

The nature of the immunologic process responsible for tolerating the presence of a fetus containing 50% foreign antigens is complex. Both autoimmune and alloimmune factors have been identified as causes of pregnancy losses.

**Autoimmune Disease.** Patients who have an autoimmune disease, such as systemic lupus erythematosus, have an increased risk of spontaneous abortion. These patients seem to form antibodies not only against their own tissue but against placental tissue, which ultimately leads to rejection of early pregnancy. Other immune factors, such as antisperm antibodies, do not cause spontaneous abortion and need not be included in evaluation of couples who have recurrent spontaneous abortion.

**Antiphospholipid Antibodies.** Attempts at identifying those patients who have systemic lupus erythematosus and who are more likely to abort resulted in the identification of a group of antibodies aimed at cellular phospholipids. The antiphospholipid antibodies, including lupus anticoagulant and anticardiolipin antibodies, were found to be elevated in patients who had this disease and who lost their pregnancies. A search for these antibodies was later extended to patients who had recurrent spontaneous abortions but did not have systemic lupus erythematosus. A prospective longitudinal study performed by the National Institutes of Health (NIH) revealed that patients who had high antiphospholipid titers and a history of spontaneous abortions were more likely to lose their pregnancies than those who had lower titers (Table 51–3). Screening patients during pregnancy reveals up to 20% of positive tests. Many of these are low level antibodies of immunoglobulin (Ig) M or Ig A isotype type and not related to pregnancy loss.

A variety of treatments have been suggested to manage patients who have positive antiphospholipid antibodies. However, no controlled prospective study has consistently shown any of these therapies to be effective. Low-dose aspirin, 75 to 80 mg per day, is commonly used to restore the equilibrium between prostacyclin and thromboxane, altered by the presence of antibodies. Subcutaneous heparin in addition to aspirin seems to add efficacy. High-dose steroids have been heavily discouraged because of the high incidence of gestational complications, such as hypertension and diabetes caused by steroids.

**Shared Parental Histocompatibility Antigens.** The fetal allograft containing foreign paternal antigens should be rejected by the mother. It is thought that the paternal antigens, which are foreign to the mother, invoke a protective blocking antibody that prevents maternal immune cells from recognizing the fetus as a foreign entity. The major histocompatibility antigens were the first antigens suggested to be involved in this recognition. However, multiple studies have now shown that parental sharing of human leukocyte antigen (HLA) does not increase the risk of spontaneous abortion.

**Passive Immunization.** Embryo rejection in animal models depends on activated natural killer (NK) cells rather than antigen-specific lymphocytes.

Some studies have suggested immunizing the mother with paternal leukocytes to suppress NK cells. In one study, immunization with paternal lymphocytes resulted in an increase in antipaternal cytotoxic antibodies protective to the fetus. After immunization, 16 of the 21 patients who developed antibodies delivered term infants compared with 2 of 7 immunized patients who did not develop the antibodies. However, based on a meta-analysis of the 19 published case series and 4 randomized controlled trials, the use of leukocyte therapy was not recommended.

**Active Immunization.** Intravenous administration of immunoglobulin (IgG) has been proposed to decrease overall maternal antibody production in an attempt to reduce fetal rejection. Theoretically, such treatment would decrease antibodies against phospholipids and foreign fetal antigens. However, any existing blocking antibody, that is protective, would also decrease. The overall effect may be assessed by examining the results of five European pilot studies involving 172 patients, in which 68 to 87% of pregnancies in patients treated with IVIG were carried to term. However, these rates were not different from pregnancy outcome in patients treated with placebo (5% albumin). Although some have argued that albumin may be immunomodulating, no convincing efficacy data exist to warrant using the expensive IVIG therapy at this time.

**Table 51–3** The Risk of Spontaneous Abortion in Patients With Antiphospholipid Antibodies

|  | Medium (%) | High (%) |
| --- | --- | --- |
| Nulligravida | 6 | 38 |
| Multigravida | 30 | 85 |

Data from Lockshin MD, Druzin ML, Goei S, et al: Antibody to cardiolipin as a predictor of fetal distress or death in pregnant patients with systemic lupus erythematosus. N Engl J Med 313:152, 1985.

## Environmental Factors

It is difficult to draw conclusions from numerous studies relating environmental factors with spontaneous abortions because of many confounding variables that are difficult to control.

**Irradiation and Antineoplastic Agent.** Radiography and antineoplastic agents are accepted abortifacients, attesting that exogenous factors during embryogenesis can cause fetal loss. In general, therapeutic radiographs or chemotherapeutic drugs are administered during pregnancy only to seriously ill women. In diagnostic doses, radiographs have not been proved to cause fetal demise. However, it would be prudent to consider radiographs as a potential teratogen.

**Cigarette Smoking and Alcohol.** Cigarette smoking and alcohol ingestion synergistically act to increase the risk of first-trimester spontaneous abortion. Cigarette smoking increases the risk of euploid pregnancy loss independent of maternal age and alcohol consumption.

A woman who smokes one pack of cigarettes a day and drinks one alcoholic beverage a day has almost a fourfold risk of spontaneous abortion compared with the patient who does not smoke or drink. It is important to advise patients of these factors without making them feel guilty about such use in previous pregnancies.

**Employment and Exercise.** Frequently, situations arise requiring patients to be at bed rest during pregnancy. There is absolutely no evidence that bed rest results in increased term pregnancies in the patient experiencing recurrent spontaneous abortions. In fact, a host of evidence does exist showing that continued employment does not increase the risk of spontaneous abortion. Epidemiologic studies, including one questionnaire study of almost 40,000 Scandinavian women, revealed no increased loss in women who continued to work during pregnancy compared with those who did not. However, it is important to ascertain chemical exposures in the workplace because these may be important risk factors in pregnancy loss.

Physically fit women can also continue to exercise. A controlled study of women who agreed to stop exercising if they were randomized to a control group revealed no increased pregnancy loss in physically fit women who continued to exercise compared with women who stopped exercising during pregnancy. Thus, women can be encouraged to continue their exercise program after conception.

**Chemical Exposure.** Exposure in the workplace to various chemicals has been shown to be associated with increased risk of spontaneous abortion. These chemicals include anesthetic gases, arsenic, aniline, benzene, ethylene oxide, formaldehyde, and lead. Tetrachloroethylene, a compound frequently found in dry cleaning and laundry establishments, increases the risk of spontaneous abortion more than threefold. Similarly, nurses who mix chemotherapeutic agents have almost twofold risk of spontaneous abortion compared with employees in oncology clinics who do not handle chemotherapeutic agents directly. Thus, it is advisable for oncology nurses and technicians to avoid the actual hands-on administration of such compounds during pregnancy. However, female medical residents have no increased risk of spontaneous abortion over the wives of male resident colleagues. Of additional note are studies showing no increased risk for either pregnant laboratory workers or pregnant pharmaceutical industry workers.

**Miscellaneous Exposure.** Exposure to electromagnetic radiation from video display terminals does not increase the risk of spontaneous abortion. Studies of women working at computers for months before pregnancy and continuing throughout pregnancy reveal no decrease in term delivery compared with women who stopped computer usage.

Women can be reassured that they can safely use hair dyes, watch television, and fly in commercial airliners during pregnancy. Although high altitude (above 11,000 feet) skiing is not advised, physically fit women can continue to ski at lower altitudes during pregnancy. These questions frequently arise in those who have experienced pregnancy loss and highlight the extreme anxiety of these patients.

## The Next Pregnancy

Perhaps more important than evaluation and treatment of the patient experiencing spontaneous pregnancy loss is the care of the patient during her next pregnancy. The psychological turmoil experienced during pregnancy by a patient with a history of miscarriages cannot be overstated. These patients derive emotional benefit from seeing their physicians weekly during the first trimester. Frequent ultrasonograms establish viability as well as allow the patient to be reassured weekly that the pregnancy is continuing. Patients who have cardiac activity demonstrated on ultrasonography at 8 weeks of gestation have a 3 to 5% risk of spontaneously aborting. This short-term goal of achieving cardiac activity at 8 weeks of gestation enables patients to have a shorter period of anxiety rather than setting a 9-month goal of a baby-in-arms. Another reason to follow the patient frequently in early pregnancy is to rule out the risk of ectopic pregnancy. Patients who are experiencing repetitive spontaneous abortions have a fourfold risk of subsequent ectopic pregnancy. After reaching 8 gestational weeks, patients may then undergo routine obstetric care.

## REFERENCES

Barlow S, Sullivan FM: Reproductive hazards of industrial chemicals: An evaluation of animal and human data. New York, Academic Press, 1982.

Carson SA, Simpson JL: Spontaneous abortion. *In* Eden RD, Boehm F (eds): Fetal assessment: Physiological, clinical and medicolegal principles. East Norwalk, CT, Appleton-Century-Crofts, 1989.

Cowchock FS, Reece EA, Balaban D, et al: Repeated fetal losses associated with antiphospholipid antibodies: A collaborative randomized trial comparing prednisone to low-dose heparin treatment. Am J Obstet Gynecol 166:1318, 1992.

Daly DC, Walters CA, Soto-Albers CE, et al: Endometrial biopsy during treatment of luteal phase defects is predictive of therapeutic outcome. Fertil Steril 40:305, 1983.

Diamond MP, Polan ML: Intrauterine synechial and leiomyomas in the evaluation and treatment of repetitive spontaneous abortions. Semin Reprod Endocrinol 7:111, 1989.

Fija-Talamanaca I, Settimi L: Occupational factors and reproductive outcome. In Hafez (ed): Spontaneous Abortion. Lancaster, NY: MTP Press, 1984, pp 61–80.

Fraser EJ, Frimes DA, Schulz KF: Immunization as therapy for recurrent spontaneous abortion: A review and meta-analysis. Obstet Gynecol 82:84, 1993.

Heinonen P, Saarikoski S, Pystynen P: Reproductive performance of women with uterine anomalies: An evaluation of 182 cases. Acta Obstet Gynecol Scand 61:157, 1982.

Kline J, Shrout P, Stein ZA, et al: Drinking during pregnancy and spontaneous abortion. Lancet 2:176, 1980.

Kutteh WH: Antiphospholipid antibody-associated recurrent pregnancy loss: Treatment with heparin and low-dose aspirin is superior to low-dose aspirin alone. Am J Obstet Gynecol 174:1584, 1996.

Lockshin MD, Druzin ML, Goei S, et al: Antibody to cardiolipin as a predictor of fetal distress or death in pregnant patients with systemic lupus erythematosus. N Engl J Med 313:152, 1985.

Malpas P: A study of abortions sequence. J Obstet Gynecol Br Commonwea 45:931, 1938.

Mueller-Eckhardt G: Immunotherapy with intravenous immunoglobulin for prevention of recurrent pregnancy loss: European experience review. Am J Reprod Immunol 32:281, 1994.

Simpson JL, Carson SA, Chesney C, et al: Lack of association between anti-phospholipid antibodies and first trimester spontaneous abortion: Prospective study of pregnancies detected within 21 days of conception. Fertil Steril 69:1998.

Stirrat GM: Recurrent miscarriage I: Clinical associations, causes and management. Lancet 336, 673, 1990.

Stray-Pedersen B, Eng J, Reikvan TM: Uterine T-mycoplasma colonization in reproductive failure. Am J Obstet Gynecol 130:307, 1978.

Thomas ML, Harger JH, Wagener DK, et al: HLA sharing and spontaneous abortion in humans. Am J Obstet Gynecol 151:1053, 1985.

US Department of Health and Human Services. Reproductive impairment among married couples. US vital and health statistics. Hyattsville, MD, National Center for Health Statistics, 1982, Series 23, No. 11, pp 5–31.

Warburton D, Fraser FC: Spontaneous abortion risks in man: Data from reproductive histories collected in a medical genetics unit. Am J Hum Gen 16:1, 1964.

Yetman DL, Kutteh WH: Antiphospholipid antibody panels and recurrent pregnancy loss: Prevalence of anticardiolipin antibodies compared with other antiphospholipid antibodies. Fertil Steril 66:540, 1996.

# 52

# Treatment of Anovulation

WILLIAM E. GIBBONS

The correction of anovulation through ovulation induction (OI) is a common therapeutic modality in the armamentarium of fertility treatment. OI may be used for the correction of a pathophysiologic state of anovulation. It is also increasingly used in assisted reproductive therapies in which supraphysiologic release of oocytes is the goal. The primary purpose of this chapter is prepare the reader to assess and produce a therapeutic management plan for the anovulatory patient.

## Incidence and Prognosis

Various estimates place the incidence of ovulatory dysfunction within the infertility population between 15 and 25%. Disorders relating to the preparation, release, fertilization, and implantation of oocytes represent a spectrum that ranges from subtle signs of a luteal phase defect that is poorly characterized through anovulation or oligomenorrhea to amenorrhea. In the majority of cases, anovulation stems from disordered or inappropriate gonadotropin secretion that falls within the spectrum of clinical abnormalities classified as polycystic ovarian syndromes (PCO) (World Health Organization, class II). Most often, there is some gonadotropin secretion with resultant ovarian production of estrogen levels higher than 40 pg/ml, which, after progesterone administration, lead to uterine bleeding (positive progesterone challenge). Follicle-stimulating hormone (FSH) levels are inadequate to sustain follicular growth, whereas luteinizing hormone (LH) levels are normal or increased. The history and physical examination should evaluate the patient for the most common observations of PCO—androgen excess and obesity—but should also be alert for the uncommon conditions associated with abnormalities of prolactin, thyroid hormone, and cortisol secretion.

Much less common is the set of conditions arising from inadequate gonadotropin secretion, which frequently appears as amenorrhea and a negative progesterone challenge test resulting from inadequate levels of serum estradiol to prime the endometrium. From a diagnostic and therapeutic standpoint, it is essential to discriminate whether amenorrhea arises from absence of gonadotropin secretion or failure of the ovary to respond (ovarian failure). In response to menopausal levels of FSH, therapeutic options include hormone replacement therapy to prevent the sequelae of hypoestrogenism or donor egg replacement, or both if fertility is the goal.

The history and physical examination are important in establishing the cause of inadequate or absent gonadotropin secretion. Is amenorrhea pri-

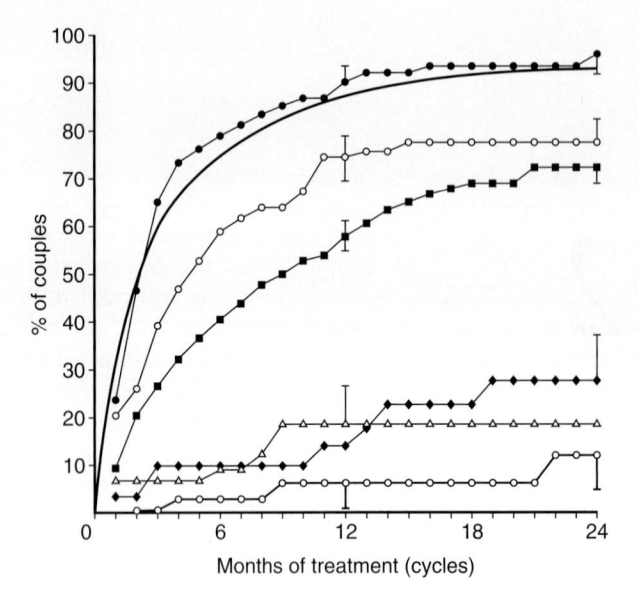

**Figure 52–1** Cumulative rates of conception in couples with single cause of infertility treated appropriately (excludes in vitro fertilization (IVF) and artificial insemination donor (AID). *solid line*, normal; *solid circles*, amenorrhea; *open circles*, oligomenorrhea; *solid squares*, unexplained infertility; *open triangles*, tubal factor; *closed diamonds*, failed sperm cervical penetration; *open diamonds*, oligospermia. (From Hull MG, Glazener CM, Kelly NJ, et al: Population study of causes, treatment, and outcomes of infertility. Br Med J 291:1693, 1985.)

mary or secondary? Do the symptoms follow postpartum hemorrhagic shock? Does the patient seek treatment for headaches or diminished optical fields? Is there evidence of congenital adrenal hyperplasia or thyroid dysfunction? Because hyperprolactinemia is an etiologic factor in conditions of inadequate gonadotropin secretion, it should be considered a routine component of the evaluation of these women.

However, rare problems are still rare, and overall, the prognosis for fertility with ovulatory dysfunction is excellent. Figure 52–1 demonstrates the cumulative rates of conception in couples with a single cause of infertility as reported by Hull and associates, who have demonstrated that the prognosis for pregnancy with treatment of anovulation approaches that of the normal population, which, in theory, it should.

Because chronic anovulation/PCO is the most common of these conditions, the emphasis of this chapter is on the therapy for patients who fit into this spectrum of conditions. Increasingly, an understanding of the expanding body of knowledge of the pathophysiology of PCO is important in managing anovulation resulting from PCO. The number of therapy plans that do not require exogenous gonadotropins is growing; therefore, it is very possible that within a decade, exogenous gonadotropin therapy will rarely be necessary for patients who have chronic anovulation/PCO. Why is this advantageous? Women who have PCO are not optimal candidates for gonadotropin therapy. They are often very sensitive to exogenous FSH stimulation and prone to hyperstimulation. Moreover, they have a higher incidence of multiple gestation than hypogonadal women, and their cycles are cancelled more often because of concern about hyperstimulation and multiple gestation.

## Evolving PCO Model

In the past, observations of elevated androgen production and an abnormal ratio of LH to FSH, resulting from lowered levels of FSH with normal, high normal, or elevated LH level, led to the vicious cycle model of anovulation associated with PCO (Fig. 52–2). LH serum concentrations are the result of an increase in the pulsatile release of LH from the pituitary with little or no change in its frequency of release. The release of LH is tied to the pulsatile release of gonadotropin-releasing hormone (GnRH) from the hypothalamus. Increased androgen production can be shown to increase the amplitude of GnRH release that suppresses gonadotropin release of FSH while increasing LH release. Because LH can stimulate thecal cells in the ovary to produce androgens, it was believed that increased LH release resulted in increased androgen production, which in turn led to alteration in gonadotropin release leading to anovulation.

What did not fit well into the theory was that most patients who have PCO also have elevated adrenal and ovarian androgen production. Furthermore, it was difficult to explain the peripubertal onset of the process.

More recently, emphasis has been placed on alterations in glucose metabolism and insulin resistance noted in women who have PCO. Increased resistance to peripheral insulin action can be partially explained by the frequent association of obesity observed in women who have PCO. However, there is a novel post–insulin-receptor defect in insulin signal trans-

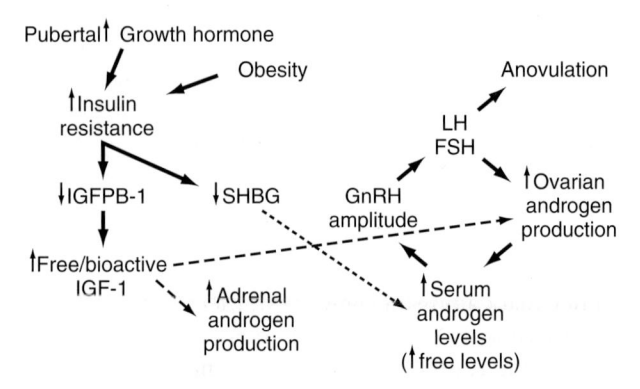

**Figure 52–2** Pathophysiologic interrelationships in polycystic ovary syndrome.

duction described between the receptor kinase and glucose transport whose etiology is not yet understood. This results in the need for a higher concentration of insulin to transport normal levels of glucose into the cell. In addition, increased resistance of insulin action also accompanies the alterations in growth hormone (GH) release in the peripubertal period.

Because steroid hormones have been associated with an increase in insulin resistance, it was postulated that the observed increase in androgen production was a significant cause of abnormal insulin function. However, GnRH analog therapy normalizes androgen levels in women affected who have PCO, but this does not correct insulin sensitivity.

Both insulin and insulin growth factor-I (IGF-I), a modulator of insulin and growth factor action, stimulate FSH-enhanced proliferation and steroidogenesis in the ovary. IGF-I circulates, like androgens, by being attached to a serum-binding protein, IGFBP-I, with the biologically active form being the free or unbound fraction. Further conditions that increase insulin concentration (e.g., obesity), result in decreases in both sex–hormone-binding proteins (SHBG) and IGFBP-I. Lowered SHBG levels result in higher concentrations of the biologically active free androgens (androgens lower SHBG levels as well). Lowered IGFBF-I levels result in higher concentrations of unbound IGF-I (see Fig. 52–2). IGF-I has been shown to enhance adrenocorticotropic hormone (ACTH)-stimulated cytochrome P-450c17 activity, which converts progesterone and pregnenolone to their C19 androgens, DHEA and androstenedione. This occurs in the ovary as well. Thus, the elevation in androgen concentrations in the blood promotes an exaggerated pulsatile release of GnRH, which suppresses FSH release in the pituitary while enhancing LH release and leading to the commonly associated alterations in the ratio of LH to FSH and the failure of folliculogenesis.

It is important to note that this process can be manipulated. If women who have PCO sustain a stringent 1000 kcal/day diet for 2 weeks, there is a two-fold increase in SHBG concentration along with parallel reductions in insulin and IGF-I concentrations. Spontaneous ovulation and pregnancy have been observed with this management, as well as increased effectiveness of clomiphene citrate administration. Data are also accumulating on new drug therapies that increase insulin sensitivity, which reverses the alterations in IGF1, SHBG, and serum androgens. Some of these agents will be discussed later. They mark a possible new era of therapy for anovulation secondary to PCO when other agents have failed. These interesting relationships do not explain every aspect of the complex spectrum of symptoms that is grouped into the classification of PCO, but they are enhancing our understanding of this most interesting process.

# Workup

The workup of the couple before therapy is begun should include a complete history and physical examination. Laboratory determinations frequently include prolactin, TSH (although the history should point to thyroid abnormalities), and FSH levels, which should alert the physician to ovarian failure or resistance. If there is clear evidence of androgen excess, baseline levels of testosterone and dihydroepiandrosterone sulfate (DHEAS) are useful in delineating a possible androgen-secreting tumor or suggesting the use of adjuvant adrenal suppressive therapy. Because of the frequency of more than one infertility factor, the male partner should be evaluated.

The physician should use his judgment concerning evaluation of tubal patency. It is acceptable to initiate ovulation induction and delay the evaluation of tubal patency until three or more ovulations have occurred without pregnancy. However, the initial evaluation of the uterine cavity and tubal patency can prevent the expense of months of therapy when other significant fertility factors are present. Methods include the standard hysterosalpingogram, and hydrosonography, which is less painful than the hysterosalpingogram. The latter method of evaluation can also be performed in the physician's office without delay.

# Diagnostic Techniques and Diagnosis of Ovulation

A necessary part of ovulation induction is confirmation that ovulation has occurred. Although pregnancy is the most stringent evidence of ovulation, there are several parameters that demonstrate presumptive evidence of ovulation. They include urinary, or serum preovulatory levels of LH, luteal levels of progesterone, endometrial biopsy, basal body temperature, and the demonstration of follicular growth and rupture by ultrasonography. In addition to detecting and timing ovulation, some techniques could be used for the purpose of timing infertility procedures, such as intrauterine insemination. Some modalities provide useful confirmation of these functions.

### BASAL BODY TEMPERATURE (BBT)

Following the midcycle LH surge in normal ovulatory cycles, granulosal cells in the ovulatory follicle luteinize and convert their steroidogenic machinery to the increased production of progesterone. This has the effect on the thermoregulatory center in the hypothalamus of increasing the core body temperature at rest by 0.5 to 1.1 degrees. This biologic shift can be used as an inexpensive marker of ovulation. The BBT rises on the day after ovulation, mirroring the rise in progesterone secretion, and falls in nonconception cycles on the days before the onset of menses as progesterone production from the corpus luteum decreases (Fig. 52–3). The normal ovulatory pattern of the BBT is labeled biphasic because there are preovulatory and postovulatory phases or patterns observed. Without ovulation and resultant progesterone production, the rise in mean BBT is not seen and the pattern is considered monophasic. Many physicians place value in the drop in the BBT that supposedly occurs just before ovulation. Because this nadir may be observed only half of the time, it is not a consistent finding.

The value of the BBT is directly proportional to how carefully the patient is instructed. An accurate BBT is dependent upon the patient's being at rest long enough for her temperature to reach its basal or resting point, unaltered by the heat from muscular activity. The patient is instructed to take her temperature immediately upon awakening each morning before rising. Any physical activity will raise her core temperature and add sufficient distortion to the BBT chart to prevent accurate assessment of her BBT pattern. Martinez and associates assessed accuracy as an index of ovulation. Of 172 records analyzed, they deemed the true positive rate was 90% in a population of carefully instructed, motivated patients who accepted technique well. It is important to note that the value of the BBT is the retrospective evaluation of the pattern of BBT change from which to make prospective predictions based on past patterns of ovulation. Grinsted and associates evaluated the positive predictive value of a positive test (PVP) for various ovulatory diagnostic methods. For the value of predicting ovulation in the current cycle, they found that the PVP of the BBT was only 25%.

Not only is the rise of the BBT curve important but the duration of the rise also provides useful information. A rise in temperature that plateaus and then falls to result in bleeding after 10 or fewer days may signal luteal insufficiency.

## DETERMINATION OF OVULATION BY ULTRASONOGRAPHIC MONITORING

The steady increase in the size of the dominant follicle along with its disappearance during ovulation can be accurately observed by ultrasonography. The ultrasonographic signs of ovulation include reduction in follicular size, appearance of intrafollicular echoes (bleeding into the corpus luteum), loss of sharp follicular margins, and appearance of cul de sac fluid resulting from the emptying of the follicular contents and postfollicular bleeding. Ovulation as stratified by the day of the menstrual cycle is demonstrated in Figure 52–4 for more than 400 natural cycles. Follic-

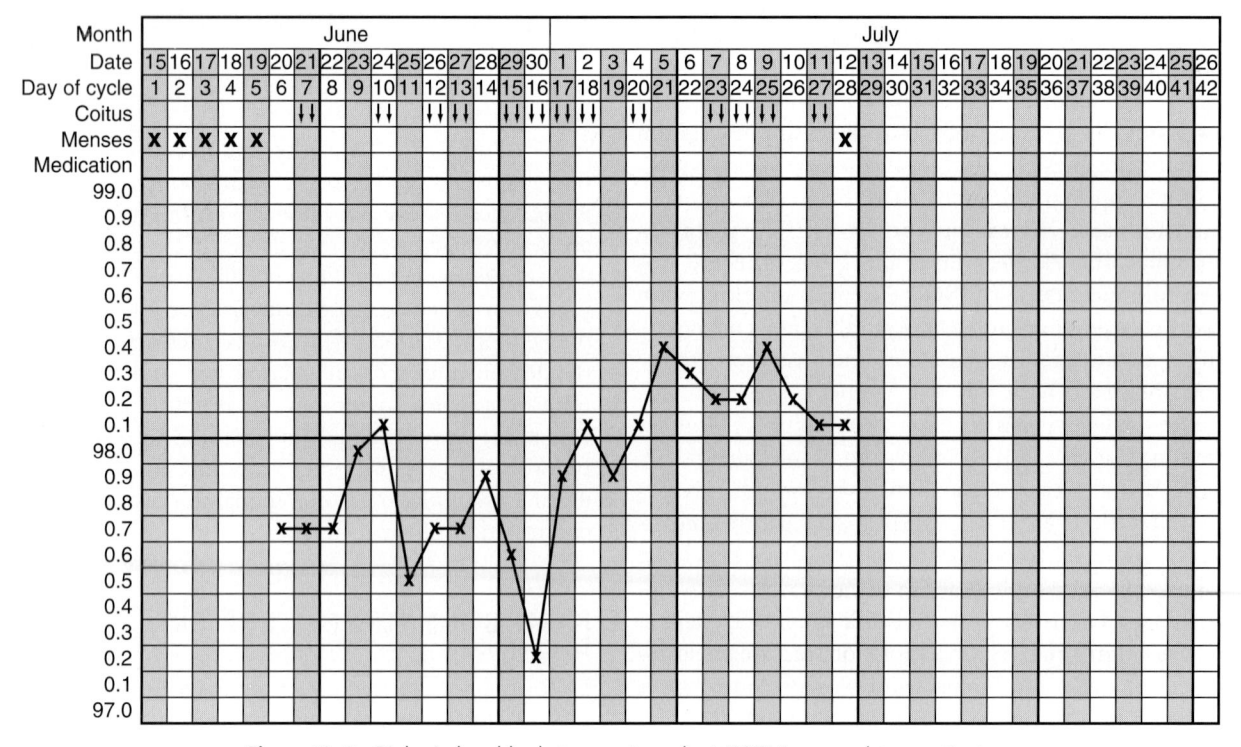

**Figure 52–3** Biphasic basal body temperature chart (BBT) in an ovulatory patient.

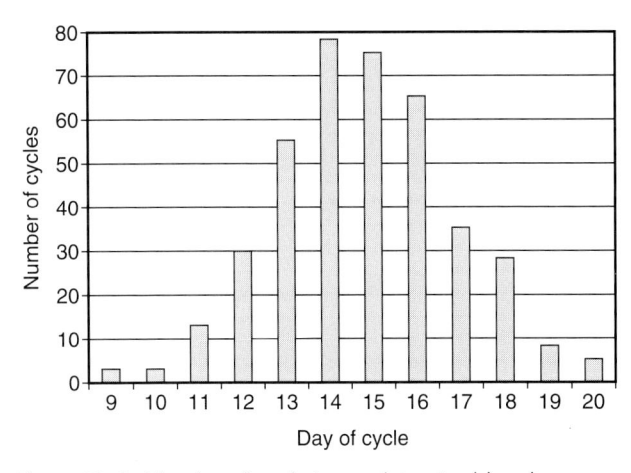

**Figure 52–4** The day of ovulation as determined by ultrasonographic monitoring of follicular development. The plot is the number of individual menstrual cycles in which ovulation was observed by a certain day of the cycle.

ular growth can be modeled most accurately with a relatively complicated volume model equation:

$$FVOL = 0.0039 \times FGA^{3.75 - 0.0529 \times FGA}$$

FVOL is the follicular volume and FGA is the follicular growth age. This complex relationship does not lend itself well to clinical use. However, follicular growth can be reasonably modeled with a more direct linear growth model:

$$MA_{ov} = (0.611 \times DO) - (18.54 \times k) + 16.52$$

$MA_{ov}$ is the menstrual age at ovulation (or the day of the cycle), DO is the day of onset of follicular growth, and k is the slope of the line of follicular growth. The net result is that by determining the size of the dominant follicle on 2 days early in follicular growth (i.e., days 10 and 12 of the cycle), the day of ovulation can be predicted within an accuracy of 1 day. This can be helpful in planning procedures, such as inseminations, or in timing the administration of human chorionic gonadotropin (hCG). Although it is very effective, the need for multiple scans and the related expense make the role of follicular ultrasonography more difficult to state in an increasingly managed-care environment.

### URINARY LH MONITORING

Since the mid-1980s, physicians and patients have had access to urinary assays to detect the preovulatory surge of LH. To assess the reliability of home urinary LH tests for timing of insemination, daily urine samples were assessed independently by both patients and physicians. In 47 cycles, agreement was seen in 42, or 89% of cycles, suggesting the usefulness of this technique. An Australian group compared urinary LH testing with serum LH levels. They found that in 82 to 88% of cases, the urinary kit predicted ovulation within 1 day, and in 89 to 96% of cases, within 2 days. In a study mentioned earlier in which positive predictive values (PVPs) were calculated for different methods, urine LH testing was found to have a PVP of 90%, which was the highest for any method. The ability of urinary LH monitoring to correlate with serum LH has been reported by multiple investigators. Monitoring of urinary LH levels to time fertility procedures, such as postcoital testing and insemination, is increasingly accepted as beneficial.

On the other hand, although it is important to determine whether ovulation induction has been successful, it is less certain that using these methods to time intercourse produces an improved cycle of fecundity. In a prospective study of carefully characterized cycles aimed at sex preselection, 91 natural cycles were evaluated for cervical mucus, BBT, hormonal characteristics, and pregnancy outcome. A fertile period of 9 to 10 days was observed with pregnancies resulting from single acts of intercourse between days −6 and +3 from ovulation. Royston, using the BBT rise as day zero, observed that although the highest probability of pregnancy occurred 2 days before the BBT rise, a significant probability of pregnancy occurred for 3 days before that (Fig. 52–5). This suggests that limiting intercourse to the day of a positive LH urine determination could adversely affect the probability of conception.

## Therapeutic Options

### CLOMIPHENE CITRATE (CC)

CC remains the first drug of choice for treatment of patients who are anovulatory. Because this drug

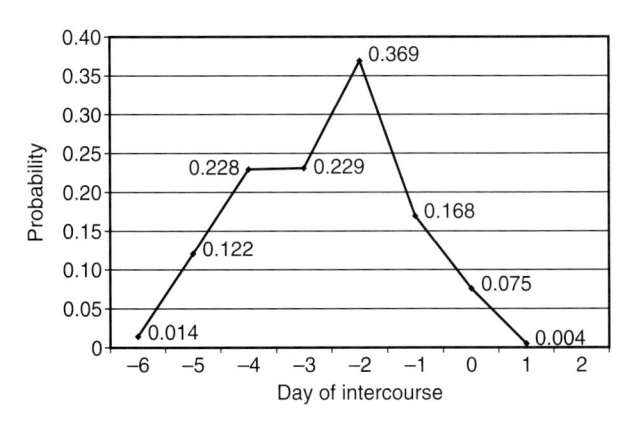

**Figure 52–5** Probability of conception based on the day of intercourse relative to the day of the rise in the basal body temperature (BBT) (day 0). (Data from Royston JP: BBT, ovulation and the risk of conception, with special reference to the lifetimes of the sperm and egg. Biometrics 38:397, 1982.)

functions by increasing endogenous levels of gonadotropins, it would not successfully produce ovulation if the pituitary-hypothalamic system were unable to secrete FSH. The treatment indications for CC use are shown in Table 52-1.

The mechanism of action of CC is not clearly understood. Adashi has reported that CC increases LH pulse frequency, which suggests an increase in GnRH pulse frequency. More important may be its effect on the pituitary as an antiestrogen in antagonizing the estrogen-promoted suppression of FSH release. Chang and associates have shown that women who have PCO are more sensitive to estrogen suppression of FSH than women who have normal ovulatory function. There is evidence that this heightened sensitivity is related to the increased amplitude of GnRH seen with PCO. However, the ovulatory response is biphasic. CC must be administered to promote increased FSH release and then it must be withdrawn so that the pituitary can recognize the ovulatory levels of estradiol necessary to trigger the LH surge.

With appropriate CC use, more than 90% of women who have oligomenorrhea and 66% who have secondary amenorrhea and progesterone withdrawal bleeding will demonstrate presumptive evidence of ovulation. However, only about half of patients who ovulate go on to conceive. This is probably more often related to other fertility factors (see Fig. 52–1). Gysler and associates reported that 85% of women who had no other infertility factors conceived, but fewer than 25% conceived when multiple fertility factors were present. Hammond and associates observed that women who had no other causes of infertility had a similar fecundity index (22%) as did a normal fertile population who stopped using barrier methods (25%). The frequency of effectiveness of CC underscores the importance of the gynecologist's gaining experience with this medication.

**Table 52-1** Indications and Contraindications of Clomiphene Citrate Therapy

**Indications**
Infertility associated with normal gonadotropic or normal prolactinemic anovulation
Infertility associated with oligo-ovulation
Infertility associated with luteal phase dysfunction
Infertility requiring improved timing of artificial insemination
Unexplained infertility requiring controlled hyperstimulation and intrauterine insemination

**Contraindications**
Ovarian cysts
Pregnancy
Liver disease
Visual symptoms

The standard therapy recommendations are to initiate 50 mg of CC on day 5 of the cycle (whether natural or induced) and continue taking it for 5 days. Ovulation usually occurs a week after the last tablet is taken (~cycle day 16). In some protocols, therapy is initiated as early as day 3. There is no clear evidence of the superiority of either a day 3 or day 5 start. Wu and Winkel evaluated 414 CC cycles in which CC was initiated from day 2 to day 5 of the cycle. They saw no difference in the rates of anovulation, luteal dysfunction, ovulation, pregnancy, or pregnancy outcome. The convention of initiating therapy on day 5 is a residual of initial CC studies, with the starting day arbitrarily selected for convenience of monitoring within the limitations of the study population.

Documentation of ovulation should be attempted. This includes BBT charting, urine LH level monitoring, follicular ultrasonography or serum testing of estrogen (cycle day 16), and monitoring of progesterone level (cycle day 23). A standard of therapy is to evaluate the patient toward the end of each treatment cycle. At this time, the documentation of ovulation should be evaluated and the patient examined for cyst formation by pelvic examination (pelvic ultrasonography is usually unnecessary unless it is difficult to assess the adnexa because of obesity). If cyst formation has occurred (~5% incidence), the medication is withheld for one cycle. The patient should be seen before initiation of the next cycle's medication. Starting CC on day 5 allows greater scheduling flexibility. If there has been no evidence of ovulation, the dosage is increased in 50-mg increments each month until ovulation occurs; a conventional maximum is 250 mg/day. The medication is then kept at the level that produces an ovulatory response through the course of therapy. The CC package insert states that a monthly dose of 500 mg should not be exceeded (or 100 mg per day for five days). This is a residual of the initial investigational new drug application (IND) filed in 1967 and does not appear to be tied to any specific adverse reaction. In a representative study, Gysler demonstrated that nearly half of patients ovulate on the 50-mg dose (Table 52–2). However, about a third of patients on each of the successively higher dosages ovulate, and once the ovulatory dose has been determined, about the same percentage of women conceive on that dose. Therefore, even though the cumulative number of women who conceive at the higher dosages is small relative to the total number of conceptions, it is worthwhile to use the higher dosages because alternative therapies are much more expensive and require much more extensive monitoring.

A course of therapy should be defined as six ovulatory cycles. In the majority of cases, if pregnancy is going to occur, it will have done so after six cycles. If

Table 52–2 Ovulation* and Pregnancy Results with Clomiphene Citrate

| Dose (mg) | Pt Cycles (N) | Ovulating (N) | (%) | Total (%) | Preg (N) | Cum Preg (%) | Preg @ This Dose (%) |
|---|---|---|---|---|---|---|---|
| 50 | 428 | 190 | 44 | 52.1 | 102 | 52.9 | 53.7 |
| 100 | 238 | 80 | 34 | 21.9 | 40 | 20.7 | 50 |
| 150 | 158 | 45 | 28 | 12.3 | 19 | 9.8 | 42 |
| 200 | 113 | 25 | 22 | 6.9 | 17 | 8.8 | 68 |
| 250 | 88 | 18 | 20 | 4.9 | 12 | 6.2 | 67 |

*Remaining subjects not ovulating = 60/428 (14%).
Cum = cumulative; Preg = pregnancies; Pt = patient.
Data from Gysler M, March CM, Mishell DR Jr, et al: A decade's experience with an individualized clomiphene treatment regimen including its effect on the postcoital test. Fertil Steril 37:161, 1982.

no pregnancy occurs, consideration must be directed at other causes of infertility (i.e., male factor or tubal factor). In the 1990s, the term "clomiphene failure" evolved. This term is indicated for those women who have failed to ovulate on any regimen of CC therapy. It is not accurately used to describe those women who ovulated, but not conceived after receiving CC therapy. Gysler's study is representative of the literature that demonstrates that failure to conceive is most often the result of associated infertility factors.

If the patient fails to ovulate on the standard 5-day regimen, CC therapy can be extended beyond the standard 5 days to 8 days of therapy or supplemental therapy can be sought that will enhance CC's effectiveness. An extended protocol using 100 mg to 150 mg of CC, administered from cycle day 3 to cycle day 9, along with 5 mg prednisone every night at bedtime has been also proposed. With this regimen, ovulation was achieved in 73% of cycles and 11 of the 24 women so treated (46%) conceived. When the serum DHEAS is at a high normal or elevated level, the addition of adrenal steroid replacement (prednisone 5 to 7.5 mg h.s. administered throughout the cycle) can improve CC responsiveness. The steroid dose is meant to be replacement therapy and is not intended to induce pharmacologic suppression.

There is evidence that CC has an effect of decreasing the quantity of cervical mucus. Randall and Templeton reported that at a dose of 150 mg/day, compared with a previous natural cycle, the cervical mucus score was significantly reduced and so was sperm mucus penetration. However, this effect was not seen at doses of 50 and 100 mg. Other investigators have noted that treatment with CC is associated with a less favorable cervical mucus score, decreased cervical mucus volume, and decreased spinnbarkeit. In the Gysler study, which reported on a group of 428 anovulatory women who were treated with CC, it was noted that the rate of abnormal postcoital tests (12%) was not different from experiences with a non–CC-treated population. Thompson and associates observed that even though cervical mucus quantity in CC-treated women was less than that in controls, CC-treated women did not demonstrate significant alterations in sperm penetration. Finally, as noted earlier in comparisons of the cycle fecundity in CC cycles vs. natural cycles, the lack of a difference suggests a minimal effect on biologically significant sperm transport.

Side effects of CC therapy include vasomotor instability, ovarian cyst formation, and visual changes. The vasomotor instability or hot flushing occurs because CC is an antiestrogen and works by blocking more potent endogenous estrogens; therefore, vasomotor instability is a common observation. Ovarian cyst formation has an incidence of about 5%. The cyst formation is transient and is expected to resolve in the next cycle. The clinical presentation may be sharp lower quadrant pain consistent with transient ovarian torsion. Most often if the patient limits physical activity, the pain resolves; rarely, the patient's condition may progress to the surgical therapy is needed to relieve the torsion, or even oophorectomy may be required if the loss of ovarian blood supply has resulted in necrosis. There are early reports on CC use in which massive ovarian cyst formation resulted when women received CC in the subsequent cycle if there was a cyst already present from the previous CC treatment cycle. Another interesting dose-related phenomenon is a visual effect in which the ability of the visual cortex to renew its image is slowed. This means that the most recent images are retained long enough to produce multiple images (i.e., passing a hand across the face can produce the effect of multiple hands moving across the face). This effect is transient. It appears to be dose-related and is usually not consistent, meaning that it may not occur every time.

## OVARIAN CANCER AND FERTILITY DRUG/CLOMIPHENE CITRATE USE

In 1994, Rossing and associates reported a case control study from the Pacific Northwest involving women who had received fertility drugs and who had an increased risk of ovarian cancer that was more pronounced when the medication was administered for longer than 12 months. Balancing this report are multiple studies suggesting that infertility itself is the major risk factor involved with—as yet—inconclusive evidence that fertility drugs were not an aggravating factor. Mosgaard and associates reported on another case control study of a population composed of all Danish women who were younger than 60 years of age and who were diagnosed with ovarian cancer between 1989 and 1994. Their findings were that nulliparity implies a 1.5 to 2.0-fold increase of ovarian cancer. Infertility *without* medical treatment increased the risk further, medical therapy decreased the risk, and pregnancy nullified the risk associated with infertility. Among parous as well as nulliparous women, treatment with fertility drugs did not increase ovarian cancer risk compared with nontreated infertile women, and there was no evidence of associated risk with longer duration of use.

## INSULIN SENSITIZERS

Expanding knowledge of the pathophysiology of PCO is leading the treatment of patients with this disorder into new directions. New classes of medications have been found by working through novel pathways, by which increased insulin sensitivity results in normalization of the menstrual cycle. These medications are not yet considered as first-line therapy, but they would be considered for those individuals who have failed treatment with clomiphene citrate and for whom the plan is to increase the sensitivity of CC and avoid the use of exogenous gonadotropins. Insulin sensitizers are not inexpensive. They require some monitoring and are associated with potentially serious side effects. However, these agents do not involve more risk than gonadotropin therapy, and they have the benefits of easier monitoring and a lowered incidence of multiple pregnancy and hyperstimulation. They also provide more targeted treatment of the pathophysiologic state.

Nestler and associates reported on a group of 61 CC-resistant women who received metformin 500 mg three times a day with or without CC. Overall, 31 of 35 women ovulated (89%) either spontaneously or with the addition of 50 mg of CC (19 of 21, 90%). Velazquez and associates noted that of 22 women who completed the 6-month trial of metformin (of 40 recruited), 21 resumed cyclic menses; of these, 4 conceived spontaneously. Of the 15 who resumed regular menses, 13 had ovulatory levels of progesterone.

Another new drug, troglitazone, is also effective. It belongs to a unique class of compounds, the thiazolidinediones, that exert direct effects on the mechanisms of insulin resistance and result in improved insulin action. The effective dosage of troglitazone is 400 mg daily. Importantly, severe liver toxicity has been reported with troglitazone. Two percent of patients have a reversible threefold elevation of serum alanine aminotransferase for which therapy should be discontinued. This requires monthly monitoring. Liver failure has been reported and appears to be an idiosyncratic response that cannot be predicted. These patients warrant close follow-up and they must give appropriate informed consent for this treatment.

Because of their recent use, experience with these agents is limited. There is some evidence that troglitazone is more effective than metformin in PCO. However, until the liver toxicity is better characterized and a larger experience is accumulated, metformin should be considered instead of troglitazone. At the present time, insulin-sensitizing agents should be selected for patients who have failed CC therapy.

It is important to reiterate the importance (and difficulty) of changing diet. A French group was able to demonstrate beneficial changes in body mass index, fasting insulin, non–SHBG-bound testosterone, SHBG, and insulin concentrations with a 1500 calorie per day diet alone. They found no additional improvement when metformin therapy was added.

## OVARIAN DIATHERMY

One of the first reported therapies for PCO was the ovarian wedge resection. In this surgical procedure, a wedge of cortical cysts and steroidogenically active stroma were removed with subsequent reductions in androgen production. Although the results were variable, an average of 80% of women resumed regular menses and about two thirds of these patients conceived. The mechanism of action is not clear, but the removal of stroma with reduced androgen production was felt to be important. Because of the frequency of postoperative adhesion formation associated with the procedure and the arrival of clomiphene citrate therapy, the wedge resection was abandoned. Additionally, the wedge was frequently of only transient benefit, particularly in more severe cases, such as ovarian hyperthecosis.

In the early 1980s, a new procedure consisting of laparoscopic ovarian electrocoagulation was reported. Initial ovulatory rates of 80+% with 60+% pregnancy rates seemed unrealistic. Multiple reports over the ensuing decade suggested pregnancy rates of 50%. There are multiple methods that use either mono- or bipolar cautery or laser therapy.

Li and associates analyzed factors that produced a more successful outcome in a retrospective review of 118 women. They observed a cumulative pregnancy rate of 54% in the year after treatment. The pregnancy rate was higher (79%) in women in whom the therapy consisted of diathermy vs. laser therapy, who had infertility of less than 3 years' duration, and who had higher LH levels. Liguori and associates performed second-look laparoscopies in a third of his 90 patients and found ovarian adhesions in 23%. In a review of these laparoscopic procedures, Cohen noted that although evaluation of different reports was complicated by lack of conformity and absence of control groups, these procedures have advantages over classic wedge resection because of their lower cost and reduced adhesion formation. He believed that they also had advantages over gonadotropin therapy, which may require serial ovulation cycles (higher cost), have the risks of ovarian hyperstimulation and multiple pregnancies, and a higher incidence of spontaneous abortion. He indicated that even with these benefits, ovarian laparoscopic therapy is not first-line therapy. Donesky and Adashi, although they pointed out the lack of long-term follow-up and operative risks of the procedure, which include ovarian failure secondary to overzealous coagulation of the ovary, also agree that the available data strongly suggest some real benefits of laparoscopic treatment for carefully selected patients who fail clomiphene citrate therapy. In conclusion, those women in whom CC therapy has failed and in whom adjunctive therapies, such as prednisone or metformin, have not improved CC responsiveness, laparoscopic ovarian cautery should be considered before gonadotropin therapy is initiated. As with any new application of operative laparoscopy, it is recommended that surgeons receive adequate training and demonstration of the technique. It is important too that understanding of the complications of a procedure be obtained before administering such treatment to patients.

## EXOGENOUS GONADOTROPIN THERAPY

Since the 1980s, the use of exogenous gonadotropins has increased almost exponentially. Instead of just limiting its use to women with primary amenorrhea (or clomiphene failures) who needed ovulatory treatment, the growth of assisted reproduction by way of in vitro fertilization (IVF) and superovulation, with or without intrauterine insemination (IUI) has resulted in large-scale use of gonadotropins in normally ovulating women for the purpose of polyfollicular development. Instead of producing a single dominant follicle for ovulation, the intent of these polyovulation protocols is the preparation of 4 to 6 oocytes compared with IUI and even higher numbers of oocytes for IVF. This has been aided by the increased availability of therapy-monitoring technologies, such as rapid, same-day serum estradiol determinations and transvaginal ultrasonography. In this section, standard exogenous gonadotropin administration to produce monofollicular development in the anovulatory woman is discussed. Hyperstimulation protocols for IVF or superovulation/IUI are presented elsewhere. This therapy is expensive and the side effects of its use (i.e., ovarian hyperstimulation and multiple pregnancy) are serious. Thus, this therapy should be performed by physicians who have experience in its use and not those who would treat only one or two patients per month. Appropriate informed consent is required in reference to intensive monitoring costs and side effects of this treatment. Informed consent should include discussions of how multiple pregnancies would be handled (including whether selective reduction is an option).

For several decades, the only gonadotropin therapy clinically available for most patients was the partially purified urinary extract of postmenopausal women. Human menopausal gonadotropins (hMG) contain equal amounts of FSH and LH. FSH is the major therapeutic component driving follicular growth. The LH component does provide stimulation of androgen production from the thecal cells. Androgen serves as a substrate for estrogen production by granulosal cells. In the 1980s, a form of urinary FSH became available in which LH was removed. This gonadotropin was administered by intramuscular injection and contains significant amounts of other urinary proteins. Further purification of urinary FSH has produced a highly purified form that allows subcutaneous injection similar to that of insulin treatment. Now, recombinant DNA technology is resulting in the synthesis of biologically active FSH macromolecules in tissue culture after the gene for FSH is cloned. Although the newer forms offer potentially higher consistency, there is not yet sufficient data from which to determine definitive superiority of any specific gonadotropin formulation.

In the spectrum of anovulation, the best candidates for gonadotropin therapy are those who are hypoestrogenic (negative progesterone challenge) and in whom there is an absence of gonadotropin secretion from the pituitary, resulting from either a loss of pituitary function or the absence of adequate pituitary stimulation by GnRH from the hypothalamus (i.e., hypogonadotropic hypogonadism or World Health Organization class I). Women who have inappropriate gonadotropin secretion (normal to elevated LH secretion with low FSH secretion) as seen in the spectrum of PCO are not optimal candidates for exogenous gonadotropin therapy because of their increased potential for polyfollicular development, aborted cycles, multifetal gestations, ovarian hyperstimulation, and lower success rates. With exogenous gonadotropin therapy that bypasses the feedback control mechanisms built into the hypothalamic-pituitary-ovarian axis to produce monofollicular development, comes the necessity for increased monitoring of drug by serial serum estradiol assay and ultrasonographic assessment of follicular growth. Women who have elevated gonadotropins are poor candidates for this therapy.

Because in women who have primary amenorrhea or gonadotropin insufficiency (or both) the pituitary may be unable to produce an ovulatory LH surge, or because with multiple follicular development there may be follicular production of peptides that may inhibit the LH surge, ovulation with gonadotropin treatment cycles is usually triggered by an alternative to the natural LH surge. This is generally human chorionic gonadotropin (hCG), but recombinant LH is another option. Therefore, one aspect of monitoring is determining the timing of administration of hCG. Another aspect of monitoring is reducing the incidence of adverse events associated with gonadotropin therapy, such as hyperstimulation and multiple pregnancy. The two major monitoring instruments are following serum estradiol concentration and follicular size through ultrasonography. Although estradiol levels are the more sensitive index of hyperstimulation, follicular ultrasonography is a superior method of determining the timing of hCG administration to trigger ovulation. Because peak follicular size varies with the method of stimulation (CC follicles at ovulation are greater than natural cycle follicles, which are greater than hMG-stimulated follicles), the timing of hCG injection is also affected. The optimal timing for hCG administration in natural cycles would be when the dominant follicle reaches a diameter of 18 mm or larger. For CC cycles, the dominant follicle size is 20 mm or larger, and for hMG, the value is larger than 16 mm.

A standard administration protocol is shown in Table 52–3. Gonadotropin stimulation cycles can be associated with a short luteal phase; therefore, luteal support with either progesterone replacement for 14 days after ovulation (50 mg progesterone intramuscularly q.d.; 200 mg progesterone vaginal suppositories q.d. or b.i.d.; or progesterone [Crinone], 8% q.d. or b.i.d.); or hCG (1500 IU q. 3 days after initial ovulatory dose × 2) is suggested, although the value of this support has not been proved.

Routine cycle fecundity rates are in the range of 7 to 28%, with higher rates associated with greater numbers of preovulatory follicles present at the time of administration of hCG and higher risk of multiple births. With conservative therapy, the multiple birth rate should not exceed 10%. The expected miscarriage rate is 25%. The etiology of increase in abortion rate is not well understood. Again, the presence of multiple fertility factors lowers overall success. In therapy cycles that are so involved, it is common to add IUI in an attempt to maximize success.

**Table 52–3** Administration Protocol for Gonadotropin (FSH) Therapy

Day 3 of cycle (spontaneous or induced) initiate 75–150 IU of Gonadotropin (IM or SC depending on medication)
Ultrasonographic monitoring
- Baseline scan before treatment (evaluate for cyst formation or underlying follicular activity)
- Ultrasonography every day until lead follicles reach 10–12 mm, then daily until hCG administration
- Scan 1 week after hCG administration to monitor ovarian volume (optional)

Serum estradiol monitoring
- Baseline value, day 3
- Value every 3 days until lead follicle size reaches 10–12 mm, then every other day
- When lead follicle reaches >14 mm, obtain daily values

Discontinue gonadotropin therapy when lead follicle reaches 16-mm size
  Administer 10,000 units hCG IM the evening of day lead follicle is >16 mm size (pending estradiol value). Ovulation is expected 36 hrs after hCG administration for reasons of timing intercourse or insemination procedures
  Increase daily gonadotropin dosage by 1.3- to 1.5-fold every 4 days should an inadequate clinical response be observed (little or no rise in serum estradiol)
  Do not administer hCG should the following be noted:
- Serum estradiol >2000 pg/ml
- >3 follicles ≥14 mm size
- >9 follicles ≥10 mm size

## OVARIAN HYPERSTIMULATION

Severe ovarian hyperstimulation syndrome (OHSS) with massive ovarian enlargement, ascites, hemoconcentration, hypovolemia, azotemia, hypercoagulability, and electrolyte imbalances can lead to cardiac arrhythmias, thromboembolism, and death. The incidence ranges from 0.01 to 4% and is more common in PCO patients. It is more common in cycles leading to pregnancy. It is avoided by careful monitoring and withholding hCG if the risk is increased by excessive numbers of follicles and high estradiol levels, as well as by avoiding coitus or IUI. When OHSS is diagnosed, judicious fluid management and paracentesis can alter its picture.

### REFERENCES

Aboulghar MA, Mansour RT, Serour GI, et al: Management of severe ovarian hyperstimulation syndrome by ascetic fluid aspiration and intensive intravenous fluid therapy. Obstet Gynecol 81:108, 1993.
Adashi EY, Rock JA, Guzick D, et al: Fertility following bilateral ovarian wedge resection: A critical analysis of 90 consecutive cases of the polycystic ovary syndrome. Fertil Steril 36:347, 1981.
Adashi EY: Clomiphene citrate-initiated ovulation: A clinical update. Semin Reprod Endocrinol 4:255, 1986.
Agarwall SK, Haney AF: Does recommending timed intercourse really help the infertile couple? Obstet Gynecol 84:307, 1994.
Artini PG, Fasciani A, Cela V, et al: Fertility drugs and ovarian cancer. Gynecol Endocrinol 11:59, 1997.
Chang RJ, Mandel FP, Lu JK, et al: Enhanced disparity of gonado-

tropin secretion by estrone in women with polycystic ovarian disease. J Clin Endocrinol Metab 54:490, 1982.

Ciaraldi TP, el Roeily A, Madar Z, et al: Cellular mechanisms of insulin resistance in polycystic ovarian syndrome. J Clin Endocrinol Metab 75:577, 1992.

Cohen J: Laparoscopic procedures for treatment of infertility related to polycystic ovarian syndrome. Hum Reprod Update. 2:337, 1996.

Crave JC, Fimbel S, Lejeune H, et al: Effects of diet and metformin administration on sex hormone-binding globulin, androgens, and insulin in hirsute and obese women. J Clin Endocrinol Metab 89:2057, 1995.

Diamond MP, Maxson WS, Vaughn WK, et al: Antiestrogenic effect of clomiphene citrate in a multiple follicular stimulation protocol. J In Vitro Fert Embryo Transfer 3:106, 1986.

Donesky BW, Adashi EY: Surgical ovulation induction: The role of ovarian diathermy in polycystic ovary syndrome. Baillieres Clin Endocrinol Metab 10:293, 1996.

Doody MC, Gibbons WE, Zamah NM: Linear regression analysis of ultrasound follicular growth: Statistical relationship of growth rate and calculated date of growth onset to total growth period. Fertil Steril 47:436, 1987.

Dunaif A, Scott D, Finegood D, et al: The insulin-sensitizing agent troglitazone improves metabolic and reproductive abnormalities in the polycystic ovary syndrome. J Clin Endocrinol Metab 81:3299, 1996.

Elkind-Hirsch K, Goldzieher JW, Gibbons WE, Besch PK: Evaluation of the OvuSTICK urinary luteinizing hormone kit in normal and stimulated menstrual cycles. Obstet Gynecol 67:450, 1986.

Ehrmann DA, Schneider DJ, Sobel BE, et al: Troglitazone improves defects in insulin action, insulin, secretion, ovarian steroidogenesis, and fibrinolysis in women with polycystic ovarian syndrome. J Clin Endocrinol Metab 82:2108, 1997.

Fluker MR, Urman B, MacKinnon M, et al: Exogenous gonadotropin therapy in World Health Organization Groups I and II ovulatory disorders. Obstet Gynecol 83:189, 1994.

France JT, Graham FM, Gosling L, et al: Characteristics of natural conceptual cycles occurring in a prospective study of sex preselection: Fertility awareness symptoms, hormone levels, sperm survival, and pregnancy outcome. Int J Fertil 37:244, 1992.

Franks S, Kiddy DS, Hamilton-Farley D, et al: The role of nutrition and insulin in the regulation of sex hormone binding globulin. J Steroid Biochem Mol Biol 39:835, 1991.

Gjonnaess H: Polycystic ovarian syndrome treated by ovarian electrocautery through the laparoscope. Fertil Steril 41:20, 1984.

Glasier AF, Irvine DS, Wickings EJ, et al: A comparison of the effects on follicular development between clomiphene citrate, its two separate isomers and spontaneous cycles. Hum Reprod 4:252, 1989.

Golddzieher JW, Green JA: The polycystic ovary: I. Clinical and histologic features. J Clin Endocrinol Metab 22:325, 1962.

Grinsted J, Jacobsen JD, Grinsted L, et al: Prediction of ovulation. Fertil Steril 52:388, 1989.

Gudgeon K, Leader L, Howard B: Med J Aust 152:344, 1990.

Gysler M, March CM, Mishell DR Jr, et al: A decade's experience with an individualized clomiphene treatment regimen includes its effect on the postcoital test. Fertil Steril 37:161, 1982.

Hammond MG, Halme JK, Talbert LM: Factors affecting the pregnancy rate in clomiphene citrate induction of ovulation. Obstet Gynecol 62:196, 1983.

Haning RV, Austin CW, Carlson IH, et al: Plasma estradiol is superior to ultrasound and urinary glucuronide as a predictor of ovarian hyperstimulation during induction of ovulation with menotropins. Fertil Steril 40:31, 1983.

Henry RR: Thiazolidinediones. Endocrinol Metab Clin North Am 26:553, 1997.

Hull MG, Glazener CM, Kelly NJ, et al: Population study of causes, treatment, and outcomes of infertility. Br Med J 291:1693, 1985.

Isaacs JD, Lincoln SR, Cowan BD: Extended clomiphene citrate (CC) and prednisone for the treatment of chronic anovulation resistant to CC alone. Fertil Steril 68:745, 1997.

Langer R, Golan A, Ron-EL R, et al: Hormonal changes related to impairment of cervical mucus in cycles stimulated by clomiphene citrate. Aust N Z J Obstet Gynecol 30:25, 1990.

Lobo RA, Paul W, March CM, et al: Clomiphene and dexamethasone in women unresponsive to clomiphene alone. Obstet Gynecol 60:497, 1982.

Li TC, Saravelos H, Chow MS, et al: Factors affecting the outcome of laparoscopic ovarian drilling for polycystic ovarian syndrome in women with anovulatory infertility. Br J Obstet Gynaecol 105:338, 1998.

Liguori G, Tolino A, Moccia G, et al: Laparoscopic ovarian treatment in infertile patients with polycystic ovarian syndrome: Endocrine changes and clinical outcome. Gynecol Endocrinol 10:257, 1996.

Marchini M, Dorta M, Bombelli F, et al: Effects of clomiphene citrate on cervical mucus: Analysis of some influencing factors. Int J Fertil 34:154, 1989.

Martinez AR, Bernardus RE, Vermeiden JP, et al: Hum Reprod 7:751, 1992.

Martinez AR, van Hooff MH, van der Meer M, et al: The reliability and applications of basal body temperature (BBT) records in the diagnosis and treatment of infertility. Eur J Obstet Gynecol Reprod Biol 47:121, 1992.

Merchant RN: Treatment of polycystic ovary disease with laparoscopic low-watt bipolar electrocoagulation of the ovaries. J Am Assoc Gynecol Laparosc 3:503, 1996.

Mosgaard BJ, Lidegaard O, Kjaer SK, et al: Infertility, fertility drugs, and invasive ovarian cancer: A case-control study. Fertil Steril 67:1005, 1997.

Nestler JE, Jakubowicz DJ, Evans WS, et al: Effects of metformin on spontaneous and clomiphene-induced ovulation in the polycystic ovary syndrome. N Engl J Med 338:1876, 1988.

Nestler JE, Jakubowicz DJ: Lean women with polycystic ovarian syndrome respond to insulin reduction with decreases in ovarian P450c17 alpha activity and serum androgens. J Clin Endocrinol Metab 82:4075, 1997.

Parazzini F, Negri E, La Vecchia C, et al: Treatment for infertility and risk of invasive epithelial ovarian cancer. Hum Reprod 12:2159, 1997.

Randall JM, Templeton A: Cervical mucus score and in vitro sperm mucus interaction in spontaneous and clomiphene cycles. Fertil Steril 56:465, 1991.

Rossavik IK, Gibbons WE: Variability of ovarian follicular growth in natural menstrual cycles. Fertil Steril 44:195, 1985.

Rossing MA, Daling JR, Weiss NS, et al: Ovarian tumors in a cohort of infertile women. N Engl J Med 331:771, 1994.

Roumen FJ, Doesburg WH, Rolland R: Treatment of infertile women with a deficient postcoital with two antiestrogens: Clomiphene and tamoxifen. Fertil Steril 41:237, 1984.

Royston JP: BBT, ovulation and the risk of conception, with special reference to the lifetimes of the sperm and egg. Biometrics 38:397, 1982.

Schenker JG, Weinstein D: Ovarian hyperstimulation syndrome: A current survey. Fertil Steril 30:255, 1978.

Schwartz M, Jewelewicz R, Dyrenfurth I, et al: The use of human menopausal gonadotropins for induction of ovulation. Am J Obstet Gynecol 138:801, 1980.

Scott RT, Hoffman GE: Prognostic assessment of ovarian reserve. Fertil Steril 63:63, 1995.

Thompson LA, Barratat CLR, Thornton SJ, et al: The effects of clomiphene citrate and cyclofenil on cervical mucus volume and receptivity over the periovulatory period. Fertil Steril 59:125, 1993.

Velazquez E, Acosta A, Mendoza SG: Menstrual cyclicity after metformin therapy in polycystic ovary syndrome. Obstet Gynecol 90:392, 1997.

Venn A, Watson L, Lumley J, et al: Breast and ovarian cancer incidence after infertility and in vitro fertilization. Lancet 346:995, 1995.

Vermesh M, Kletzky OA, Davajan V, et al: Monitoring techniques to predict and detect ovulation. Fertil Steril 47:259, 1987.

Watkins PB, Whitcomb RW: Hepatic dysfunction associated with troglitazone. N Engl J Med 338:916, 1998.

Wu CH, Winkel CA: The effect of therapy initiation day on clomiphene citrate therapy. Fertil Steril 52:564, 1989.

# 53

# Amenorrhea

RICHARD E. BLACKWELL
LISA A. FARAH

Amenorrhea is one of the most common conditions encountered in the practice of gynecology. It may be associated with a life transition, such as puberty or menopause; it may represent a physiologic condition, such as pregnancy; or it could be the result of a variety of illnesses, medications, and therapies (Tables 53–1 and 53–2).

## Definitions

Amenorrhea is an arbitrary definition that signifies failure to menstruate either primarily or secondarily by a certain age or over a period of time. It is influenced by many life transitions and states, with girls entering puberty at an average age of 11.5 years and beginning to menstruate some time thereafter, and women ending reproduction at the average age of 51.4 years with the onset of menopause. It is generally assumed that the failure of sexual development and menstruation by the age of 14 years suggests the presence of pathology and may represent the state of primary amenorrhea, whereas cessation of menstruation in the nonpregnant state earlier than 35 years of age would represent secondary amenorrhea.

## Diagnostic Strategies

The first step in the evaluation of amenorrhea is to determine whether the condition is caused by delayed puberty or early menopause. One should always remember that any woman of reproductive age who is amenorrheic is assumed to be *pregnant until proved otherwise*. Once this condition can be ruled out, a search should be conducted for the major causes of primary amenorrhea, which include genetic aberration, outflow tract obstruction, systemic illness, and secondary amenorrhea, which includes uterine trauma and ovarian, thyroid, adrenal, pituitary, or central nervous system pathology.

## History

As the clinician is dealing with myriad conditions that can influence primary or secondary amenorrhea, obtaining a thorough history is imperative. It should be determined whether the patient is the product of an uncomplicated term pregnancy, whether delivery was traumatic, and whether the neonatal period was associated with infection, hemorrhage, or drug withdrawal. A history of childhood illnesses should be obtained, including meningitis, encephalitis, and head trauma. Developmental milestones should be noted. If the patient failed to develop signs of secondary sexual characteristics by 13 or 14 years of age, it might be presumed that dysfunction of the central nervous system or ovaries exists. Interruption of the pubertal process often signifies a disruption in pro-

**Table 53–1** Causes of Amenorrhea

**PRIMARY**

**Genetic Dysfunction**

1. Gonadal dysgenesis (Turner's syndrome and its variants)
2. XX and XY gonadal dysgenesis
3. Mixed gonadal dysgenesis
4. Pseudo-Turner's syndrome
5. Galactosemia

**Systemic Disorders**

1. CNS dysfunction
   a. Tumor
   b. Malformation
   c. Radiation
   d. Infiltrative/granuloma-forming disorders
   e. Trauma and others
   f. Isolated and multiple pituitary hormone deficiency
2. Chronic diseases
3. Malnutrition
4. Stress
5. Exercise
6. Hypothyroidism
7. Cushing's disease/syndrome
8. Drug use

**Outflow Trace Dysfunction or Malformation**

1. Male pseudohermaphroditism
   a. Enzyme defects
      1. 20–22 desmolase
      2. 3β-hydroxysteroid dehydrogenase-isomerase deficiency
      3. 17α-hydroxylase deficiency
      4. 17,20-desmolase deficiency
      5. 17β-hydroxysteroid dehydrogenase deficiency
   b. Defect in androgen action
      1. Testicular feminization
      2. Incomplete testicular feminization
      3. 5α-reductase deficiency
2. Uterovaginal anomalies
   a. Vaginal agenesis
   b. Transverse septum
   c. Imperforate hymen

---

duction or delivery or both of gonadotropin-releasing hormone (GnRH). If the patient had the appropriate growth spurt and development of breasts, as well as pubic and axillary hair yet failed to menstruate, absence of the uterus or outflow tract obstruction should be considered. Inquiry should be made as to whether the patient's development was similar to that of her peers, and whether other close female family members experienced similar menstrual dysfunction.

The history should concentrate on associated systemic medical illnesses, such as sickle cell anemia, cystic fibrosis, and cardiac, pulmonary, or renal disease as well as obscure disorders, such as temporal arteritis, von Recklinghausen's disease, histiocytosis X, cavernous sinus thrombosis, syphilis, tuberculosis, and many other illnesses that may trigger endocrine dysfunction that may result in amenorrhea. Further, inquiry should be made about whether the patient has received either chemotherapy or radiation therapy for any malignancy.

A careful history should be obtained regarding the patient's physical activity and exercise levels, or whether any recreational drugs have been used. The patient should be questioned regarding any rapid alteration in body weight, either positive or negative. She should be questioned regarding breast discharge, headache, and unexpected hair growth or distribution. She should be asked about cyclic abdominal pain and any surgery involving the central nervous system, the pituitary, the thyroid, or adrenal glands, the ovaries, or the uterus. Finally, a careful history of drug exposure should be elicited, because at times these exposures interact with physiologic processes to produce amenorrhea. Examples include the individual who undergoes a miscarriage and a traumatic dilatation and curettage (D&C) and subsequently develops amenorrhea induced by weight loss secondary to stress; or the young woman who has a history of menstrual irregularity for which she was placed on a low-dose birth control pill and who subsequently lost weight and became amenorrheic after discontinuing

**Table 53–2** Causes of Amenorrhea

**SECONDARY AMENORRHEA**

**Genetic Dysfunction**

1. Gonadal dysgenesis
   a. Turner's syndrome
   b. Turner's mosaicism

**CNS Dysfunction**

1. Chronic hypothalamic anovulation
2. Hypothalamic amenorrhea
   a. Eating disorders
   b. Exercise
   c. Chronic illness
3. Tumors
4. Infiltrative/granuloma-forming diseases
5. Trauma
6. Drugs—recreational, steroids

**Pituitary Dysfunction**

1. Tumors
2. Postpartum hemorrhage (Sheehan's syndrome)
3. Empty sella syndrome
4. Radiation/surgery of pituitary tumor
5. Drugs—leuprolide acetate (Lupron Depot) medroxyprogesterone acetate (Depo-Provera)
6. Hyperprolactinemia—any cause
7. Hypothyroidism

**Adrenal Dysfunction**

1. Adrenal hyperplasias
2. Adrenal tumors

**Ovarian Dysfunction**

1. Polycystic ovary (PCO)
2. Hyperthecosis
3. Surgery
4. Tumors
5. Chemotherapy/radiation therapy
6. Premature ovarian failure—idiopathic or autoimmune
7. Savage syndrome

**Uterine**

1. Asherman's syndrome—any cause
2. Pregnancy
3. Hysterectomy
4. Uterine ablation

the pill; or the young woman who was treated with medroxyprogesterone acetate (Depo-Provera) for contraception, who may remain amenorrheic for up to 2 years after taking a single 150-mg dose.

## Physical Examination

Particular attention should be paid to the height-to-weight ratio of amenorrheic patients and the absolute amount of body fat. For example, an individual who is 5'4" in height should weigh a minimum of 114 pounds. Weight loss of 10 to 15% results in ovulatory dysfunction. In the case of the individual who has exceptional height or a short stature, further evaluation may demonstrate a 46,XY, 45,X/46,XX, or 45,X karyotype. These individuals may have abnormalities of skull shape, scoliosis, or limb defects. Attention should be turned to evaluation of the skin. In the case of hirsutism, virilism, or both, a Ferriman-Gallwey score should be established. The skin should be examined for the presence of neurofibromas, café au lait spots, dryness, and extreme alterations, such as myxedema, signs of acanthosis nigricans, and other signs associated with androgen excess, including acne and oiliness. Attention should be turned to the development of the breasts and hair distribution, and a Tanner staging should be assigned to each. The head should be evaluated for such findings as exophthalmos, high-arched palate, cleft palate, and cleft lip; the thyroid should be evaluated for masses or the presence of a goiter. The breasts should be examined for galactorrhea and symmetry, and signs of biopsy, reduction, or augmentation. Both the chest and the head should be examined for signs of trauma as well as surgery or infection. The abdomen should be inspected for organomegaly, the presence of either purple or white striae, any signs of a surgical incision, or palpable inguinal masses. The appendages should be evaluated for temperature, any malformation, such as, hypo- or hyperreflexia or vascular fragility. The whole body should be inspected for discoloration, such as the hypercarotenemia seen in patients who have anorexia nervosa and the ashen tone acquired by the skin in Addison's disease. Finally, care should always be taken to review the vital signs, because hypertension can be associated with conditions such as Cushing's disease and various forms of adrenal hyperplasia, and tachycardia may be seen with hyperthyroidism and other disorders.

On pelvic examination, the vulva should appear normal and be nonambiguous. Attempts should be made to visualize the cervix, and, if not possible, sonographic imaging should be carried out either transabdominally or transrectally. Bimanual examination should be performed to reveal whether a uterus is present, and whether the ovaries are palpable bilaterally. There should be an adult female escutcheon and no clitoromegaly should be present. The finding of a bulging blue hymenal membrane suggests imperforate hymen. A blind pouch vagina might suggest the Rokitansky-Küster-Hauser syndrome or a transverse vaginal septum. A flat perineum may be found in the various syndromes of androgen insensitivity, and genital ambiguity may be found in cases of 45,X/46,XY gonadal dysgenesis.

## Laboratory Studies and Diagnostic Evaluation

Perhaps the single key laboratory test in the evaluation of amenorrheas is a combined serum luteinizing hormone (LH) level and follicle-stimulating hormone (FSH) level. Elevation of these gonadotropins strongly suggests a genetic origin of primary amenorrhea, or it may herald the onset of perimenopause, menopause, or both in the case of secondary amenorrhea. An elevated LH/FSH ratio, particularly if associated with hyperandrogenemia, may point to polycystic ovary syndrome as the origin of the ovulatory dysfunction. A decreased LH/FSH ratio with FSH being greater than LH, strongly suggests the diagnosis of psychogenic amenorrhea associated with disorders such as anorexia nervosa, athletic amenorrhea, or stress. Normal gonadotropins with an appropriate ratio of LH greater than FSH suggest chronic hypothalamic anovulation and are also found in women who have outlet obstruction or uterine synechiae (Asherman's syndrome). If the FSH level is markedly elevated, a karyotype should be carried out to determine the genotype. If the gonadotropins are low or normal, thyroid-stimulating hormone (TSH) level and prolactin levels should be obtained; if signs of hyperandrogenemia are present, an androgen profile, including levels of total testosterone, free testosterone, and sex hormone–binding globulin should be obtained. Levels of follicular phase 17α-hydroxyprogesterone and dehydroepiandrosterone (DHEAS) should be obtained to evaluate adrenal hyperplasia; if Cushing's disease is suspected, a 24-hour urinary free cortisol and creatinine determinations should be obtained. This test does not detect adrenal failure (Addison's disease), and in the patient who has hypotension, weakness, vascular instability, and ashen skin, an adrenocorticotropic hormone (ACTH) stimulation test should be performed. In women who have galactorrhea and an elevated prolactin level, a computed tomography (CT) scan or magnetic resonance imaging (MRI) scan of the pituitary should be obtained, and if a macroadenoma is detected, a visual field examination should be carried out using Goldman-Bowl perimetry. In patients who have marked hyperandrogenemia, an ultrasonogram of the ovaries should be obtained to rule out the presence of a tumor or polycystic ovary syndrome. If a markedly elevated DHEAS level is found, a CT scan of the adrenal gland should be obtained to evaluate a potential adrenal adenoma or malignant tumor. Finally, any discharge from the breast should be evaluated by microscopic examination. If fat globules are not apparent, the discharge is most likely not associated with the amenorrhea but should be subjected to cytologic evaluation and Gram's stain to exclude breast disease.

## Differential Diagnosis of Primary Amenorrheas

The primary amenorrheas generally result from a genetic abnormality, outflow obstruction, or systemic illness. The classic 45,X gonadal dysgenesis (Turner's syndrome) is the most frequent cause of premature ovarian failure. This syndrome is caused by the absence of one of the two X chromosomes. The short arm of the X chromosome carries somatic information that affects height as well as skeletal and cardiac development, and the long arm carries the information necessary for follicle development and maturation. The patient who has Turner's syndrome frequently manifests lymphedema, shield chest, cubitus valgus, and ovarian failure at birth. However, pregnancies have been reported in patients who have 45,X gonadal dysgenesis as well as 45,X/46,XX mosaicism. In fact, not all patients who have Turner's syndrome have primary amenorrhea. Short stature is the hallmark of the syndrome. Another variant is 46,XY gonadal dysgenesis, also known as Swyer syndrome. These individuals have female external and internal genitalia, and the testicles are dysgenetic. There are a large number of other gonadal dysgenesis variants, including XO/XY, XO/XYY, XO/XY/XYY, and XO/XY, all called by the term mixed gonadal dysgenesis. These mosaics have a range of phenotypic findings, from those noted in patients who have gonadal dysgenesis to those who have marked ambiguity. There also exists a group of patients afflicted with pure gonadal dysgenesis, who have streak gonads but are of normal stature and lack other stigmata associated with Turner's syndrome. They usually have a eunuchoid habitus and primary amenorrhea; the latter condition is ordinarily their primary complaint. Finally, mention should be made of the so-called pseudo-Turner's syndrome (Noonan's syndrome). These patients have webbed neck, ptosis, short stature, cubitus valgus, and lymphedema; they tend to have triangular facies, pectus excavatum, and right-sided heart disease, including pulmonic stenosis, atrial septal defect, and mental retardation. Females with this syndrome have normal ovarian function, although sterility is generally the rule, and they have mildly elevated gonadotropins.

## Male Pseudohermaphrodism (Genetic Male and *Female-Like* Phenotype)

Patients who have this condition have either deficient androgen formation or deficiencies in androgen action. A variety of enzyme defects have been described that result in various forms of general ambiguity, including 21-hydroxylase deficiency, 3β-hydroxysteroid dehydrogenase-isomerase deficiency (which in its less severe forms occasionally appears in puberty or post puberty with hirsutism); 17α-hydroxylase deficiency, which results in a female who has negligible estrogen production and sexual infantilism, and 17,20-desmolase (lyase) deficiency (which has been reported to produce normal female external genitalia, a blind vaginal pouch, no müllerian derivatives, atrophic wolffian derivatives, and bilateral abdominal testes). The 17-β-hydroxysteroid dehydrogenase deficiency can be associated with pubertal gynecomastia and virilism. The formation of testosterone and estradiol is blocked; therefore, the gonads secrete increased levels of androstenedione and estrone, which can be converted to testosterone in extratesticular sites. Feminization occurs with this syndrome as a direct result of estrogen production directly or indirectly originating in the testes.

There are at least four defects in androgen action; the most common form of male pseudohermaphroditism is the complete form of testicular feminization. This is inherited as an X-linked recessive or X-linked dominant disorder, and it may be found in several family members. These individuals have a female habitus, normal stature, and abundant breast tissue; however, they have scant or absent pubic and axillary hair. The vagina is a blind pouch and they usually have a flat perineum, although there is no ambiguity of the external genitalia. Incomplete or partial forms of the disorder have been described, although there is some difference of opinion as to whether this may represent a 17-β-hydroxysteroid dehydrogenase deficiency. Finally, there has been a spectrum of X-linked recessive type incomplete male pseudohermaphrodite phenotypes that have been characterized under a variety of names, including Lubs, Gilbert-Dreyphus, Reifenstein's, and Rosewater's syndromes. These span the spectrum from near female phenotype to near male phenotype. There are also the autosomal recessive type 5-α-reductase deficiency patients, referred to as having pseudovaginal paraneoscrotal hypospadias. These individuals show vaginal development and are identified as females at birth; however, at puberty they undergo masculinization.

## Outflow Tract Obstruction

Müllerian ducts undergo fusion and canalization during the first 8 to 12 weeks of fetal life. Failure of formation, fusion, or canalization of these ducts, or failure of the urogenital sinus to canalize can result in primary amenorrhea. The most common outlet obstructions are the imperforate hymen and the Rokitansky-Kuster-Hauser syndrome. The imperforate hymen, as well as the mid-transverse vaginal septum, have the symptom of cyclic abdominal pain; at times, a bluish bulge can be seen in the perineum, and either excision or excision and placement of a vaginal mold establishes menstruation. Because the uterus is absent 90% of the time in müllerian agenesis, cyclic pain is not a symptom. These individuals show full secondary sexual maturation and may have cyclic ovulatory pain. As expected, they have a 46,XX karyotype and normal gonadotropin levels: A vagina can be created using the Frank or Ingram procedure, or a split-thickness skin graft can be placed according to the technique of McIndoe.

## Systemic Disorders

A great many systemic disorders can result in primary amenorrhea. For normal menstruation to occur, the arcuate nucleus must release pulses of GnRH approximately every hour. Stress or chronic illness often slows this pulse frequency to once every 3 hours. Virtually any disorder that can affect health and well-being can produce this disruption, including dysfunction of the central nervous, cardiac, endocrine, pulmonary, hematologic, or renal system. Furthermore, tumors or infiltrative disorders of the central nervous system and its appendages can result in failure to menstruate, as can the intake of recreational drugs, such as marijuana.

A well-described entity that disrupts menstruation in younger individuals is the relationship of stress and exercise to body weight. These disorders bridge the gap between primary and secondary amenorrhea; therefore, a fairly extensive discussion is warranted.

### ANOREXIA NERVOSA

This disorder is generally seen in white females younger than age 25. It is a syndrome that includes a history of weight loss, amenorrhea, and behavioral changes. This classic triad manifests the need to remain in a prepubertal body habitus, thus allowing the individual to avoid sexuality.

The incidence of anorexia nervosa has been reported to be from 1 in 100 to 1 in 200 in Caucasian girls between 12 and 18 years of age. However, there appear to be certain populations at risk. About two thirds of a sample of adolescent girls showed at least one symptom of disturbed eating behavior during adolescence before entering college, and early physical maturation presented a definite risk factor. Professional ballet dancers, for example, have an incidence ranging from 1 in 20 to 1 in 5. Many investigators consider weight loss and amenorrhea to be an early form of the disorder. Anorexia usually occurs in teenagers who lose 25% of their body weight and acquire distorted eating attitudes. These patients deny that they are ill, do not recognize their nutritional needs, and have a paralyzing sense of ineffectiveness. They hoard food, and many of them work in food processing businesses. They have no other psychological factors or obvious medical illnesses that can account for their condition. They physically manifest amenorrhea, cardiovascular dysfunction, and bulimia, although not all anorectic patients vomit. Often, patients consult a physician because they are amenorrheic, not because they feel they are underweight. They frequently have ovulatory dysfunction and may be infertile. Other patients seek medical help with the complaint of obesity, wanting medication for bloating, diuretics, or some sort of laxative to help control body weight. The serious consequence of anorexia is not amenorrhea or infertility but cardiovascular collapse, which may be lethal.

Amenorrhea occurs in almost all patients who have anorexia nervosa. It occurs before women lose weight; therefore, there is a psychological component. Most women who have anorexia do not restart their periods when they regain weight and must undergo ovulation induction with gonadotropins. These patients usually become pregnant easily because they have resting ovaries that respond readily to gonadotropins or pulsatile GnRH.

Women who have anorexia nervosa manifest the following physical findings: hypotension, hypothermia, bradycardia, cachexia, bradypnea, parotid enlargement, peripheral edema, increased body hair (lanugo), and hypercarotenemia. The skin may take on a yellowish hue, and they may have electrolyte imbalances, including metabolic alkalosis, hypokalemia, and mild azotemia. Therefore, the individual who demonstrates fear of obesity, body image disturbance, loss of 25% body weight, refusal to gain weight, and one or more physical findings described earlier should be considered for the diagnosis of psychogenic amenorrhea if not anorexia.

Typical laboratory studies in the patient who has anorexia nervosa include a decreased and inverted LH to FSH level. The evaluation of a 24-hour secretory pattern of LH level reveals lack of normal episodic variation, and the pattern may revert to a prepubertal one with episodic nocturnal LH spurts. The patient's serum cortisol level may be normal or increased, triiodothyronine (T3) production is decreased, and reverse T3 production is increased. Dehydroepiandrosterone, dehydroepiandrosterone sulfate (DHEAS), and 17β-estradiol levels are decreased, and antidiuretic hormone regulation is altered. It is suggested that when cortisol levels are elevated the response to adrenocorticotropic hormone-releasing factor (ACTH-RF) is abnormal, and the ACTH-RF level is increased in cerebrospinal fluid. Corticotropin-releasing hormone (CRH) is known to suppress LH pulses in both humans and in animals and may augment dopaminergic and opioid inhibition of GnRH. Hypothalamic dysfunction has also been described. There is a deficiency of the handling of water load, which results in a mild form of diabetes insipidus, abnormal thermoregulatory responses on exposure to temperature extremes, and a lack of shivering. The differential diagnosis of weight loss includes cancer, hypothalamic dysfunction, and various endocrine disorders, such as Addison's disease and hyperthyroidism, as well as functional disorders, including depression, schizophrenia, and chronic wasting diseases, such as tuberculosis and Crohn's disease.

## BULIMIA

A syndrome closely aligned to anorexia nervosa, which is considered part of the family of psychogenic amenorrhea, is bulimia, which is the Greek word for ox hunger. It may or may not include menstrual irregularities. A very large number of women have bulimia; more than one third of first-year college students have experienced this problem. Many women have some episodes of bulimia in their lifetime. Bulimic individuals are binge eaters, and they tend to have favorite foods, such as ice cream, cookies, pastries, and popcorn with lots of butter. They gorge and then vomit. Eating is usually done alone. The termination of the binge usually results in vomiting, which may occur over a dozen times a day. Frequently, bulimic individuals will come to the emergency room with an esophageal tear (Mallory-Weiss syndrome). Bulimic women try to lose weight and frequently seek diuretics, diets, and cathartics. Their weight may not fluctuate by more than 10 pounds, which is why they have so few problems with menstrual function. As opposed to anorectic women, they know that they have a disturbed eating behavior. Bulimic women tend to be polydrug abusers, taking diet pills, recreational drugs, and excess alcohol. Many of them have criminal records, because they are caught shoplifting food to satisfy their eating habit. The bulimic behavior pattern is often found in highly motivated young women who are under considerable family pressure to achieve social success.

Psychoneuroendocrinology is a rapidly developing field that encompasses many disorders frequently seen by the practicing gynecologist, including chronic hypothalamic anovulation, stress-related amenorrhea, amenorrhea associated with weight loss and a change in the lean body mass–to-fat ratio, athletic amenorrhea, and menstrual problems associated with eating disorders, including anorexia nervosa, bulimia, and bulimorexia. These conditions are so blended in the modern gynecologic patient, so that the practitioner is frequently faced with a young professional woman in a high-stress position who participates in a significant exercise program each week and maintains a body weight that correlates with the threshold at which menstrual dysfunction can develop. These individuals frequently have low normal gonadotropin levels and are hypoestrogenic. This can result in osteopenia, perhaps an increased incidence of stress fractures, change in status of lipoproteins, and a specific form of malnutrition.

A variety of activities can result in exercise-induced amenorrhea. This can range from ballet dancing, which may delay puberty in young women, to long distance running and certain field events. The intensity and length of training correlates directly with amenorrhea and, in fact, amenorrhea has been found to vary with types of exercise. For example, runners are much more prone to amenorrhea than swimmers, which is attributed to a difference in body composition among swimmers, who frequently have a higher fat ratio. Likewise, body bulk seems to be lower in runners than in swimmers.

It is virtually impossible to separate body weight and composition from exercise. It has been suggested that one of the events that triggers the onset of puberty is the acquisition of a body weight of 48 kg and an appropriate fat-to-lean mass ratio. It is known that malnutrition delays puberty. Fat to lean body weight changes from 1.5 to 1.3 and 22% fat is required for the maintenance of menstrual function. A loss of 10 to 15% of body weight causes cessation of menstruation. Athletic amenorrhea can occur before weight loss, as it does in anorexia nervosa. The acute interruption of exercise, mainly through injury, can also result in the restoration of menstrual function without an appreciable change in body weight.

All of these alterations result in psychic stress that inhibits GnRH release from the GnRH pulse regulator in the arcuate nucleus. This results in a sequence of events ranging from disorders of folliculogenesis to luteal phase defect, oligo-ovulation, anovulation, and amenorrhea. Individuals who are subject to high levels of exercise or stress are influenced by the conditions set forth in the general adaptation syndrome by Selye. These individuals show signs of hypercortisolism, and athletes in extreme training obliterate the 24-hour circadian rhythm of cortisol. Corticotropin-releasing factor brings about the breakdown of pro-opiomelanocortin, which releases ACTH, endorphins, and other by-products. Likewise, there are alterations in thyroid function, with a significant reduction in serum 3,5,3′-T3 and thyroxine (T4) and an elevation in growth hormone, prolactin, melatonin, epinephrine, and norepinephrine.

The management of the patient who has exercise-related amenorrhea is difficult. Frequently, these women are addicted to the physical and psychic euphoria that they achieve through exercise and are determined to maintain a trim body habitus and a competitive lifestyle. It is suggested that these women be given accurate information regarding the risk of maintaining a hypoestrogenic state and be offered replacement hormone therapy. Likewise, the use of calcium supplements and multivitamins may be beneficial.

## Secondary Amenorrhea

Many of the systemic causes of primary amenorrhea are also found in secondarily amenorrheic patients. Dysfunction of the central nervous system, decrease in gonadotropin production, eating disorders, and extremes in athletic activity or stress can produce dysfunction in the older as well as the younger patient. However, the most common cause of secondary amenorrhea is chronic hypothalamic anovulation. As noted earlier, these patients have normal gonadotropin levels with an appropriate LH-to-FSH ratio. They respond with withdrawal bleeding to the intramuscular administration of progesterone, 100 mg (Progesterone Challenge). This is opposed to the patient who has hypothalamic amenorrhea with a decreased LH-to-FSH level and an inversion of the LH-to-FSH ratio, who fails to respond to a progestogen challenge.

Pituitary dysfunction can likewise result in secondary amenorrhea. Perhaps the most common cause is functional hyperprolactinemia, which is thought by many investigators to represent a disorder of central dopamine metabolism or the presence of prolactinoma. Likewise, secondary amenorrhea can occur after resection of prolactinomas or other tumors, or in association with infarction of the pituitary gland (Sheehan's syndrome) or head trauma. In the former state, hyperprolactinemia is diagnosed by elevated prolactin levels on multiple occasions and by hypopituitarism (the finding of low normal gonadotropin levels). At times, this can be associated with hypothyroidism, although not exclusively. The patient who has hypothyroidism may have dry skin, lethargy, and constipation. Frequently, the T4 level is normal, whereas the TSH level is markedly elevated. However, hypothyroidism may be associated with a low T4 level and a low TSH level. All these conditions should be treated with replacement thyroid hormones.

Disorders of adrenal metabolism can likewise result in the development of secondary amenorrhea. Dehydroepiandrosterone sulfate may be mildly elevated in patients with polycystic ovary syndrome 50% of the time or a variation in congenital adrenal hyperplasia with either 21-hydroxylase, 17-β-hydroxylase, or 3-β-hydroxysteroid dehydrogenase deficiency. Markedly elevated DHEA-S associated with virilism is an indication of adrenal adenomas or other tumors. Hyperadrenalism is manifested in the form of Cushing's syndrome that may be dependent or independent of ACTH.

Obesity is associated with the development of menstrual dysfunction; however, it may not be associated with polycystic ovary syndrome (PCO). The relationship between excess body fat and ovulatory dysfunction appears to be stronger for early-onset obesity. A correction of ovulatory function can be achieved approximately 68% of the time with normalization of body weight.

The ovary is one of the most common sites for the development of ovulatory dysfunction. This may result from elevated androgen secretion in patients who have PCO, hyperthecosis, or ovarian tumors. Patients who have PCO manifest an elevated LH-to-FSH ratio 40% of the time; elevated DHEAS levels 50% of the time; elevated prolactin levels 20% of the time; a testosterone value at the upper limit of normal, elevated, free testosterone; and decreased sex hormone binding globulin.

Premature ovarian failure (i.e., the cessation of menses before age 35) may be hereditary, an autoimmune response, or of unknown etiology. The diagnosis is usually made by finding FSH levels higher than 40 mIU/ml in association with amenorrhea or oligoovulation. However, frequently patients manifest variable symptoms, such as mood alteration, depression, lethargy, and dysphoria, which are not associated with menstrual irregularities or hot flushes. Elevated FSH levels suggestive of the 10- to 15-year perimenopausal period may also be present. These patients are best treated with oral contraceptive agents or hormone replacement therapy to carry them through this difficult life transition.

Although it is not frequently recognized as an ovarian cause of secondary amenorrhea, surgery with either wedge resection or resection of endometriomas can result in ovulatory dysfunction or premature ovarian failure. Like patients who have premature ovarian failure, these individuals have an FSH level in the range of 25 to 40 mIU/ml. Likewise, children or young women who have been treated for leukemia, lymphoma, or other adolescent neoplasia, with drugs such as alkylating agents, may develop ovarian failure. Rarely, one sees a patient who has gonadotropin-resistant syndrome (Savage syndrome) in which ovarian follicles are present within the ovarian stroma; however, these germ cells cannot bind FSH. These individuals have elevated LH and FSH levels and should be treated with hormone replacement therapy.

Finally, disorders of the endometrium are an uncommon cause of secondary amenorrhea. Uterine synechiae may be of the unintentional or intentional (endometrial ablation) type. Asherman's syndrome is associated with uterine trauma either secondary to the presence of an infected IUD, an infected spontaneous incomplete miscarriage, or a D&C. The patient with Asherman's syndrome has normal gonadotropin and estrogen levels and deformity of the uterine cavity when evaluated by hysterosalpingography. The condition is treated surgically and followed up with estrogen priming of the endometrium.

## Treatment

The treatment of the patient who has amenorrhea is dependent upon age and whether the patient wishes to become pregnant in the near future. The younger patient who has not achieved sexual development is best treated with hormone replacement therapy consisting of cyclic estrogen and progestogen combinations. Because nausea is frequently a problem with this form of therapy, it is suggested that the patient start with a low dose of conjugated estrogen, such as 0.3 mg for 3 to 4 months before increasing the dose and adding a cyclic overlapping progestogen. Concomitantly, the patient who has a systemic illness should be treated appropriately in an attempt to restore well-being. This may involve medical or surgical therapy as determined by the particular illness. Patients who have outflow tract obstruction usually require surgical correction. These patients often have an acute abdomen, and the surgeon must establish an egress of menstruation. Patients who require a neovagina must be carefully evaluated before such surgery is attempted. This is a long and arduous therapy and requires considerable maturity and dedication. It is suggested that individuals reach at least their late teens to early twenties before undertaking such surgery. The frank technique of dilation, however, can be attempted at a younger age but may not be successful in an individual who is not highly motivated.

The approach to the patient with secondary amenorrhea again must be judged in terms of whether future pregnancy is desired. If the patient is under- or overweight, and this is determined to be the causative factor, attempts should be made to restore normal body weight. If the patient has compensated hypothyroidism, replacement thyroid hormones usually restore menstrual function. Patients who have hyperprolactinemia may be treated by surgical therapy if it is associated with a pituitary tumor, or by medical therapy in the presence or absence of a tumor. Patients who have microadenomas (i.e., tumors smaller than 1 cm) frequently have resolution of the lesion after surgery. However, approximately half of these individuals continue to have persistent ovulatory dysfunction. With larger lesions, the failure rate exceeds 70%. The medication of choice for the treatment of hyperprolactinemia is bromocriptine, in doses ranging from 1.25 to approximately 15 mg. The majority of patients respond to doses between 1.25 and 5 mg administered one to four times a day. It is suggested that bromocriptine therapy be started with a 1.25 dose at bedtime, as this produces maximum prolactin suppression. The dose should be slowly increased over several weeks until euprolactinemia has been obtained. Patients who fail to respond to bromocriptine may be treated with pergolide mesylate in doses ranging from 50 to 100 µg at bedtime. Although not approved by the FDA for the treatment of hyperprolactinemia in the United States, this drug is used widely in Europe and Canada. A third generation dopamine agonist, cabergoline, has been introduced in a dose range of 0.5 to 1 mg twice per week. All of these drugs produce normalization of serum prolactin levels and effectively shrink large or small pituitary tumors. The return to ovulation and pregnancy rate are extremely high with all forms of therapy.

The patient who has premature ovarian failure should be referred to an egg donation program if she desires pregnancy and begun on replacement cyclic overlapping hormonal therapy with estrogen and progestogen. The dose should be titrated until symptoms are resolved.

The management of the patient with hyperandrogenemia again depends upon whether or not pregnancy is desired. If the patient does not wish to be pregnant, it is suggested that oral contraceptive therapy be instituted with a monophasic pill containing a nonandrogenic progestogen. Spironolactone, 100 to 200 mg per day, can be added to this therapy to produce satisfactory control of hirsutism and other signs of androgen excess. The patient who has one of the variants of adrenal hyperplasia is best treated by replacement glucocorticoid therapy. In general, a daily dose of dexamethasone, 0.5 to 0.75 mg, is adequate for control.

The patient who desires conception and is euprolactinemic, euthyroid, and euandrogenemic is best treated with clomiphene citrate at doses ranging from 50 to 150 mg per day on cycle days 2 to 6. These patients should be given a progesterone withdrawal bleeding episode before the administration of medication, and ovulation should be monitored with a urinary LH surge kit, midluteal progesterone level test, basal body temperature chart, and sequential sonography. Individuals who do not conceive within three to five ovulatory cycles should have complete infertility workup, and other forms of ovulation induction should be contemplated. The therapy of choice for these patients would be ultrapurified or recombinant FSH administered in a customized protocol. Likewise, pulsatile GnRH may be administered either subcutaneously or intravenously. Although the pregnancy rate is satisfactory with this form of therapy, a high incidence of miscarriage has been reported.

## Summary and Conclusion

The evaluation of the patient with amenorrhea is a complex undertaking that demands a command of reproductive medicine and logical therapy. Pregnancy should be ruled out in virtually any age group whether or not the patient admits to being sexually active. Whether the amenorrhea is primary or secondary, the age of the patient helps guide the clinician through the differential diagnosis. Assays of LH, FSH, prolactin, and TSH levels usually point to the location of dysfunction. Interpretation of these values in light of a careful history and physical examination will avoid misdiagnosis and inappropriate therapy.

### REFERENCES

Asherman JG: Amenorrhea traumatica (atretica). J Obstet Gynaecol Br Emp 55:23, 1948.
Asukai K, Uemura T, Minaguchi H: Occult hyperprolactinemia in infertile women. Fertil Steril 60:423, 1993.
Blackwell RE: Diagnosis and management of prolactinomas. Fertil Steril 43:5, 1985.
Blackwell RE, Younger JB: Long-term medical therapy and follow-up of pediatric-adolescent patients with prolactin-secreting macroadenomas. Fertil Steril 45:713, 1986.
Boyar RM, Katz J, Finkelstein JW, et al: Anorexia nervosa: Immaturity of the 24-hour luteinizing hormone secretory pattern. N Engl J Med 219:861, 1974.
Bruch H: Anorexia nervosa and its differential diagnosis. N Nerv Ment Dis 141:555, 1965.
Bullen BA, Skriinar GS, Beitins IZ, et al: Induction of menstrual disorders by strenuous exercise in untrained women. N Engl J Med 312:1349, 1985.
Colover J: Sarcoidosis with involvement of the nervous system. Brain 71:451, 1948.
Costello RT: Subclinical adenoma of the pituitary gland. Am J Pathol 12:205, 1936.
Deirschke DH, Bhattarharya AN, Atkinson LE, et al: Circhoral oscillations of plasma LH levels in the ovariectomized rhesus monkey. Endocrinology 87:850, 1970.
Fisher EC, Nelson ME, Frontera WE, et al: Bone mineral content and levels of gonadotropins and estrogens in amenorrheic running women. J Clin Endocrinol Metab 62:1232, 1986.
Frisch RE, Gotz-Webergen AVE, McArthur JW, et al: Delayed menarche and amenorrhea of college athletes in relation to age of onset of training. JAMA 246:1559, 1981.
Frisch R, Wyshak G, Vincent L: Delayed menarche and amenorrhea in ballet dancers. N Engl J Med 303:17, 1980.
Griffin JE, Edwards C, Madden JD, et al: Congenital absence of the vagina. Ann Int Med 85:224, 1976.
Griffin JE, Wilson JD: The androgen resistance syndrome: 5α-reductase deficiency, testicular feminization and related disorders. In Scriver CR, Beaudet AI, Sly WS, et al (eds): The Metabolic Basis of Inherited Disease, 6th ed. New York, McGraw-Hill, 1989, pp 1919–1944.
Hsu LK: Outcome of anorexia nervosa: A review of the literature (1954–1978). Arch Gen Psychiatry 37:1041, 1980.
Klibanski A, Need RM, Bettins IZ, et al: Decreased bone density in hyperprolactinemic women. N Engl J Med 303:1511, 1980.
Klibanski A, Zervas NT: Diagnosis and management of hormone-secreting pituitary adenomas. N Engl J Med 324:822, 1991.
Knobil E, Plant TM, Wilde L, et al: Control of the rhesus monkey menstrual cycle: Permissive role of hypothalamic gonadotropin-releasing hormone. Science 207:1371, 1980.
Lamberts SWJ, Quik RPF: A comparison of the efficacy and safety of pergolide and bromocriptine in the treatment of hyperprolactinemia. J Clin Endocrinol Metab 72:635, 1991.
Marshall JC, Kelch RP: Gonadotropin-releasing hormone: Role of pulsatile secretion in the regulation of reproduction. N Engl J Med 315:1459, 1986.
Marshall WA, Tanner JM: Variation in the pattern of pubertal changes in boys. Arch Dis Child 45:13, 1970.
McDonough PG: Disorders of gonadal differentiation and sex chromosome anomalies. Semin Reprod Endocrinol 5:221, 1987.
Molitch ME, Elton RL, Blackwell RE, et al: Bromocriptine as primary therapy for prolactin-secreting macroadenomas: Results of a prospective multicenter study. J Clin Endocrinol Metab 60:698, 1985.
Morris JM: The syndrome of testicular feminization in male pseudohermaphrodites. Am J Obstet Gynecol 65:1192, 1953.
Plant TM, Krey LG, Moossy J, et al: The arcuate nucleus and the control of the gonadotropin and prolactin secretion in the female rhesus monkey (Macaca mulatta). Endocrinology 102:52, 1978.
Pugliese MT, Lipshitz F, Grad G, et al: Fear of obesity: A cause of short stature and delayed puberty. N Engl J Med 309:513, 1983.
Pyle R, Mitchell J: Bulimia, a report of 34 cases. J Clin Psychiatry 42:60, 1981.
Reindollar RH, Byrd JR, McDonough PG: Delayed sexual development: A study of 252 patients. Am J Obstet Gynecol 140:371, 1981.
Rivier C, Rivier J, Vale W: Stress-induced inhibition of reproductive functions: Role of endogenous corticotropin-releasing factor. Science 231:607, 1986.
Sanborn CF, Martin BJ, Wagner WW: Is athletic amenorrhea specific to runners? Am J Obstet Gynecol 143:859, 1982.
Serri O, Rasio E, Beauregard H, et al: Recurrence of hyperprolactinemia after selective transsphenoidal adenomectomy in women with prolactinoma. N Engl J Med 309:280, 1994.
Sheehan HL: Postpartum necrosis of the anterior pituitary. J Pathol Bacteriol 45:189, 1937.
Siris ES, Leenthal BG, Vaitukiatis JL: Effects of childhood leukemia and chemotherapy on puberty and reproductive function in girls. N Engl J Med 294:1143, 1976.
Suh BY, Liu JH, Berga SL, et al: Hypercortisolism in patients with functional hypothalamic amenorrhea. J Clin Endocrinol Metab 66:733, 1988.
Turner HH: A syndrome of infantilism, congenital webbed neck, and cubitus valgus. Endocrinology 23:566, 1938.
Vogel JM, Vogel P: Idiopathic histiocytosis: A discussion of eosinophilic granuloma, the Hand-Schuller-Christian syndrome and Letterer-Siwe syndrome. Semin Hematol 9:349, 1972.
Warren M: The effects of exercise on pubertal progression and reproductive function in girls. J Clin Endocrinol Metab 51:1150, 1980.
Weiss MH, Teal J, Gott P, et al: Natural history of microprolactinomas: Six year follow-up. Neurosurgery 12:180, 1983.
Wiser WL, Bates GW: Management of vaginal agenesis: A report of 92 cases. Surg Gynecol Obstet 159:108, 1984.
Wyshak G, Frisch RE: Evidence for a secular trend in age of menarche. N Engl J Med 306:1033, 1982.
Zacharias L, Wurtman JR: Age at menarche. N Engl J Med 280:868, 1969.

# 54

# Dysfunctional Uterine Bleeding*

LEON SPEROFF

Dysfunctional uterine bleeding is defined as a variety of bleeding manifestations of anovulatory cycles (in the absence of pathology or medical illness). It can be confidently managed without surgical intervention by therapeutic regimens founded on sound physiologic principles. This formulation is based on knowledge of how the postovulatory menstrual function is naturally controlled and uses pharmacologic application of sex steroids to reverse the abnormal tissue factors that lead to the excessive and prolonged flow typical of anovulatory cycles.

This mode of clinical management has been in regular use for many years, and failure to control vaginal bleeding with this therapy, despite appropriate application and utilization, excludes the diagnosis of dysfunctional uterine bleeding. If this occurs, attention is directed to a pathologic entity within the reproductive tract as the cause of abnormal bleeding.

Heavy but regular menstrual bleeding can be encountered in ovulating women. In the absence of a specific pathologic cause, it is presumed that this reflects subtle disturbances in the mechanisms that control bleeding from endometrial tissue. In essentially all cases, evaluation and treatment are identical to the approach detailed in this chapter.

## Normal Withdrawal (Menstrual) Bleeding

Of all the types of hormonal-endometrial relationships, the most stable endometrium and the most reproducible menstrual function in terms of quantity and duration occurs with postovulatory estrogen-progesterone withdrawal bleeding. It is so controlling that many women over the years come to expect a certain characteristic flow pattern. Any slight deviations, such as plus or minus 1 day in duration or minor deviation from expected napkin or tampon use, are causes for major concern in the patient. So ingrained is the expected flow that considerable clinician reassurance may be required in some instances of minor variability. Although variability of menstrual cycles is a common feature during teenage years and the perimenopausal transition, the characteristics of menstrual bleeding do not undergo appreciable change during the reproductive years.

The usual duration of flow is 4 to 6 days, but many women flow as little as 2 days and as much as 8 days.

---

*This chapter is adapted from the sixth edition of Clinical Gynecologic Endocrinology and Infertility written by Leon Speroff, Robert H. Glass, and Nathan G. Kase and published by Lippincott, Williams & Wilkins, Philadelphia, 1999.

The normal volume of menstrual blood loss is 30 ml. Greater than 80 ml is abnormal. Most blood loss occurs during the first 3 days of a period, so excessive flow may exist without prolongation of flow.

Although the postovulatory phase averages 14 days, greater variability in the proliferative phase produces a distribution in the duration of a menstrual cycle. Based on the normal experience, menstrual bleeding more often than every 24 days or less often than every 42 days deserves evaluation. Flow that lasts 7 or more days also deserves evaluation. A flow that totals more than 80 ml per month usually leads to anemia and should be treated. In general, however, an effort to quantitate menstrual flow beyond historical information is not necessary because evaluation and treatment are responses to a patient's own perceptions regarding duration, amount, and timing of her menstrual bleeding. Although the correlation between a patient's perceptions and actual menstrual blood loss is poor, an individual patient's anxiety and concern deserve consideration and evaluation. Midcycle bleeding can be a consequence of the preovulatory fall in estrogen; however, intermenstrual bleeding is often due to pathology.

There are three reasons for the self-limited character of estrogen-progesterone withdrawal bleeding. First, it is a universal endometrial event. Because the onset and conclusion of menses are related to a precise sequence of hormonal events, menstrual changes occur almost simultaneously in all segments of the endometrium. Second, the endometrial tissue that has responded to an appropriate sequence of estrogen and progesterone is structurally stable, and random breakdown of tissue due to fragility is avoided. The events leading to ischemic disintegration of the endometrium are orderly and progressive, being related to rhythmic waves of vasoconstriction of increasing duration. Finally, inherent in the events that start menstrual function after estrogen-progesterone are the factors involved in stopping menstrual flow. Just as waves of vasoconstriction initiate the ischemic events, prolonged vasoconstriction abetted by the stasis associated with endometrial collapse enables clotting factors to seal off the exposed bleeding sites. Additional and significant effects are obtained by resumed estrogen activity.

The withdrawal of estrogen and progesterone initiates important endometrial events: vasomotor reactions, the process of apoptosis, tissue loss, and finally menstruation. The most prominent immediate effect of this hormone withdrawal is a modest shrinking of the tissue height and remarkable spiral arteriole vasomotor responses. The following vascular sequence has been constructed from direct observations of rhesus endometrium. With shrinkage of height, blood flow within the spiral vessels diminishes, venous drainage is decreased, and vasodilatation ensues. Thereafter, the spiral arterioles undergo rhythmic vasoconstriction and relaxation. Each successive spasm is more prolonged and profound, leading eventually to endometrial blanching. Within the 24 hours immediately preceding menstruation, these reactions lead to endometrial ischemia and stasis. White cells migrate through capillary walls, at first remaining adjacent to vessels but then extending throughout the stroma. During arteriolar vasomotor changes, red blood cells escape into the interstitial space. Thrombin-platelet plugs also appear in superficial vessels. The prostaglandin content ($PGF_2$ and $PGE_2$) in the secretory endometrium reaches its highest levels at the time of menstruation. The vasoconstriction and myometrial contractions associated with the menstrual events are believed to be significantly mediated by $PGF_2$ from glandular cells and the potent vasoconstrictor, endothelin-1, derived from stromal decidual cells.

In the first half of the secretory phase, acid phosphatase and potent lytic enzymes are confined to lysosomes. Their release is inhibited by progesterone stabilization of the lysosomal membranes. With the waning of estrogen and progesterone levels, the lysosomal membranes are not maintained, and the enzymes are released into the cytoplasm of epithelial, stromal, and endothelial cells and eventually into the intercellular space. These active enzymes will digest their cellular constraints, leading to the release of prostaglandins, extravasation of red blood cells, tissue necrosis, and vascular thrombosis. This process is one of *apoptosis* (programmed cell death, characterized by a specific morphologic pattern that involves cell shrinkage and chromatin condensation culminating in cell fragmentation) mediated by cytokines.

Endometrial tissue breakdown involves a family of enzymes, matrix metalloproteinases, that degrade components (including collagens, gelatins, fibronectin, and laminin) of the extracellular matrix and basement membrane. The metalloproteinases include collagenases that degrade interstitial and basement membrane collagens, gelatinases that further degrade collagens, and stromelysins that degrade fibronectin, laminin, and glycoproteins. The expression of metalloproteinases in human endometrium follows a pattern correlated with the menstrual cycle, indicating a sex steroid response as part of the growth and remodeling of the endometrium, with a marked increase in late secretory and early menstrual endometrium. Progesterone withdrawal from endometrial cells induces matrix metalloproteinase secretion that is followed by the breakdown of cellular membranes and the dissolution of extracellular matrix. Appropriately, this enzyme expression increases in the decidualized endometrium of the late secretory phase, during the time of declining progesterone levels. With the continuing progesterone secretion of early pregnancy, the decidua is maintained and metalloproteinase expression is suppressed, in a mechanism mediated by

TFG-β. In a nonpregnant cycle, metalloproteinase expression is suppressed after menses, presumably by increasing estrogen levels. Metalloproteinase activity is restrained by specific tissue inhibitors, designated as transforming growth factor. Thus, progesterone withdrawal can lead to endometrial breakdown through a mechanism that is independent of vascular events (specifically ischemia), a mechanism that involves cytokines.

Eventually, considerable leakage occurs as a result of diapedesis, and finally, interstitial hemorrhage occurs due to breaks in superficial arterioles and capillaries. As ischemia and weakening progress, the continuous binding membrane is fragmented and intercellular blood is extruded into the endometrial cavity. New thrombin-platelet plugs form intravascularly upstream at the shedding surface, limiting blood loss. Increased blood loss is a consequence of reduced platelet numbers and inadequate hemostatic plug formation. Menstrual bleeding is influenced by activation of clotting and fibrinolysis. Fibrinolysis is principally the consequence of the potent enzyme, plasmin, formed from its inactive precursor, plasminogen. Endometrial stromal cell tissue factor (TF) and plasminogen activators and inhibitors are involved in achieving a balance in this process. TF stimulates coagulation, initially binding to factor VII. TF and plasminogen activator inhibitor-1 (PAI-1) expression accompanies decidualization, and the levels of these factors may govern the amount of bleeding. PAI-1 in particular exerts an important restraining action on fibrinolysis and proteolytic activity.

With further tissue disorganization, the endometrium shrinks even more and coiled arterioles are buckled. Additional ischemic breakdown ensues with necrosis of cells and defects in vessels, adding to the menstrual effluvium. A natural cleavage point exists between basalis and spongiosum, and once breached, the loose, vascular, edematous stroma of the spongiosum desquamates and collapses. The process is initiated in the fundus and inexorably extends throughout the uterus. In the end, the typical deflated shallow dense menstrual endometrium results. Within 13 hours, the endometrial height shrinks from 4 to 1.25 mm. Menstrual flow stops as a result of the combined effects of prolonged vasoconstriction, tissue collapse, vascular stasis, and estrogen-induced "healing." In contrast to postpartum bleeding, myometrial contractions are not important for control of menstrual bleeding. Thrombin generation in the basal endometrium in response to extravasation of blood is essential for hemostasis. Thrombin promotes the generation of fibrin, the activation of platelets and clotting cofactors, and angiogenesis.

Platelets and fibrin play a direct part in the hemostasis achieved in a bleeding menstrual endometrium. Deficiencies in these constituents cause the increased blood loss seen in von Willebrand's disease and in thrombocytopenia. The blood loss at menses in afibrinogenemia indicates the importance of fibrin-generating and fibrinolytic factors in the menstrual process. Intravascular thrombi are observed in the functional layers and are localized to the shedding surface of the tissue. These are known as impeding "plugs" in that blood may flow past these only partially occlusive barriers. Therefore, thrombi continue to develop within the menstrual blood, accounting for the platelets and large amounts of fibrin found in this effluent. Fibrinolysis occurs in the endometrial tissue, limiting fibrin deposition in the proximal still unshed layer. Despite large holes in vessel walls, with blood exposed to collagen surfaces, no occlusive surface thrombus is formed. After early dependence on thrombin plugs to restrain blood loss, later generalized vasoconstrictive hemostasis without thrombin plugs occur. The healing endometrium is pale, collapsed, and disorderly, but no thrombi and no fibrin deposits are seen.

Lockwood and associates assigned a key role to decidual cells in both the process of endometrial bleeding (menstruation) and the process of endometrial hemostasis (implantation and placentation). Implantation requires endometrial hemostasis, and the maternal uterus requires resistance to invasion. Inhibition of endometrial hemorrhage can be attributed, to a significant degree, to appropriate changes in critical factors as a consequence of decidualization (e.g., lower plasminogen activator levels, reduced expression of the enzymes that degrade the stromal extracellular matrix [such as the metalloproteinases], increased levels of PAI-1 and TF). Withdrawal of estrogen and progesterone support, however, leads to changes in the opposite directions, consistent with endometrial breakdown.

## Categories of Uterine Bleeding

Traditional definitions are as follows: oligomenorrhea, intervals greater than 42 days; polymenorrhea, intervals less than 24 days; menorrhagia, regular normal intervals, excessive flow and duration; and, metrorrhagia, irregular intervals, excessive flow and duration.

### ESTROGEN WITHDRAWAL BLEEDING

This category of uterine bleeding can occur after bilateral oophorectomy, radiation of mature follicles, or administration of estrogen to a castrate and then discontinuation of therapy. Similarly, the bleeding that occurs postcastration can be delayed by concomitant estrogen therapy. Flow will occur on discontinuation of exogenous estrogen. Midcycle bleeding can occur secondary to the decrease in estrogen that immediately precedes ovulation.

## ESTROGEN BREAKTHROUGH BLEEDING

Here a semiquantitative relationship exists between the amount of estrogen stimulating the endometrium and the type of bleeding that can ensue. Relatively low doses of estrogen yield intermittent spotting that may be prolonged but is generally light in quantity of flow. On the other hand, high levels of estrogen and sustained availability lead to prolonged periods of amenorrhea followed by acute often profuse bleeds with excessive loss of blood.

## PROGESTERONE WITHDRAWAL BLEEDING

Removal of the corpus luteum will lead to endometrial desquamation. Pharmacologically, a similar event can be achieved by administration and discontinuation of progesterone or a nonestrogenic synthetic progestin. Progesterone withdrawal bleeding occurs only if the endometrium is initially proliferated by endogenous or exogenous estrogen. If estrogen therapy is continued as progesterone is withdrawn, the progesterone withdrawal bleeding still occurs. Only if estrogen levels are increased 10- to 20-fold will progesterone withdrawal bleeding be delayed.

## PROGESTERONE BREAKTHROUGH BLEEDING

Progesterone breakthrough bleeding occurs only in the presence of an unfavorably high ratio of progesterone to estrogen. In the absence of sufficient estrogen, continuous progesterone therapy will yield intermittent bleeding of variable duration, similar to low-dose estrogen breakthrough bleeding noted above. This is the type of bleeding associated with the long-acting progestin-only contraceptive methods, levonorgestrel (Norplant) and medroxyprogesterone acetate (Depo-Provera).

# Diagnosis

Dysfunctional uterine bleeding is a diagnosis made by exclusion. A very common cause of abnormal uterine bleeding is pregnancy and pregnancy-related problems such as ectopic pregnancy or spontaneous abortion. This category of problems should always receive diagnostic consideration. Patients may be using medications unknowingly with an impact on the endometrium. For example, the use of ginseng, an herbal root, has been associated with estrogenic activity and abnormal bleeding. Pathology of the menstrual outflow tract includes cancers of the cervix and endometrium, endometrial polyps, leiomyomata uteri, and infections. Although uterine bleeding is a common problem with various contraceptive methods and postmenopausal hormonal therapy, the clinician should always be convinced no pathology is present. Abnormal menstrual cycles are occasionally the first sign of either hypothyroidism or hyperthyroidism. One should keep in mind that as many as 20% of adolescents with dysfunctional uterine bleeding will have a coagulation defect, although the most common cause is anovulation. Bleeding secondary to a blood dyscrasia is usually a heavy flow with regular cyclic menses (menorrhagia), and this same pattern can be seen in patients being treated with anticoagulants. Irregular serious bleeding is often associated with severe organ disease, such as renal failure and liver failure. Finally, careful examination is worthwhile to discover genital injury or a foreign object.

The effects of tubal ligation are still not certain. The first well-controlled studies of this issue demonstrated no change in menstrual patterns, volume, or pain. Subsequently, these same authors reported an increase in dysmenorrhea and changes in menstrual bleeding. However, these authors failed to agree in their findings (a change found by one group was not confirmed by the other). Adding to the confusion, the incidence of hysterectomy for bleeding disorders in women after tubal sterilization was reported to be increased by some, but not by others. In a large cohort of women in a group health plan, hospitalization for menstrual disorders was significantly increased; however, the authors believed this reflected bias by patient and physician preference for surgical treatment. It is possible that extensive electrocoagulation of the fallopian tubes can change ovarian steroid production. Perhaps this is why menstrual changes have been detected with longer (4 years) follow-up, whereas no changes have been noted with the use of rings or clips. However, attempts to relate poststerilization menstrual changes with extent of tissue destruction fail to find a correlation, and an increase in hospitalization for menstrual disorders after unipolar cautery cannot be documented. Still another long-term follow-up study (3 to 4.5 years) failed to document any significant changes in menstrual cycles. This inconsistency can reflect differences in sterilization techniques and the fact that a surgical solution is more likely to be chosen if continuing fertility is no longer an issue. The best answer for now is that some women experience menstrual changes, but most do not.

# Treatment

The immediate objective of medical therapy in anovulatory bleeding is to retrieve the natural controlling influences missing in this tissue: universal synchronous endometrial events, structural stability, and vasomotor rhythmicity.

## PROGESTIN THERAPY

Most women will at sometime during their reproductive years either fail to ovulate or not sustain adequate corpus luteum function or duration. But this occurs with increased frequency in adolescence and in the decade before menopause. The usual clinical presentation is oligomenorrhea with bouts of heavy bleeding. Women correctly seek medical advice promptly because these menstrual aberrations suggest unplanned pregnancy or uterine pathology. Under most circumstances, progestin therapy will suffice to control the abnormality once uterine pathology is ruled out.

Progesterone and progestins are powerful antiestrogens when given in pharmacologic doses. Progestins stimulate 17β-hydroxysteroid dehydrogenase and sulfotransferase activity, which convert estradiol to estrone sulfate (which is rapidly excreted from the cell). Progestins also diminish estrogen effects on target cells by inhibiting the augmentation of estrogen receptors that ordinarily accompanies estrogen action (receptor replenishment inhibition). In addition, progestins suppress estrogen-mediated transcription of oncogenes. These influences account for the antimitotic antigrowth impact of progestins on the endometrium (prevention and reversal of hyperplasia, limitation of growth postovulation, and the marked atrophy during pregnancy or in response to combined oral contraceptives).

In the treatment of oligomenorrhea, orderly limited withdrawal bleeding can be accomplished by administration of a progestin such as medroxyprogesterone acetate, 10 mg daily for 10 days every month. Absence of induced bleeding requires workup. In the treatment of dysfunctional menometrorrhagia or polymenorrhea, progestins are prescribed for 10 days to 2 weeks (to induce stabilizing predecidual stromal changes) followed by a withdrawal flow—the so-called medical curettage. Thereafter, repeat progestin is offered cyclically for at least the first 10 days of each month to ensure therapeutic effect. Failure of progestin to correct irregular bleeding requires diagnostic re-evaluation. If contraception is desired, the use of an oral contraceptive is a better choice.

## ORAL CONTRACEPTIVE THERAPY

In young women, anovulatory bleeding may be associated with prolonged endometrial buildup, delayed diagnosis, and heavy blood loss. In these cases, combined progestin-estrogen therapy is used in the form of combined oral contraceptives. Any low-dose oral combination monophasic tablets are useful. Whatever formulation is available or chosen, therapy is administered as one pill twice a day for 5 to 7 days. This therapy is maintained despite cessation of flow within 12 to 24 hours. If flow does not abate, other diagnostic possibilities (polyps, incomplete abortion, and neoplasia) should be re-evaluated.

If flow does diminish rapidly, the remainder of the week of treatment can be given over to the evaluation of causes of anovulation, investigation of hemorrhagic tendencies, and blood replacement or initiation of iron therapy. In addition, the week provides time to prepare the patient for the estrogen-progestin withdrawal flow that will soon be induced. For the moment, therapy has produced the structural rigidity intrinsic to the compact pseudodecidual reaction. Continued random breakdown of formerly fragile tissue is avoided and blood loss stopped. However, a large amount of tissue remains to react to estrogen-progestin withdrawal. The patient must be warned to anticipate a heavy and severely cramping flow 2 to 4 days after stopping therapy. If not prepared in this way, it is certain that the patient will view the problem as recurrent disease or failure of hormonal therapy.

In successful therapy, on the fifth day of flow or in the usual Sunday start fashion, a low-dose combination oral contraceptive medication (one pill a day) is started. This will be repeated for several (usually three) 3-week treatments, punctuated by 1-week withdrawal flow intervals. A decrease in volume and pain with each successive cycle is reassuring. Oral contraceptives reduce menstrual flow by at least 60% in normal uteri. Early application of the estrogen-progestin combination limits growth and allows orderly regression of excessive endometrial height to normal controllable levels. If the estrogen-progestin combination is not applied, abnormal endometrial height and persistent excessive flow will recur.

In the patient not requiring contraception in whom cyclic estrogen-progestin for 3 months has reduced endometrial tissue to normal height, the oral contraceptive can be discontinued and unopposed endogenous estrogen permitted to reactivate the endometrium. In the absence of spontaneous menses, the recurrence of the anovulatory state is suspected, and a brief preemptive course of an orally active progestin is administered to counter endometrial proliferation. Once pregnancy is ruled out, medroxyprogesterone acetate, 10 mg orally daily for at least 10 days, is given monthly. Reasonable flow (progestin withdrawal flow) will occur 2 to 7 days after the last pill. With this therapy, excessive endometrial buildup is avoided and an increased risk of endometrial and possibly breast cancer is avoided. If contraception is desired, routine use of oral contraception is warranted and will also be of prophylactic value.

Depot-medroxyprogesterone acetate in the dose used for contraception, 150 mg intramuscularly every 3 months, is a useful option for poorly compliant patients. Breakthrough bleeding is treated with estrogen as discussed below.

## ESTROGEN THERAPY

Intermittent vaginal spotting is frequently associated with minimal (low) estrogen stimulation (estrogen breakthrough bleeding). In this circumstance, where minimal endometrium exists, the beneficial effect of progestin treatment is not achieved, because there is insufficient tissue on which the progestin can exert action. A similar circumstance also exists in the younger anovulatory patient in whom prolonged hemorrhagic desquamation leaves little residual tissue.

In these circumstances, when bleeding is acute and heavy, high-dose estrogen therapy is applied using as much as 25 mg conjugated estrogen intravenously every 4 hours until bleeding abates or for 24 hours. This is the sign that the "healing" events are initiated to a sufficient degree. The mechanism of action for estrogen is believed to be a stimulus to clotting at the capillary level. Progestin treatment (usually an oral contraceptive) is started at the same time. Where bleeding is less, lower oral doses of estrogen (1.25 mg of conjugated estrogens or 2.0 mg estradiol daily for 7 to 10 days) can be prescribed initially. When bleeding is moderately heavy, a more intensive oral program can be used, 1.25 mg conjugated estrogens or 2 mg estradiol every 4 hours for 24 hours, followed by the single daily dose for 7 to 10 days. All estrogen therapy must be followed by progestin coverage and a withdrawal bleed.

Estrogen therapy is also useful in two examples of problems associated with progestin breakthrough bleeding. These are the breakthrough bleeding episodes occurring with use of oral contraception or with depot forms of progestational agents. In the absence of sufficient endogenous and exogenous estrogen, the endometrium shrinks by pharmacologically induced pseudoatrophy. Furthermore, it is composed almost exclusively of pseudodecidual stroma and blood vessels with minimal glands. Peculiarly, experience has shown that this type of endometrium also leads to the fragility bleeding more typical of pure estrogen stimulation.

The usual clinical story is a patient on long-standing oral contraception who, after experiencing marked diminution or absence of withdrawal flow in the pill free interval, begins to see breakthrough bleeding while on medication. Conjugated estrogens 1.25 mg or estradiol 2.0 mg daily for 7 days during, and in addition to, the usual birth control pill administration are effective. This treatment rejuvenates the endometrium and intermenstrual flow stops. Another frequently encountered problem is the progestin breakthrough bleeding experienced with chronic depot administration of progestin (Depo-Provera). This therapy is used not only for contraception but also in the treatment of endometriosis and the prevention of menses during chemotherapy. In 75% of recipients, continuous therapy is not associated with abnormal menstrual bleeding. In the remainder, breakthrough progestin bleeding occurs. Judicious use of estrogen is the appropriate and effective therapy in these instances.

Bleeding problems are common with Norplant, another example of the effect of persistent progestational influence on the endometrium. Patients who can no longer tolerate prolonged bleeding will benefit from a short course of oral estrogen as above.

### Risk Associated with Estrogen Therapy

There is concern that high doses of estrogen could precipitate a thrombotic event. More than one oral contraceptive per day and multiple doses of oral or intravenous estrogen in a 24-hour period certainly should be regarded as high doses. There are no data available, however, to verify or quantitate any risk associated with this use of hormonal therapy. This treatment must be chosen by clinician and patient after weighing the risk-benefit considerations that surround the uterine bleeding problem. As a matter of clinical judgment and prudent practice, lower doses can be used in patients with lifestyle or medical history consistent with an increased risk of vascular complications.

## USE OF ANTIPROSTAGLANDINS

There seems little doubt that prostaglandins have important actions on the endometrial vasculature and presumably on endometrial hemostasis. The concentrations of $PGE_2$ and $PGF_{2\alpha}$ increase progressively in human endometrium during the menstrual cycle, and nonsteroidal eicosanoid synthesis inhibitors decrease menstrual blood loss perhaps by also altering the balance between the platelet proaggregating vasoconstrictor thromboxane $A_2$ and the antiaggregating vasodilator prostacyclin ($PGI_2$). Excessive bleeding in women with menorrhagia can be reduced by approximately 40 to 50%. In a comparison study of ovulating women with menorrhagia, treatment during menses with a prostaglandin synthetase inhibitor was no more effective than high-dose progestin supplementation during the 7 days preceding menstruation, but both treatments were effective. Occasionally, a woman will demonstrate, for unknown reasons, an anomalous response to this treatment, with an increase in menstrual bleeding. A study of postoperative surgical specimens after mefenamic acid treatment revealed evidence of vasoconstriction and improved platelet aggregation.

Whatever the exact mechanism, prostaglandin synthetase inhibitors diminish menstrual bleeding in normal women and in the bleeding secondary to intrauterine device (IUD) use. This approach should be considered as a first line of defense in the absence of pathology in those women who are ovulatory but bleed heavily. Side effects are unusual because treatment is limited, usually beginning with the onset of bleeding and continuing for 3 to 4 days. This treatment will also relieve the other symptoms of menstrual molimina.

## TREATMENT WITH A PROGESTIN IUD

The delivery of a progestational agent directly to the endometrium in a local fashion is possible with an IUD that releases progesterone or levonorgestrel. In a comparison trial with a prostaglandin synthetase inhibitor and an antifibrinolytic agent, the levonorgestrel-releasing IUD outperformed the medical treatment dramatically. The reduction in menstrual flow reached 96% after 12 months, and some patients even become amenorrheic. This is an attractive option in patients with intractable bleeding associated with chronic illnesses (such as renal failure). A progestin-releasing IUD is also a good choice for normally ovulating women who have extremely heavy menstrual bleeding.

## TREATMENT WITH GONADOTROPIN-RELEASING HORMONE AGONISTS

Treatment with a gonadotropin-releasing hormone (GnRH) agonist can achieve short-term relief from a bleeding problem, for example, in a patient with renal failure or a blood dyscrasia. This choice is a good one for patients who experience menstrual bleeding problems after organ transplantation (especially after liver transplantation) where the toxicity of immunosuppressive drugs makes the use of sex steroids less desirable. However, the expense and long-term side effects make this an unlikely choice for chronic therapy. If long-term GnRH agonist therapy is chosen, after gonadal suppression is achieved (2 to 4 weeks), we recommend add-back treatment with a daily combination of 0.625 mg conjugated estrogens or 1.0 mg estradiol and 2.5 mg medroxyprogesterone acetate or 0.35 mg norethindrone.

## TREATMENT WITH DESMOPRESSIN

Desmopressin acetate is a synthetic analog of arginine vasopressin. It has been used to treat abnormal uterine bleeding in patients with coagulation disorders, especially in patients with von Willebrand's disease. It can be administered intranasally, but the intravenous route (0.3 µg/kg diluted in 50 ml saline and administered over 15 to 30 minutes) is more effective. Treatment is followed by a rapid increase in coagulation factor VIII and von Willebrand's factor, which lasts approximately 6 hours. This treatment should be regarded as a last resort for selected patients with coagulation problems. The nasal spray is very effective for patients with von Willebrand's disease type 1.

## ABLATION OF THE ENDOMETRIUM

Persistent bleeding despite treatment is both aggravating and concerning. Hysterectomy is an appropriate choice for some of these patients. Others would prefer to avoid a major operation, and still others have conditions that make major surgery a high-risk procedure. Patients and clinicians should consider the option of hysteroscopic endometrial ablation. Ablation of the endometrium can be accomplished with either a laser, a resectoscope with a loop or rolling ball electrode, or radio frequency-induced thermal destruction. Success with these methods is not 100%. Approximately 90% of women with menorrhagia will show improvement after an ablation procedure; only 40 to 50% will become amenorrheic. Some women will continue to have menorrhagia. In a randomized trial comparing endometrial resection and hysterectomy, subsequent surgery was required by 22% of the women after endometrial resection compared with 9% in the hysterectomy group. The best results are obtained if the endometrium is first suppressed for 4 to 6 weeks with either a high dose of a progestin, GnRH agonist treatment, or danazol. Caution must be exercised regarding the possibility of excessive absorption of irrigating fluid with subsequent fluid overload. Despite the advantages of lower risk, fewer complications, and more rapid recovery with endometrial resection, patients treated by hysterectomy tend to be more satisfied with the outcome.

There is concern that obliteration of segments of the uterine cavity can allow isolated residual endometrium to progress to carcinoma without recognition. Long-term follow-up will be necessary before we know if this is a real risk.

## LESS APPEALING CHOICES

Antifibrinolytic agents (e.g., tranexamine acid) are associated with a large number of side effects. Danazol effectively reduces menstrual blood loss, but treatment requires significant doses maintained for a long time period. The expense and androgenic side effects associated with danazol make it a poor choice.

## Summary of Key Points in Therapy of Anovulatory (Dysfunctional) Bleeding

| Teenager | Adult |
|---|---|
| *Preliminary* | *Preliminary* |
| Pelvic or rectal examination | Pelvic examination |
| | Pap smear |
| | Endometrial biopsy |

1. Intense estrogen-progestin therapy for 7 days.
2. Cyclic low-dose oral contraceptive for 3 months.
3. If contraception is desired, continue oral contraception.
4. If not exposed to pregnancy, medroxyprogesterone acetate, 10 mg daily for at least 10 days every month.

*If bleeding has been prolonged, if biopsy yields minimal tissue, if the patient is on progestin medication, or if follow-up is uncertain:*

*Conjugated estrogens (1.25 mg) or estradiol (2.0 mg) daily for 7 to 10 days, followed by the daily estrogen combined with 10 mg medroxyprogesterone acetate for 7 days. If acute bleeding is moderately heavy, the oral estrogen dose can be administered every 4 hours during the first 24 hours. For very heavy acute bleeding, conjugated estrogen, 25 mg intravenously every 4 hours until bleeding stops or significantly slows, then proceed to Step 1 above. If no response in 24 hours, proceed to dilatation and curettage (D & C).*

The clinical problem of dysfunctional bleeding is associated with either anovulation and estrogen withdrawal or breakthrough bleeding or with anovulation caused by exogenous progestin medication and bleeding due to progestational endometrial breakthrough. These categories of bleeding lack the three important characteristics of normal estrogen-progesterone withdrawal bleeding:

1. Universal simultaneous change in all segments of the endometrium.
2. An orderly progression of events involving a rigid compact structure.
3. Vasomotor rhythmicity with vasoconstriction, structural collapse, and clotting.

Questioning should be directed by the differential diagnosis of abnormal uterine bleeding. Clues to the diagnosis may be apparent on physical examination, such as hirsutism, acne, galactorrhea, thyroid enlargement, evidence of an eating disorder, bruises, and, of course, abnormalities on examination of the pelvis. Brown dark-colored bleeding is often secondary to obstruction in a müllerian anomaly. Laboratory tests that can be helpful (but not always necessary) are coagulation studies (prothrombin time, partial thromboplastin time, platelet count, bleeding time, and the ristocetin cofactor assay for the von Willebrand factor), quantitative human chorionic gonadotropin, prolactin, thyroid function tests, liver function tests, and appropriate cervical cultures.

Office aspiration biopsy of the endometrium should always be performed in patients considered to be at high risk for endometrial hyperplasia and cancer. Texts and review articles continue to emphasize that endometrial biopsy is in order if the patient is older (e.g., >35 or 40 years old). ***It is not the age of the patient that is critical; it is the duration of exposure to unopposed estrogen. Women in their 20s and even teenagers can develop endometrial cancer.*** The small flexible suction cannulas are preferred for greater patient comfort, and results are comparable to the older traditional methods. Office hysteroscopy is also useful for the direction of biopsies and the detection of polyps and submucous myomas.

Therapy involves an initial choice between intensive estrogen-progestin combination medication or relatively high doses of estrogen. The estrogen-progestin combination will be ineffective unless endometrium of sufficient quantity and responsiveness to allow the formation of pseudodecidual tissue is present. Therefore, the initial choice of therapy should be estrogen in the following situations:

1. When bleeding has been heavy for many days and it is likely that the uterine cavity is now lined only by a raw basalis layer.
2. When the endometrial curet yields minimal tissue.
3. When the patient has been on progestin medication (oral contraceptives, intramuscular progestins) and the endometrium is shallow and atrophic.
4. When follow-up is uncertain, because estrogen therapy will temporarily stop all categories of dysfunctional bleeding.

If estrogen therapy does not significantly abate flow within 24 hours, re-evaluation is mandatory, and the need for curettage is likely. It is believed that patients with coagulation disorders respond better if the uterine cavity is first evacuated with a suction curet. Consideration should be given to the empirical administration of fresh frozen plasma to adolescents who present with acute serious bleeding. It is prudent to combine hysteroscopy with curettage to achieve full accuracy in diagnosis and treatment.

Once the acute bleeding episode in an anovulatory patient is under control, the patient should not be forgotten. With persistent anovulation, recurrent hemorrhage is a common pattern, and more importantly, chronic unopposed estrogen stimulation to the endometrium can eventually lead to atypical tissue changes. It is absolutely necessary that the patient undergo periodic progestational withdrawal either with a routine oral contraceptive regimen, or if contraception is not desired, a progestational agent (medroxyprogesterone acetate, 5 to 10 mg daily for at least 10 days) should be administered every month.

Curettage is *not* the first line of defense, but rather the last. The utilization of appropriate steroids for the clinical management of dysfunctional bleeding is based on a physiologic understanding of the endometrium and its responses to hormones. Adherence to this program will avoid D&C except in a rare case of dysfunctional bleeding and except in those cases where bleeding is due to a pathologic entity within the reproductive tract where D&C is truly indicated and necessary.

If a patient has recurrent bleeding despite repeated medical therapy, submucous myomas or endometrial polyps must be suspected. Thorough curettage can miss such pathology, and further diagnostic study can be helpful. Either hysterosalpingography with slow instillation of dye and careful fluoroscopic examination or hysteroscopy may reveal a myoma or polyp; hysteroscopy can also direct a more accurate biopsy of the endometrium. A pathologic problem such as this should especially be suspected in the puzzling case of the patient who has abnormal bleeding and ovulatory cycles.

Patients who are ovulating but have a heavy menstrual flow (menorrhagia) can be effectively treated with prostaglandin inhibitors, progestins administered daily for the 7 days preceding menses, or oral contraceptives in the routine manner. If contraception is not required, we prefer the use of one of the fenamate prostaglandin inhibitors (which block both synthesis and prostaglandin receptors). Women who have menorrhagia but are ovulating should be evaluated for a coagulation disorder (prothrombin time, partial thromboplastin time, platelet count, bleeding time, and the ristocetin cofactor assay for the von Willebrand factor). The IUD that releases progesterone or a progestin is a good choice for ovulating women with menorrhagia, and it should be also considered in patients with chronic illnesses.

## REFERENCES

Belsey EM, Pinol APY, Task Force on Long-Acting Systemic Agents for Fertility Regulation: Menstrual bleeding patterns in untreated women. Contraception 55:57, 1997.

Belsey EM, Task Force on Long-Acting Systemic Agents for Fertility Regulation: Vaginal bleeding patterns among women using one natural and eight hormonal methods of contraception. Contraception 38:1812, 1988.

Bergqvist A, Rybo G: Treatment of menorrhagia with intrauterine release of progesterone. Br J Obstet Gynaecol 90:2552, 1983.

Bruner KL, Rodgers WH, Gold LI, et al: Transforming growth factor beta mediates the progesterone suppression of an epithelial metalloproteinase by adjacent stroma in the human endometrium. Proc Natl Acad Sci USA 92:7362, 1995.

Cameron IT, Haining R, Lumsden M-A, et al: The effects of mefenamic acid and norethisterone on measured menstrual blood loss. Obstet Gynecol 76:85, 1990.

Christiaens GCML, Sixma JJ, Haspels AA: Hemostasis in menstrual endometrium: A review. Obstet Gynecol Surv 1982; 37:281.

Claessens EA, Cowell CL: Acute adolescent menorrhagia. Am J Obstet Gynecol 139:377, 1981.

Cohen BJB, Gibor J: Anemia and menstrual blood loss. Obstet Gynecol Surv 35:597, 1980.

Crosignani PG, Vercellini P, Apolone G, et al: Endometrial resection versus vaginal hysterectomy for menorrhagia: Long-term clinical and quality-of-life outcomes. Am J Obstet Gynecol 177:95, 1997.

DeStafano F, Huezo CM, Peterson HB, et al: Menstrual changes after tubal sterilization. Obstet Gynecol 62:673, 1983.

DeStafano F, Perlman J, Peterson HB, et al: Long-term risk of menstrual disturbances after tubal sterilization. Am J Obstet Gynecol 152:835, 1985.

DeVore GR, Owens O, Kase N: Use of intravenous premarin in the treatment of dysfunctional uterine bleeding—a double-blind randomized control study. Obstet Gynecol 59:285, 1982.

de Ziegler D, Bergeron C, Cornel C, et al: Effects of luteal estradiol on the secretory transformation of human endometrium and plasma gonadotropins. J Clin Endocrinol Metab 74:322, 1992.

Diaz S, Croxatto HB, Pavez M, et al: Clinical assessment of treatments for prolonged bleeding in users of Norplant implants. Contraception 42:97, 1990.

Eddowes HA, Read MD, Codling BW: Pipelle: A more acceptable technique for outpatient endometrial biopsy. Br J Obstet Gynaecol 97:961, 1990.

Farhi DC, Nosanchuk J, Silverberg SG: Endometrial adenocarcinoma in women under 25 years of age. Obstet Gynecol 68:741, 1986.

Fothergill DJ, Brown VA, Hill AS: Histological sampling of the endometrium—a comparison between formal curettage and the Pipelle sampler. Br J Obstet Gynaecol 99:779, 1992.

Fraser IS: Hysteroscopy and laparoscopy in women with menorrhagia. Am J Obstet Gynecol 162:1264, 1992.

Fraser IS: Prostaglandin inhibitors in gynaecology. Aust N Z J Obstet Gynecol 25:114, 1985.

Fraser IS, McCarron G: Randomized trial of 2 hormonal and 2 prostaglandin-inhibiting agents in women with a complaint of menorrhagia. Aust N Z J Obstet Gynecol 31:66, 1991.

Fraser IS, McCarron G, Markham R: A preliminary study of factors influencing perception of menstrual blood loss volume. Am J Obstet Gynecol 149:788, 1984.

Gimpelson RJ, Rappold HD: A comparative study between panoramic hysteroscopy with directed biopsies and dilatation and curettage. Am J Obstet Gynecol 158:489, 1988.

Gurpide E, Gusberg S, Tseng L: Estradiol binding and metabolism in human endometrial hyperplasia and adenocarcinoma. J Steroid Biochem 7:891, 1976.

Hall P, Maclachlan N, Thorn N, et al: Control of menorrhagia by the cyclo-oxygenase inhibitors naproxen sodium and mefenamic acid. Br J Obstet Gynaecol 94:554, 1987.

Hallberg L, Högdahl A, Nilsson L, et al: Menstrual blood loss—a population study. Acta Obstet Gynaecol Scand 45:320–351, 1966.

Haynes PJ, Hodgson H, Anderson ABM, et al: Measurement of menstrual blood loss in patients complaining of menorrhagia. Br J Obstet Gynaecol 84:763, 1977.

Higham JM, O'Brien PMS, Shaw RM: Assessment of menstrual blood loss using a pictorial chart. Br J Obstet Gynaecol 97:734, 1990.

Higham JM, Shaw RW: A comparative study of danazol, a regimen of decreasing doses of danazol, and norethindrone in the treatment of objectively proven unexplained menorrhagia. Am J Obstet Gynecol 169:1134, 1993.

Hopkins MP, Androff L, Benninghoff AS: Ginseng face cream and unexplained vaginal bleeding. Am J Obstet Gynecol 159:1121, 1988.

Horowitz IR, Copas PR, Aarono M, et al: Endometrial adenocarcinoma following endometrial ablation for postmenopausal bleeding. Gynecol Oncol 56:460, 1995.

Irwin JC, Kirk D, Gwatkin RBL, et al: Human endometrial matrix metalloproteinase-2, a putative menstrual proteinase. Hormonal regulation in cultured stromal cells and messenger RNA expression during the menstrual cycle. J Clin Invest 97:438, 1996.

Kirkland JL, Murthy L, Stancel GM: Progesterone inhibits the estrogen-induced expression of c-*fos* messenger ribonucleic acid in the uterus. Endocrinology 130:3223, 1992.

Kjer J, Knudsen L: Hysterectomy subsequent to laparoscopic sterilization. Eur J Obstet Gynaecol 35:63, 1990.

Kubrinsky NL, Tulloch H: Treatment of refractory thrombocytopenic bleeding with desamino-8-D-arginine vasopressin (desmopressin). J Pediatr 112:993, 1998.

Livio M, Mannucci PM, Vigano G, et al: Conjugated estrogens for the management of bleeding associated with renal failure. N Engl J Med 315:731, 1986.

Lockwood C, Krikun G, Papp C, et al: The role of progestionally regulated stromal cell tissue factor and type-1 plasminogen activator inhibitor (PAI-1) in endometrial hemostasis and menstruation. Ann NY Acad Sci 734:57–79, 1994.

Lockwood CJ, Schatz F: A biological model for the regulation of periimplanttional hemostasis and menstruation. J Soc Gynecol Invest 1996; 3:159, 1996.

Loffer DD: Hysteroscopy with selective endometrial sampling compared with D&C for abnormal uterine bleeding: The value of a negative hysteroscopic view. Obstet Gynecol 73:16, 1989.

Markee JE: Menstruation in intraocular endometrial transplants in the rhesus monkey. JAMA 250:2167, 1946.

Markee JE: Morphological basis for menstrual bleeding: Relation of regression to the initiation of bleeding. Bull NY Acad Med 24:253, 1948.

Milsom I, Andersson K, Andersch B, et al: A comparison of flurbiprogen, tranexamic acid, and a levonorgestrel-releasing intrauterine contraceptive device in the treatment of idiopathic menorrhagia. Am J Obstet Gynecol 164:879, 1991.

Nelson L, Rybo G: Treatment of menorrhagia. Am J Obstet Gynecol 110:713, 1971.

O'Connor H, Broadbent JAM, Magos AL, et al: Medical Research Council randomised trial of endometrial resection versus hysterectomy in management of menorrhagia. Lancet 349:897, 1997.

O'Connor H, Magos A: Endometrial resection for the treatment of menorrhagia. N Engl J Med 335:151, 1996.

Phipps JH, Lewis BV, Prior MF, et al: Experimental and clinical studies with radio frequency-induced thermal endometrial ablation for functional menorrhagia. Obstet Gynecol 76:876, 1990.

Rodgers WH, Matrisian LM, Giudice LC, et al: Patterns of matrix metalloproteinase expression in cycling endometrium imply differential functions and regulation by steroid hormones. J Clin Invest 94:946, 1994.

Rose EH, Aledort LM: Nasal spray desmopressin (DDAVP) for mild hemophilia A and von Willebrand disease. Ann Intern Med 114:563, 1991.

Rulin MC, Davidson AR, Philliber SG, et al: Long-term effect of tubal sterilization on menstrual indices and pelvic pain. Obstet Gynecol 82:118, 1993.

Rulin MC, Davidson AR, Philliber SG, et al: Changes in menstrual symptoms among sterilized and comparison women: A prospective study. Obstet Gynecol 79:749, 1989.

Rulin MC, Turner JH, Dunworth R, et al: Post tubal sterilization syndrome: A misnomer. Obstet Gynecol 151:13, 1985.

Rybo G: Menstrual blood loss in relation to parity and menstrual pattern. Acta Obstet Gynaecol Scand 7:119, 1966.

Salamonsen LA: Matrix metalloproteinases and endometrial remodelling. Cell Biol Int 18:1139, 1994.

Schatz F, Aigner S, Papp C, et al: Plasminogen activator activity during decidualization of human endometrial stromal cells is regulated by plasminogen activator inhibitor 1. J Clin Encrinol Metab 80:1504, 1995.

Shy KK, Stergachis A, Grothaus LC, et al: Tubal sterilization and risk of subsequent hospital admission for menstrual disorders. Am J Obstet Gynecol 166:1698, 1992.

Silver MM, Miles P, Rosa C: Comparison of Novak and Pipelle endometrial biopsy instruments. Obstet Gynecol 78:828, 1991.

Stergachis A, Shy KK, Grothaus LC, et al: Tubal sterilization and the long-term risk of hysterectomy. JAMA 264:2893, 1990.

Tabibzadeh S: The signals and molecular pathways involved in human menstruation, a unique process of tissue destruction and remodelling. Mol Hum Reprod 2:77, 1996.

Thranov I, Hertz JB, Kjer JJ, et al: Hormonal and menstrual changes after laparoscopic sterilization by Falope-rings or Filshie-clips. Fertil Steril 57:751, 1992.

Townsend DE, Richart RM, Paskowitz RA, et al: Rollerball coagulation of the endometrium. Obstet Gynecol 76:310, 1990.

Treloar AE, Boynton RE, Borghild GB, et al: Variation of the human menstrual cycle through reproductive life. Int J Fertil 12:77, 1967.

van Eijkeren MA, Christianes GCML, Geuze JH, et al: Effects of mefenamic acid on menstrual hemostasis in essential menorrhagia. Am J Obstet Gynecol 166:1419, 1992.

van Eijkeren MA, Christiaens GCML, Haspels AA, et al: Measured menstrual blood loss in women with a bleeding disorder or using oral anticoagulant therapy. Am J Obstet Gynecol 162:1261, 1990.

Wilcox LS, Martinez-Schnell B, Peterson HB, et al: Menstrual function after tubal sterilization. Am J Epidemiol 135:1368, 1992.

# 55

# Hyperandrogenism

SAM S. THATCHER
MICHAEL P. DIAMOND

The definition, the diagnosis, and the therapy of hyperandrogenism (HA) are perplexing and problematic. Hyperandrogenism refers to an excess of androgen, or male hormone. However, most patients seek medical attention because of the symptoms of hyperandrogenism, and these may occur in the absence of elevated androgens as measured by standard laboratory techniques. Androgens are produced only in the gonads and the adrenal cortex but can arise as a product of steroid metabolism in many other organs, including liver, skin, fat, and muscle. Fortunately, the vast number of patients who have androgen excess can be placed along the spectrum of polycystic ovarian syndrome (PCOS). Fewer than 1% of patients who manifest signs of hyperandrogenism have a diagnosis more serious than that of their initial symptom. Indeed, most cases of medically significant hyperandrogenism are not missed. This chapter is a synopsis of the evaluation, differential diagnosis, and management of hyperandrogenism. It does not address disorders of sexual differentiation or the relative HA of menopause.

## Effects of Hyperandrogenism

HA is apparent in three different sets of symptoms:
1. Menstrual cycle disturbance and infertility.
2. Problems with self-image and appearance arising from the effect of HA on the skin.
3. Metabolic derangements, including dyslipidemia, insulin resistance, and hypertension. Often, gynecologists have concerned themselves with only the first problem and have been relatively insensitive to the latter two. A more holistic approach to HA is certainly warranted and can have a significant effect in altering the patient's quality of life.

Skin manifestations of HA are more common than menstrual cycle irregularity. As with abnormal bleeding, dichotomous etiologies for HA can span the range from a harbingers of a life-threatening process to an idiopathic functional and cosmetic problem. Disorders of the skin related to HA include acne, seborrhea, androgenic alopecia, hidradenitis suppurativa, acanthosis nigricans, and hirsutism. Hirsutism is defined as a male pattern of hair distribution in the female that is different from hypertrichosis, which is excessive growth of nonsexual hair. With the exception of hirsutism, HA manifestations are often dismissed or not recorded in the gynecologist's evaluation.

Acne and seborrhea develop rapidly after androgens rise. Androgen increases sebum production, which causes plugged pores, bacterial alteration of fatty acids, and inflammation. Closed comedones are known as whiteheads, whereas blackheads are open comedones; their characteristic blackness comes from the breakdown of keratin. HA is also related to seborrhea. Dandruff, which is caused by oily rather than dry skin, is a variety of seborrheic dermatitis.

During the luteal phase, progesterone levels are increased, and during menstruation estradiol levels are decreased, causing relative HA with resultant increased oiliness and inflammation of the skin. Perhaps the most distressing HA disorders is alopecia. The most androgen-sensitive area of the scalp is the vertex. Frontal balding and anterior hairline recession occur only in very severe cases of HA. The mechanism for hair growth (and loss) has been extensively studied, but no unified theory has emerged.

Two basic determinants of the appearance of HA are hormone and hormone receptor. There must be androgen-stimulated sexual hair growth. Sexual hair follicles contain the enzymatic machinery necessary to convert circulating androgens to testosterone. To exert its effect, testosterone must be converted to dihydrotestosterone (DHT) by the enzyme 5α-reductase. The hair follicle also contains aromatase, which can convert androgens to estrone and may serve as a potential protective mechanism (i.e., decreases hair production).

Increased steroid conversion does not seem to be a product of isolated follicles but of large areas acting in concert. As would be expected, there are greater numbers of androgen receptors in sites of greater response. A fair-skinned individual may have little excess hair growth despite high levels of testosterone because of the absence of a specific receptor, or enzyme coverting capacity, in the hair follicles. Another individual may be quite hirsute with no abnormality in circulating hormones. Some individuals may manifest HA by hirsutism, but others may have different skin problems. The most commonly used objective method of evaluating the extent and course of hirsutism is the Ferriman-Gallwey scoring system (Table 55–1). Conducting this test may be too rigorous for a routine examination, but some form of semiobjective scoring of degree and distribution of body hair should be made.

## Patient History

In no other gynecologic condition are the patient's general medical history and overall physical appear-

**Table 55–1** Ferriman-Gallwey Scoring System for Hirsutism

| Upper lip | ___ | Arm | ___ |
| Face | ___ | Chest | ___ |
| Chin | ___ | Upper abdomen | ___ |
| Jaw and neck | ___ | Lower abdomen | ___ |
| Upper back | ___ | Thigh | ___ |
| Lower back | ___ | Perineum | ___ |

1 = scant or mild coverage; 4 = marked or complete coverage; total score >8 = hirsutism.

**Table 55–2** Key Points of History

General wellness
Menstrual history since menarche
Speed of symptom progression
Contraceptive
Chronic illness
    Hypertension
    Diabetes
    Thyroid
Medication use
Similar condition in family members

ance of more importance than in HA (Table 55–2). Often, the diagnosis of HA can be made as soon as the patient enters the consulting office, and this is when the examination should begin. Never expect only a single complaint or physical finding in the hyperandrogenic patient. HA should be considered a panendocrinopathy that spares few body systems (Table 55–3).

A key point in the patient's history, and one that is especially important in the exclusion of a more serious pathology, is the rapidity of symptom progression. More ominous diagnoses usually have more rapid onset. Obviously, a detailed menstrual history, including menarche, early pattern of menses, cycle interval, and change of pattern within the preceeding year, should be obtained. Often patients who have HA have used oral contraceptives or even established a pregnancy, thus obscuring cycle abnormalities. The HA patient is frequently overweight, and the timeline of the weight gain should be noted. The amount of facial hair is usually self-evident, but a good screening question is to ask how much hair is present between the umbilicus and the pubic hairline. A particularly important point in the history is to inquire whether other family members have had similar problems. Certain enzyme deficiencies are inherited, but tumors of the adrenal gland and ovary are not.

## Physical Examination

In addition to recording customary height and weight measurements, support staff should be accustomed to recording the patient's waist-to-hip ratio and calculating the body mass index. Hirsutism is the most common physical finding of HA. In the general examination, the distinction between virilization and

**Table 55–3** Review of Endocrine Systems

| Weight/diet change | Headache/vision changes |
| Hot/cold intolerance | Polydipsia/polyuria |
| Weakness/fatigue/libido | Palpitations |

**Table 55–4** Characteristics of Virilization

| | |
|---|---|
| Extensive hirsutism | Loss of female body habitus |
| Vertex/temporal balding | Clitoromegaly |
| Deepening of voice | |

hirsutism is usually distinct, and the diagnosis is seldom questioned (Table 55–4). A side view of the face is more revealing than a frontal view. If virilization is present, there is often male pattern balding and severe hirsutism. A search for acanthosis nigricans (AN) should be a part of every exam. The signs of AN are velvety, raised skin pigmentations, usually seen on the back of the neck, the axillae, and beneath the breasts. AN is often seen in association with skin tags (acrochordons). There is an association of AN and simple obesity as well as other endocrine disorders, such as Cushing's disease, Addison's disease, and acromegaly. AN should always alert the clinician to a risk of insulin resistance, diabetes (or both), major lipid abnormalities, and hypertension. It may be a harbinger of adenocarcinoma, especially of the stomach.

Both hyper- and hypothyroidism are associated with HA. Pulse rate is usually elevated in hyperthyroidism. In the milder forms of hypothyroidism there are usually few distinguishing symptoms or physical characteristics. A thyroid examination, conducted while facing the patient and during swallowing, should be performed on all patients. The cushingoid patient is typically plethoric and rosy-faced. A usually reliable physical finding of Cushing's disease is the inability to stand from a lower sitting position, as a result of muscle wasting. An important component of the breast examination is the finding of galactorrhea (Table 55–5).

## Laboratory Evaluation

Virtually all patients who have hyperandrogenism have at least subtle laboratory abnormalities. These may not be outside the normal range as reported by the laboratory. The overall pattern and subtleties of an endocrine laboratory panel screening often are more important in evaluating hypothalamic-pituitary dysfunction, whereas significant pathology may be evidenced more by a single test. Although the value of repeated measurements could be questioned, it is recommended that every HA patient have an initial, relatively comprehensive evaluation (Table 55–6). In the following synopses, normal levels are not given because of the marked variations between laboratories and techniques. Any level that is twice the upper or lower limit of normal is significant. A marginally elevated test is almost always indicative of dysfunctional rather than pathologic conditions. As a rule, endocrine testing, other than a pregnancy test, is probably best performed on a return visit and in the morning, soon after spontaneous or induced menses. The periovulatory portion of the cycle should be avoided. Hormonal evaluation of patients who are taking an oral contraceptive often gives spurious results on levels of gonadotropin, ovarian steroid, and sex hormone–binding globulin (SHBG) concentrations and are thus of limited value. There have been a large number of tests and procedures used in the past for evaluation of HA. The following tests should provide sufficient data for a comprehensive investigation.

**Testosterone.** Testosterone is obviously a hormone to be measured in every HA patient. More than 75% of circulating testosterone comes from conversion of other steroids by the liver and skin. The decision whether to measure free or total testosterone should be based on availability and cost of the test. Total testosterone is more likely to be related to overall metabolic status and is less specific than free testosterone. Marked elevation of either free or total hormone is equally worrisome and warrants complete investigation to exclude neoplasia. Ovarian tumors are usually diagnosed by ultrasonography and adrenal tumors by magnetic resonance imaging (MRI).

**Luteinizing Hormone (LH) and Follicle-Stimulating Hormone (FSH).** The absolute levels of LH and FSH, as well as the LH to FSH ratio, can offer significant insight into the HA patient. In patients who have ovarian neoplasia, elevated testosterone production usually suppresses gonadotropin secretion with an intact hypothalamic-pituitary axis. Modestly elevated LH levels should provide reassurance that a

**Table 55–5** Key Physical Findings

| | |
|---|---|
| Weight, height | Thyroid |
| Waist-hip ratio, BMI | Galactorrhea |
| Blood pressure, pulse | External genitalia |
| Assessment of skin | |

BMI = body mass index.

**Table 55–6** Laboratory Evaluation of Hyperandrogenism

| | |
|---|---|
| Testosterone | Prolactin |
| LH/FSH ratio | SHBG |
| DHEAS | 17-hydroxyprogesterone |
| TSH | |

DHEAS = dehydroepiandrosterone sulfate; FSH = follicle-stimulating hormone; LH = luteinizing hormone; SHBG = sex hormone–binding globulin; TSH = thyroid-stimulating hormone.

steroid-secreting ovarian tumor is not present. Traditionally, the diagnosis of PCOS has been made when the LH to FSH ratio is more than three. The use of monoclonal assays, which are specific only for closely related isotypes, has reduced the validity of this ratio. Still, finding a reverse of the LH to FSH ratio, points to increased LH pulse frequency and amplitude, a hallmark of PCOS. The alteration in the LH to FSH ratio is more likely to be evident before, rather than after, a progestin challenge test.

**Dehydroepiandrosterone (DHEA) and Dehydroepiandrosterone Sulfate (DHEAS) Levels.** Both DHEA and DHEAS are relatively weak androgens and are almost exclusively of adrenal origin. Although produced in relatively large amounts, they have little potency but can be converted in the ovary and peripheral sites to more active metabolites. Adrenal tumors often produce very large amounts of DHEAS and are seldom associated with only modest elevations. A DHEAS measurement can be used to determine whether there is an adrenal component to PCOS and whether the patient may benefit from a trial of low-dose corticosteroids. Many women who have 21-hydroxylase deficiency do not have an elevated DHEAS level.

**Androstenedione Level.** Although androstenedione may be the steroid most often elevated in HA evaluation, its lack of specificity in determining the source of HA or modifying treatment probably makes its measurement unnecessary. Androstenedione is almost totally and equally produced from the adrenal gland and ovary.

**Prolactin.** Hyperprolactinemia has been associated with increased production of DHEAS, which is reversed after treatment with bromocriptine. Although a direct effect is possible, another mechanism may be indirect from conversion of DHEA to estrone in the periphery. Estrogens are known to elevate prolactin levels through a central mechanism. Despite this fact, it is still not clear that the findings of HA and hyperprolactinemia, both relatively common disorders, are not coincidental. Potential functional causes of mildly elevated prolactin levels are drug use; stress, possibly at the time of the phlebotomy; recent breast stimulation or examination; and sampling during the periovulatory phase of the cycle. Patients whose prolactin levels are more than marginally elevated on repeat examination should be referred for MRI.

**Thyroid-Stimulating Hormone (TSH).** This is the single most important measurement of thyroid function. Except in the relatively uncommon disorder of central suppression, in which both TSH and free thyroxine are suppressed, TSH is diagnostic of both hyper- and hypothyroidism. A free thyroxine level may be added to a repeat TSH measurement if the initial TSH measurement is low. There is no clinical utility in the "thyroid panel," or total thyroxine measurement, and these tests should be abandoned. TSH is the method of choice for monitoring thyroid replacement therapy. It should be noted that a 4- to 6-week period is necessary for equilibrium to be reached. Patients who are receiving replacement therapy should be titrated to the midnormal TSH range. Overly supplemented patients are at risk for osteoporosis and heart disease.

**Sex Hormone–Binding Globulin (SHBG).** This is a useful but not commonly used marker in HA. Low levels are a relatively good indicator of PCOS and an excellent indirect measurement of insulin resistance. Age, weight, and diet, as well as steroid and thyroid hormone levels, all affect the concentration of SHBG. Hypothyroidism is associated with a decrease in SHBG. There is an inverse correlation between body mass and SHBG in women but not men. Women who have high waist-to-hip ratios have lower SHBG, possibly relating to correlation with hyperinsulinemia. While there is a clear direct dose-related effect of estrogen administration, it is much less clear what effect concomitant use of progestational agents has on SHBG levels.

**17-Hydroxyprogesterone (17-OHP).** A measurement drawn between 8 and 9 AM from a patient in a fasting state in the follicular phase identifies most cases of 21-hydroxylase deficiency. Levels should be more than twice the normal range. Although not as sensitive as dynamic testing using synthetic adrenocorticotropic hormone (ACTH), it is much easier.

**Other Testing.** Many HA patients are obese, with a propensity toward hyperlipidemia, hypertension, and diabetes. Also, some therapies might have an adverse effect on hepatic or renal function. It may be reasonable to order a comprehensive biochemical profile. Other more specialized tests are described later.

## Dynamic Testing

**Adrenocorticotropic Hormone (ACTH) Stimulation.** This test is performed by measuring basal 17-OHP before and 1 hour after an intravenous infusion of one vial (250 μg) of synthetic ACTH (Cortrosyn). More than doubling base level is suggestive of 21-hydroxylase (21-OHD) deficiency. This test is also usually diagnostic for the less common 11β-hydroxylase deficiency. Measurement of desoxycortisol is the metabolite specifically indicated for 11β-hydroxylase deficiency. This same test, but instead measuring cortisol, is used to exclude adrenal insufficiency.

**Dexamethasone Suppression.** This test is simple to perform and may be used in conjunction with Cortrosyn stimulation. Dexamethasone 1 mg is given at 10:00 PM. Early the following morning, a serum cortisol level is obtained. Usually, the suppression is quite obvious. There are relatively high false-positive and false-negative rates. Obese patients can have incomplete suppression as can patients with Cushing's disease. Measurement of a 24-hour urinary free cortisol (UFC) production as a measure of hypercortisolism may be superior to suppression testing. False-positive tests may be lower with UFC and the test is arguably easier to perform. Both tests should be performed if one is positive. If a repeat test is positive, ACTH levels should be drawn.

**Glucose Tolerance Testing (GTT).** This test is familiar to most obstetric practices. Performance of GTT should be considered for all HA patients, especially those who are more than 120% of ideal weight, have first-degree relatives who have diabetes, have elevated serum lipid levels, or who have had an infant whose birth weight was more than 9 lb. The American Diabetic Association (ADA) has designated individuals who have fasting glucose levels higher than 126 mg/dl as diabetic. At present, individuals whose fasting levels are between 110 and 126 mg/dl, are described as having impaired glucose tolerance. Type 2 diabetes describes insulin resistance and has replaced the older terminology of adult onset. No distinction is made for insulin dependency. The ADA recommends a 2-hour screening after a 75-g glucose load as a definitive test.

## Diagnostic Imaging

**Ultrasonography.** Sonography of the pelvis is warranted in virtually every HA patient. Evaluation should be performed by individuals who are experienced in judging ovarian and endometrial functions. Findings of more than 10 cystic structures of less than 10 mm in either ovary meets the generally established ultrasonographic criteria of PCOS. Often, cysts of PCOS are located in a peripheral subcortical ring, leading to the reference of a "string of pearls." PCOS ovaries are typically 1.5 to 3 times larger than those of normal size. In some cases, the ovary is virtually filled with small cysts. In other cases, it is heterogeneously dense, with hardly detectable microcystic changes. It must be remembered that any hyperandrogenic state may be manifested by the ovary that appears to have PCOS. Diffusely enlarged ovaries that do not reveal a discrete mass on examination by ultrasonography and that have an absence of adrenal findings are consistent with the diagnosis of hyperthecosis, which is probably a less common variant in the PCOS spectrum.

**Magnetic Resonance Imaging (MRI).** MRI of the adrenal glands is an important procedure in cases of documented hyperadrenalism and has largely replaced selective vein catheterization. MRI of the pituitary gland is indicated when a prolactin level is more than modestly elevated, or in cases of hyperadrenalism in which Cushing's disease is a possibility. Patients who have a new history of headache, or especially vision changes, should also undergo imaging. MRI is considered superior to computed tomographic (CT) scan.

## Differential Diagnosis

The greatest fear in diagnosing HA is missing the uncommon disorder that is usually relegated to textbooks (Table 55–7). All cases of virilization or markedly elevated testosterone should be actively pursued until a definitive diagnosis is made. Once ovarian and adrenal tumor are excluded, which is relatively easy in most cases, there are a number of diagnoses that share common symptoms and laboratory findings and follow a relatively benign course.

**Ovarian Tumors.** Rapid progression of HA, and especially virilization, should raise the suspicion of an ovarian tumor. Most functional tumors occur in the second through fourth decades of life. They are usually easily diagnosed by ultrasonography and have often been palpated by the time medical attention is sought. These tumors are usually solid, or mostly solid, when viewed by ultrasonography. An exception may be the smaller hilar cell tumor that is more common in postmenopausal women and that follows an indolent growth pattern. Hilar cell tumors have hormonal characteristics of Leydig's cells and produce tetosterone. Together, functional tumors account for fewer than 1% of solid ovarian tumors. The most common is the Sertoli-Leydig cell tumor (arrhe-

**Table 55–7** Differential Diagnosis of Hyperandrogenism

| |
|---|
| OVARY |
|     Ovarian tumor |
|     PCOS |
| ADRENAL |
|     Congenital adrenal hyperplasia |
|     Adrenal tumor |
|     Cushing's disease/syndrome |
|     Dysfunctional |

PCOS = polycystic ovary syndrome.

moblastoma). This is usually unilateral and, if confined to the ovary, can be conservatively treated with a unilateral oophorectomy. Less frequently, elevated androgen levels are seen in granulosa theca tumors, but here the estrogen levels are proportionately higher than testosterone. An excellent biochemical marker for the granulosa cell tumor is inhibin. Adenocarcinoma of the ovary is associated with increased steroid production in some cases. HA is seen much less often than endometrial hyperplasia with granulosa cell tumors. Although traditionally mentioned as a diagnostic tool in difficult cases, the risks of selective ovarian vein catheterization probably preclude its use in all but the rare instance.

**Adrenal Tumors.** The adrenal gland does not normally produce testosterone but rather precursors that are converted in the periphery to testosterone. Tumors that secrete androgen only are exceedingly rare. High levels of DHEAS characterize adrenal tumors, which are usually large at the time of diagnosis and easily seen by adrenal imaging. However, some adrenal tumors have DHEAS levels that are normal or only slightly elevated. All adrenal tumors are rare and require a high index of suspicion.

**Congenital Adrenal Hyperplasia (CAH).** CAH results from an inherited enzyme deficiency causing accumulation of androgenic precursors. While these metabolites may have only weak androgenic potential, their abundance can have a significant effect after peripheral and perhaps ovarian conversion. The most common form of CAH, 21-OHD, is the subject of an enormous amount of literature as a model for gene expression. The classic form of 21-OHD, which appears in the female neonate who has ambiguous genitalia, can be an emergent life-threatening condition because of electrolyte imbalance (salt wasting). The classic form is reported in about 1 in 15,000 births, and salt wasting is seen in about two thirds of these cases. A milder form of the deficiency, referred to as nonclassic, late onset, acquired, occult, or cryptic 21-OHD, may go unrecognized until after puberty, when females manifest signs and symptoms present in a manner indistinguishable from those of PCOS. The prevalence of late-onset 21-OHD deficiency depends on the particular patient population and the aggressiveness of diagnostic testing. Frequency has been reported to be between 1 and 30% incidence in patients who have HA. Detection of 21-OHD is by measurement of 17-OHP. For prenatal diagnosis in known carriers, 17-OHP can be measured in amniotic fluid.

A less common form of COH, 11β-hydroxylase deficiency, is characterized by hypertension and found in approximately 1 out of 100,000 persons in the general population. The frequency is much higher in Jewish families of North African origin. Genital ambiguity at birth is present in the classic form. Nonclassic forms also exist. Patients have elevated levels of testosterone and deoxycortisol. Testing for both 21-OHD and 11β-deficiency can be performed by measurement of 17-OHP. If a distinction is needed, deoxycortisol can be measured. Other forms of COH have been reported, but all are exceedingly rare and more comprehensive texts should be consulted.

**Cushing's Disease and Syndrome.** HA is a common manifestation of the relatively rare Cushing's syndrome and rarer Cushing's disease. Cushing's syndrome has an insidious onset. Often, months pass before a diagnosis is made, but because of life-threatening consequences, it is a diagnosis not to be missed. It occurs mostly in women between 20 and 50 years of age. Most patients are hypertensive and obese, with menstrual and psychological alterations. Diabetes is common. Cushing's disease, the most common cause of Cushing's syndrome, results from a pituitary tumor that produces ACTH. Cushing's syndrome is a manifestation of hypercortisolism from other sources, including nonpituitary tumors, adrenal tumor, and ectopic production, usually associated with neoplasia. Either 24-hour UFC or dexamethasone suppression can effectively exclude hypercortisolism. Marked suppression of ACTH levels occurs with functioning adrenal tumors, whereas ACTH levels are normal or elevated in Cushing's syndrome. Ectopic production is most commonly observed in lung tumors. Most patients have elevated DHEAS levels. MRI of the adrenal system and skull are usually performed to evaluate the etiology of cortisol elevations.

**Hyperandrogenism, Insulin Resistance, and Acanthosis Nigricans (HAIR-AN) Syndrome.** The constellation of findings of HA, insulin resistance, and acanthosis nigricans represents a caricature of the relationship between hyperinsulinemia and HA. Earlier studies identified these patients are "bearded diabetics." Most patients have moderate hirsutism and, occasionally, virilization. Ovaries show hyperthecoses and, less often, polycystic appearance.

**Hyperthecosis.** This disorder is characterized by proliferation of the theca cells. It may cause marked elevation in testosterone and even virilization. Its association with HAIR-AN syndrome may dictate its placement along the PCOS spectrum. The ovaries are enlarged, usually more than 3 cm$^3$, and contain few follicular cysts. Treatment is the same as for PCOS.

**Idiopathic Hirsutism.** This is a largely unsatisfactory diagnosis and usually implies either an increase in receptors or an increased conversion in the hair follicles of normal levels of circulating androgens to dihydrotestosterone. To make this diagnosis valid, menstrual function, laboratory studies, and ultrasonographic scan should all be normal.

**Polycystic Ovarian Syndrome (PCOS).** PCOS is a complex hormonal disturbance that has numerous implications for general health and fertility. The most consistent feature of PCOS is HA, but there is great difficulty in isolating causes and effect. It should be remembered that any etiology of HA may induce a PCOS-like appearance in the ovaries, and that the diagnosis of PCOS represents one of exclusion of the variety of diagnoses listed earlier. Originally described as a disease, the disorder is now referred to as a syndrome to reflect its various causes and manifestations. Even this might be too restrictive a designation, and polycystic ovarian spectrum, may be more theoretically and clinicaly appropriate. The clinical presentation of PCOS is a final common pathway of a variety of disorders, and the diagnosis of PCOS remains one of exclusion. Stein and Leventhal made the association between the clinical triad of obesity, hirsutism, and menstrual cycle disturbance with the pathologic finding of sclerocystic ovaries in 1935. Later, they suggested a primary ovarian defect as an etiology because of the return of menstruation after ovarian wedge resection. There is clearly an alteration in the hypothalamic pituitary ovarian (HPO) axis, with inappropriate gonadotropin secretion and chronic anovulation, but it is unclear to what degree an active or passive role is played by the ovaries. Still, the designation of PCOS is well entrenched in the literature. Depending on the diagnostic criteria, the incidence of PCOS in the general population is between 5 and 30% in women of reproductive age. Pelvic ultrasonography has shown that approximately 20 to 30% of women in the reproductive age range have polycystic-appearing ovaries despite proven fertility and lack of other characteristic findings. The majority of hirsute women who have regular menses and those who have oligomenorrhea have PCOS. It is the most common cause of ovulatory disturbance, leading to infertility and, probably, pregnancy loss. The relative contributions of adrenal and ovarian steroid production in PCOS are disputed. ACTH levels are usually normal, and elevated LH does not seem to have a significant effect on the function of the adrenal glands. Some have suggested subtle steroid-converting enzyme alterations in PCOS, whereas others have postulated a specific but yet to be isolated cortical adrenal stimulating factor (CASH). A well-supported theory is that PCOS is an exaggerated adrenarche.

There is nearly universal agreement that PCOS is genetic, but the heritage is complex. It may be of paternal or maternal origin, with the traits passed on in various degrees. Franks and colleagues have characterized PCOS as an oligenic disorder in which genes involved in glucose homeostasis and steroid biosynthesis are both involved in the interaction of a small number of key genes with nutrient and environmental factors. A paternal origin should not be overlooked.

The relationship between obesity and PCOS is unclear, and a distinction has been made between the lean and the obese PCOS patient. The typical obesity of PCOS is characterized by "centripetal" distribution of fat in the center of the body as opposed to the thighs and hips. This type of obesity—an apple vs. a pear shape—is clearly associated with greater risk of hypertension, diabetes, and dyslipidemias. Certainly, many metabolic derangements improve with weight loss, but PCOS is not cured by weight reduction. Most often, the obese HA patient is recalcitrant to weight reduction. Too often, the obese patient has been told to exercise more or to eat less. Certainly, weight loss can only be achieved when caloric expenditure exceeds caloric intake, but genetic, metabolic, and environmental alterations make this an extremely complex equation.

The coexistence of hyperandrogenism and hyperinsulinism in many women with PCOS has led to consideration of the possibility of a cause-and-effect relationship. Potentially, an elevated insulin level caused by insulin resistance could stimulate increased synthesis of ovarian androgens. Alternatively, increased serum androgens (particularly testosterone) could directly stimulate pancreatic insulin secretion or cause insulin resistance (or both) with consequent compensatory hyperinsulinism. A third possibility also exists; namely, that hyperandrogenism and hyperinsulinism coexist but are due to another as yet unidentified factor.

At present, there is probably greater acceptance for the concept that elevated insulin levels increase ovarian androgen production. Hyperinsulinemia is usually a consequence of relative insulin resistance, which, if left uncorrected, would result in elevated glucose levels (e.g., type 2 diabetes mellitus). To prevent this occurrence, the body possesses homeostatic mechanisms that attempt to maintain normoglycemia; namely, enhanced pancreatic insulin secretion. In fact, even in a group of women who have normal glucose tolerance as assessed by a standardized glucose tolerance test, a range of serum insulin levels exist that are reciprocally related to insulin sensitivity. Such insulin resistance could be caused by obesity, type 2 diabetes mellitus, or, as will be discussed later, hyperandrogenism.

Insulin's ability to stimulate ovarian androgen production has been demonstrated by in vitro studies in many models, including porcine granulosa cells, ovarian theca cells, and human granulosa cells. It has been hypothesized that insulin may act on the ovary to increase androgen production via the insulin-like growth factor 1 (IGF-1) receptor (with which it shares considerable homology) rather than its own.

Additionally, human in vivo data have now accumulated to show that a reduction of insulin resistance or a reduction in circulating insulin levels (or both) is associated with a reduction in serum androgens. This observation has been demonstrated with three separate agents: diazoxide, metformin, and troglitazone. Importantly, in studies of the latter two agents, the reduction in androgen levels was associated with reversion of gonadotropin profiles toward those observed in cycling women, as well as resumption of spontaneous ovulation in many of the study subjects.

The ability of hyperandrogenism to cause hyperinsulinism could take place via a direct effect on pancreatic insulin secretion or an indirect effect caused by creation of an insulin-resistant state (or both). With regard to the former, during a hyperglycemic clamp study in women receiving methyltestosterone, we were unable to demonstrate significant changes in pancreatic insulin secretion.

A series of studies in animals and women have demonstrated that androgens can reduce insulin sensitivity. We have demonstrated that administering short-term methyltestosterone to women significantly reduced glucose uptake during hyperglycemic, euglycemic, and hyperinsulinemic clamp studies. Additionally, in women receiving norgestrel (the progestin with the most potent androgenic action) in the form of a long-acting implant (Norplant), a reduction in insulin-stimulated glucose uptake was identified by using the euglycemic hyperinsulinemic clamp technique. However, in studies in which androgen levels were reduced by a gonadotropin-releasing hormone (GnRH) analog, insulin sensitivity has not been shown to be improved. Furthermore, we were unable to identify a positive correlation between serum androgen levels and insulin sensitivity in women with androgen levels within the normal range.

Thus, at this time, there is evidence supporting both hypotheses, that hyperandrogenism causes hyperinsulin production and that hyperinsulinism causes hyperandrogenism. As such, conditions are present for the establishment of a self-perpetuating cycle, regardless of whether either of these was the original incising event. Alternatively, a yet unidentified factor could be the initiating event; this initiating event could be puberty, with its elevation of circulating androgens, including DHEAS. This observation would be consistent with multiple reports that have now demonstrated pancreatic insulin hypersecretion and insulin resistance during puberty.

Regardless of the factors that lead to its development, once it is present, hyperinsulinemia results in an increase in insulin-like growth factor binding protein (IGFBP-1), leading to an enhancement of IGFs. IGFs bind to pituitary cells to augment release, which in turn causes increased androgen production by the ovary. In the ovary, IGFs and insulin bind to theca cells and together with increased androgen production bring about alterations in follicle growth insulin resistance (IR) and a genetically acquired dysregulation of steroidogenesis or HPO axis abnormality (or both), probably act in concert as in the etiology of PCOS. The degree of participation of each of these etiologies varies between patients, and although a unified concept is emerging, most likely a single cause of PCOS will not be found.

## Therapy

There is no known cure for non-neoplastic causes of HA. Neither is there any medication approved for the treatment of hirsutism, although a variety provide some degree of effectiveness in treatment (Table 55–8). Although the risk of feminizing a male fetus is more speculative than substantive, no antiandrogenic agent should be used without some form of protection against pregnancy. If fertility is desired, clomiphene citrate and then gonadotropins are the choices of therapy. These agents do not provide treatment, but they can overpower the many forms of ovarian dysfunction, regardless of etiology. It appears that insulin-sensitizing agents will be increasingly used in clomiphene-resistant patients and perhaps even as first-line therapy in selected patients.

**Weight Loss.** Although dieting is certainly valuable, it is the most difficult of therapeutic regimens to administer. Obesity should be viewed as another symptom, rather than the cause of HA. With weight loss, there is often an improvement in endocrine parameters and sometimes return of menses. Plans that focus on behavioral modification and group

**Table 55–8** Medical Therapy for Hyperandrogenism

| |
|---|
| INHIBITORS OF ANDROGEN PRODUCTION |
| Oral contraceptives |
| GnRH analogs |
| Progestins |
| Costicosteroids |
| INHIBITORS OF ANDROGEN ACTION (RECEPTORS) |
| Cyproterone acetate |
| Spironolactone (Aldactone) |
| Flutamide |
| Finasteride |
| INHIBITORS OF INSULIN ACTION |
| Metformin (Glucophage) |
| Troglitazone (Rezulin) |

GnRH = gonadotropin-releasing hormone.

involvement have been the most effective. Weight loss may improve general health and menstrual regularity, but it has little effect on hirsutism.

**Oral Contraceptives (OCs).** OCs are the mainstay of treatment of HA. The estrogen component of OCs increases SHBG and thus reduces the amount of circulating free testosterone. The progestational component of OCs reduces the LH tone and, therefore, testosterone production from the ovary. The first-generation progestin, norethindrone, is the standard by which other agents are measured. The second-generation progestin, levonorgestrel, is the most potent of the progestins and has the greatest androgenic capacity, but it also may have the greatest capacity to reduce LH. The third-generation progestational agents, such as desogestrel, are the least androgenic and most estrogenic of the progestational agents. Unfortunately, there has been controversy as to whether some of the newer progestational agents are associated with an increased risk of stroke and myocardial infarction. The literature is so controversial, biased, and conflicting that meaningful conclusions cannot be made. This is unfortunate, because the individuals who would be best served by the third-generation progestins are also at highest risk for complications.

**Cyproterone Acetate (CA).** CA is a potent antiandrogen and weak progestin available only outside the United States. Its effectiveness in treatment of hirsutism is well substantiated. Most patients report decreased hair growth, and some patients become amenorrheic. Although CA is usually well tolerated, its glucocorticoid activity may cause weight gain. The usual dose in 50 mg daily in conjunction with an oral contraceptive. CA has also been compounded with ethinyl estradiol and marketed as Diane, an oral contraceptive. The efficacy of Diane in treatment of hirsutism has been questioned, but it may help to control hair growth. Drug-induced hepatitis has been reported, and it is prudent to monitor liver function in patients who take Diane.

**Spironolactone.** Spironolactone is an aldosterone antagonist used primarily as a potassium-sparing diuretic to treat hypertension. It reduces hair growth by competitively inhibiting androgens at the androgen receptor site. At high doses, spironolactone blocks the cytochrome P-450 system involved in ovarian and adrenal steroidogenesis as well as the conversion of testosterone to DHT by 5α-reductase enzyme. Some patients have a surprisingly good response to therapy whereas others seem completely resistant. In some cases, especially when OCs cannot be used, it may represent first-line therapy. The effects of OC therapy may be additive. OCs may also reduce a tendency of irregular bleeding seen in some patients who use spironolactone. The usual starting dose is 50 mg once or twice daily. This may be increased to 100 mg twice daily. It is prudent to have baseline electrolyte levels drawn and reassessed after several weeks of therapy, although hyperkalemia is rarely seen in young healthy women. Because of the hepatic metabolism of spironolactone, baseline liver function testing should be performed. The most common side effects are nausea and dyspepsia, and some patients report increased fatigue.

**Flutamide.** Flutamide is a nonsteroidal antiandrogen indicated for treatment of prostatic cancer. Its action is similar to those of spironolactone and cyproterone acetate because androgen action is competitively inhibited at the androgen receptor site. Flutamide is theoretically superior to cyproterone because of its absence of glucocorticoid activity and likewise superior to spironolactone because of its lack of renal alterations.

A majority of patients report the side effect of dry skin. Less common side effects are hot flushes, increased appetite, headache, fatigue, and nausea. Flutamide is metabolized by the liver, and fatal hepatic toxicity has been reported. The usual dose is 125 to 250 mg once or twice daily for treatment of hirsutism. Although some have reported the drug as safe and superior to spironolactone, others report a similar efficacy but avoid its use because of its high cost and potential for serious liver damage.

**Finasteride.** Finasteride is a specific inhibitor of 5α-reductase activity indicated for use in the management of benign prostatic hypertrophy. Because its action is directed at the point of peripheral conversion in the skin of testosterone to DHT, the drug shows great promise. The dose of 5 mg daily is usually prescribed. Finasteride is probably as effective as spironolactone. The safety and patient tolerance profiles appear to be very good. Despite the pregnancy warning and high cost, the theoretical advantages and excellent patient tolerance may make this a drug to consider.

**GnRH Analogs.** Long-acting GnRH agonists block LH release and reduce steroid production from the ovary. Adrenal androgen production is unaffected. The various preparations are identical in action but differ in route of administration. A 3-month depot injection of leuprolide acetate is now available. Add-back therapy with OCs, or estrogens and a progestin, offers additional advantages of increasing SHBG and reducing the risk of osteoporosis and symptoms of menopause. A great disadvantage is the high cost of this regimen.

**Corticosteroids.** Corticosteroids have the ability to suppress adrenal androgen production and may be useful in treatment of HA of adrenal origin. Overall, their use is better in theory than practice, and they are often discontinued by patients because of their side effects. The effectiveness of corticosteroids in control of hirsutism is questioned, and they should probably be considered third-line therapy. Doses as low as 0.25 mg of dexamethasone can be used chronically with little fear of overly suppressing adrenal function. Because cortisol levels are higher at night, suppression therapy is probably better given at bedtime.

**Progestins.** Progestins are indicated to induce regular withdrawal bleeding and protect against endometrial hyperplasia in the unopposed estrogen state common in HA. Almost all cases of complex hyperplasia and endometrial cancer seen in women between ages 20 and 40 years have findings of PCOS as well. Although LH may be reduced by progestins, they appear to be of little use in reduction of hair growth. The most commonly used agent is medroxyprogesterone acetate (Cycrin, Amen, Provera). A regimen of 5 to 10 mg for 10 to 14 days monthly is used for normalization of cyclic bleeding. Some prefer therapy every 3 months. It is unclear whether this is effective in reducing the risk of hyperplasia. Alternatively, norethindrone acetate (Aygestin) can be used at 5 mg daily in a similar regimen.

**Metformin (Glucophage).** This drug was introduced in 1995 and is now used by several milion patients for management of type 2 (insulin-resistant) diabetes. Metformin enhances peripheral tissue sensitivity to insulin and inhibits hepatic glucose production without the risk of hypoglycemia. Given the strong association between PCOS and hyperinsulinemia/insulin resistance, metformin and similarly acting drugs may represent the first therapies to impact on a central, perhaps causative, mechanism of PCOS. They have shown great promise in early trials in reversing many of the metabolic derangements of PCOS. Some patients have shown weight loss, improved lipid profiles, lowering of blood pressure, return of menstruation, and pregnancy. Metformin appears to have an excellent safety profile and is generally well tolerated. Gastrointestinal upset, a tendency toward loose stools, and more frequent bowel movements are the most frequent side effects. These are common in the first week and can be reduced by starting at lower doses and increasing thereafter. Lactic acidosis is a rare and potentially fatal condition that has been associated with metformin use. Its incidence is 3 out of 100,000 patients using the drug for 1 year. Almost all cases occurred in elderly patients who had other significant diseases and risk factors. Use of metformin may have the relative disadvantage of postponement of more aggressive fertility therapy. It must be emphasized that the risk during pregnancy is unknown.

These drugs have been given a class B rating by the Food and Drug Administration (FDA), indicating safety, but with insufficient data to identify a harmful effect. Studies in laboratory animals have not shown alteration in fertility, increase in rate of pregnancy loss, or birth defects. The medication has been used in a small number of pregnant patients with no apparent adverse events. At present, it is recommended that metformin (and troglitazone) be discontinued if pregnancy is established. A pregnancy test should be performed if pregnany is suspected.

**Glitazones (Rezulin).** Troglitazone (Rezulin) is a thiozolidinedione antidiabetic agent not related to either the sulfonylureas or metformin. It is used for treatment of type 2 diabetes. Justification for its use is the same as described earlier for metformin. Its mechanism of action is thought to involve binding to nuclear receptors that regulate transcription of insulin-related genes critical for glucose and lipid metabolism. Blood glucose is lowered by improving target cell response to insulin. Although it seems to be better tolerated than metformin (i.e., less gastrointestinal distress), a repeated warning has been issued by the FDA regarding the potential of serious liver damage. Liver function testing should be performed monthly for the first 6 months. The usual dose is 400 to 600 mg once daily. Rosiglitazone (Avandia) was introduced in the summer of 1999 for treatment of type 2 diabetes. Its insulin-altering action is similar to that of troglitazone. It does not contain the vitamin E moiety of troglitazone, which may be both an advantage and disadvantage. Liver toxicity has not been reported, but the cardioprotective effects may be lost and weight gain is more likely. There is very limited information on use of rosiglitazone in PCOS patients. Pioglitazone (Actos) is in the final stages of development.

**Other Medical Therapy.** Cimetidine, which was always of questionable value, is no longer listed as a potential treatment. Ketoconazole is a potent fungicide that blocks steroidogenesis and that formerly showed some promise as an antiandrogen. Its use has been abandoned because of poor patient compliance and potentially serious side effects.

**Surgical Therapy.** Except for removal of neoplasia, surgery should not be considered as first-line therapy in the treatment of HA or PCOS. Previously, ovarian wedge resection was used in the treatment of PCOS, with a significant reduction in LH and androgen production, re-establishment of regular menses in more than 75% of patients, and a pregnancy rate of about 60%. However, pelvic adhesive disease, which was often severe, occurred in about 30% of patients. There is probably no longer an indication for wedge resection by laparotomy, although electrosurgical incisions, or "ovarian drilling," has become relatively commonplace. Success rates of microcautery vary, depending on the skill of the operator, and although adhesion formation may be considerably less, it is still common. A unipolar needle is used to make 10 to 20 punctures on each ovary at a depth and diameter of 4 to 5 mm using 30 to 40 watts of cutting current. Alternatively, the $CO_2$ laser has been used, but the surface injury may be greater. Some reports have suggested adhesion barriers, such as Interceed, to reduce adhesion formation after cautery. Laparoscopic outcomes seem comparable with those achieved by traditional wedge resection. The mechanism by which surgical therapy works is not known. It is unclear whether it is surface destruction and thinning of the cortex or reduction of ovarian mass that causes the procedure to be effective. Long-term effects are largely unknown. Early menopause resulting from partial destruction of the oocyte pool is a theoretical risk.

**Cosmesis.** This is a useful if unnecessary adjunctive therapy. Permanent hair removal can be accomplished by electrolysis, which destroys the hair papillae. Contrary to popular belief, shaving and plucking does not induce faster or coarser hair growth. However, it is painful and can cause significant inflammation, infection, and scarring. If possible, medical therapy should be the first line of therapy followed by electrolysis.

## REFERENCES

Arniel SA, Sherwin RS, Simonson DC, et al: Impaired insulin action in puberty. A contributing factor to poor glycemic control in adolescents with diabetes. N Engl J Med 9:315–215, 1986.

Barnes RB: Pathophysiology of ovarian steroid secretion in polycystic ovarian syndrome. Semin Reprod Endocrinol 15:159–168, 1997.

De Leo V, Lanzetta D, D'Antona D, et al: Hormonal effects of flutamide in young women with polycystic ovarian syndrome. J Clin Endocrinol Metab 83:99–102,1988.

Diamond MP, Davis B: Menopause, ovarian and adrenal steroids, and carbohydrate metabolism. Metab Clin North Am 6:711–720, 1995.

Diamond MP, Grainger D, Diamond MC, et al: Methyltestosterone Induced Insulin Resistance. Society for Gynecologic Investigation, San Diego, CA, March 1997.

Diamond MP, Thornton K, Connolly-Diamond M, et al: Reciprocal variations in insulin-stimulator glucose uptake and pancreatic insulin secretion in women with normal glucose tolerance. J Soc Gynecol Invest 2:708–715, 1995.

Diamond MP, Wentz AC, Cherrington AD: Alterations in carbohydrate metabolism as they rate to reproductive endocrinology. Fertil Steril 50:387–397, 1988.

Dunaif A: Insulin resistance and the polycystic ovary syndrome: Mechanism and implications for pathogenesis. Endocrinol Rev 18:774–800, 1997.

Dunaif A, Givens JR, Hazeltine FP, et al (eds): Polycystic Ovarian Syndrome. Cambridge, MA, Blackwell Scientific, 1992.

Franks S, Gharani N, Waterworth D, et al: The genetic basis of polycystic ovarian syndrome. Hum Reprod 12:2641–2648, 1997.

Edwards RG, Beard HK, Bradshaw JP: Balancing risks and benefits of oral contraception. Hum Reprod 12:2339–2340, 1997.

Erenus M, Yucelten D, Durmusoglu F, et al: Comparison of finasteride versus spironolactone in the treatment of idiopathic hisutism. Fertil Steril 68:1000–1003, 1997.

Futterweit W: Pathophysiology of polycystic ovarian syndrome. In Redmond GP (ed): Androgenic Disorders. New York, Raven Press, 1995, pp 77–166.

Grainger D, DeFronzo RA, Sherwin RS, et al: Exogenous Androgens Block Insulin Action Under Hyperglycemic, Hyperinsulinemic Conditions in Women. 38th Annual Meeting of the Society for Gynecologic Investigation, San Antonio, TX, March 1991.

Grainger D, Thornton K, Rossi G, et al: Influence of basal androgen levels in euandrogenic women on glucose homeostasis. Fertil Steril 58:113–118, 1992.

New MI: Congenital adrenal hyperplasia. In Degroot LJ (ed): Endocrinology, 3rd ed. Philadelphia, WB Saunders, 1995, pp 1813–1835.

Rayuburn W: Diabetes. New recommendations for classification and diagnosis. J Reprod Med 42:585, 586, 1997.

Redmond GR: Clinical evaluation of the woman with an androgenic disorder. In Redmond GP (ed): Androgenic Disorders. New York, Raven Press, 1995, pp 1–20.

Shanti A, Murphy AA: Surgical approaches to ovulation induction. Semin Reprod Endocrinol 15:183–192, 1997.

Sharp S, Diamond MP: Sex steroids and diabetes. Diabet Rev 1:318–342, 1993.

Stein IF, Leventhal ML: Amenorrhea associated with bilateral polycystic ovaries. Am J Obstet Gynecol 29:181–191, 1935.

Velazquez E: Menstrual cyclicity after metformin therapy in polycystic ovarian syndrome. Obstet Gynecol 90:392–395, 1997.

Wong IL, Lobo RA: Ovarian androgen-producing tumors. In Adashi EY, Rock JA, Rosenwaks Z (eds): Reproductive Endocrinology, Surgery, and Technology. Philadelphia, Lippincott-Raven, 1996, pp 1571–1598.

Yen SSC: A contemporary overview. In Adashi EY, Rock JA, Rosenwaks Z (eds): Reproductive Endocrinology, Surgery, and Technology. Philadelphia, Lippincott-Raven, 1996, pp 1117–1126.

# 56

# Thyroid Disorders

NANDALAL BAGCHI

Thyroid disorders have three common presentations in clinical practice: hyperthyroidism, hypothyroidism, and diffuse or nodular goiter in an otherwise euthyroid subject. These presentations are discussed.

## Hyperthyroidism

Hyperthyroidism is a clinical syndrome resulting from excess thyroid hormone action on the tissues.

### HISTORY AND PHYSICAL EXAMINATION

Hyperthyroid patients typically exhibit signs and symptoms affecting most organ systems, as shown in Table 56–1. These features are mostly attributable to hypermetabolism (heat intolerance, increased sweating, weight loss), apparent organ hyperfunction (palpitation, gastrointestinal hypermotility, increased neuromuscular excitability), and increased catabolism leading to tissue wasting (weight loss, muscle weakness, osteoporosis), all resulting from excess thyroid hormone action. The presentation varies widely, however, and is often determined by preexisting disease. Subjects with asymptomatic heart disease, for example, often present with angina, arrhythmias, or congestive heart failure when hyperthyroidism is superimposed. Elderly subjects commonly present with loss of weight, cardiovascular symptoms, and muscle weakness. The thyroid gland is usually enlarged. This is depends, however, on the underlying etiology and does not occur in all cases.

Hyperthyroidism occasionally presents in a severe life-threatening form called thyroid storm. The condition is precipitated by trauma, surgery, or concurrent illnesses in a patient with poorly controlled hyperthyroidism, usually from Graves' disease. The clinical features include fever, altered mental status, and signs and symptoms of severe hyperthyroidism. The diagnosis is made largely on clinical grounds.

### DIAGNOSIS

Laboratory diagnosis of hyperthyroidism requires measurement of serum thyroid-stimulating hormone

**Table 56–1** Common Clinical Features of Hyperthyroidism

Goiter: Usually
Hypermetabolism: Weight loss, heat intolerance, excess sweating
Heart: Tachycardia, hyperdynamic circulation with wide pulse pressure, atrial arrhythmias
Neurologic: Nervousness, irritability, emotional lability, tremor, brisk tendon reflexes, hyperkinesia
Musculoskeletal: Proximal muscle weakness
Gastrointestinal: Frequent bowel movements
Skeletal: Osteoporosis
Reproductive: Oligo- or amenorrhea

**Table 56–2** Diagnostic Workup of Hyperthyroidism

STEP A. DIAGNOSIS
  Tests
    TSH and FT$_4$ (all cases)
    T$_3$ and/or TRH test (in selected cases only)
  Patterns
    Overt hyperthyroidism: TSH low, FT$_4$ high
    Mild hyperthyroidism: TSH low, FT$_4$ normal
                          T$_3$ high, TRH
                          response flat
    Pituitary or hypothalamic hyperthyroidism:
                          TSH normal or high
                          FT$_4$ high

STEP B. DIFFERENTIAL DIAGNOSIS
  Tests
    Radioisotope uptake and scan
    Other tests depending on presentation

FT$_4$ = free thyroxine; T$_3$ = triiodothyronine; TRH = thyroid-releasing hormone; TSH = thyroid-stimulating hormone.

(TSH) and estimation of serum free thyroxine(T$_4$), as outlined in Table 56–2. Serum TSH should be measured by one of the newer sensitive assays. Free thyroxine (FT$_4$) constitutes only 0.03% of the total circulating hormone, the remainder being bound to proteins such as thyroxine binding globulin (TBG), thyroxine binding prealbumin or transthyretin, and albumin. However, FT$_4$ is the physiologically active component. It can be measured directly by several techniques (e.g., radioimmunoassay, equilibrium dialysis, etc). It can also be indirectly estimated as free thyroxine index (FT$_4$I), calculated from total serum T$_4$ and resin triiodothyronine (T$_3$) uptake test. FT$_4$I is strongly correlated to FT$_4$ except when serum T$_4$ binding proteins are very high or very low or in the presence of abnormal binding proteins (e.g., dysalbumin, T$_4$ binding antibodies, etc). Total serum T$_4$ alone is not useful in the diagnosis of hyperthyroidism because most (99.97%) of it is bound and physiologically inactive and the levels are affected by the concentration of binding proteins.

Once hyperthyroidism is clinically suspected, one should obtain serum TSH and FT$_4$ (or FT$_4$I). In a typical patient, TSH is suppressed to undetectable levels, whereas FT$_4$ is elevated. These findings establish the diagnosis of hyperthyroidism. Further testing is then directed to the determination of the underlying cause of hyperthyroidism.

The combination of undetectable TSH and normal FT$_4$ is sometimes encountered in mild hyperthyroidism. In these cases, measurement of serum T$_3$ levels or TRH testing is quite useful. Serum T$_3$ rises to a greater degree than serum T$_4$ in most hyperthyroid patients. A relative excess of T$_3$ in relation to T$_4$ thus indicates hyperthyroidism. This is generally demonstrated by supranormal T$_3$ values in association with a T$_3$/T$_4$ (ng/μg) ratio exceeding 20. The use of serum T$_3$ is restricted by the observation that several nonthyroid conditions decrease T$_3$ production from T$_4$ and thus result in falsely low T$_3$ values. These conditions include acute and chronic illnesses (including the immediate postsurgical state), treatment with drugs (e.g., glucocorticoids, amiodarone, β-adrenergic blockers), imaging with iodinated radiocontrast media, and extremes of age (neonate, the elderly). One must be aware of these conditions in interpreting T$_3$ levels.

Thyrotropin-releasing hormone (TRH) testing is performed by intravenous (IV) injection of 500 μg TRH as a bolus and measurement of serum TSH at 15-minute intervals over 0 to 60 minutes. TRH, a hypothalamic tripeptide, stimulates pituitary thyrotrophs to release TSH. A rise of serum TSH follows with a peak (2 to 32 μU/ml over the baseline) at 15 to 30 minutes. The pituitary is suppressed by the negative feedback from excess thyroid hormones in hyperthyroidism. Serum TSH therefore does not appreciably rise after TRH in hyperthyroid subjects. A flat TRH response is thus characteristic of hyperthyroidism.

Subnormal TSH is occasionally found in clinically euthyroid subjects with normal FT$_4$ and T$_3$ concentrations. This may indicate subclinical hyperthyroidism, a condition often associated with nodular goiters. A similar laboratory profile can also occur in a number of nonthyroid conditions. These include illnesses requiring hospitalization and treatment with drugs (e.g., glucocorticoids, dopamine, phenytoin, and somatostatin analogs). Subclinical hyperthyroidism is associated with a higher incidence of atrial fibrillation, tachycardia, premature atrial contractions, and osteoporosis. However, subclinical hyperthyroidism is often transient and progression to overt hyperthyroidism is uncommon.

Rarely, serum TSH is normal or even elevated in hyperthyroid patients with elevated FT$_4$. These inappropriate TSH levels suggest pituitary hypothalamic disorders as the etiology of hyperthyroidism. These disorders include TSH secreting pituitary tumor or thyroid hormone resistance syndrome limited to the pituitary and the hypothalamus.

## DIFFERENTIAL DIAGNOSIS

Once hyperthyroidism has been diagnosed, the underlying etiology has to be identified. The various conditions causing hyperthyroidism are shown in Table 56–3. Graves' disease constitutes over 80% of the cases. It is an autoimmune disease affecting the thyroid, orbital tissue (causing exophthalmos), and other areas such as skin (causing pretibial myxedema). Thyroid stimulation results from an antibody binding to

### Table 56–3  Causes of Hyperthyroidism

| | |
|---|---|
| External thyroid stimulation | Drug induced |
|   Graves' disease |   Iodine |
|   Trophoblastic tumors |   L-Thyroxine |
|   Inappropriate TSH secretion |   Amiodarone |
| Thyroid autonomy | Ectopic hormone production |
|   Toxic nodular goiter |   Struma ovarii |
|   Hyperfunctioning adenoma |   Thyroid carcinoma |
| Thyroiditis | |
|   Subacute thyroiditis | |
|   Painless thyroiditis | |

TSH = thyroid stimulating hormone.

the TSH receptor and thereby stimulating the thyroid cell. External stimulation of the thyroid by TSH or human chorionic gonadotropin (hCG), which has weak thyrotropic activity, underlie other disorders causing hyperthyroidism. Thyroid nodules can cause hyperthyroidism through excessive and autonomous overproduction of hormone, as in toxic nodular goiter (Plummer's disease) or hyperfunctioning adenoma. Thyroid inflammation (thyroiditis) can cause hyperthyroidism by releasing preformed hormones. Thyroiditis could be painful as in subacute thyroiditis or without pain as in painless thyroiditis. Because the hormone stores are limited, hyperthyroidism from thyroiditis lasts only a few weeks. Hyperthyroidism may be followed by a short period of hypothyroidism before the euthyroid state is restored. An interesting cause of hyperthyroidism is exposure to excess iodine from diet (e.g., kelp) or drugs (e.g., amiodarone). The physiologic response to iodine excess is inhibition of thyroid hormone synthesis and release initially followed by an escape from the inhibition. Small subsets of the population fail in either of these adaptive steps. Failure of inhibition leads to iodine induced hyperthyroidism. Failure of escape causes iodine induced hypothyroidism, as described in that section below.

A thorough initial evaluation usually provides insight into the underlying cause, as indicated in Table 56–4. Of particular interest are the autoimmune features that accompany Graves' disease. An important manifestation is ophthalmopathy resulting from autoimmune inflammation affecting the orbital tissues. This leads to the clinical presentations of exophthalmos, redness, tearing, diplopia, and even blindness. Other autoimmune features include pretibial myxedema (thickening of the skin over the tibia due to deposition of glycoproteins), vitiligo, and myasthenia gravis. Hypokalemic periodic paralysis is occasionally observed in patients with Graves' disease, usually in Asians and Latin Americans, and improves with the treatment of hyperthyroidism.

Several laboratory investigations are useful in the differential diagnosis.

1. Radioiodine uptake (RAIU) by the thyroid: RAIU measures the percent orally administered radioiodine that is retained by the thyroid at specific times. The normal value is 10 to 30% at 24 hours. Although RAIU is not satisfactory in the diagnosis of hyperthyroidism, it is quite useful in the differential diagnosis, as shown in Table 56–5.
2. Thyroid scan: This is an imaging study using iodine or technetium isotope and is useful in the functional assessment of a palpable nodule. Thus, a hyperfunctioning nodule concentrates isotope to a greater extent than the surrounding thyroid tissue. A scan is quite useful in the diagnosis of hyperfunctioning adenoma ("hot nodule") and toxic nodular goiter.
3. Thyroid-stimulating immunoglobulin (TSI): Autoimmune thyroid disease is characterized by the production of various antibodies directed to the TSH receptor. Some antibodies stimulate the receptor, whereas others block its function. Presence of stimulatory antibodies (TSI) is characteristic of most patients with Graves' disease. However, TSI measurement is necessary in the management of selected cases only.
4. Other tests: These depend on the clinical background and include urinary iodine excretion, hCG, and pituitary magnetic resonance imaging (MRI).

### Table 56–4  Clinical Clues to the Etiology of Hyperthyroidism

| Feature | Etiology |
|---|---|
| Exophthalmos | Graves' disease |
| Pretibial myxedema | Graves' disease |
| Presence of other autoimmune diseases | Graves' disease |
| Tender thyroid | Subacute thyroiditis |
| Pregnancy (present or recent) | hCG-induced hyperthyroidism |
| Thyroid nodule | Toxic nodular goiter Hyperfunctioning adenoma |
| Exposure to iodine, Levo-T$_4$, amiodarone | Drug-induced hyperthyroidism |

hCG = human chorionic gonadotropin; Levo-T$_4$ = L-thyroxine.

### Table 56–5  Radioiodine Uptake in Hyperthyroidism

| Uptake | Etiology |
|---|---|
| Low | Subacute or painless thyroiditis; iodine or Levo-T$_4$–induced hyperthyroidism |
| Normal | Hyperfunctioning adenoma, toxic nodular goiter |
| High | Graves' disease; TSH or hCG-induced hyperthyroidism; toxic nodular goiter |

hCG = human chorionic gonadotropin; Levo-T$_4$ = L-thyroxine; TSH = thyroid-stimulating hormone.

## HYPERTHYROIDISM AND PREGNANCY

Pregnancy is associated with several changes in thyroid physiology. First, there is increased iodine loss due to increased renal and placental clearance. This may be of some concern in iodine-deficient countries but not in the United States. Second, the elevated estrogens cause a marked increase in circulating TBG. This is due to an increase in hepatic synthesis and a decrease in its metabolism due to increased sialylation. The TBG changes result in an increase in serum $T_4$ and a decrease in resin $T_3$ uptake. However, serum $FT_4$ and $FT_4I$ values remain normal. Finally, hCG has weak thyrotropic activity. Serum hCG increases in pregnancy particularly in the first trimester. This may cause weak thyroid stimulation and suppression of serum TSH to subnormal levels. High serum hCG, as observed in hyperemesis gravidarum and twin pregnancy, may cause mild clinical hyperthyroidism. The hyperthyroidism observed in molar pregnancy and choriocarcinoma is mediated by hCG.

Hyperthyroidism is present in about 0.1% of pregnant women. It is usually due to Graves' disease and less commonly due to thyroiditis and hyperfunctioning adenoma. However, as high as 66% cases of hyperemesis gravidarum may present with biochemical evidence of hyperthyroidism.

Graves' disease, like several other autoimmune diseases, usually has a mild course during pregnancy. In addition, the hypermetabolic state associated with pregnancy makes the clinical diagnosis of hyperthyroidism difficult. Correct diagnosis is suggested by tachycardia (>100 bpm), decreased weight gain, the presence of goiter, the specific features of Graves' disease (e.g., exophthalmos, pretibial myxedema), or a prior history of Graves' disease. Untreated Graves' disease has detrimental effects on both maternal and fetal health. The maternal complications include pregnancy-induced hypertension and heart failure. Fetal complications include stillbirth, prematurity, small for gestrational age birth weight, and congenital malformations. Hyperthyroidism at the time of conception may have detrimental effects on the fetus. However, control of hyperthyroidism improves the prognosis in both the mother and the fetus. Additional complications may arise from transplacental passage of TSIs. Such transfers may result in fetal or neonatal hyperthyroidism.

Hyperthyroidism may occur in the postpartum period. The reported incidence is 1.9% to 8.8% in the United States, but the incidence is substantially higher if the mother has insulin-dependent diabetes or is positive for serum thyroid autoantibodies during pregnancy. The hyperthyroidism occurs in the first 6 months postpartum and often is followed by a hypothyroid phase before eventual recovery. The condition may recur in subsequent pregnancies. The underlying etiology appears to be autoimmune, and the condition is likely a variant of painless thyroiditis. A significant number (20 to 25%) of patients eventually develop permanent hypothyroidism.

Diagnosis of hyperthyroidism in pregnancy uses the usual criteria of suppression of TSH and elevation of $FT_4$. $FT_4$ rather than $FT_4I$ is used as a measure of free hormone because in some subjects with very high TBG levels, $FT_4I$ may not accurately reflect $FT_4$. Serum TSH is often low in the first trimester of pregnancy. This is probably due to the thyrotropic action of hCG and, in the absence of an increase in $FT_4$, does not indicate hyperthyroidism. Fetal hyperthyroidism is diagnosed by measurement of TSH and $FT_4$ in the cord blood.

## TREATMENT

Treatment depends on the etiology. Because Graves' disease constitutes the major cause, its management is discussed in greater detail.

### Graves' Disease

There are three therapeutic options: long-term treatment with thiourea drugs, surgery, or ablation with radioiodine. The choice depends on patient characteristics and preferences and should be arrived at jointly by the physician and the patient.

The rationale for long-term drug therapy is to control hyperthyroidism until remission, expected eventually in Graves' disease, sets in. Whether such therapy hastens remission or not is not clear. It is difficult to predict remission, though factors such as a reduction in gland size, decrease in TSI levels, return of TRH response, or certain HLA (human leukocyte antigens) types appear to favor remission. The treatment is begun with thiourea drugs such as propylthiouracil (PTU) 300 to 400 mg/d in three to four divided doses or methimazole (MMI) 20 to 40 mg/d in one or two divided doses. Both drugs act by blocking hormone synthesis. PTU also inhibits the conversion of $T_4$ to $T_3$. Once the patient becomes euthyroid, usually in 1 to 3 months, a lower dose is required to maintain euthyroidism. The treatment is continued for 6 to 12 months and then stopped to determine if spontaneous remission has occurred. It relapse occurs, usually in the first 6 months, drug treatment is reinstated for another 6 to 12 months and the cycle is repeated until permanent remission is achieved. The rate of remission varies widely in different studies (14 to 80%) but increases with longer durations of treatment. The drugs are tolerated well but serious side effects such as agranulocytosis, hepatic toxicity, or vasculitis can occur and require discontinuance of the drug. It is necessary to monitor patients for these side effects with blood counts and liver function tests. Patient compliance is absolutely essential for long-term drug therapy to be successful.

Some patients require short-term drug therapy before any of the three definitive therapies are instituted. They are those with severe disease including thyroid storm, those with cardiac dysfunction, and elderly patients. Thiourea drugs are the mainstay of short-term drug therapy. However, severe conditions (e.g., thyroid storm) also require blockade of hormone release by agents such as iodine (saturated solution of potassium iodide, one drop or 60 mg every 8 hours) or, less satisfactorily, lithium carbonate. The iodine drops are begun 1 to 2 hours after thiourea drug are started. β-Adrenergic blockade (e.g., with propranolol 40 mg po every 6 to 8 hours) is quite useful and relieves symptoms like tremor, palpitation, and anxiety. Glucocorticoids (40 to 60 mg prednisone/d) are often used in the treatment of thyroid storm. These agents decrease the production $T_3$ from $T_4$ and also have immunosuppressive effects.

Surgery (subtotal thyroidectomy) is preferred by a small group of patients for definitive treatment. It requires prior control of hyperthyroidism by the use of thiourea drugs. Iodine drops are often used for a few days before surgery to reduce the vascularity of the gland. Surgical complications include persistent hyperthyroidism (too much tissue left), hypothyroidism (too much tissue removed), and, infrequently, injury to the recurrent laryngeal nerve and hypoparathyroidism.

Partial thyroid ablation with radioiodine ($^{131}$I) is the most popular treatment in the United States. Most patients respond to one treatment, but some, especially those with large nodular goiters, require additional treatment repeated after 6 months. Once euthyroidism is achieved, usually in 1 to 3 months, hyperthyroidism rarely recurs. Radiation thyroiditis induced by radioiodine may transiently increase serum thyroid hormones 1 to 2 weeks later and worsen the clinical condition in some patients (e.g., those with severe hyperthyroidism, cardiac dysfunction, and the elderly). These patients require control of hyperthyroidism, as outlined above, before $^{131}$I therapy. Radioiodine therapy is attended with a significant incidence of permanent hypothyroidism (>50% in a year and increasing thereafter) but does not have carcinogenic or teratogenic effects. The hypothyroidism requires replacement therapy with L-thyroxine. Radioiodine therapy is usually restricted to subjects who are older than 20 years of age, although studies in younger patients have not shown any detrimental effects.

Hyperthyroidism in pregnancy is treated either by surgery or thiourea drugs. Surgery is performed preferably in the second trimester after euthyroidism is achieved by treatment with drugs. This option has not been popular, and most patients are treated with thiourea drugs. Both PTU and MMI have been used successfully, although PTU may be preferable, in theory, because of greater protein binding and consequently lesser transplacental passage. The minimum dose of antithyroid drugs is used to reduce fetal exposure to these agents. This is achieved by aiming for a high normal $FT_4$ in the mother. The newborn should be checked for goiter and hypothyroidism. PTU treatment can be continued during breastfeeding because the drug appears in the milk only in small quantities and does not affect thyroid function in the infant.

Hyperthyroidism in the fetus is diagnosed by tachycardia, ultrasonographic evidence of goiter, and measurement of thyroid hormone in the cord blood. Treatment requires use of high dose of thiourea drugs in the mother so that enough drug is delivered to the fetal thyroid. The large doses may cause maternal hypothyroidism and necessitate addition of L-thyroxine to the maternal regimen.

Hyperthyroidism in the neonate is also caused by transplacental passage of TSI and may last for several months. The clinical features include tachycardia, irritability, goiter, and hepatosplenomegaly. Drugs used in the treatment include thiourea drugs, β-adrenergic blockers, and iodine.

Hyperthyroidism in the first trimester of pregnancy is mild and transient and requires no more than β-adrenergic blockade for symptomatic relief. Postpartum hyperthyroidism is usually mild and transient and due to painless thyroiditis. These mild symptoms are often treated by β-adrenergic blockers. However, it is important to remember than new-onset Graves' disease may also occur in the postpartum period.

## Toxic Nodular Goiter and Hyperfunctioning Adenoma

These conditions, unlike Graves' disease, are not self-limited. Long-term drug therapy is therefore not indicated for most patients. Short-term drug therapy may be needed in patients with cardiac disease or the elderly. Radioiodine therapy is usually used for definitive treatment. Surgery is an alternate choice. Some of these patients have atrial fibrillation. If the arrhythmia continues several months after therapy, elective cardioversion may be necessary. If arrhythmia continues, anticoagulant therapy with warfarin is indicated.

## Subacute and Painless Thyroiditis

Hyperthyroidism from these causes are of short duration. Symptomatic treatment with aspirin for pain and β-blockers for tachycardia and nervousness are usually adequate. Rare cases require glucocorticoid therapy. Thiourea drugs or iodine are of no benefit.

# Hypothyroidism

This is a clinical syndrome resulting from diminished thyroid hormone effects on the tissues. Serum thyroid hormone levels are decreased in most cases.

## HISTORY AND PHYSICAL EXAMINATION

The signs and symptoms of hypothyroidism involve multiple organs, and a careful review of all systems is important in identifying the condition. The common features are summarized in Table 56–6. The manifestations vary with the speed of development and intensity of hypothyroidism. Hypometabolism (e.g., lethargy, cold intolerance, weight gain) and sluggish organ function (e.g., bradycardia, constipation, hypokinesia, impaired memory and concentration) dominate the clinical picture. Another common feature is mucinous deposition in the skin and submucosa leading to thick skin, nonpitting edema, hoarseness of voice, periorbital puffiness, and nerve entrapment syndromes (causing paresthesia and carpal tunnel syndrome). There is only modest weight gain, and most obese patients do not have hypothyroidism.

Sometimes hypothyroidism has uncommon presentations. Although depression is common, manic symptoms ("myxedema madness") can occasionally occur. Other less common presentations include serous effusions in the pericardium, pleura and peritoneum, galactorrhea, premature puberty, and paralytic ileus. Long-standing primary hypothyroidism can result in pituitary enlargement and dysfunction.

The clinical presentation varies with the age at onset. Thyroid hormone is critical for growth and development. Hypothyroidism can lead to impaired neurologic development when it occurs before 2 years of age. Children born in endemic iodine-deficient areas have cretinism, a particularly severe form of the disease. Hypothyroidism developing during childhood can result in impaired bone growth and sexual maturation.

The clinical presentation is somewhat different if hypothyroidism is central in origin (i.e., a result of hypothalamic pituitary disease). Unlike primary hypothyroidism resulting from thyroid disease, central hypothyroidism is characterized by lack of weight gain, a small heart, lack of serous effusions, thin skin, and deficiency of other pituitary hormones. The clinical picture results from the deficiency of TSH and other pituitary hormones (e.g., ACTH [adrenocorticotropic hormone], gonadotropins, etc).

Hypothyroidism occasionally presents as myxedema coma, a life-threatening emergency with a high mortality (40 to 50%). It is precipitated usually in a patient with primary hypothyroidism by factors such as exposure to cold, sepsis, trauma, or treatment with central nervous system-depressant drugs. Besides exhibiting the usual features of severe hypothyroidism, these patients have hypothermia, altered mental state progressing to coma, respiratory acidosis, hypoglycemia, and hyponatremia. The diagnosis is made on clinical grounds because hormonal profiles do not distinguish myxedema coma from severe hypothyroidism.

## DIAGNOSIS

Laboratory diagnosis of hypothyroidism requires measurement of serum TSH and $FT_4$ or $FT_4I$ (Table 56–7). Serum $T_3$ measurements are not useful because the levels are subnormal only in advanced disease. Thyroidal radioiodine uptake measurements are also not useful in the diagnosis.

Serum TSH increases early in the course of primary hypothyroidism before a significant change in serum $FT_4$. Clinically overt disease is diagnosed by high serum TSH and subnormal serum $FT_4$. Mild hypothyroidism is characterized by increased serum TSH but a normal serum $FT_4$, albeit in the low normal range. Another group of patients with no apparent clinical disease have mild elevation of serum TSH (usually 5 to 10 µU/ml) and normal serum thyroid hormones. This condition, known as subclinical hypothyroidism, is particularly prevalent in women older than 55 to 60 years and with incidence as high as 10%.

Central (hypothalamic pituitary) hypothyroidism is diagnosed by a combination of low serum $FT_4$ and an inappropriately normal or low serum TSH. However, serum $FT_4$ may be in the low normal range early in

**Table 56–6**  Common Clinical Features of Hypothyroidism

| | |
|---|---|
| Goiter: | Variable |
| Hypometabolism: | Weight gain, cold intolerance, decreased sweating |
| Heart: | Bradycardia, decreased pulse pressure, pericardial effusion |
| Neurologic: | Lethargy, poor memory, hypokinesis |
| Musculoskeletal: | Cramps, arthralgias |
| Gastrointestinal: | Constipation |
| Reproductive: | Menorrhagia, anovulation |
| Skin and mucous membrane: | Thickening of skin, nonpitting edema, hoarseness of voice, nerve entrapment syndromes |

Table 56–7  Diagnostic Workup of Hypothyroidism

Step A. Diagnosis
  Tests: TSH, FT$_4$
  Patterns
    Overt primary hypothyroidism:     TSH high
                                      FT$_4$ low
    Mild primary hypothyroidism:      TSH high
                                      FT$_4$ normal
    Pituitary or hypothalamic hypothyroidism:  TSH normal or low
                                               FT$_4$ low
Step B. Differential diagnosis
  Tests
    Antithyroglobulin antibody
    Anti-TPO antibody
    Other tests depending on presentation

Anti-TPO = anti–thyroid peroxidase; FT$_4$ = free thyroxine; TSH = thyroid-stimulating hormone.

the course of the disease. The TSH has decreased bioactivity in this condition due to abnormal glycosylation of the molecule. Deficiencies of other pituitary hormones usually coexist.

The rare condition of thyroid hormone resistance syndrome presents with elevated serum FT$_4$ and T$_3$ and inappropriately normal or elevated serum TSH.

A number of other laboratory abnormalities are often encountered in hypothyroid patients. Hyponatremia is common and results from decreased renal blood flow and glomerular filtration and probably inappropriate antidiuretic hormone secretion. In central hypothyroidism, an additional factor is glucocorticoid deficiency. Hypoglycemia may occur particularly in myxedema coma or central hypothyroidism. Respiratory acidosis occurs characteristically in myxedema coma and results from diminished respiratory drive and mechanical factors relating to the chest wall and the airway. Primary hypothyroidism often presents with elevated serum enzymes such as aspartate aminotransferase and creatine kinase and hyperlipidemia. The enzyme elevations occur due to reduced clearance and do not necessarily indicate myocardial infarction. The lipid profile shows elevation of low-density-lipoprotein cholesterol due to reduced hepatic clearance. Finally, serum prolactin may be elevated in hypothyroidism, both primary and central.

## DIFFERENTIAL DIAGNOSIS

The common causes of hypothyroidism are listed in Table 56–8. Thyroidal causes account for most cases; whereas hormone resistance syndrome is quite rare. The most common cause is *autoimmune thyroiditis*, either the goitrous (Hashimoto's thyroiditis or atrophic (primary myxedema) form. Hypothyroidism results from destruction of the gland by the autoimmune process. A second common cause is partial or complete *ablation* of the thyroid by $^{131}$I, external radiation or surgery performed as a treatment for hyperthyroidism and thyroid carcinoma. *Iodine deficiency* is a common cause of hypothyroidism in many parts of the world. *Drugs* such as lithium, excess iodine (often in the form of iodinated drugs, e.g., amiodarone), or interferon-γ can inhibit thyroid function and cause hypothyroidism in a subset of exposed subjects. *Congenital hypothyroidism* results from thyroid dysgenesis or inheritable deficiencies of enzymes involved in the synthesis and secretion of thyroid hormone. *Transient hypothyroidism* can occur during the recovery phase of painless or subacute thyroiditis. Transient hypothyroidism can occur in the neonate due to transplacental passage of TSH receptor blocking antibody from the mother. *Central hypothyroidism* can result from pituitary or hypothalamic diseases (e.g., tumor, trauma, infarction, granuloma). Isolated TSH deficiency is rare but has been reported. *Thyroid hormone resistance* syndrome is often associated with mutation of the thyroid hormone receptor β-gene. Patients are often euthyroid. However, resistance varies among tissues so that features of hypo- and hyperthyroidism may coexist in the same patient. Usually, the brain, pituitary, and bone are more insensitive to thyroid hormone than the heart, liver, and basal metabolism.

A thorough clinical examination often provides important information regarding the underlying etiology. The history should bring out such etiologic factors as prior thyroid surgery, $^{131}$I treatment, external irradiation, or exposure to various thyroactive drugs. An enlarged firm gland is suggestive of Hashimoto's thyroiditis. Presence of an anterior neck scar is a valuable clue. Association with other autoimmune diseases (e.g., insulin-dependent diabetes, pernicious anemia, rheumatoid arthritis, systemic lupus erythematosus) supports the diagnosis of autoimmune thyroiditis. Coexistence of other pituitary hormone (e.g.,

Table 56–8  Common Causes of Hypothyroidism

Thyroid
  Autoimmune thyroiditis
    Hashimoto's thyroiditis
    Primary myxedema
  Thyroid ablation or damage
    Surgery, $^{131}$I, radiographs
  Drugs: iodine, lithium
  Iodine deficiency
  Congenital: Dysgenesis, defects in hormone biosynthesis
Central (pituitary, hypothalamus)
  Tumors, granuloma, infiltrative diseases, infarction, isolated TSH deficiency

$^{131}$I = radioactive iodine.

ACTH, gonadotropins) abnormalities is common in central hypothyroidism.

Several laboratory investigations are helpful in identifying the underlying etiology:

1. Antithyroid antibodies: These include antibodies directed against thyroglobulin and thyroid peroxidase (TPO) and, less commonly, blocking antibodies to the TSH receptor. Anti-TPO antibodies (formerly known as antimicrosomal antibodies) are most specific for the diagnosis of autoimmune thyroiditis and are present in about 70 to 80% of patients.
2. Fine-needle aspiration of the thyroid. This can reliably diagnose Hashimoto's thyroiditis. However, it is seldom necessary for clinical management.
3. Twenty-four-hour urinary iodine excretion, serum lithium concentration. These are obtained only in selected cases.
4. TRH test: This test is not necessary in the diagnosis of primary hypothyroidism. The elevated baseline TSH suffices. In central hypothyroidism, the test should, in theory, distinguish between pituitary (no response) and hypothalamic (delayed response) etiologies. However, this has not been observed consistently.
5. Tests for pituitary and hypothalamic diseases: These include baseline hormone assays, dynamic tests of function, and imaging studies (e.g., MRI).

## HYPOTHYROIDISM AND PREGNANCY

Maternal hypothyroidism is quite uncommon. This probably reflects the high prevalence of anovulatory cycles (>70%) in hypothyroid women. In addition, hypothyroid women have a high rate of fetal loss in the first trimester. As in nonpregnant women, hypothyroidism is commonly due to autoimmune thyroiditis and prior ablation of thyroid by surgery or [131]I treatment. Maternal hypothyroidism is generally due to a thyroidal cause because conception is unlikely in cases of central hypothyroidism. Demonstration of an elevated TSH is the most useful test. Mild cases may be missed by measurement of $FT_4$ alone.

Untreated hypothyroid mothers have increased maternal and fetal complications. Maternal complications include anemia, pregnancy-induced hypertension, placental abruption, and postpartum hemorrhage. Fetal complications include low birth weight, congenital anomalies, increased perinatal mortality, and impaired physical and mental development. Treatment, particularly when monitored by TSH measurements, results in far fewer complications. It has been reported that mental development was normal in newborns whose mothers were hypothyroid in the initial 5 to 10 weeks of gestation but treated to euthyroidism soon after.

Fetal hypothyroidism is usually due to thyroid disease (agenesis, enzyme deficiency) or transplacental passage of TSH receptor blocking antibody or antithyroid drugs (iodine, thiourea drugs). Fetal bradycardia and goiter, demonstrated by ultrasonography, suggest the diagnosis. However, hypothyroidism due to the transfer of maternal antibodies is not associated with fetal goiter. The possibility of such antibodies should be kept in mind in any pregnant woman with current or prior autoimmune thyroid disease, including Graves' disease. The diagnosis of fetal hypothyroidism is made by measuring TSH and $FT_4$ in the cord blood obtained by cordocentesis. Perinatal hypothyroidism due to autoimmunity or drugs are transient and resolves in a few weeks.

Transient hypothyroxinemia without TSH elevation is frequent in premature infants. The underlying pathophysiology is not clear, although hypothalamic immaturity has been suspected. The $FT_4$ levels decrease initially after birth, unlike in full-term infants. The levels increase later after a delayed TSH surge at 1 week of age. Recent studies have shown that the hypothyroxinemia is associated with an increased risk of cerebral palsy and reduced mental development at 2 years of age. Whether these complications are causally related to the hypothyroxinemia remains to be determined.

Although the placenta constitutes a barrier to maternal-fetal flux of thyroid hormone, significant quantities of the hormone are transferred to the fetus. Maternal transfer provides the only source of thyroid hormone until the fetal thyroid starts functioning at 10 weeks of gestation and continues to be a significant source thereafter. In cases of fetal hypothyroidism, further protection is afforded by adjustment of the iodotyrosine deiodinase isoenzyme activities. In the hypothyroid fetus, type II deiodinase activity, which converts $T_4$ to $T_3$ in the brain and pituitary, is increased, whereas the activities of type I and III deiodinases, which degrade $T_3$, are decreased. These changes favor maintenance of $T_3$ levels in the fetal brain.

Recent observations have shown that weight and development at birth are usually normal in hypothyroid infants, even those with thyroid agenesis. Intrauterine hypothyroidism is usually manifested by increased TSH, low or low normal $FT_4$, and often a delay in bone maturation. These data suggest that either the metabolism and development of the fetus do not depend on thyroid hormone or that the small amounts of maternal thyroid hormone transported across the placenta are sufficient to prevent most hypothyroid manifestations. Postnatal development, however, strongly depends on maintenance of an euthyroid state. Early intensive postnatal treatment of infants with intrauterine hypothyroidism usually normalizes childhood intelligence quotients. However, irreversible mental retardation has been reported in a few infants born with very high TSH, very low $T_4$, and delayed bone maturation.

## TREATMENT

Hypothyroidism is treated by replacement therapy with Levo-$T_4$. $T_4$ is converted to $T_3$ in vivo and generates a steady plasma level of $T_3$. The long half-life of $T_4$ (7 days) makes it possible to use a single daily dose. Preparations containing $T_3$ are not recommended because $T_3$ has a short half-life (approximately 1 day), requiring multiple daily dosing and leading in turn to "peaks and troughs" in serum concentration. Mean absorption of $T_4$ from tablets is 70 to 80% and is greater in empty stomach. Malabsorption of $T_4$ is rare except in patients with short bowel syndrome. Drugs such as cholesterol-binding resins, aluminum hydroxide, sucralfate, and ferrous sulfate can interfere with the absorption of $T_4$ as can soybean formula feeding in infants.

The aim of replacement therapy is to restore serum TSH values to normal in primary hypothyroidism. Most patients require 1.7 μg/kg/d $T_4$, about 100 to 200 μg. The requirement is somewhat less (by 10%) in the elderly. Doses increase by 25 to 50% during pregnancy due to a number of causes (e.g., increase in serum TBG concentrations, placental degradation of $T_4$, transfer of $T_4$ to the fetus, and increased maternal clearance of $T_4$). Drugs such as rifampin and phenytoin increase metabolic clearance of $T_4$ and increase the daily $T_4$ requirement.

The initial dose depends on the duration and severity of hypothyroidism and patient characteristics (e.g., age, cardiac status etc.). In hypothyroidism of rapid onset (e.g., after surgery or radioiodine treatment of Graves' disease), substitution therapy can be started with full dosage. In hypothyroidism of long duration, therapy is begun with 50 to 75 μg Levo-$T_4$ and gradually increased by 12.5- to 25-μg increments until TSH is normalized. Because pituitary response to $FT_4$ changes is slow, TSH measurements are performed 6 or more weeks alter a dosage change. In elderly subjects and patients with cardiovascular disease, it may be necessary to begin with a very low dose (12.5 to 25 μg/d). The dose should be increased by 12.5 μg/d every 2 to 3 weeks provided the cardiac status remains stable. It may not be possible to achieve full replacement is some patients with heart disease until coronary revascularization is carried out.

*Neonatal hypothyroidism* requires initiation of therapy as soon as possible. Initial dose of $T_4$ is 10 to 15 μg/kg/d. The dosage is adjusted to keep $FT_4$ levels in the upper half of normal range. *Fetal hypothyroidism* is treated by intra-amniotic Levo-$T_4$ injection 250 to 500 μg/wk for 2 to 4 weeks.

*Myxedema coma* is a medical emergency and requires management in an intensive care unit. Therapy should begin with an IV bolus of 250 to 500 μg/L-$T_4$, followed 24 to 48 hours later by 100 μg L-$T_4$ IV daily. It is customary to include cortisol, 100 to 300 mg daily, in the treatment regimen initially. Other measures include passive rewarming, treatment of hypoglycemia, respiratory and cardiac support, and treatment of precipitating events.

In *central hypothyroidism* complicated with adrenal insufficiency, glucocorticoid replacement should precede Levo-$T_4$ replacement to avoid precipitating adrenal crisis. The adequacy of Levo-$T_4$ replacement is determined by the clinical response and plasma $FT_4$ levels because TSH cannot be used for this purpose.

Treatment of *subclinical hypothyroidism* is controversial. Some physicians advocate Levo-$T_4$ replacement in view of studies showing improvement in psychometric testing score or systolic ejection time. The role of subclinical hypothyroidism as a cardiovascular risk factor is not known. Other physicians prefer a conservative approach delaying treatment until hypothyroidism becomes clinically manifest. Progression to clinical hypothyroidism does not occur in many patients but is more likely if there is coexistent autoimmune thyroiditis.

# Goiter and Thyroid Nodule

Goiter is an enlargement of the thyroid gland. It can be diffuse or nodular. Thyroid nodules are palpable in 4 to 7% of the adults. Smaller nonpalpable nodules occur, however, with much higher frequency. Indeed, the prevalence of thyroid nodules based on autopsy or ultrasonographic data is approximately 50% in the adult population. Nodules are more common in women. The incidence of nodules increases with the duration of goiter, advancing age, exposure to ionizing radiation, and dietary iodine deficiency.

## HISTORY AND PHYSICAL EXAMINATION

The thyroid gland is palpated by slightly flexing the neck and palpating in the area between the trachea and the sternomastoid muscle. The gland is also palpated as the patient swallows. Nodules are easy to feel when they are superficial and are more than 1.0 to 1.5 cm in diameter. Palpation is difficult when the nodules are located deep or posteriorly in the gland and in patients having a short thick neck.

Most goiters are asymptomatic though often visibly

apparent. They are usually detected by the physician during an unrelated examination. Goiters may enlarge asymmetrically and deviate the trachea to one side. Others may grow into the retrosternal space (i.e., in the superior mediastinum). Pressure on the adjacent structures may cause dysphagia, stridor, a sensation of choking, and cough. Venous congestion in the head and neck area may occur from compression of the superior vena cava. Hoarseness of voice can result from infiltration of the recurrent laryngeal nerves by thyroid carcinoma.

Painless firm enlargement of the regional lymph nodes, sometimes fixed to the adjacent tissues, may be associated with thyroid malignancy. The patient should be questioned about any prior irradiation of the head or neck area. Such treatment results in an increase in the incidence of both benign and malignant thyroid nodules 20 to 30 years later. Approximately 50% of these nodules could be malignant. Radiation-induced cancers are often multicentric. A positive family history of thyroid carcinoma may be present in medullary carcinoma of the thyroid.

## DIAGNOSIS

The following investigations are useful in the diagnosis and management of goiter:

1. Thyroid function tests: Serum TSH and $FT_4$ or $FT_4I$ should be obtained in every patient. Patients with hypo- or hyperthyroidism should be managed as indicated earlier. Most patients with diffuse or nodular goiter are euthyroid. However, hyperthyroidism may develop later in the course of nodular goiter.
2. Serum calcitonin is a marker of medullary carcinoma of the thyroid. It should be obtained in patients with a family history of thyroid carcinoma or if the fine-needle aspiration cytology (see below) is suggestive of tumor.
3. Radioisotope scanning of the thyroid is useful in assessing the function (i.e., the ability to concentrate isotope) of a palpable nodule. A hyperfunctioning nodule is unlikely to be malignant and generally does not require aspiration biopsy. Malignant nodules appear hypofunctioning as do a large number of benign nodules. The procedure is therefore of high sensitivity but poor specificity for the diagnosis of malignancy.
4. Ultrasonography is useful in determining the size and in monitoring the growth of a palpable nodule. Ultrasonography often reveals the coexistence of other smaller nonpalpable nodules. Malignant nodules often have distinct imaging characteristics (e.g., hypoechoic pattern, incomplete peripheral halo, an irregular margin, or internal microcalcifications). However, these findings lack specificity.
5. Fine-needle aspiration cytology (FNAC) is the most valuable tool in the assessment of a thyroid nodule. In experienced hands, false-negative results are less than 5% and false-positive results are less than 1% for malignancy. About 10% aspirates are nondiagnostic, which is usually insufficient. The cytology is reported as benign, malignant, follicular neoplasm, or insufficient. The report of follicular neoplasm presents a special situation. Low-grade follicular carcinoma and Hurthle cell carcinomas are usually not distinguishable from the corresponding benign adenomas on the basis of aspiration cytology. About 20% of those reported as follicular neoplasm prove to be malignant. If the aspirate is insufficient, a repeat, often ultrasonography guided, aspiration should be performed. Ultrasonography guided aspiration is particularly useful in obtaining cells from the solid component of a partly cystic lesion.
6. Computed tomography and MRI are useful in demonstrating retrosternal extension of a goiter or pressure on adjacent structures by a goiter.
7. Genetic testing for RET proto-oncogene mutation is useful in familial medullary carcinoma.

## DIFFERENTIAL DIAGNOSIS

### Diffuse Goiter

The common causes of diffuse euthyroid goiter are shown in Table 56–9. Diffuse goiter is a clinical diagnosis. Ultrasonography often reveals the presence of small nonpalpable nodules in these goiters.

The most common cause is sporadic nontoxic goiter. The pathophysiology of the goiter is not clear. Involvement of TSH has been postulated and, indeed, is the basis of therapy with Levo-$T_4$. The patients are generally euthyroid. Another common cause is Hashimoto's thyroiditis. Unlike sporadic nontoxic goiter, hypothyroidism can occur in this disease with elevation of serum TSH in about a third of the patients. Autoantibodies to thyroid peroxidase and thyroglobulin are present in 70 to 80% of patients.

**Table 56–9** Common Causes of Diffuse Euthyroid Goiter

---
Sporadic nontoxic goiter
Hashimoto's thyroiditis
Drugs: iodine, lithium
Hereditary biosynthetic defects
Iodine deficiency
---

Other tests (e.g., FNAC) or tests demonstrating defects in iodine metabolism (e.g., perchlorate discharge test) support the diagnosis of Hashimoto's thyroiditis but are not usually necessary. Iodine deficiency is a common cause worldwide but is practically unknown in the United States. Dyshormonogenesis represents a number of congenital defects of iodine metabolism and is quite rare.

## Nodular Goiter

Nodules develop increasingly with time in diffuse sporadic nontoxic goiters. The resulting nodular goiter also becomes larger with time. It may press on surrounding structures (e.g., esophagus, trachea) and also extend retrosternally. Some nodules develop TSH-independent (autonomous) function and cause clinical or subclinical hyperthyroidism. Exposure to excess iodine, usually as iodinated drugs (e.g., amiodarone), may precipitate hyperthyroidism in some patients with nodular goiter. Bleeding into a nodule can cause acute pain. There is no evidence that the rate of malignancy is increased in nodules arising in sporadic nontoxic goiter.

A major concern in the management of a nodular goiter is the possibility that a given nodule may turn out to be malignant. Solitary nodules are worked up for malignancy, as described below. In case of a multinodular goiter, attention is directed to the dominant nodule or any unusual nodule (e.g., hard, rapidly growing, etc).

The common causes underlying thyroid nodules are shown is Table 56–10. About 5% of palpable nodules prove to be malignant. Although the autopsy data show a much higher rate of thyroid malignancy (4% of the adult population), most are nonpalpable (<1 cm diameter) and do not grow to clinical significance. The risk of malignancy in a palpable nodule is increased if the nodule is very firm, rapidly growing, fixed to the adjacent structure, and accompanied by enlargement of regional lymph nodes and vocal cord paralysis. Other risk factors include a family history of thyroid carcinoma (for medullary carcinoma), history of irradiation in the head and neck area, male sex, and age less than 20 or more than 60 years.

The workup of a thyroid nodule usually begins with FNAC, although some prefer to obtain an isotope scan first and exclude the functioning nodules from FNAC. If the cytology is reported as malignant, surgical treatment is advised. If the cytology is reported as follicular neoplasm, a radioiodine scan should be obtained. "Hot" nodules are unlikely to be malignant. Surgical treatment is advised for the others. Benign nodules require follow-up for several years to guard against false-negative results. An isotope scan may be obtained at this time to exclude functioning nodules. The nodules are examined every 6 to 12 months. Any abnormal physical or growth characteristics usually require a repeat FNAC. Some physicians routinely include a repeat FNAC in the workup. The use of Levo-T$_4$ in the follow-up is discussed later.

Small thyroid nodules (<1.5 cm diameter) do not require FNAC in the absence of a family history of thyroid carcinoma or a history of irradiation to the head and neck region. They should, however, be monitored for growth. The protocol for the diagnostic workup of a thyroid nodule is shown in Table 56–11.

**Table 56–10** Common Causes of Thyroid Nodule

Thyroid carcinoma: Papillary, follicular, medullary, anaplastic
Thyroid adenoma
Nodular goiter
Thyroiditis: subacute, chronic
Cysts
Granulomas
Metastatic tumors
Developmental abnormalities (e.g., dermoid teratoma)

**Table 56–11** Suggested Workup of a Thyroid Nodule

Laboratory tests
  TSH, FT$_4$, thyroid autoantibodies,
  Calcitonin (in selected cases)
FNAC
  Suspicious for malignancy: Advise surgery
  Follicular neoplasm: Obtain radioiodine scan. Advise surgery for hypofunctioning nodules.
  Insufficient material: repeat FNAC.
  Benign: Follow-up with or without Levo-T$_4$ suppression. Radioiodine scan or repeat FNAC may be useful.

FNAC = fine needle aspiration cytology; FT$_4$ = free thyroxine; Levo-T$_4$ = L-thyroxine; TSH = thyroid-stimulating hormone.

## TREATMENT

### Diffuse Goiter

Patients with diffuse goiter are generally treated with Levo-T$_4$ for reduction of goiter size and prevention of further enlargement. The dose of Levo-T$_4$ is adjusted to the maximal amount tolerated without precipitation of overt hyperthyroidism. This is generally accomplished by keeping seum TSH levels to subnormal but detectable levels. This treatment appears to be efficacious in most patients. The goiter usually regrows upon cessation of treatment.

## Nodular Goiter

1. Euthyroid patients can be treated with Levo-$T_4$, as outlined above for diffuse goiter for similar therapeutic aims. Most patients respond favorably to this treatment. Patients with subnormal pretreatment TSH levels should be excluded from Levo-$T_4$ suppressive therapy. These patients have subclinical or clinical hyperthyroidism from autonomously functioning nodules. Levo-$T_4$ suppressive therapy for solitary thyroid nodules is more controversial. Several short-term studies have failed to demonstrate any reduction of nodule size after such therapy. However, prevention of nodule growth or any favorable effect on the usually coexistent nonpalpable nodules would be a desirable outcome. Longer term studies are needed to examine these issues.
2. Hyperthyroidism associated with nodular goiter is treated as described earlier.
3. Treatment of pressure effects: Pressure on the trachea and esophagus can be documented by ultrasonography, computed tomography, or pulmonary function tests. Retrosternal goiters are readily demonstrated by computed tomography and less satisfactorily by radioiodine scanning. Treatment requires surgical excision of the goiter. Ablation with $^{131}I$ is an option if surgery is contraindicated.
4. Bleeding into a nodule can cause acute pain. Needle aspiration may be useful in alleviating the pain.

## Thyroid Carcinoma

### Differentiated Carcinoma

These are of the papillary and follicular types and constitute most (85 to 90%) thyroid cancers. They grow slowly and generally have an excellent 20- or 30-year prognosis. They retain some capacity to concentrate iodine. This forms the basis of treatment with $^{131}I$ iodine. Unfavorable prognostic features include the presence of distant metastasis, local invasion, primary tumor size greater than 4 cm, and older age.

In most cases, differentiated thyroid cancers are treated with near total or total thyroidectomy followed 6 weeks later by $^{131}I$ ablation of residual thyroid tissue. The patients are then tested at 6-month intervals for recurrence or metastases by total body scanning with $^{131}I$ and serum thyroglobulin. Serum thyroglobulin should be very low or undetectable in cancer-free patients. Metastases and recurrences are treated with $^{131}I$. All patients require $T_4$ replacement except before the metastatic workup outlined above. Because TSH may stimulate the growth of cancer cells, serum TSH is kept below normal in most cases and even to undetectable levels in more aggressive tumors. Overt iatrogenic hyperthyroidism should, however, be avoided.

### Medullary Carcinoma

These tumors do not concentrate $^{131}I$. They should be treated by complete thyroidectomy.

### Anaplastic Carcinoma

These tumors are very aggressive and respond poorly to treatment. They do not concentrate $^{131}I$. Palliative surgery is often all that can be offered.

## REFERENCES

Berghout A, Wiersinga WM, Smits N, et al: Interrelationships between age, thyroid volume, thyroid nodularity, and thyroid function in patients with sporadic nontoxic goiter. Am J Med 89:602–608, 1990.

Cooper DS: Antithyroid drugs. N Engl J Med 311:1353–1362, 1984.

Franklyn JA: The management of hyperthyroidism. N Engl J Med 330:1731–1738, 1994.

Gharib H, Goellner JR: Fine-needle aspiration biopsy of the thyroid. Ann Intern Med 118:282–289, 1993.

Klein I. Thyroid hormone and the cardiovascular system: Am J Med 88:631–637, 1990.

Klein I, Trzepacz P, Roberts M, et al: Symptom rating scale for assessing hyperthyroidism. Arch Intern Med 148:387–390, 1988.

Lazarus JH: Investigation and treatment of hypothyroidism. Clin Endocrinol 44:129–131, 1996.

Mandell SJ, Brent GA, Larsen PR: Levothyroxine therapy in patients with thyroid disease. Ann Intern Med 119:492–502, 1993.

Rojeski MT, Gharib H: Nodular thyroid disease evaluation and management. N Engl J Med 313:428–436, 1985.

Ross DS: Thyroid hormone suppressive therapy of sporadic nontoxic goiter. Thyroid 2:263–269, 1992.

Roti E, Emerson CJ: Postpartum thyroiditis. J Clin Endocrinol Metab 74:3–5, 1992.

Roti E, Minelli R, Salvi M: Management of hyperthyroidism and hypothyroidism in the pregnant woman. J Clin Endocrinol Metab 81:1679–1682, 1996.

Sawin CT: Thyroid dysfunction in older persons. Adv Intern Med 37:223–248, 1991.

Singer PA, Cooper DS, Daniels GH, et al: Treatment guidelines for patients with thyroid nodules and well-differentiated thyroid cancer. Arch Med Intern 156:2165–2172, 1996.

Singer PA, Cooper DS, Levy EG, et al: Treatment guidelines for patients with hyperthyroidism and hypothyroidism. JAMA 273:808–812, 1995.

Surks MI, Chopra U, Mariash CN, et al: American Thyroid Association guidelines for use of laboratory tests in thyroid disorders. JAMA 263:1529–1532, 1990.

Tan GH, Gharib H: Thyroid incidentalomas: Management approaches to nonpalpable nodules discovered incidentally on thyroid imaging. Ann Intern Med 126:226–231, 1997.

Utiger RD: Follow-up of patients with thyroid carcinona [editorial]. N Engl J Med 337:928–930, 1997.

Weetman AP, McGregor AM: Autoimmune thyroid disease: Further developments in our understanding. Endocrinol Rev 15:788–830, 1994.

# 57

# Menopause

SUSAN L. HENDRIX

Menopause is a momentous time in a woman's life. The significant reduction in estrogen after menopause contributes to a variety of symptoms that can be annoying and displeasing. However, adverse long-term health effects accompany menopause, and women should be treated for both symptoms and prevention of diseases common to women.

The U.S. Bureau of the Census has estimated that by 1990 there were 36 million women in the United States older than 50 years of age. Because the median age of menopause in the United States is 50 years and the life expectancy for women is 83 years, nearly 15% of the population will live a third of their lives in an estrogen-deficient state. This population will increase, both in the United States and worldwide; thus, addressing healthier living after ovarian involution is a priority.

Emerging concepts that are helping us shape a new paradigm to understand the menopausal transition include:

1. A model that uses a gradual transition from pre- to peri- to postmenopause, including both transient and persistent signs and symptoms.
2. A hormone-based definition of menopause replacing a bleeding-based definition.
3. More sensitive and reliable assays to measure sex steroids and inhibin.

## Definitions

Although by definition, *menopause* is cessation of menstruation, this event is only one point in the continuum of declining ovarian function. It signals the time of change and loss of reproductive function in a woman's life. The process of transition has been termed the *climacteric* or *perimenopause*; however, it may more appropriately be termed *transmenopause* (Fig. 57–1). Prominent during the climacteric are the symptoms of menopause. Premature menopause, more appropriately termed *premature ovarian failure*, is the cessation of menses before 40 years of age.

The age of menopause is determined genetically and is not related to the number of prior ovulations (e.g., pregnancy, lactation, use of hormonal contra-

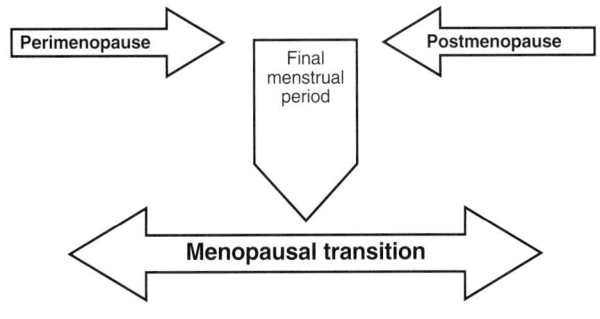

**Figure 57–1** The transmenopausal cycle.

ceptives, or anovulatory cycles). Studies also suggest that the age of menopause is unrelated to race, socioeconomic status, level of education, height, weight, age of menarche, or age at last pregnancy. However, menopause occurs earlier in women who are cigarette smokers, in women who live at high altitudes, and in women with poor nutritional status.

Because menopause is part of the normal aging process, the diagnosis and treatment approach is one of balancing the patient's risk of disease with the benefits and risks of therapy.

## History and Consideration of Health Risks

Irregular menses and intermittent symptoms of hot flushes, night sweats, and mood swings begin sometime after 40 years of age. When a patient reports the following signs and symptoms and she is older than 40 years of age, she is most likely experiencing symptoms of estrogen fluctuation and possibly estrogen deficiency. Until a patient is estrogen deficient, the approach to treatment should be directed at relieving her discomfort.

### VASOMOTOR, MOOD, AND CHANGES

- Hot flushes and night sweats
- Increased perspiration
- Sleep disturbance
- Anxiety and a feeling of tension
- Depression and irritability
- Skin changes

### REPRODUCTIVE TRACT

- Vaginal dryness
- Dyspareunia
- Urinary frequency and recurrent urinary tract infection
- Loss of libido and sexual dysfunction

### HEALTH RISKS

- Bone loss progressing to osteopenia and osteoporosis
- Cardiovascular disease

### CHANGES IN MENSTRUAL BLEEDING PATTERNS

In the earliest phase of the menopausal transition, disturbances in menstrual patterns are characteristic.

Cycle lengths may be normal or slightly shortened. Subsequently, reports of increasing length between periods with infrequent very short cycles are common. Finally, menses completely stop. This is the usual change in bleeding pattern as the transmenopause progresses. However, many women experience more frequent, heavier, or prolonged bleeding before the onset of oligomenorrhea. This is secondary to the decrease in length of the follicular phase or an anovulatory cycle.

The diagnosis of the last menstrual period is made retrospectively and requires 6 to 12 months of amenorrhea to confirm. Once elevated gonadotropin levels confirm the menopause, subsequent bleeding must be monitored for endometrial pathology.

### HOT FLUSHES AND NIGHT SWEATS

A hot flush is described commonly as a sudden perception of intense upper body warmth, which usually begins in the chest region and rises to the neck and face. Intense sweating in the upper body often follows the flushes. They can be accompanied by lightheadedness and a rapid heart beat. Hot flushes often are preceded by prodromal symptoms sometimes described as increasing head pressure. They are particularly disturbing at night, causing night sweats, insomnia, and fatigue the next day. The range of hot flushes frequency varies from every 20 minutes to once or twice per month. The duration can be as short as seconds or as long as an hour. Furthermore, more than 80% of menopausal women continue to experience hot flushes after 1 year, and 25% still experience them after 5 years.

The mechanisms responsible for the hot flush are not well understood. Therefore, identifying ways to treat them is difficult. Although skin temperature rises with the flush, the core body temperature actually falls. The vasomotor hot flush is experienced by nearly 75% of menopausal women with varying frequency, duration, and intensity.

### MOOD CHANGES AND MEMORY

The relationship between anxiety, irritability, nervousness, headaches, fatigue, joint and muscle pain, dizziness, and depression and estrogen deficiency is unknown. Certain symptoms may be the result of hot flushes at night (night sweats), causing sleep disorders and subsequent mood alteration. This may explain why some of these symptoms may improve with estrogen therapy. There have been reports of improvement of memory with hormone replacement therapy, but these small studies need confirmation before the association between estrogen loss and diminished cognitive function can be made.

Early reports from observational studies suggest that Alzheimer's disease and dementia occur less frequently in women receiving hormone replacement therapy. Additionally, women with Alzheimer's disease who were given estrogen showed improved cognitive performance. Unfortunately, these studies were too small to prove the beneficial effect of estrogen on cognitive function.

## SKIN CHANGES

There is substantial evidence that estrogen influences the epidermis and dermis. Collagen synthesis and maturation are estrogen sensitive. Estrogen may preserve collagen content and thickness. This may result in few skin wrinkles and dry skin.

## VAGINAL ATROPHY

Both estrogens and progestins influence normal vaginal moisture. Estrogens increase blood flow to the vagina, increasing the normal vaginal transudate and sensation of vaginal moisture. The absence of estrogen causes thinning of the vaginal mucosa, decreased rugae and vascularity, shortening of the vaginal canal, and changes in the normal bacterial flora. On examination, a pale, sometimes friable epithelium is present. Typically, the vaginal pH increases to greater than 4.5, whereas premenopausally it is less than 3.4. Altered vaginal pH allows recolonization of the vagina with enteric bacteria and may result in pruritus and discharge. Inflammation of the vaginal mucosa secondary to progressive estrogen loss, known as *atrophic vaginitis*, can cause the mucosa to have a "strawberry" appearance.

Atrophic changes are responsible for the common reports of dysuria (secondary to a thinned urethral mucosa), urinary frequency and urgency (caused by atrophic trigonitis), vaginal dryness, and dyspareunia. Urinary frequency can occur both during the day and at night. It commonly is accompanied by urinary urgency. Stress urinary incontinence (worsened by diminished sphincter tone) and urge incontinence due to atrophic trigonitis, which are common in this age group, can be worsened by estrogen deficiency.

## LOSS OF LIBIDO AND SEXUAL DYSFUNCTION

There are many determinants of libido and sexuality in women. Endocrine, environmental, sociocultural belief, and emotional factors all impact a woman's sexual function. The links between hormone status and sexual function are not well understood; however, clinical practice supports their relationship.

Simultaneous with the decline of estrogens in the menopause, there is a 50 to 75% decrease in the production of all four androgens: dehydroepiandrosterone sulfate (DHEAS), dehydroepiandrostenedione (DHEA), androstenedione, and testosterone. The decline in DHEAS and DHEA by the adrenal gland begins between the ages of 30 and 40 years and continues gradually throughout life. This is thought to be an age-related phenomenon and not related to the hormonal decline associated with the menopause. However, the reduction in androstenedione and testosterone do appear to be more closely related to the menopause. Androstenedione production is decreased in both the ovary and the adrenal gland. With the reduction in androstenedione, testosterone synthesis is limited.

Sexual interest is decreased, and there is a diminution of orgasmic and coital frequency. Diminished sexual sensation and dyspareunia compound the dysfunction. Determining which component of sexual desire is malfunctioning is important. The three primary components are drive (neurophysiologic), cognition (reflects expectations, beliefs, and values about sexuality), and motivation (willingness to engage in sexual activity). Often the cause for sexual dysfunction is multifactorial, and therapy involves counseling, education, and medication.

## CARDIOVASCULAR DISEASE

The most common cardiovascular complaint in the menopausal transition is heart palpitations. Their cause is unknown, but they often are benign and improve with estrogen replacement. The first symptom of coronary heart disease may be chest pain, or "angina." The chest pain, which is caused by reduced blood flow in the coronary arteries, typically occurs behind the sternum and may travel the left arm or up the neck, or be a squeezing, pressing sensation that does not change with breathing. It usually is caused and made worse by exercise and is eased by rest. The pain usually lasts 2 to 5 minutes. Reduced blood flow to the heart can cause symptoms other than chest pain. For example, some women experience atypical angina. The chest pain may linger, occur in a different location than behind the sternum, or not be worsened by exertion and eased by rest. Some women have shortness of breath or indigestion. Women who report chest symptoms should be evaluated thoroughly.

Among women older than 50 years, heart disease and stroke are responsible for more than 50% of deaths each year. Coronary heart disease in women occurs 10 to 12 years later in life than men. Because their rates approach those of men in the older ages and there are more older women than men, approximately half of all coronary deaths occur in women. Almost all these deaths occur in postmenopausal women.

There is concern that more serious consequences may develop in women after a coronary heart disease event than in men. Women also appear to have a higher incidence of certain types of cardiovascular disease, such as angina pectoris.

Observational studies have suggested that women using estrogen replacement have a 50% decrease in heart disease risk. Because the evidence is based largely on results from observational studies, they are always subject to bias. Although the addition of progestins previously was thought to attenuate the positive effects of estrogen, recent studies have confirmed a cardioprotective effect in combined regimens as well.

Multiple mechanisms have been suggested as responsible for estrogen-medicated prevention of cardiovascular disease. These include physiologic effects on lipid metabolism, blood pressure, coagulation factors, endothelial cells, and carbohydrate metabolism. The development of atherosclerosis is probably one of the main mechanisms for subsequent cardiovascular events and is related to increases in low-density lipoprotein cholesterol (LDL-C) and decreases in high-density lipoprotein cholesterol (HDL-C). Increases in total cholesterol and LDL-C and less dramatic decreases in HDL-C have been documented in postmenopausal women. The administration of conjugated estrogen, 0.625 mg daily, has been shown to decrease LDL-C as much as 10 to 15%. This translates to a 14% decrease in cardiovascular risk.

HDL-C is the best risk predictor of coronary heart disease risk in women and appears to be protective against coronary heart disease. Estrogen increases HDL-C 10 to 14%. It has been suggested that the first-pass hepatic effect may cause oral estrogen preparations to be more potent in causing the lipoprotein changes than are nonoral preparations.

Multiple studies have suggested that the addition of a progestin to estrogen replacement therapy (ERT) attenuates the beneficial effects of estrogen on lipoprotein profile, causing a decrease in HDL-C. Other studies have shown that women treated with combined estrogen and progestin have equivalent or improved levels of HDL-C. The Postmenopausal Estrogen/Progestin Intervention (PEPI) Trial provides the best evidence to date and confirms previous studies that found estrogen alone showed the greatest increase in HDL-C compared with placebo. Conjugated equine estrogens and micronized progesterone had slightly lower but similar degrees of increase in HDL-C as estrogen alone. Conjugated equine estrogens with cyclic or continuous medroxyprogesterone acetate showed an increase in HDL-C, but it was significantly lower than in either of the aforementioned groups.

Another mechanism of improved cardiovascular risk for the postmenopausal woman receiving estrogen is the evidence suggesting that natural estrogens may significantly decrease blood pressure. This contrasts the evidence in oral contraceptive users where an increase in blood pressure can be seen in a small number of women. Three of six studies on the effect of natural estrogens on blood pressure show improvement with the addition of estrogen, and three show no change in blood pressure. Other mechanisms for estrogen's presumed cardioprotective effects include favorable effects on both glucose and insulin levels and the positive effects on blood vessel wall tone and reactivity.

There is concern that estrogen use may increase a woman's risk for thromboembotic disorders. This concern initially was based on the experience of women receiving oral contraceptive therapy. Three large observational epidemiologic studies and a large clinical trial have confirmed that current postmenopausal estrogen users had a two- to three-fold increased risk of thromboembolism or thrombophlebitis. This translates into a relatively small absolute risk. The current risk for women older than 50 years for venous thromboembolism (VTE) is 10 in 100,000, which increases to 30 in 100,000 with estrogen or hormone replacement therapy. This risk is not present for past users.

The mechanism for this increase in blood rush is controversial. Aylwood and colleagues showed that natural estrogens do not increase clotting factors, as opposed to ethinyl estradiol. The PEPI study found no change in fibrinogen levels in women in the active treatment group, suggesting no increase in risk from thrombotic abnormalities.

Women at risk for coronary heart disease because of hypertension, hypercholesterolemia, obesity, or family history should be considered potential candidates for hormone replacement therapy. Smoking cessation and other lifestyle changes, such as the reduction of dietary fat intake and regular aerobic exercise, should be recommended for all women, regardless of risk status.

## OSTEOPENIA AND OSTEOPOROSIS

Osteopenia is low bone mass, and osteoporosis is a reduction in bone mass per unit volume of bone tissue and is characterized by microarchitectural deterioration of bone. This leads to increased bone fragility and fracture risk. The two most significant determinants for their development are the peak bone mass (achieved by middle to late adolescence) and the rate of bone loss after menopause.

Bone remodeling predominates after linear growth ends and helps to keep bone dynamic and elastic. After peak bone mass is achieved, remodeling ensures that the amount of bone resorbed by osteoclasts is equal to the amount formed by osteoblasts. During this time, bone mineral density (BMD) remains relatively constant. Bone remodeling is affected by various factors, including parathyroid hormone; growth hormone; 1,25 dihydroxyvitamin D; and estrogen deficiency.

Pathologic processes may include either increased resorption or decreased formation. The decline in bone mass begins sometime after 35 years of age and accelerates with estrogen deficiency. After 40 years of age, bone resorption exceeds formation by 0.5 to 5% for trabecular bone and 1.5% of cortical bone each year after menopause. The greatest loss in bone mass occurs in the first 2 to 3 years postmenopause, so early assessment and initiation of therapy are important. A combination of low BMD and a single traumatic event can result in an osteoporotic fracture of the hip, spine, or wrist. Untreated bone loss also may result in the osteoporotic syndrome of pain and disability.

Back or hip pain in a menopausal woman should alert the clinician to possible osteopenia or osteoporosis. Loss of height can be documented with regular office visits. Spontaneous vertebral fractures can result from everyday activities such as lifting, walking, or rising from a reclining position. Pain can be acute or chronic and can present as a sharp or a dull ache.

There may be other causes for bone loss during menopause. Endocrine disorders such as hyperthyroidism, primary hyperparathyroidism, hypercortisolism, and gastrointestinal disorders such as biliary cirrhosis and malabsorption syndromes may result in bone loss. Screening should be performed when bone loss is suspected to assess osteoporosis risk.

Osteoporosis remains a significant cause of morbidity and mortality in menopausal women. More than one million fractures are reported each year in menopausal women, and nearly 15% of women with hip fractures die within 3 months. Factors contributing to development of osteoporosis (Table 57–1) include age, calcium metabolism, and estrogen. Fracture risk is difficult to assess and depends on bone mass and rate of bone loss at the time of menopause. Women who decline therapy for prevention of osteoporosis in menopause can expect to shrink approximately 2.5 inches over their lifetime. Calcium supplementation alone does not completely prevent loss of bone mineral content.

BMD is the most accurate measure of bone mass and the strongest predictor of osteoporotic fracture. The two most common methods for measurement of BMD are dual energy x-ray absorptiometry (DXA) and quantitative computed tomography (QCT). DXA has a better precision than QCT and shorter scanning time and lower radiation dose. Measurement of BMD generally should be performed only when the result will affect patient management, that is, to confirm or exclude the presence of osteoporosis or allow decisions about treatment.

Using DXA, BMD usually is measured at two or three sites, namely, the lumbar spine, hip, and forearm, whereas by QCT, BMD usually is measured only in the spine. BMD measured by DXA is not a true density but rather an apparent density (g/cm²) corrected for bone length and width. The risk of fracture primarily relates to how a subject's value compares with a young, healthy population, and consequently, BMD usually is expressed as a "T score," or the number of standard deviations (SDs) from the mean of young normal values. Thus, a T score of −2 is a value 2 SDs below the young normal mean. The T score cutoff points for diagnostic categories as proposed by the World Health Organization are shown in Table 57–2.

Using these cutoffs, the term *severe osteoporosis* is used when a patient has a low BMD and already has sustained an atraumatic fracture. This latter category

**Table 57–1** Common Risk Factors for Osteoporosis

Genetic
Family history of osteoporosis
White, Asian race
Hypogonadism
Early menopause
Drugs
Corticosteroids
Anticonvulsants
Nutritional
Low dietary calcium intake
Malabsorption
Lifestyle
Smoking
Low body weight
Immobility/sedentary lifestyle
High risk of falls
History of previous fractures after 50 years of age
Other

**Table 57–2** Bone Mineral Density and Fracture Risk

| Result | T Score |
| --- | --- |
| Normal | Values > 1 SD below the young adult mean |
| Low bone density or osteopenia | Values between 1–2.5 SD below the young adult mean |
| Osteoporosis | Values > 2.5 SD below the young adult mean |

is analogous to the older term *established osteoporosis*, which should be avoided because it implies that osteoporosis is present only after a fracture occurs, whereas a markedly reduced BMD is an indication for treatment to prevent future fractures.

BMD and T score values differ between QCT and DXA machines and between different types of DXA and QCT machines. Hence, serial measurements to assess the rate of bone loss or the response to therapy should be performed optimally on the same equipment using the same software. Standard biochemical tests generally are not helpful in the diagnosis of osteoporosis but may be appropriate to exclude causes of secondary osteoporosis or other bone disorders. Newer biochemical markers of bone turnover, such as serum osteocalcin (a marker of bone formation) and urinary pyridinolines (collagen breakdown products used as markers of bone resorption), may predict response to therapy but are of limited value for routine use.

Ultrasound may be used to measure the density of the shinbone, a good predictor of general bone mass. The procedure takes only a few minutes, is safe and painless, costs less than DXA, and is less complicated to administer.

### DIAGNOSTIC STRATEGIES AND RISK ASSESSMENT

#### Laboratory Tests for Estrogen Deficiency

The first step is to determine whether the woman is estrogen deficient and in need of replacement therapy. This can be done by measuring the primary premenopausal estrogen, 17β-estradiol ($E_2$) and serum follicle-stimulating hormone (FSH). After the cessation of menses, circulating serum $E_2$ levels fall to less than 30 pg/ml (most of which is derived from the peripheral conversion of estrone), and estrone levels fall to less than 70 pg/ml (most of which is derived from the peripheral conversion of androstenedione). The androgen-to-estrogen ratio increases because of a marked decline in estrogen, and reports of mild hirsutism are common. In the period immediately preceding menopause, which can range from 2 to 10 years, estradiol levels can fluctuate widely, giving rise to the symptoms of perimenopause.

In response to the decreasing ability of the ovary to produce estradiol, inhibin FSH levels rise and then fluctuate during the perimenopausal period until menopause is established, wherein levels remain elevated greater than 40 mIU/ml. Menopause thus is characterized by declining $E_2$ levels, the loss of inhibin, and subsequent increase in FSH. FSH and estrogen assays are readily available and, although somewhat expensive, allow you to better predict when your patient needs replacement therapy.

Estrone is the major circulating estrogen in menopause. Before menopause, the estradiol-to-estrone ratio is greater than 1.0. After menopause, the adrenal gland continues to produce androstenedione, which is converted to estrone in peripheral fat and other tissues. The ovarian production of estradiol is markedly decreased, and the estradiol-to-estrone ratio is reversed to less than 1.0.

The maturation index of the vaginal smear is a measure of the ratio of superficial cells and intermediate cells over parabasal cells. Before serum estrogen testing was easily available, it was used as an indicator of relative estrogen deficiency. With estrogen depletion, there is diminution of the superficial cells and prevalence of the parabasal cells, or a "shift to the left." This cellular distribution is reversed by the addition of estrogen.

## Approach to Therapy of Specific Problems

### HOT FLUSHES AND NIGHT SWEATS

ERT is approximately 95% successful in the treatment of hot flushes. Conjugated estrogen, 0.625 mg daily or its equivalent, generally controls hot flush episodes, but higher doses may be necessary. Schiff and colleagues documented that conjugated estrogen, 0.625 mg/day, in addition to decreasing hot flushes, increased rapid eye movement (REM) sleep and improved sleep. Medroxyprogesterone acetate (MPA), 10 mg daily, also can be effective and is a reasonable alternative therapy in women for whom estrogen therapy is contraindicated. Megestrol acetate, 10 to 40 mg/day, also has been shown to be effective in the treatment of hot flushes. There are no long-term data on the effect of these drugs on bone mass. They should not be used as substitutes for proven methods unless contraindicated. Abnormal bleeding can occur in 25 to 50% of women, so this treatment is primarily of benefit in women who have previously had a hysterectomy.

Other agents have been used with varying success. Bellergal-S, a mixture of ergotamine tartrate and levorotatory alkaloids of belladonna and phenobarbital, given twice daily, has been used in the treatment of hot flushes. One study found significant reduction in the intensity of hot flushes with Bellergal-S. However, another study found relief of symptoms only in the first 4 weeks of therapy. The patient should be warned about the drug's sedative effects and its addictive potential.

Clonidine (Catapres TTS-1), an α-adrenergic agonist commonly used as an antihypertensive agent, has been shown effective in reducing the frequency and severity of hot flushes. Initiation of therapy begins with a 0.1-mg/day patch to be worn for 1 week. The dose can be increased as needed for control of hot flushes, but one must be careful to monitor the blood pressure when increasing the dosage. Side effects are mild and tend to decrease with continued therapy. Common complaints include dizziness, drowsiness, localized skin irritation, and dry mouth.

The use of propanolol to treat hot flushes has been associated with conflicting outcomes, with one study showing significant benefit; however, the study was not controlled with placebo. In a placebo-controlled trial, Coope and associates showed that reductions in hot flushes were equal to placebo. The Food and Drug Administration (FDA) approve neither clonidine nor propanolol for treatment of hot flushes.

## VAGINAL ATROPHY

Symptomatic vaginal atrophy usually is relieved with estrogen therapy. If estrogen is not an option, over-the-counter preparations are available to increase vaginal moisture, but none reverses vaginal atrophy. Available agents include glycerin compounds, such as Astroglide, Lubrin, Replens, K-Y jelly, and Moist Again.

## OTHER CHANGES

Psychological symptoms of the menopause have been one of the most contentious issues in menopause research. These symptoms include, but are not limited to, inability to concentrate, mood lability, irritability, anxiety, insomnia, mood depression, memory loss, lack of energy, aggressiveness, nervousness, and headache. Accompanying these symptoms can be myalgia, joint aches, lack of libido, and palpitations. These symptoms often are ill defined and nonspecific. Although the relationship between the biologic and psychosocial nature of these symptoms is not well understood, they nonetheless are real and need attention.

Estrogen therapy often is accompanied by decreases in insomnia, anxiety, and irritability, and improvement of memory. In decreasing hot flushes during sleep, the quality of sleep is improved, preventing chronic insomnia. Campbell and coworkers showed in a double-blind crossover study that estrogen was significantly more effective in relieving not only hot flushes, but insomnia, irritability, headaches, and urinary frequency. Thus, estrogen improves many psychological symptoms in addition to relieving hot flushes.

## OSTEOPOROSIS

ERT, if given, should start as soon as possible after natural menopause or oophorectomy because estrogen replacement slows the rate of bone loss. Menopausal estrogen replacement cannot restore bone mass to pretreatment levels. Riis and colleagues studied three groups of menopausal women who received 17β-estradiol 1 mg/day, calcium 2 g/day, or placebo. Of the three groups, only the women receiving estrogen showed stable bone mass after 2 years. Conjugated estrogen (0.625 mg), ethinyl estradiol (20 μg), and micronized estradiol (1 mg) have proved efficacious in the prevention of osteoporosis. According to one study, bone loss also can be slowed when lower doses of estrogen (0.3 mg conjugated estrogen) and higher doses of calcium (1.5 g/day) are used. Transdermal administration of 17β-estradiol has been equally effective in arresting bone loss.

Other antiresorptive agents such as calcitonin and bisphosphonates (alendronate, etidronate) have similar effects on bone density and appear to protect somewhat against fractures. Calcitonin prevents osteoblasts from causing more bone breakdown. Bisphosphonates are incorporated into the bone matrix and have a long life in bone. The question of whether this bone is of good quality and is mineralized properly will be answered with ongoing long-term studies.

There is real risk in overdoing antiresorption therapy. Prevention of osteoporosis involves slowing the process of bone breakdown and remodeling, which are critical for bone repair. If the antiresorptive effect is too strong, bone repair is arrested and microfractures and other small areas of bone damage are not repaired. The bone becomes older and less healthy. Thus, the bone's resistance is lessened and fatigue fractures can develop. Careful administration of these agents is warranted.

## POSSIBLE ADVERSE EFFECTS OF ESTROGEN

### Endometrial Hyperplasia and Cancer

Estrogen is a known cellular mitogen in the endometrium, and endometrial hyperplasia and cancer have been associated with unopposed estrogen use. This effect is both dose and duration dependent, with an increase of 1.8-fold and 12.7-fold with conjugated estrogen dosages of 0.625 mg and 1.25 mg, respectively. Furthermore, when unopposed estrogen was given for 5 to 10 years or longer, the relative risk for endometrial cancer rose from 4.1 to 11.6. However, the development of endometrial cancer while using unopposed estrogen is associated with a better prognosis. Women diagnosed with stage I, grade 1 adenocarcinoma demonstrated a 96.7% 5-year survival rate. More recently, the PEPI Trial confirmed these earlier reports associated with unstopped estrogen use and reinforced the need for the addition of a progestin to estrogen therapy for women with a uterus.

The addition of progestin to estrogen therapy has been shown to decrease the occurrence of endometrial hyperplasia and cancer. This effect also appears to be dose and duration dependent. The addition of norethindrone for 7 and 10 days each month decreased the incidence of endometrial hyperplasia from 32% in the estrogen alone group to 4 and 2%, respectively. It appears that therapy for greater than 12 days each cycle is required to reduce the rate of endometrial hyperplasia to zero. This makes intuitive sense because in ovulating women, increased progesterone secretion effects the endometrium for 13 to 14 days. The most efficacious dose and type of progestin for endometrial stabilization with minimal metabolic impact on lipoprotein profiles remains to be determined.

## Breast Cancer

Epidemiology literature since the early 1980s has attempted to determine whether there is an association between postmenopausal estrogen use and breast cancer. The determination of this relationship is difficult because of the confounding variables of estrogen type, dose, and duration of exposure. However, there is the suggestion of a 50% increase if estrogen use is longer than 20 years. The type of estrogen appears to be of importance: one European study reported an 80% increase in the breast cancer rate among women using ethinyl estradiol for longer than 9 years. Using meta-analytic techniques, data from separate investigations can be analyzed to generalize conclusions. One report using meta-analysis to review 556 articles found no significant increase in the risk of breast cancer with conjugated estrogen use. Another report that used this technique to analyze specific types of estrogen reported a 30% increase in the risk of breast cancer among women taking estradiol.

The latest report from the Nurse's Health Study (Colditz and associates, 1995) found an increased risk of 30 to 40% of breast cancer in women currently using estrogen or estrogen plus progestin for more than 5 years, as compared with menopausal women who had never used hormones. Also, the risk of breast cancer with 5 or more years of menopausal hormone therapy use was greater among women aged 60 to 64. However, the user and nonuser groups were very different. Current users had a 14% higher prevalence of mammography, more benign breast disease, less childbirths, and an earlier menarche. Differences in breast cancer risk may be related to these factors as opposed to an increased risk from using hormones.

In contrast, a large case-control study from Washington state showed that estrogen plus progestin was not associated with an increase in breast cancer risk in middle-aged women. In fact, long-term users (8 or more years) had a 60% reduction in risk.

Taken together, there is inconclusive evidence relating the causal effects of estrogen use and breast cancer, especially when considering conjugated equine estrogens. These data should be discussed with each patient before estrogen therapy is instituted.

**Table 57–3** Absolute Contraindications to Hormone Replacement Therapy

- Suspected or previously diagnosed estrogen dependent neoplasia (breast or advanced stage uterine cancer)
- Active thrombosis or embolic disease
- Undiagnosed uterine bleeding
- Active liver disease or severely impaired hepatic function

## THERAPY

Because exogenous estrogen therapy in estrogen-deficient women lessens and possibly prevents undesirable, potentially life-threatening sequelae, therapy should be considered seriously for all menopausal women. Large-scale, cross-sectional, prospective studies confirm that the benefits of replacement therapy outweigh the risks. Epidemiologic studies have estimated the number of preventable deaths to be hundreds per 100,000 estrogen users 65 to 75 years of age and the cumulative preventable deaths to be in the thousands. Therapy should be at the lowest dosage possible to maximize relief from symptoms but minimize bone resorption and slow the progression of atherosclerosis.

## Contraindications

The medical history is used to determine whether absolute contraindications are present (Table 57–3). Relative contraindications are listed in Table 57–4. Progestin-only therapy may be beneficial in patients who cannot undergo estrogen therapy. There is no

**Table 57–4** Estrogen Use in Preexisting Conditions (Relative Contraindications)

- Chronic liver dysfunction (may use smaller and less frequent doses of estrogen)
- Preexisting symptomatic uterine leiomyomas or active endometriosis
- Acute intermittent porphyria (estrogens precipitate attacks)

Table 57–5  Natural and Synthetic Estrogens

| Natural Estrogens | Synthetic Estrogens |
|---|---|
| Estrones | 17β-ethinyl estrogens |
|   Conjugated equine estrogens | Mestranol |
|   Estropipate | Diethylstilbestrol |
| Estradiols |  |
|   Micronized estradiol |  |
|   Estradiol valerate |  |

reason to deny use of hormone replacement therapy (HRT) in women with controlled hypertension, diabetes mellitus, or biliary stones. Further prospective studies need to be performed to determine whether ERT can be used without harm in patients with previously treated breast or endometrial cancer or with acute myocardial infarction. Stage I endometrial cancer recurrence rates are not increased with HRT. Stages II, III, and IV are still relative contraindications.

## Available Estrogen Preparations

Estrogen preparations commonly used for menopausal ERT or HRT are natural estrogens (found naturally in a plant or animal), whereas estrogens used in oral contraceptive preparations are synthetic (Table 57–5). Synthetic estrogens differ from natural estrogens in their increased target tissue potency.

The rationale for any medical therapy is to prescribe the lowest possible dose to achieve the desired clinical effect. Studies have shown that 5 μg of ethinyl estradiol is comparable in biologic potency to 0.625 mg of conjugated equine estrogens. Low-dose oral contraceptives for hormone replacement provides 4 to 7 times the amount of estrogen in traditional hormone replacement therapy.

Unopposed estrogen therapy is an option as long as proper precautions are taken. Therapy often is reserved for the patient who suffers intolerable adverse side effects from progestin component. If estrogen-alone therapy is ultimately desired in a woman with a uterus refusing progestin, discussion regarding the increased risk of endometrial hyperplasia and cancer should be undertaken. Pretreatment and annual endometrial biopsies are warranted. If abnormal endometrial histology is identified, then estrogen therapy should be stopped and the patient appropriately treated with observation or high-dose progestin therapy.

Conjugated equine estrogens (Premarin, PMB; Tables 57–6 to 57–8) are derived from pregnant mares' urine, which contains estrone, equilin, and a mixture of other estrogen metabolites. Equilin is a potent estrogen, and because it is stored in fat, it is also long lasting. The recommended starting dose of conjugated equine estrogen is 0.625 mg. When applied vaginally or transdermally, estrogens bypass the liver and act directly on the target tissue. After prolonged treatment with conjugated equine estrogens, serum equilin levels can remain elevated for 13 weeks or more post-treatment because of storage and slow release from adipose tissue.

Estradiol (Estrace, Estraderm, and Climara) is a synthetically produced natural 17β-estradiol. Estrace is the micronized form of estradiol. The recommended starting dose is 1 mg. Estraderm is a transdermal patch applied twice weekly (see Table 57–6). The recommended starting dose is 0.05 mg, and the patch is applied to the skin of the lower trunk and changed once every 3.5 days. Serum levels remain constant for 84 hours, then fall rapidly. Although Climara contains the same estrogen as Estraderm, the patch is manufactured differently and it is applied only once weekly.

Estropipate (Ogen, Ortho Est) is a naturally produced estrogen prepared from purified crystalline estrone. The recommended starting dose for estropipate is 0.625 mg (0.75-mg estropipate). Esterified

Table 57–6  Available Oral Estrogens

| Generic Name | Trade Name | Usual Dose | Manufacturer |
|---|---|---|---|
| Conjugated equine estrogens | Premarin | 0.625–1.25 mg | Wyeth-Ayerst |
| 17β-Estradiol | Estrace | 1–2 mg | Bristol-Myers, Squibb |
| Estropipate | Ogen, Ortho-Est | 0.625–1.25 mg | Upjohn, Ortho |
| Esterified estrogens | Estratab, Menest | 0.3, 0.625, 1.25, 2.5 mg | Solvay, Smith-Kline Beecham |
| Estrogen/progestin combinations | Prempro, Premphase | 0.625 mg Premarin, 2.5 mg or 5 mg medroxyprogesterone acetate | Wyeth-Ayerst |
| Estinyl estradiol | Estinyl | 0.02, 0.05, or 0.5 mg | Schering-Plough |
| Estrone | Estrone (no longer available) | 2 mg (no longer available) | Legere |
| Estradiol cypionate | Ecypionate | 5 mg (no longer available) | Legere |
| Quenistrol | Estrovis | 100 μg/week | Warner Lambert, Parke-Davis |

**Table 57-7** Transdermal Estrogen Replacement Therapy

| Generic Name | Trade Name | Estrogen/Gram | Usual Dose | Site | Manufacturer |
|---|---|---|---|---|---|
| 17β-Estradiol | Estraderm | 0.05, 0.1 mg/day | 0.05–0.1 mg q3.5d | Skin | Ciba |
| 17β-Estradiol Combi patch | Climara | 0.05, 0.1 mg/day | 0.05–0.1 mg once weekly | Skin | Berlex |
| Conjugated equine estrogens | Premarin vaginal cream | 0.625 mg | 1–4 g daily | Vagina | Wyeth-Ayerst |
| Estropipate | Ogen vaginal cream | 1.5 mg | 1–4 g daily | Vagina | Upjohn |
| 17β-Estradiol | Estrace vaginal cream | 1 mg | 3 g weekly | Vagina | Bristol-Myers, Squibb |
| Dienestrol | Ortho dienestrol cream | 0.1 mg | 3–18 g weekly | Vagina | Ortho |

estrogens (Estratab, Menest) are plant estrogens and have the same starting date.

Esterified estrogens and methyltestosterone (Estratest, Estratest HS described in Tables 57–9 and 57–10) are the only available estrogen/androgen combination capsules.

Vaginal creams are also available. Estrogen is absorbed readily through the vaginal epithelium; however, circulating levels of estrogen are only one fourth the levels of an equivalent oral dose. Disadvantages include messy application and variable absorption patterns resulting in widely different bioavailability.

## Estrogen Side Effects

Studies by Sherwin suggest that estrogen replacement in postmenopausal women may improve cognitive function. She prospectively studied women who underwent bilateral oophorectomy and found that women who were started on estrogen in the immediate postoperative period performed better on tests of cognitive function than did women in the placebo group. In a similar study, Sherwin also found that women with Alzheimer's disease who were receiving estrogen were able to maintain their scores on a test of short-term memory, whereas those in the placebo group were not.

Known side effects of estrogen include nausea, breast tenderness, and edema. These usually decrease in intensity and often resolve with continued therapy.

## Regimens

Before initiating therapy, a thorough discussion should include the indications for therapy, dosing schedule, possible side effects, and alternative therapy, and the possible change in recommendations as new information becomes forthcoming. If the information is presented as an issue of prophylaxis against osteoporosis and cardiovascular disease, then the patient should understand therapy as preventive health care. However, the concern about possible increased risk for breast cancer also must be presented during informed consent. The informed patient is more likely to remain compliant with the recommended therapy.

Patients who have previously undergone hysterectomy for benign tumors can be treated with estrogen therapy alone. The addition of progestin in these patients remains controversial but cannot be endorsed. Common oral therapeutic regimens include conjugated equine estrogens, 0.625 to 1.25 mg, or estradiol, 1 mg, all days. Transdermal application of estrogen 0.05 or 0.1 mg maintains a relatively constant circulatory drug level. It has added advantages of lower overall dose of estradiol with precise control, reduced frequency of dosing, and convenient administration and termination. Transdermal delivery systems avoid first-pass metabolism in the liver, thereby leaving more available to target tissues.

**Table 57-8** Injectable Estrogens

| Generic Name | Trade Name | Usual Dose | Manufacturer |
|---|---|---|---|
| Conjugated equine estrogens | Premarin injection | 25 mg/ml | Wyeth-Ayerst |
| Estradiol cypionate | Estro V injection | 0.5 mg/ml | Legere |
| Polyestradiol phosphate | Estradurin (no longer available) | 40 mg/ml IM q2–4 wk | Wyeth-Ayerst |

**Table 57-9** Oral Estrogen/Testosterone Preparations

| Generic Name | Trade Name | Usual Dose | Manufacturer |
|---|---|---|---|
| Conjugated equine estrogens and methyltestosterone | Premarin and testosterone | 0.625 mg/5 mg 1.25 mg/10 mg | Wyeth-Ayerst |
| Esterified estrogen and methyltestosterone | Estratest, Estratest H.S. | 0.625 mg/5 mg 1.25 mg/10 mg | Solvay |

Table 57-10  Oral Estrogen/Tranquilizer Therapy

| Generic Name | Trade Name | Usual Dose | Manufacturer |
|---|---|---|---|
| Esterified estrogen and chlordiaz-epoxide | Menrium (no longer available) | 0.2 mg/5 mg 0.4 mg/10 mg | Roche |

For patients with an intact uterus, progestin is added to the regimen for endometrial protection against atypical changes. A routine pretreatment endometrial biopsy is not necessary. Estrogen/progestin regimens can be sequential or continuous. The success of the therapy depends largely on the history of the patient. If the patient is bleeding monthly on a regular or semiregular schedule, sequential therapy offers a window for withdrawal bleeding and lessen the chance of intermittent abnormal uterine bleeding. Cyclic bleeding usually continues as long as therapy does. Combined continuous therapy, although having the initial disadvantage of a year or more of irregular bleeding, offers the patient eventual relief from monthly bleeding episodes. If, however, she has been amenorrheic for 6 months or more, then combined continuous therapy offers her the benefits of replacement without the added worry of monthly withdrawal bleeding and is the only logical choice.

### Sequential Combined Therapy

Sequential therapy is defined by a hormone-free period when withdrawal bleeding is allowed to occur. Estrogen therapy can be administered continuously with the addition of a progestin for 12, 14, or 25 days of the patient's cycle. Continuous daily estrogen therapy provides for patient convenience and avoids annoying cyclic postmenopausal symptoms. There is no evidence that continuous combined estrogen therapy is associated with an increase in endometrial hyperplasia when compared with a cyclic combined regimen.

Common regimens include conjugated equine estrogens, 0.625 to 1.25 mg, or estradiol, 1 mg, each day, with 12 to 14 days of MPA 5 mg or 25 days of MPA 2.5 mg. Menses usually ensue within 5 to 6 days after the progestin withdrawal.

MPA, 10 mg/day, is a commonly used progestin that can be associated with the side effects of depression, fluid retention, and bloating in nearly 25% of women. Reducing the dosage to 5 mg/day often eliminates these symptoms. Micronized progesterone for menopausal treatment was used successfully in the PEPI Trial in a cyclic fashion with minimal side effects. This progestin is often more tolerable than MPA, but patients should be forewarned of its sedative effects. Taken before bedtime it has an added advantage in patients with insomnia. Alternative progestin therapies also may be substituted to ameliorate these untoward effects (Table 57–11). Norethindrone, 0.7 mg, is endometrial protective when added to estrogen therapy and is associated less commonly with the side effects that are found with MPA. Megestrol acetate 10 mg/day also appears to have less unwanted side effects, although there is no evidence on long-term use benefits or risks.

### Continuous Combined Therapy

In continuous combined therapy, estrogen and progestin are administered on a continuous, daily basis. The major benefit of this therapy is possible avoidance of cyclic bleeding and, therefore, better compliance as well as a lower progestin dose. Daily progestin causes endometrial atrophy and protection from atypical changes. Because the progestin is administered at a lower dose, its adverse effects on lipoproteins and side effects such as breast tenderness, bloating, headache, and emotional lability are minimized.

Minimal spotting may occur during the first 12 months of therapy; however, 33% of patients do not experience bleeding at all, and 80% of patients who bleed stop within the first year. Continuous dosing may decrease the incidence of additional problems associated with cyclic premenstrual symptoms and uterine fibroids. This approach, first described by Staland, has received great attention. In a prospective, randomized study, endometrial biopsy specimens from the group receiving continuous combined therapy showed an atrophic or proliferative-inactive pat-

Table 57-11  Progesterone and Progestins

| Generic Name | Trade Name | Usual Dose | Manufacturer |
|---|---|---|---|
| Medroxyprogesterone acetate | Provera, Cycrin | 2.5, 5, or 10 mg | Upjohn, ESI, Lederle |
| Norethindrone acetate | Norlutate (no longer available) | 5 mg | Parke-Davis |
| Norethindrone tablets | Norlutin (no longer available) | 5 mg | Parke-Davis |
| Norethindrone acetate | Aygestin | 5 mg | ESI, Lederle |
| Norethindrone tablets | Micronor | 0.35 mg | Ortho |
| Micronized progesterone | Prometrium | 100 mg hs continuous 200 mg hs days 12–25 | Solvay |

tern. Five percent of the combined biopsies from the group receiving sequential therapy, however, showed cystic or adenomatous hyperplasia. Varying doses of progestin (MPA 2.5–5 mg, or norethindrone 0.35–1.45 mg) have been examined using the continuous combined regimen. In one study, women who received 2 mg of micronized estradiol and 1 mg of norethindrone continuously for 12 months had persistent decrease in LDL over the study period.

Early evidence suggests that combined continuous therapy may have similar protective effect on bone as combined sequential therapy. A combination of conjugated equine estrogens 0.625 mg with MPA 2.5 mg for combined continuous therapy currently is available. The potential advantages of continuous, daily administration of estrogen and progestin are summarized in Table 57–12.

## ALTERNATIVES TO ESTROGEN THERAPY

### Selective Estrogen Receptor Modulators

Selective estrogen receptor modulators (SERMs) are synthetic estrogen look-alikes. They act as agonist or antagonist to specific tissues and therefore promise an exciting future for the prevention and treatment of many menopausal disorders. Many are just beginning early clinical trials primarily for the treatment of osteoporosis. Some are being studied as alternatives to traditional hormone replacement therapy, being more acceptable than estrogens because of their antiestrogenic effects on the breast.

Most have beneficial effects on bone mass and lipids and are appealing as a "bleedfree" form of hormone replacement therapy (because they do not stimulate the endometrium). Raloxifene (Evista) is FDA approved for the prevention of osteoporosis. Raloxifene is half as effective on BMD as estrogen and has a side effect profile of increased hot flushes and leg cramps. Venous thromboembolism risk appears to be the same as estrogen. The increase in hot flushes remains a stumbling block for use in some women. A beneficial effect may be a reduction in breast cancer risk. Following is a review of some of the more hopeful medications in the treatment of hot flushes. Only raloxifene is available in the United States for general use.

Tibolone is a gonadomimetic synthetic steroid in the norpregnene family with combined estrogenic, progestogenic, and androgenic effects. It mainly has been studied as an agent to prevent bone loss in postmenopausal women, and it appears to relieve menopausal hot flushes and vaginal dryness as well. It causes endometrial atrophy, maintains skeletal integrity, and is antagonistic to the breast. In addition to not stimulating the endometrium, tibolone may improve symptoms of vaginal dryness, dyspareunia, sexual enjoyment, and libido. The major side effects are weight gain and bloating. In early studies, although Lp(a) lipoprotein levels were reduced, a significant reduction in HDL-C also was observed, implying that it might not have cardiovascular benefit and may even have risk.

Idoxifene is an iodinated descendant of tamoxifen that has both estrogen agonist and antagonist activity. It is in nononcologic clinical trials and, because of its long half-life, it may have fewer undesirable vasomotor side effects than other drugs in this class. It appears to have antagonist effects on the breast, as well as agonist effects on the bone and heart. Developments with this drug have shown that it use increases benign endometrial polyp formation and this will limit its usefulness if it is released. Other agonist/antagonist agents with similar profiles include droloxifene, and toremifene. Toremifene has a profile similar to tamoxifen and, because of increased vasomotor flushing, probably is not an alternative for treatment of menopausal symptoms.

### Phytoestrogens

Phytoestrogens are weak estrogens of plant origin. The precursors of the biologically active compounds originate in soybean products (mainly isoflavonoids) and whole grain cereals, seeds, and nuts (mainly ligands). These plant glycosides are converted by intestinal bacteria to weak estrogen-like compounds.

Epidemiologic investigations have suggested that they are natural anticancer compounds because the highest concentrations of these compounds are found in the diet of countries with low cancer rates. They may have antiestrogenic effects in much the same way as SERMs, competitively binding to the estrogen receptor and displacing more potent endogenous estrogens (estrone). This hypothesis is corroborated by the low rates of breast cancer in Hispanic women despite their increased adiposity, a breast cancer risk factor.

High dietary intake of these plant estrogens appears to reduce risk for breast cancer and also has been linked to fewer menopausal symptoms. In a

**Table 57–12** Potential Advantages of Continuous Dosing

- Amenorrhea
- Endometrial atrophy (protection from atypical changes and pregnancy)
- Uterine atrophy (asymptomatic fibroids)
- Less adverse effect on blood lipoproteins
- Convenience, therefore better compliance

small study of 58 postmenopausal women, soy (daidzin) and wheat (enterolactones) reduced hot flushes 40 and 25%, respectively. However, it is unclear whether these estrogens may be potent enough to stimulate the growth of estrogen-dependent tumors.

## Ongoing Research in the Field

Results from the Heart and Estrogen-Progestin Replacement Study were published in August 1998. In this trial, 2500 women with established coronary heart disease were randomized to placebo or continuous conjugated equine estrogens with MPA to look at the impact on sudden death and fatal and nonfatal myocardial infarction. If the trial has enough events, the risks and benefits of combined estrogen-progestin therapy can be studied in detail in women with known heart disease.

The Women's Health Initiative (a longitudinal clinical trail examining causes and prevention of cardiovascular disease, breast and colorectal cancer, and osteoporosis in menopausal women) is beginning follow-up, and many of these issues will be better defined with results from this study. The Women's Health Initiative Memory Study, evaluating more than 7000 women in a randomized clinical trial of estrogen vs. placebo, will look at cognitive function and estrogen. Its goal is to determine whether estrogen improves cognitive function and memory and prevents or delays the onset of Alzheimer's disease.

## Conclusion

With an ever-increasing number of women seeking health care during menopause, it is important to provide these women with a rational plan for HRT. Before any therapeutic modality can be recommended, sound medical practice demands that inherent benefits of such therapy outweigh the identifiable associated risks for each patient. This chapter has reviewed the inherent health risks associated with estrogen deficiency and the associated benefits with HRT. The risks and side effects of this therapy known in advance to the patient, with a verbalized plan to address them, fosters an understanding that will promote patient compliance.

### REFERENCES

Adlercreutz H: Phytoestrogens: Epidemiology and a possible role in cancer protection. Environ Health Perspect 103(suppl):103–112, 1995.

Albrecht BH, Schiff I, Tulchinsky D, et al: Objective evidence that placebo and oral medroxyprogesterone acetate therapy diminish menopausal vasomotor flashes. Am J Obstet Gynecol 139(6):631–635, 1981.

Alcoff JM, Campbell D, Tribble D, et al: Double blind placebo controlled cross-over trial of propanolol as treatment for menopausal vasomotor symptoms. Clin Ther 3:356–364, 1981.

Aylwood M, Maddock J, Lewis PA, et al: Oestrogen replacement therapy and blood clotting. Curr Med Res Opin 4(suppl 3): 83, 1971.

Baird DT, Frazer IS: Blood production and ovarian secretion rates of estradiol-17B and estrone in women throughout the menstrual cycle. J Clin Endocrinol Metab 38:1009–1017, 1984.

Barnes RB, Lobo RA: Pharmacology of estrogens. In Mishell DR (ed): Menopause: Physiology and Pharmacology. Chicago, Year Book Medical Publishers, 1987, p 301.

Barrett-Connor E, Brown WV, Turner J, et al: Heart disease risk factors and hormone use in postmenopausal women. JAMA 241:2167, 1979.

Barrett-Connor E, Laaksko M: Ischemic heart disease risk in postmenopausal women: Effects of estrogen use on glucose and insulin levels. Arteriosclerosis 10:531–534, 1990.

Bass KM, Newschaffer CJ, Klag MJ, et al: Plasma lipoprotein levels as predictors of cardiovascular death in women. Arch Intern Med 153:2209–2216, 1993.

Benson J, Riis BJ, Storm V, et al: Continuous oestrogen-progestogen treatment and serum lipoproteins in postmenopausal women. Br J Obstet Gynaecol 94:130, 1987.

Bergkvist L, Adami H, Persson IM, et al: The risk of breast cancer after estrogen and estrogen-progestin replacement. N Engl J Med 321:293, 1989.

Bergmans MGM, Merkus JMWM, Corby RS, et al: Effect of Bellergal retard on climacteric complaints: A double blind placebo controlled study. Maturitas 9:227, 1987.

Birkenfeld A, Kase NG: Menopause medicine: Current treatment options and trends. Comp Ther 17:36–45, 1991.

Bjarnason NH, Bjarnason K, Haarbo J, et al: Prevention of bone loss in late postmenopausal women. J Clin Endocrinol Metab 81: 2419–2422, 1996.

Bradbeer J, Stroup HS, Zhao H: Dose refining study of the effects of idoxifene (SB-223030) on bone loss, plasma cholesterol and uterine weight in the ovariectomized rat model of osteoporosis. ASBMR abstract. Internal Document, SmithKlein Beecham, No. PP1002. FDA Submission, October 1995.

Brambilla DJ, McKinlay SM: A prospective study of factors affecting the age of menopause. J Clin Epidemiol 42:1031–1039, 1989.

Brincat M, Moniz CF, Kabalan S, et al: Decline in skin collagen content and metacarpal index after the menopause and its prevention with sex hormone replacement. Br J Obstet Gynaecol 94: 126–129, 1987.

Brincat M, Moniz CF, Studd JW, et al: Long-term effects of the menopause and sex hormones on skin thickness. Br J Obstet Gynaecol 92:256–259, 1985.

Bush TL, Barrett-Connor E, Crowan L, et al: Cardiovascular mortality and noncontraceptive use of estrogen in women: Results from the Lipid Research Clinics Program Follow-up Study. Circulation 74:1102–1107, 1987.

Bush TL; Noncontraceptive estrogen use and risk of cardiovascular disease: An overview and critique of the literature. In Korenman SG (ed): The Menopause: Biological and Clinical Consequences of Ovarian Failure; Evaluation and Management. Norwell, MA, Serono Symposia, 1990, pp 221–224.

Bush TL, Barrett-Connor E: Noncontraceptive estrogen use and cardiovascular disease. Epidemiol Rev 7:89–104, 1985.

Campbell S, Whitehead M: Estrogen therapy and the postmenopausal syndrome. Clin Obstet Gynecol 4:31–47, 1977.

Campbell S, Beard RJ, McQueen J, et al: Double blind psychometric studies on the effects of natural estrogens on post-menopausal women. In Campbell S (ed): Management of the Menopause and Post-menopausal Years. Lancaster, England, MTP Press LTD, 1976, p 33.

Castelo-Branco C, Duran M, Gonzalez-Merlo J: Skin collagen changes related to age and hormone replacement therapy. Maturitas 15:113–119, 1992.

Castelli WP: Cardiovascular disease in women. Am J Obstet Gynecol 158:1553–1560, 1988.

Chander SK, McCague R, Luqmani Y, et al: Pyrrolidino-4-iodotamoxifen, new analogues of the antiestrogen tamoxifen for the treatment of breast cancer. Cancer Res 51:5851–5858, 1991.

Chetowski R, Medrum D, Steingold K, et al: Biological effects of estradiol (E2) administration by a transdermal therapeutic system (TTS) (abstract). Presented at the 32nd Annual Meeting of the Society for Gynecologic Investigation, Phoenix, AZ, 1985, p 67.

Chetkowski RJ, Meldrum DR, Steingold KA, et al: Biologic effects of transdermal estradiol. N Engl J Med 314:1615–1620, 1986.

Christiansen C, Christiansen GS, McNair P, et al: Prevention of early postmenopausal bone loss: Controlled 2 year study in 315 females. Eur J Clin Invest 10:273–279, 1980.

Christensen C: What should be done at the time of menopause? Am J Med 98:56S–59S, 1995.

Cignarelli M, Cincinelli E, Corso M, et al: Biophysical and endocrine-metabolic changes during menopausal hot flashes: Increase in plasma free fatty acid and norepinephrine levels. Gynecol Obstet Invest 27:34–37, 1989.

Clayden JR, Bell JW, Pollard P: Menopausal flushing: Double blind trial of a nonhormonal preparation. Br Med J 1:409–412, 1974.

Colditz GA, Hankinson SE, Hunter DJ, et al: The use of estrogens and progestins and the risk of breast cancer in postmenopausal women. N Engl J. Med 332:1589–1593, 1995.

Coope J, Williams S, Parreson JS: A study of the effectiveness of propanolol in the menopausal hot flash. Fr J Obstet Gynecol 85:472–475, 1978.

Crailo MD, Pike MC: Estimation of the distribution of age at natural menopause from prevalence data. Am J Epidemiol 17:356, 1983.

Creasman WT, Henderson D, Hinshaw W, et al: Estrogen replacement therapy in patients treated for endometrial cancer. Obstet Gynecol 67:326, 1986.

Creasman W: Estrogen replacement therapy: Is previously treated cancer a contraindication? Obstet Gynecol 77:308, 1991.

Cruqui MH, Suarez L, Barrett-Connor E, et al: Postmenopausal estrogen use and mortality: Results from a prospective study in a defined homogenous community. Am J Epidemiol 128:606–614, 1988.

Del Pino J, Martin-Gomez E, Martin-Rodriguez M, et al: Influence of sex, age, and menopause in serum osteocalcin (BGP) levels. Klin Wochenschr 69:1135–1138, 1991.

Dennerstein L, Burrows GD, Hyman GJ, et al: Hormone therapy and affect. Maturitas 1:247–259, 1979.

Dewhurst J: Postmenopausal bleeding from benign causes. Clin Obstet Gynecol 26:769, 1983.

Dunn LB, Damesyn M, Moore AA, et al: Does estrogen prevent skin aging? Results from the first National Health and Nutrition Examination Survey (NHANES I). Arch Dermatol 133:339–342, 1997.

Dupont WD, Page DL: Menopausal estrogen replacement therapy and breast cancer. Arch Intern Med 151:67, 1991.

Elders PJ, Netelenbos JC, Lips P, et al: Accelerated vertebral bone loss in relation to the menopause: A cross-sectional study on lumbar bone density in 286 women of 46 to 55 years of age. J Bone Miner Res 5:11–19, 1988.

Ettinger B, Genant HK, Cann CE: Postmenopausal bone loss is prevented by treatment with low-dosage estrogen with calcium. Ann Intern Med 106:40–47, 1987.

Falkeborn M, Persson I, Adami HO, et al: The risk of acute myocardial infarction after oestrogen and oestrogen-progestogen replacement. Br J Obstet Gynaecol 99:821–828, 1992.

Farish E, Barnes JF, Rolton HA, et al: Effects of tibolone on lipoprotein (a) and HDL subfractions. Maturitas 20:215–219, 1994.

Freedman RR, Norton D, Woodward S, et al. Core body temperature and circadian rhythm of hot flashes in menopausal women. J Clin Endocrinol Metab 80:2354–2358, 1995.

Frommer DJ: Changing age of the menopause. Br Med J 2:349–351, 1964.

Gambrell RD: Estrogen Replacement Therapy. Dallas, Essential Medical Information Systems, 1989.

Gambrell RD: Prevention of endometrial cancer with progestogens. Maturitas 8:159–168, 1986.

Gambrell RD: Use of progestogen therapy. Am J Obstet Gynecol 156:1304–1313, 1987.

Ginsburg J, Prelevic G, Butler D, et al: Clinical experience with tibolone (Livial) over 8 years. Maturitas 1:71–76, 1995.

Goldbourt U, Medalie JH: High density lipoprotein cholesterol and incidence of coronary heart disease: The Israeli Ischemic Heart Disease Study. Am J Epidemiol 109:296–308, 1979.

Gordon T, Kannel W, Hjortland M: Menopause and coronary heart disease. Ann Intern Med 89:157–161, 1978.

Grady D, Rubin SM, Petitti DB, et al: Hormone therapy to prevent disease and prolong life in postmenopausal women. Ann Intern Med 117:1016–1037, 1992.

Gray LS, Christopherson WM, Hoover RN: Estrogens and endometrial carcinoma. Obstet Gynecol 49:385–389, 1988.

Gruchow HW, Anderson AJ, Barboriak JJ, et al: Postmenopausal use of estrogen and occlusion of coronary arteries. Am Heart J 115:954–963, 1988.

Guy RH, Hadgraft J, Bucks DAW: Transdermal drug delivery and cutaneous metabolism. Xenobiotica 17:325, 1987.

Hammond DO: Cytological assessment of climacteric patients. Clin Obstet Gynecol 4:49–69, 1977.

Hammond CB, Maxon WS: Current status of estrogen therapy for the menopause. Fertil Steril 37:5, 1982.

Henderson BE, Ross RK, Lobo, RA, et al: Re-evaluating the role of progesterogen therapy after the menopause. Fertil Steril 49(suppl):9S–15S, 1988.

Henderson BE, Ross RK, Paganini-Hill A, et al: Estrogen use and cardiovascular disease. Am J Obstet Gynecol 154:1181–1186, 1986.

Hendrix SL, Fitts D, Watrous M, et al: Idoxifene improves menopausal symptoms in a short term, dose ranging study, NAMS Annual Meeting, Boston, September 1997.

Henneman DH: Effect of estrogen on the in vivo and in vitro collagen biosynthesis and maturation in old and young female guinea pigs. Endocrinology 83:678–690, 1968.

Horn-Ross PL. Phytoestrogens, body composition, and breast cancer. Cancer Causes Control 6:567–573, 1995.

Hulka BS: Hormone replacement therapy and the risk of breast cancer. CA Cancer J Clin 40:289, 1990.

Hunt K, Vessey M, McPherson K, Coleman M: Long-term surveillance of mortality and cancer incidence in women receiving hormone replacement therapy. Br J Obstet Gynaecol 94:620–635, 1987.

Jick H, Porter J, Morrison AS: Relation between smoking and age of natural menopause. Lancet 1:1354, 1977.

Jordan VC: Alternate antiestrogens and approaches to the prevention of breast cancer. J Cell Biochem Suppl 22:51–57, 1995.

Kao KY, Hitt WE, McGavack TH: Effect of estradiol benzoate upon collagen synthesis by sponge biopsy connective tissue. Proc Soc Exp Biol Med 119–364, 1965.

Kaplan NM: Hypertension induced by pregnancy, oral contraceptives and postmenopausal replacement therapy. Cardiol Clin 6:475–482, 1988.

Kempers R: Hormone replacement therapy: The breast-cancer controversy. Postgrad Obstet Gynecol 12:1–5, 1992.

Krailo MD, Pike MC: Estimation of the distribution of age at natural menopause from prevalence data. Am J Epidemiol 117:356–361, 1983.

Lebherz TB, French LT: Nonhormonal treatment of the menopausal syndrome: A double blind evaluation of an autonomic system stabilizer. Obstet Gynecol 33:795, 1969.

Lind T, Cameron EC, Hunter WM, et al: A prospective trial of six forms of hormone replacement therapy given to postmenopausal women. Br J Obstet Gynaecol 86(suppl 3):1–29, 1979.

Lindsay RL, Heart DM: The minimum effective dose of oestrogen for prevention of postmenopausal bone loss. Obstet Gynecol 63:759–763, 1984.

Linquist O, Bengtsson C: The effect of smoking on menopausal age. Maturitas 1:171, 1979.

Lobo RA: Effects of hormonal replacement on lipids and lipoproteins in postmenopausal women. J Clin Endocrinol Metab 73:925–930, 1991.

Lobo RA, Pickar JH, Wild RA, et al: Metabolic impact of adding medroxyprogesterone acetate to conjugated estrogen therapy in postmenopausal women. Obstet Gynecol 8:987–995, 1994.

Luciano A: Hormone replacement therapy in postmenopausal women. Infertil Reprod Med Clin North Am 3:109–128, 1992.
Luciano AA, Turkey RN, Carrel J, et al: Clinical and metabolic responses of postmenopausal women to sequential versus continuous estrogen and progestin replacement therapy. Obstet Gynecol 71:39–43, 1988.
Magos AL, Brincat M, Studd JWW, et al: Amenorrhea and endometrial atrophy with continuous oral estrogen and progesterone therapy in postmenopausal women. Obstet Gynecol 65:496–499, 1985.
Mandel FP, Geola Fl, Meldrum DR, et al: Biologic effects of various doses of vaginally administered conjugated equine estrogens in postmenopausal women. J Clin Endocrinol Metab 57:133, 1983.
Marcus R: Organization and functional aspects of skeletal health. In Marcus H (ed): Osteoporosis. Cambridge, MA, Blackwell Scientific, 1994, p 12.
Mashchack CA, Lobo RA, Dozono-Takano R, et al: Comparison of pharmacodynamic properties to various estrogen formulations. Am J Obstet Gynecol 144:511, 1982.
Matheson LA, Sammie G: Estrogen-progestogen replacement therapy in climacteric women particularly as it regards a new type of continuous regimen. Acta Obstet Gynaecol Scand 130:53–58, 1985.
McKinlay SM, Jefferys M, Thompson B: An investigation of the age of menopause. J Biosoc Sci 4:161–173, 1972.
Meuwissen JH, Wiegerinck MA, Haverkorn MJ: Regression of endometrial thickness in combination with reduced withdrawal bleeding as a progestational effect of tibolone in postmenopausal women on oestrogen replacement therapy. Maturitas 21:121–125, 1995.
Miller VT: Dyslipoproteinemia in women: Special considerations. Endocrinol Metab Clin North Am 19:381–398, 1990.
Mugglestone CJ, Swinhoe JR, Craft IL: Combined estrogen and progesterone for the menopause. Acta Obstet Gynaecol Scand 59:327, 1980.
Munk-Jensen N, Nielsen SP, Obel EB, et al: Reversal of postmenopausal vertebral bone loss by oestrogen and progestogen: A double blind placebo controlled study. Br Med J 296:1150, 1988.
Murkies AL, Lombard C, Strauss BJ, et al: Dietary flour supplementation decreases post-menopausal hot flushes: Effect of soy and wheat. Maturitas 21:189–195, 1995.
Nabulsi AA, Folsom AR, White A, et al: Association of hormone-replacement therapy with various cardiovascular risk factors in postmenopausal women. N Engl J Med 328:1069–1075, 1993.
Newnham HH: Oestrogens and artherosclerotic vascular disease: Lipid factors. Clin Endocrinol Metab 7:61–93, 1993.
Persson l, Adami HO, Bergkvist L, et al: Risk of endometrial cancer after treatment with oestrogens alone or in conjunction with progestogens: Results of a prospective study. Br Med J 298:147–151, 1989.
Pfeffer RI, Kurosaki TT, Charlton SK: Estrogen use and blood pressure in later life. Am J Epidemiol 110:469–478, 1979.
Powers MS, Schenkel L, Darley PE, et al: Pharmacokinetics and pharmacodynamics of transdermal dosage forms of 17 β-estradiol: Comparison with conventional oral estrogens used for hormone replacement. Am J Obstet Gynecol 152:1099–1106, 1985.
Psaty BM, Heckbert SR, Atkins D, et al: The risk of myocardial infarction associated with the combined use of estrogens and progestins in postmenopausal women. Arch Intern Med 154:1333–1339, 1994.
Quigley MET, Martin PL, Burnier AM, et al: Estrogen therapy arrests bone loss in elderly women. Am J Obstet Gynecol 156:1516–1523, 1987.
Quirk JG, Wendel GD: Biologic effects of natural and synthetic estrogens. In Buchsbaum HJ (ed): The Menopause. New York, Springer-Verlag, 1983, pp 55–75.
Rebar RW, Thomas MA, Gass M, et al: Problems of hormone therapy: Evaluations, follow-up, complications. In Korenman SG (ed): Menopause. Boston, Serona Symposia, 1989.
Regensteiner JG, Hiatt WR, Byyny RL, et al: Short-term effects of estrogen and progestin on blood pressure of normotensive postmenopausal women. J Clin Pharmacol 81:543–548, 1991.
Riis BJ, Johnson J, Christiansen C: Continuous oestrogen-progestogen treatment and bone metabolism in postmenopausal women. Maturitas 10:51, 1988.
Riis B, Thomsen K, Christiansen C: Does calcium supplementation prevent postmenopausal bone loss? A double-blind controlled clinical study. N Engl J Med 316:173–177, 1987.
Rijpkena AH, van der Sanden AA, Ruijis AH: Effects of postmenopausal oestrogen-progesteron replacement therapy on serum lipids and lipoproteins: A review. Maturitas 12:259–285, 1990.
Ross LA, Alder EM: Tibolone and climacteric symptoms. Maturitas 21:127–136, 1995.
Rymer J, Chapman MG, Fogelman I: Effect of tibolone on postmenopausal bone loss. Osteoporos Int 4:314–319, 1994.
Rymer J, Chapman MG, Fogelman I, et al: A study of the effect of tibolone on the vagina in postmenopausal women. Maturitas 8:127–133, 1994.
Rymer J, Fogelman I, Chapman MG: The incidence of vaginal bleeding with tibolone treatment. Br J Obstet Gynaecol 101:53–56, 1994.
Schiff I, Sela HK, Cramer D, et al: Endometrial hyperplasia in women on cyclic or continuous estrogen regimens. Fertil Steril 37:79–82, 1982.
Schiff I, Tulchinsky D, Cramer D, et al: Oral medroxyprogesterone in the treatment of postmenopausal symptoms. JAMA 242:2405–2407, 1979.
Schiff I, Regestein Q, Tulchinsky D, et al: Effects of estrogens on sleep and the psychologic state of hypogonadal women. JAMA 242:2405–2407, 1979.
Sherwin BB: Affective changes with estrogen and androgen replacement therapy in surgically menopausal women. J Affect Dis 14:177–187, 1988.
Silferstope G, Gustafsson A, Samsioe G, et al: Lipid metabolic studies in oophorectomized women: Effects on serum lipids and lipoproteins of three synthetic progestogens. Maturitas 4:103–111, 1982.
Siseles NO, Halperin H, Benencia HJ, et al: A comparative study of two hormone replacement therapy regimens on safety and efficacy variables. Maturitas 21:201–210, 1995.
Skolnick AA: At third meeting, menopause experts make the most of insufficient data [Medical News and Perspectives]. JAMA 268:2483–2485, 1992.
Smith QT, Allison DJ: Changes of collagen content in skin, femur and uterus of 17beta-estradiol benzoate-treated rats. Endocrinology 79:486, 1966.
Staland B: Continuous treatment with natural oestrogens and progestogens: A method to avoid endometrial stimulation. Maturitas 3:145–156, 1981.
Stampfer MJ, Colditz GA: Estrogen replacement and coronary heart disease: A quantitative assessment of the epidemiologic evidence. Prev Med 20:47–63, 1991.
Stanford JL, Weiss NS, Voigt LF, et al: Combined estrogen and progestin hormone replacement therapy in relation to risk of breast cancer in middle-aged women. JAMA 274:137–142, 1995.
Steinberg KK, Thacker SB, Smigh SJ, et al: A meta-analysis of the effect of estrogen replacement therapy on the risk of breast cancer. JAMA 265:1985, 1991.
Tataryn IV, Lomax P, Meldrum, et al: Objective techniques for the assessment of postmenopausal hot flashes. Obstet Gynecol 57:340–344, 1981.
Tataryn IV, Lomax P, Bajorek JG, et al: Postmenopausal hot flashes: A disorder of thermoregulation. Maturitas 2:101–107, 1980.
Thompson B, Hart SA, Durno D, et al: Menopausal age and symptomatology in general practice. J Biosoc Sci 5:71–82, 1973.
The Writing Group for the PEPI Trial: Effects of hormone replacement therapy on endometrial histology in postmenopausal women. JAMA 275:370–375, 1996.
The Writing Group for the PEPI Trial: Effects of estrogen or estrogen/progestin regimens on heart disease risk factor in postmenopausal women. JAMA 273:199–208, 1995.
Tikkanen MJ, Kuusi T, Nikklia EA, et al: Postmenopausal hormone replacement therapy: Effects of progesterons on serum lipids and lipoproteins: A review. Maturitas 8:7–17, 1986.
U.S. Bureau of the Census: Population Estimates and Projections, Series P-25, no. 937, 12. Bethesda, MD: Government Printing Office, 1983.

Voda AM: Climacteric hot flash. Maturitas 3:73–90, 1981.

Walsh BW, Schiff I, Rosner B, et al: Effects of postmenopausal estrogen replacement on the concentrations and metabolism of plasma lipoproteins. N Engl J Med 325:1196–1204, 1991.

Weinstein L, Bewtra C, Gallagher CJ: Evaluation of continuous combined low dose regimen of estrogen-progestin for treatment of the menopause patient. Am J Obstet Gynecol 162:1534–1542, 1990.

Whitehead MI, King RB, McQueen J, et al: Endometrial histology and biochemistry in the climacteric woman during estrogen and estrogen/progesterone therapy. J R Soc Med 72:322–327, 1979.

Whitehead MI, Siddle N, Lane G, et al: The pharmacology of progestogens. *In* Mishell DR Jr (ed): Menopause: Physiology and Pharmacology. Chicago, Year Book Medical Publishers, 1987, pp 317–334.

Williams SR, Frenchek B, Speroff T, et al: A study of combined continuous ethinyl estradiol and norethindrone acetate for postmenopausal hormone replacement. Am J Obstet Gynecol 162:438–446, 1990.

Wren B, Garret D: The effects of low-dose piperazine oestrogen sulphate and low-dose levonorgestrel on blood lipid levels in postmenopausal women. Maturitas 7:141–146, 1985.

Wren BG, Routledge AD: The effect of type and dose of oestrogen on the blood pressure of post-menopausal women. Maturitas 5:135, 1983.

Ziel HK, Finkle WD: Increased risk of endometrial carcinoma among users of conjugated estrogen. N Engl J Med 293:1167–1170, 1975.

Zwicke DL, Niazi I, Reeves WC, et al: Reduced transcutaneous nitroglycerin absorption in blacks. Circulation 74(suppl 2):543, 1986.

# 58

# Evaluation and Management of Infertility

JOHN Y. PHELPS
EDWARD E. WALLACH
KAMRAN S. MOGHISSI

## Definitions and Epidemiology

*Infertility* has been defined as failure of a reproductive-age couple to conceive after 12 months or more of regular coitus without using contraception. Conversely, *fertility* refers to the ability to conceive. Infertility is considered primary when it occurs in a woman who has never established a pregnancy and secondary when it occurs in a woman who has a history of one or more previous pregnancies. *Subfertility* applies to conditions that do not completely prohibit conception but rather decrease its likelihood. Examples of conditions associated with subfertility are endometriosis and oligospermia. *Sterility* is defined as the absolute inability to conceive. Examples of conditions associated with sterility are azoospermia and bilateral tubal occlusion. *Fecundability* is defined as the probability of achieving a conception within one menstrual cycle. *Fecundity* is defined as the probability of achieving a live birth within one menstrual cycle. Fecundity takes into account the full range of the reproductive process, from conception to birth of a live infant, whereas fecundability refers to conception only. Fecundity rates are lower than conception rates because of pregnancy losses once conception occurs.

Infertility is a disease that affects the couple. Male or female infertility cannot be considered in isolation. However, women frequently are first to seek care for this condition.

The contribution of male and female to infertility differs in several ways. The male must be able to develop adequate numbers of good quality sperm and deposit them in the female vagina. The role of the female, however, is more complex. In addition to developing a normal gamete (oocyte), the female must be able to transport adequate numbers of healthy sperm from the vagina to the distal portion of the fallopian tubes, provide an appropriate environment for the fertilization of the oocyte and development of a blastocyst, transport the conceptus across the oviduct, have a receptive uterus for implantation of the blastocyst and fetal development, and ultimately, carry a pregnancy to viability stage.

As of 1995, there were an estimated 60.2 million reproductive-age females between 15 and 44 years old living in the United States. Approximately 10% (6 million) of these women have impaired fecundity. However, the prevalence of subfertility may be higher because impairment of fertility in one partner may be compensated by the other one, and the couple's attempt at establishing a pregnancy may not be delayed sufficiently to be a problem. Of couples who seek infertility services, most do so from a generalist specializing in obstetrics and gynecology. As of 1997, the American Board of Obstetricians and Gynecologist estimated that there were 29,300 board-certified obstetricians and gynecologists compared with only 667 subspecialty board-certified reproductive endocrinologists. It also is estimated that 71% of generalists in obstetrics and gynecology provide infertility services without consultation from subspecialists. Obstetricians and gynecologists who provide services to infertile couples must be competent in the management of infertility. With a fundamental understanding of infertility diagnosis and treatment, generalists in obstetrics and gynecology should be able to help most infertile couples. However, generalists also must understand when it is appropriate to refer infertile couples to subspecialists so as not to compromise or delay their care.

# Etiology

## FACTORS AFFECTING STERILITY

Several important factors are known to affect fertility. They include:
- Age
- Frequency of coitus
- Nutrition
- Environmental factors
- Sexually transmitted diseases (STDs)
- Smoking
- Alcohol and drugs
- Stress

The effect of age on fertility has been documented repeatedly. Demographic studies demonstrate a consistent decline in fecundity after 30 to 35 years of age, with an incidence of involuntary infertility in women older than 40 years of age ranging from approximately 33 to 64%.

Reduced age-related fecundity is predominately the result of the decline in oocyte quality, atresia, and an increased rate of chromosomal abnormalities, and is associated with a rise in basal follicle-stimulating hormone (FSH) levels, indicative of reduced ovarian reserve, and an increased incidence of irregular menstrual function. Additionally, advancing age is associated with both a decrease in embryo viability and an exponential increase in trisomies and aneuploidics in the conceptus. Age affects the male partner as well. Declining androgen levels, decreased sexual interest, and reduced sexual activity are related to aging.

Available data indicate that with decreasing frequency of intercourse, the percentage of conception during a given interval declines.

Nutritional status of a woman appears to play an important role in her fertility. It has long been recognized that extremes of weight are associated with ovulatory disturbances and consequent infertility. At one end of the spectrum, women who significantly exceed their ideal body weight may have chronic anovulation with or without androgen excess and insulin resistance (i.e., polycystic ovarian disease). At the other end, women who are grossly below their ideal body weight experience amenorrhea and infertility. Weight gain in such women often leads to resumption of ovulation and restoration of fertility. Chronic deficiency of certain nutrients such as proteins, vitamins, and trace elements also may be a cause of reproductive failure.

Environmental and occupational factors such as radiation, anesthetic agents, toxins, and pollutants may adversely affect both male and female fertility or result in early pregnancy loss.

STDs have a significant impact on fertility. Long-term prospective studies have shown a dose response relationship between laparoscopically proven pelvic inflammatory disease (PID) and infertility. These data indicate that infertility occurs in 11% of women after one episode of PID, in 23% after two episodes, and in 54% after three episodes. Both gonorrhea and chlamydial infections may lead to tubal obstruction and infertility. Chlamydia infection rate has increased sevenfold in the past decade in the United States. It frequently is unrecognized by patients and remains untreated. Similarly, chlamydia trachomatis and *Neisseria gonorrhoeae* may result in epididymitis and scarring and obstruction of seminiferous tubules, leading to oligozoospermia.

Approximately 25% of North American women currently smoke. Cigarette smoke contains a variety of toxins that have been shown in animal studies to affect various levels of reproductive function. A recent review of relevant studies of natural conception, assisted reproduction, and spontaneous abortion concluded that there is a small but clinically significant detrimental effect of female smoking on both time to conception and spontaneous abortion risk. The effect of male smoking on fecundity is probably far less significant.

Ethanol may depress the release of gonadotropin-releasing hormone (GnRH) from the hypothalamus by activating endogenous pathways that inhibit the efflux of the releasing hormone. Chronic alcoholism has been associated with infertility and menstrual disorders and also may have severe consequences for the fetus. In men, alcohol affects testicular synthesis and secretion of testosterone, which can result in abnormal sperm morphology and sexual dysfunction. Similarly, opioids and other recreational drugs may cause an alteration of gonadotropin release and subfertility. Marijuana use brings about a suppression of gonadotropin in both sexes, resulting in shorter menstrual cycle and short luteal phase in women and a transient decrease in sperm count in men.

Prescription medication also may have an adverse effect in both sexes. Examples are the use of psychotropic drugs in the female, causing hyperprolactinemia and menstrual disorders, and sulfasalazine in the male, producing oligospermia.

The involvement of emotional factors in infertility generally has been accepted. Clinicians frequently encounter menstrual irregularities, even amenorrhea, in patients who are emotionally stressed. In the male, impairment of sperm density and quality may be observed after mental stress and psychic tension. Sexual activities and performance may be affected during periods of emotional stress and psychic disturbance. Decreased libido, impotence, and premature ejaculation commonly are induced psychologically. In the female, vaginismus, dyspareunia, and frigidity can result from emotional trauma or strain. Psychological, sexual, and marital difficulties may arise in the course of a lengthy infertility evaluation.

## Initial Interview

Every effort should be made to initiate the fertility survey by a joint interview with both partners. The couple should be encouraged to appear together at the initial consultation. This visit provides an excellent opportunity for the physician to explain basic reproductive mechanism, to outline his or her plan of infertility treatment, to allay the apprehension of the couple, and to answer their inquiries.

When a lack of motivation is sensed by the physician or the stability of the marriage is doubtful, the thoughtful physician should point out the need for appropriate marriage or psychiatric counseling before initiating diagnostic or therapeutic measures. The study of infertility should be orderly, meticulous, and comprehensive.

## History

Taking an in-depth and accurate patient history is the most important aspect of the initial patient evaluation. Information elicited from the patient's history should be used to focus the remainder of the infertility evaluation on optimizing the couple's chances of a successful pregnancy. The history should be obtained in an open and unbiased manner. Information regarding patient age, medical problems, medications, previous surgeries, hospitalizations, as well as tobacco use, should be obtained as part of any standard medical history. The gynecologic and obstetrical history should include information regarding menstrual cycle length and regularity, pelvic pain, contraceptive use, hirsutism, galactorrhea, and previous pregnancies and their outcome. A thorough sexual history also should be obtained with information regarding the length of time the couple has been trying to conceive, frequency and timing of coitus, and the use of vaginal lubricants, which may be spermicidal. History of STDs and PIDs also should be discussed. Information concerning the male partner, specifically regarding medical problems, medication use, impotence and ejaculatory dysfunction, history of STDs, and past fertility also should be obtained. Finally, the history should include the details of any previous evaluation and treatment for infertility. When available, past medical records, including clinic visits, endometrial biopsies, surgery reports, and imaging studies, should be reviewed.

## Physical Examination

After obtaining a complete history, a thorough physical examination is required. Special attention needs to be directed toward examination of the thyroid gland, breast, abdomen, and pelvis. The breast should be inspected for masses as well as nipple discharge. Cervical cultures for *N. gonorrhoeae, Chlamydia trachomatis, Mycoplasma hominis,* and *Ureaplasma urealyticum* can be obtained at the time of the initial speculum examination. If the patient is at midcycle and recently has had intercourse, a postcoital test may be performed. The cervix should be inspected for irregularities that may be indicative of previous surgical instrumentation, such as a conization, electrocautery, or cryosurgery that may impair cervical mucus production. A bimanual examination is necessary to evaluate the adnexa and uterus. A rectovaginal examination also should be performed because not infrequently it reveals masses in the posterior cul-de-sac that would have been missed if only a vaginal examination was performed. The skin also should be inspected for signs of hyperandrogenism, such as excessive hair growth and acanthosis nigricans.

In the male partner, in addition to systemic examination, the genital tract should be examined with regard to position, size, and consistency of the testes, status of vas deferens, size and consistency of the prostate, and the presence of varicocele.

# Laboratory and Diagnostic Evaluation

The cornerstone of any infertility evaluation relies on the assessment of six basic elements: (1) semen analysis, (2) ovulation, (3) tubal patency, (4) sperm-cervical mucus interaction, (5) uterine abnormalities, and (6) peritoneal abnormalities. In a recent survey, most board-certified reproductive endocrinologists indicated that as part of their infertility evaluation, they routinely order a semen analysis (99.9%), an assessment of ovulation (98%), a hysterosalpingogram (96%), laparoscopy (89%), and a postcoital test (79%). Less frequently, reproductive endocrinologists use hysteroscopy (53%), pelvic ultrasound (55%), antisperm antibody testing (24%), and cervical cultures for gonorrhea (37%), chlamydia (54%), ureaplasma (26%), and mycoplasma (24%) as part of their routine evaluation. The lack of a consistent standardized approach emphasizes the variability among infertility patients as well as practitioners. For optimal results, the infertility evaluation should be individualized based on each couple's circumstances.

## SEMEN ANALYSIS

A semen analysis is an essential part of the infertility evaluation. It does not make sense to subject the female partner to the risks associated with ovulation induction or invasive procedures before obtaining a semen analysis. Proven paternity or a normal postcoital test does not eliminate the need for a semen analysis. Failure of the male partner to agree to produce a specimen for semen analysis may be an early sign of his lack of motivation for participating in the infertility evaluation. It is customary to have the male abstain from ejaculation for at least 2 days before producing the specimen. Frequent ejaculation can lower sperm counts in some individuals. The specimen routinely is obtained by masturbation and collected in a clean glass or plastic container. If the male partner has difficulty with masturbation, the specimen can be obtained by intercourse using a silicone condom (semen-collecting pouch). Latex condoms are coated with spermicides and are to be avoided. Ideally, the specimen is produced at the same location where it is analyzed. If this arrangement is not possible, the specimen needs to be kept at body temperature during the trip to the laboratory. The World Health Organization (WHO) criteria for a normal semen analysis includes a sperm count greater than 20 million sperm/ml, with at least 50% motility and 30% normal morphology (Table 58–1).

## HYSTEROSALPINGOGRAPHY

Hysterosalpingography (HSG) refers to radiographic visualization of the uterine cavity and lumina of the fallopian tubes after instillation of an opaque contrast medium through the cervical os (Fig. 58–1). Many gynecologists consider HSG to be an integral part of the infertility evaluation, whereas others consider it unnecessary. Drawbacks to performing an HSG are that it is limited to outlining the contour of the uterine cavity and the luminal aspect of the fallopian tubes. For identification of endometriosis and pelvic adhesions, direct visualization of the peritoneal cavity is required. In addition, many patients who undergo HSG ultimately require laparoscopy and/or hysteroscopy. An advantage of performing HSG is that it allows both the gynecologist and the patient to be better informed and prepared for anticipated laparoscopic and hysteroscopic findings. Also, pregnancy rates have been thought to improve after HSG.

The therapeutic benefit of HSG in improving pregnancy rates may be related to a flushing effect created by hydrostatic pressure during the procedure. It is postulated that this could break down intraluminal adhesions and remove obstructing debris. Other proposed reasons suggested for an increase in pregnancy rates after HSG include inhibition of sperm phagocytosis by peritoneal lymphocytes and macrophages, stimulation of tubal ciliary action, and bacteriostatic effects of contrast media. The therapeutic

**Table 58–1** Normal Values of Semen Variables

| Variable | Normal Value |
| --- | --- |
| Volume | 2 ml or more |
| pH | 7.2–8.0 |
| Sperm concentration | $20 \times 10^6$ spermatozoa per ml or more |
| Total sperm count | $40 \times 10^6$ spermatozoa per ejaculate or more |
| Motility | 50% or more with forward progression or 25% or more with rapid progression within 60 minutes of ejaculation |
| Morphology | 30% or more with normal forms |
| Leukocytes | Fewer than $1 \times 10^6$ per ml |
| Immunobead test | Fewer than 20% spermatozoa with adherent particles |
| Mixed Antiglobulin Reaction test | Fewer than 10% spermatozoa with adherent particles |

From World Health Organization: WHO Laboratory Manual for the Examination of Human Semen and Sperm-Cervical Interaction. 3rd ed. New York, Cambridge University Press, 1992.

EVALUATION AND MANAGEMENT OF INFERTILITY   613

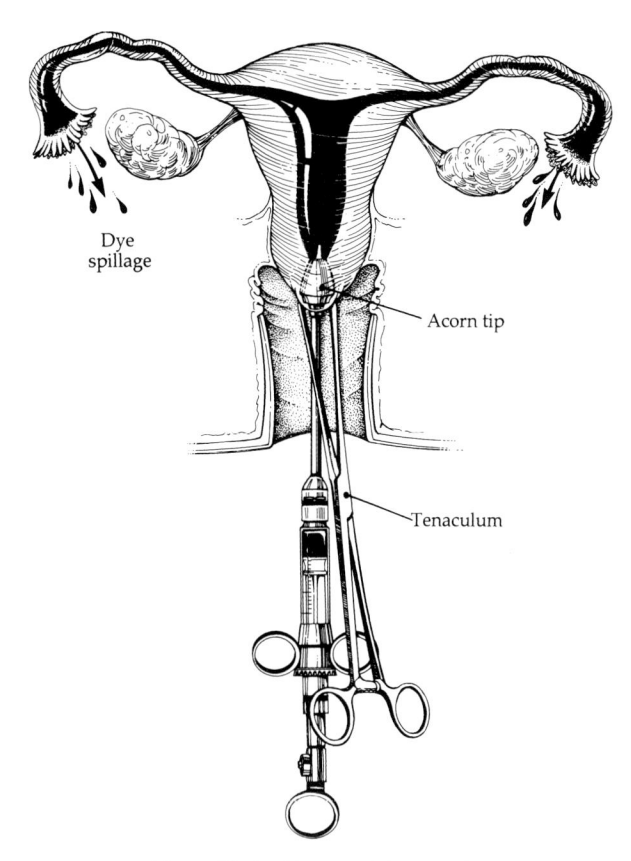

**Figure 58–1** Hysterosalpingography.

effect on pregnancy rates is greater with oil contrast media compared with that of water-soluble contrast media. However, the high viscosity of oil soluble media results in slow filling of the fallopian tubes and often necessitates a delayed film taken 24 hours later to detect and define hydrosalpinx formation and peritubal adhesions. Also, because of slow absorption, oil contrast media are associated with a higher incidence of granuloma formation. Another disadvantage is that the risk of embolization may be increased with the use of oil contrast media if intravasation occurs.

HSG is best performed during the follicular phase of the cycle after cessation of menstrual flow. Performing an HSG during menstruation could propel menstrual blood into the peritoneal cavity by retrograde flow through the fallopian tubes and lead to endometriosis. Performing an HSG after ovulation could unnecessarily expose a developing embryo to contrast media and x-rays. When performing an HSG, 6 to 10 ml of contrast medium is usually sufficient. Nonsteroidal anti-inflammatory drugs taken a few hours before the procedure can decrease discomfort related to distention of the uterus with contrast medium. The contrast medium should be injected slowly to first fill the uterine cavity and then the fallopian tubes. Tubal patency is confirmed by spillage of contrast medium into the peritoneal cavity. If the tubes are dilated, doxycycline 200 mg followed by 100 mg twice a day for 5 days is recommended as prophylaxis against salpingitis. Loculation of contrast medium around the fallopian tubes is suggestive of peritubal adhesions. In general, findings observed on HSG correlate approximately 60 to 70% of the time with those observed at laparoscopy. HSG cannot be used to diagnose peritubal adhesions and underestimates tubal patency when compared with laparoscopic chromopertubation. Plausible explanations include tubal spasm and instillation of insufficient amount of contrast medium into the uterine cavity. In addition to the diagnosis of tubal abnormalities, HSG allows for evaluation of uterine pathology, such as congenital anomalies, leiomyomas, intrauterine adhesions, and endometrial polyps. When abnormalities are identified by HSG, laparoscopy or hysteroscopy is indicated for confirmation and treatment.

## POSTCOITAL TEST

The postcoital test (PCT) is used to assess sperm-cervical mucus interaction after intercourse. The postcoital test frequently is referred to as the Sims-Huhner test and has been part of the basic infertility evaluation over the past 100 years. Despite its long history of popularity, the validity of the PCT in predicting fertility is debatable. In a literature review, Griffith and associates concluded that the PCT lacks validity as a test for infertility. Also, sperm have been recovered from peritoneal fluid in women with poor PCT results. Nevertheless, the PCT is accepted as part of the routine infertility evaluation. It documents whether intravaginal ejaculation has occurred and provides information regarding cervical mucus quality and the ability of sperm to survive in this new environment hours after intercourse.

Mucus in the cervical crypts acts as a reservoir for sperm and facilitates their gradual release into the uterus and fallopian tubes after intercourse. Motile sperm have been found in the cervical mucus up to 7 days after intercourse. Estrogen stimulates increased mucus production from the cervical epithelial cells, which provide a favorable environment for sperm survival. Immediately after menstruation, when estrogen levels are low, the cervical mucus is scant, thick, turbid, and tenacious, qualities that are detrimental for sperm penetration and survival. As ovulation approaches, with increased circulating levels of estrogen, the mucus becomes more profuse and clearer and demonstrates increased elasticity. The elasticity of cervical mucus is referred to as *spinnbarkeit*. Preovulatory cervical mucus is watery and clear and exhibits intense crystallization (ferning) when dried on a microscope slide. Within 1 to 2 days after ovulation, as estrogen levels decline and progesterone levels rise, cervical mucus production again decreases and the mucus becomes thick and cellular, exhibiting little or no spinnbarkeit or ferning and is less favorable for sperm penetration and survival (Fig. 58–2).

For optimal results, the PCT should be performed 1 to 2 days before the predicted time of ovulation, when there is maximum estrogen secretion unopposed by progesterone. The most common reason for an abnormal PCT result is poor timing. For women with 28-day menstrual cycles, the test should be scheduled around day 12 or 13 of the cycle. In women with irregular cycles or an initially abnormal PCT result, it may be necessary to repeat the test at 2-day intervals. Urinary ovulation predictor kits and basal body temperature charts obtained from previous cycles are helpful in predicting ovulation. In anovulatory patients or in women with extremely irregular cycles, the test can be performed after ovulation induction with clomiphene citrate or gonadotropins. However, clomiphene citrate has antiestrogenic effects on cervical mucus, and its use may be associated with abnormal PCT results.

It is customary to ask the couple to abstain from sex for 2 days before having intercourse for the PCT. Disagreement exists pertaining to the number of hours the PCT should be performed after intercourse. Recommendations range from 2 to 24 hours. Because the purpose of the PCT is to assess the reservoir capacity of the cervical mucus, documenting prolonged survivability of the sperm would appear to be justified. We recommend a time span of approxi-

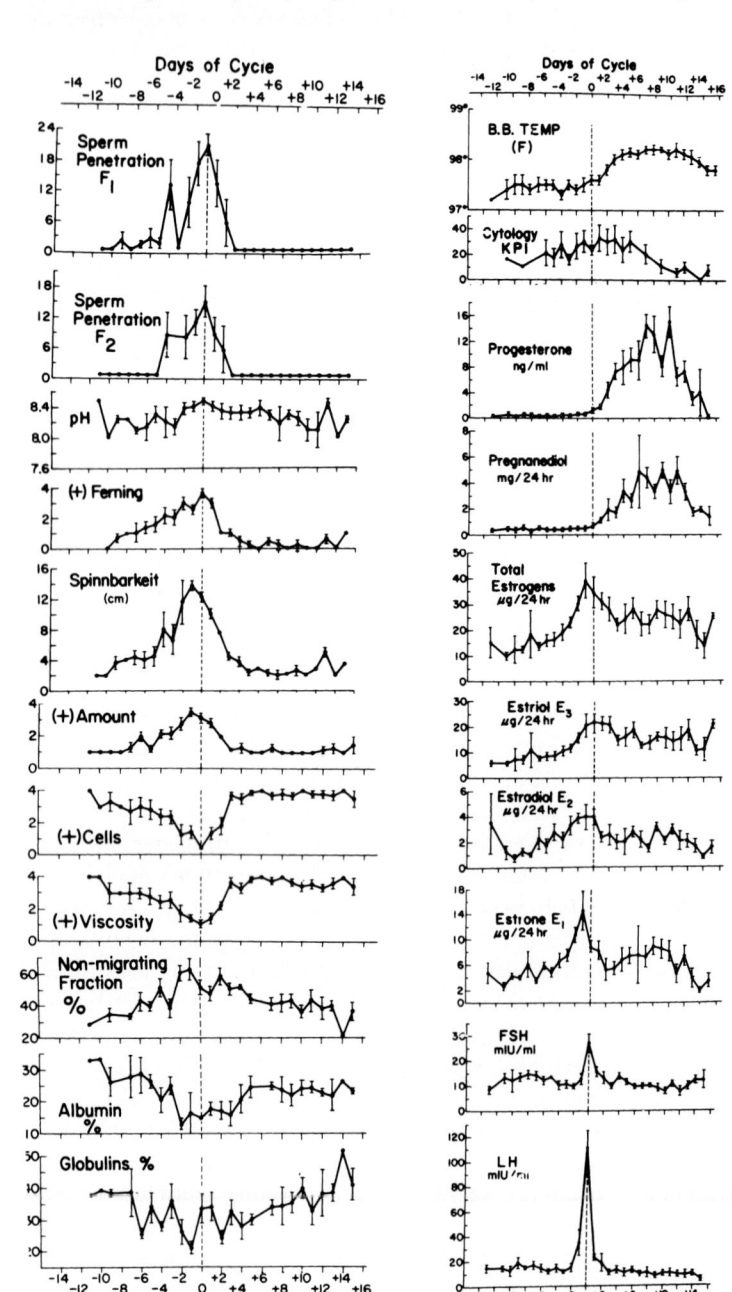

**Figure 58–2** Composite profile of serum gonadotropin and progesterone, urinary estrogens pregnanediol, basal body temperature (BBT), karyopyknotic index (KPI) of vaginal cytology, and cervical mucus properties throughout the menstrual cycle in 10 normal women. Day 0 = day of luteinizing hormone (LH) peak (*dotted line*). Vertical bars represent one standard error of the mean. $F_1$ and $F_2$ indicate the number of sperm in the first and second microscopic fields (200×) from interface, 15 minutes after the start of the in vitro sperm-cervical mucus penetration test. (Data from Moghissi KS, Syner FN, Evans TN: A composite picture of the menstrual cycle. Am J Obstet Gynecol 114:405, 1972.)

mately 8 to 12 hours after intercourse before performing the PCT. This allows for flexibility and enables the couple under normal circumstances to have intercourse anytime during the night before the scheduled PCT.

To perform a PCT, a bivalved speculum lubricated with only warm water should be inserted into the vagina. Lubricants other than water may be spermicidal. The cervical mucus should be obtained from the cervical canal using a pipette, syringe, or mucus forceps. Once the mucus is withdrawn from the cervical canal, it is placed onto a glass slide and covered by a cover slip. The mucus can be tested for its volume, spinnbarkeit, ferning, cellularity viscosity, and pH (Fig. 58–3). To evaluate objectively the properties of cervical mucus, the scoring system recommended by the WHO may be used. Normal ovulatory mucus stretches approximately 8 cm. The pH of the cervical mucus also can be tested at this time. The optimal pH for sperm survival in the cervical mucus ranges between 7.0 and 8.5. The specimen should be examined microscopically first at low-power magnification to find a representative field and then under high-power magnification (400×). Microscopic examination should assess the degree of cellularity, presence of sperm, and their motility, as well as the amount of leukocytes. The presence of a large number of leukocytes in the specimen is suggestive of cervicitis. There is no uniform agreement as to the number of motile sperm per high-powered

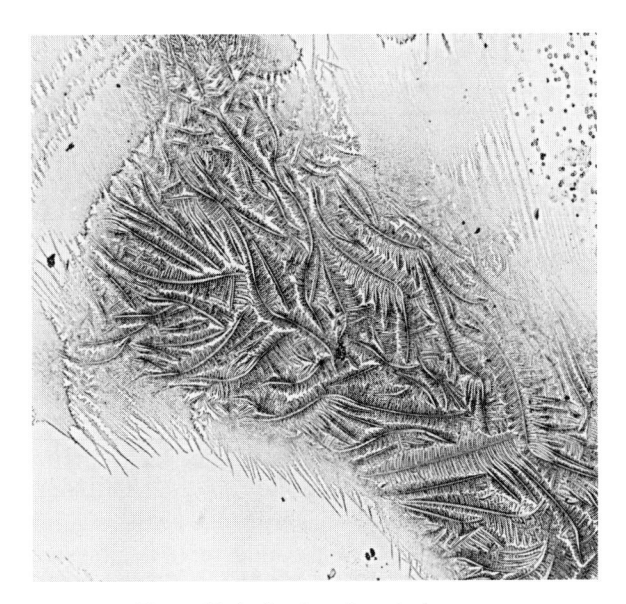

**Figure 58–4** Ferning of cervical mucus.

field (HPF), which should be seen as a prerequisite for a normal postcoital test result and ranges between 1 and 20, depending on the author. More than 10 motile sperm per HPF is considered normal by most authors. Cycle fecundity rates do not correlate with the number of motile sperm per HPF. However, one should remember that the PCT assesses only sperm transport through the cervix rather than anatomic and functional integrity of the entire reproductive tract and cannot be expected to predict pregnancy rate. After the specimen has dried, ferning can be assessed. Ferning represents crystallization of the mucus, which is dependent on the concentration of electrolytes, principally sodium chloride (Fig. 58–4).

## Assessment of Ovulation

Disorders of ovulation are believed to be responsible for infertility in approximately 20 to 25% of women. These disturbances include anovulation with or without oligoamenorrhea, oligo-ovulation, and luteal phase defect. Commonly performed techniques for documentation of ovulation are shown in Table 58–2.

### BASAL BODY TEMPERATURE CHART

The basal body temperature chart is a simple, noninvasive, and inexpensive means to acquire information regarding ovulation and the duration of the luteal phase. Patients are instructed to take their temperature on awaking each morning, before any physical activity. A temperature increase of 0.4° F (0.22° C) for 2 consecutive days is indicative of ovulation. Be-

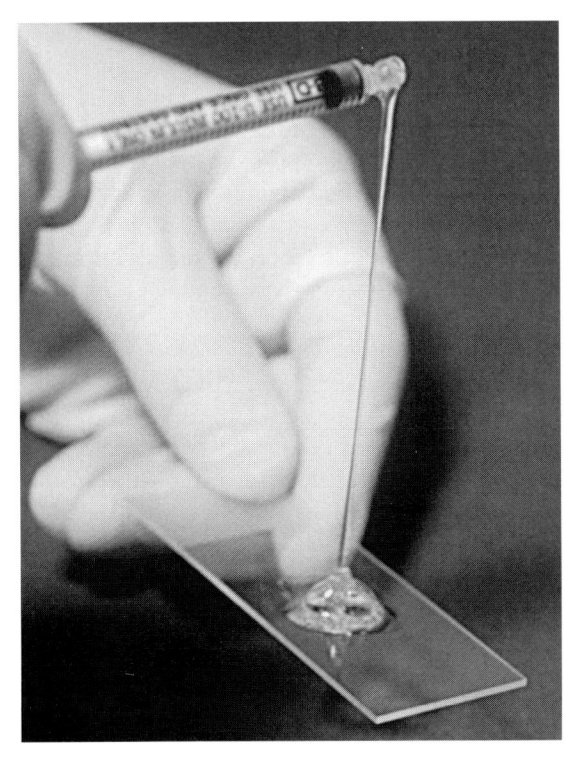

**Figure 58–3** Technique for determining spinnbarkeit (elasticity) of cervical mucus.

**Table 58–2** Methods of Ovulation Detection

Recording of BBT
Assessment of characteristics of cervical mucus (volume, spinnbarkeit, consistency, and ferning)
Testing of urinary LH
Midluteal phase progesterone level
Midluteal phase pregnanediol level
Endometrial biopsy
Serial pelvic ultrasound

BBT, basal body temperature; LH, luteinizing hormone.

cause the expected temperature increase is in the order of decimals of a degree, we recommend using a basal or digital thermometer for easier interpretation. The temperature increase is a function of the thermogenic effect of progesterone on the hypothalmus. The initial rise in serum progesterone may occur anytime between 48 hours before to 24 hours after ovulation. For this reason, an increase in temperature is useful for establishing that ovulation has occurred but should not be used to predict the onset of ovulation in a given cycle. In most women, a biphasic basal body temperature chart is indicative of ovulation, whereas a monophasic basal body temperature chart suggests anovulation or defective corpus luteum function. However, ovulation has been reported to occur in 3 to 12% of women with monophasic basal body temperature charts. Furthermore, ovulation may not occur in some patients with biphasic basal body temperature charts. Once the temperature elevation has occurred, it usually persists for 12 to 14 days. Temperature elevations that are not sustained for at least 11 days are reported to correlate with luteal phase defects. However, approximately 36% of patients with biopsy-confirmed luteal phase defects frequently have sustained temperature elevations for more than 11 days. Therefore, the diagnosis of luteal phase deficiency should rely on histologic dating of the endometrium and not on basal body temperature records.

In addition to recording their temperature each morning, patients should be instructed to mark the days on which they experience bleeding and when intercourse occurs. Reviewing the basal body temperature chart is useful for determining the frequency of intercourse and its relationship to the cycle as well as for scheduling other diagnostic tests, such as the HSG, the PCT, serum progesterone, and endometrial biopsy (Fig. 58–5).

## TESTS BASED ON CERVICAL MUCUS

Secretion of cervical mucus is regulated by ovarian hormones. Estrogen stimulates production of large amounts of thin, watery, alkaline, acellular cervical mucus with intense ferning, spinnbarkeit, and sperm receptivity. Progesterone inhibits the secretory activity of cervical epithelial and produces scanty, viscous, cellular mucus with low spinnbarkeit and absence of ferning, which is impenetrable by spermatozoa.

Changes of various properties of cervical mucus related to gonadotropins and sex steroids during a normal menstrual cycle in 10 women are shown in Figure 58–2.

Changes in the appearance of the cervix and physical properties of cervical mucus form the basis for many tests commonly used to determine the time of ovulation. These include appearance of the cervix, midcycle mucorrhea, crystallization (ferning), spinnbarkeit, and viscosity or consistency of cervical mucus.

Appearance of the cervix varies during the menstrual cycle. In midcycle, the cervix softens progressively, the os dilates, and clear, profuse mucus exudes from the os. Within a few days after ovulation, the cervix becomes firm and the os is closed and covered by scanty, turbid, tenacious mucus. Women who are adequately instructed are able to predict and identify the approximate time of ovulation by recognizing increased midcycle mucus discharge, which occurs around the time of ovulation.

## URINARY LUTEINIZING HORMONE

With the development of monoclonal antibody technology, several kits of dipstick type for rapid assay of urinary luteinizing hormone (LH) have become available. These are based on enzyme immunoassay (EIA) techniques and are designed to be used by the patient at home once or twice per day (morning and evening) beginning approximately 4 days before suspected ovulation. For optimal efficiency in identifying urinary LH surge, twice-daily testing is recommended. There are differences in manufacturer's recommendations regarding the best time of the day for urine testing. For best results, these recommendations should be followed.

It is claimed that these rapid EIAs have an accuracy of greater than 90% to detect the LH surge. These kits currently are used extensively by patients and are recommended by physicians involved in the care of infertile couples for timing of coitus, artificial insemination, PCTs, and the like. However, their efficacy relative to improvement of fecundity rate is doubtful.

## SERUM PROGESTERONE

Of all the methods to detect ovulation, midluteal phase serum progesterone is the one most frequently used by reproductive endocrinologists. A midluteal

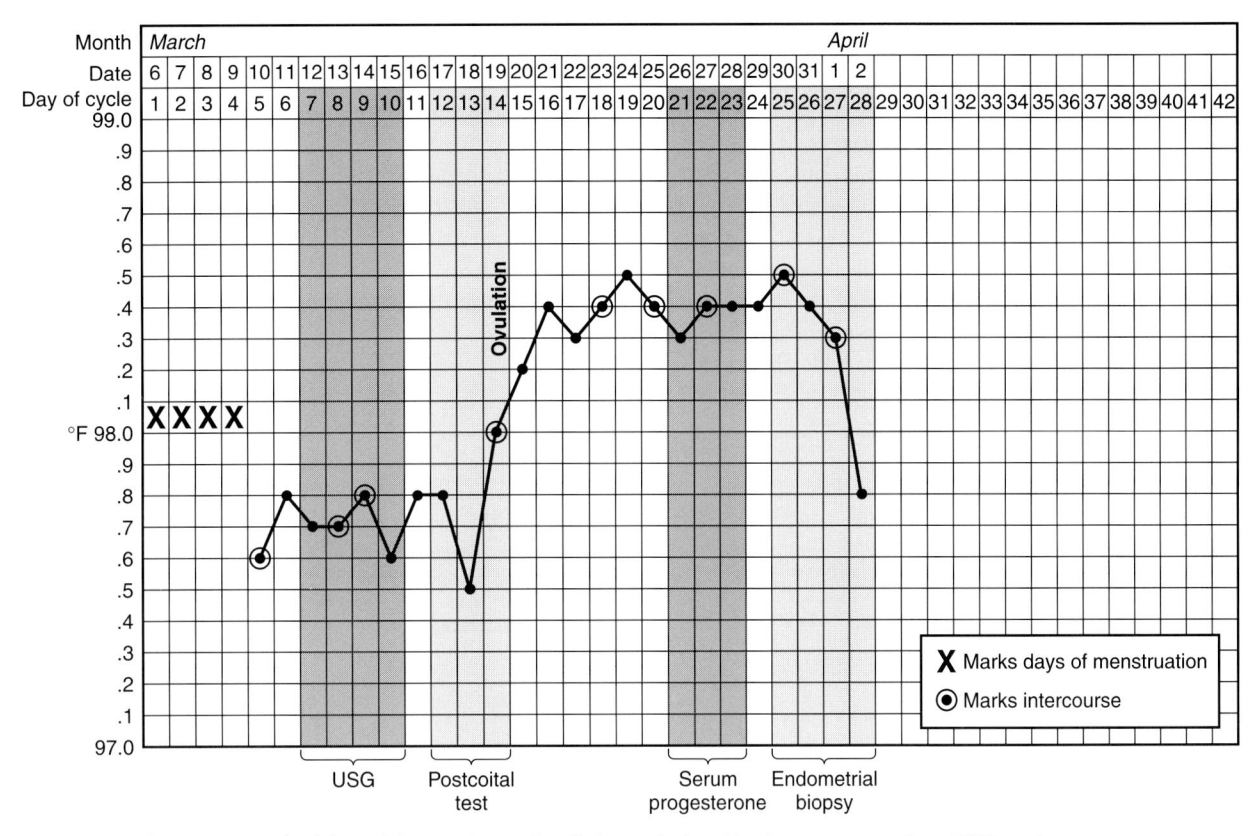

**Figure 58–5** Scheduling of diagnostic tests in relation to the basal body temperature chart. USG = ultrasonography.

phase serum progesterone level of 5 ng/ml or greater is presumptive evidence that ovulation has occurred. Luteal phase serum progesterone levels less than 10 ng/ml are presumed to be associated with luteal phase deficiency. However, this dictum is debatable and should not be relied on. Progesterone is secreted in a pulsatile manner, and normal serum levels are not necessarily indicative of an adequate endometrial response. Therefore, an endometrial biopsy is preferred over a serum progesterone level for diagnosing luteal phase deficiency. If serum progesterone is used, levels should be measured 7 days after estimated ovulation.

Urinary assay of pregnanediol, a metabolite of progesterone, also can aid in ovulation detection. In midluteal phase, pregnanediol levels reach 4 to 6 mg/24 hour. A urinary level of 2 mg or greater is thus consistent with ovulatory cycles (see Fig. 58–2). Assays of urinary pregnanediol 3α glucoronide are also available and may be used for documentation of ovulation.

## ENDOMETRIAL BIOPSY

The endometrial biopsy is performed to evaluate the adequacy of the luteal phase. It gives indirect evidence of ovulation and allows for direct histologic assessment of endometrial responsiveness to circulating levels of estrogens and progesterones. Luteal phase deficiency generally is thought to be secondary to deficiency of progesterone secretion by the corpus luteum but also may be related to an end-organ defect leading to disruption of endometrial maturation. Under normal circumstances, progesterone stimulates endometrial gland maturation and decidual transformation, alterations that support implantation and maintenance of early pregnancy. There should not be more than a 2-day discrepancy between the expected endometrial pattern according to the day on which ovulation occurred and the day of onset of menstruation and the observed endometrial pattern. Basal body temperature charts and urinary ovulation predictor kits are helpful in estimating the day of ovulation. Although the criterion for luteal phase deficiency is controversial, it often is defined as two luteal endometrial biopsies, appropriately dated, that are more than 2 days out of phase. In addition to endometrial dating, the endometrial biopsy may reveal evidence of endometritis, hyperplasia, or malignancy.

The biopsy should be scheduled 2 to 3 days before the expected day of onset of menstruation to allow for full endometrial development. Because the procedure is performed after ovulation in couples who are trying to conceive, there may be concern of interrupting an early pregnancy. The estimated risk of performing an endometrial biopsy during a cycle of conception is about 3 to 5% with a 17% incidence of spontaneous abortion after the biopsy. This figure is similar to the incidence of spontaneous abortion in infertility patients. Nevertheless, if there is concern about the possibility of interrupting an early pregnancy, the couple should abstain from intercourse or use a barrier method of contraception in the cycle during which the biopsy is to be performed. Alternatively, a sensitive pregnancy test can be obtained just before the scheduled biopsy.

## ULTRASONOGRAPHY

Ultrasonography has been described as a rapid, reliable method for monitoring follicular growth, rupture, and regression. This approach provides good presumptive, but not definitive, evidence of ovulation. Transverse and longitudinal scans are performed on both ovaries, and the mean diameter of each follicle is calculated. Ovulation is deemed to have occurred if the follicle reached a mean diameter of 18 to 25 mm and subsequently changed in size, shape, or sonographic density. Accuracy of ovulation timing with this methods is approximately 85%. Potential sources of error consist of the possibility of an oocyte being retained by an apparently ruptured and collapsed follicle and regression of an unruptured follicle, as a result of inappropriate hormonal stimulation.

The introduction of transvaginal ultrasonography has improved considerably the sensitivity of this technique for ovulation detection.

Collectively, the results of studies reported thus far indicate that ultrasonography recording of follicular size is a useful method for timing of ovulation or as a reference for this purpose. However, serial ultrasonographic determination is needed, which may be expensive. Current practice is to use other methods of ovulation timing and to perform two or three ultrasonic measurements of follicular size close to the time of ovulation for confirmation of follicular maturation or collapse.

## OTHER LABORATORY TESTS

In women with irregular menstrual cycles or galactorrhea, it is worthwhile to order serum thyroid-stimulating hormone (TSH) and prolactin levels. Hypothyroidism and hyperprolactinemia can cause ovulatory dysfunction and are readily treatable. Early follicular phase FSH levels are not a routine part of the initial evaluation but should be considered in patients suspected of having poor ovarian reserve. Patients with FSH values of ≥25 IU/L or greater, obtained on either day 2 or 3 of the menstrual cycle, respond poorly to ovulation induction and are unlikely to conceive. Screening for human immunodeficiency virus (HIV), hepatitis, rubella, and syphilis also should be offered to infertility patients. In women suspected of having polycystic ovarian syndrome or hyperandrogenism, serum LH, dehydroepiandrosterone sulfate (DHEAS), 17-hydroxyrogesterone, and testosterone levels are of diagnostic value.

## CERVICAL CULTURES

Cervical cultures can be obtained during the initial visit for *N. gonorrhoeae*, *C. trachomatis*, *M. hominis*, and *U. urealyticum*, all of which have been associated with infertility. Both *N. gonorrhoeae* and *C. trachomatis* can cause salpingitis and fallopian tube damage, leading to infertility. However, the roles of *U. urealyticum* and *M. hominis* in infertility are unclear. *U. urealyticum* has been recovered more frequently from infertile women compared with fertile women and more from spontaneous abortions compared with induced abortions. In addition, *U. urealyticum* is associated with an increased risk of preterm delivery. Whether eradication of *U. urealyticum* with antibiotic therapy enhances fertility and improves pregnancy outcome is in doubt; however, several authors report improvement with treatment. The relationship of *M. hominis* to infertility and pregnancy outcome is even more in doubt. *M. hominis* has been recovered from infertile and fertile women in similar frequencies. However, women who harbor *M. hominis* more often have a history of PID and are more likely to have the presence of *U. urealyticum* and bacterial vaginosis. Bacterial vaginosis has been associated with an increased risk of salpingitis and endometritis.

## LAPAROSCOPY AND HYSTEROSCOPY

Laparoscopy and hysteroscopy are important elements of the infertility evaluation. These procedures are part of the final steps of an infertility investigation and need not be performed until the basic workup is completed. Laparoscopy is necessary to evaluate the peritoneal cavity for endometriosis and pelvic adhesions as well as to verify when tubal disease is suspected by HSG. Hysteroscopy is necessary for confirmation and treatment of intrauterine abnormalities that may have been noted on previous imaging studies, such as HSG. If the patient has not undergone previous imaging studies, a laparoscopy with chromopertubation and hysteroscopy can be performed simultaneously.

# Differential Diagnosis

The differential diagnosis of infertility includes male (35%), pelvic (25%), ovarian (20%), cervical and uterine (10%), and unexplained (10%) factors (Fig. 58–6). The impact of immunologic factors on fertility is controversial. Immunologic-related infertility may result from destruction of gametes by antiovarian or antisperm antibodies. Antibodies also may adversely affect sperm transport, implantation, and cleavage of the embryo.

*Male factor infertility* encompasses conditions in which defects occur in mechanisms of sperm delivery or function, including abnormalities in sperm production and maturation. Conditions that prohibit adequate delivery of sperm include anatomic defects of the penis, erectile dysfunction, and ejaculatory dysfunction. The PCT is useful in documenting delivery of sperm to the cervix. A semen analysis is required, however, to accurately evaluate ejaculate volume and sperm concentration, motility, and morphology. Males with an abnormal semen analysis should undergo an evaluation by a urologist/andrologist to rule out serious medical pathology and identifiable causes of male infertility.

*Pelvic factor infertility* refers to conditions that affect the fallopian tubes, uterus, or peritoneum. Salpingitis is a common cause of tubal factor infertility. Salpingitis damages the tubal mucosa, which is composed of ciliated and secretory cells that aid in gamete transport. As a result of intrinsic tubal damage, tubal occlusion with hydrosalpinx formation often occurs. Appendicitis, ectopic pregnancy, endometriosis, and previous pelvic or abdominal surgery also can damage the fallopian tubes and cause adhesion formation. Peritubal adhesions may hinder the delivery of an oocyte into the tubal ostium, thereby preventing conception. Another condition that is associated with tubal factor infertility is salpingitis isthmica nodosa. This condition is characterized by formation of diverticula in the muscularis of the isthmic portion of the fallopian tube. Characteristically, salpingitis isthmica nodosa appears as intramural outpouchings of contrast medium on HSG (Fig. 58–7). Uterine abnormalities are responsible for infertility in approximately 2% of cases. Congenital deformities of the uterus, leiomyomas, and intrauterine adhesions (Asherman's syndrome) may be causative factors for infertility. Among uterine abnormalities, uterine leiomyomas are the most common. Submucosal myomas can interfere with implantation and lead to pregnancy loss. Intramural leiomyomas that distort the uterine cavity also may adversely affect implantation. Subserosal leiomyomas rarely cause infertility unless they distort the fallopian tube enough to interfere with sperm and oocyte transport. Asherman's syndrome may be associated with amenorrhea or hypomenorrhea. This condition characteristically follows a uterine curettage for abortion, intrauterine infection, myomectomy, metroplasty, or retained placenta. The intrauterine synechiae formation associated with Asherman's syndrome provides an unfavorable environment for implantation.

Endometriosis is a condition in which viable endometrial tissue exists outside of the uterine cavity. Endometriosis may cause pelvic pain and infertility. It is estimated that endometriosis is present in 1 to 7% of women in the United States. Among infertility patients, the prevalence of endometriosis increases to an estimated 30%. All stages of endometriosis have been associated with decreased fecundity rates. It is not entirely clear how endometriosis without tubal or pelvic adhesions impairs fecundity. There is, however, consistent evidence that peritoneal fluid in patients with endometriosis contains increased numbers of activated macrophages. It is thought that these activated macrophages promote cell-mediated cytotoxicity, leading to a progressive inflammatory reaction that inhibits gamete function, as well as early embryonic development and implantation. When endometriosis causes anatomic distortion of the pelvis or fallopian tube obstruction, fecundity rates are likely to be lower. The appearance of endometriosis is variable. Classically, endometriosis presents as a bluish-gray lesion on the ovarian or peritoneal surface. Hemolyzed menstrual blood that becomes encapsulated by fibrotic tissue is responsible for the color. Endometriosis also may appear as nonpigmented, clear vesicles, whitish plaques, or reddish petechiae. In addition, microscopic endometriosis has been identified in up to 6% of infertile women with visually normal-

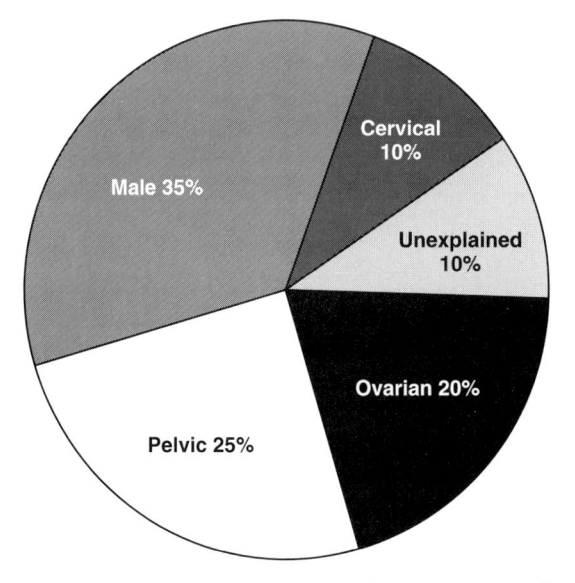

**Figure 58–6** Causes of infertility. (Data from American College of Obstetricians and Gynecologists: Infertility. ACOG Technical Bulletin No. 125. Washington, DC, ACOG, 1989.)

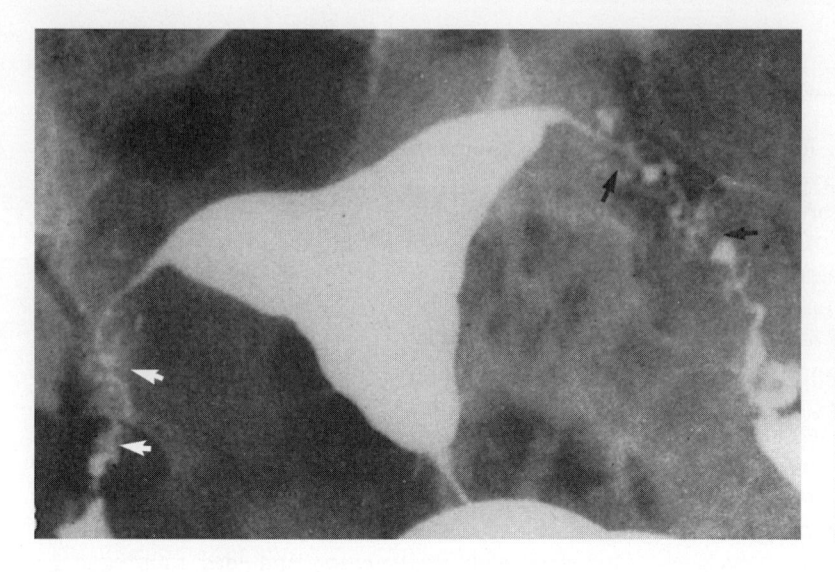

Figure 58–7 Salpingitis isthmica nodosa refers to formation of diverticula in the muscularis of the isthmic portion of the fallopian tube; diverticula characteristically appear as intramural outpouchings of contrast media on a hysterosalpingogram. (Data from Siegler AM: Hysterosalpingography. In Wallach EE, Zacur HA (eds): Reproductive Medicine and Surgery. St. Louis, Mosby–Year Book, 1995, p 501.)

appearing peritoneum. Confirmation of endometriosis relies on histological examination.

*Ovarian factor infertility* should be suspected in patients with irregular cycles, abnormal basal body temperature charts, midluteal phase serum progesterone levels less than 5 ng/ml, or luteal phase defect documented by endometrial biopsy. Ovulatory dysfunction may be intrinsic to the ovaries or secondary to thyroid, adrenal, prolactin, or central nervous system disorders. It is important to inquire about emotional stress, changes in weight, or excessive exercise, all of which can inhibit GnRH secretion from the hypothalamus and result in ovulatory dysfunction. Ovulatory dysfunction is also a common feature of polycystic ovarian syndrome. Classically, patients with polycystic ovarian syndrome present with obesity, hirsutism, oligomenorrhea, and infertility. Luteal phase deficiency also is classified under ovarian dysfunction, although in some patients it is not the result of inadequate ovarian progesterone secretion, but rather a problem with endometrial responsiveness to progesterone. It is estimated that the incidence of luteal phase deficiency in infertile women is between 5 and 10%.

*Cervical factor infertility* is suspected when well-timed PCT results are consistently abnormal in the presence of a normal semen analysis. Cervical factor infertility results from inadequate mucus production by the cervical epithelium, poor mucus quality, or the presence of antisperm antibodies. Previous surgical treatment such as conization for dysplasia may predispose patients to cervical factor infertility. Estrogen deficiency also can adversely affect the production and quality of cervical mucus. Furthermore, bacteria can interfere with mucus production and alter the pH of the cervical mucus so as to hinder sperm survivability. Patients with an abnormal PCT result should be screened for an infectious etiology. The presence of immotile sperm or sperm shaking in place and not demonstrating forward motion in cervical mucus may be associated with immunologic infertility. In vitro sperm-cervical mucus tests and antisperm antibody testing are indicated when appropriately timed PCT results are repeatedly abnormal despite normal-appearing cervical mucus and normal semen analysis.

The term *unexplained infertility* should be used only after a *thorough* infertility investigation has failed to reveal an identifiable source and the duration of infertility is 24 months or longer. The requirements of a *thorough* infertility investigation have never been established. Most protocols include history, physical examination, documentation of ovulation, endometrial biopsy, semen analyses, PTC, HSG, and laparoscopy. Interpretation of the result of these evaluations is critical to determine causality. In addition, couples without an identifiable source of infertility should have cervical cultures obtained for *N. gonorrhoeae, C. trachomatis, M. hominis,* and *U. urealyticum*, as well as immunologic and sperm penetration studies. The true incidence of unexplained infertility is probably less than 5% after a detailed and meticulous investigation has been completed. For many patients, altered ovarian function associated with aging may be the contributing factor to unexplained infertility. It also has been demonstrated that patients with unexplained infertility have subtle defects in their ovulatory function when compared with fertile controls.

# Management of Infertility

Before undergoing therapeutic interventions for infertility, couples as well as physicians must have realistic expectations. Healthy fertile couples who have intercourse regularly without contraception have a 25 to 30% chance of conceiving in a given menstrual cycle. It is difficult to surpass this rate even with aggressive intervention. With the use of assisted reproductive technologies such as in vitro fertilization (IVF), gamete intrafallopian transfer (GIFT), or zygote intrafallopian transfer (ZIFT), the overall pregnancy rate was 24% per cycle in the United States during 1995. Also, because couples with subfertility may conceive on their own, it is difficult to distinguish whether conception is the direct result of infertility treatment. In a study by Collins and associates involving 2198 couples with infertility of greater than 1 year, the cumulative rate of conceptions leading to live birth without treatment was 14, 21, and 25% at intervals of 12, 24, and 36 months, respectively (Fig. 58–8). When subdivided based on infertility diagnosis, the cumulative live birth rate at 36 months without treatment for male, tubal, endometriosis, ovarian, and unexplained factors was 22, 16, 16, 23, and 33%, respectively. Conversely, it is estimated that 85 to 90% of fertile couples will conceive on their own within 12 months (Table 58–3). Because reproductive-age couples are likely to conceive on their own, education and reassurance often is more appropriate than aggressive intervention. Couples may benefit from simply being informed as to the optimal time to have intercourse. In a series of 221 patients, a total of 625 menstrual cycles were followed by Wilcox and associates in which women had intercourse during natural cycles. There were no pregnancies when intercourse occurred the day after ovulation. All conceptions resulted from intercourse that occurred during a 6-day period preceding ovulation, with most conceptions occurring when couples had intercourse within 2 days before ovulation. To optimize timing of ovulation with intercourse, home urine LH kits are of value in predicting ovulation. For couples whose

**Table 58–3** Guttmacher's Classic Data: Normal Time Required for Conception

| Time Period | % Pregnant |
|---|---|
| 3 mo | 57 |
| 6 mo | 72 |
| 12 mo | 85 |
| 24 mo | 93 |

From Guttmacher AF: Factors affecting normal expectancy of conception. JAMA 161:855, 1956.

infertility is due to azoospermia, bilateral tubal obstruction, or prolonged amenorrhea, intervention should not be delayed because it is unlikely that they will conceive on their own. Also, intervention should not be delayed for older couples whose infertility is age-related.

The financial resources and motivation of both partners are important aspects that also need to be considered. Once the decision is made to proceed with an infertility investigation, the workup should be targeted and performed in an efficient manner so that couples are not put through unnecessary testing or inappropriate delays. Undergoing an infertility evaluation can be both emotionally and financially stressful. With appropriate timing, most of an infertility evaluation can be completed within one menstrual cycle.

## Treatment

### MALE FACTOR INFERTILITY

Intrauterine insemination (IUI) frequently is used to treat couples with male factor infertility. Intrauterine insemination refers to the process whereby processed sperm is placed directly into the intrauterine cavity. The objective of IUI is to augment the number of normal motile sperm delivered to the fallopian tube for fertilization of the ovum. Through bypassing the cervix, it is postulated that IUI with processed sperm can enhance fertility in couples with male factor infertility by increasing the concentration of motile sperm delivered to the upper female reproductive tract. Whole fresh semen should not be used for IUI for both proven practical and hypothetical reasons. The typical ejaculate of 2 to 5 ml exceeds the normal uterine capacity. Moreover, prostaglandins present in the ejaculate are potent stimulators of uterine contractions, which can be very painful to the patient. An additional hypothetical advantage of semen processing is to remove dysfunctional or dying sperm from the ejaculate to inseminate with an enriched population of healthy sperm. When performing an IUI approximately, 0.3 to 0.5 ml of prepared sperm

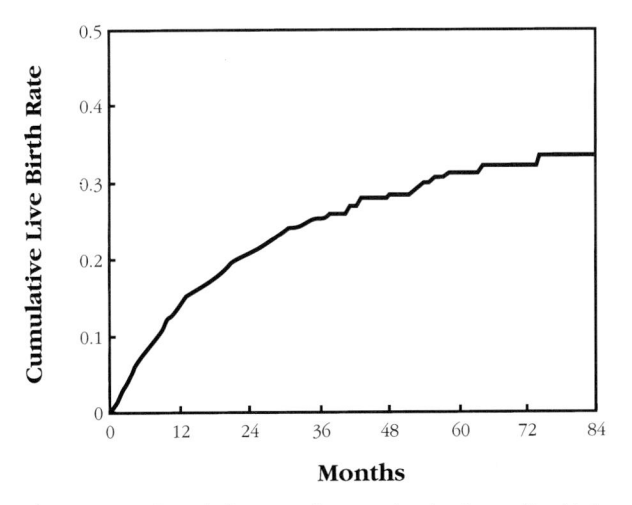

**Figure 58–8** Cumulative rate of conception leading to live births among untreated infertile couples. (From Collins JA, Burrows EA, Willan AR: The prognosis for live birth among untreated infertile couples. Reprinted by permission from the American Society for Reproductive Medicine [Fertil Steril 64:22, 1995].)

is drawn up into the catheter and slowly is injected transcervically into the uterine cavity. Instruments usually used are an Insemi-Cath (Cook Ob/Gyn, Spencer, IN) or a Tomcat catheter (Monoject, St. Louis, MO) fitted unto a 1-ml tuberculin syringe. Injecting volumes greater than 0.5 ml is to be avoided to minimize uterine cramping and sperm expulsion. Intrauterine insemination can be performed during natural or controlled ovarian hyperstimulation (COH) cycles. Agents used to induce COH include clomiphene citrate and human gonadotropin. In COH cycles, multiple eggs are released, which may increase the chance of fertilization; however, the risk of multiple pregnancies is increased. In addition to increasing chances of fertilization, increased secretion of estrogen and progesterone from hyperstimulated ovaries may help overcome subtle defects of ovulatory function.

Intrauterine insemination performed during unstimulated cycles for the treatment of male factor infertility is not recommended because pregnancy rates are relatively low, only between 3 to 6% per cycle. The addition of clomiphene citrate, in conjunction with IUI for the treatment of male factor infertility, is of little value with pregnancy rates of only 3 to 4% per cycle. However, ovulation induction with gonadotropins in conjunction with IUI does significantly increase pregnancy rates. Success rates for achieving pregnancy are between 7 to 14% per cycle when IUI is performed in conjunction with human menopausal gonadotropin (hMG)–stimulated cycles. The superiority of ovulation induction with gonadotropins in IUI cycles most likely is related to the increased number of oocytes available for fertilization as well as better control and predictability of ovulation. Therefore, to maximize results for males with impaired semen parameters, IUI should be performed in conjunction with ovulation induction using gonadotropins. However, in patients with severe oligoasthenozoospermia (sperm counts less than 5 million/ml or when linear progressive motility is 20% or less), ovulation induction combined with IUI is unlikely to lead to pregnancy. Such patients with severely impaired semen parameters are candidates for more advanced reproductive technologies, such as IVF or IVF combined with intracytoplasmic sperm injection (ICSI).

In vitro fertilization, alone or combined with ICSI, has changed dramatically the treatment of male factor infertility over the past decade. Previously, couples with severe male factor infertility refractory to treatment had to rely on donor sperm. For men with obstructive azoospermia, sperm now can be obtained by epididymal aspiration or testicular biopsy and used for ICSI.

For those couples who do not wish or cannot afford to have IVF, therapeutic donor insemination using properly screened frozen semen may be offered as an alternative to IVF.

## PELVIC FACTOR

The mainstay of treatment of pelvic factor infertility relies on laparoscopy and hysteroscopy. In many instances, tubal reconstructive surgery, lysis of adhesions, ablation, and resection of endometriosis can be accomplished laparoscopically. Endometrial polyps, submucosal myomas, and intrauterine adhesions can be resected hysteroscopically. Only rarely is a laparotomy necessary. Reconstructive tubal procedures include neosalpingostomy, fimbrioplasty, salpingolysis, and tuboplasty. Neosalpingostomy involves the surgical creation of an opening in the distal end of a fallopian tube. Fimbrioplasty entails lysis of adhesions between fimbrial folds. Salpingolysis refers to division of adhesions around a fallopian tube. Tuboplasty is a broad term that refers to any reconstructive procedure involving a fallopian tube. Candidates for tuboplasty should be selected carefully, and the operation should be performed by a knowledgeable surgeon using modern microsurgical techniques.

The goal of tubal surgery is to restore tubal patency and normal tubo-ovarian anatomy. The single most important prognostic factor in pregnancy outcome after tubal reconstructive surgery is the functional integrity of the tube. Pregnancy rates are inversely proportional, and ectopic rates are directly proportional to the extent of tubal disease. Crude pregnancy rates after neosalpingostomy vary depending on the study, most often ranging from 20 to 40%, with a 10 to 30% incidence of ectopic pregnancies. Crude pregnancy rates after fimbrioplasty are estimated at 35 to 72%, with a 7 to 10% incidence of ectopic pregnancies. Lysis of periadnexal adhesions also improves pregnancy rates. Overall, pregnancy rates are low for patients with severe tubal disease despite tubal reconstructive surgery, probably because of irreparable intrinsic tubal damage. Patients with bilateral salpingitis isthmica nodosa and infertility without any other identifiable cause are candidates for tubal resection and anastomosis. From a cost-effectiveness standpoint, IVF is superior to tubal reconstructive surgery for patients with severe tubal disease. Thus, patients with severe tubal disease should be offered IVF as the primary approach instead of tubal reconstructive surgery. Also, patients who have persistent infertility after tubal reconstructive surgery are likely to benefit from IVF. More than 70% of women with tubal factor infertility have a live birth within four cycles of treatment with IVF.

Hormonal therapy for endometriosis-related infertility is inappropriate. Although hormonal therapy relieves symptoms of pelvic pain, there is no evidence that such treatment is beneficial in women with endometriosis-associated infertility. Convincing evidence for the efficacy of surgical therapy of infertility associated with minimal to mild endometriosis also is lacking. However, a recent multicenter study using laparoscopically performed laser ablation or cauterization of endometrial implants suggests improved pregnancy rates. It is also debatable whether a relationship exists between the stage of endometriosis and pregnancy rates after treatment. A study conducted by the American Society for Reproductive Medicine found no significant differences in pregnancy rates after treatment among patients with minimal, mild, moderate, or severe endometriosis. Surgical treatment includes coagulation, laser vaporization, and resection. As an adjunct in the treatment of endometriosis, ovulation induction with gonadotropins followed by intrauterine insemination increases fecundity rates to an estimated 12 to 17%.

Uterine abnormalities such as endometrial polyps, submucosal myomas, synechiae, and septa can be resected hysteroscopically. Patients with severe uterine abnormalities refractory to treatment are candidates for a surrogate uterus.

## OVARIAN FACTOR

Clomiphene citrate is the first line of therapy for patients with ovulatory dysfunction because of its low cost, oral route, and lower rate of multiple pregnancies compared with injectable gonadotropin therapy. It should be used only after other identifiable factors that can affect ovulatory function have been excluded or treated, such as hypothyroidism, hyperprolactinemia, and adrenal hyperplasia. In most cases, ovulatory function returns once these other causes are treated. Clomiphene citrate is a nonsteroidal agent that is weakly estrogenic and works primarily by competing with endogenous estrogens at hypothalamic estrogen receptor sites. By displacing endogenous estrogens with a weaker estrogen compound at the receptor site, clomiphene citrate functions as an antiestrogen. Clomiphene citrate alleviates the negative feedback effect exerted by endogenous estrogen at the hypothalamic level thereby increasing GnRH release and, subsequently, gonadotropin release. Clomiphene citrate also has pharmacologic effects on targets other than the hypothalamus, including the pituitary, ovaries, endometrium, cervix, and fallopian tubes. Its antiestrogenic properties may be detrimental to implantation and production of cervical mucus. The use of clomiphene citrate requires the presence of an intact hypothalamic-pituitary axis capable of eliciting normal ovarian function and ovaries that contain follicles. The recognition of endogenous ovarian estrogen production is a favorable sign for a positive ovulation response to clomiphene citrate. Clomiphene citrate usually is started at a dose of 50 mg/day during days 5 to 9 of the cycle. Ovulation is expected between 7 to 10 days after the last dose of clomiphene citrate. Ovulation on a specified dosage of clomiphene citrate should be confirmed with either a midluteal phase serum progesterone assay, basal body temperature increase, pelvic ultrasonography, endometrial biopsy, or urinary ovulatory predictor kits. If ovulation does not occur with a specified dose of clomiphene citrate, the dose can be increased by 50-mg increments per day in subsequent cycles. The maximum dose of clomiphene citrate should not exceed 250 mg per day. The addition of dexamethasone has been advocated for women who remain anovulatory despite high doses of clomiphene citrate. Adrenal androgen production, which may be detrimental to ovarian follicular development, is suppressed by dexamethasone therapy. Traditionally, dexamethasone therapy has been reserved for clomiphene-resistant patients with elevated DHEAS levels. However, a 10-day course of 0.5 mg of oral dexamethasone initiated concurrently with a 5-day course of clomiphene citrate has been reported to improve pregnancy rates in anovulatory women with normal DHEAS levels who previously were resistant to clomiphene citrate. The rationale for this observation may be that dexamethasone itself enhances follicular development independent of adrenal androgen suppression. An extended course of clomiphene citrate, 100 mg daily on cycle days 3 to 12, also has been recommended for patients who fail to ovulate on conventional regimens. As an alternative to dexamethasone, prednisone given 5 mg orally each night throughout the cycle, combined with an extended course of clomiphene citrate (100 to 150 mg on cycle days 3 through 9) is reported to be efficacious in patients resistant to clomiphene citrate alone. Clomiphene citrate also can be combined with human chorionic gonadotropin (hCG) 7 days after the last dose of clomiphene citrate or, preferably, when ultrasound reveals a follicle of 22 to 24 mm in diameter. Side effects of clomiphene citrate include hot flushes (10%), abdominal bloating or pain (5.5%), nausea and vomiting (2.2%), visual disturbances (1.5%), headaches (1.3%), and dryness or loss of hair (0.3%). The incidence of multiple gestations with clomiphene citrate is 5 to 10%. Approximately 33% of anovulatory patients treated with clomiphene citrate become pregnant within five cycles of therapy. Treatment with clomiphene citrate for more than six ovulatory cycles is not recommended because of low success rates. For women with normal ovulatory function, clomiphene citrate is not efficacious and therefore not recommended.

Human gonadotropins also are used for controlled ovarian hyperstimulation. Compared with clomiphene citrate, pregnancy rates with gonadotropin therapy for management of anovulatory infertility are higher, at an estimated 25% per cycle. This is most likely the result of recruitment of more follicles with gonadotropin therapy. Human gonadotropins consist of FSH and LH. Until recently, all human gonadotropins were prepared from pooled urine specimens collected from postmenopausal women (hMG). Highly purified and recombinant FSH are currently available. Before starting a patient on gonadotropins, a baseline ultrasound is recommended to rule out ovarian follicular cyst, which may hinder follicular development. In addition, a baseline serum estradiol concentration should be obtained on day 2 or 3 of the cycle. If there are no follicular cysts greater than 10 mm and the estradiol concentration is less than 50 pg/ml, gonadotropins are started on day 3 of the menstrual cycle. The customary starting dose of gonadotropin (hMG or FSH) is 150 IU per day. Most patients require between 7 to 12 days of gonadotropins. Estradiol levels are monitored during the cycle. Estradiol levels usually are checked on the fourth, sixth, and eighth day after initiation of gonadotropin therapy. Optimal estradiol concentrations on the fourth, sixth, and eighth day of gonadotropins range from 100 to 200, 400 to 600, and 800 to 1200 pg/ml, respectively. The dosage of gonadotropins is adjusted according to the ovarian response. When the estradiol concentration reaches 600 pg/ml, a follow-up ultrasound is performed. hCG is administered intramuscularly when a single follicle or multiple follicles have reached 17 mm or greater in diameter. The usual dose of hCG is 10,000 IU. If there is concern of ovarian hyperstimulation, hCG is withheld, or only 5000 IU are prescribed. Patients are instructed to either have intercourse or intrauterine insemination performed 34 to 36 hours after the hCG injection. Progesterone frequently is prescribed for luteal phase support. A serum β-hCG determination is obtained 16 to 18 days after timed intercourse or intrauterine insemination.

The incidence of multiple gestations with hMG therapy is 25 to 30%. The increased incidence of multiple gestation is secondary to the recruitment of large numbers of follicles, all of which have the potential to become fertilized. In the event that stimulation has produced a large cohort of mature follicles, it may be appropriate to convert from IUI or timed intercourse to IVF or GIFT in an attempt to control for multiple gestations. Patients who receive gonadotropin therapy also have an estimated 1% risk of developing ovarian hyperstimulation syndrome. Extra caution is needed in patients with polycystic ovarian syndrome because they are highly sensitive to gonadotropins and are at increased risk of developing ovarian hyperstimulation and having multiple pregnancies. In addition to risks of ovarian hyperstimulation and multiple gestations, several reports have suggested an association between ovulation induction and ovarian cancer. However, infertility alone is an independent risk factor for the development of ovarian cancer. A recent case-control study by Mosgaard and associates found that ovulation induction did not increase the risk of ovarian cancer, and infertility without medical treatment increased the risk of ovarian cancer even further.

The beneficial effect of treating luteal phase deficiency is controversial. Although the existence of luteal phase deficiency is not in doubt, it is debatable whether this condition causes infertility. Luteal phase deficiency occurs in fertile women but more frequently in infertile women, and treatment is not always advantageous. Nevertheless, when an infertile patient has a documented luteal phase deficiency, it is reasonable to offer treatment. Progesterone is the standard treatment and usually is prescribed as an intravaginal suppository at a dose of 25 mg twice a day. Progesterone also can be administered as a vaginal gel or intramuscularly. Progesterone is continued until the projected luteoplacental shift occurs at approximately 8 to 10 weeks' gestation. Clomiphene citrate has been used as an alternative approach for luteal phase deficiency, with efficacy similar to progesterone. hCG and ovulation induction with hMG or FSH also may be used to overcome luteal phase defects secondary to inadequate corpus luteum secretion of progesterone.

Women with ovulatory dysfunction secondary to ovarian failure or poor ovarian reserve should consider obtaining oocytes from a donor source. Donated oocytes can be fertilized in vitro with the partner's sperm, followed by embryo transfer into the recipient's uterus.

## CERVICAL FACTOR

Patients with *N. gonorrhoeae* or *C. trachomatis* should be treated with appropriate antibiotic therapy in an attempt to avoid permanent damage to the fallopian tubes. Although the roles of *U. urealyticum* and *M. hominis* in infertility are controversial, a positive culture warrants treatment with doxycycline or tetracycline. Patients with scanty cervical mucus were treated in the past with estrogen, expectorants such as guaifenesin, and precoital alkaline douches with sodium bicarbonate. The efficacy of these agents in improving pregnancy outcome has never been confirmed. Gonadotropin therapy, as a result of increased ovarian estrogen secretion, improves cervical mucus production and quality and is associated with higher fecundity rates. The higher fecundity rates associated with gonadotropin therapy likely are more dependent on the recruitment of multiple ovarian follicles than on improvement in cervical mucus quality. Intrauterine insemination, which bypasses the cervical barrier, presently is the mainstay of treatment for cervical factor infertility, including patients with cervical mucus antisperm antibodies. For patients with cervical factor infertility, fecundity rates are estimated to be 5 to 6% when IUI is performed during natural cycles. When IUI is combined with gonadotropin therapy, fecundity rates markedly improve to an estimated 26 to 30% per cycle. Clomiphene citrate as an adjunct for the treatment of cervical factor infertility is not beneficial.

## Conclusion

Providers who offer infertility treatment must be well versed in diagnostic and treatment modalities. Infertile couples must receive impartial and realistic advice so that no false expectations or hopes are given. Couples should be informed of the anticipated benefits of treatment intervention as well as the likelihood of not conceiving. In most instances, couples will conceive without the need of assisted reproductive technologies such as IVF or GIFT. However, couples whose chances of conceiving by conventional means are remote or who fail treatment should be referred promptly to an infertility specialist. Provided infertile couples without gametes are willing to accept donated gametes and women without a functional uterus are willing to use a surrogate, all couples, regardless of their cause of infertility, can be offered treatment.

## REFERENCES

Adamson GD, Pasta DJ: Surgical treatment of endometriosis-associated infertility: Meta-analysis compared with survival analysis. Am J Obstet Gyneol 171:1488, 1994.

Adelusi B, Al-Nuaim L, Makanjoula D, et al: Accuracy of hysterosalpingography and laparoscopic hydrotubation in diagnosis of tubal patency. Fertil Steril 63:1016, 1995.

American Fertility Society. Investigation of the Infertile Couple. Birmingham, AL, American Fertility Society, 1991.

American Society for Reproductive Medicine. Age Related Infertility. Guidelines for Practice, American Society for Reproductive Medicine, 1995.

Aribarg A, Sukcharoen N: Intrauterine insemination of washed spermatozoa for treatment of oligozoospermia. Int J Androl 18:62, 1995.

Arici A, Byrd W, Bradshaw K, et al: Evaluation of clomiphene citrate and human chorionic gonadotropin treatment: A prospective, randomized, crossover study during intrauterine insemination cycles. Fertil Steril 61:314, 1994.

Balasch J, Fabregues F, Creus M, et al: The usefulness of endometrial biopsy for luteal phase evaluation in infertility. Hum Reprod 7:973, 1992.

Barad DH: Work-up of the infertile woman. Infertil Reprod Med Clin North Am 2:255–453, 1991.

Barbieri RL: Etiology and epidemiology of endometriosis. Am J Obstet Gynecol 162:565, 1990.

Batista MC, Cartledge TP, Zellmer AW, et al: A prospepctive controlled study of luteal and endometrial anbormalities in an infertile population. Fertil Steril 65:495, 1996.

Benadiva CA, Kligman I, Davis O, et al: In vitro fertilization versus tubal surgery: Is pelvic reconstructive surgery obsolete? Fertil Steril 64:1051, 1995.

Blacker CM, Ginsburg KA, Leach RE, et al: Unexplained infertility: Evaluation of the luteal phase. Results of the National Center for Infertility Research at Michigan. Fertil Steril 67:437, 1997.

Boyers SP: Evaluation and treatment of disorders of the cervix. In Keye WR, Chang JR, Rebar RW, Soules MR (eds): Infertility Evaluation and Treatment. Philadelphia, WB Saunders, 1995, p 195.

Bristow RE, Karlan BY: Ovulation induction, infertility, and ovarian cancer risk. Fertil Steril 66:499, 1996.

Bush MR, Walmer DK, Couchman GM, et al: Evaluation of the postcoital test in cycles involving exogenous gonadotropins. Obstet Gynecol 89:780, 1997.

Chaffkin LM, Nulsen JC, Luciano AA, et al: A comparative analysis of the cycle fecundity rates associated with combined human menopausal gonadotropin (hMG) and intrauterine insemination (IUI) versus either hMG or IUI alone. Fertil Steril 55:252, 1991.

Collins JA, Burrows EA, Willan AR: The prognosis for live birth among untreated infertile couples. Fertil Steril 64:22, 1995.

Crosignani PG: The defective luteal phase. Hum Reprod 3:157, 1988.

Crosignani PG, Rubin B: Guidelines to the prevalence, diagnosis, treatment and management of infertility. Hum Reprod 11:1775, 1996.

ESHRE Capri Workshop Group on ovulatory infertility. Hum Reprod 10:1549–1553, 1995.

Friberg J: Mycoplasmas and ureaplasmas in infertility and abortion. Fertil Steril 33:351, 1980.

Friedman A, Haas S, Kredentser J, et al: A controlled trial of intrauterine insemination for cervical factor and male factor: A preliminary report. Int J Fertil 34:199, 1989.

Fujii S, Fukui A, Fukushi Y, et al: The effects of clomiphene citrate on normal ovulatory women. Fertil Steril 68:1997, 1997.

Garcia C, Freeman EW, Rickels K, et al: Behavioral and emotional factors and treatment responses in a study of anovulatory infertile women. Fertil Steril 44:478, 1985.

Glatstein IZ, Harlow BL, Hornstein MD: Practice patterns among reproductive endocrinologists: The infertility evaluation. Fertil Steril 67:443, 1997.

Gnarpe H, Friberg J: Mycoplasma and human reproductive failure. Am J Obstet Gynecol 114:727, 1972.

Gregoriou O, Vitoratos C, Papadias C, et al: Pregnancy rates in gonadotropin stimulated cycles with timed intercourse or intrauterine insemination for the treatment of male subfertility. Eur J Obstet Gynecol Reprod Biol 64:213, 1996.

Griffith CS, Grimes DA: The validity of the postcoital test. Am J Obstet Gynecol 162:615, 1990.

Gruppo italiano per lo studio dell'endometriosi: Prevalence and anatomical distribution of endometriosis in women with selected gynaecological condition: Results from a multicentric Italian study. Hum Reprod 9:1158, 1994.

Guttmacher AF: Factors affecting normal expectancy of conception. JAMA 161:855, 1956.

Guzick DS, Silliman NP, Adamson GD, et al: Prediction of pregnancy in infertile women based on the American Society for Reproductive Medicine's revised classification of endometriosis. Fertil Steril 67:822, 1997.

Hammond MG, Talbert L: Infertility, A Practical Guide for Physicians. Boston, Blackwell Scientific, 1992.

Healy DL, Schenken RS, Lynch A, et al: Pulsatile progesterone secretion: Its relevance to clinical evaluation of corpus luteum function. Fertil Steril 41:114, 1984.

Hensleigh PA, Fainstat T: Corpus luteum dysfunction: serum progesterone levels in diagnosis and assessment of therapy for recurrent and threatened abortion. Fertil Steril 32:396, 1979.

Hillier SL, Kiviat NB, Hawes SE, et al: Role of bacterial vaginosis-associated microorganisms in endometritis. Am J Obstet Gynecol 175:435, 1996.

Hirama Y, Ochiai K: Estrogen and progesterone receptors of the out-of-phase endometrium in female infertile patients. Fertil Steril 63:984, 1995.

Ho PC, So WK, Chan YF, et al: Intrauterine insemination after ovarian stimulation as a treatment for subfertility because of subnormal semen: A prospective randomized controlled trial. Fertil Steril 58:995, 1992.

Huang KE: The primary treatment of luteal phase inadequacy: Progesterone versus clomiphene citrate. Am J Obstet Gynecol 155:4, 1986.

Hughes EG, Fedorkow DM, Collins JA: A quantitative overview of controlled trials in endometriosis-associated infertility. Fertil Steril 59:963, 1993.

Hughes EG, Brennan BG: Does cigarette smoking impair natural or assisted fecundity? Fertil Steril 66:679, 1996.

Isaacs JD, Lincoln SR, Cowan BD: Extended clomiphene citrate (CC) and prednisone for the treatment of chronic anovulation resistant to clomiphene citrate alone. Fertil Steril 67:641, 1997.

Jansen RPS: Spontaneous abortion incidence in the treatment of infertility. Am J Obstet Gynecol 143:196, 1982.

Jewelewicz R, Wallach EE: Evaluation of the infertile couple. In Wallach EE, Zacur HA (eds): Reproductive Medicine and Surgery. St. Louis, Mosby–Year Book, 1995, p 363.

Johannson EDB, Larsson-Cohn U, Gemzell C: Monophasic basal body temperature in ovulatory menstrual cycles. Am J Obstet Gynecol 113:933, 1972.

Jones HWR Jr, Toner JP: The infertile couple. N Engl J Med 329:1710, 1993.

Kalugdan T, Chan PJ, Seraj IM, et al: Polymerase chain reaction enzyme-linked immunosorbent assay detection of mycoplasma consensus gene in sperm with low oocyte penetration capacity. Fertil Steril 66:793, 1996.

Karamardian LM, Grimes DA: Luteal phase deficiency: Effect of treatment on pregnancy rates. Am J Obstet Gynecol 167:1391, 1992.

Kirby CA, Flaherty SP, Godfrey BM, et al: A prospective trial of intrauterine insemination of motile spermatozoa versus timed intercourse. Fertil Steril 56:102, 1991.

Kundsin RB, Leviton A, Allred E, et al: *Ureaplasma urealyticum* infection of the placenta in pregnancies that ended prematurely. Obstet Gynecol 87:122, 1996.

Kurman RJ, Mazur MT: Benign diseases of the endometrium. In Kurman RJ (ed): Blaustein's Pathology of the Female Genital Tract. 3rd ed. New York, Springer-Verlag, 1987, p 302.

Luber K, Beeson CC, Kennedy JF, et al: Results of microsurgical treatment of infertility and early tubal second-look laparoscopy in the post-pelvic inflammatory disease patient: Implications for in vitro fertilization. Am J Obstet Gynecol 154:1264, 1986.

Luciano AA, Peluso J, Koch E, et al: Temporal relationship and reliability of the clinical, hormonal, and ultrasonographic indices of ovulation in infertile women. Obstet Gynecol 75:412, 1990.

Mardh P, Elshibly S, Kallings I, et al: Vaginal flora changes associated with *Mycoplasma hominis*. Am J Obstet Gynecol 176:173, 1997.

Martinez AR, Bernardus RE, Voorhost FJ, et al: Pregnancy rates after timed intercourse or intrauterine insemination after human menopausal gonadotropin stimulation of normal ovulatory cycles: A controlled study. Fertil Steril 55:258, 1991.

McNeely MJ, Soules MR: The diagnosis of luteal phase deficiency: A critical review. Fertil Steril 50:1, 1988.

Moghissi KS: Cervical and uterine factors in infertility. Obstet Gynecol Clin North Am 14:887–904, 1987.

Moghissi KS, Syner FN, Evans TA: A composite picture of the menstrual cycle. Am J Obstet Gynecol 114:405, 1972.

Mosgaard BJ, Lidegaard O, Kjaer SK, et al: Infertility, fertility drugs, and invasive ovarian cancer: A case-controlled study. Fertil Steril 67:1005, 1997.

Murray DL, Reich L, Adashi EY: Oral clomiphene citrate and vaginal progesterone suppositories in the treatment of luteal phase dysfunction: A comparative study. Fertil Steril 51:35, 1989.

Nulsen JC, Walsh S, Dumez S, et al: A randomized and longitudinal study of human menopausal gonadotropin with intrauterine insemination in the treatment of infertility. Obstet Gynecol 82:780, 1993.

Olive DL, Schwartz LB: Endometriosis. N Engl J Med 328:1759, 1993.

Olive DL, Martin DC: Treatment of endometriosis-associated infertility with $CO_2$ laser laparoscopy: The use of one- and two-parameter exponential models. Fertil Steril 48:18, 1987.

Oral E, Arici A, Olive DL, et al: Peritoneal fluid from women with moderate or severe endometriosis inhibits sperm motility: The role of seminal fluid components. Fertil Steril 66:787, 1996.

Pearlstone AC, Fournet N, Gambone JC, et al: Ovulation induction in women age 40 and older: The importance of basal follicle-stimulating hormone level and chronological age. Fertil Steril 58:674, 1992.

Perloff WH, Steinberger E: In vivo survival of spermatozoa in cervical mucus. Am J Obstet Gynecol 88:439, 1964.

Pittaway DE, Winfield AC, Maxson W, et al: Prevention of acute pelvic inflammatory disease after hysterosalpingography: Efficacy of doxycycline prophylaxis. Am J Obstet Gynecol 147:623, 1983.

Quagliarello J, Arny M: Incracervical versus intrauterine insemination: Correlation of outcome with antecedent postcoital testing. Fertil Steril 46:870, 1986.

Rana N, Braun DP, House R, et al: Basal and stimulated secretion of cytokines by peritoneal macrophages in women with endometriosis. Fertil Steril 65:925, 1996.

Rasmussen F, Lindequist S, Larsen C, et al: Therapeutic effect of hysterosalpingography: Oil- versus water-soluble contrast media—A randomized prospective study. Radiology 179:75, 1991.

Risi GF Jr, Sanders CV: The genital mycoplasmas. Obstet Gynecol Clin North Am 16:611, 1989.

Schlaff WD, Hassiakos DK, Damewood MD, et al: Neosalpingostomy for distal tubal obstruction: Prognostic factors and impact of surgical technique. Fertil Steril 54:984, 1990.

Shushan A, Eisenberg VH, Schenker JG: Subfertility in the era of assisted reproduction: Changes and consequences. Fertil Steril 64:459, 1995.

Shushan A, Palteil O, Iscovich J, et al: Human menopausal gonadotropin and the risk of epithelial ovarian cancer. Fertil Steril 65:13, 1996.

Siegler AM: Hysterosalpingography. In Wallach EE, Zacur HA (eds): Reproductive Medicine and Surgery. St. Louis, Mosby–Year Book, 1995, p 481.

Society for Assisted Reproductive Technology. Assisted reproductive technology in the United States and Canada: 1994. Results generated for the American Society for Reproductive Medicine/Society for Assisted Reproductive Technology Registry. Fertil Steril 66:697–705, 1996.

Sompolinsky D, Solomon F, Elkina L, et al: Infections with mycoplasma and bacteria in induced midtrimester abortion and fetal loss. Am J Obstet Gynecol 121:610, 1975.

Trott EA, Plouffe L, Hansen K, et al: Ovulation induction in clomiphene-resistant anovulatory women with normal dehydroepiandrosterone sulfate levels: Beneficial effects of the addition of dexamethasone during the follicular phase. Fertil Steril 66:484, 1996.

Tulandi T, Collins JA, Burrows E, et al: Treatment dependent and treatment independent pregnancy among women with periadnexal adhesions. Am J Obstet Gynecol 162:354, 1990.

U.S. Department of Health and Human Services, Centers for Disease Control and Prevention, National Center for Health Statistics: Fertility, Family Planning and Women's Health: New Data from the 1995 National Survey of Family Growth 23:7, 1997.

Vanden Eede B: Investigation and treatment of infertile couples: ESHRE guidelines for good clinical and laboratory practice. Hum Reprod 10:1246–1272, 1995.

Van Voorhis BJ, Sparks AET, Allen BD, et al: Cost-effectiveness of infertility treatments: A cohort study. Fertil Steril 67:830, 1997.

Watson A, Vandekerckhove P, Lilford R, et al: A meta-analysis of the therapeutic role of oil soluble contract media at hysterosalpingography: A surprising result? Fertil Steril 61:470, 1994.

Weil SJ, Wang S, Perez MC, et al: Chemotaxis of macrophages by a peritoneal fluid protein in women with endometriosis. Fertil Steril 67:865, 1997.

Wentz AC, Herbert CM, Maxson WS, et al: Cycle of conception endometrial biopsy. Fertil Steril 46:196, 1986.

Wessels PH, Viljoen GJ, Marais NF, et al: The prevalence of risks, and management of *Chlamydia trachomatis* infections in fertile and infertile patients from the high socioeconomic bracket of the South African population. Fertil Steril 56:485, 1991.

Westrom L: Incidence, prevalence and trends of acute pelvic inflammatory disease and its consequences in industrialized countries. Am J Obstet Gynecol 138:880, 1980.

Whittemore AS, Harris R, Itnyre J, et al: Characteristics relating to ovarian cancer risk: Collaborative analysis of 12 US case-controlled studies. II. Invasive epithelial ovarian cancers in white women. Am J Epidemiol 136:1184, 1992.

WHO Task Force of the Prevention and Management of Infertility: Tubal infertility: Serologic relationship to past chlamydial and gonococcal infection. Sex Transm Dis 22:71, 1995.

Wichmann L, Isola J, Tuohimma P: Prognostic variables in predicting pregnancy—A prospective follow up study of 907 couples with an infertility problem. Hum Reprod 9:1102–1108, 1994.

Wilcox AJ, Weinberg CR, Baird DD: Timing of sexual intercourse in relation to ovulation. N Engl J Med 333:1517, 1995.

Wilcox AJ, Weinberg CR, O'Connor J, et al: Incidence of early loss of pregnancy. N Engl J Med 319:189, 1988.

World Health Organization: WHO Laboratory Manual for the Examination of Human Semen and Sperm-Cervical Interaction. 3rd ed. New York, Cambridge University Press, 1992.

Zinaman MJ, Clegg ED, Brown CC, et al: Estimates of human fertility and pregnancy loss. Fertil Steril 65:503, 1996.

# 59

# Andrology

PETER N. KOLETTIS
ANTHONY J. THOMAS, JR.

The field of andrology has been changing rapidly with many exciting and important new discoveries in the areas of male sexual dysfunction and infertility. The importance of andrologic investigation was recently brought to the public's attention by the Massachusetts Aging Study. It reported the probability of some degree of impotence to be over 50% in its study population of men between the ages of 40 and 70 years. Studies concerning male reproductive function have also hit the popular press when investigators reported a definite decrease in the sperm counts for fertile men during the past 50 years. The observation of declining sperm counts, though argued by some to be regional and not global, and the implications for future fertility have prompted a search for possible offending environmental toxins. The putative environmental toxins that have received much of the attention are naturally occurring compounds in plants that may have estrogen-like activity.

Although there has been an increase in the research devoted to the study of male reproductive disorders, many of the basic mechanisms of spermatogenesis and sperm function remain poorly understood. Recent advances in assisted reproductive technologies (ARTs) allow physicians to bypass both qualitative and quantitative sperm defects, thereby permitting some couples with severe male factor infertility to have their own biologic children. As a consequence of this science, there have been some reproductive specialists who have recommended that men forgo an investigation of their fertility other than a semen analysis. If the analysis proves abnormal and pregnancy is not achieved through intercourse, some have advocated that these couples go directly to ART, be it intrauterine insemination (IUI) or in the case of more severe male factor in vitro fertilization with intracytoplasmic sperm injection (IVF/ICSI). Although for some couples this may seem expedient, there are some good reasons to not have men act as only "gamete donors" but rather to give them the chance to be an active participant in finding a solution to their infertility problem. It has been estimated that 40% of infertility is due to a male factor problem, and proper evaluation and treatment may improve that percentage in at least half of these men, allowing them to establish a pregnancy through intercourse. Also, bypassing a thorough investigation of the male may fail to uncover previously unrecognized significant medical problems that should be dealt with in the best interest of the patient. If the cause for the infertility is a correctable male factor, it would not be appropriate to put his partner at risk by subjecting her to drug-induced ovarian stimulation and oocyte retrieval without first trying to correct his problem. Finally, it has been demonstrated in a number of reports that some treatments for the male are more cost effective and result in higher pregnancy rates than some of the more technically sophisticated

ARTs. This chapter focuses on the evaluation and treatment of the male partner of an infertile couple. A thorough and efficient simultaneous investigation of both partners is mandatory to minimize the cost while maximizing the effectiveness of treatment.

The clinical evaluation of the infertile male is best performed by a physician with a thorough understanding of male reproductive function and an interest in this field of endeavor. Otherwise, the investigation will generally be brief, incomplete, and unfair to the patient, his spouse, and the referring physician.

## Definition

Infertility is defined as the inability to establish a pregnancy after 12 months of unprotected frequent intercourse. Defining the male factor that is causing the infertility problem is often difficult because there can be great variation in reproductive capacity and a deficiency by one partner may be overcome by the other's higher fertility potential. It is probably better to speak in terms of male factors that may totally inhibit (i.e., azoospermia) or make it less likely for a natural pregnancy to occur. It is difficult to define what were previously thought to be *absolute* male factors (i.e., nonobstructive azoospermia) that prevent the establishment of a pregnancy because even these conditions may at times be overcome with the newer reproductive techniques.

## History

A carefully taken medical history starts with basic demographic information, including age, education, and a work history, which can provide clues to any possible toxic exposure, past or present. The duration of infertility, establishment of prior pregnancies and their outcome, and any type of fertility treatment previously rendered are documented. Exploring what evaluation has been done for his partner is important, and good communication with her reproductive specialist is essential.

Identifying specific medical problems may lead to a cause for the couple's infertility. Diabetes mellitus may cause erectile dysfunction, retrograde ejaculation, or even an absence of seminal emission. Recurrent pulmonary infections may indicate a problem with the microstructure of the cilia of the bronchial tree and reflect a similar problem with abnormal or absent flagellar movement of the sperm. Anosmia and visual field defects may be suggestive of Kallmann's syndrome (hypogonadotropic hypogonadism) or a pituitary tumor.

Recent past and current drug use—prescribed, over

**Table 59–1** Drugs that May Affect Sperm Production or Function

| | |
|---|---|
| Alcohol | Gentamicin |
| Alkylating agents | Marijuana |
| Allopurinol | Neomycin |
| Anabolic steroids | Nitrofurantoin |
| Cimetidine | Spironolactone |
| Colchicine | Sulfasalazine |
| Cyclosporine | Tetracyclines |
| Erythromycin | |

the counter, or illicit—should all be identified. A smoking and alcohol history is documented because this may be toxic to the germinal epithelium (Table 59–1). Childhood illnesses, genitourinary infections, long-term febrile illnesses, cryptorchidism, testicular torsion, or a history of surgery involving or near the genitourinary tract are important in assessing reproductive potential.

Frequency and timing of intercourse are of obvious importance. It is not uncommon for each partner to have a different perception of their pattern of sexual activity. In relationships where both partners may be working full time, intercourse four times a week may mean twice on Saturday and again on Sunday with only chance contact at the time of ovulation. Problems with libido, potency, and ejaculation need to be explored to look for an underlying cause or significant psychological problems, which may require attention.

## Physical Examination

A thorough physical examination with emphasis on the genitourinary tract is essential in the investigation of the male. Absence of typical male pattern hair and fat distribution or the presence of gynecomastia may indicate an endocrine problem. The position and caliber of the urethral meatus should be noted. Severe degrees of hypospadias can minimize the chance of sperm being deposited near the cervix during intercourse. The penis is examined for any lesions that may interfere with normal sexual function. Most testicular mass is composed of the seminiferous tubules. Testicular size, therefore, can indirectly provide an estimate of spermatogenic potential. Normal size testicles are more than 20 cm$^3$ in volume or approximately 4.5 × 2.5 × 2.5 cm when measured in three dimensions. The normal consistency of the testicle is firm and pliant, somewhat analogous to that of the cartilaginous tip of the nose. The presence or absence of vasa deferentia and any signs of thickening or tortuosity that may indicate a distal obstruction are noted. Thickening, tenderness, or induration of the epididymis may indicate an obstructive problem at that level.

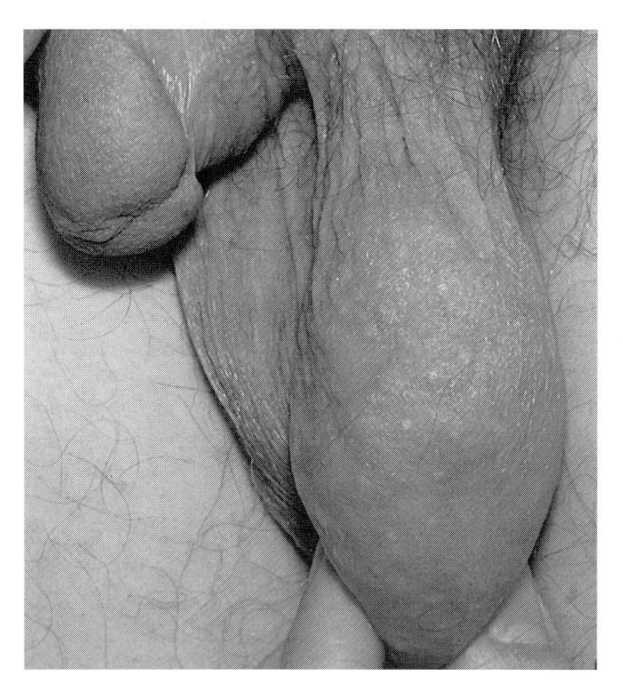

**Figure 59-1** A left varicocele, visible through the skin.

It has been reported that 40% of men presenting for fertility evaluation may have a varicocele. These dilated veins of the pampiniform plexus are more commonly seen on the left, though they can be right sided or bilateral and often are associated with poor sperm quality. A moderate or large-size varicocele is palpable and often visible when the patient is standing in a warm well-lighted examining room. (Fig. 59-1). A smaller varicocele may be better detected by palpation of the cord and the use of a Doppler stethoscope, hearing an audible venous rush with Valsalva maneuver or with color Doppler ultrasonography.

Digital rectal examination is performed to evaluate the prostate and seminal vesicles for signs of inflammation, infection, or neoplasm. In documented cases of leukocytospermia (>10$^6$ white blood cells [WBC]/ml semen), expressed prostatic secretions should be examined by light microscopy. The presence of large numbers of white cells indicates an inflammatory or infectious process within the prostate and requires further assessment and treatment. Prostatic nodules or areas of induration, particularly in men over the age of 40, should be evaluated by obtaining a serum prostate-specific antigen level and performing a transrectal ultrasonography (TRUS) and prostate biopsy, if appropriate, to rule out malignancy.

## Laboratory and Diagnostic Evaluation

### SEMEN ANALYSIS

A semen analysis is generally the first laboratory test ordered in the evaluation of the infertile male. Two or three semen samples, obtained approximately 2 weeks apart, should be requested to begin assessment of reproductive potential. Samples should be collected into sterile plastic or glass, nonspermatotoxic containers by masturbation after 2 to 3 days of sexual abstinence. The semen should be examined within 1 hour of collection. Viscosity, volume, pH, sperm concentration, motility, and morphology are the *basic* parameters that should be measured. Any samples apparently devoid of sperm should be centrifuged and the resulting pellet stained and examined for sperm.

Immature germ cells and WBC are often difficult to distinguish without special staining. Because most WBC seen in excess in the semen are almost always granulocytes, a simple method for differentiation of germ cells from granulocytes is the myeloperoxidase test or Endtz test. Acceptable semen parameters, as determined by the World Health Organization (WHO), are given in Table 59-2.

Sperm morphology is assessed and reported as a differential of normal v. abnormal either by the criteria established by WHO or the so-called strict criteria as suggested by Kruger. The clinical significance of the strict Kruger morphology is not entirely clear with respect to natural conception, but the percentage of normal forms has been shown to correlate to some degree with successful fertilization *in vitro*. The parameters for both methods are given in Table 59-3.

### HORMONE TESTING

Normal spermatogenesis depends on a proper hormonal milieu created by the hypothalamic-pituitary-testicular endocrine axis. Pure endocrine problems causing infertility make up only a small portion of the infertile male patient population, but measurement of the hormones involved with sperm production is extremely helpful whenever there is azoospermia or a moderate or severe oligospermic condition. Azoospermia or severe oligospermia, lack of normal secondary sex characteristics, gynecomastia, small testicles, and undeveloped or underdeveloped genitals can indicate an endocrine problem that needs to be addressed. The rarer endocrinopathies such as adult

**Table 59-2** Normal Semen Parameters (from WHO Criteria)

| | |
|---|---|
| Volume | ≥2.0 ml |
| pH | 7.2–8.0 |
| Sperm concentration/ml | ≥20 × 10$^6$ |
| Motility | ≥50% with forward progression |
| Morphology (WHO) | ≥30% normal forms |
| White blood cells | <1 × 10$^6$ |
| Immunobead test | ≤20% spermatozoa with adherent particles |

Table 59–3 Comparison of WHO and Kruger's Strict Criteria for Normal Sperm Morphology

| | WHO | Kruger* |
|---|---|---|
| Head shape | Oval | Oval |
| Head length | 4–5.5 μm | 5–6 μm |
| Head diameter/width | 2.5–3.5 μm | 2.5–3.5 μm |
| Acrosome | 40–70% of head | 40–70% of head |
| Cytoplasmic droplets | <1/3 of head | <1/2 of head |
| Other | No neck, midpiece or tail defect; all borderline forms abnormal | No neck, midpiece or tail defect; all borderline forms abnormal |

*Kruger TE: Strict criteria for sperm morphology. In Lipshultz LI, Howards SS (eds): Infertility in the Male. St. Louis, Mosby, 1997, p. 491.

adrenogenital syndrome, androgen insensitivity, or some of the intersex problems may not be as readily recognized. Given the abnormal basic hormonal values (follicle-stimulating hormone [FSH], luteinizing hormone [LH], and testosterone [T]), the clinical picture should initiate further study involving the endocrine pathways. Most men being evaluated for infertility will be normal in appearance and will not have a significant endocrinopathy. If their semen analyses reveal either severe oligospermia (defined as less than 2 million sperm/ml or a total of less than 10 million sperm) or azoospermia, obtaining FSH, LH, and total serum T will allow the clinician to determine if a patient has testicular failure (high FSH and LH and low T), spermatogenic failure (high FSH and normal LH and T), or is hormonally normal or under stimulated (low FSH, low or normal T). Serum prolactin is added to the testing if the patient is oligospermic, has a low serum T, and a decreased libido. These signs and symptoms may be indicative of a prolactin-producing pituitary tumor.

## SPERM FUNCTION TESTING

The results of the medical history, physical examination, semen analyses, and hormone values and input regarding any apparent female factors will begin to allow some decision-making regarding possible treatment options for the couple.

For some individuals, semen parameters may be borderline normal, demonstrate one or two parameter deficiencies, or appear to be adequate by WHO standards and still the couple cannot establish a pregnancy. These individuals may benefit from *functional* testing of their sperm to try to identify where the problems lie and to more efficiently direct the couple's treatment. Many of these functional tests have been developed to evaluate *(in vitro)* the ability of sperm to carry out those events before and at the time of fertilization. Some of these tests are highly labor intensive and study the function of only a small number of the sperm in a sample. No single test examines all processes involved in the complex interactions required for successful fertilization.

### Postcoital Test

The postcoital test (PCT) is used to evaluate sperm-cervical mucus interaction. The couple is instructed to have intercourse from 2 to 12 hours before the test during the periovulatory period. The cervical mucus is examined for the presence of motile sperm. Failure to find greater than 5 to 10 motile spermatozoa per high power field in the mucus can be interpreted as one indicator of decreased sperm quality or a cervical mucus abnormality. Interpretation of the results of the PCT can, at times, be difficult because of a multitude of variable factors involved, and it has lost favor with some gynecologists and urologists. A "normal" test still has value in the investigation of the male, because it will indicate the ability to deposit adequate numbers of motile sperm into a nonhostile environment.

### Bovine Cervical Mucus Penetration Test

This assay does not address the cervical factor per se but rather measures the ability of sperm to traverse mucus, which is in some ways similar to human cervical mucus. This test has been shown to be reproducible and reliable, measuring a property of sperm function not measured by conventional semen analysis. The distance traveled in millimeters by the farthest traveling sperm (vanguard sperm) and the first cluster of sperm is recorded and the patient's value is compared with a preset standard of 30 mm distance in 60 minutes. This test is particularly helpful to assess the quality of motility, which if poor may prompt examination of the semen for antisperm antibodies.

### Zona-Free Hamster Egg Penetration Assay

The zona-free hamster egg test can be used to assess certain aspects of sperm function, including hyperactivation, capacitation, and the acrosome reaction as well as nuclear membrane fusion and decondensation. In theory, fewer sperm from infertile men should penetrate each egg or fewer eggs will be penetrated. The percentage of hamster eggs penetrated is lower in men whose sperm cannot fertilize in vitro compared with those men whose sperm can. In some studies, a positive result (a high number of sperm penetrating when compared with a known donor sample run simultaneously) has been predictive of a successful IVF outcome. Depending on how the test is performed and interpreted, the predictive value of the results may vary from laboratory to laboratory. Disadvantages of this study include lack of a standardized protocol, measurement of interaction with a mechanically disrupted nonhuman oocyte, and the labor-intensive nature of the test.

## Mannose Ligand Receptor Assay

Capacitation is defined as the biophysiologic changes that sperm undergo, transiting the female genital tract, that allow them to bind to the zona pellucida (ZP), undergo the acrosome reaction, and prepare to fertilize the egg. Studies have demonstrated that the sugar mannose is important for sperm recognition of the ZP. When oocytes were treated with concavalin A, a mannose-binding lectin, no sperm are bound to or penetrate the ZP. To perform the assay, sperm are capacitated, washed, and then reacted with fluorescein isothiocyanate-conjugated mannosylated bovine serum albumin. The sperm are then examined for the different patterns of mannose binding sites expressed as a percentage and compared with a known donor sample run at the same time. The presence of particular patterns of D-mannose–ligand binding sites on sperm is correlated with the ability of sperm to recognize and fertilize eggs in vitro. Some investigators have recommended ICSI rather than IVF alone based on abnormal mannose binding test results.

## Acrosome Reaction

The acrosome is an organelle that is surrounded by an outer and inner membrane. The inner acrosomal membrane is adjacent to the sperm nuclear membrane and the outer acrosomal membrane is adjacent to the sperm plasma membrane. During the acrosome reaction, the plasma membrane fuses with the outer acrosomal membrane and the acrosomal contents, including hydrolytic enzymes, are released. Evaluation of the sperm's ability to undergo the acrosome reaction in vitro is a logical test of sperm function because this is one of the critical events in sperm-egg interaction. There are several different methods to evoke the acrosome reaction and measure the sperms' response, including staining procedures or monoclonal antibody-coated beads. The percentage of sperm that can be induced to undergo the acrosome reaction has been shown by some investigators to correlate with successful IVF. In addition, the induced results may be correlated with semen quality.

## Hemizona Assay

The hemizona assay was designed to evaluate the ability of a man's sperm to bind to the ZP. This assay uses the ZP of bisected nonfertilizable human oocytes. One half is used to test the patient's sperm, the other, a donor control. Washed sperm from the patient and fertile control are incubated with the matching hemizona. The hemizona index is calculated by dividing the number of sperm bound by the test subject by the number of sperm bound by the control and multiplying by 100. The results of the assay have been reported to be predictive of success with IVF. The disadvantages of this test include the lack of a consensus protocol, particularly for capacitation, and the requirement for human oocytes and a micromanipulation system. In addition, the assay does not measure postzona binding events such as membrane fusion capability. Essentially, this assay measures an interaction between sperm and a mechanically disrupted ovum, which may be different from that between a sperm and an intact oocyte.

## Antisperm Antibody

Antisperm antibodies are found in the semen of 3 to 12% of infertile men and are thought to be a contributing factor for infertility in up to 10% of infertile couples. The significance, methods of measurement, and treatment for these antibodies are controversial. Antisperm antibodies should be suspected in patients with decreased motility, sperm agglutination, or poor PCT results. Seminal immunoglobulins, IgG and IgA, bound to the head or midpiece are those that are believed to be clinically significant. Antisperm antibodies can be measured by direct or indirect means. A commonly used assay for sperm antibodies is the immunobead assay, which uses anti-human IgG- and IgA-coated beads. Conditions in which there has been a presumed breach of the blood-testis barrier such as vasectomy, testis biopsy, testicular trauma, torsion, varicocele, orchitis, testis cancer, and cryptorchidism have been associated with the presence of antisperm antibodies. Some men will be found to have sperm antibodies without antecedent cause. The significance of these antibodies as they relate to an individual's fertility varies greatly from person to person but should be considered an important factor when there is poor motility, marked

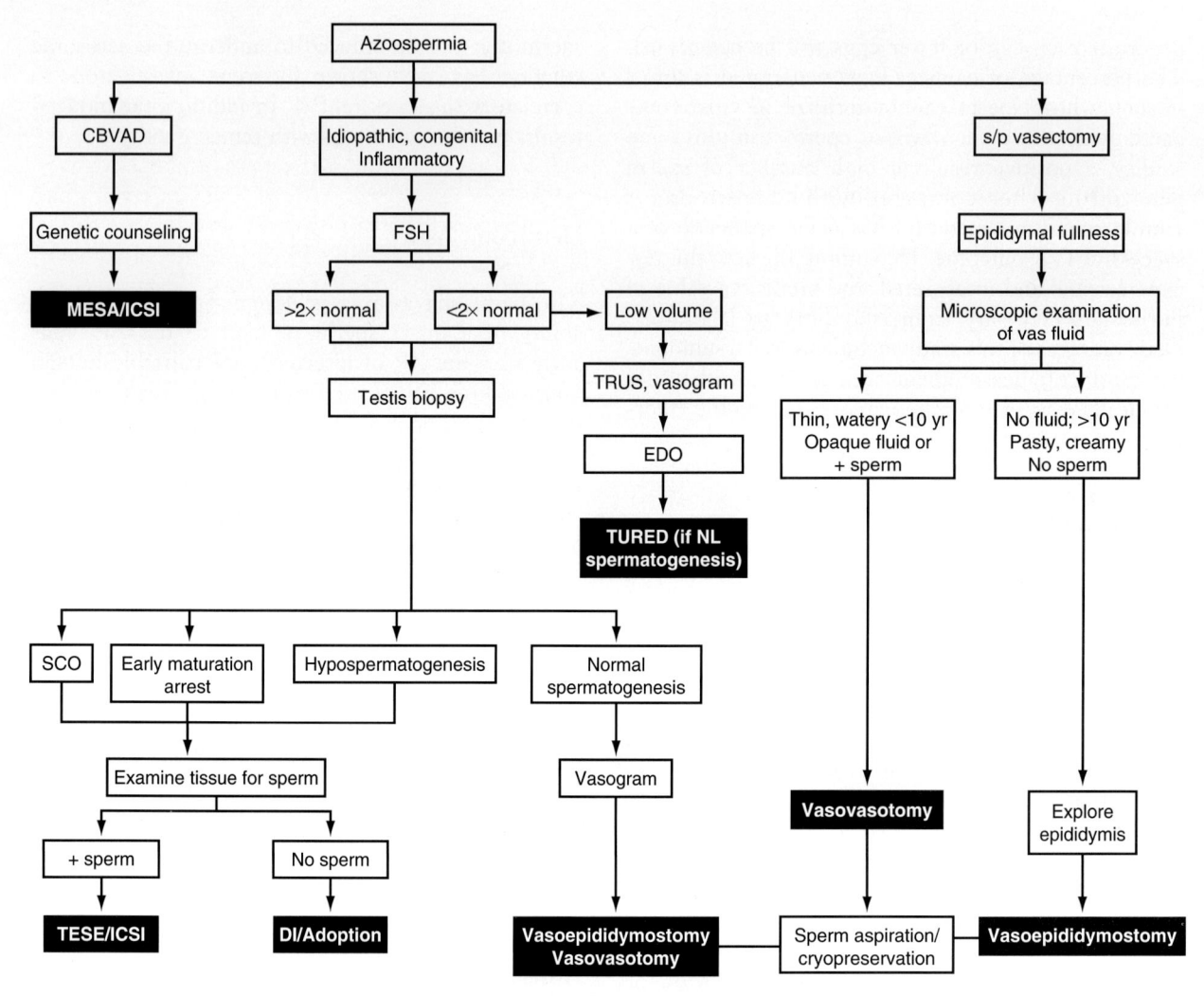

**Figure 59–2** Evaluation and management of azoospermia. CBAVD=bilateral absence of the vas deferens; DI= donor insemination; EDO-ejaculatory duct obstruction; FSH=follicle-stimulating hormone; ICSI=intracytoplasmic sperm injection; MESA=microsurgical epididymal sperm aspiration; SCO=Sertoli cell only; TESE=testicular sperm extraction; TRUS-transurethral ultrasonography; TURED=transurethral resection of the ejaculatory ducts. (Adapted from Thomas AJ, Padron O: Obstructive azoospermia and vasoepididymostomy. *In* Hellstrom JG [ed]: Male Infertility and Sexual Dysfunction. New York, Springer-Verlag, 1997, p 245)

agglutination of sperm, or poor penetration of cervical mucus.

## GENETIC TESTING AND COUNSELING

About 10% of men with nonobstructive azoospermia (NOA) and a smaller percentage with severe oligospermia have been found to have microdeletions of the Y chromosome, specifically of the *DAZ* (Deleted in AZoospermia) gene. Identifying these gene loci is an extremely important step in gaining an understanding of why some men are infertile. Of practical and immediate importance regarding the treatment of these men is the fact that some may have small islands of spermatogenesis within the testis despite having no sperm in their ejaculate. It is possible to treat some of these affected couples by isolating sperm from the testicular tissue and performing IVF/ICSI. One consequence of a successful pregnancy is the potential for passing on the same "genetic abnormality" to the male offspring. Besides these Y chromosome abnormalities, a higher incidence of karyotypic abnormalities has been shown that may have greater consequences for the offspring. Some men with azoospermia or severe oligospermia may carry an extra sex chromosome (i.e., Klinefelter's syndrome: 47,XXY) or a translocation of a portion of a chromosome that, if inherited, may play a role in the mental or physical development of the child conceived through ICSI. It would seem reasonable, therefore, that men with NOA or severe oligospermia should be offered a karyotype and genetic counseling before ICSI is attempted.

Cystic fibrosis (CF) is an autosomal recessive disorder with a carrier frequency of 1/25 in people of northern European descent. Chronic respiratory infections, exocrine pancreatic insufficiency, and Wolffian duct anomalies characterize the disease. Congenital bilateral absence of the vas deferens (CBAVD) is regarded as a genital form of CF and is believed to represent one end of a phenotypic spectrum caused by mutations in the CF transmembrane conductance regulator *(CFTR)* gene. Approximately three quarters of men with CBAVD have at least one detectable *CFTR* gene mutation. There are probably many other gene loci associated with these mutations, but all are not known. Testing is available at many centers for the most prevalent gene mutations. It is recommended that both partners undergo genetic testing for these gene mutations and genetic counseling before proceeding to sperm aspiration and IVF/ICSI.

# Refining the Diagnosis and Defining Treatment

## VARICOCELE

Approximately 15% of American men and as many as 40% of men presenting for evaluation of their fertility have a varicocele. Their predominant occurrence on the left side is probably related to the greater length of the left gonadal vein and its insertion at a right angle into the renal vein.

A varicocele may be associated with a variety of abnormalities noted on semen analysis, or in some cases, semen quality may be completely normal. The pathophysiology of varicocele-induced infertility is incompletely understood, but the most popular hypothesis suggests that the absence of valves within the testicular vein(s) results in dilatation and an increase in arterial blood flow, with elevation of testicular temperature that in turn disturbs various elements of spermatogenesis. The bilateral effects of a unilateral varicocele may be secondary to left to right venous shunting.

Many studies, mostly *uncontrolled*, have demonstrated some benefit with varicocele ablation in terms of improvement in semen quality and pregnancy. Various investigators have reported that about 60% of men will improve at least some of their semen parameters and about 40% will establish a pregnancy if their partner is reproductively normal. In one controlled trial, varicocelectomy demonstrated a benefit resulting in a 76% pregnancy rate in the treatment group compared with 10% in the control group. When the remaining patients in the control group were crossed over to surgical treatment, 12 of 18 (67%) ultimately established a pregnancy. Even some men who are azoospermic with biopsy-proven maturation arrest may respond to varicocele ablation, as will some men with severe oligospermia.

Varicocele ablation can be performed by open surgical ligation, laparoscopic clipping, or transcutaneous venous embolization. Recently, minimally invasive microsurgical ligation of the spermatic veins has gained a great deal of popularity and appears to return the patient to his normal activities as quickly as embolization and laparoscopy. A recent analysis compared the effectiveness (i.e., live delivery) and cost with patients of varicocele ablation vs. IVF/ICSI. Although these two forms of treatment had comparable live delivery rates, the cost per delivery with IVF/ICSI was over $60,000 higher.

## AZOOSPERMIA

Figure 59–2 is an algorithm detailing the evaluation and recommended treatment(s) for the azoospermic man. For those men who are amenable to correction of an obstructive problem, surgery should be performed by someone who has the requisite training and skills to perform tedious microsurgical anastomoses; otherwise, the results will be haphazard and for the most part discouraging.

Microsurgical vasovasostomy and vasoepididymostomy, when performed by practiced microsurgeons, offer a very reasonable chance of patency and pregnancy (Tables 59–4 and 59–5). These procedures have even been shown to give the couple a better chance to establish a pregnancy at a lower cost per live baby than using sperm aspiration and ICSI (Table 59–6).

Some patients that are not candidates or do not want surgical reconstruction may be offered sperm aspiration with IVF/ICSI as an option to other choices, such as donor insemination or adoption. Sperm can be retrieved from the epididymis, vas deferens, or the testis and used for ICSI. Percutaneous

**Table 59–4** Results of Microsurgical Vasovasostomy

| Author | Year | No. of Patients | Patency (%) | Pregnancy Rate |
|---|---|---|---|---|
| Owen | 1977 | 50 | 98 | 72 |
| Silber | 1977 | 126 | 90 | 76 |
| Lee, McLoughlin | 1980 | 26 | 96 | 54 |
| Cos et al | 1983 | 87 | 75 | 46 |
| Requeda et al | 1983 | 47 | 80 | 46 |
| Owen, Kapila | 1984 | 475 | 93 | 82 |
| Soonawala, Lal | 1984 | 339 | 89 | 63 |
| Lee | 1986 | 324 | 90 | 51 |
| Belker et al | 1991 | 1247 | 86 | 52 |
| Fox | 1994 | 103 | 84 | 48 |

From Thomas AJ, Howards SS: Microsurgical treatment of male infertility. *In* Lipshultz LI, Howards SS (eds): Infertility in the Male. St. Louis, Mosby, 1997, p 377.

Table 59–5  Results of Microsurgical Vasoepididymostomy

| Author | Year | No. of Patients | Patency (%) | Pregnancy Rate (%) |
|---|---|---|---|---|
| Fogdestam et al | 1986 | 41 | 85 | 37 |
| Silber | 1988 | 139 | 78 | 56 |
| Fuchs | 1991 | 39 | 60 | 36 |
| Schlegel and Goldstein | 1993 | 107 | 70 | 31 |
| Niederberger and Ross | 1993 | 22 | 48 | N/A |
| Thomas | 1993 | 153 | 76 | 42 |

Thomas AJ, Howards SS: Microsurgical treatment of male infertility. In Lipshultz LI, Howards SS (eds): Infertility in the Male. St. Louis, Mosby, 1997, p 382.

aspiration of sperm is less expensive to perform than open biopsy or microsurgical epididymal sperm aspiration, but the numbers of sperm obtained are less than with open biopsy or open aspiration and the overall pregnancy rates have reportedly been lower. With increasing experience in the processing of testicular sperm, however, the pregnancy rates using testicular sperm are approaching those for epididymal sperm.

## OLIGOASTHENOSPERMIA

Oligoasthenospermia is defined as diminished sperm concentration (<20 million sperm/ml) and motility (less than 50%). Oligospermia can be arbitrarily categorized for the purpose of prognostication as severe ($< 2 \times 10^6$/ml), moderate (2 to $10 \times 10^6$/ml), and mild (10 to $20 \times 10^6$/ml). Specific treatment is directed toward an identifiable cause for the sperm abnormalities (see below).

In many instances, however, no specific abnormality is identified, and we are left with the option of trying some form of empirical therapy or moving directly to ART. If the serum FSH level is elevated, indicating some degree of spermatogenic failure, and the patient has moderate to severe oligospermia without other abnormalities, there is little to no benefit from nonspecific hormone therapy. When the FSH is low or in the normal range, some patients have been given trials of clomiphene citrate or tamoxifen, though the response rate is very low and controlled studies have not shown any sustained benefit from these drugs. A *small* subpopulation of patients appear to benefit from this therapy, at least insofar as achieving an increase in sperm concentration. Clomiphene citrate, 50 mg, may be given on alternate days, three times a week. During the fifth week of therapy, the FSH and T levels are again measured and compared with the pretreatment levels. If the values are more than one and one half times the upper limits of normal on either test, the drug is stopped because in our experience it has not been effective in these men. If the laboratory values are normal or only slightly elevated, the drug is continued for 3 to 6 months, monitoring the patient at 3 and 6 months by examination, semen analysis, and serum FSH and T.

Asthenospermia can occur for a variety of reasons. It may not be real but apparent due to the method of sample collection such as with the use of a latex condom or an improper receptacle, the chemical makeup of which may immobilize the sperm. Exposure of the sample to cold ambient temperatures as it is being transported to the laboratory from home will also diminish the percent of motile sperm. If circumstances for collection and delivery to the laboratory are optimized and the motility is less than 40% or sluggish in character, further assessment should be carried out. Sperm antibody status should be determined. If there are less than 20% motile sperm, viability stains should be done. If there are no motile sperm but the sperm are alive, scanning and transmission electron microscopy of the sperm is recommended to identify ultrastructural abnormalities.

## ANTISPERM ANTIBODIES

The treatment of antisperm antibodies is still a highly controversial topic. Some couples may have primary immunologic infertility due to antibodies present on the sperm and/or in the partner's cervical mucus. On the other hand, approximately half the men who undergo vasectomy will have antibodies to sperm in their semen. Many of these will, however, be able to successfully establish a pregnancy after a vasectomy reversal. For those who are affected, having significant agglutination and poor motility and not achieving pregnancies, therapeutic trials using oral cortico-

Table 59–6  Postvasectomy Obstruction: Two Studies' Comparisons Between Delivery Rates and Cost per Live Delivery for Sperm Aspiration/ICSI vs. Microsurgical Reconstruction

|  | Kolettis and Thomas* | Pavlovich and Schlegel† |
|---|---|---|
| Delivery rate |  |  |
|   Sperm aspiration/ICSI | 29% | 33% |
|   Microsurgical reconstruction | 36% | 47% |
| Cost per delivery |  |  |
|   Sperm aspiration/ICSI | $51,024 | $72,521 |
|   Microsurgical reconstruction | $31,099 | $25,475 |

*Kolettis PN, Thomas AJ: Vasoepididymostomy for vasectomy reversal. A critical assessment in the era of intracytoplasmic sperm injection. J Urol 157:467–470, 1997 (vasoepididymostomy only).
†Pavlovich CP, Schlegel PN: Fertility options after vasectomy: A cost-effectiveness analysis. (Reprinted by permission from the American Society for Reproductive Medicine [Fertil Steril 67:133–141, 1997] {vasovasostomy and vasoepididymostomy}.)

steroids have yielded conflicting results with regard to pregnancies and can be associated with the potential for serious complications. Gastrointestinal bleeding and aseptic necrosis of the hips, shoulders, or other ball joints are the more significant problems reported. At present, when sperm dilution and washing with IUI fails in the presence of high antibody titers, it is suggested to consider IVF/ICSI as the most efficient means of establishing a pregnancy for this group of patients.

## HYPOGONADOTROPIC HYPOGONADISM

Hypogonadotropic hypogonadism is a rare cause of infertility but one that does have specific therapy. This entity should be suspected in the setting of low T, low gonadotropins, and oligospermia or azoospermia. Causes include Kallmann's syndrome (deficient secretion of gonadotropin-releasing hormone by the hypothalamus associated with midline defects and anosmia), pituitary tumors, pituitary trauma, and isolated gonadotropin deficiency. Treatment is gonadotropin replacement. Pregnancies can be achieved even though these patients may never reach normal sperm concentrations.

## HYPERPROLACTINEMIA

Patients with hyperprolactinemia have decreased T levels and may also have depressed gonadotropins. This condition is often associated with infertility and sexual dysfunction (erectile dysfunction and decreased libido). The causes include pituitary tumors (macro- or microadenomas), hypothyroidism, liver disease, and the use of certain medications that elevate prolactin such as the phenothiazines. Computed tomography or magnetic resonance imaging should be performed to rule out a pituitary tumor. Macroadenomas may be amenable to surgical resection, whereas microadenomas and idiopathic hyperprolactinemia can often be treated effectively with bromocriptine.

## EJACULATORY DYSFUNCTION

A low volume ejaculate raises the suspicion of ejaculatory dysfunction, either failure of emission, retrograde ejaculation, or partial or complete obstruction of the ejaculatory ducts. Problems with ejaculation are common in patients with diabetes mellitus, spinal cord injury, prior bladder neck surgery, or previous retroperitoneal lymph node dissection for testis cancer.

The presence of sperm in a postejaculate urine (PEU) confirms the diagnosis of retrograde ejaculation. Depending on the cause, some of these men may benefit from a trial of sympathomimetic medication to stimulate the sympathetic nervous system that is responsible for the emission of semen into the posterior urethra and closure of the bladder neck at the time of seminal expulsion. If antegrade ejaculation cannot be achieved, the urine must be alkalinized using oral sodium bicarbonate or other suitable drug and a PEU collected either by voiding after ejaculation or catheter drainage and washed for IUI or IVF.

Patients who have had testis tumors removed and subsequent non–nerve-sparing retroperitoneal lymph node dissection often have a failure of seminal emission (no ejaculate and a negative PEU), although erection and orgasmic sensation remain intact. These men can also be effectively treated with sympathomimetics, although it is not often successful. In those who are unable to obtain sperm by medical manipulation, other options, such as direct sperm aspiration from the testis, excurrent ducts, or use of electroejaculation, may be offered. The latter procedure will require a full general anesthetic in these otherwise neurologically normal men. Testis cancer treated with chemotheraphy may result in impaired or absent spermatogenic function. Therefore, the presence of spermatogenis must be confirmed in men who have undergone any form of chemotherapy or radiation therapy before going to electroejaculation or the more sophisticated assisted reproductive techniques. Many men with spinal cord injuries have problems with both erection and ejaculation depending on the level and completeness of the injury. Those who are anejaculatory can be offered and benefit from electrovibratory stimulation or electroejaculation.

A low volume ejaculate with normal-sized testes and a normal FSH with either azoospermia or severe oligospermia may be indicative of an ejaculatory duct obstruction, complete or partial. The diagnosis is made based on the physical examination and a TRUS that will demonstrate enlarged seminal vesicles and a dilated ejaculatory duct partially traversing the posterior lobe of the prostate. If ejaculatory duct obstruction is suspected and a testis biopsy demonstrates active spermatogenesis, the problem can be effectively dealt with by transurethral unroofing of the ejaculatory ducts.

## LEUKOCYTOSPERMIA

Leukocytospermia ($>1 \times 10^6$ WBC/ml) can indicate genital tract inflammation or infection. Leukocytes are thought to impair sperm function, in part, through the production of reactive species (ROS) that can lead to lipid peroxidation of the sperm membrane, cellular damage, and dysfunction. Leukocytospermia has been correlated with reduced fertilization in vitro. Treatment of leukocytospermia in the setting of infertility may start with a trial of antibiotics such as doxycycline or one of the varieties of quinolones along with the recommendation for frequent ejaculation because this combination has been demonstrated to be more successful than antibiotics alone. Because leukocytes produce ROS, there is a rather speculative rationale for empiric antioxidant therapy in this group of patients as well.

If leukocytospermia persists after initial treatment, the semen is sent for routine culture and for chlamydia and ureaplasma with subsequent specific antibiotic treatment being instituted again with emphasis on frequent ejaculation. If no specific organism is isolated, some success in white cell reduction has been reported with the use of nonsteroidal anti-inflammatory drugs (ibuprofen 400 mg three times a day) and, again, frequent ejaculation. If the leukocytospermia persists, TRUS is recommended to rule out any anatomic obstructive problem that may be present and correctable.

## Conclusions

Andrology is a rapidly evolving and exciting field. New therapies allow couples to have their own biologic children when it was previously not possible. The underlying pathophysiology for inadequate sperm production and function in an otherwise perfectly healthy male remains poorly understood. ARTs touted in the popular media are expensive and not guaranteed but may be the most effective form of therapy for these individuals with whom nothing else has worked. However, the use of IVF/ICSI is not without its own limitations. Live delivery rates are roughly 25 to 30% per cycle in most reported series. Significant complications such as the ovarian hyperstimulation syndrome are infrequent but real. Although it is tempting to recommend the "high tech" methods of conception to infertile couples as *efficient* answers to their problem, it would seem a disservice to them not to fully evaluate each person and offer other treatment options when possible to allow them to establish a pregnancy by the most natural means.

### REFERENCES

Agarwal A, Tolentino MV, Sidhu RS, et al: Effect of cryopreservation on semen quality in patients with testicular cancer. Urology 46:382–389, 1995.

Aitken RJ, Baker HWG: Seminal leukocytes: Passengers, terrorists or good Samaritans? Hum Reprod 10:1736–1739, 1995.

Auger J, Kunstmann JM, Cxyglik F, et al: Decline in semen quality among fertile men in Paris during the past 20 years. N Engl J Med 332:281–285, 1995.

Becker S, Berhane K: A meta-analysis of 61 sperm count studies revisited. Fertil Steril 67:1103–1108, 1997.

Belker AM, Thomas AJ, Fuchs EF, et al: Results of 1,469 microsurgical vasectomy reversals by the vasovasostomy study group. J Urol 145:505–511, 1991.

Benoff S, Cooper GW, Hurley I, et al: Human sperm fertilizing potential *in vitro* is correlated with differential expression of a head-specific mannose-ligand receptor. Fertil Steril 59:854–862, 1993.

Bonduelle M, Wilikens A, Buysse A, et al: Prospective follow-up study of 877 children born after intracytoplasmic sperm injection (ICSI), with ejaculated epididymal and testicular spermatozoa and after replacement of cryopreserved embryos obtained after ICSI. Hum Reprod 11(suppl):131–159, 1996.

Burkman LJ, Coddington CC, Franken DR, et al: The hemizona assay (HZA): Development of a diagnostic test for the binding of human spermatozoa to the human hemizona pellucida to predict fertilization potential. Fertil Steril 49:688–697, 1988.

Carlsen E, Giwerman A, Keiding N, et al: Evidence for decreasing quality of semen during past 50 years. Br Med J 305:609–613, 1992.

Cha KY, Oum KB, Kim HJ: Approaches for obtaining sperm in patients with male factor infertility. Fertil Steril 67:985–995, 1997.

Chehval MJ, Purcell MH: Deterioration of semen parameters over time in men with untreated varicocele: Evidence or progressive testicular damage. Fertil Steril 57:174–177, 1992.

Cohen J, Weber RFA, van der Vijver JCM, et al: In vitro fertilizing capacity of human spermatozoa with the use of zona-free hamster ova: Interassay variation and prognostic value. Fertil Steril 37:565–572, 1982.

Cos LR, Valvo JR, Davis RS, et al: Vasovasostomy: Current state of the art. Urology 22:567–575, 1983.

Cummins JM, Jequier AM: Treating male infertility needs more clinical andrology, not less. Hum Reprod 9:1214–1219, 1994.

De Jonge CJ, Pierce J: Intracytoplasmic sperm injection—what kind of reproduction is being assisted? Hum Reprod 10:2518–2520, 1995.

de Lamirande E, Leclerc P, Gagnon C: Capacitation as a regulatory event that primes spermatozoa for the acrosome reaction and fertilization. Mol Hum Reprod 3:175–194, 1997.

Dewire DM, Thomas AJ, Falk RM, et al: Clinical outcome and cost comparison of percutaneous embolization and surgical ligation of varicocele. J Androl 15:38s–42s, 1994.

Doyle P: The outcome of multiple pregnancy. Hum Reprod 11(suppl):110–120, 1996.

Feldman HA, Goldstein I, Hatzichristou DG, et al: Impotence and its medical and psychosocial correlates: Results of the Massachusetts male aging study. J Urol 151:54–61, 1994.

Fogdestam I, Fall M, Nillson S: Microsurgical epididymovasostomy in the treatment of occlusive azoospermia. Fertil Steril 46:925–929, 1986.

Foreman R, Cohen J, Fehilly CB, et al: The application of the zona-free hamster egg test for the prognosis of human in vitro fertilization. J In Vitro Fertil Emb Trans 1:166–171, 1984.

Fox M: Vasectomy reversal-microsurgery for best results. Br J Urol 73:449–553, 1994.

Fuchs E: Restoring fertility through vasoepididymostomy. Cont Urol 3:27, 1991.

Geva E, Bartoov B, Zabludovsky N, et al: The effect of antioxidant treatment on human spermatozoa and fertilization rate in an *in vitro* fertilization program. Fertil Steril 66:430–434, 1996.

Gilbaugh JH, Lipshultz LI: Nonsurgical treatment of male infertility. An update. Urol Clin North Am 21:531–548, 1994.

Goldstein M, Matthews GJ: Induction of spermatogenesis and pregnancy after microsurgical varicocelectomy in azoospermic men. J Urol 155(suppl):443A, 1996.

Gorelick JI, Goldstein M: Loss of fertility in men with varicocele. Fertil Steril 59:613–616, 1993.

Haas GG: Antibody-mediated causes of male infertility. Urol Clin North Am 14:539–550, 1987.

Haas GG, Manganiello P: A double-blind, placebo-controlled study of the use of ethylprednisolone in infertile men with sperm-associated immunoglobulins. Fertil Steril 47:295–301, 1987.

Halden W, White RI: Outpatient embolotherapy of varicocele. Urol Clin North Am 14:137–144, 1987.

Henkel R, Muller C, Miska W, et al: Determination of the acrosome reaction in human spermatozoa is predictive of fertilization *in vitro*. Hum Reprod 8:2128–2132, 1993.

Honig SC, Lipshultz LI, Jarow J: Significant medical pathology uncovered by a comprehensive male infertility evaluation. Fertil Steril 62:1028–1034, 1994.

Hughes EG, Brennan BG: Does cigarette smoking impair natural or assisted fecundity? Fertil Steril 66:679–689, 1996.

Jaffe T, Oates RD: Genetic aspects of infertility. In Lipshultz LI, Howards, SS (eds): Infertility in the Male. St. Louis, Mosby, 1997; p. 280.

Jarow JP: Intratesticular arterial anatomy. J Androl 11:255–259, 1990.

Jarow JP: Seminal vesicle aspiration in the management of patients with ejaculatory duct obstruction. J Urol 152:899–901, 1994.

Kessopoulou E, Powers HJ, Sharma KK, et al: A double-blind randomized placebo cross-over controlled trial using the antioxidant vitamin E to treat reactive oxygen species associated male infertility. Fertil Steril 64:825–831, 1995.

Kim ED, Gilbaugh JH, Patel VR, et al: Testis biopsies frequently demonstrate sperm in men with azoospermia and significantly elevated follicle-stimulating hormone levels. J Urol 157:144–146, 1997.

Kolettis PN, Thomas AJ: Vasoepididymostomy for vasectomy reversal: A critical assessment in the era of intracytoplasmic sperm injection. J Urol 157:467–470, 1997.

Kruger TF. Strict criteria for sperm morphology. In Lipshultz LI, Howards SS (eds): Infertility in the Male. St. Louis, Mosby, 1997, p. 491.

Kruger TF, Acosta AA, Simmons KF, et al: Predictive value of abnormal sperm morphology in in vitro fertilization. Fertil Steril 49:112–117, 1988.

Kruger TF, Menkveld R, Stander FSH, et al: Sperm morphologic features as prognostic factor in *in vitro* fertilization. Fertil Steril 46:1118–1123, 1986.

Lee HY: A 20 year experience with vasovasostomy. J Urol 136:413–415, 1986.

Lee L, McLoughlin MG: Vasovasostomy: A comparison of macroscopic and microscopic techniques at one institution. Fertil Steril 33:54–55, 1980.

Lenzi A, Culasso F, Gandini, L, et al: Placebo-controlled, double-blind, cross-over trial of glutathione therapy in male infertility. Hum Reprod 8:1657–1662, 1993.

Madgar I, Weissenberg R, Lunenfeld B, et al: Controlled trial of high spermatic vein ligation for varicocele in infertile men. Fertil Steril 63:120–124, 1995.

Mak V, Jarvi KA: The genetics of male infertility. J Urol 156:1245–1257, 1996.

McClure RD, Khoo D, Jarvi K, et al: Subclinical varicocele: The effectiveness of varicocelectomy. J Urol 145:789–791, 1991.

Moghissi KS: Postcoital test: Physiologic basis, technique, and interpretation. Fertil Steril 27:117–129, 1976.

Mulhall JP, Reijo R, Alagappan R, et al: Azoospermic men with deletion of the *DAZ* gene cluster are capable of completing spermatogenesis: Fertilization, normal embryonic development and pregnancy occur when retrieved testicular spermatozoa are used for intracytoplasmic sperm injection. Hum Reprod 12:503–508, 1997.

Niederberger C, Ross LS: Microsurgical epididymovasostomy: Predictors of success. J Urol 149:1364–1367, 1993.

Nijs M, Geerts L, van Roosendaal E, et al: Prevention of multiple pregnancies in an *in vitro* fertilization program. Fertil Steril 59:1245–1250, 1993.

Ohashi K, Saji F, Kato M, et at: Acrobeads test: A new diagnostic test for assessment of the fertilizing capacity of human spermatozoa. Fertil Steril 63:625–630, 1995.

Olsen GW, Bodner KM, Ramlow JM, et al: Have sperm counts been reduced percent in 50 years? A statistical model revisited. Fertil Steril 63:887–893, 1995.

Owen ER: Microsurgical vasovasostomy: A reliable vasectomy reversal. Aust NZ J Surg 47:305–309, 1977.

Owen ER, Kapila H: Vasectomy reversal: Review of 475 microsurgical vasovasostomies. Med J Aust 140:398–400, 1984.

Padron OF, Sharma RK, Thomas AJ, et al: Effects of cancer on spermatozoa quality after cryopreservation: A 12-year experience. Fertil Steril 67:326–331, 1997.

Patrizio P: Intracytoplasmic sperm injection (ICSI): Potential genetic concerns. Hum Reprod 10:2520–2523, 1995.

Pavlovich CP, Schlegel PN: Fertility options after vasectomy: A cost-effectiveness analysis. Fertil Steril 67:133–141, 1997.

Poland ML, Moghissi KS, Giblin PT, et al: Variation of semen measures within normal men. Fertil Steril 44:396–400, 1985.

Pryor JL, Howards SS. Varicocele. Urol Clin North Am 14:499–513, 1987.

Reijo R, Lee TY, Salo P, et al: Diverse spermatogenic defects in humans caused by Y chromosome deletions encompassing a novel RNA-binding protein gene. Nat Genet 10:383–393, 1995.

Schlegel PN: Examining the mechanics of ejaculation. Cont Urol 45–52, November 1995.

Schlegel PN, Goldstein M: Microsurgical vasoepididymostomy: Refinements and results. J Urol 150:1165–1168, 1993.

Schlegel PN, Su LM: Physiological consequences of testicular sperm extraction. Hum Reprod 12:1688–1692, 1997.

Sharma RK, Agarwal A: Role of reactive oxygen species in male infertility. Urology 48:835–850, 1996.

Sherins RJ, Thorsell LP, Doffmann A, et al: Intracytoplasmic sperm injection facilitates fertilization even in the most severe forms of male infertility: Pregnancy outcome correlates with maternal age and number of eggs available. Fertil Steril 64:369–375, 1995.

Sigman M, Lipshultz LI, Howards SS: Evaluation of the subfertile male. *In* Lipshultz LI, Howards SS (eds): Infertility in the Male. St. Louis, Mosby, 1997; p. 173.

Silber SJ: Microscopic vasectomy reversal. Fertil Steril 28:1191–1202, 1977.

Silber SJ: Specific tubule vasoepididymostomy. Paper presented at the 43rd annual meeting of the America Fertility Society, Reno, September 28–30, 1987.

Smith KD, Rodriguez-Rigau LJ, Steinberger E: Relationship between indices of semen analysis and pregnancy rate of infertile couples. Fertil Steril 28:1314–1319, 1977.

Soonawalla FB, Lal SS: Microsurgery in vasovasostomy. Ind J Urol 1:104–108, 1984.

Stillman RJ, Rosenberg MJ, Sachs BP: Smoking and reproduction. Fertil Steril 46:545–566, 1986.

Sukcharoen N, Keith J, Irvine DS, et al: Predicting the fertilizing potential of human sperm suspensions in vitro: Importance of sperm morphology and leukocyte contamination. Fertil Steril 63:1293–1300, 1995.

Suleiman SA, Ali ME, Zaki ZMS, et al: Lipid peroxidation and human sperm motility: Protective role of vitamin E. J Androl 17:530–537, 1996.

Thomas AJ: Microsurgical end-to-side vasoepididymostomy: An analysis of 153 procedures. Paper presented at the 88th annual meeting of the American Urological Society, San Antonio, TX, May 1993.

Thomas AJ, Howards SS: Microsurgical treatment of male infertility. *In* Lipshultz LI, Howards SS (eds): Infertility in the Male. St. Louis, Mosby, 1997, p. 371.

Thomas AJ, Padron O: Obstructive azoospermia and vasoepididymostomy. *In* Hellstrom WJG (ed): Male Infertility and Sexual Dysfunction. New York, Springer-Verlag, 1997; p. 244.

Thomas AJ, Pontes JE, Rose NR, et al: Microsurgical vasovasostomy: Immunologic consequences and subsequent fertility. Fertil Steril 35:447–450, 1981.

Thompson ST: Prevention of male infertility: An update. Urol Clin North Am 21:365–376, 1994.

Tripp BM, Gagnon C: Advanced sperm fertility tests. *In* Lipshultz LI, Howards SS (eds): Infertility in the Male. St. Louis, Mosby, 1997; p. 194.

Turek PJ: Immunopathology and infertility. *In* Lipshultz LI, Howards SS (eds): Infertility in the Male. St. Louis, Mosby, 1997; p 305.

Urry RL, Carrel DT, Hull DB, et al: Penetration of zona-free hamster and bovine cervical mucus by fresh and frozen human spermatozoa. Fertil Steril 39:690–694, 1983.

Van Asssche E, Bonduelle M, Tournaye H, et al: Cytogenetics of infertile men. Hum Reprod 11(suppl):1–26, 1996.

van der Ven K, Montag M, Peschka B, et al: Combined cytogenetic and Y chromosome microdeletion screening in males undergoing intracytoplasmic sperm injection. Mol Hum Reprod 3:699–704, 1997.

Vine MF, Tse CKJ, Hu PC, et al: Cigarette smoking and semen quality. Fertil Steril 65:835–842, 1996.

Vogt PH: Genetic aspects of artificial fertilization. Hum Reprod 10(suppl):128–137, 1995.

Wilcox AJ, Weinberg CR, Baird DD: Timing of sexual intercourse in relation to ovulation. Effects on the probability of conception, survival of the pregnancy, and sex of the baby. N Engl J Med 333:1517–1521, 1995.

Witt MA, Lipshultz LI: Varicocele: A progressive or static lesion? Urology 42:541–543, 1993.

Wolf DP, Sokoloski JE, Quigley MM, et al: Correlation of human *in vitro* fertilization with the hamster egg bioassy. Feril Steril 40:53–59, 1983.

Wolff H: The biologic significance of white blood cells in semen. Fertil Steril 63:1143–1157, 1995.

World Health Organization: The influence of varicocele on parameters of fertility in a large group of men presenting to infertility clinics. Fertil Steril 57:1289–1293, 1992.

World Health Organization: *In vivo* test (postcoital test). *In* WHO Manual for the Examination of Human Semen and Sperm-Cervical Mucus Interaction. Cambridge, England, Cambridge University Press, 1992; p 34.

World Health Organization: Morphological classification of human spermatozoa. *In* WHO Manual for the Examination of Human Semen and Sperm-Cervical Mucus Interaction. Cambridge, Cambridge University Press, 1992; p 14.

Yamamoto M, Hibi H, Katsuno S, et al: Antibiotic and ejaculation treatments improve resolution rate of leukocytospermia in infertile men with prostatitis. Nagoya J Med Sci 58:41–45, 1995.

Yanushpolsky EH, Politch JA, Hill JA, et al: Is leukocytospermia clinically relevant? Fertil Steril 66:822–825, 1996.

Yanushpolsky EH, Politch JA, Hill JA, et al: Antibiotic therapy and leukocytospermia: A prospective, randomized, controlled study. Fertil Steril 63:142–147, 1995.

# 60

# Assisted Reproductive Technologies

CHARLA M. BLACKER

Before 1978, couples with severe tubal infertility or male factor infertility had little hope of becoming biological parents. Few scientific advances have revolutionized medical therapy as much as the assisted reproductive technologies (ARTs), which have changed infertility therapy. Currently, there are few couples who do not have a chance to achieve a pregnancy by use of one or more of these techniques. In fact, the science has progressed more rapidly than has our ability to deal with the ethical implications of some of the procedures. Nonetheless, there has never been a better time to be infertile.

ARTs were developed initially to treat women with irreparable fallopian tubes; however, many variants on the basic in vitro fertilization methodology have been introduced and have increased options available to infertile men and women. The proliferation of these procedures has led to a new lexicon of names and acronyms in the medical literature. Table 60-1 describes the currently accepted procedures among the ARTs and the generally accepted acronym for each. An overview of the commonly used ARTs is described. The choice of appropriate ART should be made together with the patient after careful consideration of the patient's age, etiology of infertility, tubal status, and the success of an individual ART program with the procedure.

This chapter serves to discuss the various ART procedures, how they are performed, indications, and results. A practical management scheme for patients is presented, realizing that care must be individualized, as previously noted.

## Referral of Patients for Assisted Reproductive Technology

Infertile couples should undergo complete infertility evaluation, and conventional treatments for infertility generally should be exhausted before consideration of ART. In many cases, there are simpler, less expensive therapies that can offer outcomes equal to those of ART procedures. An appropriate trial of therapy should be instituted before ART. This usually includes at least six ovulatory cycles, correcting any factors that have been diagnosed. Because the background conception rate is high during the second year of unprotected intercourse for couples with no significant tubal or male factors, a conservative approach to the use of ART is indicated. The older the female partner, however, the more expeditious should be the evaluation and treatment and referral for ART because the success with ART decreases rapidly in the late 30s and particularly after 40 years of age.

**Table 60–1** Assisted Reproductive Technologies: Procedures

| Description | Term |
|---|---|
| Infertility therapy procedures that have in common the manipulation of oocytes, spermatozoa, and/or embryos | Assisted reproductive technologies |
| Ovulation stimulation with monitoring in normal ovulatory women with the intent to induce multiple follicles | Controlled ovarian hyperstimulation |
| Ovulation induction combined with timed intrauterine insemination | Controlled ovarian hyperstimulation/intrauterine insemination |
| Laboratory culture of aspirated oocyte(s) and spermatozoa followed by transcervical embryo transfer | In vitro fertilization<br>Embryo transfer |
| Placement of aspirated oocyte(s) and spermatozoa into the fallopian tube(s) | Gamete intrafallopian transfer |
| Laboratory culture of aspirated oocytes with spermatozoa followed by placement of fertilized zygote(s) or embryo(s) into the fallopian tube(s) | Zygote intrafallopian transfer<br>Tubal embryo transfer |
| Removal of a portion of the zona pellucida from the oocyte in order to facilitate fertilization by spermatozoa with lower fertility potential | Partial zona dissection |
| Insertion of several spermatozoa into the perivitelline space to facilitate fertilization | Subzonal insertion |
| Injection of a single spermatozoa into the oocyte cytoplasm to facilitate fertilization | Intracytoplasmic sperm injection |
| Creation of a gap in the zona pellucida of cleaved embryos to enhance implantation | Assisted hatching |
| Laboratory culture of aspirated oocytes from a donor woman followed by culture of sperm/oocyte (in vitro fertilization) or placement of oocyte/sperm mixture into the fallopian tube (gamete intrafallopian transfer) | Oocyte donation |

Performing a complete evaluation before consideration of ART not only aids in choosing the appropriate therapeutic approach, it also serves to determine the prognosis for pregnancy. The three most important issues in deciding whether a form of ART is appropriate are (1) the woman's age, (2) the woman's follicle-stimulating hormone (FSH) level, and (3) the male partner's semen quality. Outcomes-based analysis has indicated several diagnostic categories that benefit from aggressive use of ART. Couples with poor-prognosis tubal disease should be offered immediate access to ART because in vitro fertilization–embryo transfer (IVF-ET) has been demonstrated to be more cost-effective than tubal surgery. Couples with severe oligoasthenozoospermia are less likely to conceive with inseminations than other diagnostic groups, even with controlled ovarian hyperstimulation, and should be offered donor insemination or intracytoplasmic sperm injection early in therapy. Also, cumulative and clinical pregnancy rates are substantially lower in women older than 35 years of age, regardless of ovulatory status, and these women may benefit from aggressive use of ART. Controlled ovarian hyperstimulation with intrauterine insemination (COH/IUI) is associated with ongoing cycle fecundity rates of 9.6%, 5.2%, and 2.4% at 40, 41, and 42 years of age respectively; pregnancies are rare with COH/IUI in women ≥ 43 years of age or older. Women who are older than 40 years of age or in whom the FSH level is greater than 25 mIU/ml have a very poor chance of conceiving through IVF, however, and probably are treated better by use of donor oocytes.

The unexplained infertility patient remains a dilemma. Age and duration of infertility must be considered in planning therapy. A prospective, nonrandomized study by Peterson and colleagues suggested that two cycles of menotropin ovulation induction with intrauterine inseminations were comparable with a single cycle of IVF or zygote intrafallopian transfer (ZIFT) and inferior to gamete intrafallopian transfer (GIFT), whereas four cycles of menotropins with intrauterine inseminations were superior to all techniques. Because the expense of a cycle of IVF in their program was greater than four cycles of human menopausal gonadotropin (hMG)/IUI, a cost-benefit analysis favored using COH/IUI for four cycles before resorting to other forms of ART. In women with normal fallopian tubes, either GIFT or IVF is an appropriate choice if male factor is not an issue. Even in women who have failed to conceive after three cycles of ovarian stimulation and IUI, satisfactory pregnancy rates occur with the use of either IVF and GIFT with no significant difference in the two techniques. Because IVF is less invasive and offers diagnostic information regarding sperm-oocyte interaction, we generally would recommend it in women after failure of COH. A management scheme demonstrating how ART fits into an infertility therapy regimen is shown in Figure 60–1.

## Controlled Ovarian Hyperstimulation

It generally is accepted that the cycle fecundity of normal couples is approximately 20%, whereas the cycle fecundity of couples with a history of infertility may be only 1 to 3%. Strategies to improve cycle fecundity rely on increasing the chances of sperm-oocyte interaction and/or improving the quality of ovulation when no other infertility factors have been diagnosed. The goal is to approximate or exceed the cycle fecundity of normal couples and treatment strategies should be evaluated with this goal in mind.

COH/IUI of capacitated sperm has been used to treat a subset of infertile couples in whom no tubal or peritoneal factors exist. The proposed mechanisms of enhanced fertility with COH/IUI include: (1) increased numbers of oocytes available for fertilization; (2) increased levels of follicular and luteal phases gonadal steroids; (3) optimizing the chance of gamete interaction by ensuring that oocyte(s) and spermatozoa are present in the reproductive tract simultaneously; and (4) providing large numbers of highly motile capacitated spermatozoa at the site of fertilization in the distal fallopian tubes.

The primary fertility enhancing effect of COH is probably secondary to the increase in number of oocytes released. The ovulation induction regimens used for this purpose have included clomiphene citrate, hMGs with human chorionic gonadotropin (hCG), clomiphene citrate and hMG-hCG, purified follicle-stimulating hormone (pFSH)-hCG, and hMG or pFSH-hCG after pretreatment with a gonadotropin-releasing hormone (GnRH) agonist. No well-designed comparative trials have been performed to determine the regimen of choice. Although clomiphene citrate has been documented to increase fecundity in women with unexplained infertility or with minimal endometriosis, lower cycle fecundity has been observed with clomiphene citrate–induced cycles in women with unexplained infertility compared with cycles induced with hMG. Nonetheless, because clomiphene citrate is less expensive than gonadotropin preparations and requires less monitoring, it often is used together with IUI for several cycles before hMG is tried. Further research is necessary to determine the most cost-effective approach for COH yielding the maximum cycle fecundity.

For the ovulatory infertile woman, a pFSH-hCG regimen comparable to that used for IVF-ET commonly is used (see Table 60–3). The selection of the initial dosage is determined by the woman's weight and age, typically 2 or 3 ampules (75 to 150 IU) per day. Cycles are monitored using ultrasound and rapid estradiol, and hCG is administered to trigger oocyte release when the dominant follicle measures approximately 18 mm in mean diameter and estradiol is greater than 500 pg/ml. Compared with IVF-ET, it is generally advisable to lower the maximum number of dominant preovulatory follicles acceptable for COH/IUI because of the increased risk of clinically significant ovarian hyperstimulation syndrome and multiple gestation. Low incidence of ovarian hyperstimulation syndrome has been observed when peak serum estradiol before hCG is less than 2000 pg/ml;

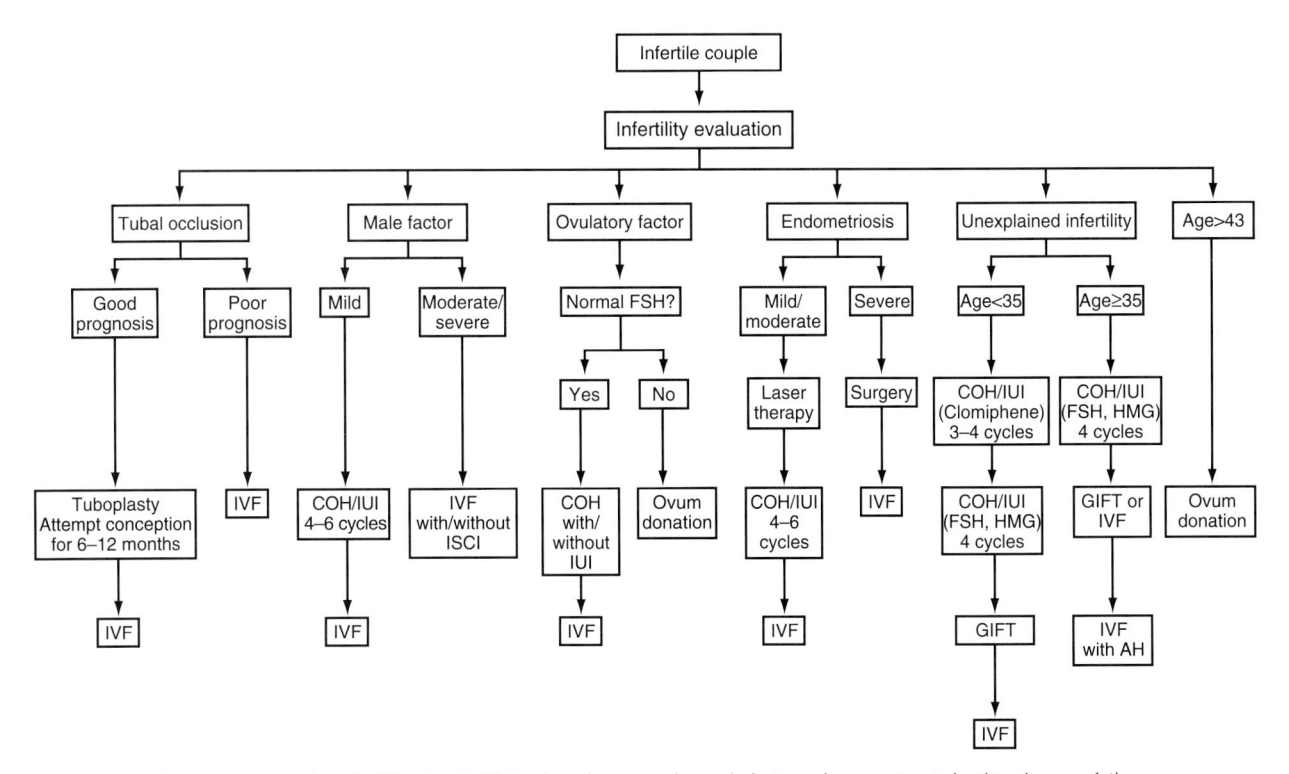

**Figure 60–1** In vitro fertilization (IVF) is often the procedure of choice when routine infertility therapy fails. This procedure should be performed promptly in women who have poor prognosis tubal disease and in severe male factor cases. Assisted reproductive techniques should also be employed expeditiously in women who are older than 35 years of age.

however, there is no specific level of estradiol or number of large preovulatory and small follicles that can guarantee that ovarian hyperstimulation or multiple gestation will not occur. Pretreatment with GnRH agonists has been used in an attempt to decrease hyperstimulation rates while improving fecundity rates by prevention of premature luteinizing hormone (LH) surge. Gagliardi and associates concluded from their retrospective study that adjunctive use of a GnRH agonist during COH/IUI cycles improved cycle fecundity; however, their series included couples with ovulatory dysfunction. Women with endometriosis also may benefit from pretreatment with a GnRH agonist for 6 weeks before initiation of menotropins. Conversely, a prospective study by Dodson and colleagues found that GnRH agonists were not cost-effective in unexplained infertility because they increased gonadotropin requirement without improving cycle fecundity. The detrimental effects of premature luteinization described in in vitro fertilization cycles does not seem as problematic during IUI cycles, which require less precise timing.

The use of IUI reduces the attrition of sperm as they ascend through the female reproductive tract and ensures that large numbers of capacitated spermatozoa reach the site of fertilization in the distal ampulla of the fallopian tube. Wash techniques are used to separate effectively the sperm from the liquid portion of the ejaculate. Resuspension of this highly motile fraction in a small volume of sterile fluid allows introduction of the specimen into the uterine cavity without the severe uterine contractions and risk of infection associated with the use of the raw ejaculate.

The impact of IUI alone in enhancing the cycle fecundity remains unsettled. Improved pregnancy rates have been noted in some reports but not in others. Therefore, IUI alone rarely is used when the only identifiable infertility factor is oligoasthenozoospermia. The contribution of IUI to improved fecundity rates during COH cycles is also controversial. Improved fecundity rates during COH cycles have been reported when IUI was performed compared with either IUI or COH alone. Johnson and associates demonstrated a cycle fecundity of 18% in COH cycles with timed intercourse compared with 20% in those couples also undergoing IUI; not a significant difference. A recent randomized prospective study demonstrated a cycle fecundity rate of 10% in patients who underwent superovulation alone and 19% in those treated with superovulation plus IUI.

Cycle fecundity approaching that of normally fertile couples has been observed in many subsets of the infertile population treated with COH/IUI (Table 60–2). The reported success rates with COH/IUI vary significantly between different centers, probably secondary to patient selection biases, differing COH regimens, and degree of hyperstimulation and multiple pregnancy that the center is willing to accept. One of the most frequent diagnoses selected for COH/IUI is male factor infertility. Comparison of the different studies is hampered by differing definitions of what constitutes significant male factor. However, the overall fecundity of 9% in couples using hMG usually is expected. A minimum of 1 million sperm in the inseminate appears necessary to achieve pregnancy. However, other factors affecting semen quality, such as teratozoospermia and immunologic factors, can result in failure to achieve pregnancy despite otherwise excellent sperm recovery. Couples with unexplained infertility generally have the best prognosis for pregnancy using COH/IUI (Table 60–2), and cycle fecundity approaches that of normal fertile couples, approximately 15 to 20% per cycle. Likewise, women with minimal and mild endometriosis have excellent results using COH/IUI with cycle fecundity virtually identical to that observed with unexplained infertility. Although COH/IUI has been used in peritoneal factor infertility in an effort to increase number of oocytes available for tubal pickup, women with severe pelvic adhesive disease or hydrosalpinges secondary to endometriosis or pelvic inflammatory disease are not good candidates and should be encouraged to consider IVF-ET. Similarly, couples who do not conceive within the first four cycles of COH/IUI are unlikely to conceive in subsequent cycles and should use alternative therapies.

Although severe ovarian hyperstimulation syndrome is uncommon, occurring in less than 1% of gonadotropin-stimulated cycles, mild to moderate hyperstimulation is frequent, with some degree of ovarian enlargement occurring in all gonadotropin-stimulated cycles. Unfortunately, the greater the degree of follicular stimulation, the greater the chance of pregnancy and the higher the incidence of complications. Therefore, a balance must be achieved between the risks and potential for pregnancy for every patient in each cycle. Unexplained variations in cycle to cycle and individual patient response mean that

**Table 60–2** Cycle Fecundity by Diagnosis

| Diagnosis | Pregnancies/Cycle | Fecundity |
|---|---|---|
| Male | 13/85 | 0.15 |
| Unexplained | 17/116 | 0.15 |
| Endometriosis | 63/474 | 0.13 |
| Minimal | 41/263 | 0.16 |
| Mild | 13/146 | 0.09 |
| Moderate | 9/51 | 0.18 |
| Severe | 0/14 | 0 |
| Adnexal adhesions | 13/131 | 0.10 |
| Cervical | 5/25 | 0.20 |

Data from Dodson WC, Haney AF: Controlled ovarian hyperstimulation and intrauterine insemination for treatment of infertility. Fertil Steril 55:457–467, 1991.

**Table 60–3** Typical Menotropin Stimulation Protocol for Controlled Ovarian Stimulation/Intrauterine Insemination

| Protocol | Day of Cycle | | | | | | | | | | | | | |
|---|---|---|---|---|---|---|---|---|---|---|---|---|---|---|
| | 1 | 2 | 3 | 4 | 5 | 6 | 7 | 8 | 9 | 10 | 11 | 12 | 13 | 14 |
| hpFSH | — | — | 150 IU | 150 IU | 150 IU | 150 IU | 150 IU | 150 IU | 150 IU | 150 IU | 150 IU | 150 IU | | |
| Serum estradiol | — | — | + | — | — | — | — | + | — | + | — | + | | |
| Vaginal ultrasonography | — | — | + | — | — | — | — | — | — | + | — | + | | |
| hCG* | — | — | — | — | — | — | — | — | — | — | — | + | | |
| IUI† | | | | | | | | | | | | | * | * |

*10,000 IU intramuscularly if mean follicular diameter is 18 mm.
†Intrauterine insemination (IUI) is performed approximately 18 and 40 hr after the human chorionic gonadotropin (hCG) injection. Coitus should be encouraged.
hpFSH = human pituitary follicle-stimulating hormone.

each cycle must be monitored carefully. Considerable experience is required to achieve maximal cycle fecundity safely. Despite careful monitoring, multiple gestation rate is high, with approximately 20% of cycles resulting in multiple gestation. Of these, 15% are usually twin gestation (often considered a desirable event by couples with long-standing infertility), 3% are triplet gestation, and 2% represent quadruplets and higher order. Triplet gestation and higher are associated with significant risk of prematurity, fetal demise, or compromise, as well as representing a major medical hazard for the mother. Although maternal age is directly related to spontaneous abortion rate and inversely related to implantation rate, there is no age at which a woman can be guaranteed that hyperstimulation or multiple gestation cannot occur. Because advanced maternal age increases the chance of pregnancy complications, high-order pregnancies in older women are especially serious, and couples should be counseled carefully regarding these risks.

## Intrauterine Insemination Technique

Various protocols for sperm preparation have yielded good results; however, most successful andrology programs individualize the technique based on the male's semen characteristics. Although no difference in pregnancy rates have been attributed to different sperm preparation methods, a method usually is chosen that yields greater numbers of motile sperm and reduces the amount of debris present in the inseminate. Inseminations are timed to coincide with the presence of the oocyte in the female reproductive tract, approximately 36 to 40 hours after the ovulating dose of hCG. Although data on timing of inseminations is scant, in a prospective, randomized trial, Silverberg and colleagues observed a higher cycle fecundity (52.2%) associated with two inseminations compared with a single insemination (8.7%).

Inseminations usually are performed in the dorsal lithotomy position, visualizing the cervix using a standard bivalve speculum. A sterile narrow-gauge catheter usually passes easily through the periovulatory cervix and is advanced into the upper uterine corpus. A tenaculum occasionally is required when cervical stenosis or a circuitous endocervical canal is encountered. The insemination volume is usually small, typically 0.2 to 0.5 ml, to minimize reflux and maximize sperm concentration. Reflux does not seem to decrease the chance of conception. Endometrial trauma and bleeding may reduce sperm viability; knowing the uterine position before attempting insemination is essential for easy, atraumatic insemination.

The primary risk of IUI is the risk of infection. Freshly ejaculated semen is not sterile, and there is no way to prepare a semen sample to completely eliminate genital tract pathogens. Use of a double-column discontinuous Percoll gradient reduces the number and spectrum of bacteria isolated. However, *Escherichia coli* still can be present in the final specimen. The infection rate, however, is low after IUI and is estimated to be comparable with the rate of pelvic infection after endometrial biopsy or hysterosalpingography (less than 1 in 500 procedures). It is recommended that the separated sperm sample be viewed microscopically by a trained observer before every IUI to exclude the presence of significant numbers of round cells (leukocytes). If numerous round cells are present, the sample should not be used for IUI, although coitus potentially may be used because the cervical mucus may filter out the seminal microbial flora while allowing sperm penetration into the upper genital tract.

Other concerns about IUI include the effects of components of the seminal plasma, such as prostaglandins within the upper female reproductive tract. Prostaglandins can cause severe uterine contractions and, theoretically, anaphylactic reactions. For this reason, "washing" the semen is used to separate seminal plasma from the cellular components. Suspension of the concentrated sperm pellet into a small volume of sterile, nonirritating medium allows delivery of a highly concentrated, highly motile cohort of sperm into the uterine cavity while avoiding the prostaglandin contamination. Theoretical concerns about induction of antisperm antibodies after IUI have not been validated. Fewer than 5% of women developed antibodies after IUI.

In the absence of male factor, improvement of cycle fecundity with the addition of IUI to COH has not been established unequivocally. However, several studies suggest improved rates. Because the risks associated with IUI are low and it is reasonably inexpensive, in the absence of large, prospective randomized trials, it is appropriate to offer IUI to couples undergoing COH.

# In Vitro Fertilization

In vitro fertilization (IVF) has dramatically changed the management of infertility. Since the first successful human pregnancy after IVF was reported in 1978, more than 11,000 live deliveries in the United States alone result from IVF procedures each year.

Although IVF originally was used for women with tubal occlusion, it currently is used for almost every etiology of infertility. A normal uterus in a woman with no contraindication to pregnancy, functioning ovaries (or availability of preovulatory oocytes), and availability of spermatozoa are minimal requirements for successful IVF. Recent technologic advances allow IVF to be used even when obstructive azoospermia or severe oligozoospermia prevent fertilization using traditional IVF techniques.

## INDICATIONS FOR IN VITRO FERTILIZATION

**Tubal Factor.** Approximately 25% of infertility is caused by tubal pathology. Although pregnancy rates after microsurgical tubal anastomosis after tubal ligation may exceed 60%, surgery for more significant tubal pathology is far less successful. Pregnancy rates after surgical repair of severe hydrosalpinges, after bipolar tubal disease, or after previous failed tuboplasty have been reported to be as low as 5%. IVF should be considered as primary therapy for poor-prognosis tubal disease and after bilateral salpingectomy. Outcome for these patients is favorable, with clinical pregnancy rates exceeding 25% per embryo transfer (ET) at most successful programs.

**Male Factor.** Male factor is the primary diagnosis in approximately 40% of infertile couples. Thorough evaluation of the male partner is imperative to diagnose conditions amenable to medical or surgical therapy. Unfortunately, surgical or medical therapy using IUI with or without COH is often unsuccessful in cases of a severe male factor. IVF has become increasingly useful in the management of male factor infertility, being both diagnostic and therapeutic. IVF offers the unique ability to observe sperm-oocyte interaction, in many cases giving insight into reasons for unexplained failure to conceive. Exposure of multiple oocytes to a high density of motile sperm in a small volume of culture media enhances the possibility of fertilization. Microsurgical fertilization techniques may improve the chances of fertilization in cases of previously failed fertilization or in cases in which the sperm quality is so poor as to predict a low probability of fertilization with conventional IVF.

Fertilization rates are reduced in male factor IVF cases, with ET rates of approximately 50% in most units. Use of microfertilization techniques may increase this rate to approximately that of those couples in whom male factor does not exist. Once fertilization has occurred, however, implantation rates are similar to those achieved in other diagnostic groups. Delivery rates approaching 40% are not unusual in couples undergoing IVF with microfertilization for male factor.

**Endometriosis.** Approximately 50% of women with endometriosis do not conceive after standard surgical or medical therapy. IVF in women with endometriosis results in ongoing pregnancy rates similar to those with tubal factor infertility. Disease stage may affect success rates by reducing the number or quality of oocytes recovered. Medical therapy before the IVF attempt may improve results.

**Immunologic Infertility.** Immunologic infertility is suggested by the presence of antisperm antibodies in semen, serum, or cervical mucus. Treatment options include washed IUIs with or without COH, immunosuppression (not recommended secondary to unproved efficacy and significant side effects), or ARTs. IVF pregnancy rates for couples with immunologic infertility are similar to those of other IVF-treated populations. However, fertilization rates decrease as the titer of antibody increases. When antibodies are detected in seminal plasma, ejaculation directly into the insemination medium may diminish sperm binding before the processing of the sample and may increase fertilization rate. The presence of high titers of antisperm antibodies in semen generally are accepted as an indication for use of intracytoplasmic sperm injection (ICSI), which yields results comparable with tubal factor infertility.

**Idiopathic Infertility.** For those couples in whom no etiology for infertility can be determined, treatment is largely empiric. COH/IUI often is attempted before consideration of ART. IVF may be diagnostic as well as therapeutic for this group, allowing evaluation of sperm-oocyte interaction. Unexpectedly low fertilization rates may indicate an intrinsic gamete defect, undetectable through routine infertility testing. IVF pregnancy rates for these couples generally exceed those for patients with pure tubal factor infertility.

# Predictive Tests in Assisted Reproductive Technology

Patient screening is an essential component of the ART process and allows selection of the most appropriate technique for the individual couple as well as tailoring of the regimen to provide the best results. Screening and selection criteria vary from program to program based on the program's experience and results with various ART procedures.

The single most important factor in predicting success through IVF is the female partner's age. Women older than 40 years of age have a poorer prognosis than younger women. The 1996 U.S. IVF Registry reported only an overall delivery rate of 8% per cycle in women older than 39 years, compared with 28.7% delivery rate in women younger than 35 years of age. Whereas women younger than 35 years who conceived had an adverse outcome in approximately 14% of conception cycles, women older than 40 years of age had a loss rate of greater than 35%. Preconceptual genetic testing of pre-embryos suggests that the decreased implantation and increased pregnancy loss rate reflects increased numbers of aneuploidic embryos with increasing maternal age. This is supported clinically by excellent implantation and delivery rates in older women conceiving through oocyte donation. For this reason, many programs discourage IVF attempts in women older than 40 years of age.

In addition to age, "ovarian reserve" may reflect an individual woman's potential for pregnancy during an ART cycle. Evaluation of baseline (cycle day 3) peripheral FSH and estradiol ($E_2$) may predict response to ovarian stimulation. An elevated day 3 FSH or $E_2$ may be indicative of incipient ovarian failure and reduced chance for success after IVF-ET. Dynamic testing of the hypothalamic-pituitary-ovarian axis using the clomiphene citrate challenge test may further detect subtle signs of occult ovarian dysfunction by an exaggerated increase in the FSH level on cycle day 10.

# TECHNIQUE OF IN VITRO FERTILIZATION–EMBRYO TRANSFER

In vitro fertilization consists of several discrete steps: (1) controlled ovarian hyperstimulation; (2) retrieval of oocytes, usually by transvaginal ultrasound guidance; (3) insemination of oocytes; (4) culture of pre-embryos; (5) pre-embryo transfer, and (6) luteal phase support.

**Ovarian Stimulation.** Although the first successful IVF attempt occurred during a spontaneous menstrual cycle, low efficiency has resulted in almost universal use of ovarian stimulation before IVF attempts. Likewise, the use of clomiphene citrate is uncommon secondary to high cancellation rates and reduced numbers of embryos available for transfer. Most successful IVF programs use gonadotropin to achieve controlled ovarian hyperstimulation. Down-regulation of pituitary function using a GnRH agonist such as leuprolide acetate before initiation of gonadotropin stimulation seems to result in increased conception rates. This improvement appears to be the result of decreased cancellation rates, although some authors have suggested improved embryo quality and increased window of implantation in leuprolide cycles.

A GnRH agonist generally is administered in a single daily subcutaneous dose of 0.5 to 1 mg, beginning either in the midluteal phase of the preceding cycle (long protocol) (Table 60–4) or day 2 or 3 of the follicular phase ("flare" protocol). In the long protocol, ovarian suppression generally is achieved by the onset of menses, before the onset of menotropin therapy. In the "flare" protocol, exogenous menotropins are initiated at the peak of the agonist-induced increase of endogenous gonadotropins. No significant differences were noted in cancellation or pregnancy rates between the two protocols. In either case, luteal phase support using exogenous progesterone or hCG is important to prevent luteal insufficiency.

Currently available gonadotropin preparations include hMG, pFSH consisting of 75 IU of FSH with less than 1 IU of LH per ampule; and recombinant FSH (rFSH), which consists of 75 IU of FSH per ampoule. Gonadotropin therapy generally is initiated at a daily dose of 150 to 300 IU. Monitoring is similar to that used during COH/IUI cycles and includes transvaginal ultrasound and measurement of serum $E_2$. Timing of hCG administration is determined by a number of variables, including serum $E_2$, diameter of lead follicles, and pattern of follicular growth. Typically, 5,000 to 10,000 IU of hCG is administered when the two lead follicles are 17 to 18 mm with a serum $E_2$ greater than 500 pg/ml. Oocyte retrieval is performed approximately 35 hours after hCG administration, an interval designed to stimulate the re-

Table 60–4 Long Protocol for In Vitro Fertilization

| Protocol | Day of Cycle | | | | | | | | | | | | |
|---|---|---|---|---|---|---|---|---|---|---|---|---|---|
| | 21 | — | 3 | 4 | 5 | 6 | 7 | 8 | 9 | 10 | 11 | 12 | 13 | 14 |
| Leuprolide Acetate (SC) | 1 mg | 1 mg | 0.5 mg | 0.5 mg | 0.5 mg | 0.5 mg | 0.5 mg | 0.5 mg | 0.5 mg | 0.5 mg | — | | | |
| hpFSH | — | — | 225 IU | 225 IU | 225 IU | 150 IU | 150 IU | 150 IU | 150 IU | 150 IU | — | | | |
| Serum estradiol | — | — | + | — | — | — | — | — | — | — | + | + | | |
| Vaginal ultrasonography | — | — | + | — | — | — | — | + | — | + | + | — | | |
| hCG* | — | — | — | — | — | — | — | — | — | — | + | — | | |
| Progesterone (Crinone 8%)† | | | | | | | | | | | | | + | +† |

*10,000 IU intramuscularly when mean follicular diameter of the two lead follicles are 18 mm. Ovum retrieval is scheduled 35 hours after administration of human chorionic gonadotropin (hCG).
†Progesterone intravaginal gel is administered daily from retrieval until β-hCG is obtained 12 days after embryo transfer (ET). If a pregnancy results, the progesterone is continued until gestational age of 9 wk.
SC = subcutaneous.

sumption of meiosis and extrusion of the first polar body.

**Oocyte Retrieval.** Although oocyte retrievals first were performed laparoscopically, currently more than 95% of aspirations are performed using an ultrasound-guided transvaginal approach under light sedation. Ovarian follicles are aspirated and preovulatory oocytes isolated by an experienced embryologist. Oocytes are graded for maturity to improve timing of hCG administration in future cycles and to determine the incubation interval before insemination.

**Insemination and Culture.** Approximately 100,000 to 200,000 washed, capacitated spermatozoa are used to inseminate each oocyte; however, the concentration of added sperm may be increased to as high as 500,000/oocyte to enhance the probability of fertilization. Gametes then are co-incubated in the fertilization medium for 12 to 18 hours before examination for evidence of normal fertilization (identification of 2 pronuclei or extrusion of the second polar body). Fertilization rates usually exceed 70% for mature oocytes but usually are reduced to about 50% for immature oocytes. Fertilization rates also may be compromised in male factor cases. The resulting embryos are cultured for an additional 24 to 48 hours in growth medium, allowing cleavage to the four- to eight-cell stage.

**Embryo Transfer.** This can be performed 1 to 3 days after oocyte retrieval, with embryos from the 1- to 12-cell stage. Success rates increase if more embryos are transferred but plateau at approximately six embryos. Multiple gestation risk increases with the number of embryos transferred, so the number of embryos usually is restricted, especially in younger women with a higher per embryo implantation rate. Excellent results have occurred from development of culture to blastocyst stage and transfer 5 to 6 days after oocyte retrieval allowed transfer of one to two embryos. ET is performed with a transcervical catheter. The embryos are loaded into a sterile transfer catheter in a small volume of transfer medium (20 to 50 μl). The catheter is advanced atraumatically to approximately 1 cm from the uterine fundus, and the embryos gently injected using a small syringe attached to the proximal end of the catheter. To optimize placement, the catheter may be advanced by ultrasound guidance. Atraumatic and accurate placement seems to improve implantation rates. Patients usually remain recumbent for a short interval after transfer, although there are little data about the effects of ambulation on outcome.

**Luteal Phase Support.** Although multiple corpora lutea are formed after IVF retrieval, luteal phase support is necessary to achieve optimal conception rates secondary to aspiration of many of the progesterone-producing granulosa cells. Exogenous progesterone supplementation usually is initiated on the day of oocyte retrieval. Progesterone may be administered intramuscularly, orally using micronized progesterone preparations, or vaginally with progesterone suppositories or a gel-based preparation. Vaginal progesterone gel and intramuscular progesterone injections yield similar conception and ongoing pregnancy rates. Some programs support the luteal phase with additional injections of hCG, but this may increase the risk of developing ovarian hyperstimulation syndrome.

A successful IVF-ET cycle is documented by a positive hCG level 12 to 14 days after retrieval. Normally rising serial hCG levels confirm pregnancy. Because ectopic pregnancy occurs in approximately 2% or more of IVF pregnancies, ultrasonography should be performed early. Ultrasound also is used to document the number of gestational sacs and fetal viability. Luteal support usually is continued to at least 6 weeks gestational age.

## PREGNANCY OUTCOME AFTER IN VITRO FERTILIZATION

Success rates can be reported in a variety of ways, and it is important to know which rates a program is using. *Clinical* pregnancy means that the pregnancy has progressed, at a minimum, to the stage at which the gestational sac and fetal heart motion can be visualized. *Ongoing* pregnancies are comprised of currently viable gestations and successfully delivered babies. Pregnancy rates also can be expressed per stimulation commenced, per egg retrieval, or per ET. Because the major economic investment for most couples is oocyte retrieval, the most meaningful way of reporting the results of IVF-ET is deliveries (or ongoing pregnancies for recent data) per oocyte retrieval.

Data generated by clinics in the United States and Canada in 1996 indicated that 58,913 cycles of IVF were performed, resulting in 13,314 live births. IVF had a success rate of 22.6% live births per cycle start and a live birth rate of 25.9% per retrieval procedure. Spontaneous abortion rate was approximately 13% but was significantly higher in older women. Ectopic pregnancies occurred in less than 1% of pregnancies, and heterotopic pregnancies were significantly increased secondary to the transfer of multiple embryos. There appears to be no increased risk of congenital malformations or other perinatal morbidity, when controlling for maternal age and multifetal pregnancies, as compared with spontaneously conceived children. The most common complication of IVF-ET is multiple gestation, representing approximately 32% of ART deliveries, of which 26% were twins and 6% were triplets or higher-order multiple gestations. Because multiple gestation is associated with increased risk of preterm labor and delivery, improving the per embryo implantation rate sufficiently to produce acceptable pregnancy rates while reducing risk of multiple gestation remains a major challenge for IVF programs.

## Gamete Intrafallopian Transfer

The fallopian tubes function both as site of fertilization and transporter for gametes and embryos. After spontaneous ovulation, the earliest that the oocyte could be recovered from the endometrial cavity was 80 hours after ovulation. Synchronization of endometrial maturation with embryo development is a significant factor affecting the chances of implantation. Gamete intrafallopian transfer (GIFT) was developed as an alternative to IVF-ET for infertility that was not related to tubal or male factors. GIFT consists of discrete steps similar to those of IVF-ET: (1) COH; (2) retrieval of oocytes, usually by transvaginal ultrasound guidance or laparoscopically; (3) preparation of spermatozoa; and (4) luteal phase support. GIFT differs from IVF because oocytes and spermatozoa are transferred into the fallopian tube(s) immediately after retrieval, usually laparoscopically. GIFT requires normal tubal transport mechanisms; therefore, it is limited to women with at least one normal fallopian tube.

## INDICATIONS FOR GAMETE INTRAFALLOPIAN TRANSFER

The main indications for GIFT are unexplained infertility and endometriosis. GIFT has yielded disappointing results for immunologic or significant male factor infertility. However, it has proved useful when there is minor impairment of semen characteristics, in cervical factor, and iatrogenic pelvic adhesions. GIFT generally is not recommended for women with significant adhesions resulting from pelvic inflammatory disease even with one apparently normal tube because of the possible presence of intratubal pathology.

GIFT can be performed simultaneously with diagnostic laparoscopy. Results in women undergoing combined diagnostic and operative laparoscopy were similar to those undergoing GIFT alone. It is not recommended that these procedures be combined in women with significant adhesive disease or endometriosis because the multiple ovarian follicles achieved with COH may prevent the complete visualization of the pelvic organs, and there is potential for excessive bleeding.

## PREGNANCY OUTCOME AFTER GAMETE INTRAFALLOPIAN TRANSFER

Originally, GIFT overall pregnancy and delivery rates of 27.5 and 20.2% were significantly better than those of IVF-ET (16.4 and 11.9%). The lowest success rates were reported for male factor (15% pregnancy rate) and immunologic factor (16% pregnancy rate). Higher success rates were reported in women with idiopathic infertility (31%) or endometriosis (32%). Spontaneous abortion rates were similar to those of women undergoing IVF-ET, approximately 17%. Surprisingly, the ectopic pregnancy rates is only about 4% in most series, with higher rates reported in women with tubal pathology.

GIFT success rates have remained fairly steady since its inception. The ART success rate report produced by the Society for Assisted Reproductive Technology (SART) in 1996 lists a 29% live birth rate per retrieval for GIFT. Because GIFT is significantly more invasive and the success rates of IVF-ET and GIFT currently are more similar, GIFT was only used in approximately 6% of ART cycles in 1995. Multiple gestations occurred in 35% of pregnancies, with triplets or higher-order pregnancies in 6.4% of deliveries. As seen in IVF-ET, GIFT conception rate increases along with the number of oocytes transferred, but so does the multiple gestation rate. When four oocytes are transferred, an 8% multiple delivery rate was observed, whereas multiple delivery rate increased to 12.7% when more than six oocytes were transferred. Also, success rates decrease with increasing age, and women older than 40 year of age can expect a less than 9% chance of a live birth.

Initial attempts at transcervical approach to tubal cannulation for GIFT reported results inferior to those achieved by transabdominal tubal transfers with both decreased pregnancy rate and increased ectopic pregnancy rate. More recent reports have used an approach by which the catheter is advanced blindly by "feel." Pregnancy rates have approached those achieved laparoscopically. Because of the less invasive nature of the technique, this may be an alternative to conventional GIFT, especially for those couples for whom IVF-ET is not an acceptable option.

## Zygote Intrafallopian Transfer

The inability of GIFT to document the fertilization process in vitro represents a major drawback to using the procedure for male factor or immunologic factor infertility. Zygote intrafallopian transfer (ZIFT) was developed to combine the advantages inherent in IVF with those of GIFT. The steps of ZIFT include: (1) controlled ovarian stimulation regimens similar to those used for IVF-ET; (2) oocyte retrieval under ultrasound guidance; (3) oocyte culture and insemination in vitro or by intracytoplasmic sperm injection; (4) transfer of pronuclear or cleaved embryos by transfimbrial tubal cannulation, usually laparoscopically; and (5) luteal phase support similar to IVF-ET and GIFT. The ideal time for transfer has not been clearly established. Initial studies involved the transfer of pronuclear stage zygotes, 18 to 24 hours after insemination (ZIFT). Transfer of cleaved embryos 40 to 50 hours postinsemination allows further observation of embryonic development and is described as tubal embryo transfer (TET). There have been no controlled comparative studies assessing the relative efficacy of the two different transfer times.

ZIFT is indicated predominantly for male factor or immunologic factor infertility, but it also has been used for treatment of other causes of nontubal factor infertility, including endometriosis and unexplained infertility. In 1996, ZIFT was used in only 2% of the cases reported by SART. ZIFT was associated with a 30.3% ongoing pregnancy rate per retrieval; however, there was no differentiation made for TET or ZIFT. In several prospective studies with patients randomly assigned to IVF-ET, TET, or GIFT, pregnancy rates were not significantly different among the treatment groups. Although there is a theoretical advantage in replacing zygotes into the more physiologic environment of the fallopian tube, the additional cost and requirement for an invasive procedure has limited the use of ZIFT.

## Oocyte Donation

Early attempts at donor ovum–recipient transfer involved in in vivo fertilization (insemination) and attempted nonsurgical recovery of the early conceptus by lavaging the uterus of the donor with a transcervical catheter. Efficacy was poor, and there was risk of an unwanted pregnancy as well as transmission of sexually transmitted diseases for the ovum donor. Instead, modification of conventional IVF techniques to oocyte donors has been very successful in providing a whole cohort of women the opportunity to carry and deliver a baby.

### INDICATIONS FOR OOCYTE DONATION

The primary indication for ova donation is premature menopause, attributable to ovarian failure; surgical removal of the ovaries; or gonadal dysgenesis. Other accepted indications include avoiding transmission of a genetic defect, increasing the chance of pregnancy in women with "declining fertility," and enhancing the success rate in women with poor oocyte or embryo quality after autologous oocyte retrieval.

Although oocyte donation can be performed successfully in women beyond their natural reproductive years, careful evaluation of such women, including psychological evaluation, cardiovascular assessment, and high-risk obstetric consultation, should precede acceptance into an oocyte donation program.

### OOCYTE DONATION METHODS

Current oocyte donation methods use techniques established for in vitro fertilization. Steps include (1) selection of oocyte donors, (2) COH of donor synchronized to recipient, (3) hormone replacement in the recipient, (4) oocyte retrieval by ultrasound-guided follicular aspiration, (5) insemination of oocytes with recipient partner's spermatozoa, (6) culture of pre-embryos, (7) transfer of embryos into recipient, and (8) luteal-phase support. Ovum donation can be anonymous or by known donor. Screening of the donor is similar in both cases and should include psychological evaluation as well as genetic screening, as detailed in the 1993 American Fertility Society guidelines. In addition, infectious screening is mandatory.

Synchronization of donor and recipient cycles is important to the success of oocyte donation cycles. Menopausal patients are easier to synchronize because hormone replacement medications to develop the endometrium can be started without reference to the recipient's cycles. Ovarian suppression of the donor with a GnRH agonist while the recipient also is suppressed permits coordination of the initiation of gonadotropins with that of estrogen in the recipient. In one typical regimen, the recipient starts hormone replacement 16 days before the anticipated oocyte retrieval. The donor undergoes COH by routine protocol. Progesterone is started in the recipient on the day after hCG is given to the donor to ensure that the embryo transfer occurs on the fourth day of progesterone exposure. The follicular phase can be adjusted as needed to refine the timing of transfer. Various hormone replacement regimens have been used, with the goal of producing physiologic systemic $E_2$ level and endometrial effects. Whereas nonoral routes of estrogen administration result in more physiologic serum $E_2$ and estrone ($E_1$) levels, no difference in pregnancy rates between oral and nonoral regimens has been reported. Luteal-phase support is critical for conception and maintenance of pregnancy in oocyte donation cycles because endogenous steroid production is deficient or nonexistent in the recipient. Both estrogen and progesterone are required until the placenta initiates steroidogenesis, typically until at least 10 weeks of pregnancy.

## PREGNANCY OUTCOME AFTER OOCYTE DONATION

Because oocyte donors are younger than the average IVF patient, frequently of proven fertility, and are selected for good reproductive and general health, it would be expected that pregnancy rates would be optimal in women conceiving through the use of donated oocytes. In addition, the uterine environment is optimized by avoiding antiestrogens such as clomiphene citrate or exposure to supraphysiologic levels of estrogen and/or progesterone. In 1995, there were 3,352 transfers from oocyte donation, resulting in a 35.5% live birth rate per transfer. Multiple gestations were common, occuring in 41% of conceptions. Spontaneous abortion rate was not reported, but in previous publications have been similar to that of other assisted reproductive techniques.

## Gestational Surrogacy

Gestational surrogacy uses techniques developed through oocyte donation cycles and involves transfer of embryos to a gestational surrogate, or "host uterus," who then relinquishes the ensuing child to the genetic parents after delivery. The process differs from surrogacy, in which a normal fertile woman is inseminated for the purposes of conceiving and subsequently relinquishing a child that is partially genetically hers to an infertile couple. It primarily is indicated for couples in which the woman has normal ovarian function but cannot carry a pregnancy, either because of hysterectomy or uterine abnormalities. Other indications would include severe medical conditions that would potentially be life-threatening during a pregnancy. The infertile woman undergoes COH and oocyte retrieval. Oocytes are inseminated with her partner's sperm, and the resulting embryos then are transferred into a gestational surrogate. Synchrony usually is achieved using a GnRH agonist with subsequent hormone replacement in the gestational surrogate, a regimen identical to that used by oocyte donation recipients.

In the largest series of gestational surrogacy reported, 28 couples underwent 39 cycles with a pregnancy rate of 18% per retrieval. Subsequent experience suggested that synchronized exogenous hormone stimulation of the gestational surrogate's endometrium improved the success rate with pregnancy rates greater than 60% in one series. As expected, the commissioning mother's age was closely related to implantation and spontaneous abortion rates in the host. Ethical and legal issues involved in oocyte donation and gestational surrogacy are beyond the scope of this discussion but have been reviewed elsewhere. These issues are important and illustrate the truism that medical technology progresses more quickly than our ability to deal with the resulting ethical implications.

# Micromanipulation of Gametes and Embryos

The application of micromanipulation in the assisted reproduction laboratory has revolutionized the treatment of infertility almost as much as IVF-ET did in the 1980s. Micromanipulation is both therapeutic and, increasingly, diagnostic. It can be used to facilitate the fertilization process, enhance implantation through assisted hatching or cytoplasmic transfer, restore diploidy by pronuclear extraction, and perform preimplantation genetic diagnosis, such as polar body or blastomere biopsy. Although it is beyond the scope of this chapter to discuss these topics in depth, an overview of the recent developments in the field of clinical gamete and embryo micromanipulation is presented.

## ASSISTED FERTILIZATION

Assisted fertilization offers men with impaired sperm function secondary to oligozoospermia, teratozoospermia, or asthenozoospermia the potential to father a biological child. Certain oocyte abnormalities also can be treated through micromanipulation. Assisted fertilization involves several techniques that can be applied to patients in whom the fertilization process is inhibited and enables the laboratory to circumvent specific stages of fertilization without attempting to correct the actual defect. Historically, there have been three major techniques of assisted fertilization, all of which bypass to some extent the barrier provided by the zona pellucida. Partial zona dissection (PZD) uses a mechanical procedure to introduce a gap in the zona after shrinking the oocyte by exposing it to a high molarity sucrose solution. Fertilization requires low numbers (0.2 to 0.5 × $10^5$/ml) of motile sperm per oocyte. The first human births from assisted fertilization occurred through the use of PZD. The second technique developed was subzonal sperm insertion (SZI), in which the zona is bypassed entirely and small numbers (1–5) of capacitated, acrosome-reacted sperm are deposited into the perivitelline space. Although both techniques were successful in achieving fertilization rates of up to 30% of oocytes in severe cases of male factor infertility, both fertilization and delivery rates remained below those expected.

Intracytoplasmic sperm injection (ICSI) has become the preferred technique for assisted fertilization. It can be applied to the most severe cases of oligozoospermia, even to men with azoospermia secondary to congenital blockage of the vas or failed spermatogenesis. With ICSI, a single spermatozoan is injected using a micropipette into the cytoplasm of each preovulatory oocyte. In 1995, nearly 11% of ART cycles used ICSI, for a 27.2% live birth rate per retrieval.

## ASSISTED HATCHING

The inefficiency of IVF is largely the result of implantation failure. Possible causes of this failure include genetic abnormalities of the embryos, suboptimal culture conditions, impaired uterine receptivity, and abnormalities of the zona pellucida. Munne and colleagues reported that at least 27% of normally growing embryos contain mitotic errors for selected chromosomes. Suboptimal culture conditions are evidenced by the fact that less than 25% of human blastocysts hatch in culture. Improvements in culture systems, including the use of serum-free media and coculture with a variety of human and nonhuman cells, appear to increase the average implantation rate per embryo. Zona hardening is known to occur as a result of fertilization, cryopreservation, in vitro culture, and in vivo aging. Embryos with a good prognosis for implantation have been observed to spontaneously thin their zonas in vitro, and embryos with artificial gaps in their zona secondary to assisted fertilization demonstrate a very high rate of implantation.

Assisted hatching (AH) first was performed in the zona of day 2 or 4 cell embryos mechanically using the techniques developed during PZD. Although initial results were encouraging, embryo trapping, in which only part of the cell mass is extruded, was observed secondary to the difficulty in consistently creating a hole of adequate size. Most current programs use Tyrode's solution for drilling a hole through the zona pellucida of day 3 embryos. Laser technology also has been used successfully for this purpose. No significant difference in implantation rates has been noted in randomly selected women with normal basal FSH levels between a group undergoing zona drilling (67 of 239; 28%) and a control group (49 of 229; 21%). However, when AH was performed only on embryos with thick zona or poor embryonic morphology, the implantation rate with selective AH was 25%, significantly higher than the control group (18%). In women with elevated basal FSH levels, the improvement in clinical pregnancy rate (47% vs. 13%) and implantation rate (26% vs. 10%) was even more impressive.

The indications developed for AH thus far include advanced maternal age, elevated basal FSH levels, increased zona thickness, unexplained implantation failure in a prior IVF cycle, reduced embryonic cleavage or excess fragmentation, and the use of in vitro oocyte maturation in conjunction with IVF. Successful use of AH requires excellent laboratory conditions, technical proficiency of the embryologist, and atraumatic transfer techniques because the resulting embryos are more fragile. AH remains controversial because some laboratories have failed to demonstrate improved implantation rates and possible embryo damage. However, no increase in congenital malformations has been reported in groups using AH, and when used properly, it appears to improve significantly the prognosis for difficult IVF patients.

## PREIMPLANTATION GENETIC DIAGNOSIS

Preimplantation genetic diagnosis is indicated for couples, infertile or not, at risk of transmitting a genetic disease. It is based on the genetic analysis of one or a few cells biopsied from an embryo obtained by IVF and the transfer of only presumed normal embryos to the maternal uterus. It offers an alternative to current practice, which requires a pregnant woman to carry a fetus at risk for a genetic disease and to terminate an established pregnancy. Successful preimplantation genetic diagnosis has been performed and healthy babies have been born after diagnosis of a number of X-linked diseases and single-gene defects. Additionally, these techniques can be applied to diagnose numerical chromosome abnormalities, specifically aneuploidy, and allow replacement of normal embryos, with resulting improvement in implantation and ongoing pregnancy rates.

Preimplantation genetic diagnosis requires a laboratory and personnel with excellent micromanipulative skills in addition to the ability to perform polymerase chain reaction (PCR) and fluorescent in situ hybridization (FISH). For couples at risk for transmitting X-linked genetic disease for which no specific PCR probes are yet available, FISH is the method of choice. In this case, FISH, with X- and Y-chromosome specific probes, is used to determine the gender of the embryos, so that only those with the gender that cannot express the disease are transferred. For single-gene disease for which specific PCR primers are available, PCR is performed for both X-linked and autosomal genes. For women with advanced age or who are otherwise at risk for nondisjunction undergoing IVF, FISH can be used to screen embryos for the most common aneuploidies—X, Y, 13, 16, 18, and 21—not only to prevent the birth of abnormal babies but also to increase the chances of pregnancy.

Several methods of obtaining cells exist. Preconception genetic analysis of oocytes for maternally inherited genetic defects has been performed using first polar body biopsy. The first polar body is extruded from the oocyte during the first meiotic division and is not required for normal fertilization or embryo development. Analysis also can be performed using one or more blastomeres from a cleaved embryo. In this case, the eight-cell stage (postinsemination day 3) has been shown to be the best in which to perform a biopsy; up to three cells can be removed for analysis without compromising the embryo's developmental capacity. Blastocyst biopsy offers advantages over the two previous techniques because it can yield 5 to 20 cells, enough to do metaphase chromosome spreads and reduce the chance of contamination during PCR. However, it currently is not practical because of the reduced numbers of embryos surviving to blastocyst stage. Further developments in blastocyst culture techniques may make blastocyst biopsy the method of choice. Although preimplantation genetic diagnosis currently is limited by the small number of probes available, it is a powerful tool that promises increasing future applications.

## Conclusion

Couples presenting with infertility should undergo thorough evaluation to determine the etiology of infertility. Therapy should be based on diagnosis, and traditional therapies should be used before couples are referred for the more involved reproductive technologies. Women with significant tubal disease and couples with male factor infertility should be referred promptly to a specialist for IVF because surgery or homologous inseminations are unlikely to be successful in these groups. When the appropriate assisted reproductive procedure is selected, the potential for pregnancy is excellent and dependent mostly on the female's age.

Women younger than 35 years of age have a very good prognosis, whereas women older than 39 years of age have a very limited chance of conceiving using any form of ART. For this reason, women in their late 30s who present for infertility evaluation and therapy should be referred promptly to a specialist who can discuss the benefits and risks associated with the available therapeutic options, including COH/IUI, IVF, GIFT, ZIFT, and oocyte donation. The use of ART has increased dramatically in the past several years, and conception and implantation rates have likewise improved largely because of laboratory advances. The development of micromanipulation techniques, particularly ICSI, has increased our ability to help more couples than with any technique since the development of IVF itself for the treatment of tubal infertility. Preimplantation genetic diagnosis has become a reality because of micromanipulation techniques developed for treatment of male infertility. The various ART techniques increasingly are becoming the cornerstone in the treatment of infertility of all etiologies.

## REFERENCES

Agarwal SK, Buyalos RP: Clomiphene citrate with intrauterine insemination: Is it effective therapy above the age of 35 years? Fertil Steril 65:759–763, 1996.

American Fertility Society: Guidelines for gamete donation: 1993. Fertil Steril 59:5S–9S, 1993.

Arcaini L, Bianchi S, Baglioni A, et al: Superovulation and intrauterine insemination vs. superovulation alone in the treatment of unexplained infertility: A randomized study. J Reprod Med 41:614–618, 1996.

Asch RH, Ellsworth LR, Balmaceda JP, et al: Pregnancy after laparoscopic gamete intrafallopian transfer (GIFT). Lancet 2:1034–1035, 1984.

Balasch J, Jove I, Marquez M, et al: Hormonal and histological evaluation of the luteal phase after combined GnRH-agonist/gonadotropin treatment for superovulation and luteal phase support in in vitro fertilization. Hum Reprod 6:914–917, 1991.

Balmaceda JP, Gonzales J, Benardini L: Gamete and zygote intrafallopian transfers and related techniques. Curr Opin Obstet Gynecol 4:743–749, 1992.

Bolton VN, Warren RE, Braude PR: Removal of bacterial contaminants for in vitro fertilization or artificial insemination by the use of buoyant density centrifugation. Fertil Steril 46:1128–1132, 1986.

Buster JE, Bustillo M, Rodi IA, et al: Biologic and morphologic development of donated human ova recovered by nonsurgical uterine lavage. Am J Obstet Gynecol 153:211–217, 1985.

Bustillo M, Schulman JD: Transcervical ultrasound-guided intrafallopian placement of gametes, zygotes, and embryos. J IVF ET 6:321–324, 1989.

Chetkowski RJ, Kruse LR, Nass TE: Improved pregnancy outcome with the addition of leuprolide acetate to gonadotropins for in vitro fertilization. Fertil Steril 52:250–255, 1989.

Cohen J, Elsner C, Kort H, et al: Impairment of the hatching process following IVF in the human and improvement of implantation by assisting hatching using micromanipulation. Hum Reprod 5:7–13, 1990.

Cohen J, Alikani M, Malter HE, et al: Partial zona dissection or subzonal sperm insertion: Microsurgical fertilization alternatives based on evaluation of sperm and embryo morphology. Fertil Steril 56:696–706, 1991.

Cohen J, Alikani M, Trowbridge J, et al: Implantation enhancement by selective assisted hatching using zona drilling of embryos with poor prognosis. Hum Reprod 7:685–691, 1992.

Cohen J, Malter H, Wright G, et al: Partial zona dissection of human oocytes when failure of zona pellucida penetration is anticipated. Hum Reprod 4:435–442, 1989.

Collins JA: Unexplained infertility: A review of diagnosis, prognosis, treatment efficacy and management. Int J Gynecol Obstet 39:267–275, 1992.

Corsan G, Trias A, Trout S, et al: Ovulation induction combined with intrauterine insemination in women 40 years of age and older: Is it worthwhile? Hum Reprod 11:1109–1112, 1996.

Deaton JL, Gibson M, Blackmer KM, et al: A randomized, controlled trial of clomiphene citrate and intrauterine insemination in couples with unexplained infertility or surgically corrected endometriosis. Fertil Steril 54:1083–1088, 1990.

Diaz S, Ortiz ME, Croxatto HB: Studies on the duration of ovum transport by the human oviduct: III. Time interval between the luteinizing hormone peak and recovery of ova by transcervical flushing of the uterus in normal women. Am J Obstet Gynecol 137:116–121, 1980.

Dodson WC, Haney AF: Controlled ovarian hyperstimulation and intrauterine insemination for treatment of infertility. Fertil Steril 55:457–467, 1991.

Dodson WC, Walmer DK, Hughes Jr CL, et al: Adjunctive leuprolide therapy does not improve cycle fecundity in controlled ovarian hyperstimulation and intrauterine insemination of subfertile women. Obstet Gynecol 78:187–190, 1991.

Ferraiolo A, Croce S, Anserini P, et al: "Blind" transcervical transfer of gametes in the fallopian tube: A preliminary study. Hum Reprod 6:537–540, 1991.

FIVNAT: Pregnancies and births resulting from in vitro fertilization: French national registry, analysis of data 1986 to 1990. Fertil Steril 64:746–756, 1995.

Ford WC, Williams KM, McLaughlin EA, et al: The indirect immunobead test for seminal antisperm antibodies and fertilization rates at in-vitro fertilization. Hum Reprod 11:1418, 1996.

Friedler S, Mashiach S, Laufer N: Births in Israel resulting from in-vitro fertilization/embryo transfer, 1982–1989: National Registry of the Israeli Association for Fertility Research. Hum Reprod 7:1159–1163, 1992.

Gagliardi CL, Emmi AM, Weiss G, et al: Gonadotropin-releasing hormone agonist improves the efficiency of controlled ovarian hyperstimulation/intrauterine insemination. Fertil Steril 55:939–944, 1991.

Gindoff PR, Hall JL, Nelson LM, et al: Efficacy of assisted reproductive technology during diagnostic and operative infertility laparoscopy. Obstet Gynecol 75:299–301, 1990.

Gocial B: Primary therapy for tubal disease: Surgery versus IVF. Int J Fertil Menopausal Stud 40:297–302, 1995.

Herman A, Ron-El R, Golan A, et al: Pregnancy rate and ovarian hyperstimulation after luteal human chorionic gonadotropin in in vitro fertilization stimulated with gonadotropin-releasing hormone analog and menotropins. Fertil Steril 53:92–96, 1990.

Horvath PM, Beck M, Bohrer MK, et al: A prospective study on the lack of development of antisperm antibodies in women undergoing intrauterine insemination. Am J Obstet Gynecol 160:631, 1989.

Hughes EG, Fedorkow DM, Daya S, et al: The routine use of gonadotropin-releasing hormone agonists prior to in vitro fertilization and gamete intrafallopian transfer: A meta-analysis of randomized controlled trials. Fertil Steril 58:888–896, 1992.

Jaeger AS: Legal and ethical challenges of medically assisted reproduction. In Keye WR, Change RJ, Rebar RW, Soules MR (eds): Infertility: Evaluation and Treatment. Philadelphia, WB Saunders, 1995, pp 886–899.

Jansen RPS, Anderson JC: Catheterization of the fallopian tube from the vagina. Lancet 2:309–310, 1987.

Janssen HJ, Bastiaans BA, Goverde HJ, et al: Antisperm antibodies and in vitro fertilization. J Assist Reprod Genet 9:345–349, 1992.

Johns DA. Clomiphene citrate–induced gamete intrafallopian transfer with diagnostic and operative laparoscopy. Fertil Steril 56:311–313, 1991.

Johnson L, Hemmings R, Tulandi T: Comparison of intrauterine insemination, intracervical insemination, and timed intercourse in women treated with human menopausal gonadotropin. Int J Fertil 37:218–221, 1992.

Kerin JFP, Peek J, Warnes GM, et al: Improved conception rate after intrauterine insemination of washed spermatozoa from men with poor quality semen. Lancet 1:533–534, 1984.

Kim CH, Cho YK, Mok JE: Simplified ultralong protocol of gonadotrophin-releasing hormone agonist for ovulation induction with intrauterine insemination in patients with endometriosis. Hum Reprod 11:398–402, 1996.

Kirby CA, Flaherty SP, Godfrey BM, et al: A prospective trial of intrauterine insemination of motile spermatozoa versus timed intercourse. Fertil Steril 56:102–107, 1991.

Lahteenmaki A, Reima I, Hovatta O: Treatment of severe male immunological infertility by intracytoplasmic sperm injection. Hum Reprod 10:2824–2828, 1995.

Licciardi FL, Liu HC, Berkeley AS, et al: Day 3 estradiol levels as prognosticators of pregnancy outcome in in vitro fertilization, both alone and in conjunction with day 3 FSH levels. Presented at the 38th Annual Meeting of the Society for Gynecologic Investigation, San Antonio, TX, 1991; 141, p 169.

Lisse K, Sydow P: Transvaginal gamete intrafallopian transfer: Abstract of the II Joint ESCO-ESHRE Meeting, Milan. Hum Reprod 5(suppl):99, 1990.

Manganiello PD, Stern JE, Stukel TA, et al: A comparison of clomiphene citrate and human menopausal gonadotropin for use in conjunction with intrauterine insemination. Fertil Steril 68:405–412, 1997.

Marcus SF, Edwards RG: High rates of pregnancy after long-term down-regulation of women with severe endometriosis. Am J Obstet Gynecol 171:812–817, 1994.

Meniru GI, Craft IL: Experience with gestational surrogacy as a treatment for sterility resulting from hysterectomy. Hum Reprod 12:51–54, 1997.

Moretti-Rojas I, Rohas FJ, Leisure M, et al: Intrauterine inseminations with washed human spermatozoa does not induce formation of antisperm antibodies. Fertil Steril 53:180–182, 1990.

Munne S, Alikani M, Tomkin G, et al: Embryo morphology, developmental rates, and maternal age are correlated with chromosome abnormalities. Fertil Steril 64:382–391, 1995.

Munne S, Xu K, Cohen J, et al: Preimplantation diagnosis. In Adashi EY, Rock JA, Rosenwaks Z (eds): Reproductive Endocrinology, Surgery, and Technology. Vol II. Philadelphia, Lippincott-Raven, 1996, pp 2386–2399.

Munne S, Lee A, Rosenwaks Z, et al: Diagnosis of major chromosome aneuploidies in human preimplantation embryos. Hum Reprod 8:2185–2191, 1993.

Nagy ZP, Verheyen G, Liu J, et al: Results of 55 intracytoplasmic sperm injection cycles in the treatment of male-immunological infertility. Hum Reprod 10:1775–1780, 1995.

Obruca A, Strohmer H, Sakkas D, et al: Use of lasers in assisted fertilization and hatching. Hum Reprod 9:1723–1726, 1994.

Ombelet W, Vandeput H, Van de Putte G, et al: Intrauterine insemination after ovarian stimulation with clomiphene citrate: Predictive potential of inseminating motile count and sperm morphology. Hum Reprod 12:1458–1463, 1997.

Palermo GD, Cohen J, Rosenwaks Z: Intracytoplasmic sperm injection: A powerful tool to overcome fertilization failure. Fertil Steril 65:899–908, 1996.

Peterson CM, Hatasaka HH, Jones KP, et al: Ovulation induction with gonadotropins and intrauterine insemination compared with in vitro fertilization and no therapy: A prospective, nonrandomized, cohort study and meta-analysis. Fertil Steril 62:535–544, 1994.

Pouly JL, Bassil S, Frydman R, et al: Luteal support after in-vitro fertilization: Crinone 8%, a sustained progesterone gel, versus

Utrogestan, an oral micronized progesterone. Hum Reprod 11:2085–2089, 1996.
Ranieri M, Beckett VA, Marchant S, et al: Gamete intra-fallopian transfer or in-vitro fertilization after failed ovarian stimulation and intrauterine insemination in unexplained infertility? Hum Reprod 10:2023–2026, 1995.
Rizk B, Doyle P, Tan SL, et al: Perinatal outcome and congenital malformations in in-vitro fertilization babies from the Bourn-Hallam group. Hum Reprod 69:1259–1264, 1991.
Schoolcraft WB, Schlenker T, Gee M, et al: Assisted hatching in the treatment of poor prognosis in vitro fertilization candidates. Fertil Steril 62:551–554, 1994.
Scott RT, Toner JP, Muasher SJ, et al: Follicle stimulating hormone levels on cycle day 3 are predictive of in vitro fertilization outcome. Fertil Steril 51:651–654, 1989.
Serhal PH, Katz M, Little V, et al: Unexplained infertility—The value of Pergonal superovulation combined with intrauterine insemination. Fertil Steril 49:602–606, 1988.
Serono Laboratories: Pergonal Prescribing Information. Physicians Desk Reference, 1996.
Shalev E, Geslevich Y, Matilsky M, et al: Superovulation and intrauterine insemination in the treatment of male factor infertility. Gynecol Obstet Invest 39:50–53, 1995.
Silverberg KM, Johnson JV, Olive DL, et al: A prospective, randomized trial comparing two different intrauterine insemination regimens in controlled ovarian hyperstimulation cycles. Fertil Steril 57:357–361, 1992.
Society for Assisted Reproductive Technology (SART), The American Fertility Society: In vitro fertilization–embryo transfer (IVF-ET) in the United States: 1990 results from the IVF-ET Registry. Fertil Steril 57:15–24, 1992.
Society for Assisted Reproductive Technology (SART), The American Society for Reproductive Medicine: Assisted reproductive technology in the United States and Canada: 1993 results generated from the American Society for Reproductive Medicine/Society for Assisted Reproductive Technology Registry. Fertil Steril 64:13–21, 1995.
Society for Assisted Reproductive Technology and the American Society for Reproductive Medicine: Assisted reproductive technology in the United States and Canada: 1996 results generated from the American Society for Reproductive Medicine/Society for Assisted Reproductive Technology Registry. Fertil Steril 71:798–807, 1999.
Tanbo T, Dale PO, Lunde O, et al: Prediction of response to controlled ovarian hyperstimulation: A comparison of basal and clomiphene citrate–stimulated follicle-stimulating hormone levels. Fertil Steril 57:819–824, 1992.
Tanbo T, Dale PO, Abyholm T: Assisted fertilization in infertile women with patent fallopian tubes: A comparison of in-vitro fertilization, gamete intra-fallopian transfer, and tubal embryo stage transfer. Hum Reprod 3:266–270, 1990.
Testart J, Plachot M, Mandelbaum J, et al: World collaborative report on IVF-ET and GIFT: 1989 results. Hum Reprod 7:362–369, 1992.
te Velde ER, van Kooy RJ, Waterreus JJH: Intrauterine insemination of husband's washed spermatozoa: A controlled study. Fertil Steril 51:182–185, 1989.
Toth TL, Oehninger S, Toner JP, et al: Embryo transfer to the uterus or the fallopian tube after in vitro fertilization yields similar results. Fertil Steril 57:1110–1113, 1992.
Utian WH, Goldfarb JM, Kiwi R, et al: Preliminary experience with in vitro fertilization—surrogate gestational pregnancy. Fertil Steril 42:633–638, 1989.
Ziegler WF, Russell JB: High success with gestational carriers and oocyte donors using synchronized cycles. J Assist Reprod Genet 12:297–300, 1995.
Van Voorhis BJ, Sparks AE, Allen BD, et al: Cost-effectiveness of infertility treatments: A cohort study. Fertil Steril 67:830–836, 1997.
Verlinsky Y, Ginsberg N, Lifchez A, et al: Analysis of the first polar body: Preconception genetic diagnosis. Hum Reprod 5:826–829, 1990.
Weckstein LN, Goldsman MP, Asch RH: Gamete/zygote intrafallopian tube transfer. *In* Adashi EY, Rock JA, Rosenwaks Z (eds): Reproductive Endocrinology, Surgery, and Technology. Vol II. Philadelphia, Lippincott-Raven, 1996, pp 2335–2352.

# 61

# Unexplained Infertility

KAMRAN S. MOGHISSI

Unexplained infertility (UI), or idiopathic infertility, refers to the failure of a couple to establish a pregnancy despite a comprehensive evaluation uncovering no cause. There are, however, controversies as to what constitutes a thorough evaluation of infertility. The prevalence of UI has been reported as approximately 15% among couples who have been thoroughly evaluated. In studies reported before 1970, the incidence of unexplained infertility varied between 7 and 20%, whereas in series published after 1970, it has varied between 6 and 27%. Taylor and Collins reviewed 10 series reporting on 5129 couples after 1970 and found a prevalence of 14%. In another study conducted at a multicenter Canadian infertility clinic, 2106 couples were evaluated with a uniform protocol. The percentage of unexplained infertility ranged from 8 to 37%, with a mean of 22%. The percentage difference among these centers was attributed to differences in the age of the female partner, duration of infertility, age of the male partner, occupation, and coital frequency.

Clearly, evaluation varies considerably from center to center and depends to a large extent on the competence and expertise of the physicians, the availability of clinical and laboratory facilities, and the perseverance of patients. Furthermore, there is no agreement on which studies should be performed before this diagnosis is made. Admittedly, the more exhaustive the evaluation of the infertile couple, the more likely the opportunity of detecting etiologic factors responsible for the couple's inability to achieve pregnancy. This concept emphasizes one of the major difficulties in identifying couples who are truly afflicted with UI infertility. For example, in one report, a comprehensive study of 1885 infertile couples, only 12 were identified who met the rigorously defined criteria for UI.

Logically, to establish the diagnosis of UI, the clinician should consider the following important issues:

1. *Was the infertility evaluation complete in terms of modern standards?*
2. *Were the results of studies and observations interpreted appropriately?*
3. *Has a factor that was considered within normal limits and compatible with fertility at the outset of the workup changed during the course of evaluation?*

## Infertility Evaluation

Infertility evaluation must be completed before the diagnosis of UI can be considered. In published series of patients with UI infertility, basic infertility tests have frequently been omitted and the strict criteria for the diagnosis of UI have not been met. Basic infertility evaluation is shown in Figure 61–1. Additionally, numerous other diagnostic tests are available to investigate causes of infertility, but their validity has not been established.

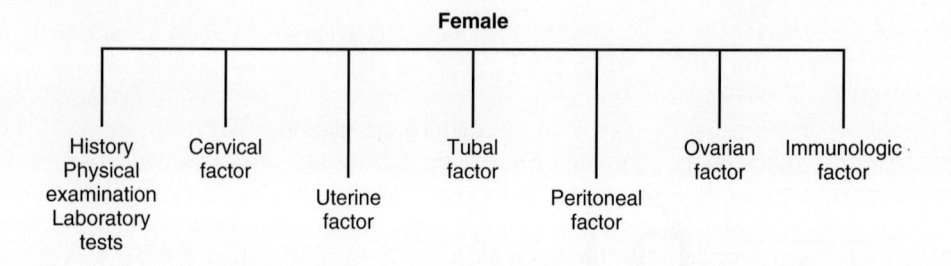

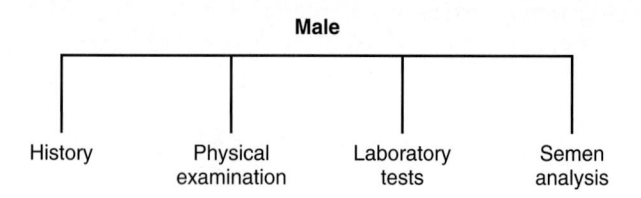

**Figure 61–1** Basic infertility survey.

The European Society for Human Reproduction and Embryology (ESHRE) Workshop on Unexplained Infertility has recommended categorizing infertility testing into three different groups based upon correlation with pregnancy rates (Table 61–1). The categories are as follows: Tests that have an established correlation with pregnancy; tests that are not consistently correlated with pregnancy but which frequently demonstrate abnormal results in association with fertility, even without therapy; and (3) tests that are not correlated with pregnancy.

Although this approach has some practical validity, it is somewhat arbitrary and questionable from the standpoint of physiologic and clinical considerations. For example, it is true that a postcoital test is not consistently correlated with pregnancy. However, the test detects only sperm–cervical mucus interaction, and to some extent sperm travel through the lower genital tract. The test may be positive in women who have tubal obstruction with no chance of pregnancy and negative when performed in anovulatory patients or at an inappropriate time; hence there is lack of correlation with pregnancy. Yet the test remains invaluable to detect the ability of sperm to gain access to the upper reproductive tract. Taylor and Collins reviewed diagnostic protocols of couples with UI in 20 studies conducted between 1960 and 1989. They found that a hysterosalpingogram or postcoital test was performed in only 13 of these protocols; laparoscopy was performed in 16; and sperm-directed antibody tests were obtained in only one study.

At present, basic infertility studies include a thorough history and physical examination and pertinent laboratory tests in both woman and man.

Specific studies consist of investigation of the male factor and evaluation of cervical, uterine, tubal, peritoneal, ovarian, psychogenic, and immunologic factors in the woman, as well as assessment of coital techniques and patterns in the couple (see Fig. 61–1). The care and expertise shown in performing and interpreting these procedures are instrumental in identifying the factor or factors responsible for infertility and often spell the difference between success and failure.

**Table 61–1** Reliability of Infertility Diagnostic Tests to Predict Pregnancy

| | |
|---|---|
| Tests that have an established association with pregnancy | • Semen analysis<br>• Tubal patency by HSG or laparoscopy<br>• Tests of ovulation |
| Tests that are not consistently associated with pregnancy | • SPA<br>• PCT<br>• Sperm antibody tests |
| Tests with no association to pregnancy | • Endometrial dating<br>• Varicocele assessment<br>• Chlamydia testing |

HSG = hysterosalpingography; PCT = postcoital test; SPA = sperm penetration assay.
Van den Eede B: Investigation and treatment of infertile couples: ESHRE guidelines for good clinical and laboratory practice. European Society of Human Reproduction and Embryology. Hum Reprod 10:1251, 1995.

## WERE RESULTS OF STUDIES AND OBSERVATIONS APPROPRIATELY INTERPRETED?

To document the cause or causes of infertility, a variety of data are accumulated, ranging from objective material, such as basal body temperature (BBT) charts, semen analysis reports, and endometrial histologic studies, to more subjective data, including results of postcoital testing and laparoscopic findings. In many cases, a second review of the results of these tests is advisable. Laparoscopic observations are subjective and findings are dependent upon the skill and orientation of the operating surgeon. The vehicle for communication of observations is the surgeon's dictated operative note. The consultant relies upon the operative report, occasionally incorporating diagrams or photographs and, rarely, videotapes of the pelvic structures, which in themselves may not be representative. With these precautionary considerations, it is essential for the consultant to review each study performed when all aspects of the investigation have been reported as within normal limits. It is even prudent to repeat some of the studies whenever doubt exists regarding the original interpretation.

## HAS A FACTOR THAT WAS CONSIDERED WITHIN NORMAL LIMITS AND COMPATIBLE WITH FERTILITY AT THE OUTSET OF THE WORKUP CHANGED DURING THE COURSE OF THE EVALUATION?

An intercurrent infection may cause obstruction of fallopian tubes that were previously found to be patent. Ovulatory patients may become oligo-ovulatory or even anovulatory during the stress of an infertility evaluation. Variations in semen quality are known to occur over a period of time. Infertility evaluation may consume considerable time and is sometimes performed in several centers by different physicians. Therefore, periodic appraisal of factors previously considered normal is prudent.

Infertility evaluation should not be considered complete unless the various factors outlined previously have been thoroughly investigated. Commonly neglected areas and the usual errors of omission include failure to obtain adequate history from the couple and omitting essential fertility tests to establish proper diagnosis.

## History and Physical Examination

Obtaining a detailed history is the most important step in the screening process of the infertile couple. Frequently, patients may not volunteer information of considerable importance, or the physician may neglect to ask leading questions regarding sexual habits, coital frequency and patterns, the stability of the couple's relationship, motivation, and psychogenic makeup. Anecdotal stories abound of patients who have proceeded through infertility studies, yet have knowingly prevented conception by various means, such as postcoital douching or avoidance of coitus at midcycle. Many problems related to sexual dysfunction (i.e., premature ejaculation, relative impotence, and nonejaculatory sexual intercourse) go unreported unlesss disclosure is specifically elicited by the physician.

Other important information consists of a history of possible exposure to physical and toxic agents and any or all of the following practices: the use of drugs, excessive smoking, and drinking alcoholic beverages—all of which may influence male or female fertility. In studies reporting on the pregnancy rate in couples undergoing in vitro fertilization–embryo transfer (IVF-ET) or therapeutic donor insemination, it has been clearly established that fecundity in women declines progressively with age. This is believed to be due to the senescence of the ova rather than an impairment of implantation because oocytes donated by young women, when fertilized and transferred to older women and even postmenopausal recipients, result in pregnancy rates identical to those of younger women.

## Male Factors

The variability of semen parameters, which are age dependent, or deterioration resulting from external or internal factors, may affect the couple's chance of successfully establishing a pregnancy.

Traditionally, semen analysis has been used to evaluate male fertility. It is now appreciated that serial semen analyses in some men may show considerable fluctuation in sperm concentration, motility, and morphologic features. During or following periods of stress, febrile reactions, and inflammatory conditions involving the reproductive tract, temporary deterioration in the quality of semen is not uncommon. For these reasons, it is important to examine several semen samples collected at 2- to 3-week intervals following a period of at least 2 days' abstinence to establish a pattern of semen quality for a given man. A past history of paternity does not eliminate the need for semen analysis because alteration of male reproductive functions and semen characteristics may have occurred since the last pregnancy was established. Sperm production is closely correlated with testicular weight. The number of spermatozoa in an ejaculate is also influenced by many factors, including age, season, the degree of sexual arousal (sexual preparation), and ejaculation frequency, or the interval since the preceding ejaculation. Ejaculation frequency profoundly influences both concentration of spermatozoa and total number of spermatozoa per ejaculate, but it does not influence daily sperm production.

Both quantitative and qualitative characteristics of the ejaculate must be evaluated to obtain a reasonable understanding of testicular function. Whenever possible, semen should be collected by masturbation.

Spermatozoa have the remarkable ability to penetrate cervical mucus, traverse the uterine cavity, gain entrance to the oviduct, and reach the site of fertilization in the distal portion of the fallopian tube in less than 15 minutes. At the end of this perilous journey, the spermatozoa must preserve their activity and fertilizing capacity.

The fertile life span of human spermatozoa is uncertain. It is generally estimated that spermatozoa maintain their fertilizing capacity for at least 48 and possibly 72 hours. Because coitus and ovulation rarely coincide, spermatozoa should be capable of surviving for at least 48 hours within the female reproductive tract and be available in the ampulla of the oviduct to accomplish fertilization.

In man, motility is the parameter of semen quality that correlates best with fertility. Motility is essential for the passage of sperm through the cervix. Visual estimation of the percentage of motile sperm is the most widely used and most abused test of sperm quality. Quantitative methods for evaluating motility of spermatozoa have been developed and include the techniques of track motility and laser-Doppler spectroscopy. These techniques are currently beyond the capacity of the average laboratory.

Morphologic evaluation of spermatozoa is critical. It provides information on testicular function and also aids in predicting a man's potential fertility. Morphologic evaluation is frequently overlooked by many laboratories and poorly performed when the advantages and disadvantages of different techniques are not considered. Various methods used to prepare and stain the seminal smear influence the number and types of abnormalities detected. The physician should insist that an accepted standard, such as that established by the World Health Organization (WHO) be enforced in the laboratory where the test is performed.

With few exceptions, the biochemical components of semen do not reflect testicular function but rather the functional integrity and relative contributions of the epididymides and accessory glands. Optional tests, such as assays of fructose, acid phosphatase, zinc, and citric acid, may be performed when disorders of these glands are suspected.

Sperm characteristics should not be considered in isolation but rather as a composite. The ideal of total morphologically normal, motile sperm that are eventually deposited in the vagina and that penetrate the cervical mucus is obviously of prime importance and may be one of the factors that determines occurrence of pregnancy.

## Establishing the Diagnosis of Unexplained Infertility: Advances and Additional Studies

Central issues in any discussion of UI are the definition of this condition and the extent of testing required to establish this diagnostic category. Some clinicians believe that it is appropriate to make the diagnosis of UI if no identifiable etiology has been detected after basic infertility evaluation, whereas others think more comprehensive and exhaustive studies are required to establish such a diagnosis.

Additionally, many of the essential steps in the reproductive process occur in the innermost recesses of the reproductive tract, where for ethical as well as practical reasons, invasion for investigational purposes is not feasible. For example, although we rely upon indirect diagnostic evidence for the occurrence of ovulation (e.g., thermal shift, secretory endometrium, elevated plasma progesterone [P] and sonographic evidence of follicular collapse), we can only assume that ovulation has occurred. Furthermore, whether the ovulated ovum is normal and reaches the oviductal lumen must be at best a matter of conjecture. Similarly, an excellent result in a postcoital test is no guarantee that the spermatozoa observed in the endocervical canal ever reach the oviducts. If the spermatozoa do gain access to the oviducts, are they capable of achieving ovum penetration and fertilization? Are the patient's fallopian tubes functional? Is a blastocyst that reaches the endometrial cavity able to implant? At present, the answers to these and many other questions are not known and many individual processes remain to be explored among the vital steps leading to conception. Even our advanced state of diagnostic sophistication is limited in the extent to which each process involved in human reproduction can be reliably evaluated. Therefore, a review of newer advances and results of modern studies is deemed appropriate to narrow down the diagnosis of UI (Table 61–2).

**Table 61–2** Newer Tests for the Diagnosis of Male Factor Infertility

- Computerized assisted semen analysis (CASA)
- Sperm penetration assay (SPA)
- Two-stage in vitro fertilization test
- Acrosin assay

# NEWER ADVANCES

## Male Factor

### Computerized Assisted Semen Analysis (CASA)

Standardized, accurate, and precise analysis of sperm motion in semen is likely to improve the prognostic and possibly the diagnostic accuracy of the andrology laboratory. Video and computer vision technology have produced new instruments that are able to identify and track individual sperm cells, and thence to calculate a number of parameters characterizing the "kinematics" (i.e., the time-dependent geometry) of sperm motion. When properly used, Computer-Assisted Semen Analysis (CASA) provides improved precision of sperm motion analysis compared with subjective visual assessments.

Additionally, CASA systems are designed to obtain measurements of sperm concentration, the percentage of motile sperm, and parameters characterizing the pattern and vigor of sperm-head motion along the swimming trajectory. Some systems can also be extended to measure sperm head morphology. The value of CASA systems is in delineating details of sperm head kinematics from which a number of kinematic parameters can be computed. Semen analysis allows an assessment of sperm production rather than sperm function. Many function tests for spermatozoa are described to assess their fertilizing ability. In general, these assays determine biological integrity of the sperm or different steps in the process of fertilization in which the spermatozoa participate. Briefly, these consist of capacitation, acrosome reaction, zona penetration, fusion with ova plasma membrane, and pronuclei formation. Tests designed to assess these functions include hypo-osmotic swelling test, which assesses both the functional and physical integrity of spermatozoa plasma membrane; acrosome reaction test, which evaluates the ability of the spermatozoa to undergo acrosome reaction, spermatozoon–zona pellucida binding assay, sperm zona-free hamster ova penetration assay (SPA), and several biochemical measurements.

### Penetration of Zona-Free Hamster Eggs by Human Sperm

The zona-free hamster egg penetration, often called the sperm penetration assay (SPA), measures the ability of the sperm to undergo capacitation and the acrosome reaction and to fuse with oocytes. Early studies indicated that the penetration rates of zona-free hamster egg by sperm from both fertile and infertile men correlated with sperm morphology but not sperm concentration.

Although SPA has been used clinically for over two decades, controversies remain with regard to standardization of the test and interpretation of its results. There is, however, agreement that the most significant outcome of SPA is a repeated 0% penetration rate. The SPA has also been a common method for screening semen before in vitro fertilization-embryo transfer (IVF-ET). Variable results have been reported from correlating SPA and IVF outcome. In general most studies have found that in males who have normal semen measurers and SPA, the results are predictive of successful IVF. A negative SPA score with a normal semen analysis suggests a lessened chance of successful IVF.

### Two-Stage In Vitro Fertilization Test

This test consists of an in vitro assay of human sperm function to evaluate two initial stages of sperm-ovum interaction: first, penetration through the zona pellucida and second, sperm entry into the ooplasm. The former stage is assessed using immature human oocytes, whereas the latter uses mature zona-free hamster eggs. The two gamete populations are incubated together in the same suspension of capacitated spermatozoa. Several types of sperm dysfunction are usually observed during gamete interaction in patients who have suspected infertility: failure to bind to the zona pellucida; zona binding with failure to penetrate the zona; incomplete zona penetration; and zona penetration with poor sperm entry into the ooplasm. Some men who have normal semen and unexplained infertility have apparent dysfunction of gamete interaction, whereas others have positive results.

### Acrosin Assay

In another approach, the level of acrosin, a trypsin-like enzyme contained in the acrosomal cap, has been correlated with fertility. Acrosin is believed to be essential for sperm penetration into the zona pellucida.

Acrosin activity level is significantly higher in the sperm of fertile men than in those who remain infertile. Also, the average sperm acrosin activity levels of ejaculates whose spermatozoa successfully fertilize human eggs in vitro are significantly higher than those of ejaculates that do not fertilize eggs.

### Male Hyperprolactinemia

More than 90% of males who have hyperprolactinemia have evidence of sexual or reproductive dysfunction or both. Hyperprolactinemia may be manifested by varying degrees of hypogonadism, impotence, and impairment or loss of libido. Among infertile men, however, hyperprolactinemia is an uncommon finding. Measurement of prolactin (PRL) serum levels should be included in the assessment of patients who have persistent infertility. PRL is found in human semen and its levels are reported to correlate positively with sperm count and motility.

## FEMALE FACTORS

Thorough and systematic investigation of female reproductive function obviates oversight and identifies treatable infertility factors, thus avoiding the often unjustified classification of idiopathic infertility. Physicians who are involved in evaluating infertile couples should have a predetermined plan, such as that proposed by The American Society for Reproductive Medicine, for investigating these patients.

Referral to a reproductive endocrinologist with special competence in infertility management should be considered when basic infertility evaluation fails to identify a specific cause for failure to achieve pregnancy.

# Evaluation of Ovulation

Disorders of ovulation are relatively common and are believed to be responsible for infertility in approximately 20 to 25% of patients. These disorders include anovulation with or without oligomenorrhea, oligoovulation, luteal phase defect, and subtle anomalies of ovulation.

Routine techniques of documenting ovulation include recording BBT, evaluating cyclic changes in cervical mucus properties and constituents, assaying serum or salivary P or urinary pregnanediol, testing urinary luteinizing hormone (LH), obtaining an endometrial biopsy, performing serial ultrasonography, and directly visualizing a corpus luteum by laparoscopy. For practical purposes, several of these techniques should be used simultaneously to document possible ovulation. None of these techniques is perfect and all are associated with specific pitfalls. Many physicians are unfamiliar with the shortcomings of BBT recordings. Generally, a biphasic BBT curve, with elevation of approximately 1°F extending over 12 days in the latter portion of the cycle suggests normal ovulation. Common patient errors include misinterpretation of the thermometer reading, inadequate rest or engaging in physical activity before recording the temperature, skipping days, and recording the BBT inappropriately on the chart. Physicians may be unaccustomed to instructing patients or interpreting such records. Inherent problems with this technique include the possibility of a monophasic BBT recording, in otherwise ovulatory women and the inability of the technique to demonstrate ovulation prospectively.

Assay of serum or salivary P has largely replaced urinary pregnanediol determination. Either assay serves as an index of corpus luteum function by assessing its ability to produce P. Some investigators consider a serum P level in excess of 3 ng/ml compatible with ovulation. However, in most normal ovulatory cycles, P levels greater than 8 ng/ml are commonly observed when blood samples are collected at the midluteal phase. A slight rise of serum P (about 2 to 3 ng/ml) may be observed in anovulatory cycles when luteinization of follicles has occurred. A recent study of salivary P levels in women with UI found a variety of disturbances including lower overall secretion of or preovulatory rise in P, decline of P secretion during the luteal phase and abnormal elevations at the beginning of menstruation. Seventy percent of cycles in patients with UI in this study had some abnormality in the progesterone profile compared to only 15% of the control cycles.

The development of enzyme immunoassay (EIA) has allowed measurements of urinary luteinizing hormone (LH) using self-administered dipstick-type test kits. When these test kits are used once or twice a day, they are accurate in determining the timing and occurrence of ovulation in more than 85% of cycles. Daily testing allows detection of the LH surge within 12 to 24 hours after its onset. Combining BBT recording and LH test may narrow the period of urinary testing and bring about accurate timing of ovulation.

Endometrial biopsy has diagnostic value only when obtained adequately and dated histologically, with reference to LH surge as well as the time of onset of the next menstrual period. Early secretory changes may occasionally be observed in the absence of ovulation as a consequence of follicular luteinization.

When ovulation-inducing agents are used to correct anovulation, the occurrence and adequacy of ovulatory cycles should be carefully monitored by the use of the previously mentioned techniques.

## LUTEAL PHASE DEFICIENCY

The term luteal phase deficiency (LPD) is defined as abnormal ovarian function leading to inadequate P production during the postovulatory phase of the cycle. A more appropriate definition may be abnormal corpus luteum (CL) function during the luteal phase. This entity, estimated to occur in 3 to 10% of infertile women, is especially prevalent among women who have received clomiphene citrate for ovulation induction, very young women, older women, and patients who have repetitive pregnancy wastage. One study reported a 4.4% prevalence of LPD in normal fertile women, whereas couples with UI had a 21% prevalence of LPD. In addition to inadequate P secretion in spontaneous LPD in infertile women, decreased levels of inhibin, estradiol, and relaxin have also been reported. Therefore, LPD may be viewed as CL dysfunction, involving all hormones that are secreted by this structure.

There is no gold standard for diagnosis of LPD that is based on solid physiologic ground. However, LPD can be diagnosed by evaluating several parameters of corpus luteum function, including the length of the postovulatory phase, the serum P levels, and the histologic features of the endometrium. To be of clinical significance, histologic evidence for luteal insufficiency must be found consistently and repetitively. In clinical practice, the simplest approach is histologic dating and interpretation of endometrial biopsy specimens in conjunction with a BBT chart, urinary LH surge, or serial pelvic ultrasonographic evaluation. The biopsy should be obtained on the 26th day of an ideal 28-day cycle (e.g., 2 days before the onset of menses) to reflect the maximal steroidogenic function of the corpus luteum. Endometrial histologic changes that are 2 or more days out of phase suggest a diagnosis of LPD, but it must be confirmed by a similarly timed biopsy in a subsequent cycle. BBT by itself is not a satisfactory diagnostic technique for quantitative evaluation of corpus luteum function because it tends to reveal an all-or-none response. However, it can be applied to detect a short luteal phase and does on occasion alert the physician to the possibility of a luteal phase dysfunction.

It is more accurate to determine the optimal time for performing the biopsy from the time of the thermal shift and the urinary LH surge than from the first day of the next cycle. Endometrial morphology represents an end-organ response to sequential and synergistic effects of estrogen and P produced respectively by the preovulatory follicle and the corpus luteum. Circulating levels of sex steroids regulate the concentration of endometrial receptors and, ultimately, the endometrial response to these steroids. For women in whom the time of ovulation can be established with reasonable accuracy, a correlation of 89% between biopsy findings and serum P has been repeated. The result of a single assay for serum P has limited value because of its short half-life and the pulsatile release of P. Daily measurement of serum P can provide a more accurate indication of corpus luteum function, but because of expense and inconvenience, this approach is clinically impractical. An integrated P level that is calculated over the duration of the luteal phase has been proposed as a suitable diagnostic criterion of LPD. An integrated P level lower than 80 ng/ml per day may be used to indicate LPD. P levels in excess of 10 ng/ml have been recommended for documentation of ovulation. Another approach is to obtain three P level determinations approximately 4, 6, and 8 days before the next expected menstrual period. In normal cycles, the sum of these three determinations should be more than 15 ng/ml, whereas the aggregate value in abnormal cycles is less than 15 ng/ml. Even this approach has shortcomings, however, in that the short luteal phase may escape diagnosis unless the entire postovulatory phase is carefully monitored.

The aluteal cycle represents a severe form of LPD. This condition is characterized by cycles terminating with menstrual bleeding at fairly regular intervals without demonstrable evidence of luteal function. In some of these cycles, hormonal evidence of ovulation, such as elevation of LH or elevated estrogen levels at midcycle may occasionally be observed; however, an increase in P levels in the second half of these cycles cannot be detected. BBT charts are usually monophasic, and endometrial biopsy specimens obtained before the onset of menses fail to demonstrate evidence of secretory activity. Although the observation of an occasional anovulatory cycle in such regularly menstruating women is not uncommon, persistent anovulation with cyclic menstrual bleeding is an unusual occurrence. Unless ovulation is carefully sought by the use of techniques previously described, this particular ovulatory defect will be missed.

The short luteal phase represents still another variant of LPD. This condition has been defined as a luteal phase of 8 days or less in otherwise healthy women. These cycles are commonly characterized by lower than normal follicular phase follicle-stimulating hormone (FSH) levels, a low midcycle estradiol ($E_2$) peak, diminished luteal phase P secretion, and an absence of the expected rise of plasma $E_2$. These hormonal deficiencies are attributed to defective follicular maturation secondary to a defect in gonadotropin secretion. Some authorities consider a luteal phase of less than 12 days to be a short luteal phase. A distinction should be made, however, between the inadequate luteal phase in which P secretion is lower than expected but the length of the postovulatory phase is of normal duration and the shortened luteal phase in which the pattern of P output may be normal but the length of the postovulatory interval is abbreviated. On occasion, the two conditions (i.e., short and deficient luteal phase) may coexist.

The extent to which LPD contributes to the etiology of unexplained infertility is not known. Furthermore, pregnancy occurs with similar frequency in women who have a normal endometrium and in those who have delayed endometrial development. This may, however, be caused by sporadic occurrence of LPD.

The etiology of luteal phase dysfunction is incompletely understood. Corpus luteum function represents a fine balance between luteotrophic and luteolytic factors that compete during a normal luteal phase. Undoubtedly, a variety of factors may be responsible for defects in corpus luteum function. Inappropriate preovulatory patterns in pituitary gonadotropin levels, a well-described shift in LH pulse frequency and amplitude, or higher amplitude in the second half of the cycle are associated with abnormalities in the developing dominant follicle and subsequent inadequacies in the function of the corpus luteum. These inappropriate patterns may be secondary to a disturbance in the pulsatile release of gonadotropin-releasing hormone (GnRH). Factors that are known to influence hypothalamic release of GnRH and pituitary function include hyperprolactinemia and excess androgen states. In addition, hyperprolactinemia and hyperandrogenism have been shown to alter the follicular microenvironment and adversely affect steroidogenesis.

Levels of $E_2$ and P receptors in human endometrial tissues are known to change throughout the menstrual cycle and are primarily responsive to fluctuations in serum steroid levels. Defects in receptor synthesis and endometrial tissue response to presumably normal circulating steroid levels have also been reported. Luteal phase defects may occur recurrently or sporadically. An occult pregnancy (chemical pregnancy), which terminates so quickly after blastocyst formation that its occurrence is not clinically suspected, may represent an early demise of the blastocyst as a result of luteal deficiency. Subtle anomaly of the luteal phase has been found to be associated with UI.

## HYPERPROLACTINEMIA AND OVULATORY DISORDERS

Hyperprolactinemia as a cause of (or in association with) amenorrhea and anovulation has been well documented. Short or inadequate luteal phase or even unexplained infertility with normal luteal function may also be associated with overt or transient hyperprolactinemia. Elevation in circulating levels of PRL may interfere with synthesis or release of GnRH or with P production in the ovary. Because of the important role that PRL plays in the secretion of GnRH and synthesis of sex steroids in the ovary, attempts have been made to treat UI with dopamine agonists. However, these attempts have generally been unsuccessful. Therefore, in the absence of hyperprolactinemia, the use of ergoline derivatives in the management of idiopathic infertility is not recommended.

## ANDROGEN EXCESS AND OVULATORY DISORDERS

A marked increase in endogenous androgen production is usually associated with oligomenorrhea, anovulation, virilization, and infertility. The central nervous system is influenced by elevated circulating androgens, leading to a functional discordance of the hypothalamic-pituitary-ovarian axis. Significant prolongation of the follicular phase and shortening of the luteal phase may be associated with elevated plasma T levels. Association of androgen excess with prolongation of the follicular phase and shortening of the luteal phase of the menstrual cycle, may explain the frequency of infertility and menstrual irregularity in hyperandrogenic women. A study of a group of 23 follicular fluids (FF) measured levels of estradiol ($E_2$) P, T, androstenedione (A), immunoactive, inhibin-like growth factor-binding protein-1, $\alpha_1$-antitrypsin and placenta protein-14. Each FF yielded an oocyte known to result in a clinical pregnancy after in vitro fertilization (IVF). The characteristics of these pregnancy-associated follicles were compared with those of FF obtained from women who failed to conceive after embryo transfer. Pregnancy was associated with follicles showing a significantly higher $E_2$ to T ratio than follicles in which the oocyte failed to implant or did not cleave in vitro. No difference was found when pregnancy-associated follicles and follicles not associated with pregnancy were compared with respect to the levels of other previously mentioned substances.

## LUTEINIZED UNRUPTURED FOLLICLE (LUF) SYNDROME

Ovulation should be defined as the disruption of a mature graafian follicle with the release of an ovum from the follicle. For many years, it has been postulated that the follicle may occasionally proceed through its preliminary stages of development without disruption and ovum release. Subsequently, the follicle undergoes luteinization and produces P. The term "luteinized unruptured follicle" is used to describe this condition. This abnormality is characterized by endocrinologic patterns that yield presumptive signs of ovulation (i.e., biphasic BBT, secretory endometrium, and other laboratory evidence of P production).

Advances in ultrasonographic technology have made it possible to monitor follicular development. Using this technique, an incidence of 4.9% of LUF in patients with unexplained infertility has been reported. The local factors responsible for follicular disruption are not completely understood, but prostaglandins, proteolytic enzymes, and ovarian contractility have all been considered as participants in the mechanical process of ovulation. Luteinization normally occurs spontaneously thereafter in the LH-primed granulosa cells.

Collectively, current information suggests that luteinization of the unruptured follicle may occur sporadically, but little evidence exists to substantiate this phenomenon as a frequent event.

## OVARIAN RESERVE

Fertility is age-related and declines in older women. Experience gained from IVF indicates that older women respond poorly to an ovarian stimulation regimen and produce fewer oocytes with low fertilization and pregnancy rates. However, when these women receive eggs from young women, their pregnancy rate is similar to that of younger women.

Women with unexplained infertility may share a decline of ovarian reserve with older women. Basal follicle-stimulating hormone (FSH) levels on day 3 of the menstrual cycle have been found to be a useful predictor of ovarian reserve. Several studies have documented that elevation of FSH levels on cycle day 3 (>15 mIU/ml) is associated with marked decrease in pregnancy rates of IVF cycles and is indicative of diminished ovarian reserve as defined by poor gonadotropin responsiveness and pregnancy rate in patients undergoing ovarian stimulation.

Another test of ovarian reserve is the clomiphene challenge test. This test consists of measuring FSH levels on cycle day 3 (basal) and then again on cycle day 10 following the administration of 100 mg of clomiphene citrate from cycle days 5 through 9. An abnormal test is defined by an elevated level in sample taken on day 3.

## SUBTLE OVULATORY ABNORMALITIES

Standard tests may fail to detect subtle anomalies of the ovulatory process. In carefully selected women with UI who had serial hormonal evaluations, several abnormal patterns of ovulatory disorders were reported. These patterns include elevation of mean $E_2$ concentrations in the early through late follicular phase, elevation of prolactin across the menstrual cycle, decline of midluteal mean P levels, elevation of FSH levels in early follicular phase and other anomalies of FSH and LH patterns. Considered together, these findings support the hypothesis that women with unexplained infertility have subtle disturbances in the hypothalamic-pituitary-ovarian axis compared with their fertile counterparts. These women may, in fact, exhibit hormonal aberrations that represent very early stages of a continuum that leads to ovarian senescence. Thus, it is reasonable to assume that these hormonal alterations may play a role in the etiology of UI.

# Uterine Abnormalities

Both congenital and acquired uterine abnormalities are usually identified by HSG. However, other imaging techniques such as ultrasonography or MRI and hysteroscopy may be required to diagnose those that are missed by hysterosalpingography (HSG). Furthermore, the role of some of these abnormalities (e.g., myoma, congenital anomalies) in infertility is unclear.

Implantation failure is an important cause of unexplained infertility. Traditionally, the evaluation of endometrial receptivity to blastocyst implantation has been limited to assessment of endometrial morphology.

More recently, an increasing number of biochemical factors (e.g., extracellular matrix, integrins, prolactin, relaxin) are being found to contribute to the growth and differentiation of the endometrium in response to steroid hormones. Intense molecular interactions at the maternal-fetal interface, both cell to cell and tissue to tissue, participate in the process of implantation. Occult defects in the expression or action of these biochemical principles may account for at least some cases of UI that stem from implantation failure. Recognition of these endometrial factors and development of clinical tests to diagnose them will assist clinicians to treat occult defects in the endometrium and to optimize implantation of blastocysts in women with UI.

# Tubal and Peritoneal Factors

Customary procedures employed for evaluation of uterus and oviducts include sonosalpingography, hysterosalpingography (HSG), hysteroscopy, and pelvic endoscopy with chromopertubation or tubal lavage. Carbon dioxide insufflation has long been relegated to history as an unreliable procedure for evaluation of tubal patency. HSG provides a reasonable evaluation of the contour of the uterine cavity and oviducts. It is a simple procedure whose major deficiencies are an inability to demonstrate integrity of the uterine cavity and the anatomic relationship between tubal ostium and ovary, and failure to identify peritubal adhesions and peritoneal disease. Both false-positive and false-negative findings are associated with hysterosalpingography as determined by pelvic endoscopy. An infertility investigation must be considered incomplete without final direct visualization of the pelvic anomalies by endoscopy.

A review and careful analysis of 18 studies that compared the result of HSG with those of laparoscopy indicated that, in the average practice, a normal HSG is followed by an abnormal laparoscopy in about

3% of cases. This provides 97% confidence that an immediate laparoscopy is not required. A normal test result would occur in 77% of patients. In the remaining 23% of patients, an abnormal test result requires follow-up with laparoscopy. Other major infertility-associated pathologies that have been observed during laparoscopy include endometriosis, pelvic adhesions, and leiomyomata. The weighted mean of total defects in a review of 2803 cases reported in the literature was 54%, of which 38% were tubal defects, 11% were endometriosis, 2% were leiomyomata, and 4% were other defects. Falloposcopy has been introduced for evaluation of intratubal lesions. The technique consists of the introduction of the falloposcope into the uterotubal ostium via the operating channel of the flexible hysterscope under video monitoring for diagnostic purpose or operative procedures. One study showed an incidence of 54% endotubal lesions in a group of 119 patients with infertility. In patients who have UI, falloposcopy may be indicated when conventional tests for tubal potency have not revealed an endotubal lesion. Falloposcopy may isolate areas of epithelial damage or other intratubal pathology that may cause abnormal tubal function and predispose to ongoing infertility.

Laparoscopy in patients who have persistent unexplained infertility may reveal endometriosis in approximately one third of cases and tubal or peritoneal disease in another 15 to 30% of subjects. Laparoscopy is obviously required before the diagnosis of unexplained infertility is considered.

Periadnexal adhesions may result from pelvic surgery, pelvic inflammation, endometriosis, inflammatory bowel disorders, or adnexal accidents. The location of adhesions may be more significant than their extent. For example, adhesions may act as a barrier to ovum transport from follicle to tubal ostium, restrict fimbrial function by a process of bridging, distort the location of the fimbriae, or interfere with normal oviductal motility. Their presence cannot be detected by pelvic examination or HSG. Pelvic endoscopy serves as the optimal diagnostic procedure for identifying periadnexal adhesions.

## Occult Infections

### MYCOPLASMA AND UREAPLASMA INFECTIONS

*Mycoplasma* microorganisms are approximately the size of large viruses, have no cell wall, and contain both RNA and DNA. One of the organisms belonging to this group, *Ureaplasma urealyticum*, has been implicated in reproductive failure (i.e., infertility and repeated spontaneous abortion). In a carefully selected group of infertile couples, 85% of men and 91% of women were found to harbor *Ureaplasma*, whereas, in a control group of pregnant women and their consorts, *Ureaplasma* was found in 23% of men and 22% of women.

Doxycycline treatment of 55 infertile couples infected with *Ureaplasma* resulted in a conception rate of 27%. This number was considered much higher than would be anticipated in a selected group of couples with more than 5 years of UI. A higher frequency of cervical and endometrial *Ureaplasma* has also been observed in couples with UI than in fertile control subjects. In another prospective study of women with reproductive failure, a positive correlation between endometrial changes and positive *Ureaplasma* culture was observed.

The frequency with which *U. urealyticum* appears in cervical mucus of fertile women and those with explained and UI varies considerably (Table 61–3). However, the highest frequency has been observed among patients with UI. Similarly, a higher frequency of positive culture was found in the semen of infertile men.

Several studies have indicated decreased sperm motility in ejaculates containing *Ureaplasma* organisms. A significant increase in the number of tapering forms and spermatoblasts with a stress pattern has also been reported to be found in the semen of infected men who have nongonococcal urethritis. Treatment of *Ureaplasma* infection in infertile couples has been reported to result in successful pregnancies in 5 to 23% of patients. A higher conception rate (17 to 46%) has been observed after treatment of couples with UI. Similar conception rates, however, have been reported in untreated couples who served as control subjects.

These conflicting reports lead to the conclusion that couples with UI have a greater yield of positive cultures for *U. urealyticum* than normal control subjects or those who have infertility with identifiable factors. Furthermore, in selected groups of patients with positive cultures, treatment of *U. urealyticum* may be associated with an increased rate of conception. Remaining, however, is a relatively large percentage of couples who have *Ureaplasma* infection and who apparently suffer no deleterious effect on

Table 61–3 Frequency of *Ureaplasma urealyticum* in Semen and Cervical Mucus of Fertile and Infertile Patients

|  | Men | Women |
|---|---|---|
| Fertile controls | 19–36 | 23–68 |
| Infertile controls | 29–47 | 35–52 |
| Couples with unexplained infertility | 39–85 | 52–91 |

reproductive function, or, if they are infertile, the colonization is not responsible for their inability to achieve conception.

## CHLAMYDIA INFECTION

*Chlamydia trachomatis* is a major etiologic agent in salpingitis. Several studies have reported isolation of *Chlamydia* from the fallopian tubes and endocervix of 20 to 30% of patients who have acute salpingitis. Serologic studies in Scandinavian countries suggest that *C. trachomatis* is associated with 40 to 60% of cases of acute salpingitis. Based upon available serologic data, approximately 20% of acute salpingitis cases in the United States are associated with *Chlamydia*. *Chlamydia* infection may be associated with subclinical or asymptomatic tubal or peritoneal diseases and thus should be considered as a cause of unexplained infertility.

## TUBERCULOSIS

In many developing countries, genital tuberculosis is a significant factor in infertility and is observed in 5 to 20% of couples evaluated. In contrast, in the United States, the comparable figure is less than 1%. Although clinical manifestations may include amenorrhea or other menstrual disorders and salpingitis, asymptomatic pelvic tuberculosis is not uncommon. In more than 90% of women who have genital tuberculosis, the oviducts are involved. Asymptomatic and unsuspected cases of tuberculous endometritis are also frequent. Histologic findings include isolated small tubercles scattered irregularly through the endometrium, infiltration with round cells, and characteristic Langhans' giant cells. The diagnosis may be established by histologic examination and bacteriologic evaluation of the endometrium, HSG, and pelvic endoscopy. Histologic evidence of chronic endometritis should alert the physician to the possibility of tuberculous endometritis.

# Endometriosis

Endometriosis and infertility are closely associated. In asymptomatic patients who have otherwise UI, varying degrees of endometriosis may be observed frequently during laparoscopy.

The precise reasons for infertility in women with endometriosis may vary, depending upon location and extent of the disease. Peritubal and tubo-ovarian adhesions are frequently found. Ovarian function is usually preserved, and the speculation that endometriosis may be responsible for luteinization of unruptured follicles has not been substantiated by direct endoscopic visualization of ovaries. The uterine endometrium is usually uninvolved, and biopsy specimens obtained in the luteal phase customarily demonstrate secretory endometrium with progestational maturity. It has been suggested that luteal phase defects may be associated with pelvic endometriosis. Although this association requires further confirmation, luteal defects should be specifically sought in infertile patients who have minimal endometriosis. Dysfunction of oviductal motility, secondary to fibrosis, scarring, and interference with ovum pickup, may be responsible for infertility in some cases. However, in many cases, infertility associated with mild or moderate endometriosis cannot be explained on an anatomic basis. Increased levels of prostaglandins (PGs) contained in the peritoneal fluid may adversely affect tubo-ovarian function. Other studies have identified humoral antibodies in the serum of women who have endometriosis. It is suggested but not proved that these antibodies may interfere with normal development of eutopic endometrium and implantation process. Several investigations have shown that the number of peritoneal macrophages and their phagolytic activity are increased in women who have endometriosis. It is unclear whether macrophage activity represent a cause or an effect of endometriosis.

A few reports have documented alteration of prolactin and gonadotropin metabolism in patients who have endometriosis. However, the accuracy of these findings has been questioned. Another interesting observation is the result of therapeutic evaluation of patients who have mild to moderate endometriosis (stage I and II R-AFS). In at least six clinical trials, medical treatment of minimal endometriosis did not improve the cumulative pregnancy rate when compared with that of control subjects. The combined odds ratio for five of these studies using steroid hormones for treatment was 0.9 (95% CI −0.6 to 1.2) This suggests that even though mild endometriosis is associated with a decline in fecundity rate, ovulation suppression therapy, which induces amenorrhea and reduces the extent of visible endometriosis, does not improve fertility.

# Assessment of the Cervical Factor and Sperm Transport

The uterine cervix functions as a biologic valve that at certain periods during the reproductive cycle permits the entry of sperm into the uterus and at other times bars their admission. In approximately 5 to 10% of infertile women, cervical abnormalities may be partially or totally responsible for continued infertility. The cervical role in infertility has been extensively reviewed by several authorities and is usually assessed by postcoital testing and by in vitro sperm–cervical mucus penetration tests. These simple tests are often omitted totally from an evaluation, or they are ill-timed, inadequately performed, or misinterpreted. Because interpretation of these tests may be subjective, the experience and expertise of the physician performing them is of considerable importance.

Soon after ejaculation, spermatozoa are transferred from seminal plasma to female genital tract fluid, in which they are suspended. The migration, survival, and fertilizing potential of spermatozoa depend to a large extent on their ability to adapt to this new environment. The postcoital test (PCT) provides valuable insight into sperm–cervical mucus interaction. The quality of the cervical mucus significantly influences sperm receptivity; therefore, mucus characteristics should be evaluated thoroughly before a PCT is performed. Similarly, sperm motility, morphology, and concentration within the ejaculate can each influence sperm migration through cervix and should be studied prior to attempting in vivo or in vitro sperm–cervical mucus tests.

Interpreting the postcoital test requires an understanding of cervical function and sperm transport. Cervical mucus protects sperm from the hostile environment of the vagina and from phagocytosis. The mucus may provide a substrate to help meet the spermatozoa's energy requirements and also serve as a filter to retain abnormal and sluggish sperm. Generally, 6 to 8 hours after coitus, more than 10 sperm with adequate motility (3+) should be found per high-power field ($\times$ 400) in cervical mucus.

Once within the uterine cavity, the spermatozoa depend principally on uterine contractions for their transport. The intrinsic sperm motility is of secondary importance. Factors responsible for sperm transport through the oviducts include the following:

1. Tubal motility
2. Ciliary activity of the epithelial cells lining the endosalpinx
3. Circulation of tubal fluid
4. Sperm motility

None of these functions is amenable to clinical evaluation. Thus, it is reasonable to assume that UI in certain individuals may be secondary to a disturbance in the normal function of one of these processes.

Because of its accessibility, evaluation of cervical function should not be neglected. No couple should be considered to have UI unless abnormalities in the cervix and sperm–cervical mucus interaction have been excluded. It is recommended that the standards developed by WHO be followed when performing the PCT. To assess the adequacy of sperm transport, attempts have been made to develop a clinical test of sperm migration using sperm recovery from the pelvic cavity during laparoscopy. This approach is based upon the assumption that sperm recovered from the peritoneal cavity have already demonstrated their ability to reach the site of fertilization in the fallopian tube.

## Sperm Antibodies and Unexplained Infertility

The antigenicity of spermatozoa and seminal plasma components has been recognized since the turn of the century. Numerous studies have revealed that antigens found in the seminal plasma constituents or bound to spermatozoa have the ability to induce specific autoimmunity with resulting infertility. When this phenomenon occurs, spermatozoa may be unable to penetrate cervical mucus or retain motility during sperm transport in sensitized women. Men may also produce autoantibodies against seminal or sperm components. Spermatozoa coated with such antibodies may show agglutination in the ejaculate or fail to migrate through the cervix, reach the site of fertilization, or fertilize the oocyte. Sperm antibodies belong almost exclusively to Ig(immunoglobulin)A and IgG immunological classes. IgA antibodies found in semen or cervical mucus have greater clinical impact than do IgG antibodies.

The most commonly used tests for antisperm activity are the immunobead test and the mixed antiglobulin reaction test (MAR). Quantitative tests include microagglutination, macroagglutination, and immobilization (complement-dependent cytotoxicity). The first two tests detect sperm-agglutinating antibodies, whereas the latter procedure identifies immobilizing antibodies. The results of the immunobead test and the MRI test do not always agree. The immunobead test, however, correlates well with sperm agglutination and immobilization tests performed on serum.

Most previous studies have attempted to detect the presence of sperm antibodies in the sera of infertile couples. Such antibodies have been reported in 7 to 17% of infertile women, varying with the type of test performed and the population screened. When classified as to the type of infertility, the frequency figures change considerably.

In couples with UI 14 to 40% have been considered to have an immunologic basis. Unfortunately, most reports present few data with respect to the selection of these cases and the thoroughness of the infertility evaluation.

The human reproductive tract, especially that of the female, is capable of a local immune response to foreign antigens, including those associated with spermatozoa. Serum titers of sperm antibodies are not indicative of the presence and concentration of antibodies at local sites.

In recent years, studies of sperm antibodies in the female and their relationship to infertility have been shifted from assays of serum to analyses of reproductive tract fluids. In a study of 200 carefully selected couples with persistent infertility who were comprehensively evaluated, sperm antibodies were found in 12 and 6% of the sera of women and men, respectively. In cervical mucus, agglutinating or immobilizing sperm antibodies were present in 23.6%. Interestingly, in 19% of females, sperm antibodies were present exclusively in the cervical mucus, and in 7.5%, exclusively in the serum. These data indicate that sperm antibodies can occur in cervical mucus independent of their presence in the serum.

Collectively, the available data may be summarized as follows:
1. Sperm antibodies are in some way related to persistent infertility.
2. A higher proportion of couples with persistent UI are found to have sperm antibodies in sera, reproductive tract fluids, or both.
3. A high correlation is found between the presence of high sperm antibody titers and continuing infertility of more than 3 years.

## Zona Antibodies

The zona pellucida is a noncellular, gelatin-like layer surrounding the oocyte and preimplantation embryo, which is probably composed of glycoproteins. Major functions of the zona pellucida in fertilization include sperm recognition (species-specific) and prevention of polyspermia. Species-specific sperm receptor sites located on the surface of the zona are responsible for preventing sperm of one species from fertilizing eggs of another species.

Antibodies to the zona pellucida have been produced experimentally in several species in an attempt to achieve immunocontraception. A few studies have also been undertaken to detect autoantibodies to the zona in sera obtained from infertile women. In these investigations, the indirect fluorescent antibody method is used with pig zona (human and pig zonae share a common antigen) as the target antigen, because adequate numbers of human zonae are not available for testing purposes.

Autoantibodies against the zona may be responsible for continuing UI infertility in some cases. However, at the present time, many questions regarding both the existence of autoantibodies to the zona and their alleged role as causative agents in human infertility have not been adequately resolved and require further investigation.

## Emotional Factors

Some older reports suggested that 40 to 50% of infertility cases might be caused by emotional factors. Infertile couples were described as having typical personality traits that may have resulted in their inability to conceive. Currently, it is believed that emotional factors constitute a causative factor in less than 5% of all cases of infertility. In a study that matched 20 infertile women and 20 fertile control subjects, it was found that more emotional disturbances were identified among the infertile women than among the controls. Others studies have reported that infertile women exhibited various psychosexual maladjustments. Similar reports have appeared concerning infertile men. Infertility itself may also provoke emotional problems, rather than serve as the result. The degree of stress and desperation experienced by infertile couples is emphasized by the fact that suicide among childless couples is approximately twice as frequent as among couples with offspring. In men, emotional stress might add to oligospermia and psychosexual disturbances. Four types of disturbances associated with psychological factors may be observed in male infertility: impotence, sham ejaculation, retrograde ejaculation, and oligospermia. Impotence may be induced as a result of the demands for sexual performance during an infertility investigation, such as the need to submit semen samples for evaluation and to perform coitus for postcoital testing. Couples who have had normal sexual function before their seeking treatment for their infertility problem may develop decreased coital frequency, orgasmic dysfunction, midcycle male impotence, and the inability to achieve coitus for postcoital examination. Emotional stress associated with the infertile state or resulting from a long and demanding infertility evaluation may exert its influence through autonomic or neuroendocrine control of the reproductive process. Excessive catecholamines resulting from stress may in some way affect ovulation, either directly or by increasing adrenal stimulation, by release of adrenocorticotropic hormone, or by inducing hyperprolactinemia. A number of studies have shown that psychological trauma can lead to alterations in central catecholamines and endorphins, resulting in anovulation and amenorrhea. Stress-related catecholamine excess might also affect oviductal activity and gamete transport.

The conclusion to be derived from the previously described studies and many others is that an awareness of the intense, often overwhelming emotional turmoil that infertile couples frequently face is essential. Regardless of whether psychological factors and emotional stress are the cause or the result of infertility problems, they deserve to be managed equally and in parallel with organic and functional causes of infertility by an astute and empathetic physician. Careful attention to the sexual history and a sympathetic approach to diagnosis and management of emotional difficulties and psychological disturbances of couples with persistent identified infertility or UI may not only lead to resolution of these problems but favorable outcome of the infertility issue.

## Treatment of Unexplained Infertility

The diagnosis of UI is usually made by exclusion of any detectable pathology after a standard infertility evaluation. As previously stated, with more comprehensive investigation, subtle anatomic or functional disorders in the man, the woman, or both may be elicited. When such anomalies are found they are usually treated. However, it is unclear whether any pregnancy ensuing is the result of treatment or chance. Unfortunately, controlled clinical trials are not available to document the effectiveness of several modalities of therapy and clinicians may have to resort to empiric treatment with questionable outcome. Ideally, before any treatment of UI is chosen, it should be demonstrably superior to the no-treatment option.

The prognosis for untreated UI can vary depending on the characteristics of each individual couple. Factors affecting the pregnancy rate include the duration of infertility, age of the female (and possibly the male) partner, previous reproductive history, and coital frequency.

Duration of infertility and female partner's age have powerful effects on pregnancy rates. With increasing duration of infertility and advancement of female age, there is a gradual decline in pregnancy rate. It is estimated that pregnancy rate is reduced by 26% for every additional year of infertility. For example, a couple has a 51% change of pregnancy after 2 years, but only 39% after 3 years' duration of infertility. With secondary infertility, the prognosis is 2.4 times better at a given duration of infertility. With respect to female age, favorable prognosis is reduced by 9% for each added year of the female partner's age. Thus, if a couple has primary infertility of 4 years' duration and the female partner is 36 years of age, the likelihood of pregnancy is 25%.

### TREATMENT OF MALE FACTOR ABNORMALITIES

#### Anatomic Abnormalities

Among male anatomic disorders, the most controversial one is the varicocele. Semen analysis of men with varicocele frequently shows a typical stress pattern consisting of a high percentage of immature and tapering spermatozoa. However, other men with varicocele do not show these changes and seem to have no difficulty fathering a child.

The results of varicocele ligation on pregnancy rates vary significantly. Improvement in semen parameter is usually seen within 6 to 18 months. Pregnancy rates of 20 to 60% have been reported following varicocelectomy. However, controlled trials are required to substantiate these results.

### Medical Treatment

Medical management of subtle anomalies or idiopathic infertility in males detected by semen analysis or functional tests is not satisfactory. In the past, a variety of nonspecific regimens were tried and rejected. Clomiphene citrate has been successful in some cases but not in all reported series. Furthermore, it is not known how to select the best candidates for this treatment. Currently, the most promising results are obtained by intrauterine insemination (IUI), therapeutic donor insemination (TDI), in vitro fertilization (IVF), and intracytoplasmic sperm injection (ICSI).

### Management of Female Idiopathic Infertility

Once again, there are no controlled data to document that management of minor anatomic disorders of the female reproductive tract lead to an improved pregnancy rate. However, most clinicians attempt to correct any anatomic abnormalities while they are investigating the etiology of infertility. These include removal of submucous myomas and uterine polyps lysis of intrauterine synechiae by hysteroscopy; lysis of tubo-ovarian adhesions by laser ablation or cauterization of endometrial implants during laparoscopy. There is evidence that the latter treatment in fact improves the pregnancy rate.

Currently, the most effective treatment of idiopathic infertility is assisted reproduction. Initially, controlled ovarian hyperstimulation with or without IUI is attempted. Considering that a substantial percentage of cases of idiopathic infertility are caused by ovulatory disorders, it is reasonable to try this procedure for up to four cycles. Cycle fecundity rate of 18.6 (range 15 to 42%) has been reported with this procedure. IVF, gamete intrafallopian transfer (GIFT), and zygote intrafallopian transfer (ZIFT) have all been successfully used to treat UI (see Chapter 60). ICSI is used when fertilization fails to occur during IVF procedure.

## Summary

To recapitulate, three questions must be raised when the couple has been evaluated and found to be normal:

1. Was the infertility evaluation complete in terms of modern standards?
2. Were the results of studies and observations appropriately interpreted?
3. Has a factor that was considered within normal limits and compatible with fertility at the outset of the workup changed during the course of the evaluation?

Both the couple and the managing physician are frustrated and plagued by feelings of inadequacy when no positive findings can be identified during the course of an infertility evaluation. This situation obviously requires of the physician a combination of delicacy, patience, expertise, and considerable attention to each detail of the evaluation that has just been completed.

## REFERENCES

Aksel S: Sporadic and recurrent luteal phase defects in cyclic women: Comparison with normal cycles. Fertil Steril 33:372, 1980.
Amann RP: A critical review of methods for evaluation of spermatogenesis from seminal characteristics. J Androl 2:37, 1981.
Andersen CY: Characteristics of human follicular fluid associated with successful conception after in vitro fertilization. J Clin Endocrinol Metab 77:1227, 1993.
Badaway SZA, Cuena V, Steitzel A, et al: Autoimmune phenomena in infertile patients with endometriosis. Obstet Gynecol 63:271, 1984.
Belonoschkin B: Determination of fertilizing ability of sperm. Int J Fertil 4:1, 1959.
Blacker CM, Ginsburg KA, Leach RE, et al: Unexplained infertility: Evaluation of the luteal phase; results of the National Center for Infertility Research in Michigan. Fertil Steril 67:437, 1997.
Burkman LJ, Kruger TF, Coddington CC, et al: The hemizona assay (HZA): Development of a diagnostic test for the binding of human spermatozoa to human hemizona pellucida to predict fertilization potential. Fertil Steril 49:688, 1988.
Cedars MI: Controlled ovarian hyperstimulation as therapy for unexplained infertility. Infertil Reprod Med Clin 8:649, 1997.
Collins JA, Crosigriani PG: Unexplained infertility: A review of diagnosis, prognosis, treatment efficacy and management. Int J Symbol Obstet 39:267, 1992.
Collins JA, Milner RA, Row TC: The effect of treatment on pregnancy among couples with unexplained infertility. Int J Fertil 36:140, 1991.
Davis RO, Katz DF: Standardization and comparability of CASA instruments. J Androl 13:81, 1992.
diZerega GS, Hodgen GD: Luteal phase dysfunction infertility: A sequel to aberrant folliculogenesis. Fertil Steril 35:489, 1981.
Eistein M: Effect of infertility on psycho-sexual function. Br Med J 5:295, 1975.
Friberg J: Mycoplasmas and ureaplasmas in infertility and abortion. Fertil Steril 33:351, 1978.
Gnarpe H, Friberg J: Mycoplasma and human reproductive failure. I. The occurrence of 7 different mycoplasmas in couples with reproductive failure. Am J Obstet Gynecol 114:727, 1972.
Hafez ESE: Transport and survival of spermatozoa in the female reproductive tract. In Hafez ESE (ed): Human Semen and Fertility Regulation in Men. St. Louis, C. V. Mosby, 1976, p 107.
Haney AF, Muscato JJ, Weinbert JB: Peritoneal fluid cell populations in infertile patients. Fertil Steril 35:696, 1981.
Harrison RF, Blades M, DeLouvois J, et al: Doxycycline treatment and human infertility. Lancet 1:605, 1975.
Hembree WC, Overstreet JW: Defects in human sperm penetration in vitro. In Troen P, Nankin HR (eds): The Testis in Normal and Infertile Men. New York, Raven Press, 1977, p 513.
Hesla JS, Schoolcraft WB: Treatment of idiopathic infertility with assisted reproductive technologies. Infertil Reprod Med Clin North Am 8:665, 1997.
Horne HW, Hertig AT, Kundsin RB, et al: Sub-clinical endometrial inflammation and T-mycoplasma: A possible cause of human reproductive failure. Int J Fertil 18:226, 1973.
Kennedy WP, Kaminski JM, Vandervan HH, et al: A simple clinical assay to evaluate the acrosin activity of human spermatozoa. J Androl 10:221, 1989.
Kerin JF, Kirby E, Morris D, et al: Incidence of luteinized unruptured follicle phenomenon in cycling women. Fertil Steril 40:620, 1983.
Kerin JF, Pearlstone AC, Surrey ES: Tubal microendoscopy: Salpingoscopy and falloscopy Keye WR, Chang RJ, Rebar RW, et al (eds): In Infertility: Evaluation and Treatment. Philadelphia, WB Saunders Co, 1995, pp 372–386.
Kim AH, Adamson GD: Does therapy for minimal/mild endometriosis enhance conception? Infertil Reprod Med Clin North Am 8:623, 1997.
Leach RE, Moghissi KS, Randolph JF, et al: Intensive hormone monitoring in women with unexplained infertility: Evidence for subtle abnormalities suggestive of diminished ovarian reserve. Fertil Steril 68:413, 1997.
Li TC, Dockery P, Cooke ID: Endometrial development in the luteal phase of women with various types of infertility: Comparison with women of normal fertility. Hum Reprod 6:325, 1991.
Liu DY, Clarck GY, Lopata A, et al: Sperm zona pellucida binding test and in vitro fertilization. Fertil Steril 50:281, 1989.
Moghissi KS: Basic workup and evaluation of infertile couples. Clin Obstet Gynecol 22:11, 1979.
Moghissi KS: The cervix in infertility. Clin Obstet Gynecol 22:27, 1979.
Moghissi KS, Sacco AG, Borin K: Immunologic infertility. II Pregnancies in patients with sperm antibody activity. In Insler V, Bettendorf G (eds): Advances in Diagnosis and Treatment of Infertility, Amsterdam, Elsevier-North 1982, p 235.
Moghissi KS: Prediction and detection of ovulation. Fertil Steril 34:89, 1980.
Mohsenian M, Syner FN, Moghissi KS: A study of sperm acrosin in patients with unexplained infertility. Fertil Steril 37:223, 1982.
Mortimer D: Objective analysis of sperm motility and kinematics. In Keel B, Webster BW: Handbook of Laboratory Diagnosis and Treatment of Infertility. Boca Raton, CRC Press 1990, p 97–133.
Overstreet JW, Yanagimachi R, Katz DF, et al: Penetration of human spermatozoa into the human zona pellucida and the zona-free hamster egg: A study of fertile donors and infertile patients. Fertil Steril 33:534, 1980.
Perryman RL, Thorner MO: The effects of hyperprolactinemia on sexual and reproductive function in men. Am J Androl 5:233, 1981.
Sacco AG: Immunocontraception: Consideration of the zona pellucida as a target antigen. In Wynn R (ed): Obstetrics and Gynecology Annual, New York, Appleton-Century-Crofts, 1981, p 1.
Segal S, Polishuk WZ, Ben-David M: Hyperprolactinemic male infertility. Fertil Steril 27:1425, 1976.
Seibel MM, Taymor ML: Emotional aspects of infertility. Fertil Steril 37:137, 1982.
Soules MR, McLachlan RI, EKM, et al: Luteal phase deficiency characterization of reproductive hormones over the menstrual cycle. J Clin Endocrinol Metab 69:804, 1989.
Stray-Pedersen B, Eng J, Reikvan TM: Uterine T *Mycoplasma* colonization in reproductive failure. Am J Obstet Gynecol 130:307, 1978.
Taylor PJ, Collins JA: Unexplained infertility. Oxford, Oxford University Press, 1992, pp 4–8.
Templeton AA, Penney GC: The incidence, characteristics, and prognosis of patients whose infertility is unexplained. Fertil Steril 37:175, 1982.

Treharne JD, Ripa KT, Mardh PA, et al: Antibodies to *Chlamydia trachomatis* in acute salpingitis. Br J Venereal Dis 55:26, 1979.

Trounson AO, Leeton J-F, Wood C, et al: The investigation of idiopathic infertility by in vitro fertilization. Fertil Steril. 34:431, 1980.

Varma TR: Tuberculosis of the Male Genital Tract. *In* Sciarra JJ (ed): Gynecology and Obstetrics. Vol. 8. Philadelphia, Lippincott-Raven, 1998, pp 1–21.

World Health Organization: WHO laboratory manual for the examination of human semen and sperm cervical mucus interaction, 3rd ed. Cambridge, England, Cambridge University Press, 1992.

# 62

# Surgery of the Fallopian Tube

CARLA P. ROBERTS
ANA A. MURPHY

Assisted reproductive technologies have drastically changed decisions as to the appropriate treatment for tubal disease. Certainly, couples with severe tubal factor should be counseled about the poor pregnancy rates seen after tubal reconstruction and about extracorporeal fertilization. Additionally, laparoscopic operative techniques have become increasingly more accepted vs. traditional microsurgical laparotomy. The significant decreases in morbidity and cost of laparoscopic surgery have been well documented. Additionally, pregnancy rates are similar in those achieved by laparotomy.

The following discussion of surgical technique is not intended to be an extensive review of the literature; rather, it is intended to present the surgical techniques used by the authors.

## Tubal Factors in Infertility

The physiologic significance of the fallopian tubes is evidenced by their transport of sperm to the newly released ovum, development of an appropriate fertilization milieu, and transport of the zygote to the uterine cavity. Several developments have made a significant impact on plastic surgery of the fallopian tube. Alterations in this process either by ciliated movement disorders or tubal occlusion may lead to implantation abnormalities or infertility. The anatomic relationship of the fallopian tube to the ovary appears to be important in ovum pickup. The ciliated lining of the fimbria embraces the ovary and transports the oocyte to the ampulla for fertilization.

Tubal infections generally alter the anatomy and function of the fallopian tube. Endosalpingitis may produce tubal occlusion along the entire course of the fallopian tube but most commonly results in distal obstruction with formation of hydrosalpinx or fimbrial agglutination. Westrom has estimated that 17.4% of patients become infertile because of pelvic inflammatory disease (PID) tubal damage. Multiple infection, increasing age at first infection, and severe infection worsen fertility prognosis. PID can be divided into exogenous (sexually transmitted diseases) and endogenous agents. Sexually transmitted diseases account for 60 to 80% of PID in women younger than 25 years of age. Gonococcal endosalpingitis is likely the best studied single cause; however, it has become clear that PID is more commonly polymicrobial. Furthermore, subclinical infections such as chlamydia also may cause irreparable damage to the tubal mucosa. Impairment of ciliary activity may interfere with tubal motility and ovum pickup. Peritubal

**Table 62-1** Classification of Tubal Procedures

1. Lysis of periadnexal adhesions (salpingolysis-ovariolysis): Classified according to adnexa with least pathology.
   a. Minimal: 1 cm of tube or ovary involved
   b. Moderate: partially surround tube or ovary
   c. Severe: encapsulating peritubal and/or periovarian adhesions
2. Lysis of extra-adnexal adhesions
   a. Minimal
   b. Moderate
   c. Severe
3. Tubouterine implantation
   a. Isthmic: implantation of isthmic segment
   b. Ampullary: implantation of ampullary segment
   c. Combination: different type implantation on right and left sides
4. Tubotubal anastomosis
   a. Interstitial (intramural)-isthmic
   b. Interstitial (intramural)-ampullary
   c. Isthmic-isthmic
   d. Isthmic-ampullary
   e. Ampullary-ampullary
   f. Ampullary-infundibular (fimbrial)
   g. Combination: different type anastomosis on right and left sides
5. Salpingostomy (salpingoneostomy): Surgical creation of a new tubal ostium
   a. Terminal
   b. Ampullary
   c. Isthmic
   d. Combination: different type salpingostomy on right and left tubes
6. Fimbrioplasty: Reconstruction of existent fimbriae
   a. By deagglutination and dilatation
   b. With serosal incision (for completely occluded tube)
   c. Combination: different type fimbrioplasty on right and left tubes
7. Other reconstructive tubal operations (specify)
8. Combination of different types of operations
   a. Bipolar: for occlusion at both proximal and terminal end of tube (specify)
   b. Bilateral: different operations on the right and left sides (specify)

adhesions with impaired tubal transport also may occur in association with endometriosis and from prior abdominopelvic surgery.

Diagnostic modalities most commonly used to evaluate tubal function are hysterosalpingography (HSG), laparoscopy, and salpingoscopy. The most complete evaluation is likely a combination of laparoscopy and either HSG or salpingoscopy. Although laparoscopy is the most important method of assessing fallopian tubes, it cannot evaluate the endosalpinx, and the presence of rugal folds on HSG is a favorable prognostic sign. Young and associates noted a significant decrease in pregnancy rates from 60.7% in patients with good rugal markings to 7% when none were seen. Changes in salpingoscopy, such as adhesions, flattened mucosa, and agglutination, are predictive of subsequent pregnancy rates.

Microsurgery is a philosophy of gentle operative technique using delicate instruments, fine needles, sutures only when necessary, minimal coagulation for meticulous hemostasis, and magnification. Most often, this is achieved with the operating microscope, although loupe and laparoscopic magnification also are used. Lasers became popular at the time of tuboplasty. The $CO_2$ laser currently is the most commonly used laser, although potassium-titanyl-phosphate (KTP) 532 and neodymium:yttrium-aluminum-garnet (Na:YAG) lasers are gaining popularity. The reported advantages of lasers include precise lysis of adhesions and minimal tissue damage and bleeding. There is no evidence, however, of decreased adhesion formation and subsequent increases in pregnancy rates.

An important issue facing reproductive surgeons is the lack of generally accepted classification system for tubal surgery. The Ad Hoc Committee of the International Federation of Fertility and Sterility introduced a classification that was modified last in 1980 (Table 62-1). International use of this classification may create some uniformity in reporting reliable success rates. The American Society for Reproductive Medicine also has proposed classifications of tubal procedures based on the extent of disease (Table 62-2). Usefulness of these classification systems remains to be established because there are few series that examine them compared with pregnancy success rates.

In general, tubal surgery deals with four main areas of disease. Tubolysis or salpingolysis is performed for peritubal adhesion. Quite frequently, the ovary may be adhered to the sidewall, fixed to the fallopian tube, or enveloped in adhesions, and ovariolysis is

**Table 62-2** Classification of the Extent of Tubal Disease with Distal Fimbrial Obstruction

| | |
|---|---|
| *Mild* | 1. Absent or small hydrosalpinx <15 mm diameter |
| | 2. Inverted fimbriae easily recognized when patency achieved |
| | 3. No significant peritubal or periovarian adhesions |
| | 4. Preoperative hysterogram reveals a rugal pattern |
| *Moderate* | 1. Hydrosalpinx 15–30 mm in diameter |
| | 2. Fragments of fimbriae not easily identified |
| | 3. Periovarian and/or peritubular adhesions without fixation, minimal cul-de-sac adhesions |
| | 4. Absence of a rugal pattern on preoperative hysterogram |
| *Severe* | 1. Large hydrosalpinx >30 mm in diameter |
| | 2. No fimbriae |
| | 3. Dense pelvic or adnexal adhesions with fixation of the ovary and tube to either the broad ligament, pelvic sidewall, omentum, and/or bowel |
| | 4. Obliteration of the cul-de-sac |
| | 5. Frozen pelvis (adhesion formation so dense that limits of organs are difficult to define) |

performed as well. Neosalpingostomy or fimbrioplasty is performed for distal obstruction, depending on the severity of disease. Segmental obstruction most commonly, but not exclusively secondary to previously ligated tubes, is treated with end-to-end anastomosis. Proximal obstruction may be treated with tubocornual anastomosis; uterotubal implantation rarely is used because pregnancy rates are lower than with anastomosis. New nonsurgical therapies for proximal obstruction include hysteroscopic or fluoroscopic cannulation.

## SALPINGOLYSIS

Patients with peritubular adhesions as a sole factor are uncommon. The infundibulum is by definition uninvolved, and the incidence is approximately 4 to 5%. In general, these adhesions are the result of salpingitis or prior abdominal surgery. Endometriosis frequently spares the infundibulum, yet endometriosis should not be included in this series because the pathogenesis is thought to be different.

Inspection of anatomic landmarks of the oviduct and ovary is necessary before undertaking adhesiolysis to avoid inadvertent incision of the fimbriated end, ovarian/mesosalpingeal vasculature, or tubal serosa. Tubal surgery requires careful mobilization, elevation of the adnexa, and excision of adhesions. If extensive adhesion formation is present, careful, painstaking removal of individual adhesions is required to prevent damage to underlying structures. At the time of laparotomy, gentle dissection of a densely adherent adnexa with the finger allows elevation to a platform made from lint-free packs placed in the cul-de-sac. Once the adnexa are mobilized, the surgeon should carefully excise all adhesions at their origin and insertion. Plastic or insulated metal rods may be used to elevate adhesions so that their insertion and origin are delineated clearly. The adhesion should be placed on tension before excision, using fine-needle monopolar cautery or laser. The adhesion should be lysed completely at the junction of the adhesion and the organ with meticulous technique to avoid trauma to serosal surfaces. Large, fibrous vascular adhesions between ovary, fallopian tube, and small bowel are particularly difficult to remove without damage to serosal surfaces. An appropriately insulated manipulator may help to prevent this damage. Once all adhesions are removed and the anatomy is normalized, careful, magnified inspection of the fimbriae should be performed. Tear duct probes are often quite helpful in combing the fimbria for adhesions.

Gomel reported fertility-enhancing laparoscopic surgery in 1977. Good results depend on the use of microsurgical technique. As discussed with laparotomy surgery, the adhesion should be removed at both its origin and insertion point. This is best accomplished by using the uterine manipulator or placing a probe or forceps through an ancillary port. Excision may be accomplished with microscissors, fine-point needle cautery, knife, or laser. The scissors or knife may be combined with electrocautery as well. Once the adhesion is lysed, it may be grasped and rolled to completely excise the other end (Fig. 62–1). Multilayered adhesions should be lysed layer by layer to prevent trauma to underlying structures, especially to the ureter or the bowel. The most important maneuver is countertraction with visualization of tissue planes. Vascular adhesions should be coagulated before sharp lysis to maintain meticulous hemostasis. If $CO_2$ laser is used, a beam with the smallest spot size possible in superpulse mode is applied with a sweeping motion to vaporize the tissue. Care must be taken to provide gentle traction without tearing the tissue because this is traumatic and causes bleeding.

Ovarian adhesions also should be lysed in the aforementioned manner. A different method, however, may be needed to remove ovarian adhesions that encapsulate the ovary. If the adhesions cannot be dissected free, they can be vaporized using a defocused beam and low-power density. Copious irriga-

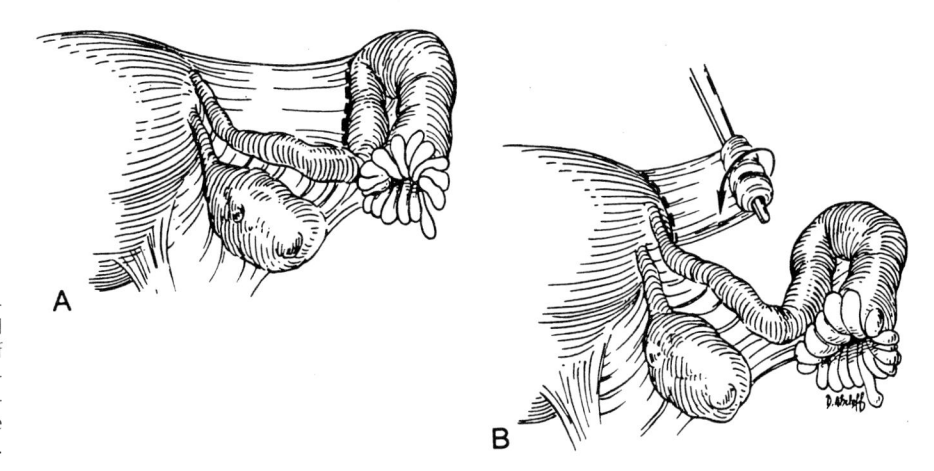

**Figure 62–1** Salpingolysis. *A,* Adhesions are placed on tension and lysed at their insertion. A polytef (Teflon) probe may facilitate exposure and protect underlying structures. *B,* Adhesions should be placed on tension to facilitate lysis.

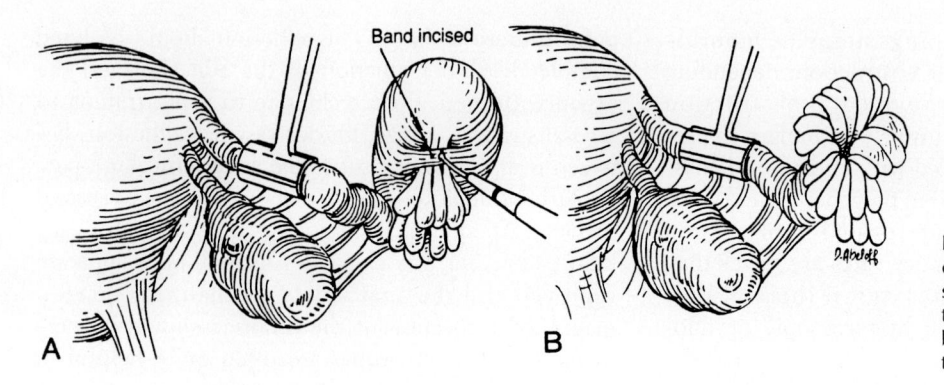

**Figure 62–2** Fimbrioplasty. *A,* Incomplete tubal obstruction resulting from a tubal band. *B,* When the band is removed, normal fimbriae appear. One or two fine sutures help maintain patency.

tion to remove the carbonized tissue and other debris is necessary.

Hydrodissection is an alternative technique involving the application of irrigant at high pressures to develop cleavage planes between adherent structures. This is particularly effective with early second-look laparoscopic lysis of adhesions. Denuded areas may result, even with careful dissection. Careful consideration should be given to covering denuded areas with an adhesion barrier such as Interceed (Johnson & Johnson, Raritan, NJ), Gortex (W. L. Gore and Associates, Flagstaff, AZ), or a chemically modified hyaluronic acid and carboxymethylcellulose (Seprafilm). Reperitonealizing no longer is recommended. Sutures are foreign substances that can cause anoxia if tied too tightly and can lead to adhesion formation. In addition, the peritoneum may be placed on tension and cause anatomic distortion.

Postoperative pregnancy rates are quite good after salpingolysis by laparotomy. Most series quote term pregnancy rates ranging from 30 to 68%. Gomel reported that of a series of 92 women who underwent laparoscopic salpingo-ovariolysis for moderate to severe adnexal adhesions, 57 (62%) achieved a term pregnancy. A 5% ectopic pregnancy rate was noted. Fayez reported a 67% pregnancy rate with laparoscopic tubolysis, 72% with ovariolysis, and 50% with salpingo-ovariolysis. These results are comparable to the intrauterine pregnancy rates after salpingo-ovariolysis via laparotomy (30–60%).

## SALPINGOPLASTY

Salpingoplasty is a collective term that describes procedures that are performed on the tubal infundibulum, including fimbrioplasty and neosalpingostomy. The normal anatomy must be restored before repairing the distal oviduct. Complete restoration of tubo-ovarian relationships should be the goal of reconstruction. In particular, the fimbria ovarica should be identified carefully because it is a very important landmark in the tubo-ovarian anatomy.

## FIMBRIOPLASTY

Fimbrioplasty is defined as the lysis of fimbrial adhesions or dilatation of fimbrial phimosis. On occasion, a peritoneal ring results in an obstruction of the distal portion of the fallopian tube such that simple lysis of this tissue uncovers normal-appearing fimbriae (Fig. 62–2). In most instances, periadnexal adhesions are also present. The shaft of the tube and ovary must be mobilized before attempting patency by fimbriolysis.

If agglutination is present at laparotomy, a fine delicate mosquito forceps can be introduced into the phimotic opening of the tube and gently opened. The forceps then are withdrawn gently, causing dilatation of the tubal ostia. By repeating this procedure in several directions, even dilatation of the fimbrial os is accomplished. In some instances, a small incision over scarred tissue may be necessary. Long-term patency may be aided by a few sutures of 8–0 polyglactic suture to maintain established eversion.

Phimotic or clubbed fimbria may be released through the laparoscope. The distal portion of the tube must be free of adhesions. The tube is distended to identify the lumen, and the fallopian tube is stabilized with atraumatic forceps. Occasionally, the anterior cul-de-sac may be used to provide a platform for dissection. It is understood that, as in laparotomy surgery, periadnexal adhesions are lysed and removed before fimbrial reconstruction. Fibrous tissue covering the terminal end of the tube is excised with fine-needle unipolar cautery, microscissors, or laser. If the fimbriae are agglutinated, forceps or tongs may be introduced into the opening and then gently withdrawn (Fig. 62–3). Gentleness is necessary to avoid excessive trauma and bleeding.

The fimbria then should be explored carefully for fimbrial adhesions that can be freed with fine-needle cautery, fine scissors, or laser. Care should be taken not to damage the fragile mucosa because this may lead to complete fimbrial occlusion postoperatively.

Prefimbrial phimosis may be released by incising the fibrous band that constricts the infundibulum with laser or fine-needle cautery. A very shallow inci-

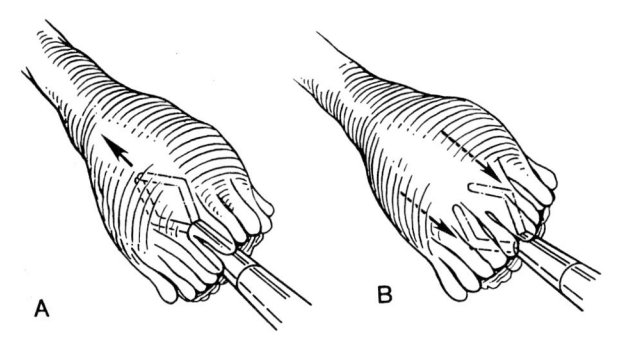

**Figure 62–3** Fimbrial agglutination. *A,* The tongs or ampullary dilator may be inserted into the phimotic tube in the closed position. *B,* The instrument is opened and carefully withdrawn. This may be repeated at various angles to allow symmetric dilatation. The fimbriae then should be examined for interfimbrial adhesions, which should be lysed carefully.

sion should be made along the avascular scarred area from the fimbriated end and extending just beyond the region of phimosis. If appropriate, the tubal mucosa can be everted with a defocused laser or very low-power cautery to the serosal surface.

The most recent series of microsurgical fimbrioplasty through laparotomy demonstrate pregnancy rates of 30 to 70%. Similar rates (20–50%) have been reported for laparoscopic fimbrioplasty. A 5% ectopic pregnancy rate is reported for both laparotomy and laparoscopic series.

## NEOSALPINGOSTOMY

Neosalpingostomy is the creation of a new tubal ostium in which the fimbrial end is totally occluded. Terminal neosalpingostomy is the procedure of choice for establishing tubal patency in any case. Ampullary and isthmic salpingostomy are largely historical procedures that result in abysmal pregnancy success rates.

A successful neosalpingostomy requires complete understanding of the tubo-ovarian relationships, specifically, the fimbria ovarica and the relationship of the shaft of the oviduct to the ovary. Although there is some variation in the length of the fimbria ovarica, it is always present and provides a clue as to the normal axis of the oviduct. It always should be identified before an ostia is created.

With a monopolar microelectrode, laser, or fine, sharp scissors, adhesions are excised and the ovaries mobilized. The cul-de-sac then may be packed with lint-free laparotomy packs and the adnexa placed on an appropriate platform before establishing tubo-ovarian relationships. Once lysis of adhesions has restored normal anatomy, attention is turned to the distal fallopian tube. The tubes are distended by injection of methylene blue or indigo carmine dye through the fundus or cervix. Under magnification, a distinct vascular pattern with a white avascular area may be identified. As this scar is incised, the colored fluid escapes. A glass rod then is placed into the tube to explore the ampullary portion of the fallopian tube. A salpingoscope is inserted if desired. Complete distal obstruction may occur without significant hydrosalpinx or fimbrial destruction (Fig. 62–4). In this case, normal-appearing fimbriae may protrude through the opening; however, more often than not, the fimbriae are severely damaged. In this case, an initial incision at the 6 o'clock position is performed in the direction of the fimbria ovarica and in a stellate pattern over scarred areas (Fig. 62–5). The mucosa then is everted carefully with a minimal number of sutures of 7–0 or 8–0 polygalactin (Vicryl). Tiny bleeding areas may be visualized by irrigation and are coagulated with microtip bipolar forceps or laser.

The magnification of the laparoscope may be augmented by a loupe attachment to the eyepiece or through the video monitor. Neosalpingostomy requires that the end of the tube be free of adhesions. Two to three ancillary puncture sites are necessary to properly manipulate the tube. Transcervical installation of dilute indigo carmine dye distends the hydrosalpinx and aids in the identification of the scarred ostium, fimbria ovarica, and adjacent structures. As with laparotomy microsurgery, it is imperative to establish correct anatomy. The area of the dimple is incised with scissors, needle-point cautery, or laser (high-power density). The tube can be scored superficially with laser or cautery before perforating the wall and collapsing the hydrosalpinx. This facilitates completion of the dissection after collapse of the hydrosalpinx. The atraumatic forceps then may be repositioned to stabilize the margins of the incision. In cases in which normal fimbriae are released, a single incision extended at the 6 o'clock position is usually sufficient to release the band and evert the tube. In most cases, two relaxing incisions to complete the shape of a "Y" may be necessary to achieve sufficient exposure of the residual fimbriae.

When using a $CO_2$ laser, great care is necessary to avoid damage to the epithelium on the other side of the lumen. The "flowering" $CO_2$ laser technique consists of applying a defocused beam of low-power density to the serosal surface. The beam is moved continuously over the serosal area to limit damage to the tube. Absorption of water causes contraction of the serosal surface and a "flowering," thus exposing more mucosal area. The same technique can be accomplished using very low-power electrocoagulation or thermocoagulation. Eversion also may be accomplished by grasping the luminal surface gently and using another forceps to evert the edges. Sutures of 4-0 PDS (polydioxanone suture) may be placed using intraabdominal or extracorporeal endoscopic suture technique. This technique is particularly helpful for

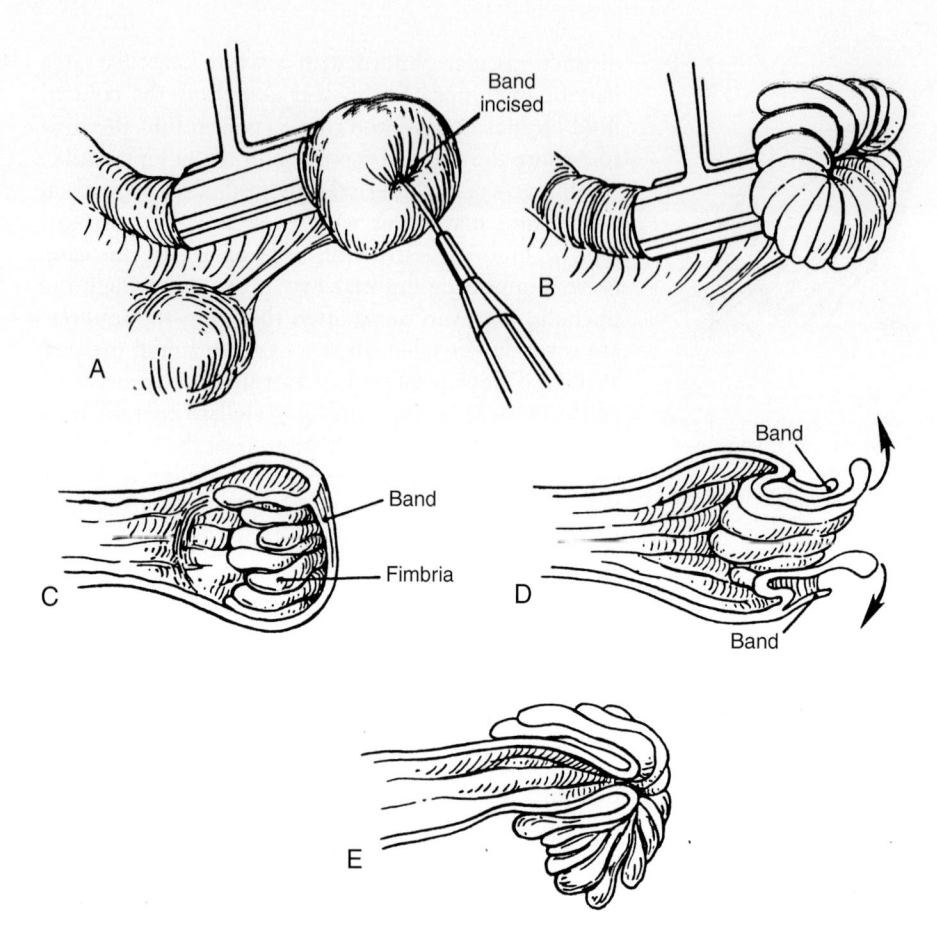

**Figure 62–4** Complete distal fimbrial obstruction without significant hydrosalpinx or fimbrial destruction. *A*, The whitish scar is incised. *B*, Fimbrial strands are revealed. A small forceps may be used to dilate the os. *C*, A cross-section reveals the peritoneal band. *D*, When the band is incised, the fimbriae are released. *E*, Fimbriae assume their normal position.

thick-walled sclerotic tubes, in which the serosal coagulation technique is not useful. An alternative technique involves placement of absorbable clips to everted edges of the tube.

Results of salpingostomy have been discouraging. Salpingostomy performed with a microscope has resulted in similar intrauterine pregnancy rates compared with conventional techniques, although an increase in ectopic pregnancy rate has been observed. The efficacy of the use of the microscope to perform this surgery remains to be established. Using minimal magnification with the loupe, pregnancy rates have not been different from rates previously reported. Schlaff and coworkers recently reported the Johns Hopkins experience with distal obstruction treated by salpingoneostomy using microsurgical technique. The pregnancy rate in patients with mild disease was 80% (70% intrauterine, 10% ectopic), whereas those with severe disease had a pregnancy rate of 16% (12% intrauterine, 4% ectopic). With the classification systems proposed by Mage and Boer-Meisel, patients in the better prognostic category had a 58.8% pregnancy rate (50% intrauterine, 8.8% ectopic) in Mage's series and 81% pregnancy rate (77% intrauterine, 4% ectopic) in that of Boer-Meisel. By comparison, those patients in the poor prognostic category had a 16.5% overall rate (7% intrauterine, 4% ectopic) and a 19% rate (3% intrauterine, 16% ectopic) in the two studies. These observations support the contention that the major determinant of successful outcome of distal tubal surgery is the severity of preexisting tubal pathology and the extent of adhesion formation.

## CONGENITAL TUBAL ANOMALIES

Women with infertility may have congenital anomalies or anatomic distortion of otherwise healthy tubes. Cohen and others have studied the alterations of the fimbrial-gonadal mechanisms related to congenital accessory ostia, elongated fimbria ovarica, and distal distortion caused by intervening paratubal cysts. Defects in canalization of the müllerian ducts may result in duplication of the ostia. The ovum may be lost after pickup by the primary ostium through the accessory ostia, or this opening may allow a loss of important ampullary secretions or fluid transport through the oviduct. Elongation of the fimbria ovarica has been reported in association with polycystic ovaries. Interestingly, Cohen and Katz speculate that the larger, heavier gonad may pull and stretch supporting muscular ligaments.

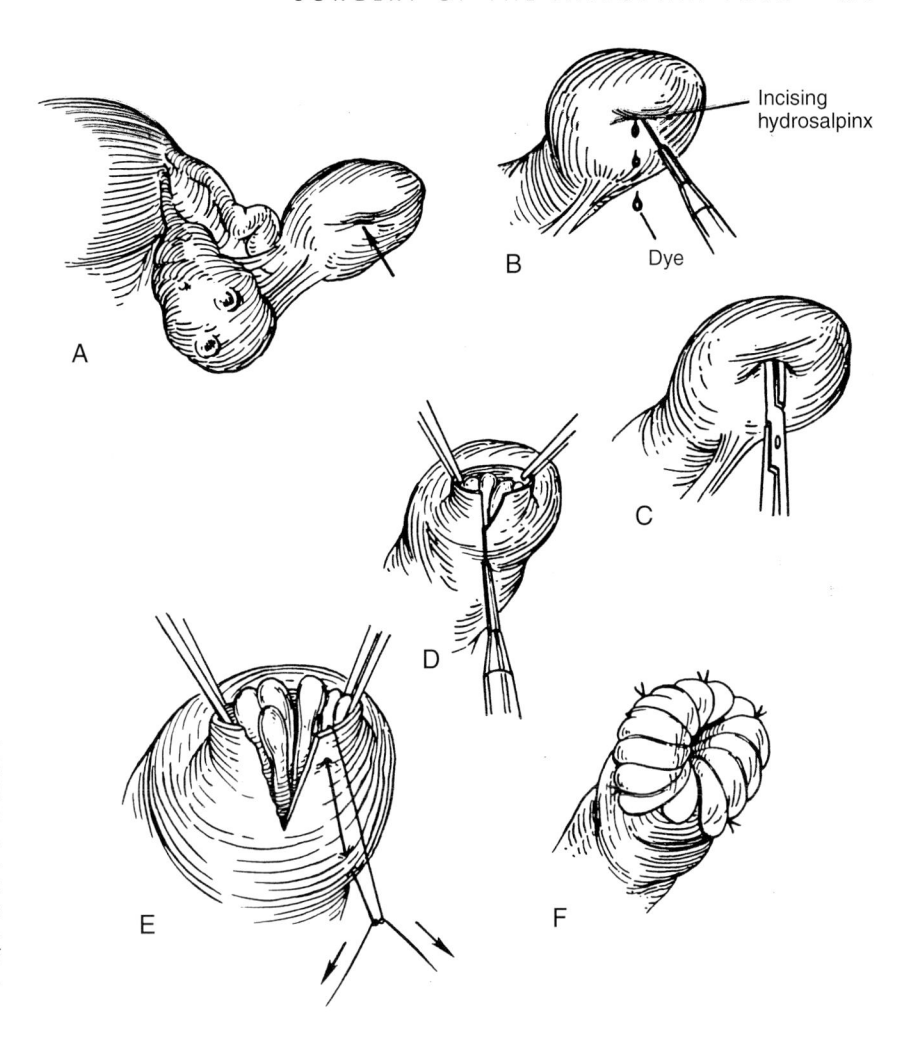

**Figure 62-5** Distal fimbrial obstruction with moderate hydrosalpinx and complete fimbrial destruction. *A* and *B*, Incision is made over the whitish scar on the distended hydrosalpinx. *C*, The ostium is dilated with a fine forceps. *D*, The incision is extended at the 6 o'clock position toward the fimbria ovarica. *E* and *F*, A cuff salpingostomy is achieved after eversion of the mucosa using 7-0 polyglactic suture.

## TUBAL ANASTOMOSIS

Microsurgical technique received a great deal of interest as a result of the enhanced pregnancy rates reported after reversal of sterilization.

Several types of tubal procedures may be reversed. Depending on the extent of tubal destruction, different segments are anastomosed. Therefore, it is difficult to separate these variables when discussing sterilization procedures in general. Unipolar cautery is associated with destruction of a large amount of tube, especially when the triple burn technique is used. As a result of the high variability of tubal destruction, preoperative laparoscopy may be indicated in patients who have undergone sterilization by unipolar cautery to determine the amount of distal fallopian tube available for the anastomosis. A copy of the operative note is essential to assess the type of procedure planned, and then one must adequately discuss options with the infertile couple. The amount of proximal tube is known from the preoperative HSG; however, proximal obstruction on HSG is usually from tubal spasm rather than obstruction of the intramural portion of the fallopian tube.

It is extremely rare for the entire intramural portion of the fallopian tube to be destroyed by a sterilization procedure. Moreover, proximal isthmus, the distal interstitial oviduct, or both are usually the regions affected. Many diverse but relatively rare disease processes also may damage the proximal oviduct. Infections such as endometritis or salpingitis may lead to obstruction; cornual polyps, a manifestation of tubal polyposis, are recognized less frequently as a cause of obstruction. Salpingitis isthmica nodosa shows a predilection for the proximal oviduct. In such cases, a tubocornual anastomosis as opposed to an implantation is the procedure of choice. Although it is apparent that the uterotubal junction is not required for human intrauterine pregnancy, improved pregnancy success rates are seen with tubocornual anastomosis when compared with uterotubal implantation.

### Technique of Tubal Anastomosis

A loupe, visor, or microscope may be used to obtain magnification. Magnification with loupes ranges from

1.5 to 6×, whereas the microscope may provide magnification from 3 to 40×. In a randomized trial, Rock showed that pregnancy rates were not different with loupe magnification vs. the operating microscope.

## Isthmic-Isthmic Anastomosis

The proximal portion of the fallopian tube is identified and its distal tip resected from the mesosalpinx. The occluded tip is resected with straight fine scissors and a 2–0 nylon suture of 40" is introduced into the lumen with fine forceps. The distention of the uterine cavity and the interstitial portion of the oviduct facilitate its passage with indigo carmine dye injected through the uterine fundus (with cervical obstruction by suitable instruments) as well as by stretching the stump.

There should be no discrepancy in luminal size if the distal segment is truly part of the isthmus. The proximal portion of the distal obstructed tube is resected in the same manner, and the nylon stent is passed through the oviduct and out the fimbriated end. The mesosalpinx is approximated carefully using 6–0 Vicryl to eliminate knot tension at the anastomotic site. The knot should be tied anteriorly to decrease chances for adhesion formation involving the ovary. The lumina of the two ends are approximated with 7–0 or 8–0 Vicryl or nylon on a ⅜" circle taper. The needle is passed through the muscularis of the proximal tube and distal segment. The sutures are tied securely but not tightly. Three to four sutures are usually necessary to approximate the muscularis, and a second layer of three additional sutures may be placed to approximate the tubal serosa. Then the nylon stent is removed.

## Isthmic-Ampullary Anastomosis

The proximal tube is prepared in a manner similar to aforementioned description. A major difficulty is encountered in the isthmic-ampullary anastomosis because there is a large discrepancy in the diameter of the lumen of the isthmus as compared with the ampullary portion of the tube. To prevent too large an opening in the ampulla, a needle technique for opening the ampulla has been described. An obturator of an intravenous placement unit of Teflon (#16) is introduced through the fimbriated end of the ampullary segment of the oviduct and advanced to the obstructed site. The needle is inserted through the Teflon obturator, and the obstructed end is perforated by the needle and the Teflon sheath. After the needle is removed, the 2–0 nylon is passed in a retrograde manner through the Teflon obturator. The mesosalpinx is approximated to reduce tension at the anastomotic site. Approximately three to four 7–0 or 8–0 Vicryl sutures are placed through the serosa and muscularis of the proximal oviduct and then through the distal tube. The tip of the needle may be introduced into the ampullary lumen by being placed in the tip of the lumen of the Teflon obturator; next, the tip of the obturator is withdrawn into the ampullary portion of the tube. In some instances, an additional, second layer of suture is placed to approximate the tubal serosa. The nylon stents are removed intraoperatively.

## Ampullary-Ampullary Anastomosis

The muscularis of the ampullary region is relatively delicate. A single layer of suture easily approximates the tubal lumina. Four to eight sutures are placed around the circumference of the ampulla (Fig. 62–6). These sutures are placed through the serosa and muscularis. The endosalpinx is spared, if possible, when approximating the lumen. No stents are used.

## Interstitial-Ampullary Anastomosis

Interstitial or cornual-ampullary anastomosis is needed if a proximal portion of the interstitial oviduct is occluded. A fine knife is used to core out the obstructed portion of the fallopian tube and create a crater around the intramural tube (Fig. 62–7). The isthmic or ampullary distal tube then is approximated to the intramural portion of the fallopian tube. Luminal proportions must be equal. This is the only procedure that requires high magnification and in which the microscope is most useful. These procedures usually are performed at 10–20×. If the distal portion is ampulla, the catheter technique previously described for an isthmic-ampullary anastomosis is necessary to obtain an ampullary lumen similar in size to the cornual lumen. Functional success of this procedure

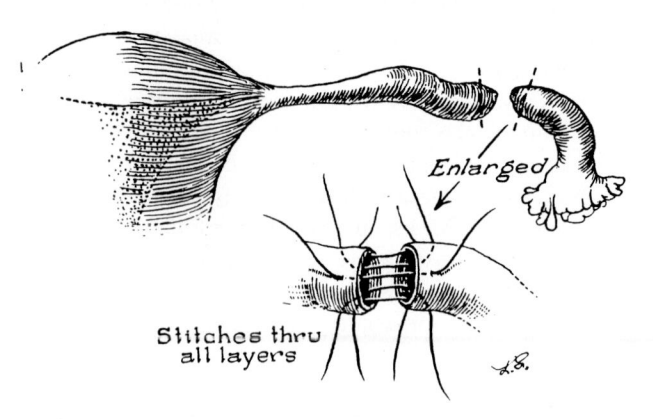

**Figure 62–6** Ampullary-ampullary anastomosis. Anastomosis of the lumen requires 6 to 8 sutures of 7-0 or 8-0 absorbable suture placed circumferentially, equidistant around the lumen.

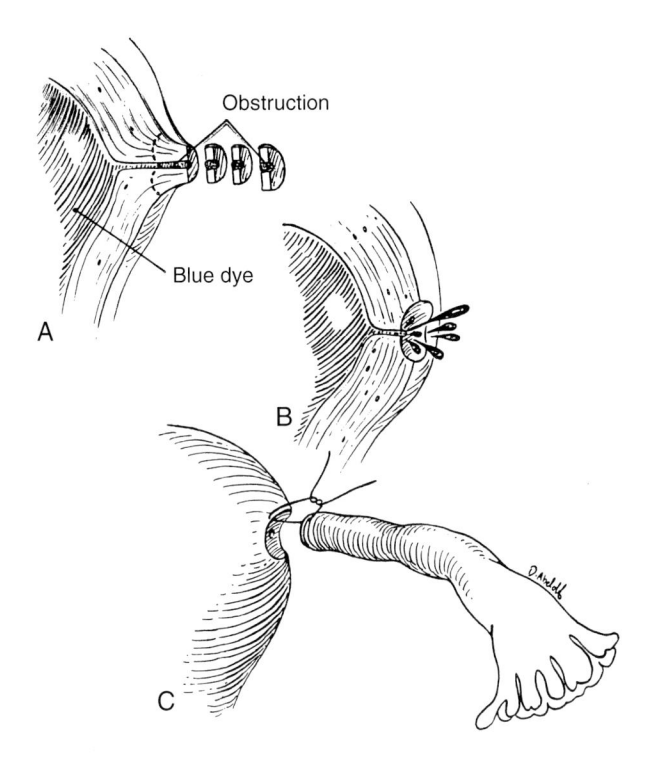

**Figure 62–7** Tubointerstitial anastomosis. *A,* The proximal tube is incised serially until the obstruction is relieved and blue dye is seen. Incision of the cornual area may require a "crater" into the myometrium. *B,* Once absolute hemostasis is achieved, three sutures are placed in the muscular layer just within the serosal surface to the interstitial portion, avoiding the endosalpinx of the cornua. It then is continued through the muscularis of the distal segment. The serosa may be closed with approximated interrupted sutures or continuous sutures of 7-0 or 8-0 absorbable material.

is maximized if the luminal portions are equal. A two-layer closure usually is required for an interstitial-isthmic anastomosis.

## UTEROTUBAL IMPLANTATION

Although this procedure is essentially obsolete, a brief description is provided. Preparation of the distal oviduct for implantation consists of either slitting its antimesenteric border or performing bilateral incisions to "fish-mouth" the tube to help preserve patency. Preparation of the uterus has varied widely. The uterine incisions for implantation techniques include a sharp cornual wedge excision, a reamer, and the posterior fundal technique. Bonney incised the uterine fundus to implant the oviductal segments under direct visualization. Holden and Sovak preferred to use a reamer to make a cornual passage. Von Csaba and colleagues reported implantation through a posterior fundal incision between the utero-ovarian ligaments. The fallopian tube (either isthmus or ampulla) then is inserted into the uterine cavity, and a nonreactive absorbable suture is brought out through the uterus, superior and inferior to the incision, and tied securely. The myometrium then is closed in two layers.

## TRANSCERVICAL FALLOPIAN TUBE CATHETERIZATION

Relief of proximal obstruction not secondary to tubal ligation may be attempted by the transcervical approach. Failure of the transcervical approach would lead to a microsurgical tubointerstitial anastomosis. As noted previously, uterotubal implantation rarely is used. Placement of the catheters may be performed under fluoroscopic guidance or hysteroscopic control. The catheter set consists of coaxial catheters introduced through the cervix with a vacuum adaptor or hysteroscope. The 5.5-F catheter is wedged into the cornua, the 3-F catheter with wire guide is introduced, and the wire guide is advanced through the obstruction. The 3-F soft tube then is advanced over the wire. Balloon-tip catheters also have been developed and dilate the proximal portion of the oviduct once canalization is achieved.

There are no data to document pregnancy success rates after transcervical fallopian tube catheterization or canalization procedures. However, patency of the proximal portion of the oviducts may be accomplished in approximately 60% of patients. These procedures are less invasive than the traditional exploratory laparotomy with anastomosis.

The pregnancy rates for tubal surgery depend on the length of viable tube, the extent of pelvic adhesions, the underlying cause of tubal disease, patient age, and other infertility factors present. In the patient with a straightforward isthmic-isthmic anastomosis and at least 4 cm of fallopian tube remaining, pregnancy rates may be as high as 81%. The pregnancy rates and time to conception decrease proportionally to the length of viable tube remaining. In addition, a disparity among luminal segments, such as with isthmic-ampullary anastomosis, has been found to result in lower pregnancy rates.

In the hands of an experienced microsurgeon, tubocornual anastomosis yields live birth rates of 32.7 to 53.8%. Its advantages to uterine implantation include maintained integrity of the uterine cornua, preservation of a longer tubal segment, decreased adhesion formation, and elimination of the need for cesarean section except for obstetric reasons.

# Conclusion

Fallopian tube disease constitutes at least 25% of female infertility. Although advanced reproductive technologies (ARTs) have become increasingly successful, they should not replace the appropriately selected surgical candidate for tubal repair. With refined technique and use of magnification, one can improve pregnancy success by reducing postoperative adhesion formation. This is particularly true for reversal of sterilization. The reproductive surgeon can establish tubal patency and minimize adhesion formation; however, this is of little benefit for the patient with severely damaged tubal mucosa and multiple factors of infertility. Pelvic surgery is the appropriate approach for women with pelvic adhesions unless they are exceedingly extensive and dense surrounding the tube and ovaries. When disease is mild or moderate, fimbrioplasty is approached surgically. Salpingostomy is appropriate for younger patients who do not have other infertility factors, particularly male factor. Sterilization reversal carries significantly higher pregnancy rates than in vitro fertilization (IVF). Tubocornual anastomosis also carries higher success rates than IVF unless extremely extensive disease is present. Bipolar procedures rarely are indicated because there is minimal chance for success. These recommendations need to be altered in older patients, in patients with male factor or multiple factor infertility, and in patients who may have other indications for surgery, such as endometriosis, pelvic pain, or symptomatic leiomyomas.

Patients must be evaluated with a day 3 follicle-stimulating hormone (FSH) and semen analysis because significant defects in either of these areas render tubal surgery unsuccessful. Duration of time to pregnancy is important because reconstructive surgery for severe distal tubal occlusion may well require several years until most chances for conception have been exhausted. The emphasis needs to be on better preoperative assessment of subsequent pregnancy success so that we can limit surgical treatment by laparoscopy or laparotomy to those who truly can benefit from it. Those patients with poor surgical prognosis should be counseled with regard to ART unless practical, financial, or religious constraints prevent it. The experience of the surgeon is, of course, a major factor in this decision, underscoring the importance of adequate training. Honest objectivity with respect to creating the most favorable situation leading to successful pregnancy should lead to referral for in vitro fertilization–embryo transfer (IVF-ET) for patients presenting with absent or minimally preserved tubal mucosa or for patients with multiple factors, especially those with male factor infertility and the older women.

## REFERENCES

American Fertility Society: The FAS classification of adnexal adhesions, distal tube occlusion, tubal occlusion secondary to tubal ligation, tubal pregnancies, müllerian anomalies and intrauterine adhesions. Fertil Steril 49:944, 1988.
Beyth Y, Kopolovic: Accessory tubes: A possible contributing factor in infertility. Fertil Steril 38:382, 1982.
Boer-Meisel ME, teVelde ER, Habbena JDF, et al: Predicting the pregnancy outcome in patients treated for hydrosalpinx: A prospective study. Fertil Steril 45:23, 1986.
Bonney V: The fruits of conservatism. J Obstet Gynaecol Br Commonw 44:1, 1937.
Bruhat MA, Mage G, Manhes H, et al: Laparoscopic procedures to promote fertility. Ovariolysis and salpingolysis: Results of 93 selected cases. Acta Eur Fertil 113:95, 1986.
Caspi E, Halperin Y, Bukovsky I: The importance of periadnexal adhesions in tubal reconstructive surgery for infertility. Fertil Steril 31:296, 1979.
Cognat M, Rochet Y: Salpingostomy. J Fr Gynecol Obstet Biol Reprod 6:839, 1977.
Cohen BM, Katz M: The significance of the convoluted oviduct in the infertile women. J Reprod Med 25:33, 1980.
Cohen BM: Microsurgical reconstruction of congenital tubal anomalies. Microsurgery 8:68, 1987.
Confino E, Friberg J, Gleicher W: Preliminary experience with transcervical balloon tuboplasty. Am J Obstet Gynecol 159:370, 1988.
Crane M, Woodruff JD: Factors influencing the success of tuboplastic procedures. Fertil Steril 19:810, 1968.
DeBruyne F, Puttermans P, Boeckx W, et al: The clinical value of salpingoscopy in tubal infertility. Fertil Steril 51:339, 1989.
Donnez J, Casanas-Roux F: Prognostic factors influencing the pregnancy rate after microsurgical cornual anastomosis. Fertil Steril 46:1089, 1986.
Donnez J: $CO_2$ laser laparoscopy in infertile women with endometriosis and women with adnexal adhesions. Fertil Steril 48:390, 1987.
Dubuisson JB, deJoliniere JB, Aubriot FX, et al: Terminal tuboplasties by laparoscopy: 65 consecutive cases. Fertil Steril 54:401, 1990.
Fayez JA: An assessment of the role of operative laparoscopy in tuboplasty. Fertil Steril 39:476, 1983.
Gomel V: Salpingo-ovariolysis by laparoscopy in infertility. Fertil Steril 40:607, 1983.
Gomel V: Microsurgical reversal of female sterilization: A reappraisal. Fertil Steril 33:587, 1980.
Gomel V: Salpingostomy by laparoscopy. J Reprod Med 18:265, 1977.
Gomel V: Salpingo-ovariolysis by laparoscopy in infertility. Fertil Steril 40:607, 1984.
Gomel V: Salpingostomy by microsurgery. Fertil Steril 29:380, 1978.
Grant A: Infertility surgery of the oviduct. Fertil Steril 22:496, 1971.
Hesla JS, Rock JA: Laparoscopic tubal surgery and adhesiolysis. *In* Azziz RA, Murphy AM (eds): Practice Manual of Operative Laparoscopy & Hysteroscopy. 2nd ed. New York, Springer Verlag, 1997.
Holden FC, Sovak FW: Reconstruction of the oviduct: An improved technique with report of cases. Am J Obstet Gynecol 24:684, 1932.
Hulka JF: Adnexal adhesions: A prognostic staging and classification system based on a five-year survey of fertility surgery results at Chapel Hill, North Carolina. Am J Obstet Gynecol 144:141, 1982.
Jansen RPS: Surgery-pregnancy time intervals after salpingolysis, unilateral salpingostomy and bilateral salpingostomy. Fertil Steril 34:222, 1980.
Mage G, Pouly JL, deJoliniere JB, et al: A preoperative classification to predict the intrauterine and ectopic pregnancy rates after distal tubal microsurgery. Fertil Steril 46:807, 1986.
McComb P, Gomel V: Cornual occlusion and its microsurgical reconstruction. Clin Obstet Gynecol 23:1229, 1980.
McComb P: Microsurgical tubocornual anastomosis for occlusive disease: Reproducible results without the need for tubouterine implantation. Fertil Steril 46:571, 1986.
Mettler L, Giesel H, Semm K: Treatment of female infertility due to tubal obstruction by operative laparoscopy. Fertil Steril 32:384, 1979.
Nezhat C, Winer WK, Cooper JD, et al: Endoscopic infertility surgery. J Reprod Med 34:127, 1989.
Novy MJ, Thurmond AS, Patton P, et al: Diagnosis of cornual obstruction by transcervical fallopian tube cannulation. Fertil Steril 50:434, 1988.

O'Brien JR, Arronet GH, Eduljee SY: Operative treatment of fallopian tube pathology in human fertility. Am J Obstet Gynecol 103:520, 1969.

Patterson PJ: Factors influencing the success of microsurgical tuboplasty for sterilization reversal. Clin Reprod Fertil 3:57, 1985.

Patton PE, Williams TJ, Coulam CB: Results of microsurgical reconstruction in patients with combined proximal and distal tubal occlusion: Double obstruction. Fertil Steril 48:670, 1987.

Puttermans P, Brosens I, Dlahin P, et al: Salpingoscopy vs. hysterosalpingography in hydrosalpinges. Hum Reprod 2:535, 1987.

Raj SG, Hulka JF: Second look laparoscopy after reconstructive pelvic surgery for infertility. Fertil Steril 38:325, 1982.

Reich H: Laparoscopic treatment of extensive pelvic adhesions, including hydrosalpinx. J Reprod Med 32:736, 1987.

Rock JA, Berquist CA, Kimball AW Jr, et al: Comparison of the operating microscope and loupe for microsurgical tubal anastomosis—A randomized clinical trial. Fertil Steril 41:229, 1984.

Rock JA, Guzick DS, Katz E, et al: Tubal anastomosis: Pregnancy success following reversal of Falope ring or monopolar cautery sterilization. Fertil Steril 48:13, 1987.

Rock JA, Katayama PK, Jones HW Jr: Tubal reanastomosis: A comparisons of Hellman's approach without magnification and a microsurgical technique. In Phillips JM (ed): Microsurgery in Gynecology. 32nd ed. Los Angeles, American Association of Gynecologic Laparoscopists, 1981, p 176.

Rock JA, Katayama P, Martin EJ, et al: Factors influencing the success of salpingostomy techniques for distal fimbrial obstruction. Obstet Gynecol 52:591, 1978.

Rock JA: Reconstruction of the fallopian tube. In Thompson J, Rock J (eds): TeLinde's Operative Gynecology. Philadelphia, Lippincott-Raven, 1997.

Schlaff WD, Hossiokos D, Damewood, MD et al: Neosalpingostomy for distal tubal obstruction: Prognostic factors and impact of surgical technique. Fertil Steril 54:984, 1991.

Seiler JC: Factors influencing the outcome of microsurgical tubal ligation reversals. Am J Obstet Gynecol 146:292, 1983.

Swolin K: Electromicrosurgery and salpingostomy: Long term results. Am J Obstet Gynecol 121:418, 1975.

Tulandi T, Falcone T, Kafka I: Second-look operative laparoscopy 1 year following reproductive surgery. Fertil Steril 52:421, 1989.

Tulandi T, Vilos GA: A comparison between laser surgery and electrosurgery for bilateral hydrosalpinx: A 2-year follow-up. Fertil Steril 44:846, 1985.

Vasquez G, Winston RML, Boeckx W, et al: Tubal lesions subsequent to sterilization and their relation to fertility after attempts at reversal. Am J Obstet Gynecol 138:86, 1980.

Von Csaba I, Keller G, Magi P, et al: Chirurgiche behandbling der weiblichen Steriletat tubenimplantation. Zentralbl Gynaekol 96:490, 1974.

Westrom L: Pelvic inflammatory disease: Bacteriology and sequelae. Contraception 36:111, 1987.

Young PE, Egan JE, Barlow JA, et al: Reconstructive surgery for infertility at the Boston Hospital for Women. Am J Obstet Gynecol 108:1092, 1970.

# 63

# Premenstrual Syndrome

KENNETH A. GINSBURG
ROSELYN DINSAY

## Definition of Premenstrual Syndrome

Although the term *premenstrual syndrome* (PMS) was first introduced by Dalton in 1953, Frank is credited with the original description in 1931 of the menstrual mood condition that later came to be known as PMS. Over 60 years ago, the syndrome was characterized as a state of indescribable tension during the premenstrual phase of the cycle, 7 to 10 days immediately preceding menstruation. The definition has changed relatively little since then. PMS is currently defined as the cyclic recurrence of a constellation of nonspecific somatic, psychological, or behavioral symptoms that are entrained with the luteal and premenstrual phases of the menstrual cycle and are of sufficient severity to result in deterioration of interpersonal relationships, interference with normal activities, or both. In 1987, the term *late luteal phase dysphoric disorder* (LPDD) was introduced to provide a systematic set of diagnostic criteria for a premenstrual mood disorder. This clinical entity was later renamed *premenstrual dysphoric disorder* (PMDD), although there were few changes in the diagnostic criteria employed. This psychiatrically oriented definition requires that PMDD include recurrence of at least five luteal or premenstrual symptoms that cause some degree of functional impairment of the individual during most cycles of the year. In this chapter, the term PMS will be used synonymously with LPDD and PMDD unless otherwise noted in the text.

Agreement by investigators on the criteria for defining PMS is important. Because historically investigators have used their own working definitions of PMS when recruiting patients into clinical protocols for studying the etiology, pathogenesis, and response to treatment, comparison and generalization of observations and conclusions have become problematic. Often one investigator's criteria used to define patients with PMS exclude patients studied by another investigator. Hence, different studies were not comparable and observations could not be transferred to other study groups. At present, there has begun to be general agreement on the diagnostic criteria used to define this condition. This fact alone may have much to do with the current inability to describe both the causes of PMS and optimal treatment of patients who have this disorder.

The timing of the appearance of symptoms is important. Symptoms begin or considerably exacerbate either in the periovulatory phase of the cycle or later, in the luteal phase, and then must either considerably improve or resolve by the onset of, or during, menstruation. Some writers further distinguish primary from secondary PMS: Patients who have *primary PMS* have a symptom-free interval at or after menses until symptoms resume at or after ovulation, whereas patients who have *secondary PMS* always have some symptoms at all stages of the cycle, even during the postmenstrual phase. The important distinction is that patients who have secondary PMS never have a symptom-free interval. However, this distinction results in considerable debate, because some experts in this area contend that women who have secondary PMS have some other underlying (usually psychiatric) condition that cyclically exacerbates symptoms present during the ovarian cycle. Thus, women who have secondary PMS are distinct from individuals who do not have underlying psychopathology and whose clinical manifestations of PMS appear during each cycle. These definitions involve more than just a semantic distinction. They are important both in considering the etiology and possible pathophysiologic mechanisms of PMS and in evaluating the efficacy of various (empiric) treatment strategies. When examining the literature regarding PMS, it is important to discern whether the study in question includes patients in the PMS cohort who have underlying psychopathology.

Premenstrual *molimina* should not be confused with PMS. Molimina refers to the premenstrual discomfort experienced by most women; these symptoms are not considered as severe as those of PMS and do not disrupt a woman's life in the same way or to the same degree. Another associated term is *dysmenorrhea*, which refers only to painful menstruation. The pain of dysmenorrhea is highly variable but is classically described as cramps, aches, or pressure of varying intensity in the midpelvic, suprapubic, or lumbosacral regions. Patients who have PMS often have dysmenorrhea as a major component of the symptom complex.

## Prevalence of Premenstrual Syndrome

Epidemiologic surveys have estimated that 70 to 90% of women of reproductive age have some symptoms associated with menstruation. These women have menstrual molimina. Twenty to forty percent of these women believe that they experience premenstrual syndrome. Generally, many women who are self-referred for treatment of PMS meet only some of the criteria for diagnosis of this condition, failing to have recurrent symptoms, a symptom-free interval, or demonstrably significant interference with their activities of daily living or their relationships. Thus, using strict criteria, only 3 to 8% of women in the reproductive age group have symptoms of sufficient severity and cyclic regularity to qualify for the diagnosis of PMDD.

Although clinical manifestations of PMS may appear at any time after the onset of ovulatory function (shortly after the menarche), women usually first seek treatment for their symptoms between the ages of 25 and 35 years. Perhaps not surprisingly, an inverse relationship of symptom severity with age has been reported, such that women who first seek treatment at a younger age have more severe symptoms. However, despite these reports, many clinicians who care for patients who have PMS can anecdotally report the patient with disabling PMS whose symptoms first began in her later reproductive years.

Cross-cultural studies have identified PMS in all racial and ethnic groups, with insignificant differences in prevalence apparently reflecting unequal access to health care and consequent reporting bias rather than true differences in the incidence and prevalence of PMS itself. In support of this apparent explanation, the study reported by Woods and associates in 1982 found a negative correlation between incidence and prevalence of PMS and socioeconomic status. One difference between sociocultural groups is apparent: Certain symptoms are identified more frequently and/or with greater severity in one culture than in another. For example, premenstrual depressive symptoms were reported four times more often in white than in black women, and tension was reported four times more often in spouses of graduate students in the United States compared with college students in Scotland. There is no correlation between marital status and parity and the presence or severity of PMS symptoms. However, there is an apparent high familial incidence of PMS in at least some groups. Daughters of mothers who have PMS (defined as premenstrual tension) are more likely to complain of PMS than daughters of mothers who are symptom-free. The underlying basis of this observation is unknown and could involve similar triggers within the environment, learned behavioral responses on the part of daughters, similar biochemical abnormalities that result in the PMS complex, or some other explanation. However, an observation that lends credence to the possibility that a biological mechanism may be responsible for PMS symptoms involves a study of twins: The concordance of PMS diagnosis was significantly higher in monozygotic twins (94%) than in either dizygotic twins (44%) or members of control populations.

## Etiology and Pathogenesis of Premenstrual Syndrome

### BIOCHEMICAL MECHANISMS OF PREMENSTRUAL SYNDROME

The etiology and pathogenesis of PMS is not known. Until recently, a potentially confounding factor was the heterogeneity of populations studied, because of the lack of uniform diagnostic criteria. With the universal adoption of the diagnostic criteria defined later in this chapter, this concern will be obviated. Hence, observations from different studies will be combined to create a broad understanding of the etiology and pathogenesis of PMS in the future. Several selected theories that have been proposed in an attempt to explain the etiology and pathogenesis of PMS (Table 63–1) are described in this chapter.

Historically, the earliest explanations of the mechanisms of PMS attempted to implicate basal or other static reproductive hormone alterations. Estrogen excess or deficiency, progesterone deficiency, estrogen-progesterone imbalance, abnormal androgen levels, and gonadotropin abnormalities have been implicated. However, studies of basal hormone levels in women who were defined as having PMS compared with control subjects have not shown consistent differences in levels of gonadotropins, gonadal steroids, or their metabolites. Isolated hormone sampling may fail to identify alterations in secretory patterns (e.g., pulse frequency, pulse amplitude, diurnal variation). Therefore, frequent sampling protocols (with or without provocative or suppressive stimuli), which were used originally to study pituitary disease, have more recently been employed to evaluate reproductive hormone dynamics in PMS patients. These dynamic endocrine studies have also failed to show abnormal secretory patterns of these hormones in PMS patients.

Other potential classic endocrine causes of PMS include prolactin excess, thyroid dysfunction, excess production of aldosterone, antidiuretic hormone, or both, and low levels of sex hormone–binding globulin. Again, studies have failed to find conclusive evidence for differences in basal hormone concentration between women with PMS and asymptomatic control women.

More recently, attention has been focused on the role of central neurotransmitters and the complex interaction of these substances with steroid hormones. Endogenous opiate peptides, including endorphins, enkephalins, and dynorphins, are important in the physiology and pathophysiology of both pain and mood changes. Cyclic changes in endorphin activity throughout the menstrual cycle have been demonstrated. β-endorphin levels have been documented to be at maximal levels during the midluteal phase when ovarian estrogen and progesterone production is maximal and are undetectable at the onset of menstruation when ovarian steroid production returns to basal levels. Based on these findings, opiate withdrawal has been suggested as a mechanism for some symptoms of PMS. Because many of the manifestations of PMS involve alterations of behavior, mood, or both, the search for the potential role of endogenous opiates in PMS seems reasonable. Conceivably, endogenous opiates may be modulators of steroid-dependent alterations in mood and behavior in PMS, or they may be acting independently of reproductive steroid hormones in the pathogenesis of PMS.

Another neurotransmitter, γ-aminobutyric acid (GABA), is known to interact with steroid hormones. GABA levels have been shown to be affected by luteal phase concentrations of progesterone and its metabolites. Evidence supports marked potentiation of GABA-containing neuron transmission by progesterone metabolites through binding to the GABA receptor complex. Because the GABA receptor complex is the major site of action of benzodiazepines (medications with known sedative and anxiolytic effects), it seems reasonable to hypothesize that progesterone-induced GABA alterations could participate in the pathogenesis or relief of PMS symptoms. There is preliminary evidence that the GABA system may be altered in PMS. We hope future studies will define this alteration further and suggest potential approaches to treatment.

Numerous studies have also suggested serotonin as a possible etiologic factor in PMS. Alterations (probably resulting from deficiency in serotonin pathways) have been found to cause disturbances in mood, sleep, food craving, and sexual interest. In vivo studies in both animals and humans have demonstrated that fluctuations in gonadal steroid levels can influence the serotonergic systems. Several lines of compelling evidence (e.g., animal models, human pharmacologic trials with serotonergic drugs) confirm the apparent causal association between serotonin alterations and various affective conditions, such as PMS, depression, and perimenopausal symptoms.

Vitamin $B_6$ (pyridoxine) deficiency has been implicated by some investigators in the pathogenesis of premenstrual syndrome. Vitamin $B_6$ is a cofactor in the synthesis of biogenic amines, such as dopamine and serotonin. It has been suggested that estrogens deplete pyridoxine availability by inducing hepatic enzymes that metabolize available vitamin $B_6$. Pyri-

**Table 63–1** Contemporary Theories of Etiology and Pathophysiologic Mechanisms in Premenstrual Syndrome

---

Reproductive and nonreproductive hormone abnormalities (including altered secretory dynamics)
    Gonadotropins
    Gonadal steroids and their metabolites
    Prolactin and the thyroid axis
    Aldosterone, antidiuretic hormone, and sex hormone–binding globulin
Altered concentration or action of central neurotransmitters
    Endogenous opiates
    γ-Aminobutyric acid (GABA)
    Serotonin and other biogenic amines, including cofactors (pyridoxine)
Prostaglandin secretion or action

doxine deficiency then causes disordered central amine production, the proximate cause of PMS symptoms. However, investigations examining this theory have so far yielded contradictory findings, and no conclusion is available.

Prostaglandins have also been hypothesized to have an etiologic role in PMS. Prostaglandins are involved in fluid balance and act as neurotransmitters centrally. Again, data are contradictory and inconsistent. Some studies suggest excess prostaglandins are found in PMS patients, whereas others have documented lower circulating levels of prostaglandin E (PGE), as well as the essential fatty acid precursors, as possible explanations for PMS.

## SUMMARY—A BIOPSYCHOSOCIAL MODEL OF PREMENSTRUAL SYNDROME

A biopsychosocial approach has been proposed to explain PMS. According to this model, premenstrual symptoms result from the interactions of various psychological (personal) and social (family, culture, society) factors in a susceptible individual. The biology involves the direct or indirect interaction of the ovarian cycle on key hormones, neurotransmitters, or other substances that render a particular patient susceptible. The expression of this as yet undefined underlying biochemical defect can be influenced by sociocultural and individual experiences, accounting for the various types and degrees of severity of symptoms. It is possible, and even probable, that various biochemical triggers can act to render different individuals susceptible to these external factors. Thus, there may *not* be one cause of PMS, but rather *a number of causes*, each unique to a different individual. For example, PMS could be viewed as any other familiar symptom complex, such as a cough. A cough can be caused by a host of underlying pathophysiologic processes (e.g., viral bronchitis, bacterial pneumonia, bronchiectasis, bronchogenic carcinoma) indistinguishable from each other on the basis of their external manifestation. Similarly, PMS may also be a condition in which various unique biochemical, social, and psychological triggers interact to produce a defined clinical syndrome in one patient that appears indistinguishable from the clinical syndrome in another patient.

# History and Physical Examination

## SYMPTOMS

Over 150 nonspecific symptoms have been associated with PMS. Most often, patients complain of a combination of symptoms. As in Table 63–2, it is convenient to consider them in two groups: psychological or behavioral symptoms and physical or somatic symptoms.

Irritability and aggression are among the most frequently reported of the psychological symptoms. Such symptoms may lead to an inability to tolerate the most trivial of social encounters, leading in turn to interpersonal and intrafamilial conflicts. The irritability and aggression may extend to a woman's place of work. Other psychological or behavioral symptoms frequently reported include depression, anxiety, inability to concentrate, poor coordination, nervous tension, emotional lability, fatigue, lethargy, insomnia, spontaneous crying spells, change in appetite (especially cravings for sweet and salty foods), increased thirst, and changes in libido.

**Table 63–2** Common Symptoms of Premenstrual Syndrome

| Psychological | Somatic |
|---|---|
| Aggression | Prone to accidents |
| Agitation | Acne |
| Anorexia | Asthma |
| Anxiety | Bloatedness (feeling of) |
| Argumentativeness | Blurred vision |
| Confusion | Breast swelling |
| Crying bouts | Breast tenderness |
| Decreased alertness | Constipation |
| Decreased libido | Diarrhea |
| Depression | Diminished activity |
| Diminished self-esteem | Diminished efficiency |
| Drowsiness | Diminished performance |
| Emotional lability | Dizziness |
| High energy level | Edema |
| Fatigue | Epilepsy |
| Food craving | Flushes |
| Hopelessness | Formication |
| Restricted to the house | Headache |
| Hunger | Joint pain |
| Hypersomnia | Mastodynia |
| Impulsive behavior | Migraine |
| Increased libido | Muscle pain |
| Insomnia | Nausea |
| Irritability | Oliguria |
| Lack of inspiration | Pain, iliac fossa |
| Lack of volition | Pain, lower abdomen |
| Lethargy | Pain, pelvic |
| Listlessness | Polyuria |
| Loss of attention to appearance | Poor coordination |
| Loss of concentration | Premenstrual dysmenorrhea |
| Loss of confidence | Pruritus |
| Loss of judgment | Puffiness |
| Loss of self-control | Rhinorrhea |
| Malaise | Sinusitis |
| Moodiness | Skin lesions |
| Pessimism | Sore eyes |
| Sadness | Sweating |
| Social isolation | Vaginal discharge |
| Suicidal tendency | Vertigo |
| Tension | Vomiting |
| Thirst | Weakness |
| Violence | Weight increase (perceived or actual) |

Data from O'Brien PMS: Premenstrual Syndrome. Oxford, Blackwell Scientific Publications, 1987.

Regarding somatic symptoms, a feeling of abdominal bloating accompanying the *perception* of weight increase is common. Often, women note that their clothes fit differently, reinforcing the feeling that they have gained weight. However, the symptoms appear to occur in virtual absence of weight increase or change in body dimensions. Other common somatic symptoms include breast swelling and tenderness, pelvic pain, skin changes, change in bowel habits, menstrual migraine and other types of headaches.

## HISTORY

The diagnostic process begins with a detailed patient history. Important in this regard is the characterization of the patient's chief complaint, assessment of the timing of symptoms throughout the menstrual cycle, ranking of symptoms according to severity, and assessment of the impact of PMS on lifestyle, daily routine, family, and friends. Establishing the age of onset of symptoms and the pattern or regularity of recurrence of symptoms each month should be attempted. The patient should be asked to describe and evaluate the results of any treatment that she initiated or any treatment given by her provider in an attempts to relieve symptoms.

The gynecologic history should include assessment of the menstrual cycle with regard to length, regularity, amount and duration of blood loss, and presence or absence of dysmenorrhea and other molimina. Current contraceptive practice should be determined. A history of gynecologic surgery should be elicited; because PMS symptoms appear to be related to endocrine ovarian function and not to menstruation per se, symptoms continue after hysterectomy in women who have ovarian function. Data regarding reproductive problems, such as infertility, spontaneous abortion, luteal phase defect, and desire for future pregnancy should be obtained to evaluate the apparent normality of ovulatory function and to aid in establishing treatment options. The goal is to confirm the presence of cyclic ovarian function, which is required for the diagnosis of PMS.

A detailed psychiatric history is also sought. Information should be gathered on previous and current psychiatric symptoms (e.g., anxiety, depression, suicidal ideation or intent, paranoia, introversion, passivity, defense mechanisms), diagnoses, hospitalization, and treatment. The history should also attempt to evaluate the presence of psychological, physical, or psychosexual abuse because these are known triggers of PMS symptoms in susceptible individuals. In the family history, information should be elicited regarding alcoholism and other drug addiction, depression and other psychiatric disorders, PMS, and parental discord and abuse. An analysis of the patient's marital and social interaction is important. The presence of stressful life events, including conflicts in marriage or other relationships, problems at work, difficulties with children, and other concerns that might contribute to PMS, should be determined. Finally, a review of systems, although usually noncontributory, may reveal underlying disorders that may either exacerbate or rarely mimic PMS.

## PHYSICAL EXAMINATION

A general physical examination is essential to rule out other conditions that may either be confused with or coexist with PMS. Emphasis should be placed on the organ systems that may account for the patient's symptoms as elicited in the history. In particular, the clinician should palpate the thyroid to check for thyromegaly or nodules that may suggest the presence of thyroid disease; perform a breast examination to exclude other causes of mastalgia; perform an abdominal examination to rule out abdominal mass or ascites, which could account for pelvic pain or abdominal bloating; and perform a pelvic examination, including a Papanicolaou smear, to exclude other gynecologic conditions.

An abbreviated mental status examination should be performed during the follicular phase of the menstrual cycle (when PMS symptoms are absent) to assess baseline level of consciousness, cognition, and mood. If a mental status alteration is suggested, referral for a more formal assessment by a psychiatrist is warranted.

## LABORATORY, RADIOLOGIC, AND OTHER DIAGNOSTIC TESTING

Further investigation—including simple hormone tests, dynamic (provocative or suppressive) endocrine evaluation, blood hematologic or chemistry tests, radiologic or sonographic imaging, mammography, or laparoscopy—is rarely needed. Indeed, their use is limited to unusual patients in whom some other underlying condition, which may be causing or aggravating the apparent cyclic symptoms, must be excluded. Because no laboratory tests are yet known that confirm or refute the diagnosis of PMS, diagnostic studies should be chosen on the basis of each patient's symptoms only to exclude medical or psychiatric conditions that could produce some or all of the patient's PMS symptom complex.

# Diagnostic Considerations and Strategies

In 1983, attempts were made to promulgate uniform diagnostic criteria for the condition we now call PMS.

The National Institute of Mental Health recommended that a diagnosis of PMS be made if prospective rating scales showed at least a 30% increase in severity of symptoms in the 5 days before menses compared with the 5 days following menses. In addition, these symptoms had to be present during at least two consecutive cycles.

In an attempt to develop a more rigorous definition of PMS that excluded other conditions, the American Psychiatric Association (APA) included diagnostic criteria for PMDD (Table 63–3). These diagnostic criteria resulted in a much narrower definition of PMS. The PMDD diagnosis emphasizes affective symptoms, the most common of which include depression, anxiety, affective lability, tension, irritability, anger, and sleep and appetite disturbances. The patient must demonstrate a clear worsening of symptoms premenstrually, with remission in the ovarian follicular phase, within a few days after the onset of menstruation. Using these criteria (i.e., at least 50% worsening of symptoms between the follicular and luteal phases of the cycle), most women who are diagnosed as having PMS or PMMD require pharmacologic treatment. Women who have PMDD usually do not respond to conservative, nonpharmacologic interventions discussed later.

## DIAGNOSTIC EVALUATION

Prospective daily rating of symptoms has been widely accepted as a means of confirming a provisional diagnosis of PMS. Retrospective questionnaires overestimate the severity and degree of cyclicity of symptoms, providing less accurate information. However, even prospective accounts can introduce bias and reflect stereotypic expectations rather than providing correct data regarding the patient's condition. In an interesting study of college women who were deliberately deceived about which phase of the menstrual cycle they were experiencing, higher symptom ratings were reported by women who thought they were in the premenstrual phase of the cycle. It is thus important that the patient not be provided with clues as to what pattern is expected for a diagnosis of PMS if the practitioner is to rely upon self-administered prospective symptom records.

More than 65 different questionnaires and scales are available for the assessment and diagnosis of PMS. The Premenstrual Assessment Form (PAF) and Menstrual Distress Questionnaire (MDQ) are well known. These forms group the individual symptoms into clusters based upon organ system involvement, presumed mechanism, and so forth, in an attempt to classify the premenstrual syndrome. Other instruments devised include the visual analog scale, premenstrual tension scale (PMTS), and the PMT-CATOR, wherein a simple rotating disc, on which dominant symptoms can be selected and recorded, is used for analysis. Because lengthy scales can be cumbersome for practical use, calendars and diaries were created for clinical purposes. An example is the PRISM calendar, which is set up to include information such as measurement of menstrual bleeding, daily weight, and basal body temperature to assess ovulation and a number of symptoms that can be semiquantitatively rated by the patient each day. This type of chart is easy to use and interpret, because the characteristics, timing, and severity of symptoms can be assessed at a glance. The classical PMS pattern shows a biphasic ovulatory temperature graph with menstrual bleeding as the temperature returns to baseline and clustering of PMS symptoms (both in terms of severity and number of symptoms recorded) during the luteal phase of the cycle. A symptom-free interval beginning with or after the onset of menstrual bleeding and continuing until or after ovulation

---

**Table 63–3** Diagnostic Criteria for Premenstrual Dysphoric Disorder (PMDD)

A. In most menstrual cycles during the past year, five (or more) of the following symptoms were present for most of the time during the last week of the luteal phase, began to remit within a few days after onset of the follicular phase, and were absent in the week after menses, with at least one of the symptoms being either (1), (2), (3), or (4):
  (1) Markedly depressed mood, feelings of hopelessness, or self-deprecating thoughts
  (2) Marked anxiety, tension, feelings of being "keyed up" or "on edge"
  (3) Marked affective lability (e.g., feeling suddenly sad or tearful or increased sensitivity to rejection)
  (4) Persistent and marked anger or irritability or increased interpersonal conflicts
  (5) Decreased interest in usual activities (e.g., work, school, friends, hobbies)
  (6) Subjective sense of difficulty in concentrating
  (7) Lethargy, easy fatigability, or marked lack of energy
  (8) Marked change in appetite, overeating, or specific food cravings
  (9) Hypersomnia or insomnia
  (10) A subjective sense of being overwhelmed or out of control
  (11) Other physical symptoms, such as breast tenderness or swelling, headaches, joint or muscle pain, a sensation of "bloating," weight gain
B. The disturbance markedly interferes with work or school or with usual social activities and relationships with others (e.g., avoidance of social activities, decreased productivity and efficiency at work or school).
C. The disturbance is not merely an exacerbation of the symptoms of another disorder, such as major depression, panic disorder, dysthymic disorder, or a personality disorder (although it may be superimposed on any of these disorders).
D. Criteria A, B, and C must be confirmed by prospective daily ratings during at least two consecutive symptomatic cycles. (The diagnosis may be made provisionally before this confirmation.)

From Diagnostic and Statistical Manual of Mental Disorders, 4th ed. Washington, DC, American Psychiatric Association, 1994.

is typical. A minimum of two months of prospective charting should be used by the clinician to establish the diagnosis of PMS.

## Differential Diagnosis

PMS is a diagnosis of exclusion. It is important to differentiate other psychiatric and medical disorders with similar symptoms because these other conditions warrant specific intervention.

The first concern is to exclude the presence of other psychiatric illness. The patient may have an underlying psychiatric problem, such as depression, anxiety, eating disorder, or personality disorder. Each of these may be exacerbated premenstrually by unknown mechanisms. Prospective charting becomes useful in these individuals because symptoms will be noted throughout the cycle in women who have chronic psychiatric disease. If further testing is needed, various psychometric tests, such as the Minnesota Multiphasic Personality Inventory (MMPI), Beck Depression Inventory, Carroll rating scale for depression, and Hamilton Depression scale are available. Some tests are self-administered, whereas others are given by the investigator. If suggested by the history, referral for psychological or psychiatric evaluation (or both) may be critical in excluding other psychopathology.

Medical conditions that may need to be considered—again, depending upon the physical, behavioral, or psychological symptoms present—include thyroid disease, anemia, diabetes, obesity, liver disease, lupus erythematosus, or other collagen vascular disease. PMS may exacerbate migraine, asthma, allergies, irritable bowel syndrome, arthritis, and seizure disorders. For patients who have breast symptoms, fibrocystic disease, galactorrhea, and breast cancer must be excluded. Of the gynecologic conditions, endometriosis, pelvic infection, dysmenorrhea, ovarian cysts, and uterine fibroids must be considered. Usually, these potential medical or gynecologic conditions can be excluded by using a careful history, performing physical and pelvic examination, and evaluating appropriate laboratory tests.

## Treatment

Despite the many unanswered questions about the etiology and pathogenesis of premenstrual syndrome, an effective program of medical therapy can be devised for the majority of women who have this syndrome. Individualization of therapy by a multidisciplinary approach is important, because the interaction of biologic triggers and psychosocial factors that cause the PMS symptom complex is unique to each woman.

Because the biological cause (e.g., hormone, neurotransmitter, prostaglandin, or other biomolecule) of PMS is not known, *specific* treatment for PMS is not available. Currently, all treatments employed for PMS involve one of two strategies: (1) agents that are used to suppress ovulation and hence remove the biological trigger, or (2) treatment attempts to alleviate certain symptoms. For this discussion, treatment options will be categorized as either nonpharmacologic or pharmacologic.

### NONPHARMACOLOGIC STRATEGIES

Initial management of all PMS patients should include education and lifestyle modifications, such as exercise, dietary manipulation, and stress reduction. Acknowledgment of the patient's experience, education about the menstrual cycle and symptoms commonly associated with PMS, and reassurance that the premenstrual changes and behavior patterns are temporary and reversible can be therapeutic in many patients. Prospective charting of symptoms is beneficial not only in confirming the diagnosis but also in providing the woman with validation and hence a sense of control over her condition. Indeed, in some patients, this alone may be sufficient to relieve much of their distress and make other interventions unnecessary.

Regular aerobic exercise may ease the severity of premenstrual symptoms and increase a woman's sense of well-being. Experience has confirmed the therapeutic benefit of aerobic exercise for many women who have PMS. Aerobic exercise is recommended for periods of 20 to 30 minutes per day for at least 3 days each week. The rationale for this recommendation is the finding that aerobic exercise leads to the release of endorphins within the central nervous system (CNS), associated with the so-called "runner's high." A decline in circulating endorphins in the late luteal phase of the menstrual cycle has been suggested as a pathophysiologic mechanism in some women who have PMS.

Although no controlled studies have shown their benefit, several dietary changes have been recommended in an attempt to control onset and severity of PMS symptoms. These modifications include elimination of refined sugar, salt, caffeine, and alcohol from the diet, and increased ingestion of foods rich in protein, fiber, and complex carbohydrates. Intake of carbohydrate-rich food has been found to increase availability of tryptophan for serotonin synthesis, which in turn leads to improved mood and decreased depression, anger, confusion, and food craving. Frequent meals, or appropriate snacks between meals, have also been found to be beneficial, suggesting that transient hypoglycemia may be responsible for at least some PMS symptoms.

Avoiding simple sugar and decreasing salt intake can minimize weight gain, premenstrual bloating, and physical discomfort. Decreasing caffeine consumption premenstrually can minimize irritability, insomnia, and breast pain. As depressants and disinhibitors, alcohol and recreational drugs frequently worsen emotional liability, and avoidance of these substances is prudent.

Cognitive, behavioral, and relaxation techniques have been suggested as treatment modalities for PMS. Various techniques, such as anger management, stress inoculation training, and audiotaped relaxation instructions, have been employed with some positive results. The success of these techniques appears to be highly related to the motivation of the patient toward use of these strategies. Although further studies are needed, these approaches appear promising in the treatment of premenstrual symptoms in some patients.

Finally, it is important to involve the patient's significant relatives in the therapeutic process. Support, encouragement, and understanding from spouse or partner and family are of therapeutic benefit to many women who have PMS. PMS support groups and group therapy may also be useful. Some women report deriving tremendous satisfaction from meeting and talking with other women who have similar problems, thereby sharing experiences and developing beneficial relationships.

## PHARMACOLOGIC STRATEGIES

If symptoms persist after the use of these nonpharmacologic measures, or when the severity of symptoms mandates a more aggressive approach, medication aimed at treatment of patients who have PMS can be initiated. Pharmacologic approaches attempt to provide therapeutic benefit by specific symptom management or by ablation of the ovarian cycle, thereby suppressing the biological or chemical trigger of PMS symptoms. It should be emphasized that few randomized, prospective, placebo-controlled pharmacologic trials exist in the PMS literature. Therefore, the substantial placebo effect of any of these drugs cannot be excluded, and hence the therapeutic effect may be totally unrelated to the pharmacologic action of the compound in question.

Oral contraceptives (OCs) may effectively treat symptoms of PMS. Some women who receive combination low-dose estrogen and progestin OCs report less premenstrual moodiness and irritability and less difficulty concentrating as well as improved affect and diminished water retention. Others, however, may experience worsening of symptoms or develop new symptoms on combination OCs. Depression, irritability, and exacerbation of migraine are common reasons for discontinuing OC pills in PMS patients. Instead of contraceptive OCs, some investigators have recommended the use of combinations of estrogen and progesteron as found in postmenopausal hormone replacement therapy. In these regimens, either oral conjugated estrogens, oral 17-β-estradiol, or transdermal 17-β-estradiol are combined with a 21-carbon progestin, such as oral medroxyprogesterone acetate or micronized progesterone. However, the superiority of this steroid therapy compared with low-dose combination OCs has never been demonstrated, and the choice of which estrogen-progestin regimen to employ must, therefore, be made based upon patient or physician preference.

Progesterone, prescribed either as a vaginal suppository or as the micronized oral form, was once widely used as a treatment for patients who had PMS. This treatment involves administration of progesterone starting in the ovulatory phase of the cycle and continuing through the luteal phase until the establishment of menstrual bleeding. Reports of improvement in PMS symptoms have appeared in the literature for over 30 years. However, the superiority of progesterone over placebo for relief of PMS symptoms has never been demonstrated in comparative trials. Other steroid remedies that are thought to potentially have some efficacy for PMS treatment include tocopherol (vitamin E) 400 U/day and evening primrose oil (EPO), a source of free fatty acids that are prostaglandin precursors, administered 500 mg/day up to a maximal dosage of 1000 mg three times daily. Improvement of PMS symptoms with EPO suggests that prostaglandin deficiency may be related to the pathogenesis of PMS symptoms in at least some patients. In direct contrast, however, other PMS patients receive some therapeutic benefit from administration of nonsteroidal anti-inflammatory drugs (NSAIDs), known to act by suppressing synthesis or release of prostaglandins in certain target tissues. In particular, NSAIDs have demonstrated efficacy in treating breast, joint, and pelvic pain, as well as headache in PMS patients. Because they have no effect on emotional or behavioral symptoms, their benefit is apparently limited to their analgesic action.

Bromocriptine has been shown to be useful for the treatment of premenstrual mastalgia, which is sometimes found in PMS patients. Doses of 2.5 to 5 mg daily have been employed. Adverse effects reported include nausea, headache, and fatigue. Interestingly, some clinicians who employ bromocriptine for treatment of PMS patients who have significant breast symptoms have also noted improvement in affective or behavioral symptoms in these individuals.

This beneficial effect of bromocriptine on mood and behavior of PMS patients may be related to the known dopaminergic actions of this drug.

Vitamin and mineral supplementation has been advocated in the treatment of PMS. Patients who have complaints of fatigue, irritability, and depression may respond to Vitamin $B_6$ (pyridoxine) therapy. Although no controlled PMS trials are conclusive, supplemental doses of 50 to 125 mg/day seem to be effective in some patients and appear safe. However, because of the possible occurrence of irreversible sensory neuropathy in women receiving excessive doses of pyridoxine, its use must be carefully monitored and large doses (>200 mg/day) should be avoided. Patients are also warned to discontinue therapy and immediately report if distal paresthesias develop while they are receiving therapy.

Danazol, a synthetic steroid with androgenic activity, has been used to treat women who have PMS. In one study, a marked decrease in the severity of symptoms of patients treated with Danazol compared with control subjects treated with placebo was reported. Danazol, administered at 200 mg/day from the onset of symptoms to the onset of menstruation, was well tolerated. Breast symptoms and bloating in particular appear to respond well to low-dose danazol use. Side effects are generally minimal when these doses are prescribed.

Therapeutic benefit has been demonstrated for women who have PMS with use of spironolactone, an aldosterone receptor antagonist. Classically, this drug was only prescribed to PMS patients with documented weight gain in an attempt to reverse the water retention thought to be the cause of their other symptoms. However, the use of relatively low doses of spironolactone (100 mg/day during the 14 premenstrual days) is associated with improvement in negative mood and somatic symptoms, such as irritability, depression, fluid retention, breast tenderness, and food craving, even in some women without documented cyclic fluid retention and weight gain. The efficacy of spironolactone may, therefore, be the result of something other than its diuretic action because significant changes in body water and fluid composition are usually not found in women who have PMS. Thus, it has been suggested that the mechanism of action involves a direct inhibition of angiotensin function, which in turn affects central cholinergic and adrenergic activity. Alternatively, in women who have PMS symptoms, improvement with use of spironolactone has been shown to be associated with higher luteal phase androgen levels. This latter observation suggests that the beneficial effect of spironolactone may be caused by blockade of a peripheral or central androgen receptor because androgen receptor actions have already been ascribed to this drug relative to treatment of hirsutism.

Well-controlled studies have consistently shown selective serotonin reuptake inhibitors (SSRIs) to be effective in the treatment of affective symptoms of PMS. Symptoms that have been shown to improve with SSRIs include depression, anxiety, nervous tension, emotional lability, aggression, and so forth. Some of the drugs evaluated in PMS trials and their recommended dosages are listed in Table 63–4. The fast-acting SSRIs, such as sertraline, have the advantage of shorter half lives and more rapid metabolism; sertraline in particular has been shown to be useful for treatment of PMS, even when administered cyclically during the menstrual cycle. For example, low doses of sertraline (25 to 50 mg daily) administered in the luteal phase of the cycle and discontinued with the onset of menses have proved beneficial in some patients. Adverse effects, such as dizziness, nausea, headache, insomnia, agitation, and decreased libido may be minimized by starting with lower doses and increasing as needed to control symptoms. The SSRI should be employed for at least two to three cycles before switching to another drug because of therapeutic failure. Other antidepressants, such as tricyclics and monoamine oxidase inhibitors, have, in general, less therapeutic efficacy in PMS. However, occasional patients obtain benefit even from these therapeutic alternatives.

Alprazolam, a benzodiazepine, has also proved to be effective therapy for some PMS patients, particularly when anxiety or agitation predominates. Alprazolam is started at 0.25 mg three times a day and titrated to a maximum of 4 mg/day, with an average dose of 2.25 mg. Because the substance can be abused, dosage is limited to the luteal phase and tapered over 2 or 3 days once the patient's menstrual period starts in an attempt to limit exposure while avoiding withdrawal symptoms from abrupt discontinuation. Other related drugs, such as diazepam (Valium), lorazepam (Ativan), or buspirone (Buspar) have been employed successfully in continuous or cyclic fashion to treat various anxiety-related symptoms in PMS patients. Again, the addictive potential of these drugs warrants

**Table 63–4** Selective Serotonin Reuptake Inhibitors for Treatment of Premenstrual Syndrome

| Agent | Trade Name | Dose |
|---|---|---|
| Fluoxetine | Prozac | 20 mg/d |
| Sertraline | Zoloft | 25–150 mg/d |
| Clomipramine* | Anafranil | 25–75 mg/d |
| Paroxetine | Paxil | 20 mg/d |
| Nefazadone | Serzone | 100–200 mg/d |

*Clomipramine has both SSRI and tricyclic antidepressant properties.
Data from Barnhart KT, Freeman EW, Sondheimer ST: A clinician's guide to the premenstrual syndrome. Med Clin North Am 79:1457–1472, 1995.

caution when using them in these susceptible patients.

Even though the pathogenic mechanisms of PMS are poorly understood, the causal relationship (at least on some level) between cyclic ovarian function and PMS is clear. Consequently, when severe PMS symptoms fail to respond to other medical therapy in a woman who is not concerned with future fertility, castration by bilateral oophorectomy has been recommended as a curative procedure. However, many practitioners are reluctant to perform bilateral oophorectomy as treatment for PMS. Reasons include the possibility that the patient will fail to obtain symptom resolution, the risks inherent in the surgical procedure, the probable need for concomitant hysterectomy (especially when steroid replacement therapy is contemplated), and the deleterious clinical and metabolic effects that result from prolonged hypoestrogenism. These effects include vasomotor instability, emotional lability, cognitive dysfunction, genital tract atrophy, sleep disturbance, osteopenia and osteoporosis, accelerated atherogenesis, and other actions. Thus, although bilateral oophorectomy can be viewed as curative of PMS, in all but extreme cases both physician and patient may be reluctant to resort to this irreversible treatment.

Gonadotropin-releasing hormone (GnRH) agonists are peptide hormones that reversibly inhibit pituitary gonadotrophs; shortly after therapy is begun, circulating follicle-stimulating hormone (FSH) and luteinizing hormone (LH) levels decline and follicular growth ceases. Ovulation and corpus luteum function are inhibited, and cyclic ovarian steroid and peptide hormone production reach base levels. With the exception of circulating gonadotropin levels, the endocrine milieu of these patients is similar to that of a surgically or naturally castrated woman. Indeed, many view the endocrine state reached to be equivalent to a "medical castration."

GnRH agonists have been documented to relieve the symptoms of PMS, presumably by inducing medical oophorectomy. Resolution of both physical and behavioral symptoms has been observed in a significant proportion of women. However, because prolonged hypoestrogenism as a result of long-term GnRH analog use increases the risk of osteoporosis and cardiovascular disease, add-back therapy with either cyclic or continuous estrogen and progesterone has been employed. Estrogens used in either regimen include conjugated equine estrogen 0.625 mg/day, oral 17-β-estradiol 0.5–1.0 mg/day, or transdermal 17-β-estradiol 0.5–1.0 mg/day. A progestin such as medroxyprogesterone acetate (2.5–5 mg/day for continuous regimens or 5 to 10 mg/day for cyclic regimens), oral micronized progesterone (100 to 300 mg/day) or norethindrone (0.35 to 0.5 mg/day) is added to antagonize the estrogen at the endometrium in an attempt to prevent endometrial hyperplasia and carcinoma. The beneficial effects seen with GnRH agonist therapy alone in PMS have been maintained when steroid hormone replacement is added, and worsening of either mood or physical symptoms was not observed. GnRH analog ovarian suppression combined with estrogen-progestin replacement has been shown to be a viable long-term treatment alternative, and, in addition, can be used to gauge anticipated response to bilateral oophorectomy before this irreversible procedure is undertaken. Used alone, GnRH analogs are generally avoided in patients who have a history of depressive disorders and in some patients who have migraine because the hypoestrogenic state they induce has been noted to precipitate depressive episodes and severe headache in some patients.

## Summary

Although the causes and pathophysiologic mechanisms responsible for PMS have not been elucidated, considerable attention has been focused on the complex interactions between ovarian hormones and central amine neurotransmitters and endogenous opiate peptides. A model is emerging in which these various biochemical and hormonal interactions render women susceptible to various psychological and social pressures, the end result of which is the clinical picture known as PMS. Despite our inability to describe the exact nature of ovarian-central nervous system interactions that are responsible for PMS, empiric observations have demonstrated several efficacious treatment alternatives. Among these, SSRIs and GnRH analogs with steroid add-back therapy have shown considerable promise in treating these patients. More effective therapy will await further clarification of the mechanisms involved in PMS symptom development.

### REFERENCES

American College of Obstetricians and Gynecologists Committee Opinion: Premenstrual Syndrome. Washington, DC. The American College of Obstetricians and Gynecologists, 66, 1989.

American Psychiatric Association: Diagnostic and Statistical Manual of Mental Disorders, 4th ed. (DSM-IV). American Psychiatric Association, Washington DC, 1994.

Andersch B, Wenderstam C, Hahn L, et al: Premenstrual complaints: I. Prevalence of premenstrual symptoms in a Swedish urban population. J Psychosom Obstet Gynaecol 5:39–49, 1986.

Arpels JC: The female brain hypoestrogenic continuum from the premenstrual syndrome to menopause. J Reprod Med 41:633–639, 1996.

Bancroft J. The premenstrual syndrome—a reappraisal of the concept and the evidence. Psychol Med (Suppl)24:1–47, 1993.

Barnhart KT, Freeman EW, Sondheimer SJ: A clinician's guide to the premenstrual syndrome. Med Clin North Am 79: 1457–1472, 1995.

Bloch M, Schmidt PJ, Rubinow DR: Clinical aspects of premenstrual syndrome. Infertil Reprod Med Clin North Am 7:315–330, 1996.

Budeiri DJ, Li Wan Po A, Dorman JC: Clinical trials of treatments of premenstrual syndrome: Entry criteria and scales for measuring treatment outcomes. Br J Obstet Gynecol 101:689–695, 1994.

Freeman EW: Premenstrual syndrome: Current perspectives on treatment and etiology. Curr Opin Obstet Gynecol 9:147–153, 1997.

Freeman E, Rickels K, Sondheimer SJ, et al: Ineffectiveness of progesterone suppository treatment for premenstrual syndrome. JAMA 264:349–353, 1990.

Freeman EW, Rickles, Sondheimer SJ, et al: A double blind trial of oral progesterone, alprazolam, and placebo in treatment of severe premenstrual syndrome. JAMA 274:51–57, 1995.

Halbreich U: Reflections on the cause of PMS. Psychiatr Ann 26:581–584, 1996.

Halbreich U, Endicott J, Lesser J: The clinical diagnosis and classification of premenstrual changes. Can J Psychiatr 30:489–496, 1985.

Johnson SR, McChesney C, Bean JA: Epidemiology of premenstrual symptoms in a nonclinical sample. I. prevalence, natural history and help-seeking behavior. J Reprod Med 33:340–346, 1988.

Keye WR Jr. The Premenstrual Syndrome. Philadelphia, WB Saunders, 1988.

MacGregor EA: "Menstrual" migraine: Towards a definition. Cephalalgia 16:11–21, 1996.

Moline ML: Pharmacologic strategies for managing premenstrual syndrome. Clin Pharm 12:181–196, 1993.

Mortola JF: Applications of gonadotropin-releasing hormone analogues in the treatment of premenstrual syndrome. Clin Obstet Gynecol 36:753–763, 1993.

Mortola JF, Girton L, Beck L, et al: Diagnosis of premenstrual syndrome by a simple prospective and reliable instrument: The Calendar of Premenstrual Experiences. Obstet Gynecol 76:302–307, 1990.

Muse KN, Cetel NS, Futterman LA, et al: The premenstrual syndrome: Effects of medical 'ovariectomy.' N Engl J Med 311:1345–1373, 1984.

National Institute of Mental Health: NIMH Premenstrual Syndrome Workshop Guidelines. National Institute of Mental Health, Rockville, Md 1983 April 14, 15.

O'Brien PMS: The premenstrual syndrome: A review. J Reprod Med 1985;30: 113–126, 1985.

O'Brien PMS: Premenstrual Syndrome. Oxford, Blackwell Scientific Publications, 1987.

Pearlstein T: Nonpharmacologic treatment of premenstrual syndrome. Psychiatr Ann 26:590–594, 1996.

Pearlstein T, Frank E, Rivera-Tovar, et al: Prevalence of axis I and axis II disorders in women with late luteal phase dysphoric disorder. J Affect Dis 20:129–134, 1990.

Price WA, Dimarzio LR, Gardner PR: Biopsychosocial approach to premenstrual syndrome. Am Fam Phys 33:117–122, 1986.

Ramcharan S, Love EJ, Fick GH, et al: The epidemiology of premenstrual symptoms in a population based sample of 2650 urban women. J Clin Epidemiol 45:377–381, 1992.

Reid RL: Premenstrual Syndrome. Current Problems in Obstetrics, Gynecology, and Fertility. Chicago, Yearbook Medical Publishers, 1985;8(2): 2–57.

Reid RL: Etiology of PMS: Medical theories. In Keye WR Jr (ed): The Premenstrual Syndrome. Philadelphia, WB Saunders, 1988.

Reid RL: Premenstrual syndrome: Theories of pathophysiology. In Demers LM, McGuire JL, Phillips A, et al (eds): Premenstrual, Postpartum, and Menopausal Mood Disorders. Baltimore, Urban & Schwarzenberg, 1989.

Reid RL, Yen SC: Premenstrual syndrome. Am J Obstet Gynecol 139:85–104, 1981.

Roca CA, Schmidt PJ, Bloch M, et al: Implications of endocrine studies of premenstrual syndrome. Psychiatr Ann 26:576–580, 1996.

Rubinow DR, Roy-Byrne P: Premenstrual syndromes: Overview from a methodologic perspective. Am J Psychiatr 141:163–172, 1984.

Rubinow DR, Schmidt PJ: The treatment of premenstrual syndrome—forward into the past. N Engl J Med 332:1574–1575, 1995.

Ruble DN: Premenstrual symptoms: A reinterpretation: Science 197:291–292, 1977.

Sarno AP Jr, Miller EJ Jr, Lundblad EG: Premenstrual syndrome: Beneficial effects of periodic, low dose danazol. Obstet Gynecol 70:30–36, 1987.

Sayegh R, Schiff I, Wurtman J, et al: The effect of a carbohydrate rich beverage on mood, appetite, and cognitive function in women with premenstrual syndrome. Obstet Gynecol 86:520–528, 1995.

Schmidt PJ, Nieman LK, Danaceau MA, et al: Differential behavioral effects of gonadal steroids in women with and in those without premenstrual syndrome. N Engl J Med 338:209–216, 1998.

Severino S, Moline M: Premenstrual syndrome. A clinician's guide. New York, Guilford Press, 1989.

Severino S, Moline M: Premenstrual syndrome: Identification and management. Drugs 49:71–82, 1995.

Steiner M: Premenstrual syndromes. Ann Rev Med 48:447–455, 1997.

Steiner M, Steinberg S, Stewart D, et al. Fluoxetine in the treatment of premenstrual syndrome N Engl J Med 332:1529–1534, 1995.

Steiner M, Wilkins A: Diagnosis and assessment of premenstrual dysphoria. Psychiatr Ann 26:571–575, 1996.

Wang M, Hammarback S, Lindhe BA, et al: Treatment of premenstrual syndrome by spironolactone: A double-blind, placebo-controlled study. Acta Obstet Gynecol Scand 74:803–808, 1995.

Woods NF, Most A, Dery GK: Prevalence of perimenstrual symptoms. Am J Public Health 72:1257–1263, 1982.

Yonkers KA, Halbreich U, Freeman EW, et al: Sertaline in the treatment of premenstrual dysphoric disorder. Psychopharmacol Bull 32:41–46, 1996.

Yonkers KA, Brown WA: Pharmacologic treatments for premenstrual dysphoric disorder. Psychiatr Ann 26:586–594, 1996.

# 64

# Endometriosis

CARLA P. ROBERTS
JOHN A. ROCK

## Definition

Endometriosis is a common condition in women of reproductive age in which abnormal growths of endometrial tissue are present in locations other than the uterine cavity. No reliable markers are available for endometriosis and, consequently, surgical procedures are necessary for diagnosis. Endometriosis is present in at least 1% of all women of reproductive age. It is a principal factor in 15% of infertile women and is found in 20% of women operated on for pelvic pain.

Many years of spontaneous cyclic menstruation appear to predispose women toward endometriosis. Regression occurs during prolonged amenorrhea, such as pregnancy and menopause, giving credence to retrograde menstruation as a risk factor. Also, certain menstrual patterns, such as early age of menarche, higher than average frequency of menses, and longer than usual duration of flow are risks for endometriosis. Defects in outflow tracts have been found to be common in teenagers who have severe endometriosis. Hereditary factors and possible immune system alterations are suggested because women who have a first-degree relative with endometriosis have a sevenfold risk of developing disease, and investigators have linked endometriosis to the presence of particular human leukocyte antigens (HLA).

The most common sites of disease are the ovary (approximately 50% of all cases), cul-de-sac, uterosacral ligaments, posterior uterine surface, broad ligament, and the remaining pelvic peritoneum (Fig. 64–1). Implants may occur over the bowel, bladder, and ureters; rarely, they may erode into underlying tissue and cause blood in the urine or stool, and their associated adhesions may result in stricture and obstruction. Implants can occur deep in the tissue, especially in the cervix or the posterior vaginal fornix, or within wounds contaminated by endometrial tissue. Very rarely, endometriosis is found in distant sites, such as lung, brain, or kidney. Pleural implantations are associated with recurrent right-sided pneumothoraces at the time of menses; these are termed catamenial pneumothoraces. Similarly, lesions in the central nervous system can cause catamenial seizures.

## Clinical Findings and Differential Diagnosis

The diagnosis of endometriosis is unfailingly obtained from a patient's history, with pelvic pain as the cardinal symptom. Most patients complain of constant pelvic pain or a low sacral backache that occurs premenstrually and subsides after menses begins. Dyspareunia is often present, particularly with deep penetration. Lesions within the urinary tract or bowel may result in bloody urine or stool in the perimen-

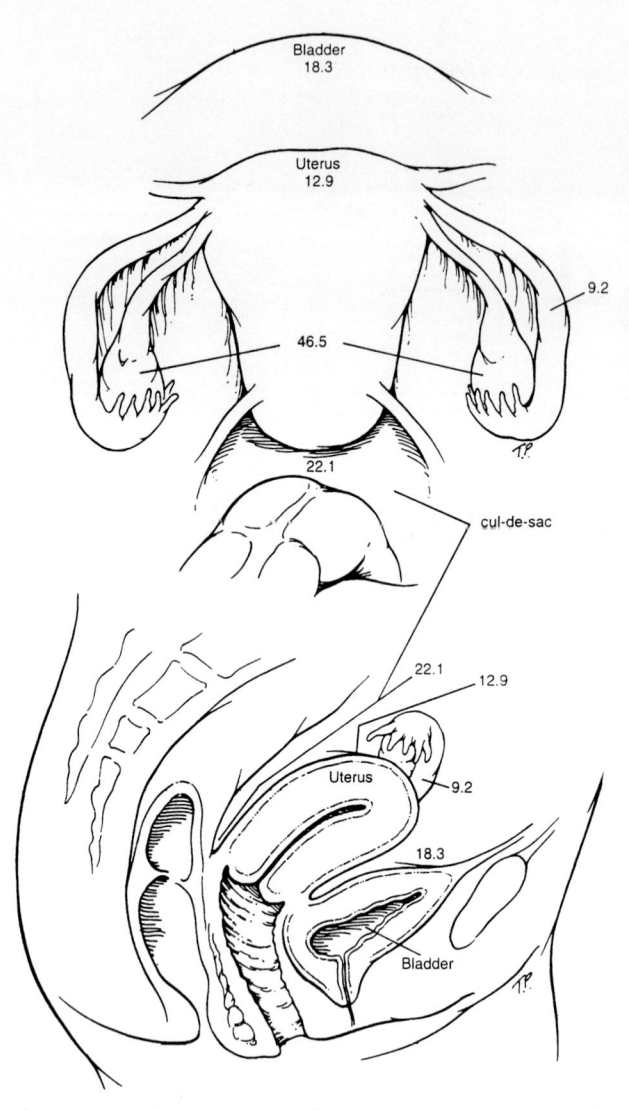

**Figure 64–1** The most common locations (percentages given) of pelvic endometriosis. (Modified from Halme J, Stovall D: Endometriosis and its Medical Management. *In* Wallach EE, Zacur HA (eds): Reproductive Medicine and Surgery. Baltimore, Mosby, 1995, p. 697.)

strual period. Implantations on or near the external surfaces of cervix, vagina, rectum, or urethra may cause pain and bleeding with defecation, urination, or intercourse at any time of the menstrual cycle, and a sensation of pelvic pressure may result if large masses are present. Premenstrual spotting may occur and is more likely to be associated with endometriosis accompanied by luteal-phase inadequacy.

Classically, the pelvic examination reveals tender nodules in the posterior vaginal fornix and pain upon uterine motion. The uterus may be fixed and retroverted as a result of cul-de-sac adhesions, and tender adnexal masses may be felt if endometriomas are present. Careful inspection may reveal implants in healed wounds—especially in episiotomy and cesarean section incisions—in the vaginal fornix or on the cervix. Biopsy may be required to prove the lesions are caused by endometriosis.

Endometriosis should be suspected in any patient of reproductive age who complains of pain and infertility. Medical treatment can be given for treatment of patients who have pelvic pain thought to be endometriosis, but the specific diagnosis of endometriosis should not be made unless documented by operative visualization.

The high incidence of endometriosis makes it an important consideration in all differential diagnosis of pelvic disease. In fact, the pain, infertility, and adhesions associated with endometriosis must be distinguished from similar accompanying pelvic inflammatory disease, pelvic tumors, and dysmenorrhea, which usually necessitate operative assessment. A persistent adnexal mass larger than 5 cm should never be presumed to be an endometrioma, even if endometriosis has been documented previously and requires operative intervention.

Several classifications have been used to describe the anatomic location and severity of disease. The scoring systems are useful for reporting operative findings and comparing results after various treatment protocols. The staging system most commonly used is the revised (R)-American Fertility Society (AFS) shown in Figure 64–2. An Endometriosis Classification Subcommittee appointed by the American Society for Reproductive Medicine (formerly the American Fertility Society) evaluated the dose-response relationship between pregnancy and the R-AFS. Interestingly, although trends were evident that the revised R-AFS was not able to predict pregnancy after treatment for any stage of endometriosis, several reasons have been postulated for the insensitivity of the R-AFS system toward pregnancy rates at all stages:

1. Anatomic features that impair fertility are not qualitatively or quantitatively identified.
2. Surgery may remove all endometriosis-related obstacles to fertility.
3. Factors other than anatomic involvement may be the mechanism for infertility.
4. Endometriosis and infertility may not be related in a cause-and-effect manner.

The point system for the R-AFS is heavily weighted toward ovarian and peritoneal involvement and adhesions as indicators of more severe disease. Although it is known that peritoneal, ovarian, and retroperitoneal disease are three distinct endometriotic lesions, the current classification system does not incorporate retroperitoneal disease into the staging process.

## Treatment

### MEDICAL MANAGEMENT

In patients who have minimal disease, expectant management is appropriate, with frequent examinations

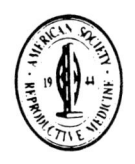

## AMERICAN SOCIETY FOR REPRODUCTIVE MEDICINE
## REVISED CLASSIFICATION OF ENDOMETRIOSIS

Patient's Name _____ Date _____
Stage I (Minimal) - 1-5
Stage II (Mild) - 6-15
Stage III (Moderate) - 16-40
Stage IV (Severe) - >40
Total _____

Laparoscopy _____ Laparotomy _____ Photography _____
Recommended Treatment _____

Prognosis _____

| PERITONEUM | ENDOMETRIOSIS | <1cm | 1-3cm | >3cm |
|---|---|---|---|---|
| | Superficial | 1 | 2 | 4 |
| | Deep | 2 | 4 | 6 |
| OVARY | R Superficial | 1 | 2 | 4 |
| | Deep | 4 | 16 | 20 |
| | L Superficial | 1 | 2 | 4 |
| | Deep | 4 | 16 | 20 |

| | POSTERIOR CULDESAC OBLITERATION | Partial | Complete |
|---|---|---|---|
| | | 4 | 40 |

| | ADHESIONS | <1/3 Enclosure | 1/3-2/3 Enclosure | >2/3 Enclosure |
|---|---|---|---|---|
| OVARY | R Filmy | 1 | 2 | 4 |
| | Dense | 4 | 8 | 16 |
| | L Filmy | 1 | 2 | 4 |
| | Dense | 4 | 8 | 16 |
| TUBE | R Filmy | 1 | 2 | 4 |
| | Dense | 4* | 8* | 16 |
| | L Filmy | 1 | 2 | 4 |
| | Dense | 4* | 8* | 16 |

*If the fimbriated end of the fallopian tube is completely enclosed, change the point assignment to 16.
Denote appearance of superficial implant types as red [(R), red, red-pink, flamelike, vesicular blobs, clear vesicles], white [(W), opacifications, peritoneal defects, yellow-brown], or black [(B) black, hemosiderin deposits, blue]. Denote percent of total described as R___%, W___% and B___%. Total should equal 100%.

Additional Endometriosis: _____ Associated Pathology: _____

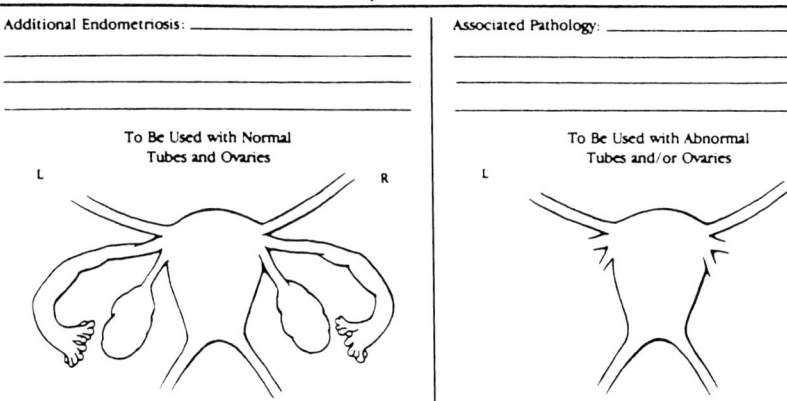

To Be Used with Normal Tubes and Ovaries

To Be Used with Abnormal Tubes and/or Ovaries

**Figure 64–2** Revised American Fertility Society staging for endometriosis. (From Fertil Steril 67:815, 1997.)

and institution of further therapy if progression of disease is noted.

Analgesic therapy includes nonsteroidal antiinflammatory agents and prostaglandin synthetase-inhibiting drugs. These drugs are appropriate as single-agent therapy for endometriosis if the patient has mild premenstrual pain caused by minimal endometriosis, no abnormalities on pelvic examination, and no desire for immediate pregnancy.

Hormonal regulatory treatment aims to create constant high levels of gonadal steroids and to "burn out" the endometriotic lesions which, historically, have been noted to regress during pregnancy. These regimens involve either constant daily administration of estrogen, progestin, or combination oral contraceptives. This regimen relieves pelvic pain in most patients, but the resultant pregnancy rates of 20 to 40% are less than ideal. Depression and significant breakthrough bleeding are found with these treatments, and thus patients are often unhappy with the results. Currently, this regimen is best reserved for patients who have milder disease, who do not require immediate fertility, and who are unable to undergo other treatments.

Endometriosis is known to regress after surgical castration or menopause; this is the basis for medications that reversibly reduce endogenous estrogen and progesterone production to constant low levels.

Danazol is a weak androgen that is the isoxazole derivative of 17α-ethinyl testosterone (ethisterone). Danazol acts at the hypothalamic level to prevent the rise in gonadotropins that would normally occur when estrogen and progesterone levels are low without affecting basal gonadotropin concentrations. Danazol binds to androgen receptors, stimulating them and thus inhibiting implant growth. In addition, danazol binds strongly to sex hormone–binding globulin and corticosteroid-binding globulin, thus displacing native testosterone and allowing it to act against the implants as well. Danazol inhibits the steroidogenic enzymes in the ovary that synthesize estrogen. Together, these actions decrease estrogen receptor stimulation within the lesions and inhibit implant growth.

The dose of danazol is 400 to 800 mg per day in divided doses over 6 months. Side effects of danazol include acne, oily skin, deepening of the voice, weight gain, edema, and adverse lipoprotein changes.

Progestational agents have been used to treat pelvic endometriosis. These agents are believed to induce initial deciduation and eventual atrophy of endometrial tissue. Vercellini and associates examined the effects of progestins and found that they were effective in treating patients who had endometriosis-associated pelvic pain; no differences were found when compared with treatment with danazol and gonadotropin-releasing hormone (GnRH) analogs.

Progestational agents are administered in various forms, but oral administration is preferable because of the rapid reversibility of its effects. The most commonly used medication in the United States is medroxyprogesterone acetate (MPA) in a dosage of 10 mg three times daily for 3 to 6 months. Side effects of the progestational agents are dependent upon the specific progestin used, the duration, and the route of administration. The most common side effect—irregular bleeding—occurs in up to 50% of patients. Other side effects include nausea, breast tenderness, fluid retention, and depression. These side effects are normally well tolerated and few patients discontinue treatment because of undesirable side effects. Progestins also adversely affect lipoprotein levels. Significant decreases in high-density lypoprotein (HDL) are reported with 19-nortestosterone derivatives. The effects of MPA on HDL suggest either no effect or a slight decrease. There are currently insufficient data on the reversibility of this effect.

There is little information on the effect of progestins on endometriotic implants. One controlled human trial demonstrated that high-dose MPA for 6 months resulted in a complete resolution of implants in 50% of patients and partial resolution in 13%. Placebo effects were 12% and 6%, respectively.

Hull and associates reported on a controlled comparative trial with oral MPA, danazol, and expectant management in women with stages I and II endometriosis. No significant differences were found among the different treatment groups when pregnancy rates were used as an endpoint (71%, 46%, and 55%, respectively). This suggests that progesterone therapy is no more effective than expectant management in the infertile patient with endometriosis.

GnRH agonists are at present the newest medical approach to the treatment of endometriosis. These medications have specific amino acid substitutions of the native GnRH peptide, resulting in compounds with longer half lives and greater receptor binding affinity. The net result is downregulation of pituitary GnRH receptors and resultant medical oophorectomy from the hypogonadotropic state.

Three agonists—goserelin, nafarelin acetate, and leuprolide acetate—are approved for treatment of pelvic pain associated with endometriosis. Nafarelin is administered as a nasal spray in a dosage of 200 or 400 mg twice daily. Leuprolide acetate is usually administered in a depot form in a dose of 3.75 mg monthly. Goserelin is administered as a subcutaneous injection of 3.6 mg monthly. Six months of therapy is the standard regimen for both compounds. Numerous side effects are associated with GnRH agonist treatments. These are transvaginal bleeding, hot flushes, vaginal dryness, decreased libido, breast tenderness, insomnia, depression, irritability and fatigue, headache, joint stiffness, and skin changes. Hypoestrogenic side effects, such as hot flushes, are more common with GnRH agonists than with danazol. Two significant concerns are the effect of GnRH agonists on lipoprotein levels and bone loss. Studies indicate that GnRH agonists do not have the same adverse effect on lipoproteins as danazol or progestins. A 6% loss of trabecular bone density, however, has been demonstrated after 6 months' use of GnRH agonists. There does not appear to be any significant decrease in cortical bone density. Most studies indicate that the trabecular bone density decrease is reversible after discontinuation of therapy.

Several GnRH agonists have been demonstrated to be effective in inducing atrophy of the ectopic endometriotic tissue and stroma. Reductions in the R-AFS classification score have been reported with the use of GnRH agonist therapy. The degree of regression is similar to that caused by danazol, but, although these implants do appear inactive after treatment with GnRH agonists, they are capable of growth later.

Five recent studies have compared GnRH agonists with danazol in the treatment of endometriosis-associated infertility. Most of these studies were laparoscopic diagnosis of endometriosis followed by randomization to agonist or danazol treatment. Cumulative pregnancy rates were 25 to 60% and 13 to 63%, respectively. There were no statistically significant differences between treatments in any study. In summary, GnRH agonists have not been shown to enhance fertility in patients who have endometriosis.

## SURGICAL MANAGEMENT

Endometriosis is diagnosed by visualizing lesions at the time of operation or after finding the characteristic histologic appearance in resected or biopsied tissue. The gross appearance of endometriosis at operation is quite characteristic and, to an experienced surgeon, is sufficient for diagnosis. The smallest and earliest implants are red, petechial lesions on the peritoneal surface. With further growth, menstrual-like debris accumulates within the lesion, giving it a cystic, dark brown, dark blue, or black appearance. The surrounding peritoneal surface becomes thickened and scarred. These "powder burn" implants typically attain a size of 5 to 10 mm in diameter. With progression of disease, the number and size of lesions increase and extensive adhesions may develop. Ovarian cysts may enlarge to several centimeters in size and are called endometriomas or "chocolate cysts." Severe disease can erode into underlying tissues and distort the remaining organs with extensive adhesions. Surgery is useful not only for diagnosis but is an ideal therapeutic means to remove endometriosis and restore normal pelvic anatomy.

When endometriosis is diagnosed during laparoscopy or laparotomy, staging should be performed. Staging requires a meticulous, systematic exploration of the entire pelvis for lesions. Extent of disease at each point of involvement is assessed, and pelvic structures involved are noted, along with number and size of endometriotic implants or endometriomas. Special attention is given to documenting involvement of peritoneum, uterus, tubes, and ovaries. Finally, a thorough staging requires documentation of the location and extent of any adhesions.

Some surgeons advocate the use of laparoscopic ovarian puncture for accurate staging of endometriosis when the ovaries appear somewhat enlarged. A 16-gauge needle can be used to puncture the ovarian capsule. Quantification of the fluid may accurately assess the size of the endometrioma. Also, preoperative ultrasonography in patients with endometriosis may be useful in screening for occult endometriomas.

## LAPAROSCOPIC THERAPY

Operative laparoscopy gives immediate diagnosis, and therapy should begin at the time of laparoscopy. Initiation of treatment during laparoscopy optimizes patient recovery and medical resources and decreases the patient's overall expense.

Laparoscopy is optimally performed during the follicular phase of the menstrual cycle when tissues are less hyperemic and recognition of endometriotic lesions is easier. During the luteal phase, there is risk of damage to the corpus luteum, which may bleed. Another reason for choosing the follicular phase is that there is decreased risk of operating during an unrecognized pregnancy and interrupting it. Although short-term suppression of ovarian function by agents like danazol or GnRH agonists is acceptable, long-term use of agents that suppress ovarian steroidogenesis should be avoided before surgery because they make endometriotic lesions much more difficult to identify and staging is then inaccurate. Because therapy for infertile patients begins at the time of laparoscopy, it is necessary to perform a complete evaluation of all infertility factors before surgery. Many clinicians believe that the highest fecundity rate occurs in the 6 to 18 months after the ablation of endometriosis. An unrecognized male factor or ovulatory factor should be diagnosed and evaluated before surgery, because post-surgery workups only delay conception.

Treatment of endometriotic implants through the laparoscope can be accomplished by a variety of techniques. Small implants may be electrosurgically ablated with unipolar or bipolar cautery. Cautery is applied until the lesion and surrounding tissue blanch. Bipolar cautery is usually safer. With this method, the implant is picked up between the two paddles and current is applied. Tissue necrosis is much more controlled, but implants deeper than 1 or 2 mm are difficult to remove. Unipolar cautery may be more beneficial in deeper lesions because of deeper penetration, but this carries a greater risk of damaging adjacent structures, such as the ureter, bladder, bowel, or vessels, by causing a greater area of thermal destruction.

Carbon dioxide ($CO_2$) laser ablation is a method of endometrial ablation that allows great precision in removing the disease with minimal bleeding and damage to surrounding tissue. Sutton and associates demonstrated that of patients who have pain caused by endometriosis and who improved 6 months after laser laparoscopy, 90% had continued relief for at least 1 year postoperatively. In addition, it was demonstrated that laparoscopic ablation of minimal and mild endometriosis enhances pregnancy rates in infertile women. One of the most appealing features of $CO_2$ laser therapy is that energy does not penetrate much beyond the surface of the tissue being removed. Thermal damage is usually limited to 0.2 mm beyond visible damage. Therefore, ablation by the $CO_2$ laser may be safer because of greater accuracy. The zone of thermal necrosis for $CO_2$ laser vaporization is minimal, especially when it is in superpulse mode. For implant ablation, the standard $CO_2$ laser laparoscope uses a focal point approximately 2 cm from the end of the delivery port. Depending on the area to be coagulated or vaporized, spot sizes vary from 0.5 to 2.5 mm. In the continuous firing mode, power densities of 2500 to 5000 $W/cm^2$ are used. Lesions that are close to vital structures may be ablated with single-pulse or superpulse modes of 0.05 to 0.1 seconds to limit the extent of tissue vaporization.

Endometrial implants should be vaporized completely with copious irrigation to remove carbon debris and to expose the base of the lesion. Repeated vaporization may be necessary to eradicate the implant completely. Argon, potassium-titanyl-phosphate (KTP), and neodymium:yttrium-aluminum-garnet (Nd:YAG) fiber lasers are also used for ablating endometriosis.

When a larger lesion is encountered, excision is recommended. With excision, the lesion can be sent for histologic confirmation; the lesion is grasped at the center, the peritoneum is tented, and the lesion is carefully circumscribed and removed. Care must always be taken to dissect the implant away from underlying healthy tissue and to identify underlying structures that can be damaged.

Entering the retroperitoneal space is occasionally required to remove endometriosis near the ureters or pelvic vessels. When laser therapy is being used, hydrodissection is a useful technique. The tip of the irrigator is placed in the subperitoneal space, and fluid is then delivered to distend and elevate the peritoneum. The fluid provides a mechanical separation of the lesion from the surrounding tissues. When the $CO_2$ laser is used, fluid provides a thermal buffer, because the $CO_2$ laser does not penetrate water. It is wise to remember that when hydrodissection is used near the broad ligaments or the pelvic side wall, the fluid may escape through the inguinal ring and resultant edema of the external genitals may occur.

Adhesions associated with endometriosis may be removed through the laparoscope. Transparent, avascular adhesions may be excised with scissors, laser, or hydrodissection. Dense adhesions need both blunt and sharp dissection. If bleeding occurs, hemostasis should be meticulously achieved with defocused laser beam or bipolar cautery. Additional ports may be needed to achieve proper visualization and countertraction. If difficulty is encountered, laparatomy should be considered immediately.

Laparoscopic treatment of endometriomas can be performed safely and effectively by laparoscopy, but this should be reserved for endometriomas smaller than 5 cm (Fig. 64–3). Initially the ovary should be

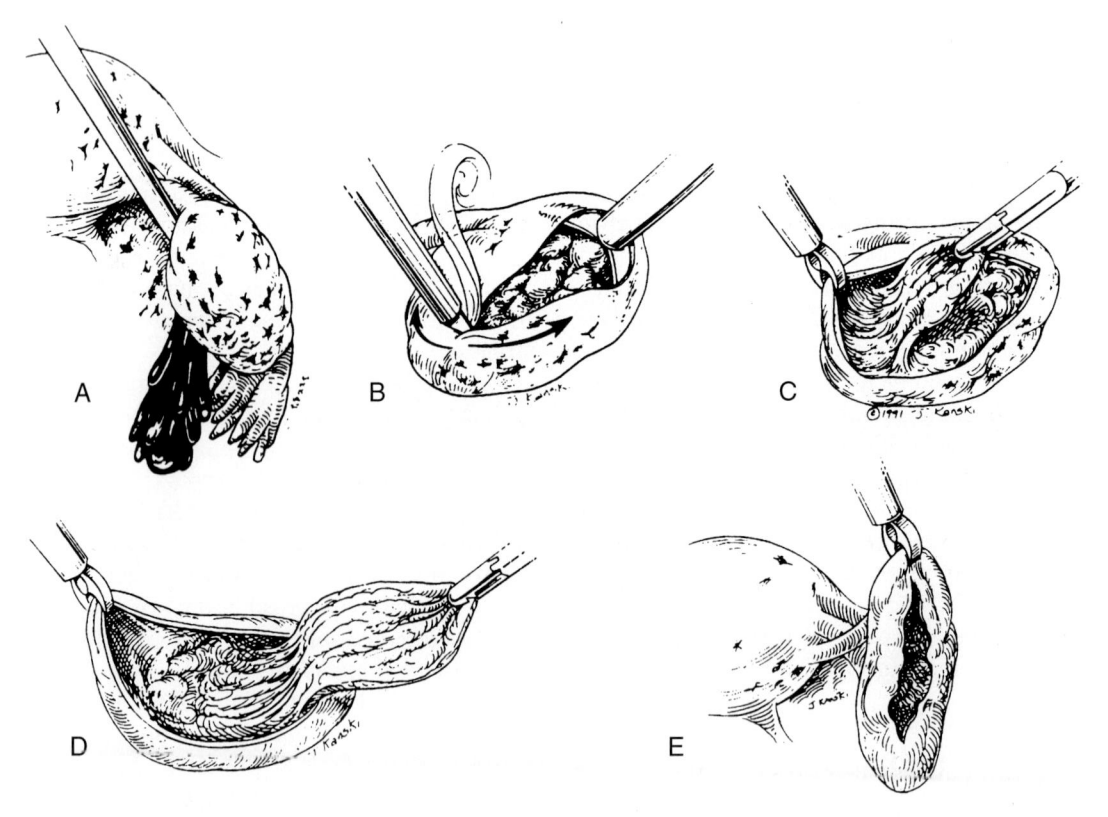

**Figure 64–3** Laparoscopic resection of an ovarian endometrioma. *A.* The ovary is mobilized. *B,* Excise the cortex superficially over the endometrioma, lave the endometrioma and inspect the cyst lining. *C,* Grasp the cyst wall. *D,* Strip the cyst wall from the ovary. *E,* Close the defect with laparoscopic suturing or let heal by secondary intention. (From Reich H, Hunt RB: Advanced laparoscopic surgery. *In* Hunt RB (ed): Atlas of Female Infertility surgery, Baltimore, Mosby, 1992.)

mobilized with lysis of adhesions. A small lesion may represent the superficial portion of a much larger endometrioma. First, the cyst is punctured, aspirated, opened, and irrigated. The cyst lining is examined to confirm the diagnosis of endometrioma; the lining is smooth and without papillary excrescences. If the cyst is confirmed as an endometrioma, the wall can be ablated with electrocauterization or laser vaporization. Secondly, the wall can be removed by grasping the cyst lining and stripping it from the ovary in a corkscrew manner. Any portions of the cyst wall remaining can then be ablated. The defect is closed with laparoscopic suturing or may be left to heal by secondary intention.

## CONSERVATIVE SURGERY WITH LAPAROTOMY

Laparotomy is required for any patient who has persistent pain or infertility after a trial of expectant management, medical management, or laparoscopic treatment. It is also indicated when severe disease has invaded the bowels, ureters, or other surrounding structures. Moreover, it is necessary when the extent of disease exceeds the operative skill of the surgeon or the availability of laparoscopic instrumentation.

Adequate exposure is a must with resection of endometriosis. Most surgeons use a transverse incision, such as the Maylard, unless there is a previous vertical incision or significant obesity. After the peritoneal cavity has been entered, staging of endometriosis is performed and then restoration of normal pelvic anatomy. Adhesions are removed and the ovaries are visualized in an atraumatic manner.

Conservative surgery is best accomplished with the use of a microsurgical technique. The pelvis is copiously irrigated throughout the operation to maintain moist tissues. Ringer's lactate solution with 5000 IU of heparin and 1 g hydrocortisone added to each liter is recommended. Adhesions are removed without damage to underlying tissues and sent for pathologic documentation of endometriosis. If hemostasis cannot be maintained by bipolar cautery, a bioabsorbable suture should be used.

Palpation is often necessary for deeper lesions, and these should be excised rather than ablated to avoid damage to surrounding healthy tissue and to enable complete resection. The focus is, once again, grasped and elevated, and the lesion is removed with a 2- to 4-mm margin.

Deep nodules of endometriosis are not uncommon; in one study, 25% of patients who had clinical disease had lesions that penetrated deeper than 5 mm. The pouch of Douglas and the uterosacral ligaments are two areas that need careful inspection and palpation for deeper implants of endometriosis. Deep infiltration (more than 5 mm) with active disease has been reported in 55% of patients who have cul-de-sac involvement and in 34% of patients who have uterosacral involvement. Endometriosis infiltrates until the level of the retroperitoneal fat is reached. Therefore, it is necessary to dissect well into the retroperitoneal fat to adequately remove the entire lesion. There is little retroperitoneal fat in the ovarian fossae and deep infiltrating lesions are found rarely.

Once the implant is excised, the defect may be left open if it is small and hemostatic. If not, the peritoneum should be closed with a 5.0 polyglycolic acid suture. Care should be taken not to close the tissues too tightly because greater tissue necrosis and risk of adhesion formation result.

Adhesiolysis is always important. Each individual adhesion should be isolated and cut with care so as not to damage the adjacent peritoneum. Although there are no studies on efficacy, most surgeons attempt to remove adhesions, if possible. The most effective manner is to fan the adhesions by gentle traction with atraumatic forceps. A tapered Teflon-covered probe is useful if held behind the adhesion to tent it away from normal structures. When two structures adhere, care must be taken to separate the structures completely and establish a well-defined plane for transection. A needle or microelectrode is optimal for cutting. Also, operating loupes (1.5 to 2.5 ×) aid in precise excision.

## Ovarian Endometriosis

Removal of ovarian endometriosis during laparotomy is similar to the technique used during laparoscopy. First, careful inspection of the ovary is performed to identify all endometriotic lesions. Next, ovarian adhesiolysis is performed. Filmy adhesions of the ovary can be lifted and excised without cutting into the ovary. It is curious to note that 40 to 50% of subovarian adhesions contain endometriosis. If the ovary is adherent to the ovarian fossae, great care should be used in the dissection so as to avoid damage to the ureter. Once the ovaries are mobilized, a Silastic platform behind the uterus aids in elevating the adnexal structures for better visualization. Superficial lesions of the ovary can be ablated with electrocautery, bipolar cautery, or laser, using copious irrigation.

As seen in Figure 64–4, an elliptic incision is made over the endometrioma, with the longitudinal axis of the ellipse parallel to the line between the fimbria ovarica and the ovarian ligament. The electromicrosurgical needle is used to make the incision approximately 0.1 to 0.2 mm deep. Next, the capsule of the endometrioma is identified. A cleavage plane is then developed with blunt, curved scissors to shell out

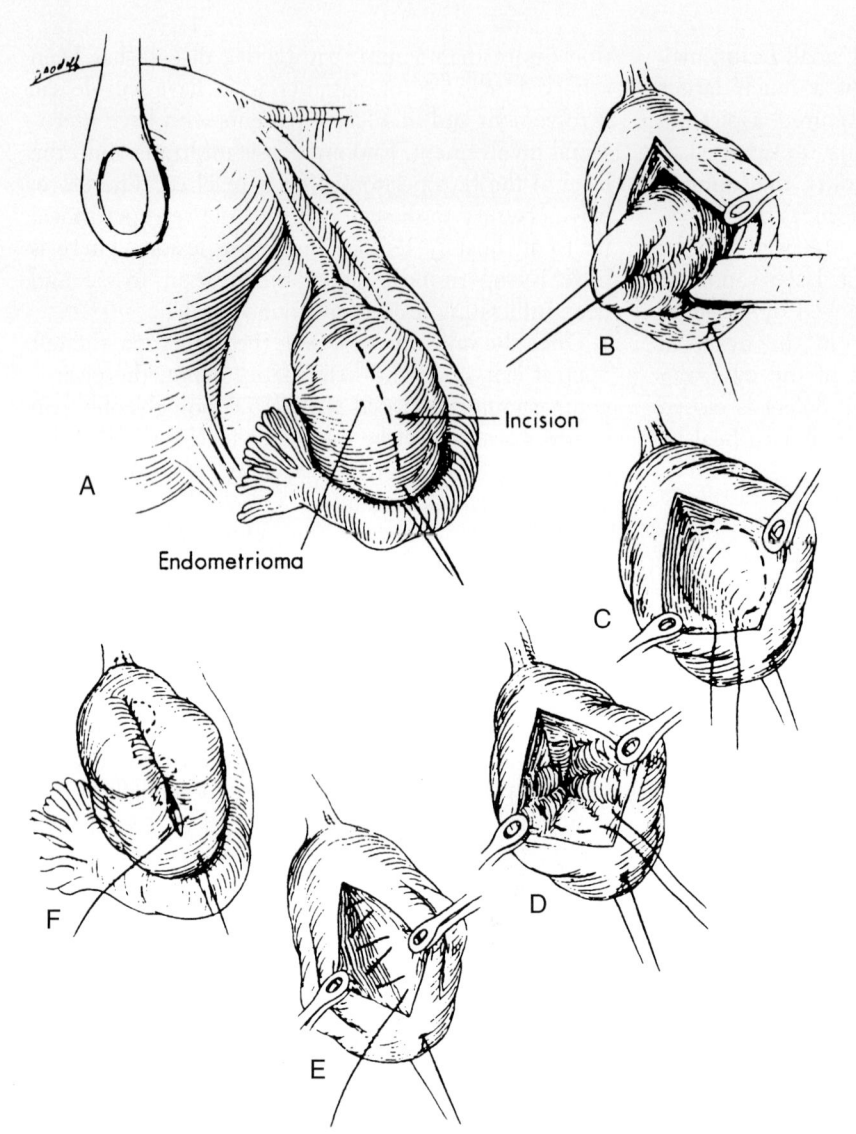

**Figure 64–4** Removal of an ovarian endometrioma at laparotomy. *A*, Make an incision over the endometrioma. *B*, Identify the capsule of the endometrioma and develop a plane to shell out the endometrioma. *C–E*, Deep portions of the ovary are closed using mattress sutures of a nonreactive absorbable suture. *F*, The ovarian surface is closed with a subcortical layer of 6-0 delayed absorbable material. (From Hesla JS, Rock JA: Endometriosis. *In* Rock JA, Murphy AA, Jones HW (eds): Female Reproductive Surgery. Baltimore, William & Wilkins, 1992.)

the endometrioma. Ideally, the cyst wall is removed without rupture. It is also useful to place lint-free lap packs around the ovary with the endometrioma to contain any spillage that may occur.

Once the endometrioma is removed, bipolar cautery is used to achieve hemostasis before ovarian reconstruction is performed. Mattress sutures of 5.0 nonreactive absorbable suture are used to close the deep portions of the ovary in layers to eliminate dead space. The ovarian surface is closed with a subcortical layer of 6.0 delayed, absorbable, polyglycolic acid suture to decrease exposure to suture material and decrease adhesion formation. Laparotomy has the advantage of enabling the surgeon to detect by palpation smaller deep lesions that may be undetected laparoscopically.

Previously, if disease appeared unilateral, the diseased adnexa was removed. Now, with assisted reproductive technology, surgery has become much more conservative and oocyte retrieval from small ovarian remnants has been successful.

## Fallopian Tube Endometriosis

Endometriosis of the fallopian tube leads to peritubal adhesion formation and tubal damage. Adhesiolysis should be performed by microsurgical techniques with attention to restoring normal anatomy. Tubal obstruction is usually the result of extensive adhesion formation rather than an obstructing endometriotic nodule. When the cause is a nodule, a preoperative hysterosalpingogram and laparoscopy can yield the diagnosis. Often, medical management with danazol or GnRH agonists is useful to shrink the lesion until patency is re-established. If medical management fails, tubal excision and anastomosis may be considered.

## Retroperitoneal Endometriosis

Retroperitoneal endometriosis usually causes severe pain, dysmenorrhea, and dyspareunia in patients. A typical examination reveals tender nodules in the cul-de-sac, the uterosacral ligaments, the rectosigmoid junction, and the rectovaginal septum. Often, the uterus is retroverted and fixed posteriorly.

Extensive retroperitoneal disease is not easily accessible by the laparoscope. Removal of disease requires retroperitoneal dissection, which may be facilitated by placing a bougie in the rectum, sponge forceps in the vagina, and a Foley catheter in the bladder. The pararectal and paravaginal spaces may be exposed by applying traction in the appropriate direction.

## Endometriosis of the Bowel

Primary endometriosis of the bowel is rare, but it occurs in up to 25% of women who have pelvic endometriosis. Location of disease (rectosigmoid, large bowel, small bowel, or appendix) determines the type of surgery necessary. Endometriosis of the gastrointestinal tract commonly involves segments that are close in proximity to the uterus, the fallopian tubes, and the ovaries. One study revealed the resulting distribution: 72.4% sigmoid, rectosigmoid, or rectal cases; 13.5% rectovaginal septum; 7% small bowel; 3.6% cecum; 3% appendix.

Before choosing a treatment modality, the patient's symptoms need to be evaluated. These symptoms include rectal pain (74%), dyspareunia (46%), constipation (49%), and rectal bleeding (31%). Complete intestinal obstruction is rare but mandates a laparotomy and resection when it occurs. If clinical symptoms are present before surgery, it is prudent to assess the bowel for evidence of involvement. A barium enema is very useful and reveals a smooth (nonmalignant) crater if disease involves the mucosa. Endovaginal ultrasonography has been helpful in diagnosing disease of the anterior rectal wall. Colonoscopy with biopsies confirms endometriosis if there is mucosal involvement and provides information that is helpful when the appropriate procedure is being planned.

Any patient who has suspected bowel involvement should have a complete mechanical and antibiotic bowel preparation before surgery. With laparotomy, superficial lesions of the bowel may be excised, fulgurated, or laser vaporized. Lesions that are deeper are best treated with segmental bowel resection. If childbearing is complete, a total abdominal hysterectomy with bilateral salpingo-oophorectomy should be considered. Alternatively, ovarian preservation may be possible if the lesion can be resected completely.

It is still unclear whether an appendectomy should be performed in patients who are undergoing bowel resection for endometriosis. In a study of 926 patients who underwent laparotomy with bowel resection for endometriosis, 126 patients (13.6%) underwent incidental appendectomy. Only 2 patients were shown to have microscopic involvement. It is believed that unless involvement of the appendix is evident, appendectomy is optional.

## Endometriosis of the Urinary Tract

Urinary tract endometriosis is rare, affecting only 1.2% of women who have endometriosis. Diagnosis begins with clinical suspicion; symptoms include frequency, dysuria, and hematuria. Cystoscopy is very useful for diagnosing vesicle endometriosis. Radiographic studies are useful in determining any ureteral involvement. An intravenous pyelogram is probably indicated for all patients who undergo surgery for extensive endometriosis.

Treatment of urinary tract endometriosis should begin with medical management with danazol or a GnRH agonist, but close surveillance of renal function is necessary. Endometriosis of the bladder may be ablated during surgery if it is superficial. More extensive disease may need partial cystectomy. Endometriosis of the ureter requires ureterolysis or resection of the involved segment with accompanying ureteroneocystostomy or ureteroureterostomy. Nephrostomy urinary diversion is considered when severe hydronephrosis is present and ureterolysis is not possible.

## Extrapelvic Endometriosis

Extrapelvic endometriosis is rare but can cause significant disease. Diagnosis needs biopsy confirmation. If complete excision is not possible, hormonal suppression may be necessary. Table 64–1 represents a staging system for extrapelvic endometriosis.

## Adjunctive Procedures for Pain Relief

The dysmenorrhea and pelvic pain associated with endometriosis are most commonly treated with medi-

**Table 64–1** Staging System for Extrapelvic Endometriosis

CLASSIFICATION
Class I:   Endometriosis involving the intestinal tract
Class U:   Endometriosis involving the urinary tract
Class L:   Endometriosis involving the lung and thoracic cage
Class O:   Endometriosis involving other sites outside the abdominal cavity

STAGING OF EXTRAPELVIC ENDOMETRIOSIS
Stage I   No organ defect
1. Extrinsic: surface of organ (serosa, pleura)
    <1 cm lesion
    1- to 4-cm lesion
    >4-cm lesion
2. Intrinsic: mucosal, muscle, parenchyma
    <1cm lesion
    1- to 4-cm lesion
    >4 cm lesion
Stage II   Organ defect*
1. Extrinsic: surface of organ (serosa, pleura)
    <1-cm lesion
    1- to 4-cm lesion
    >4-cm lesion
2. Intrinsic: mucosal, muscle, parenchyma
    <1 cm lesion
    1- to 4-cm lesion
    >4-cm lesion

*Organ defect would include—but not be limited to—obstruction and partial obstruction of the urinary tract and the intestinal tract and hemothorax, hemoptysis, and pneumothorax.

cal management of hormonal suppressive therapy or nonsteroidal anti-inflammatory drugs. There are a group of patients, however, who receive no relief from medical management, and they may need adjunctive surgical procedures.

## Laparoscopic Uterine Nerve Ablation (LUNA)

LUNA interrupts the uterosacral ligament at the insertion into the cervix and destroys a large amount of sensory nerve fibers that innervate the cervix and lower uterine segment (Fig. 64–5). LUNA can be accomplished with laser or electrocoagulation but this procedure is controversial because the uterosacral ligament is rarely completely incised. Exposure of the uterosacral ligament, is, of course, the key. This is achieved by flexing the uterus forward by a uterine manipulator. The ureters should be fully identified before ablation to prevent damage. The $CO_2$ laser is used with a power density of 5000 to 15,000 W/cm² to ablate a 2- to 5-cm segment of each uterosacral ligament adjacent to the cervix to a depth of 1 cm. The area of the posterior cervix between the uterosacral insertion points may also be ablated superficially to destroy fibers that cross to innervate contralateral sides. Some surgeons prefer to use bipolar cautery. If so, the uterosacral ligament is grasped with the bipolar forceps. Once the segment has been coagulated, laparoscopic scissors are used to transect the ligament.

## Presacral Neurectomy

Presacral neurectomy is a procedure adjunctive to laparotomy for treatment of dysmenorrhea caused by endometriosis. Patient selection is important for effectiveness of the procedure. One study showed that patients who had midline pain had excellent results after presacral neurectomy, but patients who had adnexal pain had quite variable relief of pain. This procedure has not been shown to increase pregnancy rates.

Presacral neurectomy requires an incision that allows adequate exposure by vertical midline or a Maylard transverse incision (Fig. 64–6). The intestines are easily displaced, and the bifurcation of the aorta is then identified. The posterior parietal peritoneum over the sacral promontory is then opened with Metzenbaum scissors about 6 cm beginning caudally just below the bifurcation of the aorta and extending over the ventral surface of the sacrum. The edges of the peritoneum are held outward by 3–0 silk sutures.

Dissection begins with the right edge of the posterior peritoneum. With meticuolous care, using fine-pointed scissors or a Kittner sponge, the areolar tissue containing nerve fibers is dissected off the posterior peritoneal flap. The blood vessels in this area should not be disturbed. The right ureter is identified and

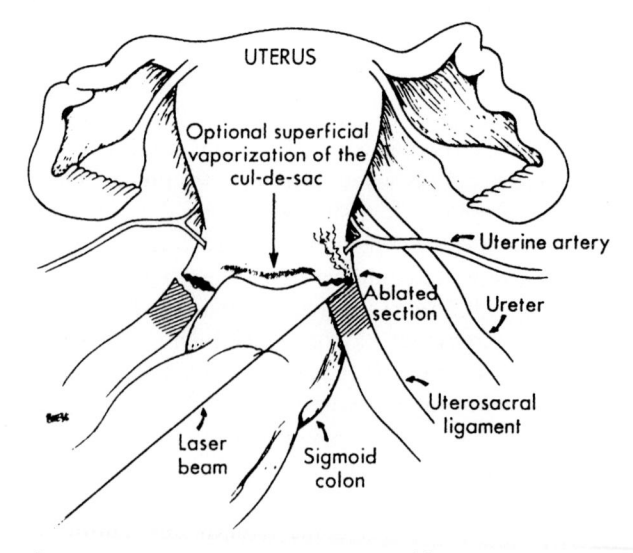

**Figure 64–5** Laparoscopic uterine nerve ablation (LUNA). (From Perry P, Azziz R: Laparoscopic uterine nerve ablation, presacral neurectomy and appendectomy. *In* Azziz R, Murphy AA (eds): Practical Manual of Operative Laparoscopy and Endoscopy. New York, Springer-Verlag, 1992.)

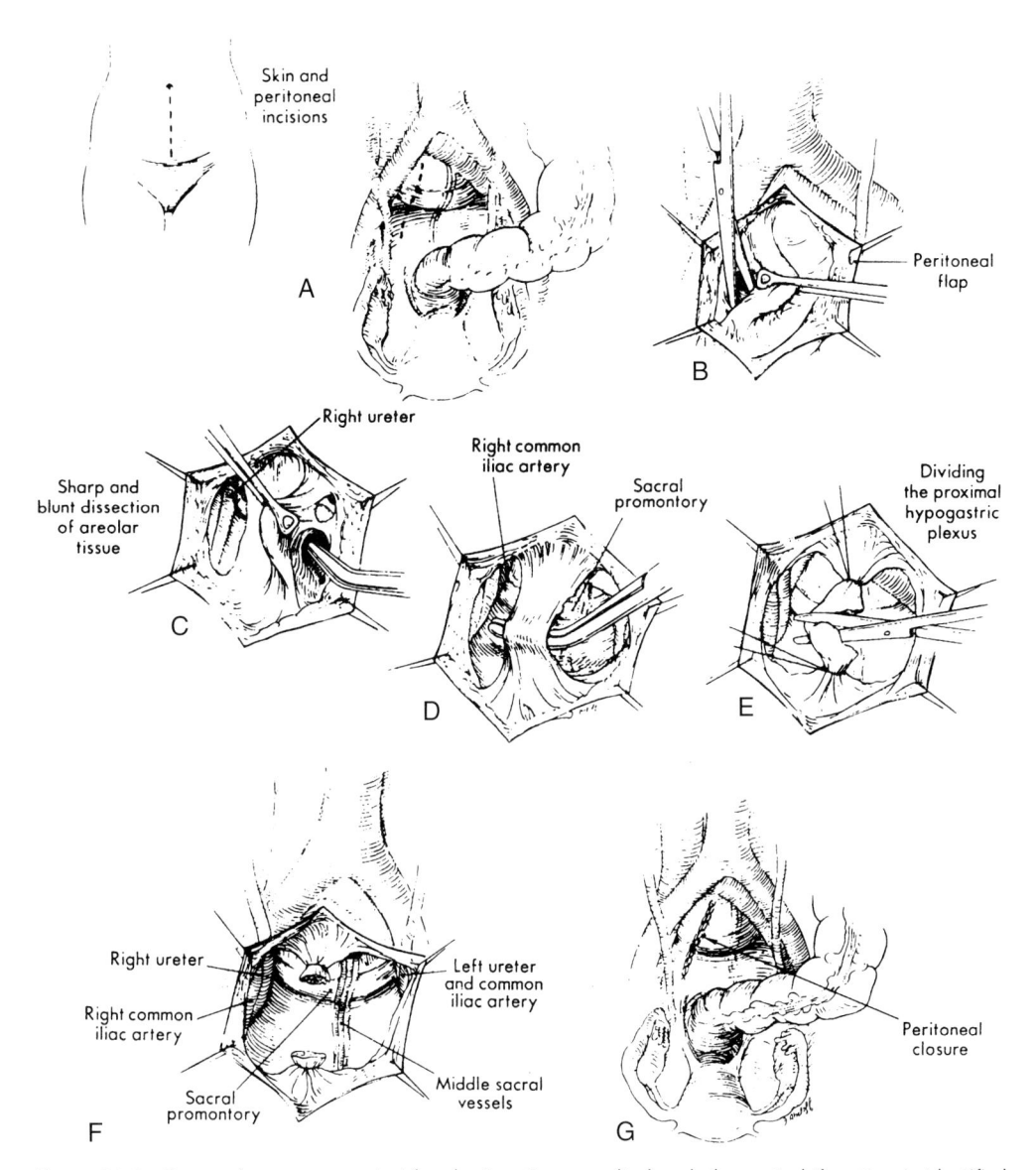

**Figure 64–6** Presacral neurectomy. *A,* After the intestines are displaced, the aortic bifurcation is identified. The posterior parietal peritoneum is opened over the sacral promontory. *B,* The peritoneal edges are held outward with silk stay sutures. *C,* The right ureter is identified and retracted laterally. *D,* The superior hypogastric nerve plexus is isolated. *E,* The hypogastric plexus is divided. *F,* The retroperitoneal space is inspected for hemostasis. *G,* The peritoneum is closed. (From Perry P, Azziz R: Laparoscopic uterine nerve ablation, presacral neurectomy and appendectomy. *In* Azziz R, Murphy AA (eds): Practical Manual of Operative Laparoscopy and Endoscopy. New York, Springer-Verlag, 1992.)

retracted laterally. The common iliac artery, which lies immediately beneath the ureter, is identified. Areolar tissue is bluntly freed from the ureter and artery. A right-angle clamp is then inserted under the sheath until the glistening white of the sacral periosteum is reached. A window is made. Care should be taken at this point to avoid the middle sacral vessels located on the surface of the promontory, because bleeding from these vessels is significant and quite difficult to stop.

Similarly, beginning on the left peritoneal flap, areolar tissue is bluntly dissected off the posterior peritoneum. Dissection is carried down until the superior hemorrhoidal vessels are encountered, and they should be ligated or clipped to avoid blood loss. The superior hypogastric nerve plexus is now isolated and bluntly dissected and lifted off the periosteum with blunt dissection. Two ties of 2–0 silk are placed proximally and distally around the nerve bundle leaving a 5- to 6-cm length of segment for excision. Once the nerve bundle is removed, the posterior peritoneum is closed with a running suture.

The immediate but rare complications of presacral neurectomy include damage to ureter and blood vessels, but the risk is greatly diminished with proper surgical technique. Side effects include constipation, vaginal dryness, and bladder dysfunction. As a rule, these symptoms resolve over several months. Laparoscopic presacral neurectomy is an effective alternative for patients wishing to avoid laparotomy.

## Postoperative Adhesion Prevention

The mainstays for preventing postoperative adhesion formation are meticulous hemostasis, minimal tissue trauma, proper suture selection, and peritoneal irrigation; the last avoids tissue trauma, anoxia, and ischemia. Some adhesions always form, however, and can undo the reconstructive work performed after resection of endometriosis.

Multiple agents have been used intraperitoneally and intravenously after resection of endometriosis to prevent adhesions, and these include dextran, nonsteroidal anti-inflammatory agents, corticosteroids, promethazine, and heparin. Briefly, three mechanical barrier agents are discussed here: modified hyaluronic acid with carboxymethylcellulose (Seprafilm), oxidized regenerated cellulose (Interceed), and expanded polytetrafluoroethylene (PTFE)(Gore-Tex). These products may be placed between the ovary and the pelvic side wall to prevent adhesion formation.

Oxidized regenerated cellulose designed in a knitted weave is known as TC-7. It is applied to a hemostatic peritoneal surface and will form a continuous gel covering within approximately 8 hours. This forms a mechanical barrier to prevent opposing raw surfaces from adhering to each other and is resorbed in 3 to 4 days.

PTFE has been evaluated on the development of postsurgical adhesions in patients who served as their own controls, and was found to have greatly decreased adhesions and was superior to oxidized regenerated cellulose. One disadvantage of this surgical membrane is that it is nonabsorbable and requires a second-look laparoscopy for removal.

Several major academic centers have been involved in the study of a chemically modified hyaluronic acid and carboxymethylcellulose (Seprafilm). It has been found to be safe and effective in human trials but did not completely eliminate adhesions in all patients. Efficacy relies on the area that requires full covering. Randomized patients who had undergone these trials were myomectomy assessed, and it was found that Seprafilm significantly reduced the incidence, severity, extent, and area of postoperative uterine adhesions when second-look laparoscopy was performed.

## Uterine Suspension

Uterine suspension has been proposed as a method of reducing adhesion formation, especially over the posterior uterus or in the cul-de-sac. Also, there is a theoretically decreased risk for tubes and ovaries to adhere to sites of resection when they are elevated. This procedure may also benefit patients who have retroflexed or retroverted uterus. We recommend a modified method of Gilliam's suspension, in which the round ligament is shortened by pulling it through the internal ring and suturing it to the rectus sheath.

## Second-Look Laparoscopy

Second-look laparoscopy is recommended by some surgeons for patients who have widespread endometriosis that requires extensive dissection. Patients who have ovaries that are dissected from the cul-de-sac or posterior uterus are thought to benefit from this procedure. If laparoscopy is performed within 4 to 12 weeks after laparotomy, adhesions are thin, filmy, and thus easy to remove. The effectiveness of this procedure in improving pregnancy outcome has yet to be proved.

## Semiconservative and Radical Surgery

Some cases are refractory to conservative management, and when childbearing is no longer an issue, the last resort is to proceed with total abdominal hysterectomy, with or without bilateral salpingo-oophorectomy. The surgical premise is to remove all visible endometriosis, or complete cytoreduction.

Radical surgery requires careful counseling of the patient and significant preoperative preparation by the surgeon. Initial evaluation involves pelvic imaging studies to rule out the presence of other entities with similar clinical presentations. A large endometrioma may present as a pelvic mass consistent with an ovarian malignancy. In these situations, the mass should be treated as a malignancy until proved otherwise. Pelvic washings are obtained for cytologic analysis. An intravenous pyelogram may be helpful if previous surgery or pelvic adhesions are suspected to have modified the course of the ureters and also to rule out the presence of a duplicated collecting system. Bowel preparation is necessary in cases in which any bowel involvement is suspected. Bowel preparation allows primary repair rather than the need for colostomy placement.

Once the decision has been made to proceed with hysterectomy, the patient and the surgeon must decide between semiconservative surgery (preservation of the ovaries) and radical surgery (removing all ovarian tissue). This decision involves consideration of the patient's age, severity of disease, and previous surgical history. Namnoum and associates demonstrated that women who had endometriosis and who underwent hysterectomy with ovarian conservation had a 6.1 times greater risk of developing recurrent pain and an 8.1 times greater risk of reoperation.

Although bilateral oophorectomy has the advantage of decreasing the risk of recurrent symptoms of endometriosis, there are several significant side effects, including severe menopausal symptoms and future risk of cardiovascular disease and osteoporosis. Although estrogen replacement should address these risks, there is a high level of patient noncompliance with long-term users and the patient requires careful and extensive counseling before surgery.

Most investigators support starting estrogen replacement therapy immediately after surgery for endometriosis. Successful use of estrogen add-back therapy with GnRH agonists in the medical management of endometriosis also supports the contention that the amount of estrogen in replacement therapy is not enough to stimulate endometriosis.

# Combination Therapy

Many gynecologists treat patients who have endometriosis with a combined medical and surgical approach. Pre- and postoperative therapies have been proposed to enhance fertility rates. There is no cure for endometriosis, and recurrence is the rule, because medical therapy only suppresses disease and surgical treatment only removes visible implants, leaving multiple microscopic implants in the peritoneum.

The rationale behind preoperative medical therapy is achieving less vascularity in the pelvis, better hemostasis, less adhesion formation, and a theoretically improved pregnancy rate. Also, ovarian suppression allows ovarian reconstruction without the presence of a follicular cyst or corpus luteum.

The rationale for postoperative medical therapy is maximal cytoreduction. Any residual disease is suppressed with chemotherapy (i.e., danazol, GnRH agonists).

The objections to combination medical therapy are many. One criticism is that preoperative therapy makes operative visualization of disease more difficult and thus harder to remove. Another is that addition of medical treatment increases the cost of treatment. Finally, the treatment time span is increased when combination therapies are used. This is very important with infertile patients, who must complete medical combination therapy before attempting to conceive and who may become distressed at missing even one potential cycle. Preoperative therapy requires two surgical procedures: diagnostic laparoscopy and definitive surgical therapy. An interval of 3 to 6 months between the two procedures is needed to complete medical therapy. In postoperative therapy, conception may be delayed 3 to 6 months while medical therapy is completed. As most clinicians believe that the best chance for postsurgical conception is within the first 6 months after conservative surgery, the infertile patient should attempt pregnancy immediately after surgery for 6 months before initiation of postoperative medical therapy. Alternatively, a 3-month course of postoperative medical therapy may be tried to decrease delay toward conception to a lesser extent.

# Summary

Endometriosis remains a challenging disease. It has captured years of study and yet remains an enigma. Its elusive nature indicates that there are subtypes of disease that are yet unclassified and encompass infertility and pain for women of childbearing ages. Surgery has played a vital role in reducing pain, especially when combined with adjunctive measures, such as presacral neurectomy. Pregnancy rates have been improved by medical management in the milder forms of endometriosis, but surgery has only proved helpful with the severest forms, which have distorted the pelvic anatomy.

Efforts are under way to reclassify the disease and its various presentations. Also necessary are further animal models to simulate the various presentations of disease because we have been able to slow the disease process with suppressive, ablating, and resecting techniques; however, a total cure is not available yet.

## REFERENCES

American Fertility Society: Classification of endometriosis. Fertil Steril 32:633, 1979.

American Fertility Society: Revised American Fertility Society classification of endometriosis, American Society for Reproductive Medicine: Revised American Society for Reproductive Medicine classification of endometriosis. Fertil Steril 67:815, 1997.

Buyalos RP: Principles of endoscopic laser surgery. In Azziz R, Murphy AA (eds): Practical Manual of Operative Laparoscopy and Hysteroscopy. New York, Springer-Verlag, 1992.

Chen FP, Soong YK. The efficacy and complications of laparoscopic presacral neurectomy in pelvic pain. Obstet Gynecol 90:974, 1997.

Counseller VS: Endometriosis. A clinical and surgical review. Am J Obstet Gynecol 65:930, 1951

Cramer DW, Wilson E, Stillman RJ, et al: The relation of endometriosis to menstrual characteristics, smoking and exercise. JAMA 255:1904, 1986.

Damario MA, Rock JA: Classification of endometriosis. Semin Reprod Endocrinol 15:235, 1997.

Davis GD, Brooks RA: Excision of pelvic endometriosis with the carbon dioxide laser laparoscope. Obstet Gynecol 72:816, 1988.

Diamond MP, Linsky CB, Cunningham T, et al: A model for sidewall adhesions in the rabbit: Reduction by an absorbable barrier. Microsurgery 8:197, 1987.

Diamond MP: Reduction of adhesions after uterine myomectomy by Seprafilm membrane (HAL-F): A blinded, prospective, randomized, multicenter clinical study. Seprafilm Adhesion Study Group. Fertil Steril 66(6):904, 1996.

Donnez J, Nisolle M, Gillerot S, et al: Rectovaginal septum adenomyotic nodules: A series of 500 cases. Br J Obstet Gynaecol 104:1014, 1997.

Dmowski WP, Radwanska E, Binor Z, et al: Ovarian suppression induced with buserelin or danazol in the management of endometriosis: A randomized, comparative study. Fertil Steril 51:395, 1989.

Fraser IS, Shearman RP, Jansen RPS, et al: A comparative treatment trial of endometriosis using the gonadotropin-releasing hormone agonist, nafarelin, and the synthetic steroid, danazol. Aust N Z J Obstet Gynaecol 31:158, 1991.

Guzick DS, Silliman NP, Adamson GD, et al: Prediction of pregnancy in infertile women based on the American Society for Reproductive Medicine's revised classification of endometriosis. Fertil Steril 67:822, 1997.

Haney AF, Hesla J, Hurst BS, et al: Expanded polytetrafluoroethylene (Gore-Tex Surgical Membrane) is superior to oxidized regenerated cellulose (Interceed TC7) in preventing adhesions. Fertil Steril 64:668, 1995.

Henderson AF, Studd JWW: The role of definitive surgery and hormone replacement therapy in the treatment of endometriosis. In Thomas E, Rock JA: Modern Approaches to Endometriosis. Boston, Kluwer Academic Publishers, 1991.

Henzl MR, Corson SL, Moghissi K, et al: Administration of nasal nafarelin as compared with oral danazol for endometriosis. A multicenter double-blind comparative clinical trial. N Engl J Med 318:485, 1988.

Hull ME, Moghissi KS, Magyar DF, et al: Comparison of different treatment modalities of endometriosis in infertile women. Fertil Steril 47:40, 1987.

Ichida M, Gomi A, Hiranouchi N, et al: A case of cerebral endometriosis causing catamenial epilepsy. Neurology 43:2708, 1993.

Interceed (TC-7) Adhesion Barrier Study Group: Prevention of postsurgical adhesions by Interceed (TC-7), an absorbable adhesion barrier; a prospective randomized multicenter clinical study. Fertil Steril 51:933, 1989.

Joseph J, Sahn SA: Thoracic endometriosis syndrome: New observations from an analysis of 110 cases. Am J Med 100:164, 1996.

Markham SM, Carpenter SE, Rock JA: Extrapelvic endometriosis. Obstet Gynecol Clin North Am 16:193, 1989.

Marcoux S, Maheux R, Berube S, et al: Laparoscopic surgery in infertile women with minimal or mild endometriosis. N Engl J Med 337:217, 1997.

Moghissi KS, Boyce CR: Management of endometriosis with oral medroxyprogesterone acetate. Obstet Gynecol 47:265, 1976.

Murphy AA, Schlaff WD, Hassiakos D, et al: Laparoscopic cautery in the treatment of endometriosis-related infertility. Fertil Steril 55:246, 1991.

Namnoum AB, Hickman TN, Goodman, SB, et al: Incidence of symptom recurrence after hysterectomy for endometriosis. Fertil Steril 64:898, 1995.

Nisolle M and Donnez J: Peritoneal endometriosis, ovarian endometriosis and adenomyotic nodules of the rectovaginal septum are three different entities. Fertil Steril 68:585, 1997.

Olive, DL: Medical treatment: Alternatives to danazol. In Schenken RS (ed): Endometriosis: Contemporary Concepts in Clinical Management. Philadelphia, JB Lippincott, 1989.

Revised American Fertility Society classification of endometriosis: 1985. Fertil Steril 43:351, 1985.

Rock JA, Truglia JA, Caplan RJ, et al: Zoladex (Goserelin Acetate Implant) in the treatment of endometriosis: A randomized comparison with danazol. Obstet Gynecol 82:198, 1993.

Rock JA, Markham SM: Pathogenesis of endometriosis. Lancet 340:1264, 1992.

Rock JA, Hurst BS: Clinical significance of prostanoid concentration in women with endometriosis. Prog Clin Biol Res 323:61, 1990.

Rock JA, Guzick DS, Sengos C, et al: The conservative surgical treatment of endometriosis: Evaluation of pregnancy success with respect to the extent of disease as categorized using contemporary classification systems. Fertil Steril 35:131, 1981.

Shock TE, Nyberg LM: Endometriosis of the urinary tract. Urology 31:1, 1988.

Simpson JL, Elias S, Malinak LR, et al: Heritable aspects of endometriosis, I: Genetic studies. Am J Obstet Gynecol 137:327, 1980.

Speroff T, Dawson NV, Speroff L, et al: A risk-benefit analysis of elective bilateral oophorectomy: Effect of changes in compliance with estrogen therapy on outcome. Am J Obstet Gynecol 164:165, 1991.

Sutton CJG, Pooley AS, Ewen SP, et al: Follow-up report on a randomized controlled trial of laser laparoscopy in the treatment of pelvic pain associated with minimal to moderate endometriosis. Fertil Steril 68:1070, 1997.

Thomas EJ: Combining medical and surgical treatment for endometriosis: The best of both worlds? Br J Obstet Gynaecol 99(suppl):5, 1992.

Tjaden B, Schlaff WD, Kimball A, et al: The efficacy of presacral neurectomy for the relief of midline dysmenorrhea. Obstet Gynecol 76:89, 1990.

Vercellini P, Cortesi I, Crosignani PG: Progestins for symptomatic endometriosis: A critical analysis of the evidence. Fertil Steril 68:393, 1997.

Walters MD: Definitive surgery. In Schenken RS (ed): Endometriosis: Contemporary Concepts in Clinical Management. Philadelphia, JB Lippincott, 1989.

Wheeler JM, Malinak LR: Combined medical and surgical therapy for endometriosis: Incidence and management. Am J Obstet Gynecol 129:245, 1997.

# 65

# Postoperative Adhesion Formation in Gynecologic Surgery: Etiology and Treatment

RICHARD E. LEACH
MICHAEL P. DIAMOND

Postoperative adhesion formation remains an enigma to the obstetrician-gynecologist. This frustration was voiced by Boys in 1942, "The peritoneal adhesion has been recognized as a surgical entity for nearly 150 years, its etiologic factors and pathologic characteristics have been understood for over 50 years and, yet, no satisfactory major prophylaxis has been developed." In 1988, there were 282,000 hospitalizations for adhesiolysis in the United States, averaging 116 hospitalizations per 100,000 population. Of these, 58% were performed on the female reproductive tract. Age distribution was bimodal, with the highest rates between 26 and 50 years and greater than 65 years of age. The mean period of hospitalization was 11 days, for a total of 608,000 inpatient days. The cost for adhesiolysis hospitalizations was $1.2 billion 1988 dollars, which included $900 million for hospitalization costs and $300 million for surgeons' fees. This rather significant financial burden does not take into account outpatient laparoscopic lysis of adhesions that were not determined in this analysis. Further, the morbidity and mortality associated with small bowel obstruction, pelvic pain, and infertility are additional causes of concern. This chapter attempts to dispel the commonly held notions that microsurgical technique alone does not result in postoperative adhesion formation and that currently there are no available surgical adjuvants to reduce them.

## Incidence

The most common cause of pelvic adhesions is surgery. The true incidence can be estimated best from postmortem examinations and second-look laparoscopy. The presence of abdominal adhesions was determined in 752 autopsies and analyzed by organ-specific involvement. These data correlated to surgical history, which excluded cancer. Analysis revealed 69% of women and 65% of men had adhesions. Cadavers with no history of surgery had 25% adhesions, with no sex differences noted. This is unexpected because one would expect women to have a higher incidence secondary to pelvic inflammatory disease. One explanation is that the epidemic of pelvic inflammatory disease did not affect these subjects because their mean age was 59 years. If this study was repeated today, one could speculate that a sex difference would be found. There is a graded increase in adhesion occurrence from single to multiple surgeries ranging from 65 to 95%. Previous gynecologic surgery, including hysterectomy and adnexal surgery, was associated with adhesions 74% of the time. In study of 325 patients undergoing exploratory laparotomy, 93% and 10% had adhesions present in repeat vs. first-time operated patients, respectively. Adhesion formation after reproductive preservation or infertility surgery, determined by second-look laparoscopy, ranges from 55 to 100% (Table 65–1). These data support the fact that most pelvic surgery results in adhesion formation even when microsurgical principles are used. The opinion that laparoscopic surgery decreases the rate of adhesion is not completely supported by the literature. The Operative Laparoscopy Study Group evaluated patients by second-look laparoscopy after laparoscopic lysis of adhesions. Sixty-six of 68 patients were found to have adhesions at the site of the initial operation. However, there was a dramatic decrease in de novo adhesion formation of 12%—that is, adhesions that form at sites outside the area of primary operation. Therefore, one can assume that most of gynecologic surgery results in adhesion formation regardless of the operative techniques used.

## Pathophysiology

The peritoneum is the most extensive serous membrane in the body. The surface area in the adult equals that of skin and consists of two layers: (1) a loose connective tissue and (2) the mesothelium, which serves to facilitate free movement of the intraabdominal contents. The mesothelial cells therefore form a continuous layer that rests on a loose mesenchymal connective tissue, a basal lamina, and a basement membrane. The minimum volume of fluid to coat the peritoneum is roughly 200 ml. Peritoneal fluid volume is highest after ovulation ranging from 5 to 20 ml. Peritoneal fluid is both filtered and absorbed through the mesothelium. Absorption of colloid and particles occurs actively through lymphatic pores, water, and electrolytes across the peritoneum. In patients undergoing peritoneal dialysis, the rate of fluid absorption is roughly 35 ml/hr. The fluid contains a variety of cells, including lymphocytes, eosinophils, mast cells, and polymorphonuclear cells.

Trauma to the peritoneum initiates a complex and yet to be completely described cascade of cellular and protein tissue repair responses (Fig. 65–1). The resulting inflammatory response, including fibrin deposition, ultimately results in reperitonealization of the injured region. However, there is evidence that tissue ischemia compromises fibrinolysis of the normally transient fibrin band formation after injury. The likely causes of ischemia are peritoneal abrasion, tense occluding ligatures, and tissue desiccation and necrosis. The resulting ischemia of the peritoneum has been shown to result directly in adhesion formation in rodents. Specifically, ischemic mesothelial cells secrete much less tissue plasminogen activator and increased levels of plasminogen activator inhibitor, resulting in the localized deposition of fibrin. The preponderance of fibrin formation vs. fibrinolysis ultimately forms the matrix on which mature adhesion develops. Although this homeostatic mechanism encompasses much of the available data regarding the contribution of fibrinolysis to adhesion formation, it falls short of incorporating the evolving data in describing the coordinated activation or inhibition of inflammatory cells, growth factors, proteases, and cytokines.

The transient influx and efflux of various cell types from the injured site is well characterized. Two cell groups in particular, peritoneal leukocytes and mesothelial cells, appear to play a fundamental role in peritoneal repair. Polymorphonucleocytes are the first cells that invade the injured site and, in the absence of infection, egress 2 days later. Peritoneal and recruited

**Table 65–1** Adhesion Formation After Reproductive Preservation or Infertility Surgery

| Study | Time from Initial Procedure | Total No. of Patients | Total No. with Adhesions | % with Adhesions |
|---|---|---|---|---|
| Diamond et al. (1987) | 1 wk–12 wk | 106 | 91 | 86 |
| Decherney and Mezer (1984) | 4 wk–16 wk | 20 | 15 | 75 |
| Surrey and Friedman (1982) | 6 wk–8 wk | 31 | 22 | 71 |
| Pittaway et al. (1985) | 4 wk–6 wk | 23 | 23 | 100 |
| Trimbos-Kemper et al. (1985) | 8 days | 188 | 104 | 55 |
| Daniell and Pittaway (1983) | 4 wk–6 wk | 25 | 24 | 96 |

Diamond MP: Surgical Aspects of Infertility. *In* Sciarra JJ (ed): Gynecology and Obstetrics. Vol. 5. Philadelphia, Harper & Row, 1988, pp 1–23.

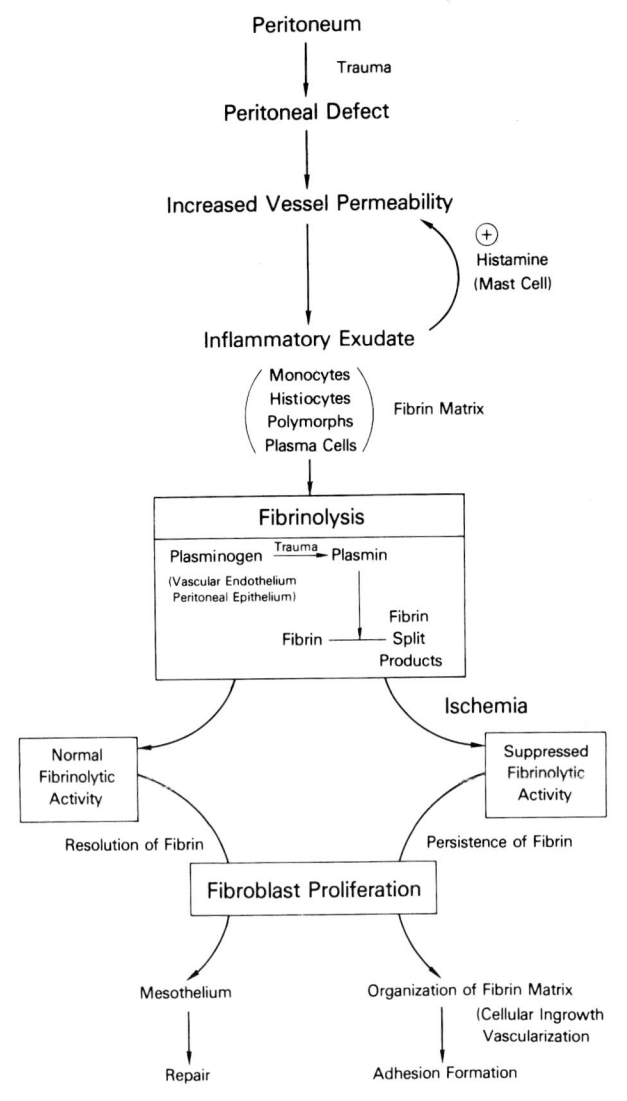

**Figure 65–1** Cascade of cellular and protein tissue repair responses to trauma of the peritoneum. (From diZerega GS, Rodgers KE [eds]: The Peritoneum. New York, Springer-Verlag, 1992, p 281.)

peripheral monocytes rapidly differentiate into tissue macrophages, which phagocytose wound debris and bacteria. Macrophages also modulate wound healing by secreting superoxide anion, interleukin-1 and tumor necrosis factor which, contributes to overall tissue remodeling.

Histologically, the injured peritoneum heals differently than the keratinized squamous epithelium of skin. Skin heals from the edge of the injury in contrast to the peritoneum, which heals from the base by the coalescing of islands of mesothelium. The net effect of this pattern of healing is that different-sized surface areas of injury are re-epithelialized completely over approximately the same length of time. By 4 days after injury, the mesothelial cells proliferate at the base of the injury under paracrine control of resident macrophages. The coordinated secretion of extracellular matrix by mesothelial cells appears to be required for angiogenesis and completion of reperitonealization.

## Etiology

As stated previously, several factors that arise during surgery, including serosal drying and abrasion, presence of blood, ischemic suture lines, foreign bodies, and peritoneal closure, have been demonstrated primarily in animal models to result in adhesion formation. Although the tenets of microsurgical techniques have evolved and been used by infertility surgical subspecialists, many of these principles may be practiced by the generalist who typically performs the initial surgery, which often is complicated by adhesion formation. Surgical techniques to minimize these factors should result in diminished adhesion formation, although none have been evaluated in prospective human clinical trials.

The presence of blood in the face of serosal injury has been shown in the rat to be a very adhesiogenic combination. Serosal drying of the cecum with compressed air alone or with the addition of autologous blood alone did not manifest in significant adhesion formation. However, the combination of both consistently resulted in adhesion formation. Further, the addition of defibrinated blood, plasma, washed erythrocytes, and heparinized blood products did not form adhesions in the presence of serosal drying, implying the role of fibrin. This is consistent with the homeostatic fibrinolytic role that mesothelial cells play in degrading immature fibrinous adhesions.

Peritoneal suturing of deperitonealized defects after tissue extirpation and abdominal wall closure generally is performed during gynecologic surgery. There is evidence that this practice may in fact increase adhesion formation. Early reports from Brunschwig found that with an early second laparotomy following pelvic exenteration, the pelvic floor was reperitonealized completely as early as 7 days after surgery. This was observed despite the fact that no peritoneum initially was present to suture together. Since then, several human studies have found that the denuded peritoneum forms less adhesions when left to heal by secondary intention rather than when attempts are made to close it primarily. Whether the adhesion-promoting action of peritoneal closure is the result of tissue ischemia from tense suture lines or foreign body reaction remains to be determined. In general, there is sufficient evidence to support the practice of allowing the parietal peritoneum to heal by secondary intention.

## Treatment

The use of surgical adjuvants to reduce adhesion formation is not a modern concept. In the beginning of the 20th century, gels, metal foil, paraffin, and tissue grafts were proposed as devices to separate injured peritoneum to reduce adhesion formation. However, in small observational series, these grafts were not found to be efficacious and were abandoned. The notion that a single pharmacologic agent could dramatically reduce adhesion formation is not reasonable because of the cascade of cellular and molecular events that are activated or inhibited after injury. Therefore, the use of barrier devices to separate injured surfaces until reperitonealization occurs theoretically is a more practical approach. Ideally, the barrier should fulfill several criteria, including not interfering with the reperitonealization process—reabsorbed after this process is complete—and not supporting bacterial growth. Two Food and Drug Administration (FDA) approved devices, Interceed and Seprafilm, fulfill these requirements. Both have been shown in prospective, randomized trials to be efficacious in reducing adhesion formation after pelvic surgery.

## INTERCEED

Interceed is composed of oxidized regenerated cellulose fibers woven into a pattern that, when hydrated, forms a continuous sheet with the consistency of a gel. This process is complete 8 hours after application to the injured surface and does not require suturing for the fabric to remain in place. The residence time of Interceed is dependent on the total amount of material placed in the cavity. It is reabsorbed both by enzymatic degradation and by macrophage-directed processes. Interceed remnant was identified in 1 of 105 patients at the time of second-look laparoscopy within 28 days of ovarian cystectomy for endometriomas.

There have been multiple clinical reports on the efficacy of Interceed in reducing adhesion formation in pelvic surgery. In one study (n = 368), patients given Interceed treatment were compared with untreated controls, and Interceed was found to be twice as effective in preventing adhesions than surgery alone.

The rate of adhesion formation involving the ovary ranged from 65 to 80%. The efficacy of Interceed after ovarian surgery was evaluated in four controlled studies. Entry criteria included bilateral ovarian disease, including adhesions and/or endometriosis. After surgery, one ovary was wrapped with Interceed, and the contralateral ovary served as control. At second-look laparoscopy, the presence and degree of adhesion formation was scored. Results indicated that of those ovaries treated with Interceed, 48% (76 of 158 cases) were free of adhesions compared with 25% of untreated ovaries (40 of 158).

A multicenter evaluation of Interceed in fallopian tube adhesiolysis by microsurgery used second-look laparoscopy to determine the effect of treatment on adhesion formation. Of the Interceed-treated fallopian tubes, 33 of 66 were free of adhesions compared with 16 of 66 treated with microsurgery alone. A similar result was observed when evaluating efficacy of treatment of the fimbria. The beneficial effect of Interceed was extended to the treatment of pelvic sidewall adhesion in two clinical trials. After adhesiolysis of both pelvic sidewalls, the deperitonealized surface was measured, and Interceed was applied to one side. The Interceed-treated sidewalls were free of adhesions in a total of 103 of 197 cases compared with 37 of 197 of the untreated sidewalls. Sekiba and associates reported that a subgroup of the 63 cases were analyzed further for efficacy of Interceed treatment after removal of severe endometriosis Stage III and IV of the American Fertility Society classification. Fifty percent of patients with severe endometriosis were free of adhesions on the Interceed-treated sidewalls compared with 18% of controls.

It is remarkable that in the multiple clinical reports performed by different surgeons the use of Interceed increased the adhesion-free rate at different surgical sites to approximately 50%, twice that found when surgery alone was performed on the contralateral side. This successful use of Interceed adds a proven surgical adjuvant to the armamentarium of the pelvic surgeon in addition to established surgical technique. To achieve this level of efficacy, the technical aspects of surgical case selection and method of application must be understood.

There are several technical details that require close scrutiny in the application of Interceed for efficacy to be achieved. Interceed should be placed on the injured site dry and in a single layer because additional layers only increase the residence time without a proven increase in efficacy. The fabric can be trimmed to fit the injured site, maintaining a 5-mm margin. If additional sheets are necessary to cover the injured site, a 3- to 5-mm margin of overlap should be maintained. The choice of surgical cases in which to use Interceed and its proper application are Fundamental to the desired result. The presence of blood in the injured site has been shown to negate the efficacy of Interceed in a rabbit model. Surgical cases such as myomectomies and severe endometriosis, in which continued oozing from the injured site can be anticipated, are not candidates for Interceed application. If the Interceed membrane is placed and the white fabric turns black, it should be removed.

Typically, the fabric turns brown when applied to properly selected surgical sites after hydration with irrigation fluid. Although Interceed adheres to the surgical site after hydration without the need of sutures, careful removal of all irrigation fluid from the abdomen is necessary to maintain placement. The patient should be placed in the reverse Trendelenburg position to collect the fluid that has accumulated in the upper abdomen during the operation. If this is not done, residual fluid in the abdomen may separate the barrier from its site when it becomes dependent in the pelvis, negating any beneficial effect. The application of Interceed to flat surfaces overlying the uterus and pelvic side wall can be achieved readily using the aforementioned techniques. Following are additional technical considerations for application over the ovary and fallopian tube.

## Ovarian Surgery

Included in ovarian surgery are cystectomy, ablation of endometriosis, lysis of adhesions, and mobilization from the ovarian fossa. These are superb indications for the use of Interceed (Fig. 65–2). The ovarian fossa and ovary application can be achieved by lifting the ovary, placing the sheet behind the ovary, and allowing it to return to its normal position. The remaining surface of Interceed then is allowed to wrap the rest of the exposed ovarian surface. The weight of the ovary against the fossa assists in maintaining the position of the barrier. The fabric then is moistened with irrigation fluid to promote adherence to the ovary.

## Tubal Surgery

The distal end of the fallopian tube is lifted and placed on the Interceed sheet and wrapped to cover the remaining surface (Fig. 65–3). The fabric then is moistened with irrigation fluid to promote adherence to the tube. The fallopian tube is placed in its normal anatomic position ensuring that the barrier has remained in place.

## SEPRAFILM

Seprafilm is a translucent membrane composed of chemically derivatized hyaluronic acid and carboxymethyl cellulose. The combined polymer results in a longer residence time than with each separately, with resorption occurring within 7 days and excretion from the body by 28 days. There are several technical details that are important in the application of Seprafilm. In general, Seprafilm requires very careful handling for proper placement (Fig. 65–4).

The efficacy of Seprafilm in gynecologic surgery was evaluated in a multicenter clinical trial that enrolled 127 women, 59 of whom received treatment. The prospective, randomized, blind study tested the efficacy of Seprafilm to reduce adhesions after myomectomy. Myomectomy previously was shown to be an extremely adhesiogenic operation, there was 94% adhesion formation involving the adnexa to the posterior uterine incision, and every patient had an adhesion present at second-look laparoscopy. In the Seprafilm study, each patient was required to have at least one posterior uterine incision greater than 1 cm in length and was randomized to receive Seprafilm

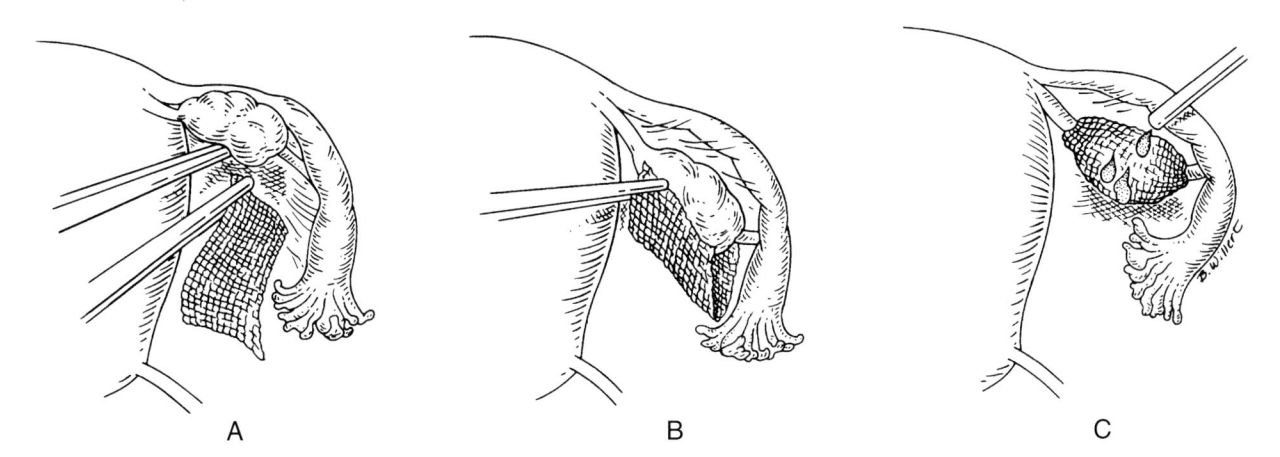

**Figure 65–2** The ovary is completely wrapped with Interceed. A, By lifting the ovary away from the ovarian fossa and placing a corner of Interceed (half piece) up into the fossa. B, The ovary is allowed to return to the normal position, thereby holding the Interceed in place. C, Moistening with a few drops of irrigating solution ensures adherence of the barrier to the ovary. (From diZerega GS, DeCherney AH, Diamond MP, et al: Pelvic Surgery: Adhesion Formation and Prevention. In diZerega GS, DeCherney AH, Diamond, et al [eds]: Pelvic Surgery: Adhesion Formation and Prevention. New York, Springer-Verlag, 1997, p 192.)

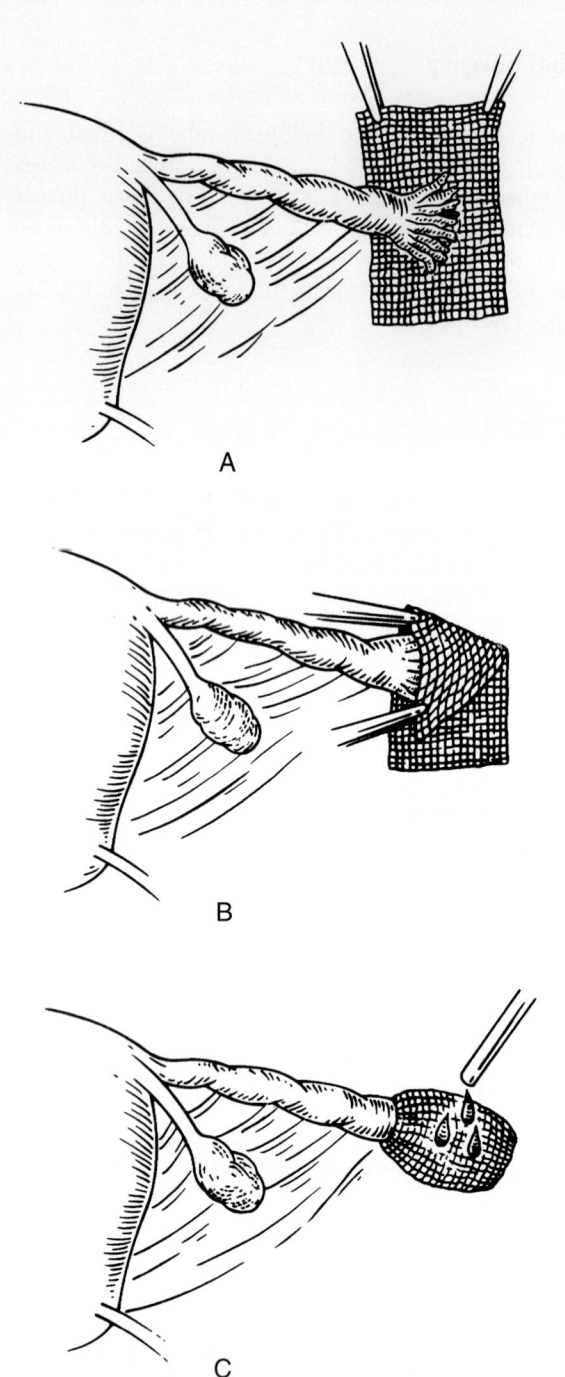

**Figure 65-3** For use after salpingostomy, the Interceed barrier is *A*, suspended by two grasping instruments and *B*, brought into contact with the salpingostomy site. The barrier is then *C*, folded over the surgical site until the four corners of the barrier are in contact with the isthmic portion of the fallopian tube. Irrigating solution (3 to 5 ml) is placed over the Interceed, thereby "sealing" an Interceed bag around the fimbria. (From diZerega GS, DeCherney AH, Diamond MP, et al [eds]: Pelvic Surgery: Adhesion Formation and Prevention. *In* diZerega GS, DeCherney AH, Diamond MP, et al: Pelvic Surgery: Adhesion Formation and Prevention. New York, Springer-Verlag, 1997, p 199.)

membrane or not. Second-look laparoscopy was videotaped and scored by an independent evaluator.

Seprafilm was shown to be safe, with no adverse events attributable to its use. In those patients with both anterior and posterior incisions, 39% of the Seprafilm group were free of adhesions to the anterior incision compared with 6% of the control group. Although the same trend existed for the posterior incision, it did not reach statistical significance (13% vs. 8%). At least one adnexa was free from adhesion to the uterus in 48% of the Seprafilm group vs. 31% in the surgery-only group. The application of Seprafilm requires the understanding of several technical considerations that relate to membrane handling.

Seprafilm is enclosed in a paper sleeve so that the barrier can be handled without direct contact before placement. Seprafilm must be placed dry to the injured site in a single layer. If it is hydrated before placement, it becomes gel-like and difficult to handle. The general strategy is to place the barrier as close to the intended site while in the sleeve. Once the sleeve is removed, the barrier must be manipulated gently with dry gloves and instruments. It does not require suture to keep in place. The presence of blood in the injured site, unlike Interceed, does not

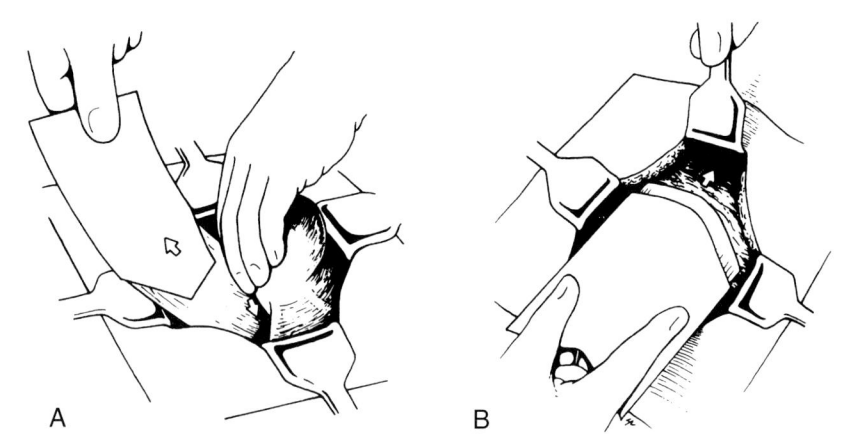

**Figure 65–4** Seprafilm membrane application is shown *A*, to the posterior uterus and *B*, beneath an anterior abdominal wall incision. To apply Seprafilm, a 2-cm leading edge of the membrane is advanced beyond the holder. The membrane is applied to the posterior side of the uterus by gently raising the uterus and advancing the exposed membrane edge. The leading edge of the membrane is applied to the tissue and the holder is pulled away, exposing the membrane to the uterine surface. Entry into the abdominal cavity and placement beneath the abdominal wall can be facilitated by slightly arching the membrane and holder. (From diZerega GS, DeCherney AH, Diamond MP, et al: Pelvic Surgery: Adhesion Formation and Prevention. *In* diZerega GS, DeCherney AH, Diamond MP, et al [eds]: Pelvic Surgery: Adhesion Formation and Prevention. New York, Springer-Verlag, 1997, p. 204.)

preclude its application. Therefore, it can be used in myomectomies and severe endometriosis, in which complete hemostasis cannot be achieved. Like Interceed, Seprafilm must be applied into an operative field free of irrigation fluid. Repositioning the patient is necessary to collect the irrigation fluid used during the operation. The application sleeve should be purposefully discarded before closure of the abdomen.

# Conclusion

The pelvic surgeon is faced with the realization that most operations will be complicated by adhesion formation. Despite the development of established macro-or microsurgical techniques, adhesion formation may result in infertility, pelvic pain, and small bowel obstruction. The use of the surgical adjuvants Interceed and Seprafilm can increase the number of adhesion-free sites up to 100% in some cases, thus justifying their use when considering this fact alone.

### REFERENCES

Altemeier WA, Culbertson WR, Fidler JP: Giant horseshoe intraabdominal abscess. Ann Surg 181:716–725, 1975.

Azziz R, Interceed adhesion Barrier Study Group: Microsurgery alone or with interceed absorbable adhesion barrier for pelvic sidewall adhesion. Surg Gynecol Obstet 177:135–139, 1993.

Boys F: The prophylaxis of peritoneal adhesions. Surgery 11:118, 1942.

Brunschwig A, Robbins GF: Regeneration of the peritoneum: Experimental observations and clinical experience in radical resections of intraobdominal cancer. *In* XV Congr Soc Int Chir, Lisbonne 1953. Bruxelles, Henri de Smedt, 1954, pp 756–765.

Buckman RF Jr, Maj MC, Buckman PD, et al: A physiologic basis for the adhesion-free healing of deperitonealized surfaces. J Surg Res 21:61–76, 1976.

Cromack DT, Cromack TR, Pretorius G, et al: Development of a predictive value equation for the minimum fluid volume to completely coat the intraperitoneal surface of rodents. Surg Forum 36:477–478, 1985.

Crone C: Does "restricted diffusion" occur in muscle capillaries? Proc Soc Exp Biol Med 112:435–455, 1963.

Diamond MP, The Seprafilm Adhesion Study Group: Reduction of adhesions after uterine myomectomy by Seprafilm membrane [HAL-F]: A blinded, prospective, randomized multicenter clinical study. Fertil Steril 6:904–910, 1996.

Diamond MP, Linsky C: Interceed absorbable adhesion barrier. *In* Diamond MP, Dechemey AH (eds): Infertility and Reproductive Medicine Clinics of North America. Philadelphia, WB Saunders, 1994.

Diamond MP, Nezhat F: Letter to the editor: Adhesions after resection of ovarian endometrioma. Fertil Steril 59:934–935, 1993.

diZerega GS, DeCherney AH, Diamond MP, et al (eds): Pelvic Surgery: Adhesion Formation and Prevention. New York, Springer Verlag, 1997.

diZerega GS, Rodgers KE: The Peritoneum. New York, Springer Verlag, 1992.

Ellis H, Harrison W, Hugh TB: The healing of the peritoneum under normal and pathological conditions. Br J Surg 52:4371–4376, 1965.

Fox Ray N, Larsen Jr JW, Stillman RJ, et al: Economic impact of hospitalization for lower abdominal adhesiolysis in the United States in 1988. Surg Gynecol Obstet 176:271–276, 1993.

Franklin RR, Ovarian Adhesion Study Group: Reduction of ovarian adhesions by the use of Interceed. Obstet Gynecol 86:335–338, 1995.

Gervin AS, Puckett CI, Silver D: Serosal hypofibrinolysis: A cause of postoperative adhesions. Am J Surg 125:80–88, 1973.

Hertzler AE: The Peritoneum. St Louis, CV Mosby, 1919.

Keckstein J: Reduction of postoperative formation after laparoscopic ovarian cystectomy. Presented at the 14th World Congress of Gynecology and Obstetrics, Montreal, 1994.

Larsson B, Efficacy of Interceed in Adhesion Prevention in Gynecologic Surgery: A Review of 13 clinical studies. J Reprod Med 41:27–35, 1996.

Menzies D, Ellis H: Intestinal obstruction form adhesions—How big is the problem? Ann R Coll Surg Engl 72:60–63, 1990.

Nordic Adhesion Prevention Study Group: The efficacy of Interceed for reformation of postoperative adhesions on ovaries, fallopian tubes, and fimbriae in microsurgical operations for infertility. Fertil Steril 63:709–714, 1995.

Odel HM, Ferris DO, Power MH: Clinical considerations of the problem of extra renal excretion: Peritoneal lavage. Med Clin North Am 32:989–1076, 1948.

Operative Laparoscopy Study Group: Postoperative adhesion development after operative laparoscopy: Evaluation at early second-look procedures. Fertil Steril 5:700, 1991.

Raferty AT: Regeneration of parietal and visceral peritoneum: An electron microscopical study. J Anat 115:375–392, 1973a.

Raferty AT: Regeneration of parietal and visceral peritoneum: A light microscopical study. Br J Surg 60:293–299, 1973b.

Raferty AT: Effect of peritoneal trauma on peritoneal fibrinolytic activity and intraperitoneal adhesion formation. Eur Surg Res 13:397–401, 1981a.

Raferty AT: A method for measuring fibrinolytic activity in a single layer of cells. J Clin Pathol 34:625–629, 1981b.

Sekiba K: Use of Interceed absorbable adhesion barrier to reduce postoperative adhesion reformation in infertility and endometriosis surgery. Obstet Gynecol 79:518–522, 1992.

Shear L, Swartz C, Shiraberger JA: Kinetics of peritoneal fluid absorption in adult man. N Engl J Med 272:123–127, 1965.

Tulandi T, Murray C, Guralnick M: Adhesion formation and reproductive outcome after myomectomy and second look laparoscopy. Obstet Gynecol 82:213–215, 1993.

Vipond MN, Whawell SA, Thompson JN, et al: Peritoneal fibrinolytic activity and intra-abdominal adhesions. Lancet 335:1120–1122, 1990.

Von Geldrop HJ: Interceed absorbable adhesion barrier reduces the formation of postsurgical adhesion after ovarian surgery. Abstract P273 American Fertility Society, 1994.

Weibel M-A, Majno G: Peritoneal adhesions and their relation to abdominal surgery. Am J Surg 126:345–353, 1973.

Wiseman DM, Kamp LF, Saferstein L: Improving the efficacy of Interceed barrier in the presence of blood using thrombin, heparin, or a blood insensitive barrier, modified Interceed. Prog Clin Biol Res 381:205–212, 1993.

# BUSINESS PRINCIPLES IN OBSTETRICS AND GYNECOLOGY

# 66

# The Economics of Obstetrics and Gynecology

GAIL A. JENSEN
ALLEN C. GOODMAN

## Economics in Obstetrics and Gynecology

The health-care sector is a large and growing portion of the U.S. economy as well as economies around the world. Slightly more than $1 of every $8 (13.6%) spent on goods and services in the U.S. economy goes to the health sector. For perspective, note that in 1950, this share was less than $1 in $20, and as recently as 1976, it was $1 in $12.[1]

Other expenditure categories are as large as health-care expenditures. As recently as 1960, food represented approximately 25% of spending, housing about 15%, and medical care only 5%. Table 66–1 indicates that in 1995, the most recent year for which data are available, medical care had supplanted food and tobacco as the largest category of personal consumption expenditures. Consumers spent 17.9% of their budgets on medical care, compared with 16.1% on food and tobacco and 15.1% on housing. The $383.6 billion spent on hospitals and nursing homes constituted 7.8% of all personal consumption expenditures, a larger share than was spent on clothing, and almost as large a share as was spent on recreational activities.

## WHY IS ECONOMICS RELEVANT?

Well into the 1970s, and possibly later than that, many health-care practitioners were comfortable dismissing economic analysis, arguing that it was irrelevant. Economics is the study of how scarce resources are used to produce goods and services. Economists observe how the scarce goods and services are distributed. If health-care goods and services previously were not thought to be scarce, their increasing costs in the 1980s and 1990s certainly suggests growing problems of scarcity.

It is nonetheless appropriate to address whether the characteristic approaches used by economists apply to health care. Are health-care consumers rational—in fact, are they the ones who make the decisions at all? Do consumers and/or their physicians, as their

---

[1]This share has leveled off in the mid 1990s amid fears that it might rise even higher.

**Table 66-1** Personal Consumption Expenditures, 1995

| Category | Expenditures (in $billions) | Share (in %) |
|---|---|---|
| Total | 4924.9 | 100.0% |
| Food and tobacco | 794.4 | 16.1% |
| Clothing, accessories, and jewelry | 320.2 | 6.5% |
| Housing | 743.7 | 15.1% |
| Household operation | 554.3 | 11.3% |
| Medical care | 883.1 | 17.9% |
|   Drugs/sundries | 85.7 | 1.7% |
|   Physicians | 189.8 | 3.9% |
|   Dentists | 46.6 | 0.9% |
|   Hospitals/nursing homes | 383.6 | 7.8% |
|   Health insurance | 61.3 | 1.2% |
|   Other | 116.1 | 2.4% |
| Transportation | 554.8 | 11.3% |
| Recreation | 401.7 | 8.2% |
| Education and research | 110.7 | 2.2% |
| Religious and welfare activities | 137.4 | 2.8% |
| Other categories | 424.6 | 8.6% |

Source: Statistical Abstract of the United States, 1997. Washington, DC, U.S. Government Printing Office, 1998.

agents, calculate optimally at the margin, as economists believe they do? Imagine a loved one suffering a cardiac arrest. Is there time or reasoning power left to calculate? Would anyone question the price of emergency services under such circumstances?

Much of health care, however, does not fit this emergency image. A considerable amount of health care is elective, meaning that the patient has and will perceive some choice over whether and when to have the diagnostics or treatment involved. Obstetric and gynecologic care provide prime examples. Women schedule regular gynecologic examinations, including screening procedures such as Papanicolaou (Pap) smear tests or mammographies. Even if such test results are positive, suggesting the need for further care, there is considerable choice involved. Radical mastectomies are performed less frequently because of better understanding of survival rates with less invasive procedures and improved technologies. The use of less invasive techniques also reflects issues of patient preferences and of cost-efficiency.

Obstetric care represents yet another example of rational choice in many cases. The decision to initiate obstetric care and the approach toward birthing represent consumer choices. Mothers' nutrition and lifestyle choices, although not explicitly medical in scope, also fall into this category. Fertility treatments for women who have difficulty becoming pregnant or carrying to term may represent very explicit economic decisions, in part because they often are not covered by insurance plans that might buffer expenditures for other procedures.

## FUNDAMENTAL ANALYSES OF ECONOMICS

The fundamental contribution of health economics is an analytical method that permits the evaluation of choices by consumers and/or their providers. Any choice, health-related or otherwise, entails the comparisons of incremental costs and incremental benefits. The benign-sounding principle states that an activity is of social benefit if the incremental (economists use the term *marginal*) benefits exceed the incremental (again, *marginal*) costs.

Consider, for example, the decision to seek provider services by a woman who has just discovered that she is pregnant. Assume, for simplicity, that the quantity of services can be summarized adequately by the number of visits that she makes to the provider in the remaining 7 to 8 months before the expected birth. Assume further that there are no particular risk factors that would indicate the need for specialized regimens of care. Such risk factors include age older than 35 years, history of pregnancies, including miscarriages, stillbirths, and prematurity, current health status, such as diabetes or hypertension, or family history of such potential problems.

The costs of visits are relatively simple to enumerate, but they are not trivial. Even with insurance, there are some out-of-pocket (money) costs. These often are exceeded by the costs of traveling to the provider's office, particularly if one does not have a car or if one lives far away. Added to these money costs are the time costs of traveling, waiting, and undergoing an examination.

Consider then a visit to the provider. Suppose that the woman must drive 10 miles each way. Government standards provide remuneration of 32.5 cents per mile, reflecting incremental costs of $6.50. Assume that the visit would cost $25, for which the patient would pay a 20%, or $5 copayment, and $2 for parking. Thus, the money costs are $13.50.

Valuing the time costs requires enumerating the time spent on various activities and then valuing the time. For simplicity again, assume a half-hour drive each way to the provider, 15 minutes to and from parking, 15 minutes of waiting in the provider's office and 1 half-hour with the provider (including time with assistants). This adds up to 2 hours spent in the office. This time has value to the woman—she could be doing something else instead of traveling, parking, and sitting in the office. Even if one argues that at best she could be working at the minimum wage (currently slightly more than $5 per hour), putting that value on her time indicates an additional cost of $10 per visit. Thus, in this example, the costs per visit are $23.50—$13.50 out-of-pocket expenses and $10 in time.

Almost everyone would agree that the incremental

benefits of even one early visit would be enormous. The provider would check the mother's health, would inform her of appropriate nutrition, would prescribe prenatal vitamins containing folic acid, would warn her against drinking alcohol or smoking, would investigate which prescription and nonprescription drugs she is taking, and would warn her against taking illicit or addictive drugs. The provider also might suggest genetic counseling and, depending on the woman's risk factors, might recommend some screening tests. We will return to that issue later in this chapter.

Clearly, the incremental benefits of the first visit exceed $23.50. One also could argue that a number of well-spaced visits (again, assuming no extraordinary conditions) would provide incremental benefits that exceed the incremental costs per visit. A second visit a month or so later would be useful, as would some number of subsequent visits leading up to the birth. However, the analysis also provides further insights. Although we have agreed that the first (and likely the second and third) visit(s) would have incremental benefits that dwarf their incremental costs, it would argue against daily visits to the provider. Why? Because the incremental visit would not likely provide more benefits. If the provider told the woman that she is fine on Tuesday, barring any problems, it is unlikely that there would be much change by Wednesday. Thus, the incremental benefits of a next-day visit would be 0 compared with incremental costs of $23.50. Simply put, the time and money would be better spent on something else—food, clothing, or housing, for example.[2]

Does this analysis argue that the incremental visits have *no* value? Absolutely not. A woman may need reassurance that certain feelings or sensations are normal, or that certain activities are appropriate or inappropriate. Assuaging such concerns is beneficial to her, but at a cost of $23.50 per day, the marginal cost exceeds the marginal benefit. A telephone call to an assistant or to a trained counselor could provide the incremental benefits of assurance at far lower cost—once again, the marginal benefits would exceed the marginal costs.

## IS HEALTH CARE DIFFERENT?

There are several dimensions of health care that raise legitimate concerns about the applicability of economics. We look at four of these—rationality, need, information, and insurance. These features are distinctive to health care, although health care is not unique in any of them. What may be unique, perhaps, is the combination of features and even the sheer number of them. In each case, where health is distinctive in economic terms, there is nonetheless a body of economic theory and empirical work that helps illuminate the issue.

One may question whether all choice is rational and well thought-out. Clearly it is not. There are emergencies, and there are uncertainties. As aforementioned however, we believe that much of the care in obstetrics/gynecology is outside of the emergency category.

A second issue with the economic model concerns the role of "need." The economic model implicitly relates the delivery of care to the ability to pay for it. Many advocates believe that people should get the health care that they need regardless of whether they can afford it. Few would deny prenatal care to poor women based on ability to pay, yet they might feel different about fertility treatment. In practice, need is difficult to define, and distributing care under certain definitions of need may cause more economic harm than good.

Informational problems in health-care markets raise many economic concerns. For example, neither the gynecologist nor his or her patient may recognize the early stages of cervical cancer without a Pap smear. At other times, the information in question is known to some parties but not to all, and this *asymmetry* of information is problematic.

The analyses described previously assume that consumers know what is necessary to know about health care, physician quality, or the benefits of nutrition. In fact, consumers do not necessarily know who is a good physician or which is a good hospital. They may not know whether they are ill or what should be done if they are. This lack of information often makes the consumer, sometimes referred to as the *principal*, depending on the provider, as an agent, in a particular way. The provider supplies both the information and the service, leading to possible conflicts of interests. Health economics must address the provision of health services in this context.

Finally, insurance plays a major role in health care. Unlike the purchase of most other goods, average Americans, and indeed citizens of other countries, do not pay directly for the costs of their health care. Rather, much is paid indirectly through an insurance company or other program, with the consumer paying directly only a portion of the bill, or coinsurance.

Return to the aforementioned example, in which the patient was incurring money costs of $13.50 per visit, of which $5 represented a 20% copayment on a visit cost of $25—recall that we added $10 in time costs, for a total of $23.50 per visit. Suppose that, as a result of a change in insurance coverage, the patient was forced to pay a 50%, or $12.50, copayment. Total

---

[2]Note, of course, that some treatments might require very frequent visits. Women with gestational diabetes may need frequent fetal monitoring. Women undergoing fertility drug treatments are often *required* to make daily visits to check hormone levels and development of eggs.

visit costs would increase from $23.50 to $31.00. At this higher price, the woman might think twice about her last visit to the provider.

This example illustrates an important feature of insurance—that the very availability of insurance may affect how people behave. In this case, more generous insurance led to more visits to the provider. More generous insurance also might lead to the use of treatments or drugs that otherwise might not have been used. The very decision to extend insurance coverage to some treatments and not to others may determine the financial viability of offering these treatments. Debates regarding the appropriate coverages for fertility treatments fall into this category.

How the insurers pay the health-care firm or provider also has become a critical fact of economic life. Whether a procedure or a professional's services are accepted for coverage by insurers may determine whether providers use the procedure. Furthermore, changes in insurance payment procedures can change substantially provider behavior and provider concerns, as evidenced by Medicare's decision to change their hospital payment system during the 1980s to control costs more effectively.

## INCOME AND PRACTICE CHARACTERISTICS OF OBSTETRICS/GYNECOLOGY

A general discussion of the field of obstetrics/gynecology (OB/GYN) suggests that since 1980 the numbers, practices and incomes of physicians in that field have mirrored the more general medical field. The total number of physicians grew from approximately 467,700 to 720,300 in 1995, or an increase of approximately 54.0%. Numbers of practitioners in the OB/GYN field grew from 19,500 in 1980 to 29,100 in 1995, or by approximately 49.2%.[3]

OB/GYN practice patterns, in the aggregate, again have tracked the more general pattern. Mean patient visits per week for all physicians stood at 117.1 per week in 1985, decreasing slightly to 109.6 per week, or by 6.4%, by 1994. OB/GYN visits per week were 112.0 in 1985, decreasing to 102.9, or by 8.1%, by 1994. Mean weekly hours in patient care for all physicians increased 1.6% from 51.3 to 52.1. Mean weekly hours in patient care for those in OB/GYN practices rose by 2.1% from 56.9 to 58.1.

Over the past 15 years, OB/GYN practitioners have maintained net income advantages over all other major groups, with the exception of surgeons. Mean net income for OB/GYN practitioners in 1994 was approximately $200,400 per year, compared with $182,400 for all physicians (and $255,200 for surgeons). The higher income comes with higher liability. OB/GYN practitioners in 1994 paid $37,400 on average in liability premiums. This was 67.7% higher than surgeons (at $22,300 per year) and 147.4% higher than the figure averaged over all physicians.

## OVERVIEW OF THE CHAPTER

Thus far, we have established an economic model of decision making that has considerable relevance to a wide range of health-care decisions. We have related it to the health-care industry with particular examples relating to the practices of obstetrics and gynecology. We also have established the income and practice characteristics of practitioners in the field. The remainder of the chapter builds on this base by addressing three substantive topics (among many). Section 2 provides an overview of health insurance in the 1990s. Three particular features are investigated. The first is health insurance coverage for women. The second concerns trends in managed care arrangements, both for women with private insurance as well as for women who rely on Medicaid. The third feature involves physician contracts with insurers, comparing different types of managed-care contracts. Section 3 investigates practice patterns among obstetricians/gynecologists. We look at two particular features. The first involves physician practice patterns, or the choice between inpatient and outpatient care. The second concerns cost-effectiveness analysis, with particular emphasis on screening initiatives. Section 4 addresses topics related to physician remuneration and patient care. The means of remunerating physicians may have substantive impacts on how patient care is delivered. This section addresses what is known about how care varies under capitated and fee-for-service arrangements. The general health economics literature is discussed, and studies specific to obstetric/gynecologic care also are examined.

# Health Insurance in the 1990s

Reimbursements for health-care services are central to the practice of medicine. Without adequate revenue, no health-care supplier would be able to stay in business very long. Employees of a physician's practice must be paid, supplies must be purchased, the rent or mortgage on office space must be covered, other costs of operating the business must be paid, and there must be enough revenue left after all these expenses to provide the physician(s) an income.

Unlike the purchase of most other goods, health care generally is paid for indirectly, through insurance

---

[3]These, and other figures, are from the *Statistical Abstract*, 1997, Tables 175 and 182.

plans sponsored by employers and through government programs such as Medicaid and Medicare. Thus, most of a physician's revenue is derived from these sources.

What are the current sources of health insurance among women? How has their coverage been changing? How do different insurance plans pay for healthcare services? And what do these trends mean for obstetricians/gynecologists? These issues are discussed in this section.

## WOMEN AND THEIR HEALTH COVERAGE

### Health Insurance Among Women

In 1995, there were 135.5 million women in the U.S. population. Eighty-six percent had either private or public health insurance to help cover the costs of medical care (Table 66–2.) Fourteen percent had no health insurance, that is, they were uninsured.

Most women have private coverage. In 1995, 70% of women were covered by private health insurance, typically group-based employer-sponsored coverage obtained either through their own employer or that of their spouse. Access to private health insurance is related to income. In general, individuals with higher household incomes are more likely to be covered by private health insurance, whereas those with lower income are more likely to be covered by either Medicaid or Medicare, two publicly sponsored health insurance programs in the United States. For example, only 18.9% of families with incomes of less than $5,000 were covered by private health insurance, compared with 91.3% among families with incomes of $50,000 or more.

Approximately 14% of women relied on Medicaid for their health coverage. Medicaid programs are run by individual states to finance health services for persons whose poor economic status is seen as largely beyond their control. The nature of benefits and the eligibility standards are determined by each state (within certain broad federal parameters); some states have relatively generous programs, others have more narrow ones. One common feature is that all states allow women and their children who are receiving benefits under their Aid to Families with Dependent Children (AFDC) program to participate in Medicaid. This group makes up most of the entire Medicaid-covered population, approximately 70%. The rest who receive Medicaid have met other (non–AFDC-related) eligibility criteria for the program—for example, they are considered disabled or otherwise "medically needy" by their state or are pregnant and have household income that places them near poverty.

Some states began extending eligibility to this last group beginning in 1986. Currently, 34 states allow pregnant women with household incomes near poverty to enroll in Medicaid. The specific threshold is either 133% or 185% of the poverty level; states vary in which of these they have chosen. (For a family of 3 in 1996, the poverty level was $12,980 in annual income.) These expansions were intended to increase prenatal and other health services available to pregnant women who otherwise might postpone care during their pregnancy because of few personal resources and, possibly, a lack of private health insurance.

Medicare, which covers 15% of all women, is the federal program that covers the elderly in the United States, although some persons younger than 65 years of age are also eligible, for example, persons who receive federal disability insurance benefits or have end-stage kidney disease. Most Medicare-covered women, however, are elderly.

### Health Insurance Among Pregnant Women

The insurance coverage of pregnant women, who obviously need the services of obstetricians, was examined most recently for 1992 (Fig. 66–1). One third of all pregnant women in that year had Medicaid coverage, and 54% had employer-sponsored health insurance. Approximately 8% of all pregnant women were uninsured. This is a considerably lower rate of uninsured than among women generally (14%) and reflects primarily the expansions of Medicaid in the late 1980s to very low-income pregnant women.

The pie chart on the right of Figure 66–1 describes insurance coverage among pregnant women living below the poverty level, illustrating the important role of Medicaid for these women. Seventy-nine percent relied entirely on Medicaid for their obstetric care and other health services that year.

Few pregnant women had Medicare. This is not surprising because this program mainly covers elderly

Table 66–2  Health Insurance Coverage in the United States by Gender, 1995

| Type of Coverage | Females | Males | Total |
| --- | --- | --- | --- |
| Total number of persons (million) | 135.5 | 129.1 | 264.3 |
| % with health insurance | 86.0% | 83.2% | 84.6% |
| % with private insurance | 70.0 | 70.7 | 70.3 |
| % with group insurance | 59.7 | 62.5 | 61.1 |
| % with Medicare | 14.6 | 11.5 | 13.1 |
| % with Medicaid | 13.7 | 10.4 | 12.1 |
| % uninsured | 14.0 | 16.8 | 15.4 |

Source: U.S. Bureau of the Census Tabulations of the 1996 Current Population Survey.

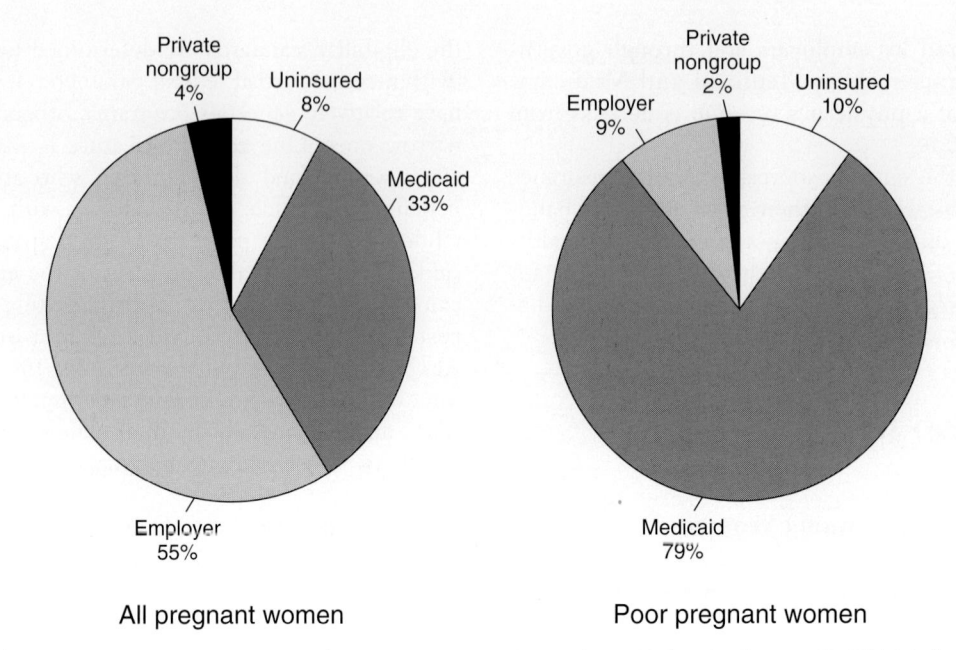

**Figure 66–1** Insurance coverage of pregnant women, 1992. (From Dubay L, Kenney G: Did Medicaid expansions for pregnant women crowd out private coverage? Health Affairs 16:185–193, 1997.)

persons. Rather, the primary sources for reimbursement of obstetric care are employer plans and Medicaid. According to the pie chart on the left in Figure 66–1, Medicaid paid for a full third of all births nationally in 1992. This rate, however, varies by state—from 20% of births in New Hampshire to half of all births in Tennessee and West Virginia.

Apparently not all pregnant women who are eligible for Medicaid take advantage of the program. Dubay and Kenny found that in 1992 only two thirds of those who could have enrolled in the program actually signed up. Participation rates varied by eligibility category. Although nearly all pregnant women with current AFDC status were enrolled in Medicaid, fewer than half of those made eligible only by virtue of their having low income participated in the program. Although some of the women in this second group had employer coverage, even among those without employer coverage, more than half (56%) failed to enroll in Medicaid. They may have been unaware of their eligibility for state-sponsored insurance.

Among pregnant women without health insurance, 41% had incomes below the poverty level, and 30% had incomes of 100 to 185% of poverty. However, four fifths of uninsured pregnant women were eligible for Medicaid. They simply had failed to sign up for it.

## THE EMERGENCE OF MANAGED-CARE PLANS

Over the past decade, women (as well as men) have been moving into managed-care plans in record numbers. So many, in fact, that by 1995, managed care had become the dominant form of health insurance in the United States. Managed care encompasses a variety of insurance arrangements; there is no one single model for these plans. However, what they all have in common is the following: much, if not all, of the patient's care is provided through *a specific network of hospitals, physicians, and other health-care providers.*

### Employer-Sponsored Managed Care

Managed care currently accounts for about three quarters of all employer-sponsored health insurance, with traditional fee-for-service plans making up the rest. There are three types of managed-care plans that we see among women with employer-sponsored coverage:

- The first type are *health maintenance organizations* (HMOs). These provide women with relatively comprehensive health care and entail few out-of-pocket expenses, but they require that all care be delivered through the plan's network, and that the patient's "primary care physician" authorize any services provided. Each subscriber is assigned a primary care physician on enrollment in the HMO. If health-care services are provided but not authorized by a primary care physician, they are not covered by the HMO. The patient is personally liable for payment of the unauthorized services.

Collectively, HMOs cover approximately 28% of all women with employer coverage. HMOs that directly employ physicians in their network are called *staff model* plans. Their network physicians simply are paid a salary by the HMO. Alternatively, plans that set up their network by contracting with physicians in geographically spread-out, independent, solo or small group practices are called *independent practice associations* (IPAs). Both types assign primary care physicians as gatekeepers for covered services. IPAs are more common than staff model HMOs and are also the fastest growing type of HMO.

- The second type are *preferred provider organizations* (PPOs). These plans give their subscribers two distinct tiers of insurance coverage. When the woman uses a provider in the PPO's "preferred provider network," then her required cost-sharing (e.g., deductible and coinsurance) is lower than when she uses non-network providers. Although there is a network, there are no physician gatekeepers. Rather, the patient simply has to pay more out of pocket if she chooses to go outside the plan's network. In this way, PPOs create a financial incentive for the patient to use network providers rather than go outside the network for her care.

The contracts that PPOs set up with physicians and hospitals generally refer to the prices providers charge. In return for promising to charge a lower-than-average price under the plan, selected providers become part of the PPO's preferred network. There is no guarantee that the provider will see patients under the plan, but if the network is not too large and the PPO's cost-sharing provisions for subscribers are network-favorable, then the provider may see a large increase in patient care business by becoming part of the network. Prompt payment for their services may be another advantage.

Providers also often agree to submit themselves to some form of utilization review under the contract. Most PPOs (88%) require pre-admission certification for a hospital stay and concurrent utilization review for such stays (83%), and about half (47%) require a mandatory second opinion for a recommendation of surgery.

Of all the managed-care plans that employers sponsor, PPOs currently are the most common. In 1995, PPOs covered approximately 27% of all women who had employer coverage.

- The third type are *point-of-service* (POS) *plans*. These plans are a hybrid of HMOs and PPOs. Like PPOs, there are two tiers of insurance benefits in a POS plan. Coverage is greater (i.e., out-of-pocket costs are lower) when members use network providers and less generous (i.e., out-of-pocket costs are higher) when they use non-network providers. Like an HMO, however, POS plans assign each member a physician gatekeeper who must authorize in-network care in order for it to be covered on in-network terms. Most POS plans generally do not require authorization for a member to use out-of-network services; such care simply is covered on less generous terms.

Loosely speaking, POS plans are the new kid on the block. As recently as 1993, they were relatively rare, but by 1995, they had increased their market share to 20% of the group coverage market nationwide. Some POS plans have been developed by HMOs, and others have been developed by existing PPOs.

## Medicaid Managed-Care Plans

In the past few years, many states have adopted managed-care models for the Medicaid coverage that they provide to their AFDC enrollees and pregnant women who meet their low-income criteria for Medicaid eligibility. The reason is a belief that in so doing, they may help contain program costs, which are a major part of most states' budget. As of June 1996, 13.3 million Medicaid beneficiaries nationwide were enrolled in some form of managed care. This represents a sharp increase from the 2.7 million in 1991.

As with employer plans, there is no one model for Medicaid managed care. Rather, programs vary considerably across the states. In some areas, states have contracted directly with HMOs that already exist in their local markets. In others, states have created their own loosely structured provider networks, which in turn contract with selected providers for discounted services, and which use physician-gatekeeping to control utilization. Some Medicaid programs, such as the one in Michigan, use combinations of both of these approaches.

## MANAGED-CARE CONTRACTS WITH PHYSICIANS

Managed-care contracts with physicians vary considerably. Most HMO and POS plans pay their network physicians on a capitation basis. Under capitation, the plan pays the physician's practice a fixed fee, generally an actuarial per-member-per-month (PMPM) dollar amount in return for the treatments that they provide to members of the insurance plan. Physicians also may be responsible for the costs of referrals, laboratory tests, and hospital services. Thus, HMOs and POS plans shift the costs of care, as well as the risk associated with those costs, directly onto physician practices. In so doing, these contracts put physician earnings at risk. If the care provided to a woman under this arrangement turns out to cost less than the fixed dollars received from the plan, then the practice makes a profit. Likewise, if her care turns out to cost more than the dollars received, then the practice must take a loss.

In contrast, PPO contracts with physicians (as noted earlier) rarely involve capitation. Instead, they specify the discounted fees for various service that the plan pays, in exchange for the privilege of being in that plan's network. If a physician joins the PPO's network and happens to provide services to one of that plan's subscribers, then the practice must accept the prenegotiated fees as payment in full. "Balance billing" of the patient is not allowed.

Plan utilization review procedures also are commonly covered in managed-care contracts, whether they are HMOs, PPOs, or POS plans. Physicians must be willing to subject themselves to the particular care-review procedures to be followed under that plan. Most managed-care contracts also require a certain degree of physician record-keeping on their enrollees, for example, patient encounter forms (plan-specific) may have to be filed with the insurer each time care is provided to the woman.

Medicaid managed-care contracts with physicians parallel those of private managed-care plans, although the specific package of services covered is determined heavily by the state's preferences. In some of the states that have set up their own Medicaid provider networks, the state contracts directly with individual gatekeeper physicians, agreeing to pay them a small fixed fee (e.g., $3.00 per month) for each Medicaid enrollee under their "control." In return for this payment, the physician serves as the woman's gatekeeper for Medicaid-covered services, hopefully authorizing only those services that are medically necessary or prudent.

## Physician Participation in Capitated Plans

Primary care physicians, because they more often have a gatekeeper role in HMO and POS plans, exhibit the highest prevalence of capitation contracts, based on a 1995 nationwide survey of physicians. General family practitioners (50%), general internists (48%) and pediatricians (64%) have capitated contracts.

Apparently even though the American Medical Association (AMA) has long considered obstetricians/gynecologists (OB/GYNs) to be primary care physicians, some insurers still do not. Only 21% of OB/GYNs have one or more capitated contracts with insurance plans. Among OB/GYNs who had entered into these agreements, they reported that they are receiving slightly more than one sixth (16.3%) of their total practice revenue from these contracts. They also reported having two to three capitation contracts (2.7 on average). Capitation was more common among larger practices.

Some plans, however, are beginning to allow direct access to OB/GYNs. In these plans, women may see their OB/GYNs without having to obtain prior authorization from their primary care physician. But to do this, women first must notify the plan that they are designating their OB/GYN as their "direct contact" for OB/GYN-related services. It may be that these plans have decided to "unbundle" the PMPM they are paying for women's primary care services into those which are OB/GYN-related and those which are not—in essence, creating two primary care providers for women enrollees. Whether this is an emerging trend is unclear.

## Limiting the Financial Risks

Some physicians are able to limit the risk associated with capitation by obtaining stop-loss provisions in their contracts or by purchasing reinsurance against large losses. A stop-loss provision limits the physician's liability per enrollee under the plan. An example would be $25,000 per year for any single enrollee. With stop-loss protection, once the cost of services provided to any one patient reaches a certain threshold (e.g., $25,000 over 12 months), the insurer would cover all additional expenses. Reinsurance works the same way, although the coverage need not be part of the explicit contract with the insurer; it may be purchased separately from a reinsurance company. Reinsurance for physician practices may specify either a stop-loss threshold per patient, or a stop-loss for all patients (collectively) with that insurer. Once incurred expenses reach the specified threshold, all or most of any additional expenses would be paid by another party, the reinsurer.

Amazingly, in 1995, just over half of all primary care physicians who had capitation contracts *did not even know* whether they had stop-loss or reinsurance protection. Among those who did know, 86% reported that neither they nor their practice had either of these sources of risk protection. Only 14% reported having such coverage. Small practices were especially likely to be without stop-loss or reinsurance provisions.

Have physicians been entering into these contractual arrangements without limits to their downside losses? These data suggest that many may well be doing so. This raises a real concern for the way that physician practices are being managed. If imprudent risks are being borne by physicians, especially among solo or small practices, financial distress eventually may result for some of them.

# Physician Practice

The model in Section 1 established an important principle of economic analysis—that one should provide services to the point at which marginal benefits equal marginal costs. This section concentrates on two particular issues relating to practice. The first example examines appropriate levels of care for women's conditions. The second examines cost-effectiveness of interventions—particular examples involve screening tests such as Pap smears for cervical cancer or mammography for breast cancer.

## APPROPRIATE CARE

The comparison of marginal benefits to marginal costs is an important one. If treatment stops at levels of treatment (numbers of visits for outpatient care or number of days for inpatient) at which the incremental benefit exceeds the incremental cost, then we have not provided "enough" treatment. An extra day or visit (or alternatively an extra dollar spent) would provide extra benefits exceeding their costs, and the patients and society would be better off.

A prime example rests in the appropriate length of stay for a mother who has had a normal childbirth. As recently as 1980, almost 70% of mothers experiencing vaginal delivery had hospital stays of 3 days or more.[4]

Inpatient care is expensive, costing several hundred dollars per day. As long as hospitals were reimbursed for what they charged, however, there was no incentive to send the woman home earlier. Such practices almost certainly failed the comparison of marginal benefits to marginal costs. Almost certainly the marginal benefits to the woman of being in the hospital for a third day did not measure up to the costs of keeping her there.

Under managed care, it became apparent that such was the case. There has been considerable pressure to reduce the stay, and by 1995, the average length of stay for a mother with a vaginal delivery was 1.7 days, with 46.8% of all mothers staying 1 day or less. For the majority, home care (starting the second day) along with appropriate outpatient follow-up, has become the alternative. Home care is not without cost, however, requiring the woman's time, and probably assistance from neighbors, friends, or hired care-givers. Nonetheless, it provides an appropriate level of care at a far lower cost than the inpatient care that it replaces.

Although the economics would seem to be transparent, there has been a continued debate over the policy. Medical care is not exact, and mistakes are made. The key phrase in describing the model was a "normal" childbirth. Opponents of managed care have been quick to seize on cases in which a child who was sent home the second day after birth developed an ailment and needed to return to the hospital or, worse still, died. Keeping the child an extra day, the argument goes, would avoid these problems.

Legislation has been passed to require that insurers guarantee at least 2 nights of hospital stay to all mothers with normal deliveries. For example, the 1996 Early Discharge of Mothers and Babies Bill passed in Maryland guaranteed that mothers and babies have coverage in the hospital for 48 hours for a normal vaginal delivery and 96 hours for a normal cesarean delivery.

This is very expensive insurance against potential ills. The incremental cost of a hospital stay must be compared with the prevalence of newborn infant problems and the cost of treating them. With approximately 4,000,000 children born each year in the United States, an incremental day of stay at a cost of $500 per day implies additional costs of more than $2 billion per year. Improved care while in the hospital, as well as improved newborn screening methods while in the hospital, could provide similar benefits and far lower costs, freeing up extra resources for the rest of society. To its credit, the Maryland law recognizes such substitutions, indicating that if the mother, in consultation with her physician, requests to leave early, she receives one home visit within 24 hours of discharge and a second home visit if ordered by her provider.[5]

## SCREENING

Over the past several years, there has been a considerable debate over the conduct of disease-screening procedures. Particularly salient examples have come from the field of obstetrics/gynecology, with examples such as mammography (for breast cancer) and the Pap smear test (for cervical cancer). To discuss these issues, it is again essential to frame the analyses in the vernacular of marginal benefits and marginal costs, and to show how careful analyses can lead to controversial findings.

### Efficacy of Screening

Disease screening involves various types of tests carried out by the patient and/or the provider to detect the earliest stages of potentially life-threatening diseases. Women are urged to conduct breast self-examinations on a routine basis and to contact a provider if suspicious lumps are found. If so, the provider is contacted, and a well-defined set of procedures are initiated.

---

[4]For these and other figures, see Gillum et al, Table R.

[5]For further information, see Summary of the final version of the 1996 Early Discharge of Mothers and Babies Bill, http://www.med.jhu.edu/mdaap/legis/archives/earlydc.html

Screening *programs* involve the administration of tests to asymptomatic patients for a wide range of diseases. Generally simple, and replicable, tests may examine blood, urine, or cells, or may take images using radiation (such as x-rays or mammography). Screening results in four possibilities:

- True-positive—The patient has the disease, and the test has found it.
- True-negative—The patient does not have the disease, and the test verifies that fact.
- False-positive—The patient does not have the disease, but the test indicates that she does.
- False-negative—The patient has the disease, and the test does not find it.

Two measures typically are used to measure the strength of a screening test. *Sensitivity* indicates the percentage of those with the disease who are diagnosed accurately, the true-positives. *Specificity* indicates the percentage of those without the disease who also are diagnosed accurately.

What are the marginal benefits, and what are the marginal costs? There are three fundamental benefits from the successful treatment of an ailment. First, the patient may be more productive at her job. Second, regardless of productivity on the job, she would feel better. Third, she would live longer, which would allow her either to be more productive on the job or to feel better. A successful screening program identifies those patients for whom treatment will be efficacious.

## Example—Pap Smears

The Pap smear screening for cervical cancer fulfills several criteria for a potentially successful screening intervention. There must be a stage before symptoms develop during which the disease, or its precursor, is detectable. There must be a test that can detect the disease or its precursor with reasonable accuracy. There must be a treatment that, if delivered early, leads to better results than waiting until symptoms develop. The Pap smear meets these conditions.[6]

What are the marginal costs of a screening program? Screening tests take time, and the tests cost money. The screening tests may cause some physical discomfort and possibly may entail risks of its own. For example, mammography exposes the patient to radiation; amniocentesis carries the risk of spontaneous abortion of the pregnancy. If subsequent treatment is indicated, then that treatment costs time and money, although the early detection may permit less radical forms of therapy, thus reducing the costs (and the cost reduction is treated as a benefit to the patient).

The fundamental analysis of marginal benefits vs. marginal costs with the Pap smear, as with other screening examinations, compares the prevalence of the disease with the possibility of a false-positive finding. In economic terms, the false-positive result represents the worst of all possible worlds because every dollar spent on treatment after the false-positive finding is *wasted*. Had there been no test, there would have been no false-positive finding and no treatment.

Russell cites studies that indicate that false-positive findings occur more than 1% but less than 10% of the time. If 5% represents an appropriate value, then repeated testing increases the chance that a woman will have a false-positive finding at some point in her life. Suppose that 100 women are tested in Round 1. In a randomly selected population, 5 of them will have false-positive results—95 will not. In Round 2, 5% of the 95 who previously tested negative will have false positives findings. This provides a probability of 9.75 women per 100 (5 in Round 1 and another 4.75 in Round 2) who register false-positive findings at some time. Thus, further tests increase the numbers of false-positive results, correspondingly.[7]

Without screening, the average woman's chance of developing invasive cervical cancer is 2.5% over her lifetime, and the chance of dying of it is 1.2%. Russell emphasizes that of every 100 women, cervical cancer eventually develops in 2 or 3 at most, whereas all 100 are vulnerable to the probability of a false-positive result.

Clearly the marginal benefit—marginal cost trade-off for screening relates the prevalence of the condition to the possibility of false-positive results. The more sensitive the test, the less likely one is to have wasteful false-positive findings. The higher the disease prevalence, the more likely one is to find it with a screening test. The effectiveness of looking for needles in haystacks depends on how good one's search methods are and how many needles are in the haystacks.

Marginal benefits vs. marginal cost analyses also tell us about resource allocation in screening programs. Russell calculates that for women with regular Pap smears, increasing the frequency of testing from every 2 years to annually brings an additional year of life at the cost of $1 million and an "uncounted" number of false-positive findings. This high incremental cost results because incremental tests are only likely to find small numbers of incremental cancers.

In contrast, one quarter of the women in the United States are not screened even every 3 years—screening them may provide substantial marginal benefits. Testing these women is likely to find incrementally more cancers, yielding higher marginal

---

[6]This analysis and discussion follows from Russell (1994).

[7]With a series of 10 tests, 40.1 women per 100 would have at least one false-positive test result.

benefits. Although the marginal costs of educating, finding, and screening them may exceed the costs of screening women who currently receive regular treatment, reallocating the dollars according to the principle of marginal benefits and marginal costs likely would result in net improvements in health, at constant or even reduced total costs.

## Physician Remuneration and Patient Care

Earlier in this chapter, we discussed how the payment policies for physician services are changing dramatically with the rapid growth of managed care. Although physician decision-making is influenced by many factors, economic theory, as well as a growing body of empirical studies, suggest that the methods by which physicians are paid also play a role. Health economists have addressed two basic questions in this area:

- How are a physician's decisions regarding a patient's treatment influenced by the way he or she is remunerated? When he or she no longer is paid a fee for each service, but rather a lump sum with the expectation that he or she will provide "appropriate" care, does the patient's course of care change, and if so, how?
- How effective is managed care at controlling health-care costs?

A few studies have addressed these for conditions that OB/GYNs treat—for pregnancy and delivery, elective sterilization, hysterectomy, and breast cancer, for example. We first review what research has found generally regarding the relationship between physician payment methods, the care received by patients, and the costs of their care, and then summarize the studies specific to women's services.

### GENERAL STUDIES

There are only a few studies that have examined the effects of either salary arrangements or capitation, per se, on patients' use of services. A large body of literature, however, has examined differences in service utilization among HMO, fee-for-service (FFS), and PPO enrollees—and salary or capitation, indeed, is often characteristic of HMOs. For example, nearly all staff model HMOs pay their physicians on either a salary or capitation basis, and just over half of IPA model HMOs also pay physicians on a capitation basis.

Existing studies fall into three categories: (1) controlled experiments and demonstrations that compare health-care utilization and the cost of patient care under different insurance arrangement; (2) analyses of actual utilization differences by type of insurance plan based on non-experimental data; and (3) evaluations of true "natural experiments," in which hospitals or other organizations changed the way their physicians were remunerated. Before reviewing each of these branches of the literature, a few general remarks are in order.

### General Comments About the Literature

Many studies have shown that HMO and PPO enrollees use significantly fewer health-care services and that their costs of health care are also substantially lower compared with enrollees in conventional FFS plans. Should we conclude, therefore, that managed care is a more cost-effective delivery system? Not necessarily. There are two phenomena that may be occurring in the market—"patient self-selection" and "provider self-selection"—and both may account for at least some of the differences researchers have observed across plans. Unless a study adequately controls for *both* sources of self-selection, it may overstate the potential cost savings associated with managed care.

Patient self-selection is well-documented: HMOs and PPOs tend to attract healthier populations.[8] Thus, the lower rates of health care utilization observed among patients in these plans may partly be due to reduced patient demand for services to begin with.

Physician self-selection is a matter for speculation. There are no studies to date that have examined whether managed-care plans are, in fact, contracting with physicians who have a natural tendency or preference toward less invasive or expensive treatments. But they may well be doing so, if they are using economic criteria for the selection of their network physicians and hospitals. Most insurers certainly have the capacity to discern physician practice styles, if they wanted to, using claims data from their FFS plans. Physician litigation records for medical malpractice are also accessible to any health insurer through the National Practitioner Data Bank, maintained by the federal government.

Most studies in the first category (described previously) have controlled effectively for patient self-selection by randomly assigning individuals to insurance plans, but they have not dealt with potential "physician self-selection" into managed-care plans. Studies in the second category have had difficulty

---
[8]For evidence, see Dowd and Feldman (1985), Hellinger (1987), Langwell and Hadley (1989), Strumwasser et al (1989), and Dowd et al (1991).

controlling for either source of self-selection. The studies in the last category are the only ones that control for *both* patient and physician self-selection.

## Controlled Experiments and Demonstrations

The Rand Health Insurance Experiment included a controlled trial of the differences in health service utilization between HMO and FFS enrollees. PPO plan enrollees were not examined. Families in Seattle who participated in the study were assigned randomly to different insurance plans that varied the price of services to them. One of the plans was a staff model HMO, specifically the Group Health Cooperative of Puget Sound. The others were various FFS plans: a "free care" plan (no out-of-pocket costs to families), a 25% coinsurance plan, a 50% coinsurance plan, a 95% coinsurance plan, and a "deductible" plan, which covered inpatient care in full, but required a $150 deductible per individual ($450 per family) for outpatient care. Families were assigned to these plans in 1974, and their health-care utilization then was tracked for several years. The study found that compared with persons in the free care plan, HMO enrollees (men and women alike) had health-care expenditures that were 30% less. These savings primarily were the result of fewer hospitalizations among the HMO enrollees.

The strength of the Rand Experiment was that families were randomized into the different health plans, thereby controlling for insurance selection effects among patients. However, the researchers were unable to control for physician self-selection into Group Health Cooperative. Thus, we do not know whether the findings are actually the result of the HMO's payment policies for its physicians or possible self-sorting of physicians in the Seattle area into that HMO.

Another important study in this category was a recent randomized trial of AFDC Medicaid-eligible women to a Medicaid HMO vs. standard FFS Medicaid, conducted by Leibowitz and colleagues. Their study is unique because women who self-selected Medicaid HMO coverage also were studied and compared with those women who actually were randomized into the HMO.

During the time that they were enrolled in the HMO, AFDC women used significantly less medical care than those under FFS Medicaid. Within the HMO, both the randomized and self-selected enrollees used 30% fewer services than the average Medicaid-eligible woman under FFS Medicaid. However, women who eventually chose to "drop out" of the HMO (i.e., the HMO disenrollees) had significantly greater health care use than either those who remained with the HMO or than the average FFS enrollee. Thus, the study found strong evidence of self-selection in who disenrolled, rather than in who signed-up initially for the HMO. Heavy users tended to leave the HMO to go back to the FFS system.

Apparently, the lower health-care utilization of HMO enrollees stemmed largely from the HMO's retention of women with less "need for care," rather than from technical efficiency, per se. Their finding of self-selection favorable to HMOs is consistent with the patterns observed for non-Medicaid populations mentioned earlier—namely, that medically high-risk persons tend to prefer FFS insurance. Some explanations offered for this finding are that heavy users already have well-established relationships with FFS physician(s), and the wait for appointments is shorter under FFS.

## Inferences from Nonexperimental Data

Most studies have examined the effects of managed care on health-care utilization using nonexperimental data. As aforementioned, their methodologic challenge is to control adequately for favorable self-selection into managed-care plans on the part of both patients and physicians. In the best studies, researchers have acknowledged the issue of patient self-selection, and have attempted to control for it by using a "sample selection model" to explain service utilization. These models seek to correct econometrically for the potential bias introduced by endogenous insurance plan choice. With a sample selection model, an investigator may be able to separate effects of type of health plan from the effects of differences in the populations enrolled in those plans. We say "may" because it is difficult to do in practice and depends heavily on having detailed demographic and health status information about enrollees within the data set being analyzed. None of the studies based on nonexperimental data have controlled for potential physician self-selection into various types of plans.

There are more than 100 studies in this category. Most have compared care under HMOs to care under FFS. A recent excellent review of this literature by Miller and Luft concluded that HMO enrollees clearly have significantly lower health-care expenditures than do enrollees in traditional FFS plans, but also that a portion of their lower costs are the result of favorable self-selection. HMOs have drawn a healthier risk-mix of the population. Where HMOs have achieved "true savings" is in the area of hospital care. HMOs have achieved lower rates of hospital admission and shorter hospital stays for those patients who are admitted.

Only a few studies have examined the use and cost of health services within PPOs. This is somewhat surprising because these plans account for about half of all enrollment in managed-care plans (HMOs and POS plans account for the other half). PPOs, like HMOs, are associated with significantly lower healthcare expenses relative to traditional FFS plans.[9] Their savings have been achieved mainly through lower care utilization rates for their members, not through lower negotiated prices with network providers. Rates of hospital admission are lower among PPO enrollees, as one might expect. Also, rates for physician office visits are lower. On balance, however, PPOs have not achieved the level of savings found for HMOs.

### Real-World Changes in Payment Methods

A few studies have been able to isolate the role of physician reimbursement methods on treatment patterns by evaluating "what happened" after a particular group of physicians experienced a change in the way that they were paid. Unlike those in the previous two categories, these studies are unique because it is highly unlikely that patient or physician self-selection could account for their findings. All of them are based a pre–post evaluation design, in which the patient and physician pools were similar in both periods; the only thing that changed was some aspect of how the physicians were paid.

Studies in this group that examined an increase in the patients' coinsurance rate, under a FFS system both before and after the change in the rate, reveal a high level of price sensitivity among patients: when their out-of-pocket price was raised (because of an increase in their required coinsurance), physician office visit rates declined significantly.[10]

Similar results have been observed for increases in the per-visit copays charged by HMOs. Cherkin and associates, for example, found that when Group Health Cooperative of Puget Sound introduced a $5 copay for physician office visits (where previously there was no copay), federal government enrollees decreased their office visits for primary care by 11%. Patient visits to specialists, however, were unchanged. An earlier study by Hankin and coworkers, involving a different HMO, found that when the visit copay was raised from $5 to $10, visits per 1000 plan enrollees declined from 414.4 to 404.7.

A study by Sterns and colleagues examined how patterns of resource use changed among a group of physicians when they no longer were paid on an FFS basis, but rather through capitation by the medical center at which they practiced. In this study, the insurance coverage of the patients seen by the physicians did not actually change—the medical center still received a fee for each service, it only altered the way that it compensated the physicians. The primary care physicians were capitated, and specialists were paid according to a reduced fee schedule. The analysis found that after the change in compensation methods, there was a substitution of outpatient for inpatient care among the patients. Their rate of hospitalization declined, their rate of physician office visits increased, particularly referrals, and their use of clinic services also increased.

## STUDIES SPECIFIC TO OBSTETRICS/GYNECOLOGY

A few studies have examined how managed-care plans treat specific medical conditions among women.

### Maternity Services

Does prenatal care differ under managed care, and do women giving birth receive a different style of care on admission to the hospital? The answers to these questions provided by the literature are somewhat mixed.

Among privately insured women, prenatal care and birth outcomes have not been found to vary under managed care, although the length of hospital stay, after delivery, is clearly shorter for women and newborns who have managed-care coverage. In 1994, for example, 82% of women privately insured by an HMO were discharged within 1 day of delivery, compared with 61% of POS and 48% of indemnity-insured women. The pattern for their newborns is about the same, as one might expect: the percentage discharged after one day was 79%, 60%, and 47%, respectively. These shorter stays under managed care, however, do not appear to be having any adverse effects on either the mothers or their newborns, at least when measured by hospital readmission rates postdischarge. Readmission rates are the same across insurance plans, both for women delivering and their infants. Generally, however, these studies have not controlled for patient self-selection. If women who are healthier or otherwise "better equipped" to produce healthy babies (e.g., more educated) tend to enroll in managed-care plans, then it is possible that on adjusting for such self-selection, we might see differences in care patterns and birth outcomes.

Studies that have examined women covered by Medicaid who are rapidly being moved into managed-care arrangements, however, suggest that maternity services and birth outcomes have not been improving with the advent of manage care—if anything,

---
[9] See Hosek et al (1990) and Smith (1997/98) for analyses of care under PPOs.
[10] See Scitovsky and Snyder (1972), Scitovsky and McCall (1977), and Scheffler (1984).

they may be suffering. A recent evaluation of Iowa's Medicaid program during the period 1989–1992 by Schulman and associates, for example, found that compared with women covered by Medicaid FFS plans, women covered by Medicaid managed-care plans tended to initiate prenatal care later in their pregnancies, and their care was more frequently judged as "inadequate," measured by the Kessner (adequacy-of-prenatal-care) Index. Perhaps as a result, the women covered by managed care delivered more low-birth-weight (1500–2499 g) and twice as many very-low-birth-weight (< 1500 g) newborns.

In Washington state, Medicaid women covered by managed care also have been initiating their prenatal care later than women covered by FFS plans. However, unlike the women in Iowa, they have had fewer instances of "inadequate" care and have delivered slightly fewer low-birth-weight infants. Another study by Goldfarb and colleagues of Medicaid managed care in Philadelphia reported no difference in the adequacy of prenatal care or birth outcomes for women covered by managed care. Thus, there is no clear pattern.

## Other Conditions Exclusive to Women

Ransom and associates examined how the care provided by a group of gynecologists changed after they no longer could bill for their services on an FFS basis, but instead received a salary from the medical center at which they were based. The study's design was similar to that of Sterns and colleagues (discussed earlier), except the focus was on gynecologists. The study found that the physicians' use of more elective procedures, such as sterilization by laparoscopy, was significantly greater under FFS reimbursement, but that severe gynecologic conditions tended to be treated the same way, regardless of the reimbursement method.

Treatments for breast cancer and decisions for hysterectomy also have been studied as a function of insurance coverage. Breast cancer patients in HMOs have been found to be less likely to receive breast-conserving surgery compared with those in non-HMOs. Also, among women who had a mastectomy, those with HMO coverage tended to have shorter lengths of hospital stay. Decisions for hysterectomy are less likely among uninsured women, but do not appear to vary for women with either HMO or commercial FFS coverage. Both of these studies, however, were based on nonexperimental data, with no controls for patient or physician self-selection. As noted throughout this section, research findings can vary when one accounts for these.

Thus, both the general literature and the few studies that have examined medical conditions unique to women suggest that physician payment methods influence the care received by patients. When physicians are either paid on a salary or capitation basis, patients tend to receive less hospital care and overall, their costs of health care are lower as a result. Both their rate of hospitalization and the duration of their hospital stays are lower.

There is evidence, however, that healthier persons have tended to enroll in managed-care plans. Thus, the lower utilization we observe under managed-care plans, when we examine nonexperimental data (as most studies have), is only *partly* the result of the payment policies of these plans. Some of the lower utilization is attributable to managed-care enrollees being healthier to begin with. Nonetheless, holding patient mix constant, salary and capitation payment methods for physicians have been found to help lower health-care costs.

## REFERENCES

Cherkin DC, Grothaus L, Wagner EH: The effect of office visit copayments on utilization in a health maintenance organization. Med Care 27:669–679, 1989.

Dowd B, Feldman R: Biased selection in twin cities health plans. *In* Scheffler RM, Rossiter LF (eds): Advances in Health Economics and Health Services Research 1985. Greenwich, CT, JAI Press, 1985.

Dowd B, Feldman R, Cassou S, et al: Health plan choice and the utilization of health care services. Rev Econ Stat 73:85–93, 1991.

Dubay L, Kenney G: Did Medicaid expansions for pregnant women crowd out private coverage? Health Affairs 16:185–193, 1997.

Employee Benefit Research Institute: Sources of health insurance and characteristics of the uninsured. EBRI Issue Brief 179. Washington, DC, Employee Benefit Research Institute, Nov 1996.

Gazmararian JA, Koplan JP: Length-of-stay after delivery: Managed care versus fee-for-service. Health Affairs 15:74–80, 1996.

Geller SE, Burns LR, Brailer DJ: The impact of nonclinical factors on practice variations: The case of hysterectomies. Health Serv Res 30(6):729–750, 1996.

Gillum BS, Graves EJ, Wood E: National Hospital Discharge Survey: Annual summary, 1995. National Center for Health Statistics. Vital Health Stat 13(133), 1998.

Goldfarb NI, Hillman AL, Eisenberg JM, et al: Impact of a mandatory Medicaid case management program on prenatal care and birth outcomes: A retrospective analysis. Med Care 29:64–71, 1991.

Hadley J, Mitchell JM: Breast cancer treatment choice and mastectomy length of stay: A comparison of HMO and other privately insured women. Inquiry 34:288–301, 1997.

Hankin JR, Steinwachs DM, Charmain E: The impact of a copayment increase for ambulatory psychiatric care. Med Care 18:807–815, 1980.

Hellinger FJ: Selection bias in health maintenance organizations: Analysis of recent evidence. Health Care Financing Rev 9:55–63, 1987.

Hellinger FJ: Selection bias in HMOs and PPOs: A review of the evidence. Inquiry 32:135–142, 1995.

Hosek SD, Marquis MS, Wells K: Health care utilization in employer plans with preferred provider organization options. Santa Monica, CA, Rand Corporation R-3800-HHS/NIMH, 1990.

Jensen GA, Morrisey MA, Gaffney S, et al: The new dominance of managed care: Insurance trends in the 1990s. Health Aff 17(1):125–136, 1997.

The Kaiser Family Foundation: Fact sheet on Medicaid's role for children. Washington, DC, The Kaiser Commission on the Future of Medicaid, May 1997.

Krieger JW, Connell FA, LoGerfo JP: Medicaid prenatal care: A comparison of use and outcomes in fee-for-service and managed care. Am J Public Health 82:185–190, 1992.

Langwell KM, Hadley JP: Evaluation of the medicare competition demonstrations. Health Care Financing Rev 11:65–80, 1989.

Leibowitz A, Buchanan JL, Mann J: A randomized trial to evaluate the effectiveness of a Medicaid HMO. J Health Econ 11:235–257, 1992.

Maddala GS: Limited Dependent Variables and Qualitative Variables in Econometrics. Cambridge, MA, Cambridge University Press, 1983.

Miller RH, Luft HA: Managed care plan performance since 1980: A literature analysis. JAMA 271:1512–1519, 1994.

Newhouse JP, the Insurance Experiment Group: Free for All? Lessons From the Rand Health Insurance Experiment. Cambridge, MA, Harvard University Press, 1993.

Ransom SB, McNeeley SG, Doot G, et al: The effect of capitated and fee-for-service reimbursement on physician decision making in gynecology. Obstet Gynecol 87:707–710, 1996.

Russell LB: Educated Guesses: Making Policy About Medical Screening Tests. Berkeley, University of California Press, 1994.

Scheffler RM: The united mine workers' health plan. Med Care 22:247–254, 1984.

Schulman ED, Sheriff DJ, Momany ET: Primary care case management and birth outcomes in the Iowa Medicaid program. Am J Public Health 87:80–84, 1997.

Scitovsky AA, Snyder NM: Effects of coinsurance on the use of physician services. Soc Sec Bull 35:3–19, 1972.

Scitovsky AA, McCall N: Coinsurance and the demand for physician services four years later. Soc Sec Bull 40:19–27, 1977.

Simon CJ, Emmons DW: Physician earnings at risk: An examination of capitated contracts. Health Aff 16:120–126, 1997.

Smith DG: The effects of preferred provider organizations on health care use and costs. Inquiry 34:278–287, 1997/98.

Statistical Abstract of the United States. Washington, DC, U.S. Government Printing Office, 1997.

Sterns SC, Wolfe BL, Kindig DA: Physician responses to fee-for-service and capitation payment. Inquiry 29:416–425, 1992.

Strumwasser I, Paranjpe NV, Ronis DL, et al: The triple option choice: Self-selection bias in traditional coverage, HMOs, and PPOs. Inquiry 26:432–441, 1989.

# 67

# Managed Care

KENNETH CHANG

DAVID NASH

Managed care has become the dominant form of health-care delivery in the United States, replacing the old fee-for-service (FFS) system. Regarded as a means of controlling rising health-care costs, managed care encompasses a variety of incentives—namely, reimbursement mechanisms and other factors that are distinctly different from FFS care. This chapter provides the practicing obstetrician and gynecologist with an overview of managed care which includes the history, typology, reimbursement mechanism for providers, comparison of managed care vs. traditional FFS based on cost and quality, and the potential future of managed care. In addition, a section concerning obstetric and gynecologic (OB/GYN) issues in managed care is discussed.

## History of Managed Care

The concepts underlying what we call managed care today can be found to have been in existence for more than 4000 years. The Codex Hammurabi, inscribed on clay tablets from ancient Babylon, revealed a health-care system that used a sliding fee schedule for services, promoted outcome measurements, required medical records to document disease and treatments, offered prescription benefits, documented a patient's bill of rights, and disseminated advertising. Though managed care did not grow directly from these ancient origins, some of the concepts remain universal today.

The beginnings of managed care in the United States can be traced to the 19th century. Large industries such as lumber, mining, and railroad needed mechanisms to ensure adequate health care for their worker populations, who were defined groups with fairly specific medical needs. Physicians were employed directly by these companies in a prepaid fashion to provide necessary care for the company's workers. Although these arrangements were small and basic compared with managed care today, they marked the beginning of limited access of physicians to patients.

Prepaid practice groups were likely the more formal forerunners of managed care. Community Hospital Association of Elk City, Oklahoma, founded in 1929, was the first prepaid medical cooperative. The 1930s and 1940s saw the proliferation of more well-known precursors to managed care, with the formation of such institutions as the Group Health Association, the Kaiser-Permanente Medical Care Program, the Health Insurance Plan of Greater New York, and Group Health Cooperative of Puget Sound. The growth of these plans was spurred by the fact that employers wanted to offer employees a small additional benefit without having to increase their salaries. This was especially true during World War II, when the government set limits on wage increases. Although these plans grew steadily from their inception, their more remarkable growth would come later.

The next stage of growth for Managed Care Organizations (MCOs) took place from the 1970s to the early 1980s, catalyzed by the passage of the Health Maintenance Organization Act in 1973. This act was designed to foster the growth of health maintenance organizations (HMOs), giving them a competitive marketing advantage by requiring all large employers and union health and welfare funds to offer employees the option of enrolling in a federally qualified HMO. In addition, grants for feasibility studies, planning funds, initial development funds, and loans were made to provide incentives for growth of HMOs. More than $200 million dollars were spent in this way. In this time frame, the enrollment in HMOs grew from 3 million to nearly 12 million members.

Despite the push for HMOs, health-care costs continued to skyrocket throughout the 1980s. Costs were increasing at double-digit rates, outpacing inflation. The biggest surge in managed care occurred during this time period. Employers viewed managed care as a way of controlling these costs. They shifted their coverage from predominantly FFS plans to the lower priced managed care plans. In the past, FFS was the dominant payment mechanism; today, managed care covers more than 85% of employer-sponsored plans. The fastest growing managed care populations are members of Medicare and Medicaid, which were traditionally FFS plans. Currently, more than 60% of the population of the United States is covered by some type of managed care arrangement.

## Definition of Managed Care

Definitions of managed care abound, but the basic concepts have been well defined by Inglehart as a system that integrates the financing and delivery of appropriate medical care by means of the following features:
1. Contracts with selected physicians and hospitals furnish a comprehensive set of health-care services to enrolled members, usually for a predetermined monthly premium.
2. Some financial risk is assumed by physicians, which fundamentally alters their role from serving as agents for patient's welfare to balancing patient's individual needs against the need for cost control, or the greater good of the whole.

The different structural arrangements used to implement these concepts are further delineated.

Managed care comes in many forms and can be divided into three major classifications: HMO, preferred provider organization (PPO), and point of service (POS) plan. An HMO can then be further subclassified as staff model, group model, network model, or independent practice association (IPA). The original type of HMO was the staff model. In this type of organization, the plan owns and operates all health-care facilities required for the care of an enrollee and directly employs physicians to work at these facilities. The enrollee is restricted to using only hospitals the plan owns and physicians directly employed by the plan. This model accounts for about 10% of all HMOs today.

The group model is a variation on the staff model. Instead of the health plan's directly employing a physician and paying him or her a salary, the plan contracts with a physician group to care for the plan's members. The groups are managed independently and reimbursed on a capitated basis. The group model accounts for about 13% of all HMOs.

The third HMO model is the IPA. This plan contracts with individual physicians or networks of independent physicians who practice in their own offices and who care for the plan's members. The payment mechanism can be either discounted FFS or capitation. The advantage to this system is that a plan can expand its geographic coverage and increase members' choices of physicians without a great expenditure of capital. IPAs are the most common type of HMO, accounting for approximately 65% of all HMO plans.

The final type of HMO is the network model plan. This is similar to the IPA model except that it contracts with only networks of independent physicians. This is an advantage for the plan, because there is no need for contracts with many physicians in small individual practices. Instead, contracts are made with a few networks to obtain the same geographic coverage. This can be a disadvantage because large physician networks can have more economies of scale and can demand more generous provider contracts.

HMOs are in a constant state of change, making increasing numbers of different arrangements with providers and employers. In an attempt to appeal to a larger market, the lines between the types of HMOs have become less clear. Mixed model HMOs (those that incorporate multiple models in their plan) will become even more prevalent in the future.

The second type of managed care arrangement is the preferred physician organization (PPO). This plan contracts with individual physicians or networks to provide health care at a discounted FFS rate. Physicians accept a lower rate of compensation in exchange for expansion of their patient base. The plan makes no effort to match a member with a primary care provider or gatekeeper. The member also retains the freedom to go to a specialist without a primary care provider's referral. Typically, the patient must still use the network of providers created by this system, but the patient retains autonomy in choosing an appropriate health-care provider (generalist or specialist).

The final type of managed care arrangement is the POS plan. Currently, this is the fastest growing managed care type. It can function within an HMO or PPO or independently. The plan typically couples the patient with a primary care provider. The coverage is similar to that of the HMO or PPO plans listed previously. The main difference is that members have the option of accessing another provider directly by paying a higher copayment, usually at lower coverage. This is a hybrid type of plan, which allows the consumer to have more freedom of choice.

The numbers of acronyms and different managed care types seem to increase daily. As managed care continues to evolve, new models continue to form. Different and more complex arrangements are created, which will likely not fit neatly into any single one of the above categories. In fact, some believe that PPO and POS plans are merely transitions for funneling members into more restrictive and less costly HMO plans. It is important to understand the framework and concepts of these managed care types and how they affect a medical practice.

## Cost of Health Care

The cost of health care in the United States increased at a rapid rate from the 1980s to the early 1990s. The annual average inflation rate of health care during this period of time was more than 10%; in fact, at its highest point, the annual inflation rate was 16% in 1981. The employer-sponsored premium rates escalated even more rapidly. In 1990 alone, the average premium rate increased by 18.1%. In 1996, more than a trillion dollars was spent for health care in the United States, accounting for approximately 14% of the gross national product. Managed care was established in an effort to help control the rapid increase in health-care spending by employers and the government. Early studies from the Health Care Financing Agency (HCFA) have shown that this may have been accomplished. With the increased penetration of managed care, the health-care inflation rate has had a steady downward trend. In fact, figures released by the HCFA for 1996 show that health-care inflation increased by only 4.4%, its lowest rate in 37 years. The sharpest drop occurred in employer-sponsored health insurance. In the past, 20% increases in premium were not an uncommon occurrence for this type of insurance. In 1996, the growth of employer-sponsored health insurance premiums fell to a low of 3.6%. This decrease in premium growth coincides with the shift in the marketplace from the traditional FFS indemnity plans to managed care plans.

The managed care plans that are more restrictive in their cost-saving strategies, such as HMOs, have shown the greatest cost savings vs. indemnity insurance, but the other managed care arrangements, which are not as restrictive, have also shown cost savings. In a study conducted by A. Foster Higgins, an employee-benefit consulting firm, employers who had HMO coverage for their employees saved an average of 14.6% per employee compared with the cost of traditional indemnity coverage. PPO and POS savings in relation to indemnity insurance were 6.1 and 7.9%, respectively.

Managed care plans attempt to control health-care costs by preventing overutilization of resources through a number of different methods, but primarily through capitation. FFS plans invited overutilization of services by offering physicians the incentive of "getting paid more for doing more procedures." By its nature, capitation promotes decreased utilization because the physician is at risk for some of his income, depending on the number of service he or she uses.

## Managed Care Utilization

Chernew reviewed 24 studies that compare the use of diagnostic tests between HMO and FFS populations. Data from these studies revealed that patients in HMOs received fewer inpatient tests and fewer tests ordered per admission. This is partially accounted for by the fact that testing has shifted to an outpatient basis. The results of the evaluation of outpatient testing were mixed. HMO patients who had chronic diseases were more likely to receive testing than similar FFS patients, but testing for acute care situations was similar between the two groups. The conclusion was that although no definitive statement regarding the overall testing rates can be made, it seems reasonable to conclude that HMOs reduce the aggregate use of diagnostic testing services.

Ransom and associates conducted a study on the variation of gynecologic services between capitated and FFS populations. The results revealed a 15% overall decrease in the number of surgical procedures performed under capitation compared with FFS. Their conclusion was that capitation seemed to discourage overuse of surgical procedures, especially elective procedures.

In addition, the number of inpatient hospital days under managed care compared with FFS are dramatically fewer. In California, where managed care has a major market share, the number of Medicare hospital days is less than 1000 days per 1000 members per year. The national Medicare average is 2835 days per 1000 members per year. Most commercial managed care plans in California have inpatient days of less than 200 per 1000 members per year, whereas the national average is approximately 500 days per 1000 members per year.

These studies and others reveal that managed care through capitation tends to favor decreased use of services, whereas FFS favors overuse of services. Though the cost of health care through managed care may be lower than traditional FFS, cost is not the only factor that needs to be compared between the two delivery systems.

## Quality of Care

One of the criticisms of managed care is that it is too driven by costs. The prevailing argument made by many of its opponents is that managed care, through capitation and other measures, is preventing patients from receiving appropriate treatment for the sake of cost-containment and that the treatment received through FFS is the gold standard by which all plans should be measured. Many studies have been conducted to compare the quality of care between managed care and FFS. These studies compared the two systems across different populations and against a spectrum of quality factors that range from immunization rates, clinical outcomes, and preventive care rates to patient satisfaction, morbidity, and mortality. Many of the results of these health services research studies revealed no significant difference in the quality of care received through the two systems. In fact, managed care performs better in some of the quality measures, most notably preventive care.

Numerous studies comparing the rates of preventive services show that managed care has a high performance level in many of these areas. Managed care emphasizes that preventing illness is more cost-effective than treating patients who have acute exacerbations of disease. Improved rates for preventive services are achieved through physician education, report cards, and financial incentives, whereas FFS offers little incentive to provide these services. A survey in Southeastern Pennsylvania revealed that patients enrolled in HMOs were more likely to receive the appropriate preventive services, such as mammogram, Papanicolaou smear, and colorectal cancer screening, than their FFS counterparts. Several studies of influenza vaccination rates among Medicare beneficiaries found that elderly patients enrolled in HMO plans had higher rates of immunization than those in FFS plans. The studies also recommended that other plans try to emulate these HMO benchmark plans to achieve these rates. In general, preventive services are more often performed in managed care than in FFS settings.

A comparison of processes and outcomes of care between FFS and managed care systems has been performed in myriad health services research studies. Managed care and FFS were compared across a large range of conditions, which included congestive heart failure, acute myocardial infarction, hypertension, diabetes, mental health, colon cancer, stroke, joint pain, and pregnancy, among many others. These studies in aggregate have generally revealed that quality of care in terms of process and clinical outcomes is the same in both systems, with neither system showing superior performance in the majority of these measures. Some examples comparing FFS and managed care in particular disease states are as follows:

1. Comparing inpatient hospitalization among patients with congestive heart failure on FFS versus managed care plans revealed that the process of care received was the same, but patients enrolled in managed care had better follow-up after discharge.
2. Comparing perioperative management of colon cancer between FFS and managed care revealed that use of perioperative services was decreased in managed care, but no difference in clinical outcomes was found after surgery.
3. Comparing treatment and outcomes of stroke patients revealed that managed care patients were less likely than FFS patients to be discharged to a rehabilitation facility, but survival patterns of the two patient populations were similar.

The other studies listed previously also show that no difference in quality of results can be measured between the two systems.

The highly respected Medical Outcomes Study by Ware and associates does present evidence that quality of care in some at-risk managed care populations may be inferior to that provided in FFS plans. This study revealed that certain managed care populations among the poor, the elderly, and those who are chronically ill may receive worse care than their FFS counterparts in terms of quality and patient satisfaction. However, other populations in the same study, such as nonelderly chronically ill patients, were found to have better quality of care under managed care. This may be explained by the fact that some populations benefit from the more structured treatment delivered by managed care, whereas others dislike the decrease in access to physicians.

A recent meta-analysis by Miller and Luft evaluated the process and outcomes of care between FFS and managed care across a spectrum of measures, including utilization, quality of care, and patient satisfaction. The conclusion of this study was that although utilization of services is decreased with managed care, the quality of care evaluated by process and outcomes measures was roughly equivalent, with neither system showing superior results. In other words, according to the article, "HMOs produce better, the same, and worse quality of care, depending on the particular organization and particular disease." The study by Chernow cited earlier also reiterated that utilization of diagnostic tests was lower in managed care but the quality of care was not diminished.

Studies that directly compared overall satisfaction among different populations covered managed care and FFS plans have revealed mixed results, although predominantly these studies show that patient satisfaction with FFS is higher than that of similar populations in managed care. Although satisfaction of patients in managed care is lower than in those in FFS, members of managed care plans are still generally satisfied with the care they receive. This is an area in which managed care groups can take large strides toward improving their performance by providing better education and meeting the expectations of their members.

In combination, all these studies show that the quality of care delivered by managed care is at least equivalent in most aspects—and sometimes superior—to that delivered by FFS plans. This can be explained by three reasons. First, Quality of care, despite decreased use of procedures, is not affected since the rates of procedures that were most affected were those of elective procedures as well as those whose clinical benefits have not been clearly shown. Second, managed care encourages more reliance on preventive care. This likely prevents or delays the more serious complications of disease that increase the use of services. Finally, managed care sets up a framework for clinicians to improve their performance through report cards, network of ancillary personnel and services, management of large databases, and commitment to continuous quality improvement activities. Managed care needs to perform research continuously to improve the quality of care provided to the populations it serves.

In addition, managed care systems are also being held accountable for their quality of care by the National Committee on Quality Assurance (NCQA). The NCQA is a foundation that performs process and outcomes measurements of managed care companies. This group was created to standardize process and outcomes measurements so that results can be comparable. Managed care companies are evaluated and they must meet a minimum standard to obtain accreditation. In addition, the NCQA has created the Healthplan Employer Data and Information Set (HEDIS), a tool that standardizes data collection and analysis methods so that outcome results from different managed care companies can be compared. For instance, HEDIS has set a standard method of collecting data on childhood immunization rates, thereby making direct comparisons between managed care companies more valid.

## Obstetrics/Gynecology and Managed Care

Managed care now covers more of the population; inevitably, OB/GYNs will be affected in many different ways. The managed care foundation of the gatekeeper model and capitation payment mechanism force OB/GYNs to practice in an ever changing health-care environment. Some of the changes that have already occurred shift responsibilities, so that OB/GYNs—who have traditionally been specialists—are becoming primary care physicians; increasing financial risk through capitation; and employing increasing numbers of nonphysician ancillary providers.

By the very nature of their specialty, OB/GYNs are very suitable as providers for primary and preventive care to women. This notion is supported by patients, the American College of Obstetricians and Gynecologists (ACOG), and managed care. Women currently receive a majority of their health care from OB/GYNs. In a survey of women patients, 54% considered their OB/GYN as their primary care physician. The same study revealed that 31% of women exclusively consulted an OB/GYN for their health care.

The Executive Board of the ACOG recognized this back in 1986 by stating "The specialty of Obstetrics and Gynecology is devoted to the health care of women throughout their lifetime. It encompasses the care of the whole patient in addition to focusing on the normal and abnormal processes of the female reproductive system, including the breast. Care provided by the OB/GYN includes preventive and primary care, care during pregnancy and childbirth, and medical and surgical management of reproductive-related disorders and diseases." More recently, in 1994, the Executive Board of ACOG defined a primary care OB/GYN as "...a physician directly accessible to patients for their initial contact. This physician will see patients who have a specific or an undifferentiated complaint or patients who desire health maintenance through periodic health check-ups. The primary care physician also provides continuity of care and is readily available to the patient when he or she has either a specific or nonspecific complaint. Such physicians perform initial evaluation and management within their expertise. The primary care physician advises when referral to another physician is indicated, coordinating subsequent and continuing care to assure the patient of appropriate comprehensive care."

In many aspects, OB/GYNs deliver services in the same framework as primary care providers. Currently, many OB/GYNs provide primary and preventive care services. In a survey by the ACOG in 1992, 53% of the OB/GYNs surveyed provided these services during more than 50% of their practice time. This study also revealed that a majority of OB/GYNs were providing blood pressure screening, breast cancer screening, Papanicolaou testing, and cholesterol screening. The study concluded that a majority of OB/GYNs deliver primary and preventive care to their patients.

In 1993, a survey of women patients corroborated the previously mentioned findings. In fact, OB/GYNs were found to perform more complete physical examinations than any other type of physician. OB/GYNs were more likely to provide primary care and preventive screening in the following areas: gynecologic evaluation, Papanicolaou smear, breast examination, mammogram, family planning, sexually transmitted diseases and human immunodeficiency virus (HIV), and hormone replacement therapy. OB/GYNs performed as well as their primary care counterparts in conducting blood pressure screening and in providing education and care in smoking cessation, drug and alcohol abuse, physical abuse, and osteoporosis. OB/GYNs were less likely to perform or discuss cholesterol screening, nutrition, exercise, medication use, and mental health issues. As the OB/GYN practice of primary care continues to expand, the providers' performance in these areas will likely improve with the increased use of these services.

To better prepare the OB/GYN for primary care practice in the future, the ACOG created a comprehensive set of guidelines that are matched for a patient's age and risk factors. This provides a framework for the practice of primary care by the OB/GYN. Also, the ACOG Residency Review Committee responded to the changes in medical practice by implementing several changes to the requirements of OB/GYN training programs. These changes include at least 6 months of direct training in primary and preventive care as well as continuity ambulatory clinics for 3 years to emphasize primary care. These changes should allow the OB/GYN to be better prepared for the practice of primary and preventive care in the future.

Capitation as a payment method has continued to grow as managed care penetrates the marketplace. Capitation is not the only payment method available and not always the best to solve some of the healthcare problems, but it will likely be the dominant reimbursement model of the future because its incentives are to control costs. OB/GYNs need to learn about this payment mechanism and how it will affect their practices. Capitation is a method of payment by which a provider accepts a monthly payment to perform services for a defined population. The payment remains fixed, regardless of whether a member uses these services or not.

There are two reasons for the impetus for use of capitation by managed care. First, capitation aligns incentives so that providers deliver only necessary services in the most efficient manner to keep covered populations healthy. Physicians should provide cost-effective ambulatory care with the goal of preventing acute exacerbations of disease, which necessitate expensive inpatient hospitalizations. Second, some of the financial risk is shifted from the insurer to the physician. Capitation fixes some of the cost for delivering health care for the insurance companies and places that financial risk on physicians. This is a powerful incentive for physicians to manage patient care as efficiently as possible.

Currently, most capitated physicians are primary care providers, not including OB/GYNs. In the future, more physicians, including OB/GYNs, will be compensated by a capitated system. Physicians who are unable or unwilling to work with this type of payment mechanism may have a difficult time continuing to practice, with constantly eroding patient base as more patients are shifted to managed care and capitation. Physicians must know how to manage their practices efficiently. They must learn about cost-effective treatments and understand population management. This new subset of skills is essential for physicians to be successful in a capitated market.

A concept related to capitation is bundled payment, or global fees. A hospital and provider are paid a set amount for an episode of care instead of a fixed monthly payment for a patient population. There are several OB/GYN areas, such as pregnancy and obstetric care, dysfunctional uterine bleeding, and infertility treatment, that lend themselves to the bundled payment method. These episodes of care are models for this payment method because they are well-contained episodes with a definitive beginning and end. In addition, these episodes have well-defined treatment interventions as well as clinical practice guidelines for standardized treatment. Such a setup allows payment to be bundled together, which motivates physicians to provide only necessary care.

Managed obstetric care during pregnancy is likely the most common episode of care that uses bundled payments, although its use is still limited. The current model of care focuses on numerous nonintegrated cost centers that act independently to deliver their services. Cost-containment methods are not maximally effective because each cost center has its own interests. This system requires infrequently occurring disease states at an ever-increasing cost, because most pregnancies are without complications and constitute an issue of wellness care. Bundled rates align the incentive of all providers and services to deliver cost-effective care because everyone benefits from any cost saving achieved. This also promotes wellness care, because aggressive prenatal care decreases obstetric complications, and this in turn will most likely decrease costs. This can be accomplished through increased integration of care, which benefits outcomes because communication will be better among all providers. In short, the goals of this approach are to improve patient care and outcomes while simultaneously controlling costs.

In addition to different payment methods being used by managed care, the services of physician extenders, such as nurse practitioners, physician assistants, and nurse-midwives, are becoming increasingly important. In fact, the demand for these nonphysician providers is growing faster than the supply and will continue to increase as managed care penetration increases. Capitation and other managed care strategies that force physicians to work more efficiently will create an increasing demand for nonphysician providers who will provide triage and preventive care, thus freeing the physician to deal with the more difficult aspects of patient management. It is often cost-effective for physician extenders to provide services that are within their scope of competency. It is generally more expensive to have such services performed by physicians, who have more training. Such an approach also allows physician groups to care for a larger population of patients.

Certified nurse midwives (CNMs) in the United States currently number 5200. In 1975, CNMs delivered 19,686 babies. In 1994, that number had increased 10-fold to 196,977 deliveries. Even with such a large increase, the number of midwife deliveries accounts for less than 5% of all births in the United States. There are data to support that in low-risk pregnancies CNMs provide cost-effective care, with decreased incidence of cesarean sections or instrument-assisted deliveries. A study showed no significant differences in outcomes of either the mother or baby when comparing patients of midwives with those of physicians. This shows that at least in low-risk pregnancies, it may be cost-effective to use the services of CNMs, leaving the more complicated cases for the obstetrician. In the future, physicians must be able to work effectively with these nonphysician providers in an effort to provide health care more efficiently to a larger population at a controlled cost.

## Possible Future of Managed Care

It is difficult to predict what changes will occur in the future. Managed care has currently been able to slow down the increasing cost of health care in the United States. It has yet to be shown that managed care will be able to control costs on a long-term basis. The tremendous profitability of managed care companies in the early to mid-1990s was caused by remarkable growth and favorable contracting with providers. Now that the majority of employers have already shifted their employees to managed care, the managed care companies will not be able to earn money on the basis of membership growth. To be profitable, they will have to deliver and manage the health care even more effectively. The cost savings realized by the shift of employees from the more expensive FFS plans to managed care may be only a temporary cost control. In fact, in 1998, employers budgeted average increases of 7% in health-care costs, which is higher than the figure in the immediately preceding years.

Maintaining profitability of managed care companies will become more difficult in the future. Increasing competition among managed care plans, increased government regulations (e.g., mandates on covered services, anti–managed-care legislation, increased employer demands for lower premiums, and increased contracting powers from physician groups have led to decreasing profit margins.) These factors have caused many managed care companies to become unprofitable. In 1996, it is estimated that only 35% of HMOs were profitable. This was down from 90% of profitable HMOs in 1990.

There will likely be a greater consolidation of the market and a decreasing number of managed care organizations in the future. The only organizations that will prosper will be those that are able to deliver cost-effective care at a reasonable price. These will continue to grow and gain a share of the market in the future. Managed care must continually strive to improve the delivery of care with consequent improved patient outcomes at a value to the system. Otherwise, another delivery system may take its place and offer these services in the market. A possible future is that the numerous managed care groups that are currently in existence will—through competition and consolidation—become a few large managed care companies that will deliver care to a large geographic population. This will enable the managed care groups to distribute their risk over even larger populations. In fact, the market seems to be consolidating in that direction. At their peak in the late 1980s, more than 600 managed care companies were in existence. Currently, this number has decreased to approximately 500.

Increased penetration of managed care into most marketplaces will cause providers to change the way they practice medicine. The physicians' percentage of income from managed care is increasing. In 1990, revenues from managed care accounted for 28% of total revenues. That had increased to 44% in 1996. Practices with at least one managed care contract increased from 61 to 88% over the same time period. With the growth of MCOs, physicians are forming larger and larger groups to be able to provide care more efficiently. In addition to providing care more efficiently, larger groups are able to offer a wider variety of services and specialties for a given population. The consolidation of physicians in these larger groups also allows them to have greater economies of scale and increased leverage in contracting to make more favorable arrangements with managed care companies. The size of physician groups has increased from 10.6 physicians in 1990 to 14.5 physicians in 1996. The benefits of practicing in larger groups make this trend likely to increase in the future.

As the profit margin for managed care companies becomes smaller and smaller, managed care groups will likely try to shift more of the financial risk to the providers. Providers and hospitals must learn how to manage this financial risk. They must be accountable to patients, payers, and themselves for providing cost-effective, evidence-based, efficient medicine. To accomplish this, physician groups must be able to manage the physician members of their groups or networks to decrease the unexplained variation in treatment. They will have to inspire use of cost-effective care among their providers. Those providers who are unable or unwilling to change their practice habits to a more cost-effective manner will have their compensation affected by other providers in the group or they may not be welcome to practice in these groups. In essence, the management and compensation systems in practices will be decided by other physicians in the group as opposed to the managed care company.

## Summary

Managed care has experienced tremendous growth in the past decade spurred by the need to control rapidly increasing health-care costs. It has been shown that in the short term, managed care can slow the rapid increases in health-care expenditures, but it has yet to be shown if managed care can sustain long-term cost savings to the system. It is certain that more and more constraints will be placed on managed care from all parties, including payers, members, providers, and government. Currently, cost is the most important factor considered by most employers. With increasing competition and narrowing margins, the factors differentiating one managed care group from another will shift from cost to quality of care delivered. Members and payers will then choose plans based on the service offered because prices of these plans should be similar.

It is impossible to predict the changes that may occur in the future. Managed care will face new challenges in an attempt to keep health-care costs under control while delivering quality care. If managed care can show prolonged cost control with no detriment to the quality of care, it will flourish in the 21st century. If managed care does not change and improve, it will be replaced by the next health-care delivery system in much the same way as it has replaced FFS systems.

## *Glossary*

**bundled fees:** Lump-sum payment that covers several health-care services in an episode of care.

**capitation:** Fixed dollar amount that covers the cost of health-care services based on the membership of the health-care services plan; usually refers to a negotiated per capita rate paid periodically to providers; often expressed in units of per member per month.

**carve-out plan:** Stand-alone program that covers a specific health-care benefit or service (e.g., dental care or mental health-care; often requires separate premium from basic health-care plan's fees.)

**case rate:** Method for controlling hospital costs in which health maintenance organizations (HMOs) and hospitals negotiate a fixed fee for all care associated with a specific procedure, regardless of the length of the hospital stay.

**coinsurance:** Provision in managed health-care member coverage that limits the plan's coverage to a certain percentage of the cost of services; the member pays the remainder.

**credentialing:** The assessment, documentation, and affirmation of a physician's competence to practice medicine.

**deductible:** Portion of health-care expenses that a plan member must pay before insurance coverage applies.

**fee-for-service (FFS):** Traditional health-care payment system in which physicians and hospitals receive a direct payment for their billed charge, either from patients or an insurance company; also called indemnity.

**gatekeeper:** Primary care physician who serves as a patient's initial contact for medical care; coordinates the patient's overall care, and makes specialty referrals; predominant feature of most managed care plans, particularly HMOs.

**global fees:** See bundled fees.

**group model HMO:** HMO that contracts with a medical group for health-care services and compensates the group for contracted services at negotiated rates; group that compensates its physicians and contracts with hospitals for patient care.

**health care financing administration:** Federal

agency responsible for administering Medicare and overseeing states' administration of Medicaid.

**health maintenance organization:** Type of managed care organization that provides or arranges coverage of specific health-care services by in-network providers needed by plan members for a fixed, prepaid premium. The four major types include staff model, group model, independent practice association (IPA) model, and network model.

**independent practice association model HMO:** Type of (HMO) network that contracts with individual physicians who see HMO members plus their own patients; the physicians are members of the independent practice association (IPA) but remain independent practitioners with their own offices, medical records, and support staff.

**managed care:** Health-care system, including HMO, PPO, and point of service POS plans that influences the use and cost of health-care services, with the goal of providing high-quality, cost-effective health-care.

**network model HMO:** HMO that contracts with multiple physician groups, including single or multispecialty groups.

**nonphysician practitioner:** Health-care provider (e.g., nurse practitioner, physician assistant, or nurse midwife) who is not a physician but can provide primary care or other medical services.

**point-of-service plan:** Managed care plan in which members have the option to choose from an HMO, PPO, or indemnity plan at the time service is required. Ideally, a POS plan offers the cost control of an HMO and the choice of FFS plan.

**preferred provider organization:** Managed care plan that contracts with independent providers who provide services for plan members at discounted rates; plan members can use in-network or out-of-network providers, although out-of-network services result in higher patient out-of-pocket costs.

**premium:** Amount paid to an insurer or health-care plan for providing coverage for a specified level of services during a set time period; can be paid by patient, employer, government, or any combination of the three.

**staff model HMO:** HMO that employs providers directly; providers see members in the HMO's own facilities; HMO pays providers a salary and usually incentives.

**utilization:** Use of goods and services by enrollees of a managed care plan.

**utilization management:** Strategy used by health-care plans to control the use of costly medical interventions by ensuring that physicians reserve expensive interventions for appropriate patients. Examples include case management, preadmission certification, and second opinions.

## REFERENCES

American College of Obstetricians and Gynecologists: Obstetrician-gynecologist specialists in reproductive health care and primary physicians for women. ACOG Statement of Policy. Washington, DC, American College of Obstetricians and Gynecologists, 1986.

American College of Obstetricians and Gynecologists: Educational Objectives: Core Curriculum in Obstetrics and Gynecology, 5th ed. Washington, DC, Council on Resident Education in Obstetrics and Gynecology, 1996.

American College of Obstetricians and Gynecologists: Guidelines for Women's Health Care. Washington, DC, American College of Obstetricians and Gynecologists, 1996.

Aston G: Managed care cited for slowdown in spending. Am Med News 41:3,10,14, 1998.

Ballard JE, Liu J, Uberuagua D, et al: Assessing influenza immunization rates in Medicare managed care plans: A comparison of three methods. J Comm J Qual Improv 23:434–442, 1997.

Carey TS, Weis K, Homer C: Prepaid versus traditional Medicaid plans: Lack of effect on pregnancy outcomes and prenatal care. Health Serv Res 26:165–181, 1991.

Carlisle DM, Siu AL, Keeler EB, et al: HMO vs. fee-for-service care of older persons with acute myocardial infarction. Am J Public Health 82:1626–1630, 1992.

Center for Studying Health System Change: Issue brief Washington, DC, CSHSC, 1997, p 9.

Chernew M: HMO use of diagnostic tests: A review of the evidence. Med Care Res Rev 52:196–222, 1995.

Clement D, Retchin SM, Brown RS, et al: Access and outcomes of elderly patients enrolled in managed care. JAMA 271:1487–1492, 1994.

Eisenberg JM, Kabcenell A: Organized practice and the quality of medical care. Inquiry 25:78–89, 1988.

Emmons D, Simon C: Managed Care: Evolving Contractual Arrangements. Socioeconomic Characteristics of Medical Practice, 1996. Chicago, American Medical Association 1996, pp 15–25.

Emmons D, Kletke P: An Examination of Practice Size. Socioeconomic Characteristics of Medical Practice, 1997. Chicago, American Medical Association 1997, pp 21–30.

Emmons D, Wozniak G: Physicians' Contractual Arrangements With Managed Care Organizations. Socioeconomic Characteristics of Medical Practice, 1997. Chicago, American Medical Association, 1997, pp 7–20.

Erb JC: 1991 Health care benefits survey: Managed care plans. Report 2. Princeton, NJ: A. Foster Higgins, 1992.

Fabius R: The spectrum of managed care model types. Clin Obstet Gynecol 40:391–394, 1997.

Gabay M, Wolfe SM: Nurse-midwifery. The beneficial alternative. Public Health Rep 112:386–394, 1997.

Ginzberg E, Ostow M: Managed care—A look back and a look ahead. N Engl J Med 336:1018–1020, 1997.

Greenfield S, Rogers W, Mangotich M, et al: Outcomes of patients with hypertension and non-insulin-dependent diabetes mellitus treated by different systems and specialty: Results from the Medical Outcomes Study. JAMA 274:1436–1444, 1995.

Hanchak NA, Murray JF, Harmon-Weiss S, et al: The effectiveness of an influenza vaccination program in an HMO setting. Am J Managed Care 2:661–666, 1996.

Horton JA, Murphy MS, Hale RW: Obstetrician-gynecologists as primary care providers: A national survey of women. Primary Care Update. Obstet Gynecol 1:212–215, 1994.

Horton JA, Cruess DF, Pearse WH: Primary and preventive care services provided by obstetrician-gynecologists. Obstet Gynecol 82:723–726, 1993.

Huey JR Jr, Astles PD: Preparing obstetricians and gynecologists for capitation. Clin Obstet Gynecol 40:427–436, 1997.

Hunter LP, Lops V: Clinical nurse midwives. JAMA 277:1095, 1997.

Inglehart JK: Health Policy Report: The American health care system managed care. N Engl J Med 327:742–747, 1992.

Jatulis DE, Bundek NI, Legorreta AD. Identifying predictors of satisfaction with access to medical care and quality of care. Am J Med Qual 12:11–18, 1997.

Kearney PR, Engh CA: History of the American health care system: Its cost control programs and incremental reform. Orthopedics 20:236–47, 1997.

Kongstvedt P: Essentials of Managed Healthcare, 2nd ed. Gaithersburg, MD, Aspen Publisher, 1997.

Levit KR, Lazenby HC, Braden BR, et al: National health spending trends in 1996. Health Aff 17:35–51, 1998.

Lurie N, Moscovice IS, Finch M, et al: Does capitation affect the health of the chronically mentally ill? Results from a randomized trial. JAMA 267:3300–3304, 1992.

Miller RH, Luft HS: Does managed care lead to better or worse quality of care? Health Aff 16:7–25, 1997.

Newcomer R, Preston S, Harrington C: Health plan satisfaction and risk of disenrollment among social/HMO and fee-for-service recipients. Inquiry 33:144–154, 1996.

O'Keeffe DF, Mayes J: Managed obstetrical care. Clin Obstet Gynecol 40:414–419, 1997.

Philadelphia Health Management Corporation: Southeastern Pennsylvania Household Health Survey. 1994.

Ransom SB, McNeeley SG, Kruger ML, et al: The effect of capitation and fee-for-service remuneration on physician decision making in gynecology. Obstet Gynecol 87:707–710, 1996.

Retchin SM, Brown B: Elderly patients with congestive heart failure under prepaid care. Am J Med 90:236–242, 1991.

Retchin SM, Brown RS, Yeh SC, et al: Outcomes of stroke patients in Medicare fee-for-service and managed care. JAMA 278:119–124, 1997.

Retchin SM, Penberthy L, Desch C, et al: Perioperative management of colon cancer under Medicare risk programs. Arch Intern Med 157:1878–1884, 1997.

Rosenblatt RA, Dobie SA, Hart GL, et al: Interspecialty differences in the obstetric care in low-risk women. Am J of Public Health 87:344–351, 1997.

Rutkow IM: Railway surgery: Traumatology and managed health care in 19th-century United States. Arch Surg 128:458–463, 1993.

Seubold FH: HMO's: The view from the program. Public Health Rep 90:99–103, 1975.

Shapiro S: An historical perspective on the roots of managed care. Curr Opin Pediatr 8:159–163, 1996.

Sisk JE, Gorman SA, Reisinger AL, et al. Evaluation of Medicaid managed care. Satisfaction, access, and use. JAMA 276:50–55, 1996.

Spiegel AD, Springer CR: Babylonian medicine, managed care, and Codex Hammurabi, Circa 1700 B.C. J Commun Health 22:69–89, 1997.

Visscher HA: The role of the obstetrician/gynecologist in primary health care. Clin Obstet Gynecol 38:206–212, 1995.

Ware JE Jr, Bayliss MS, Rogers WH, et al: Differences in 4 year health outcomes for elderly and poor, chronically ill patients treated in HMO and fee-for-service systems. Results from the Medical Outcomes Study. JAMA 276:1039–1047, 1996.

Weiss B: Managed care: There's no stopping it now. Med Econ (Managed Care Suppl):26–43, 1995.

Welch WP, Hillman AL, Pauly MV: Toward new typologies for HMOs. Milbank Q 68:221–243, 1990.

Wyn R, Collins KS, Brown ER: Women and managed care: Satisfaction with provider choice, access to care, plan cost, and coverage. JAMWA 52:60–64, 1997.

Yurkowski W: The use of nonphysician providers in managed care settings. JAMA 277:1095, 1997.

# 68

# Clinical Epidemiology

ANNETTE CASOGLOS
KULMEET S. DANG
JODY L. MEINKE
R. MICHAEL MASSANARI

The practice of medicine has been described as a mixture of art and science. As society attempts to constrain the rising costs of health care, the medical profession has been compelled to provide more scientific evidence to support its decisions regarding use of resources—to practice evidence-based decision-making. When considering the scientific evidence that supports medical practice, one often looks to laboratory research for support of clinical decisions. However, much of the evidence for sound decision-making is generated by scientific methods that use observations among groups of people or patients, rather than laboratory observations. Several methodologic paradigms are employed in the study of effectiveness of medical care; most depend on epidemiologic methods. Although knowledge of epidemiologic methods is essential for improving effective clinical decision-making, most schools of medicine offer minimal instruction in the application of these methods. The purpose of this chapter is to provide an elementary knowledge of epidemiology and how these scientific tools are used to improve health care.

Epidemiologic tools were used to study causation and treatment of disease decades before meaningful laboratory investigation. One of the early examples in which epidemiologic techniques were used to study a clinical problem was reported by an obstetrician.

Ignaz Semmelweis practiced in Vienna and later in Pest in the mid to late 19th century. Semmelweis was intrigued and distressed by the disparity in mortality rates in two different groups of obstetric patients admitted to a lying-in hospital. The mortality rate was 16% among obstetric patients admitted to a teaching unit that was attended by medical professors and medical students. In contrast, the mortality rate was much lower among obstetric patients admitted to a unit attended by midwives. Puerperal sepsis (a postpartum infection probably caused by Group A β-hemolytic streptococcus) accounted for most of the deaths. Semmelweis observed an important difference in the process of care on the two units. Autopsies routinely were conducted by medical students on the teaching unit, whereas no autopsies were performed on the midwifery unit. Medical students moved back and forth between autopsy suite and labor room without attention to handwashing or other barrier interventions. Semmelweis hypothesized that a "contagium" from the dead bodies was transmitted to otherwise healthy patients in labor. Based on his hypothesis, Semmelweis implemented an intervention consisting of handwashing in chlorinated lime water before leaving the autopsy suite. Using mortality rates as a metric to assess outcomes, he demonstrated that the handwashing intervention reduced the mortality rate from 16 to 1.27% on his teaching service, even surpassing the mortality rate of the midwifery unit. This important observation among groups of patients was deduced at a time when there still was no laboratory evidence for the "germ theory" of disease. Semmelweis used epidemiologic, scientific methods to confirm a hypothesis regarding causation and treatment, an observation that had significant impact on the well-being of obstetric patients in that era.

In this chapter, we propose to inform readers about basic epidemiologic techniques by addressing the following questions: (1) What is epidemiology? (2) Which methods are used to conduct epidemiologic studies? and (3) How do epidemiologic studies impact the practice of obstetrics and gynecology? We use examples from the obstetric and gynecologic literature to illustrate epidemiologic methods and applications in practice. The chapter focuses on descriptive statistics used to describe samples and populations of patients and on study designs used to assess causation and treatment interventions. Because epidemiology and biostatistics represent independent academic disciplines, this chapter provides only an elementary overview. For a more thorough understanding of these disciplines, the reader is referred to readings located within the references.

# What Is Epidemiology?

The term *epidemiology* is derived from several Greek terms: epi- (upon), demos (people), and -ology (the study of). Historically, epidemiology was the study of the distribution and causation of disease in populations. In recent decades, epidemiologic methods have been used to study phenomena other than disease in groups of people, for example, the distribution and utilization of healthcare resources. The investigative process consists of categorizing disease distributions across time, place, and people. Variations in the distribution of disease or other phenomena over time, place, and populations offer important clues to cause-and-effect relationships. Epidemiologists also use tools from other disciplines, such as biology, statistics, psychology, and sociology, to expand the knowledge of disease.

A clinician's charge to diagnose and treat disease in an individual demands different tools and skills. However, epidemiologic methods are invaluable for informing clinicians regarding the optimal application of diagnostic and therapeutic tools. *Clinical epidemiologists* employ epidemiologic methods to examine disease etiologies, attributes of diagnostic tests (sensitivity, specificity), and efficacy of preventive and therapeutic interventions (efficacy, effectiveness, and outcomes).

# Which Methods Are Used to Conduct Epidemiologic Studies?

## POPULATIONS AND SAMPLES

If groups of patients serve as a laboratory for clinical epidemiologic studies, it is apparent that unique methods or tools are required to describe and analyze observational and experimental studies. Before describing these methods, we first must define the groups of subjects from which the data are derived. Physicians generally are interested in observations that are applicable to a broad group of patients or population. A *population* is made up of subjects that share common characteristics. Common characteristics may be geographic or political boundaries; however, for the clinician, the distinction more likely applies to characteristics such as gender differences or age differences.

Populations usually include large groups of subjects and are not readily amenable to epidemiologic study. To facilitate the study of populations, epidemiologists select smaller samples of the populations. If properly selected, inferences from studies of samples can be extrapolated to the larger population. An appropriate *sample*, therefore, provides a reasonably accurate reflection of the characteristics of the population of interest. Thus, when selecting a sample of subjects for study and analysis, the clinician should consider two critical questions:

1. How many subjects (sample size) must be included to ensure a reliable answer to the hypothesis under consideration?
2. How will subjects be chosen?

Planning these steps in the study is as important as the statistical analysis following data collection. This overview does not allow elaboration of these important steps in study design. For purposes of this discussion, the optimal method for selecting subjects in a sample is random sampling. *Random sampling* ensures that every individual subject in a population has an equal probability of being chosen in the sample. However, it is not always convenient or practical to obtain a random sample (e.g., the study of infrequent events or disease). In this instance, the investigator may choose to include all subjects with the condition of interest identified in a given period of time or location. This is referred to as *convenience sampling*. Extrapolating from a convenience sample to populations of presumed similar individuals must be done with caution because obscure biases may have contributed to a greater or lesser probability of being included in the sample. For the generalizations that follow, we assume that samples have been selected appropriately.

## VARIABLES

When a sample has been selected appropriately, the study may begin and data may be collected. The data that are collected for the sample may include only a few or multiple variables. A *variable* is any quality, characteristic, or constituent of a person or thing that can be measured or observed. Variables reflect attributes that "vary" between and sometimes within individual subjects. Variables can either be qualitative or quantitative in nature. Typical examples of *qualitative variables* include gender, hair color, eye color, nationality, and death/survival at a certain point in time. *Quantitative variables* are those that can be expressed by numeric quantities, such as weight, height, diastolic/systolic blood pressure, age, or number of siblings. Quantitative variables can be broken down further into discrete or continuous variables. *Discrete* measurements are those for which the possible values are quite distinct and separate. Discrete measurements are either counts (e.g., number of siblings) or subjective grading (ordinal), such as Apgar scores for newborns. Apgar scores are based on the subjective characteristics of a newborn and scaled as ordinals from 0 to 2. The total score ranges from 0 to 10, where 7–10 is considered normal, requiring no resuscitation, and 4–6 is poorly responsive and may require some resuscitative measures. A score of 3 or less necessitates immediate resuscitation. These numbers do not provide any explicit value but rather are a subjective score of infant viability. *Continuous* measurements are those for which an approximate value along a continuous, uninterrupted scale is assigned. An example is height, weight, age or blood pressure. Note that continuous variables may have an upper or lower limit. Height, for example, theoretically has no upward bound but cannot be negative or less than zero.

## QUALITATIVE DATA: FREQUENCY TABLES AND BAR CHARTS

After collecting qualitative and quantitative data for a study, it is often useful and recommended that the investigator "look at" his or her data. The purpose is to configure and present the data in ways that provide enlightening descriptions of the sample. Analysis of descriptive statistics can be performed in a number of ways depending on whether the data are quantitative or qualitative. Qualitative data often are viewed by creating frequency tables. Frequency tables show the number and/or percentage of individuals in each category. For example, using hypothetical data, we can summarize in a frequency table the distribution of primary cancer sites for 1150 patients visiting an oncology clinic, as shown in Table 68–1. Note that for the sake of illustration, the category "other" in Table 68–1 was not included in Figure 68–1.

**Table 68–1** Distribution of Primary Cancer Sites

| Diagnosis | Frequency | Percentage |
|---|---|---|
| Cervix | 10 | 0.94 |
| Ovary | 16 | 1.5 |
| Uterus | 24 | 2.3 |
| Other | 1010 | 95.3 |
| Total | 1060 | |

The categoric data in Table 68–1 also can be represented in a graphical manner using a bar chart. The bar chart in Figure 68–1 corresponds to the data in the frequency table. The frequency or number of patients is displayed on the y-axis.

These graphic reporting techniques can be applied to two or more qualitative variables simultaneously. For example, the bar chart in Figure 68–2 displays the frequency of each cancer site for two age groups, younger than 50 years old and 50 years of age or older.

## RATES AND PROPORTIONS

Qualitative data also may be summarized with numeric descriptors, such as proportions, rates, or ratios, instead of graphical or tabular representations. The value of such a descriptor is the ability to compare across samples using statistical methods. Each of these descriptors is expressed mathematically as a fraction.

A *proportion* is the number of individuals or items in the category of interest divided by the total number of individuals in the set of observations. Therefore, the numerator is included in the denominator of the

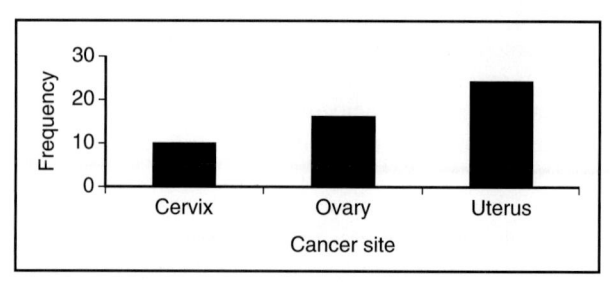

**Figure 68–1** Distribution of primary cancer sites.

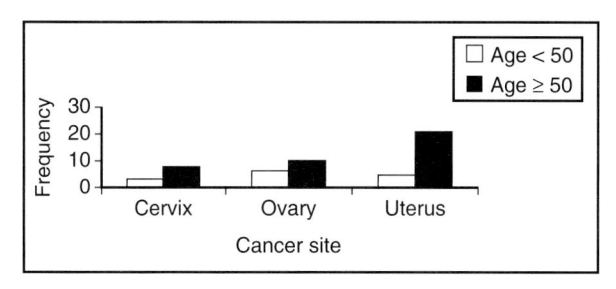

**Figure 68–2** Distribution of primary cancer sites by age.

fraction. For example, if the proportion of cesarean section (C-section) procedures that acquire surgical site infections is 4 in 250 procedures, the four infected patients are included among the 250 C-section procedures.

A *rate* constitutes a more complex fraction in which there is a measure of change of one quantity per unit change in another, usually time. Theoretically, a rate may vary between 0 and infinity. Denominators often are standardized to 1000 or 10,000 to facilitate the comparison of rates. The number of infections per 1000 patient days of stay in a hospital or the number of cases of pneumonia per ventilation days in an intensive care unit are examples of rates.

A *ratio* is also a fraction but differs from a proportion because the numerator is not included in its denominator. An example of this fraction would be the ratio of males to females admitted to a hospital or the ratio of surgical patients from a sample in whom surgical site infections develop to the number of patients from the same sample in whom surgical site infections do not develop.

## PREVALENCE AND INCIDENCE

The above description and formulation for rates illustrates the term in the general sense; however, there are two specific types of rates that should be defined further. The first commonly used rate is *prevalence*. This proportion is a static measure that provides a cross-sectional look at a sample at a single point in time. To calculate prevalence, the number of incidents or events during the specified period of time (e.g., the day of the survey) must be identified for the numerator of the fraction. The total number of patients or items studied during the time period must be accounted for in the denominator of the fraction. Because prevalence is confined to a brief period of time, conclusions regarding causal relationships and risk of disease are limited and should be made with caution.

The second commonly reported rate is *incidence*. Incidence is the rate at which a new case or event occurs over a specified period of time. Two methods for determining incidence are cumulative incidence and incidence density. *Cumulative incidence* is an *estimate* of the risk of an event during a specified period of time among individuals without disease and therefore is expressed as a proportion. Because cumulative incidence is reported as a proportion, it is only an estimate of the frequency of new events relative to the total patients at risk and does not relate the duration of exposure with the risk of occurrence of the event. The actual calculation of cumulative incidence is understood more easily when one examines the numerator and denominator separately. The numerator is the number of patients who were free of the disease or incident before the specified period but who had the incident occur or acquired the disease during the period. The denominator is the total number of patients who were free of the incident before the specified period but presumably were at risk of having the incident occur.

*Incidence density* is a measure of the *actual* rate of an event among patients without disease. Incidence density is expressed as the number of new events that occur per unit of exposure time. The unit of time is arbitrary and depends on the nature of the incident being studied. To illustrate the calculation of incidence density, consider the numerator and the denominator separately. The numerator is the number of incidents that occurred during the specified period of time. The denominator, assuming days is the unit of time, is the total number of days of exposure to the risk factor. If we are counting exposure days for patients, the total number of exposure days for all patients included in the study is termed *patient days*. The final calculation of incidence density then can be expressed as "incidents per 1000 patient days" by simply multiplying the calculated rate by 1000.

To help distinguish cumulative incidence from prevalence, consider the following example. Figure 68–3 depicts 20 patients observed for 6 months to study the development of an acute, short-lived disease lasting 5 days. The distinction between prevalence and incidence can be observed when we look at the situation at the 3-month mark. The *prevalence* at this point in time is 0/20, or 0%, because no patient among the 20 patients had the disease at that specified point in time. The *cumulative incidence* over these 3 months is 5 new cases in 20 patients, or 5/20 for 3 months, or 25/100/3 months. Note that if we had looked at the 2-month point in time, the prevalence would have been 2/20, or 10%, and the cumulative incidence would have been 25/100/2 months.

## RELATIVE RISK AND ODDS RATIO

Because we often are interested in comparing variables or attributes (i.e., incidence of disease) across

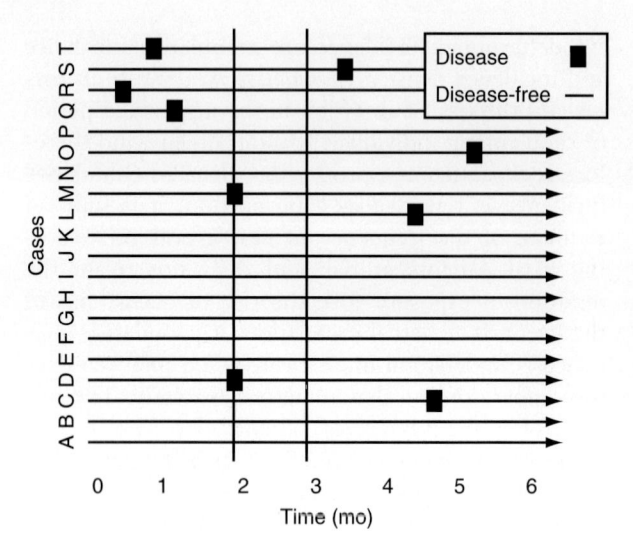

**Figure 68–3** Hypothetical acute disease data.

samples and populations, alternative methods are required to summarize data. These analyses are important in medical practice because it is often of interest to describe the risk of a particular outcome relative to the presence or absence of a predisposing factor. For example, it may be of interest to report the association between maternal height as a predictor for C-section or to report the risk of benign ovarian teratomas relative to whether the patient has a history of infertility. Two different ratios can be used to describe such risks. The first is termed the relative risk, the second, the odds ratio.

The *relative risk*, usually symbolized as RR, is a ratio of the incidence of an outcome of interest in exposed patients vis-à-vis unexposed patients. The risk ratio can be determined only in a cohort study (for description of study designs, refer to a later section in this chapter) in which a sample of patients is identified as either exposed or unexposed to the risk factor and then observed through time until the outcome of interest is seen. The value of the RR always is positive. An RR of 1 indicates an equal risk regardless of exposure in the two cohorts. An RR of less than 1 suggests a lower risk of the outcome associated with exposure, or a protective effect. An RR greater than 1 reveals a higher risk or incidence of that outcome associated with exposure to the risk factor. To illustrate, if one is interested in evaluating the association between maternal height (exposure) and risk of C-section (outcome), one would identify a sample of pregnant women, measure their height, and observe them until they deliver vaginally or by C-section. To understand the actual calculation of the RR, consider the data in Table 68–2, in which the sample of women has been divided into two groups based on height: those shorter than 150 cm and those greater than or equal to 150 cm or taller.

For simplification, RR is calculated in two steps; first the numerator and then the denominator. The numerator describes the incidence of vaginal delivery in tall women and is calculated as the number of women with height greater than or equal to 150 cm who delivered vaginally (466) divided by the total number of women with a height greater than or equal to 150 cm (470), or 466/470, which equates to 0.991. The denominator is the incidence of vaginal delivery in short women and is calculated as the number of women with height less than 150 cm who delivered vaginally (27) divided by the total number of women with height less than 150 cm (68), or 27/68, which equates to 0.397. Therefore, the relative risk is

$$RR = \frac{466/470}{27/68} = \frac{0.991}{0.397} = 2.496$$

These results can be interpreted as "a pregnant woman who is at least 150 cm tall is 2.496 times more likely to have a normal vaginal delivery than a pregnant woman who is less than 150 cm tall."

The *odds ratio*, usually symbolized as OR, is an estimate of the relative risk of the exposed group and is used when the study of interest is a case-control study. For further information on study designs, see the related discussion in this chapter. The OR also can be used to describe cohort studies but typically is used for case-control studies in which the relative risk cannot be determined because the incidence cannot be estimated. In other words, the study of interest is one in which the patient sample is selected based on the outcome of interest, and then medical histories are examined to determine exposure or risk factors.

For example, consider a case-control study designed to examine the risk factors for benign ovarian teratomas. One of the variables or risk factors of interest to the investigators was the history of infertility. The patients were selected based on their development of ovarian teratomas. The authors also selected a sample of controls in whom teratomas did not develop. The medical histories of each of the patients and controls were examined to determine whether the subject had a history of infertility. The OR was calculated as the odds that a patient was exposed to the risk factor, divided by the odds that a

**Table 68–2** Maternal Height and Delivery Method Data

|  | Vaginal Delivery | Cesarean Section |  |
| --- | --- | --- | --- |
| Maternal height < 150 cm | 27 | 41 | 68 |
| Maternal height ≥ 150 cm | 466 | 4 | 470 |
|  | 493 | 45 | 538 |

**Table 68–3** Ovarian Teratoma and Infertility Data

|  | Ovarian Teratomas | No Ovarian Teratomas |
|---|---|---|
| History of infertility | 4 | 2 |
| No history of infertility | 73 | 229 |
|  | 77 | 231 |

control was exposed. To understand the actual calculation of this ratio, consider the data in Table 68–3.

For simplification, OR is calculated in two steps, the numerator and the denominator, each of which is a ratio. The numerator is the odds that a patient with ovarian teratomas has a history of infertility and is calculated as (4/77)/(73/77), or 0.055. The denominator is the odds that a control without ovarian teratomas has a history of infertility and is calculated as (2/231)/(229/231), or 0.009. Therefore, the odds ratio is

$$OR = \frac{\frac{4/77}{73/77}}{\frac{2/231}{229/231}} = \frac{0.055}{0.009} = 6.11$$

These results can be interpreted as "the odds of benign ovarian teratomas are 6.11 times greater for a patient with history of infertility compared with a patient without history of infertility."

The OR, similar to the RR, is always positive. An odds ratio of 1 indicates equal odds of the outcome regardless of exposure in the two cohorts. An odds ratio of less than 1 suggests lower odds of the outcome associated with exposure, or a protective effect. An odds ratio of greater than 1 reveals higher odds of the outcome associated with exposure to the risk factor.

## QUANTITATIVE DATA: CENTRAL TENDENCY

*Quantitative*, or numeric, data obtained from a sample of patients can be summarized in several ways. Because each patient in a sample is reflected by a numeric value that itself may vary along a continuum, quantitative variables have unique distributions. For example, serum estradiol levels for 20 females may vary on a theoretical continuum from 0 to 300 pg/ml or greater. A *distribution* is the pattern of variation that the quantitative variables display for the sample. This variation or distribution can be presented as individual numeric values or using several types of graphs. The graphs include stem-and-leaf plots, bar graphs, dot plots, histograms, boxplots, and scatterplots. This chapter does not include descriptions of each of the types of graphical representations (see References).

Quantitative variables also can be summarized using numeric measures. The most common of these measures is an index of central tendency or the center of the distribution. The three measures of central tendency are the mean, median, and mode. The *mean* is calculated as a simple, arithmetic average of the observations and represents the numerical center of the distribution. It is symbolized by $\bar{X}$ and is calculated as follows:
1. Sum the observations.
2. Divide the sum by the total number of observations.

Using the following hypothetical values:

9.1, 5.0, 12.8, 6.8, 4.3, 7.6, 8.4, 3.2, 11.3, 5.0,

the mean of this set can be calculated as:

$$\bar{X} = \frac{\sum X_i}{n} = \frac{9.1 + 5.0 + 12.8 \ldots + 11.3 + 5.0}{10} = \frac{73.5}{10} = 7.35$$

This summary measure should only be used with quantitative data. The reason it never is used with qualitative data is because its meaning is lost. For example, taking the mean of the number of siblings each patient has and concluding that the mean is 3.4 is meaningless because no one can have 0.4 of a sibling.

The *median* is the middle observation of a set of data, that is, half of the observations are smaller and half of the observations are larger than the median value. Therefore, calculating the median follows this procedure:
1. Arrange all the observations from smallest to largest.
2. Identify the middle value. With an odd number of observations, the median is the middle value. If there are an even number of observations, the median is the arithmetic mean of the two middle values.

For example, ranking the previous hypothetical dataset from smallest to largest results in:

3.2, 4.3, 5.0, 5.0, 6.8, 7.6, 8.4, 9.1, 11.3, 12.8

Because our dataset consists of 10 values, the median is the arithmetic mean of the two middle values, 6.8 and 7.6, or 7.2, as follows:

median = 7.2

3.2, 4.3, 5.0, 5.0, 6.8,    7.6, 8.4, 9.1, 11.3, 12.8

One of the advantages of the median is that it is less sensitive to extreme values, or outliers. For example, consider if there had been a final value of 25 in the previous example. The median would be the sixth value, 7.6, not far from the median of 7.2. However, the mean of this dataset would be 8.95, which is quite different from the original mean of 7.35.

$$\bar{X} = \frac{\sum X_i}{n} = \frac{9.1 + 5.0 + 12.8 \ldots + 11.3 + 5.0 + 25}{11} = \frac{98.5}{11} = 8.95$$

Another advantage of the median is that it can be used for summarizing qualitative data because its determination does not involve the actual numeric values of the observations.

The *mode* of a set of data is the value that appears most often, or has the highest frequency. Note that a set of data could have more than one mode if two or more values appear with the same high frequency (bimodal, trimodal, etc.). The use of this summary statistic is applied best to large quantities of data when the most frequent value is of interest. Using the data from the previous example, we see that the mode of this set is 5.0 because it occurs twice whereas all other values appear only once.

## VARIATION

Previously, we introduced the term *distribution* and defined it as the pattern of variation for a set of variables from a sample of interest. One statistic used to describe variation is the range of a set of observations. The *range* is defined as the difference between the maximum value and the minimum value of the observed set of data. Therefore, the range is a numeric value that takes on the same unit as that used with the original observations. Using our previous dataset, shown as follows, it is apparent that the range of this set is 12.8 − 3.2, or 9.6.

3.2, 4.3, 5.0, 5.0, 6.8, 7.6, 8.4, 9.1, 11.3, 12.8

As useful as it is to know the range of a set of data, this information does not capture all that we need to know. The range takes into consideration only two values from the entire set of data and ignores the remainder. For example, the following are two sets of data, both with a range of 45.

40, 40.5, 41, 41, 42, 43, 60, 80, 82, 85

15, 20, 25, 30, 35, 40, 45, 50, 55, 60

Note that the first set of data appears to have the bulk of its observations close to the minimum value, whereas the second set of data has observations evenly spaced between the minimum and maximum values. If the range is the only reported measure of variation, the sets of data would look similar, when in fact, they are quite different.

An alternative measure of variation is *quartiles*. If the data are not too numerous, the lower quartile and the upper quartile can be calculated easily. Assuming that the data are in ascending order, the lower quartile is the first one quarter of the ordered observations, and the upper quartile is the last one quarter of the observations. To locate the upper boundary of the first quartile, find the value that is halfway between the minimum value and the median. To locate the lower boundary of the fourth quartile, find the value that is halfway between the median and the maximum value. To illustrate, consider the following set of ascending values, which we will divide into four groups or quartiles.

2.4, 2.7, 3.5, 5.6, 5.9, 6.2, 6.5, 7.0, 9.3, 12.9, 13.2,

14.1, 14.5, 19.8, 23.4, 28.0, 36.1

Note that the median of the dataset is 9.3. The value that is halfway between the median (9.3) and the minimum value (2.4) is 5.9. Therefore the *lower quartile* of this dataset consists of all the values that fall below 5.9. The value that is halfway between the median (9.3) and the maximum value (36.1) is 14.5. Therefore the *upper quartile* of this dataset consists of all the values that are above 14.5, as illustrated at bottom of page.

The distance between the lower and upper quartiles is termed the *interquartile range* or *interquartile distance*. This measure of variation accounts for more values than the range, but it is of limited utility when working with few observations.

A better measure of variation is the *variance*. This

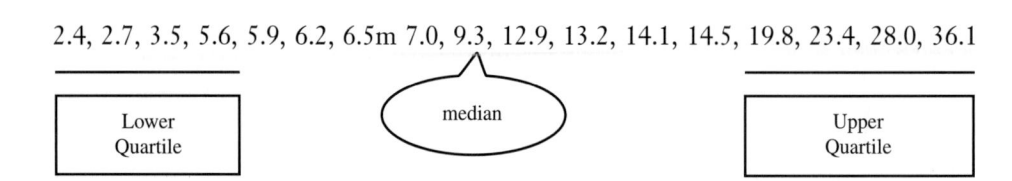

---

2.4, 2.7, 3.5, 5.6, 5.9, 6.2, 6.5m 7.0, 9.3, 12.9, 13.2, 14.1, 14.5, 19.8, 23.4, 28.0, 36.1

Lower Quartile — median — Upper Quartile

measure takes into account each value by calculating its deviation from the mean. The variance involves squaring the deviations, summing the resulting squares and then dividing by the total number of observations. Thus, the variance can be written as:

$$\text{Variance} = \frac{\sum \left(X_i - \overline{X}\right)^2}{n}$$

where $\Sigma$ is the Greek symbol for summation, $X_i$ represents each observation, $\overline{X}$ represents the mean, and n represents the total number of observations. The formula for the variance usually substitutes (n-1) for n, as follows:

$$\text{Variance} = \frac{\sum \left(X_i - \overline{X}\right)^2}{n - 1}$$

The reasons for this minor adjustment are beyond the scope of this text; however, the adjusted formula is a better estimate of the overall population variance from which the sample was originally drawn. Because it is more convenient to talk about a measure of variation that takes on the units of the original set of data and because the variance includes squared units, variation often is reported as the *standard deviation*. The standard deviation is the square root of the variance and thus has units identical to those of the original set of data.

$$\text{Standard Deviation} = \sqrt{\frac{\sum \left(X_i - \overline{X}\right)^2}{n - 1}}$$

Estimating the variance is essential before proceeding to the next step in the analysis of samples. For example, most analytical studies using epidemiologic methods compare samples of patients from one population with samples from another, for example, cases and controls or exposed and unexposed cohorts. To conclude that one sample differs from another requires the application of inferential statistics, such as the student's $T$ test, chi-squared test, or analysis of variance (ANOVA). Analyses using any inferential statistical test requires an estimate of the variance of the sample.

## METHODS FOR STUDYING POPULATIONS

The previous section illustrated measures for describing populations and samples. These tools provide the basis for comparing groups or populations, for example, cases and controls. This section describes clinical study designs commonly used to examine hypotheses by comparing two or more groups and provides examples of how descriptive measures are used to support the investigator's conclusions.

Figure 68–4 represents a classification of study designs used in epidemiologic studies to describe or compare groups of subjects. Classification of designs can vary from one textbook to another; only those designs described in this chapter are represented in the figure. Nonexperimental studies can be dichotomized into descriptive and analytical studies. Case reports and case series are examples of descriptive study designs. Analytical studies include cross-sectional and longitudinal studies. Longitudinal studies include case-control and cohort studies. A clinical trial is the only type of experimental study that is illustrated in this chapter.

## NONEXPERIMENTAL STUDIES

A *nonexperimental study* is a study in which the investigator does not play an active part in the study but

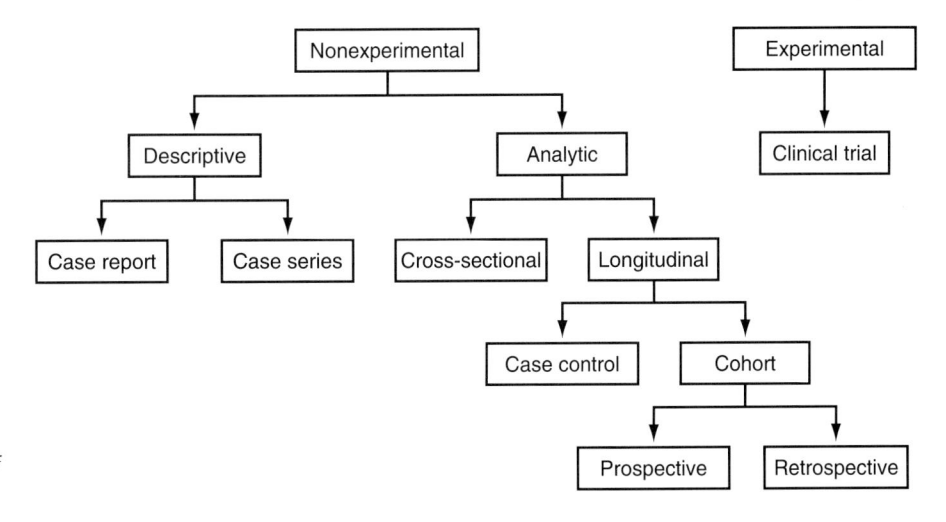

**Figure 68–4** Classification of study designs.

only records data as they occur. These studies also are designated as *observational* studies and can be broken down into two types, descriptive and analytical.

The simplest form of a descriptive study is the case report. A *case report* provides detailed documentation of a single case, or in some instances, a few cases. It is a common tool used to convey information to clinical professionals and describes rare cases or events. In a case report, information regarding exposure to the causal agent is not available, and one can make no inference regarding linkages between treatment and outcome.

*Example:*

Necrotizing fasciitis is a rare condition in which a bacterial infection occurs after trauma or a surgical break in skin integrity. Necrotizing fasciitis has been described previously in the literature after various surgical procedures. In a recent publication, the authors documented necrotizing fasciitis in a woman after postpartum tubal ligation. A 43-year-old woman, gravida 9 para 6, presented in labor at 39 weeks gestation. After delivery, a bilateral tubal ligation was performed. The procedure was considered routine, and there were no abnormal findings or misadventures. The patient presented to the emergency room 3 days postsurgery exhibiting signs of infection at the site of the incision. The necrotic area was debrided surgically, and the pathology report confirmed necrotizing fasciitis.

The preceding example is a simple description of an interesting, unusual event. In a case report, the author cannot make causal inferences or generalizations to a larger population. For the reader, a case report provides little value for facilitating diagnostic or therapeutic decisions.

Another tool for describing rare events is the case series. The *case series* is similar in design to the case report but typically describes several cases linked by common diagnoses or clinical characteristics. Like the case report, it is useful only for descriptive purposes. Because case series usually are uncontrolled and consist of convenience samples, little useful information is generated that can inform decisions in populations.

The first type of analytical study examined is the *cross-sectional* study. This is a study in which the investigator plays an active role from the beginning, and subjects are selected without prior knowledge of whether they have the disease in question. The sample then is surveyed, and an estimation of prevalence is calculated as a proportion. Cross-sectional studies are also known as *prevalence studies*. Prevalence studies have the advantage of being relatively low in cost and easy to manage. In choosing this type of study design, the investigator may describe associations between the disease and other exposure factors. However, one can make no inferences about causal relationships because there is no information on the chronologic association between presumed cause and outcome.

*Example:*

Investigators from Finland conducted a study to determine whether hospitals of different levels provide comparable obstetrical care. A cross-sectional survey, composed of data from the Finish Medical Birth Registry, was completed on all women who gave birth in Finland from 1987–1988. Hospitals were stratified into different levels of care according to official administrative categories, staffing, and access to technical equipment. The investigators found that perinatal mortality rates were not significantly different across the levels of hospitals. This study is classified as cross-sectional because it is a report of data collected at one point in time for each hospital. No follow-up occurred with the patients, and therefore, no inferences can be extrapolated to a large population.

In contrast to the cross-sectional study, a *longitudinal study* involves the collection of data from more than one subject over an extended period of time. *Case-control studies* are one of the most common epidemiologic study designs for the purpose of examining causation. *Cases* are classified as subjects who have been diagnosed with the disease of interest, whereas *controls* are those persons who are free of the disease. The investigator must take steps to ensure that the two groups are comparable, except for the presence of disease. The investigator then examines both groups for previous exposure to the agent(s) suspected of causing the disease. Figure 68–5 depicts the case-control study. The frequency of exposure is compared across the two groups and typically is reported as an OR.

*Example:*

A case-control study was conducted in Milan, Italy to determine the risk factors for benign ovarian teratomas. Cases included 77 women, aged 16–64 years, with a confirmed diagnosis of ovarian teratoma. Controls included 231 women, of the same age range, admitted to area hospitals and clinics for nongynecologic, nonhormonal, and non-neoplastic conditions. Demographic information, including reproductive histories, was collected for each of the women in the study. A history of infertility (OR = 8.3) and higher education (OR = 2.5) were associated with a higher risk for benign ovarian teratomas. The results indicated no significant relationship between cases and controls with regard to menstrual or reproductive factors.

A *cohort study* is a study of a group(s) of subjects over time. The most common cohort studies are the prospective cohort and the retrospective cohort study designs. In a *prospective cohort study*, subjects (cases) who are free of disease are selected to participate. Controls often are selected based on different levels

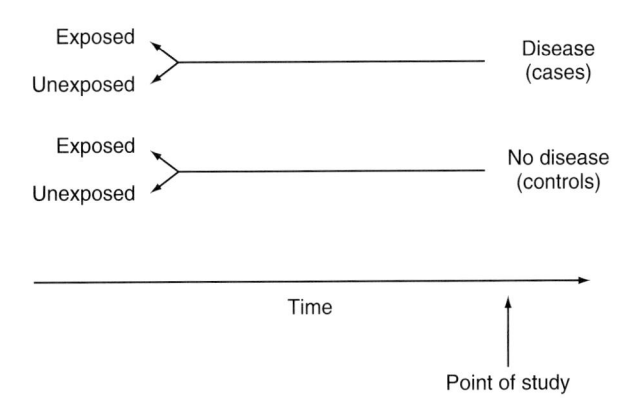

**Figure 68-5** Design of a case-control study.

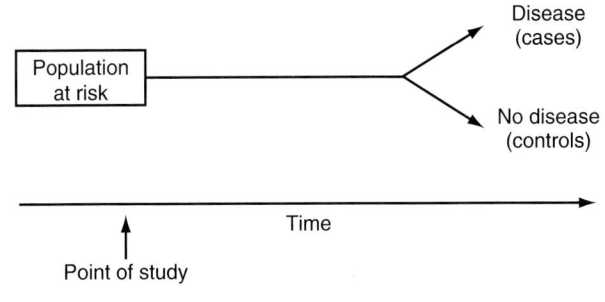

**Figure 68-6** Design of a prospective cohort study.

of exposure to presumed causal agents. Figure 68-6 depicts the design of a prospective cohort study. The cohorts are followed over time to determine which subjects develop the disease, while information regarding exposure to risk factors is collected concurrently. For those hypotheses that cannot be tested in an experimental setting because of the nature of the disease, the prospective cohort study—a natural experiment—is a good substitute. Generally, these studies tend to be more costly because the investigator must enroll large numbers of subjects who ultimately will not experience the outcome of interest, and all subjects must be followed over a long period of time.

*Example:*

To examine maternal height as a predictor of vaginal delivery, investigators in Ghana used a prospective cohort study design. The study included 538 primigravida women who reported to the department of obstetrics and gynecology in a local teaching hospital between November 1991 and January 1992. Women delivering premature babies and multiple births were among those excluded from the sample. Maternal height was measured shortly after delivery. Mothers who delivered vaginally had a mean height of 161.3 cm ± 5.7 (standard deviation) compared with 150.4 cm ± 8.8 for mothers who delivered by C-section. The investigators concluded that women less than 150 cm in height are more likely to fail spontaneous vaginal delivery and should be monitored closely for possible delivery by C-section.

In contrast to a prospective cohort study, a *retrospective cohort study* is less expensive and can be completed in a relatively short period of time. In this type of study, subjects who are known to have been exposed to a particular agent are identified from past records and followed to the present time or into the future to determine which subjects develop the disease. Figure 68-7 demonstrates the study design of a retrospective cohort study.

## EXPERIMENTAL STUDIES

*Experimental studies* are designed and managed by the investigator to examine specific hypotheses. Experimental studies often are performed in laboratories. Investigators use experimental studies to identify causation of a disease or condition, as well as to assess the efficacy of prevention and treatment. Experimental studies in human populations usually are designed to evaluate treatment for disease. The latter experimental studies are referred to as clinical trials.

A *clinical trial* is defined as a planned experiment designed to assess the efficacy of a treatment for a population by comparing the outcomes in samples of patients. One sample is treated with the agent of interest and is compared with one or more control samples receiving a placebo or standard treatment. In a randomized clinical trial, patients are assigned to either a treatment or placebo group using a randomization technique to ensure that each patient has an equal chance of being assigned to the treatment group. The randomization allows for an unbiased comparison of the treatment and placebo groups.

Clinical trials are used among pharmaceutical or manufacturing companies as a means of achieving approval by the Food and Drug Administration (FDA) for the sale of a drug, treatment, or device in the United States. For approval to be granted, the item must demonstrate both safety and efficacy

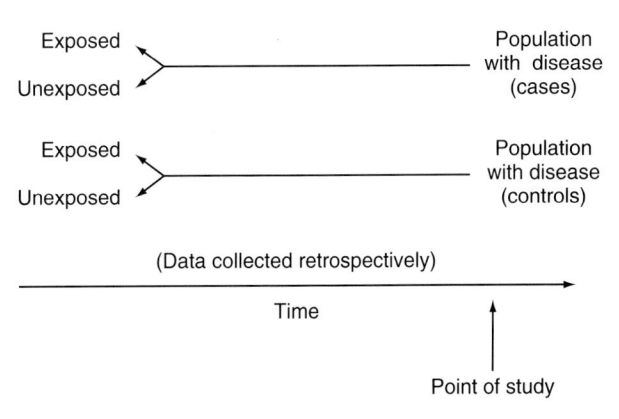

**Figure 68-7** Design of a retrospective cohort study.

through a controlled trial. This generally is achieved through the systemic conduct of four primary phases of experimentation, outlined in Figure 68–8.

*Example:*

In an effort to determine whether feedback improves the quality of cervical Papanicolaou (Pap) smears, 183 physicians were randomized to one of four intervention groups in a clinical trial. The first group served as the control group, receiving no intervention. The second group received a comment with each laboratory report based on the quality of the cervical Pap smear. The third group received a comment of the quality of their Pap smears compared with the rest of the physicians in the sample (peer comparison). Finally, the fourth group was given specific advice about how to improve on deficiencies in their procedure. The authors determined that as the intensity of the feedback increased, a correlational decrease in the number of Pap smears lacking endocervical cells was noted, but this was not found to be statistically significant. This study is an example of an experimental trial of feedback interventions.

Phase I — Clinical pharmacology and toxicity studies
Phase II — Initial clinical investigation for treatment effect
Phase III — Full-scale evaluation of treatment
Phase IV — Postmarketing surveillance

**Figure 68–8** Phases of clinical trials.

## How Do Epidemiologic Studies Impact the Practice of Obstetrics and Gynecology?

The science of clinical medicine relies heavily on epidemiologic techniques. In the following section, we provide selected examples that illustrate how the aforementioned tools can be used to evaluate and improve clinical decision-making regarding diagnosis, treatment, and management of practice. Several excellent texts are available that elaborate on these techniques as well as describe more advanced methods for informing clinical decision-making. The reader is referred to two texts: *Clinical Epidemiology: The Essentials*, 2nd ed., by Fletcher and associates, and *Clinical Epidemiology: A Basic Service for Clinical Medicine* by Sackett and colleagues.

## Applications of Epidemiologic Methods in the Evaluation of Screening and Diagnostic Tools

The effectiveness of screening and diagnostic tools is based on performance in populations of subjects. How accurately does the procedure distinguish between subjects with and without a disease or condition of interest? To answer this important question requires epidemiologic methods that describe and analyze categoric data. The attributes of screening and diagnostic methods include measures of sensitivity, specificity, predictive values, and likelihood ratios. In the following examples, sensitivity and specificity are introduced.

The terms sensitivity and specificity are used to describe the association between a diagnostic test and an individual's disease status. *Sensitivity* refers to the proportion of patients with a particular disease who have a positive diagnostic test result for the disease. The goal of a sensitive test is to reduce the number of false-negative test results. *Specificity* is the proportion of patients without disease who have a negative diagnostic test result for the disease. A test that is highly specific is unlikely to classify a person as having a disease when they actually are disease free. Figure 68–9 provides a 2 × 2 table that categorized these terms. Special attention must be given to false-negative and false-positive results.

A clinician ultimately wants a diagnostic test that has both high sensitivity and specificity. However, because of the limitations of screening and diagnostic tests, the researcher often maximizes one attribute at the expense of the alternative. Whether a clinician decides to choose a test with high sensitivity or specificity depends on the disease in question and the objectives of the user. For example, a blood bank desires a highly sensitive test for human immunodeficiency virus (HIV) to ensure that the fewest possible contaminated samples enter the blood supply. In contrast, a highly specific test would be desirable to the practitioner caring for the individual patient to avoid the emotional distress of a false-positive diagnosis for HIV.

Figure 68–10 portrays the model for calculating sensitivity and specificity for all patients tested for a certain disease. Patients may or may not have the disease and may have either a positive or negative test result. Each cell represents a mutually exclusive group of patients that share similar disease status and test result. Sensitivity and specificity can be calculated from the cells as follows:

$$\text{Sensitivity} = A/(A+C)$$

$$\text{Specificity} = D/(B+D)$$

*Example:*

To illustrate the process of validation of cervical cytology, researchers examined a database containing

748,871 cytologic screening results representing 277,842 women. There are several techniques that can be used to validate the results of the initial screening. In this study, the authors chose a long-term follow-up of initial results. Women who tested negative for cervical cancer were classified as truly negative only if a minimum of two negative cytologic examination results were documented within 3 years. Validation of positive cytologic findings was performed by subsequent histologic examination performed within 1 year. As shown in Figure 68–11, the results from their validation process revealed sensitivity of 79.98% and specificity of 99.95% for the overall population.

|  | Disease + | Disease − |
|---|---|---|
| Test result + | A | B |
| Test result − | C | D |

Sensitivity = A/(A+C)
Specificity = D/(B+D)

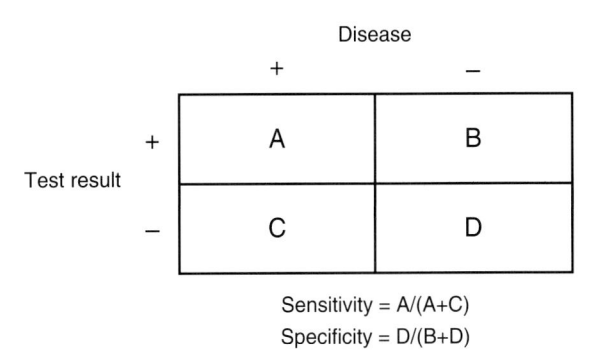

**Figure 68–10** Sensitivity and specificity 2 × 2 table.

## APPLICATIONS OF CLINICAL EPIDEMIOLOGY IN TREATMENT DECISIONS

The literature describing studies of the effectiveness of aspirin for preventing pregnancy-induced hypertension (PIH) and preeclampsia provides a good example of how clinical epidemiology intersects with the practice of obstetrics and gynecology.

An early study of drug ingestion by pregnant women reported aspirin to be one of the most commonly consumed drugs. Investigators randomly selected 911 mothers in Scotland and retrospectively surveyed their complete drug use during pregnancy. Fifty-four percent of the women admitted to using aspirin during pregnancy. The purpose of the study was to describe the frequency of drug consumption during pregnancy. No specific hypotheses were tested.

The first study to examine the specific hypothesis that the frequency of PIH is reduced among women who ingested aspirin was a case-control study of 146 primigravida women. In this retrospective analytical study, it was reported that preeclampsia developed in only 4% of women who ingested aspirin during pregnancy vs. 16% of the control group (women who took no aspirin). The study design provided evidence for a potential beneficial effect of aspirin for preventing preeclampsia. However, this study did not indicate dosages or gestational age at which the women took aspirin. In addition, one cannot be certain in this study that controls were comparable to cases. However, the case-control study did generate interest in aspirin as a potential prophylactic agent for preeclampsia.

A number of small clinical trials were conducted to examine the potential of low-dose aspirin therapy to reduce the incidence of preeclampsia. These studies consisted of small sample sizes varying from 33 to 102 patients. These clinical trials were not comparable in study design—differences included methods of randomization, blinding patients to the intervention, aspirin dosage, time of gestation that prophylaxis commenced, normotensive or hypertensive status at recruitment, and parity. The results for some of the key studies are summarized in Table 68–4. The selected studies in Table 68–4 all have a RR of less than 1, indicating a protective effect of aspirin in the development of PIH. For further explanation of RR, refer to the earlier section in this chapter. Overall, the combined literature from the several small studies suggested that aspirin reduced the risk of PIH among pregnant women by 65%.

Practitioners should recognize an important limitation in drawing conclusions from these small clinical trials. There is a tendency or bias for studies with positive results to be reported in the literature. It is likely that there were other studies of comparable sample size that were not reported because of negative findings. Thus, there is a publication bias for positive findings.

|  | Disease + | Disease − |
|---|---|---|
| Test result + | True positive | False positive |
| Test result − | False negative | True negative |

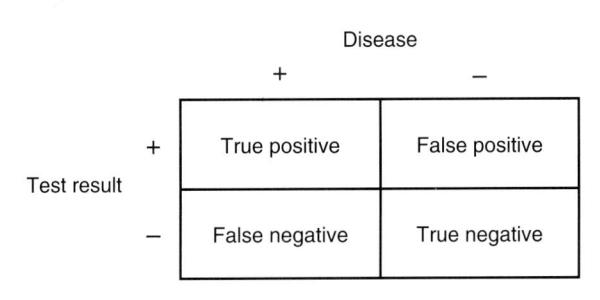

**Figure 68–9** Sensitivity and specificity model.

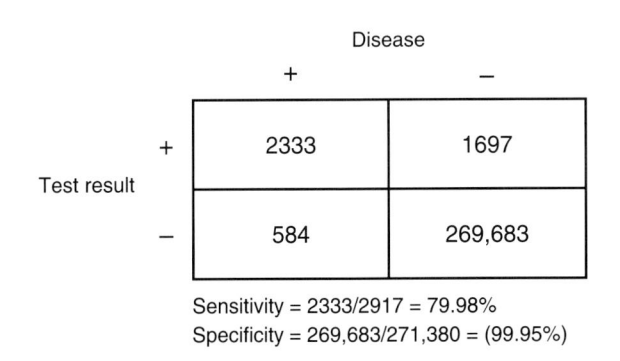

|  | Disease + | Disease − |
|---|---|---|
| Test result + | 2333 | 1697 |
| Test result − | 584 | 269,683 |

Sensitivity = 2333/2917 = 79.98%
Specificity = 269,683/271,380 = (99.95%)

**Figure 68–11** Sensitivity and specificity example.

**Table 68–4** Summary of the Controlled Trials

| Reference | Sample Size (N) | Aspirin (PIH/N) | Control (PIH/N) | Effect Size (RR) |
|---|---|---|---|---|
| Beaufils et al, 1985 | 102 | 4/48 | 9/45 | 0.42 |
| Wallenburg et al, 1986 | 46 | 3/23 | 12/23 | 0.25 |
| Wallenburg and Rotmans, 1987 | 48 | 2/24 | 4/24 | 0.13 |
| Schiff et al, 1989 | 65 | 4/34 | 11/31 | 0.33 |
| Benigni et al, 1989 | 33 | 0/17 | 3/16 | 0.00 |
| McParland et al, 1990 | 100 | 7/48 | 23/52 | 0.33 |

PIH/N, cases of pregnancy-induced hypertension/total sample size; RR, relative risk.

Recently, a number of large experimental clinical trials were conducted to address the limitations of earlier studies. The largest study was the Collaborative Low-dose Aspirin Study in Pregnancy (CLASP). The CLASP study randomized 9364 women between 12 and 32 weeks gestation from 16 countries to receive 60 mg of aspirin or a placebo every day. This is an example of a clinical trial, described earlier in this chapter. Figure 68–12 summarizes the findings of the CLASP trial for the effects of aspirin on the risk of preeclampsia. Preeclampsia developed in only 6.7% of the women in the aspirin treatment group vs. 7.6% in the control or placebo group. Using the OR to compare the outcomes in the treatment and control groups, authors reported an OR of 0.88. For an explanation of OR, the reader should refer to the discussion earlier in this chapter. Recall that when the OR is less than 1, results imply a protective effect, that is aspirin afforded some measurable protection against PIH. Earlier in this chapter, we suggested that for a cohort or experimental study, investigators may use ORs to estimate differences in cohorts; however, a preferred estimate of differences is the RR. Although it is not clear why the authors elected to report the OR rather than RR, we can estimate the RR for this study. From Figure 68–12 we see that the incidence of preeclampsia for those exposed to aspirin is 313/4659. The incidence among the unexposed is 352/4650. Thus, the RR can be calculated as:

$$RR = \frac{313/4659}{352/4650} = \frac{0.067}{0.076} = 0.88$$

The OR in this instance is a close approximation of the RR. Whether one uses the RR or OR has little impact on the interpretation of the overall results.

Having established an estimate of the difference in the risk of PIH after aspirin prophylaxis relative to placebo-treated controls, the clinician must ask whether the difference has sufficient benefit to patients to justify adoption into his or her practice. To answer this question, the clinician must address at least three additional questions, all of which depend on additional epidemiologic evidence.

1. Is the difference in the treatment effect likely to have occurred by chance, suggesting that the intervention will not benefit my patients?

Inferential statistics are used to answer this question. Based on the assumptions and statistical tools used in the CLASP study, we cannot eliminate the possibility that an OR of 0.88 occurred by chance. Therefore, the CLASP study does not support the general use of aspirin as prophylaxis against PIH in pregnant women. But let us suppose that the OR was slightly

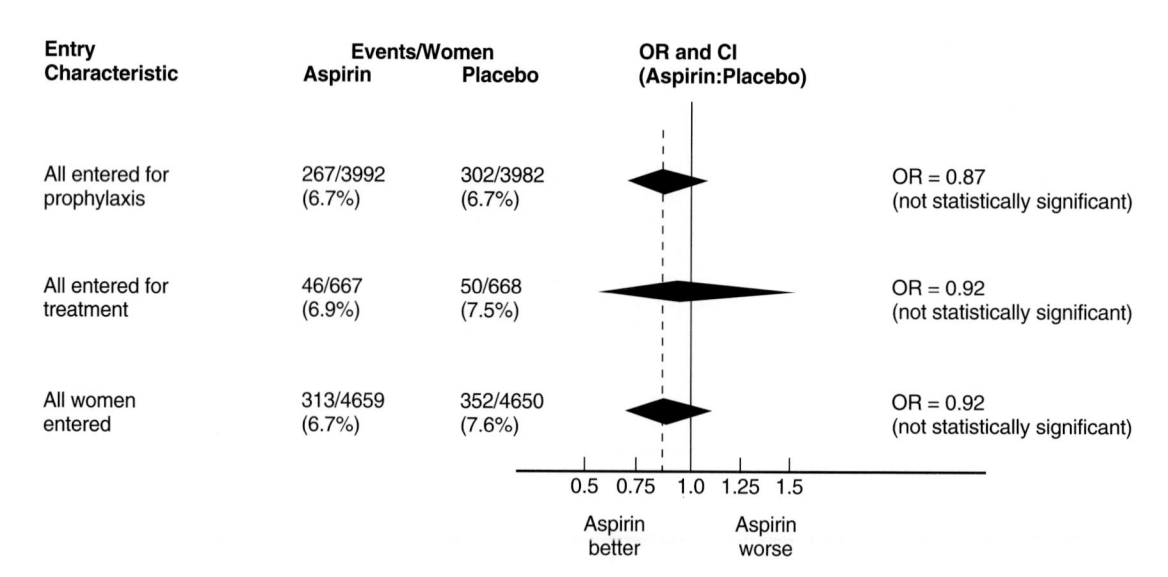

| Entry Characteristic | Events/Women Aspirin | Placebo | OR and CI (Aspirin:Placebo) | |
|---|---|---|---|---|
| All entered for prophylaxis | 267/3992 (6.7%) | 302/3982 (6.7%) | | OR = 0.87 (not statistically significant) |
| All entered for treatment | 46/667 (6.9%) | 50/668 (7.5%) | | OR = 0.92 (not statistically significant) |
| All women entered | 313/4659 (6.7%) | 352/4650 (7.6%) | | OR = 0.92 (not statistically significant) |

0.5  0.75  1.0  1.25  1.5
Aspirin better — Aspirin worse

**Figure 68–12** Effects of aspirin on proteinuric pre-eclampsia that develops after randomization. The black diamonds represent the odds ratio (OR) for developing pre-eclampsia. The stretch in the diamond is a reflection of the variation (confidence interval [CI]) for the OR at the 95% level. If the diamond is to the left of the solid vertical line, it indicates a protective effect.

greater such that inferential statistics confirmed that the benefit did not occur by chance.

2. Do the estimated benefits exceed the estimated risks of the intervention?

The answer to this question depends on the same clinical epidemiologic tools. The decision to treat with aspirin must be weighed against the frequency and severity of the potential adverse outcomes of the treatment, that is, benefits of treatment should exceed risks. If the clinician is comfortable that the benefits of the intervention outweigh the risks, a third question should be addressed before adopting it into practice.

3. What is the likelihood that the treatment, or prophylaxis, will be effective in my patients, given current circumstances, and at what cost?

The reader should not assume that when a clinical study—even when well designed—demonstrates a statistically significant effect of therapy that it necessarily will be effective in practice. If the proportion of patients who will benefit from treatment is relatively small whereas the cost of the intervention is relatively high, there may be insufficient justification for adopting the technology into practice. In addition to epidemiologic tools, answers to the third question require the application of cost-benefit analysis (or cost-effectiveness analysis).

## APPLICATIONS OF EPIDEMIOLOGIC TOOLS IN PRACTICE MANAGEMENT

Previous sections described how epidemiologic tools have been used to generate evidence supporting clinical decisions regarding screening, diagnostic testing, and selection of therapy. These epidemiologic applications have guided clinical practice for decades, although they often are transparent to the clinician. With the emergence of managed care and new integrated information technologies that facilitate access to aggregate data on processes and outcomes of medical care, epidemiologic tools are being used to generate new sources of information that challenge assumptions about the "art and science" of medical practices. The new sources of information offer opportunities to better inform decision-making and the management of clinical practice. However, physicians often are unfamiliar with this information and perceive it as threatening because it exposes personal practice patterns to managers, purchasers, and even patients. Because it is unlikely that these new sources of information on practice patterns will disappear, the clinician should use this new source of information to her or his advantage. Information describing disease profiles, technologic resource use, and individual practitioner profiles can be invaluable in improving current practice.

It has become routine to report C-section rates as a reflection of obstetric practices across health systems, hospitals, and practitioners. C-section rates provide a view of the process of obstetric care and a measure of resource use. Figure 68–13 summarizes hypothetical data reporting C-section rates (cumulative incidence) across nine obstetricians. The rates vary from 12 to 32 per 100 deliveries per annum. The generation of this report uses aforementioned tools in the section describing *rates*. In this example, the attribute or condition of interest is the performance of a C-section. The patients "at risk" of C-section are all pregnant women who present for delivery. Because we are interested in rates that can be compared across clinicians, we gather data on C-sections among pregnant women for a designated period of time. In the example in Figure 68–13, data were collected from the nine physicians during the same 12-month period. Using Physician E as an example, the practitioner

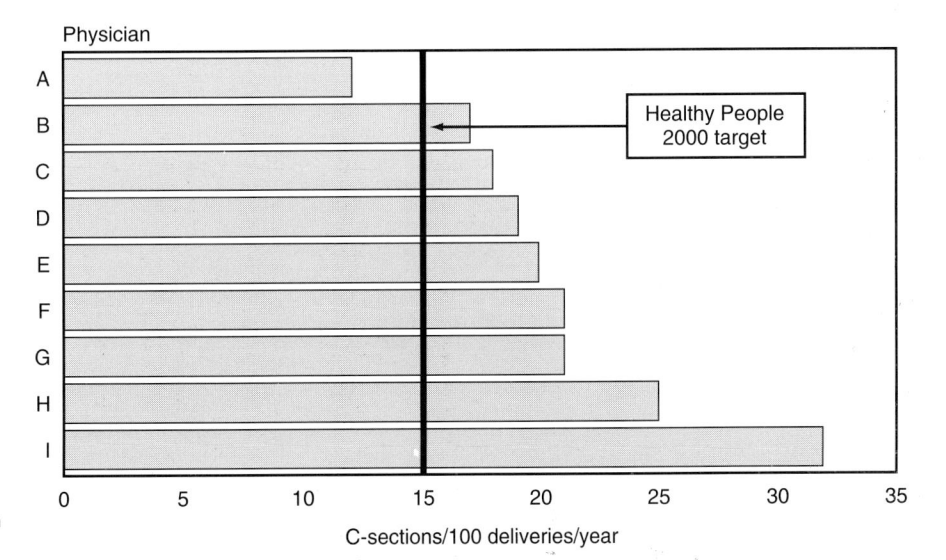

**Figure 68–13** Cesarean section rates for a sample of physicians.

attended 165 deliveries during the 12-month period of the analysis. She performed 33 C-sections among the 165 deliveries. Therefore, the C-section incidence rate for Physician E is calculated as follows:

$$\text{Incidence rate} = \frac{33 \text{ cesarean sections}}{165 \text{ total deliveries (12 months)}}$$

$$= 0.2 \text{ C-sections/delivery/annum} * \frac{100}{100}$$

$$= 20 \text{ C-sections/100 deliveries/annum}$$

Multiplication of the incidence rate of 0.2 by 100 (numerator and denominator) is a convention used to convert the rate into a quantity that makes more intuitive sense to practitioners.

Use of explicit, identical methods across all obstetricians can generate rates that can be compared across physicians (or hospitals, health systems). Figure 68–13 provides two anchors against which to compare C-section rates: (1) comparison across obstetricians in the same practice and (2) comparison against a national "target," that is, Healthy People 2000 target of approximately 15 C-sections per 100 deliveries.

How epidemiologic methods are used to generate information profiling obstetric practice is illustrated in Figure 68–13. Knowledge of epidemiology and of the strengths and weaknesses of the information must be used in the analysis of the information. On first reviewing the report in Figure 68–13, one might conclude that Physician I, with a C-section rate of 32 per 100 deliveries per annum—more than double the Healthy People 2000 target and higher than any of his colleagues—is inappropriate. However, our interpretation is limited by lack of information describing the conditions of the pregnancy and the indications for C-section. If Physician I cares for complicated, high-risk pregnant females, his C-section rate may be entirely appropriate. The information reported in Figure 68–13 should be used to raise questions. Why is there such wide variation between Physician A and I and their colleagues? There is no information in the figure that allows us to make a judgment about the appropriateness of the rates of either physician. Conversely, the information should provide a strong incentive for each individual practitioner to review her or his practice and to adjust or manage practice patterns if there is no clear indication for the high C-section rates.

There is another important limitation in the information reported in Figure 68–13. Reports of C-section rates provide a measure of process and resource use. There is no information in the figure that describes outcomes. For example, Physician A has a low C-section rate; but suppose that we reported in addition to C-section rates, rates of complications of vaginal delivery (i.e., rates of prolonged labor, infants with low APGAR scores, infants suffering consequences of hypoxemia). Also suppose that rates of adverse outcomes for Physician A were higher than her colleagues. In the latter scenario, C-section rates for Physician A may be too low.

The purpose of this discussion is to illustrate both the strengths and potential weaknesses of epidemiologic data for improving the management of our clinical practice. We add a note of caution for the practitioner. In the hands of a clinician who is knowledgeable in the strengths and weaknesses of epidemiology, the information can provide a valuable tool for improving the quality of medical care. In the hands of an uninformed manager, epidemiologic information can be misused and can compromise the quality of care. It is incumbent on physicians practicing in the current milieu to be knowledgeable in epidemiologic methods and to employ them appropriately in the improvement of current practice.

We have provided a simple example of C-section rates to illustrate the utility of epidemiologic methods in managing clinical practice. It should be apparent to the reader that the generation of other rate-based data would enhance the practitioners ability to manage care. Examples include:

## Process Measures

- VBAC (vaginal birth after C-section) rates
- Rate of physician encounters during the first trimester of pregnancy

## Outcomes Measures

- Complication rates including rates of third-and fourth-degree lacerations after vaginal delivery
- Postoperative surgical wound infection rates

All the aforementioned rates provide information on processes of clinical care that are manageable by the physician.

The epidemiologic methods described in this chapter make up some of the tools that enable clinicians to better manage practice improvement and to practice evidence-based medicine.

## REFERENCES

Beaufils M, Uzan S, Donsimoni R, Colau J: Prevention of preeclampsia by early antiplatelet therapy. Lancet 1:840–842, 1985.

Benigni A, Gregorini G, Frusca T, et al: Effect of low-dose aspirin on fetal and maternal generation of thromboxane by platelets in women at risk for pregnancy-induced hypertension. N Engl J Med 321:357–362, 1989.

Buntinx F, Knottnerus J, Crebolder H, et al: Does feedback improve the quality of cervical smears? A randomized controlled trial. Br J Gen Pract 43:194–198, 1992.

Choi S: Introductory Applied Statistics in Science. Englewood Cliffs, NJ, Prentice-Hall, 1978.

CLASP: CLASP: A randomized trial of low-dose aspirin for the prevention and treatment of pre-eclampsia among 9364 pregnant women. Lancet 343:619–629, 1994.

Crandon A, Isherwood D: Effect of aspirin on incidence of pre-eclampsia. Lancet 1:1356, 1979.

Dawson-Saunders B, Trapp R: Basic and Clinical Biostatistics. Norwalk, CT, Appleton & Lange, 1990.

Fletcher R, Fletcher S, Wagner E: Clinical Epidemiology: The Essentials. 3rd ed. Baltimore, MD, Williams & Wilkins, 1996.

Forfar J, Nelson M: Epidemiology of drugs taken by pregnant women: Drugs that may affect the fetus adversely. Clin Pharmacol Ther 14:632–642, 1973.

Gold MR, Siegel J, Russell L, et al: Cost-Effectiveness in Health and Medicine. New York, Oxford University Press, 1996.

Imperiale T, Petrulis A: A meta-analysis of low-dose aspirin for the prevention of pregnancy-induced hypertensive disease. JAMA 266:261–265, 1991.

Kuwawukume E, Ghosh T, Wilson J: Maternal height as a predictor of vaginal delivery. Int J Gynaecol Obstet 41:27–30, 1993.

Lilienfeld D, Stolley P: Fundamentals of Epidemiology. New York, Oxford University Press, 1994.

McParland P, Pearce J, Chamberlain G: Doppler ultrasound and aspirin in recognition and prevention of pregnancy-induced hypertension. Lancet 335:1552–1555, 1990.

Meinert C: Clinical Trials: Design, Conduct, and Analysis. New York: Oxford University Press, 1986.

Parazzini F, La Vecchia C, Negri E, et al: Risk factors for benign ovarian teratomas. Br J Cancer 71:644–646, 1995.

Piper J, West P: Necrotizing fasciitis following postpartum tubal ligation: A case report and review of the literature. Arch Gynecol Obstet 256:35–38, 1995.

Pocock S. Clinical Trials: A Practical Approach. New York: John Wiley & Sons, 1983.

Rimm A, Hartz A, Kalbfleisch J, et al: Basic Biostatistics in Medicine and Epidemiology. New York, Appleton-Century-Crofts, 1980.

Sackett DC, Haynes RB, Guyatt EH, et al: Clinical Epidemiology: A Basic Service for Clinical Medicine. Boston, Little Brown, 1991.

Schiff E, Peleg E, Goldenberg M, et al: The use of aspirin to prevent pregnancy-induced hypertension and lower the ratio of thromboxane $A_2$ to prostacyclin in relatively high-risk pregnancies. N Eng J Med 321:351–356, 1989.

Semmelweis I: Die aetiologie, der begriff und die prophylaxis des kindbettfieber. Pest, Wien und Leipzig, C.A. Hartleben's Verlags-Expedition, 1861.

Soost H, Lange H, Lehmacher W, et al: The validation of cervical cytology: Sensitivity, specificity and predictive values. Acta Cytol 35:8–14, 1991.

Viisainen K, Gissler M, Hemminki E: Birth outcomes by level of obstetric care in Finland: A catchment area based analysis. J Epidemiol Community Health 48:400–405, 1994.

Wallenburg H, Rotmans N: Prevention of recurrent idiopathic fetal growth retardation by low-dose aspirin and dipyridamole. Am J Obstet Gynecol 157:1230–1235, 1987.

Wallenburg H, Dekker G, Makovitz J, et al: Low-dose aspirin prevents pregnancy-induced hypertension and preeclampsia in angiotensin-sensitive primigravidae. Lancet 1:1–3, 1986.

# 69

# Clinical Integration and Quality Management

## LESTER SILBERMAN

## Quality Is in the Eyes of the Beholder

In today's health-care system, what is meant by quality depends upon the vantage point from which one is looking. For the physician, quality means doing the right things and doing them correctly. That implies appropriate decision-making and excellence in technical performance leading to good outcomes and a satisfied patient. For the patient, quality means having easy access to her health-care provider, a good patient-physician interaction, the meeting of her expectations regarding her health care, and the desired health-care outcomes. The health-care plans sees quality as satisfied payers and employees and health-care providers who cause them little or no trouble and are aware of issues of cost containment. Finally, from the vantage point of the payer, quality is satisfied employees, low and predictable costs, and, perhaps, a health plan that meets the requirements of certifying agencies.

## Advantages of Quality Management

There are many obvious advantages to quality management, including the fact that we expect it of ourselves and our patients expect it of us. In addition, quality management decreases organizational frustration and is often required to meet the standards of certifying agencies. Finally, the achievement of quality is cost-effective or, to say it another way, poor quality costs money. Preventable wound infections, incorrect billing, and delayed initiation of medication may all result in complications or additional work to right the incorrect initial effort, and those complications or additional work add unnecessary cost to the system of health care.

There are several aspects of quality management. The first is quality planning. When a new program is considered, especially in response to a particular health or administrative need, appropriate planning is required to ensure that the program is successful and meets the needs for which it was designed. The second aspect is quality control. For many things that we monitor, we work within a zone of acceptance or quality control; that is, we accept a certain rate of wound infections in clean cases, a certain rate of patient satisfaction, and certain rates of cesarean sections, and vaginal births after cesarean sections (VBACs); as long as our rates fall within the "acceptable" range, we take no action to change them. This acceptable range may be defined locally or by rates published in the literature or promulgated by national agencies. When, on the other hand, the rate falls outside the accepted range, or the accepted range is changed by current literature, or there is a realization that performance might be significantly improved and that better patient care or cost-savings will result, the third aspect of quality management is initiated—quality improvement. The three aspects of quality management are illustrated in Figure 69–1. The area under the lower range of the quality control zone can be thought of as the cost of poor quality. Lowering the quality control zone by a quality improvement effort also decreases the cost of poor quality.

## Evaluating Quality

The evaluation of quality encompasses evaluation of three components of the system: structure, processes, and outcomes. Structure includes not only the physical facilities and equipment but also the presence and training of the personnel who work there. For example, to be able to provide anesthesia for emergency cesarean deliveries an institution needs an appropriate operating room with adequate anesthesia equipment. This room is, however, worthless unless there are also anesthesiology personnel readily available to attend the cesarean delivery.

The second component of the system comprises the processes by which things get done. These may include the flow of patients through the system, the diagnostic and therapeutic efforts that are performed, and even how a department monitors adherence to standards of care. Every aspect of patient care can be looked at as a process made up of multiple steps. Again, using the anesthesia example, once the need for an emergency cesarean section is recognized, how is the anesthesiologist contacted? Is he or she always in the labor and delivery area? Is he or she paged? Is there a telephone number that is always monitored? What happens if the anesthesiologist is busy with a case in the operating room? What is the process for ensuring that an anesthesiologist will always be immediately available, 24 hours a day, to attend an emergency cesarean delivery? The better and more complete the process, the less likely that it will fail.

The last component of the system is evaluation of outcome(s). Outcomes may be the result of medical and surgical therapy or administrative efforts to improve the admission or discharge process or any other aspect of patient care. Outcomes are evaluated by the physician, the patient, the insurance company, and the payer, all of whom may be looking for something different.

In our example, outcome may be defined as how long it takes the anesthesiologist to arrive at the emergency cesarean delivery once the call is made or, perhaps, how many times it takes more than 10 minutes for the anesthesiologist to arrive at the labor and delivery area, or any other measure of the outcome of the process.

An institution may decide that it is acceptable for anesthesia to be administered within 20 minutes of the decision to do a cesarean section. The institution monitors to make sure that all cases fall within this zone of quality control. An unfortunate obstetric outcome might suggest that a time of 10 minutes from the decision point to the initiation of anesthesia is more appropriate. A quality improvement effort might then be set up to improve the process and bring anesthesia services to the patient more quickly. If this is accomplished, monitoring will ensure that the new zone of quality control is maintained.

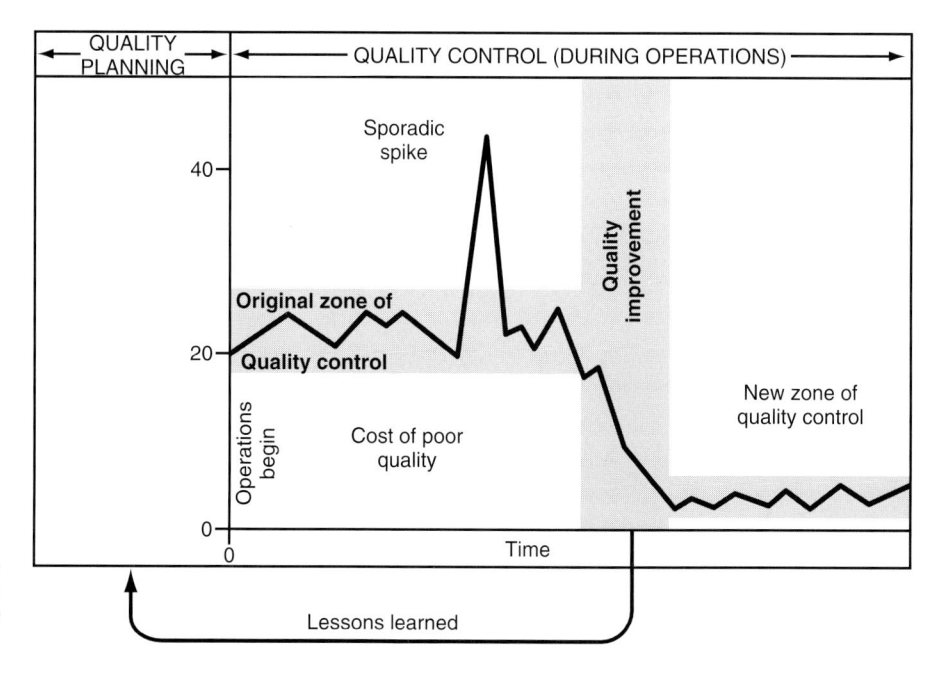

**Figure 69–1** The Juran Trilogy diagram. (From Juran JM: Juran on Quality by Design. New York, The Free Press, 1992, p 17.)

## Measurement of Quality

Process and outcome are appropriate areas for measurement of quality. Once a process is set up, adherence to that process can be evaluated. For example, the care of the pregnant diabetic patient may be the subject of a set of guidelines that define frequency of visits, how blood glucose levels are monitored, and what the acceptable range of values is, dietary and lifestyle counseling that should be performed, when fetal testing should be initiated, and timing of delivery. This process of care can then be evaluated by chart audit to determine whether or not the clinician has adhered to the guidelines. Outcomes for the pregnant woman with diabetes may also be assessed. These can include the number and length of antepartum admissions, the rate of cesarean sections, infant birth weights, maternal and neonatal lengths of hospital stay, and number of days the newborn spends in the neonatal intensive care unit (NICU). Outcomes may provide information on the adequacy of the guidelines and whether or not they are being followed. If, for example, the birth weights of infants of diabetic mothers are significantly above average, or NICU admissions are frequent, adherence to the guidelines can be studied. If compliance in the use of the guidelines is satisfactory, the guidelines themselves may require change. Other measurements of quality include patient satisfaction and cost-effectiveness.

The measurement of quality requires some sort of comparison standard. The first may be clinical, that is, a good clinician can review a record and recognize good (or bad) care and can answer the questions as to whether better care might have improved the outcome in a particular case and whether overall care was acceptable. Many peer review activities use this measurement technique. A second is to use benchmark data. These data may include evidence-based practice guidelines, best results in the literature, or even the performance of model hospitals similar to the hospital or department being evaluated.

There is, however, a problem with outcome evaluation. In simple terms, you can do everything wrong and still have a good outcome, and you can do everything right and still have an adverse outcome. The presumption is that over time, doing things right will show an advantage over not doing things right.

## Types of Quality Management

The old form of quality assurance (QA) management is well known, often used, and still useful. It involves the review of a chart after a bad outcome, the potential assignment of blame for that outcome, and some communication with the physician, either requesting additional information or indicating that care did not meet acceptable standards. For example, Dr. Jones is awakened by the nurse at 3 AM to review what the nurse considers to be an ominous fetal heart rate tracing. He tells the nurse that the pattern is all right and returns to bed. The patient subsequently delivers an obviously distressed and potentially compromised baby. The chart goes to peer review, the deficit in care is identified, and the committee indicates to the physician that care is considered substandard and refers the case to the department chairperson. The chairperson meets with the physician, reviews the case, and suggests some educational process or behavioral change in an attempt to forestall a similar episode in the future.

Using current methods of quality improvement (QI) and the same scenario as previously discussed, not only would the peer review process be concerned with the physician's faulty management of the case but it would also examine the system that allowed the physician to ignore the ominous fetal heart pattern. The question might be asked: To whom does the nurse go if a physician ignores what the nurse believes to be an abnormal pattern? Does the nurse speak to his or her supervisor, another physician, or the departmental chairperson? How does the system protect the fetus from the possible neglect of the physician? If there is no procedure in place to provide that protection, who will put it in place and monitor it to make sure it works? The QI process asks these questions and is concerned with the answers.

The system is the process or sequence of events by which things are accomplished. In any process, something is passed along. This may be information such as laboratory results, bills, or communication of policies or safety procedures. It may be materials, such as medication, linen, or food. The hospitalized patient, too, is passed along via processes of care that encompass admission, diagnostic studies, therapeutic interventions, and, finally, discharge. There are a multitude of processes that take place in the care of a patient, and each process consists of a large number of individual steps. Finally, decision-making is a process. Think of how long it takes to analyze problems and implement solutions in a large institution as opposed to how long it might take in an individual physician's office. A process involves a sequence of steps that can be modified, and that modification is the subject of total quality management.

A process should not exist unless it is of benefit to someone. That individual or group of individuals is called the customer. In a real sense, our patients are our customers, as physicians are the customers of the hospital, the nursing unit is the customer of the in-house pharmacy, and so on. The goal is to provide the greatest possible benefit to the customer within the range of resources available. Another way of stating this is that we wish to provide value, which can be further defined as quality divided by cost.

## Requirements for Quality Management

To develop a plan for quality management, there must be a clear statement detailing who are your customers, the nature and scope of services offered and how your department or organization fits into the community and the region, and any other issue of importance. This mission statement is the standard by which all planning and quality improvement efforts are measured. Quality management in a highly technical tertiary center differs from quality management in a high-touch community hospital, even though many aspects of care are similar. The other requirement is a commitment to positive change. This commitment is demonstrated by a willingness to examine processes and outcomes; provide time, resources, and training; support recommendations for change; and acknowledge the efforts of those who have worked for quality improvement.

The tools required include the following:
- Data collection and analysis
- Clinical indicators
- Clinical practice guidelines
- Medical review criteria
- Continuous quality improvement (CQI) process

## Data Collection and Analysis

The collection of data is a key part of any effort to improve quality. Anecdotal information is insufficient and leads to inadequate efforts for change. In a hospital setting, there are many sources of data (e.g., medical records department, pharmacy and therapeutics committee, blood bank, departmental peer review committees, infection control office). All may provide useful information on outcomes, rates of therapeutic interventions, and specific complications. State health departments and insurance companies can also be repositories of important information. Data obtained from these sources must be evaluated carefully for accuracy and completeness. Another potential source of data is a departmental database. This is particularly valuable for obstetrics in which the outcomes in terms of maternal, fetal, and neonatal problems are usually the results of outpatient care. As discussed previously, the adequacy of the system of ambulatory care for the pregnant diabetic patient is likely to be reflected in the number of antepartum admissions, estimated gestational age at delivery, birth weight, requirement for cesarean delivery, neonatal intensive care unit (NICU) admission, and neonatal length of stay. The development of a departmental database allows collection of data important to the provision of care in a particular department and in a particular hospital setting. The content of this database depends on the uses to which it will be applied. These are likely to include the compilation of monthly, quarterly, or annual statistics, profiling of physician activities, and quality assurance activities, such as comparative cesarean section and VBAC rates and, perhaps, clinical research. The departmental cost of collecting this data is balanced against its accuracy and completeness and its utility in pointing out problems and monitoring any improvements put into place. An example of a one-page data collection form is shown in Figure 69–2. Review of charts at the time of patient or neonatal discharge allows this form to be filled out with subsequent computer input and analysis. It may take an experienced secretary 3 to 5 minutes to identify the data elements in a chart and another minute to record the information in a computerized database manager. This process is aided significantly by standard chart format and nomenclature, a QI process in itself. At a minimum the information provided in the single-page database provides the statistical information found in Table 69–1. The database may have

Table 69–1 Example of Statistics Available From the One-Page Obstetric Database

| GENERAL STATISTICS | MATERNAL COMPLICATIONS |
|---|---|
| Total deliveries | Hypertension |
| Total births | Diabetes/gestational diabetes |
| Stillbirths | Pre-eclampsia/eclampsia |
| Neonatal deaths | Placenta previa |
| Multiple births | Abruptio placenta |
| Vaginal deliveries | Preterm PROM |
| Total cesarean deliveries | Excessive blood loss |
| Primary cesarean deliveries | |
| Repeat cesarean deliveries | |
| Low forceps deliveries | NEONATAL COMPLICATIONS |
| Midforceps deliveries | Transferred out |
| Vaginal breech deliveries | Major anomalies |
| Attempted VBAC | Preterm (<38 wks) |
| Successful VBAC | Post-term (>42 wks) |
| Indication for cesarean delivery | 5-min Apgar <5 |
| Birth weights | Respiratory distress syndrome |

PROM = premature rupture of membranes; VBAC = vaginal birth after cesarean section.

PATIENT'S NAME_____
HOSPITAL NUMBER_____ AGE_____
ADMITTED_____ DISCHARGED_____
PHYSICIAN_____ NEONATAL HOSPITAL NUMBER_____

MED/SURG HX
  0 Normal
  11 Diabetes mellitus
  12 Hypertension
  13 Cardiac disease
  14 Asthma
  15 HIV

ANTEPARTUM COMPS
  0 None
  11 Gestational diabetes
  12 Hypertension
  13 Isoimmunization
  14 Premature labor treated
  15 Fetal demise
  16 Pre-eclampsia
  17 GBBS
  18 Placenta previa
  19 Abruptio placenta

MEMBRANE STATUS
  0 No PROM
  11 PROM < 1 hour
  12 PROM > 1 hour

ONSET OB CARE
  0 No prenatal care
  1 First trimester
  2 Second trimester
  3 Third trimester

DATE DELIVERED_____
TIME DELIVERED_____
EGA AT DELIVERY_____
IMMEDIATE NEONATAL
  CONDITION
  11 Liveborn
  12 Stillborn

LABOR
  0 Spontaneous
  11 Induced
  12 Augmented

INTRAPARTUM EVENTS
  0 None
  11 Pre-eclampsia
  12 Eclampsia
  13 Chorioamnionitis
  14 Cardiopulmonary arrest
  15 Fetal demise
  16 Shoulder dystocia
  17 Abruptio placenta

METHOD OF DELIVERY
  11 Spontanous vaginal
  12 Outlet forceps
  13 Low forceps
  14 Midforceps
  15 Vaginal breech
  16 Vacuum
  21 Primary cesarean
  22 Repeat cesarean
VBAC
  0 Not applicable
  11 Successful VBAC
  12 Failed BVAC

CESAREAN INDICATION_____
  0 No cesarean
  10 Repeat
  11 Lack of progress
  12 Abruptio placenta
  13 Placenta previa
  14 Repeat + other indication
  17 Other maternal indication

  20 Macrosomia
  21 Fetal jeopardy
  22 Breech
  23 Other malposition
  24 Twins (sole indication)
  25 Twins with malposition
  26 Herpes
  27 Second twin (uncomplicated)
  29 Other fetal indication

POSTPARTUM COMPS
  0 None
  11 Infectious morbidity
  12 Cardiopulmonary arrest
  13 Pre-eclampsia/Eclampsia
  14 PP hemorrhage
  15 Blood transfusion(s)
  16 Thrombophlebitis

OPERATIVE PROCEDURES
  0 None
  11 Tubal ligation
  20 Curettage
  21 Oophorectomy
  22 Hysterectomy
  23 Other laparotomy
  24 Evacuation hematoma
  25 Operative injury

NEONATAL INFORMATION
  Birthweight_____
  BirOrd (F,S,ST,T)_____
  Apgar 5_____
  Birth Order
  _____ of _____

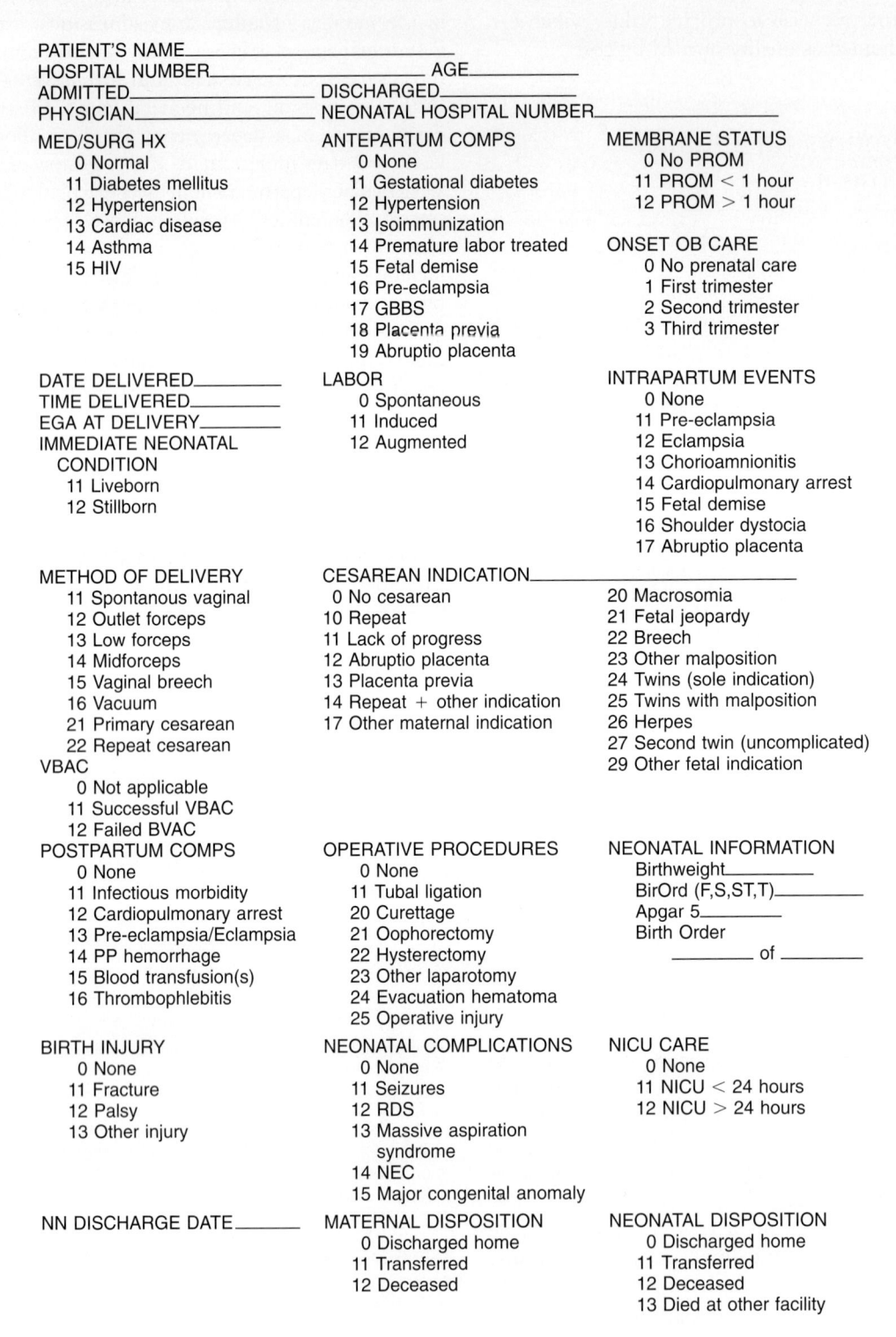

BIRTH INJURY
  0 None
  11 Fracture
  12 Palsy
  13 Other injury

NEONATAL COMPLICATIONS
  0 None
  11 Seizures
  12 RDS
  13 Massive aspiration
    syndrome
  14 NEC
  15 Major congenital anomaly

NICU CARE
  0 None
  11 NICU < 24 hours
  12 NICU > 24 hours

NN DISCHARGE DATE_____

MATERNAL DISPOSITION
  0 Discharged home
  11 Transferred
  12 Deceased

NEONATAL DISPOSITION
  0 Discharged home
  11 Transferred
  12 Deceased
  13 Died at other facility

**Figure 69–2** Example of single-page data collection form.

elements added or subtracted, depending upon the statistical needs of the department.

## Clinical Indicators

A clinical indicator is a medical event that can be counted or monitored. Monitoring of indicators allows evaluation of processes and outcomes. The original list of 21 obstetric indicators was published by the Joint Commission of Accredited Healthcare Organizations (JCAHO) in 1988, with a somewhat different list of 25 indicators published by the American College of Obstetricians and Gynecologists (ACOG) the following year. Since that time, the JCAHO list of indicators has been reduced to 5 and the ACOG list to 15. The indicators selected by a hospital department, for example, should include those that are important to the provision of quality care and which can be monitored effectively and efficiently. Indicators should be selected because they are sentinel events or because they monitor conditions or interventions that are high volume, high risk, or problem prone. Simply because a record meets the criteria of an indicator does not mean that care was below acceptable standards; it simply means that some degree of evaluation may be required, including chart review, trending, or comparison of rates with a benchmark.

Sentinel events are complications that need to be evaluated whenever they occur. These include maternal, fetal, or neonatal mortality, and operative mortality or unexpected morbidity, birth injuries, or readmission after early discharge. Cesarean section and VBAC rates, clean wound infections, and even expected operative morbidity rates are all appropriate quality control monitors. Other indicators may include adherence to established policies or guidelines, such as protocols, admission criteria, or standards set by certifying agencies. Monitoring the outcomes of clinical interventions may provide information on the appropriateness of those interventions and whether or not the interventions were used correctly. Guidelines for the evaluation and management of group B streptococcal infection can be assessed by setting up a clinical indicator to monitor neonatal or maternal infection. Excessive rates or lack of adherence to guidelines or policies may then become the subjects for QI activities.

There are two ways to choose charts that meet the criteria for an indicator. In the first, a medically sophisticated reviewer evaluates a record and determines whether it falls under any of the indicators the organization wishes to monitor. In the second, data are extracted from every record, and a computer program identifies those records that meet criteria for an indicator. The presence of a database is also helpful in choosing records that meet the criteria for indicators. Each method requires chart review, but the latter method does not require the reviewer to have the sophistication needed by the former reviewer and is therefore somewhat more cost-effective. The previous example of a one-page database allows monitoring, at a minimum, of the indicators listed in Table 69–2.

Once a record has been selected as meeting the criteria for a particular indicator, that record can be reviewed for specific predetermined characteristics. For example, if the performance of a cesarean section for dystocia is selected as an indicator, the initial review might include whether cervical dilatation was equal to or greater than 6 cm with no further progress, or whether there was full cervical dilatation without descent for 2 hours, and whether oxytocin augmentation was instituted. If these features are found, no further action need be taken. If they are not found, the chart might be forwarded to a peer review committee or department chairperson for further evaluation.

The responsibilities of a department peer review committee may include chart reviews in which unexpected occurrences are identified (e.g., postoperative infection, pulmonary embolus), evaluation of surgical cases in which the procedure or the tissue removed is not in accord with the preoperative diagnosis or in which normal tissue is removed, and investigation of referrals from utilization review or other department peer review committees. In addition, the peer review committee evaluates records identified by the monitoring of indicators.

The peer review committee has a number of options after a chart is reviewed. The medical record may be judged to reflect appropriate care, with no

**Table 69–2** Example of Obstetric Indicators Available From One-Page Obstetric Database

| Maternal Indicators | Neonatal Indicators |
| --- | --- |
| Maternal mortality | Stillbirths |
| Cardiopulmonary arrest | Neonatal deaths |
| Infectious morbidity | Transfer to NICU/other facility |
| Unplanned organ injury/removal/repair | 5-min Apgar <4 |
| | Birth trauma |
| Excessive blood loss | Massive aspiration syndrome |
| Excessive length of stay | Seizures |
| Eclampsia | Sepsis |
| Unplanned return to DR/OR | |
| Cesarean delivery for dystocia | |
| Cesarean delivery for uncertain fetal status | |

DR = delivery room; NICU = neonatal intensive care unit; OR = operating room.

further action required. The committee may elect to trend certain complications or care outcomes to track whether a particular provider's rate of these complications deviates from the rates of other members of the department or from some other identified benchmark. A letter can be sent to the responsible physician requesting further information or clarification of the particulars of the care and of the decision-making process. The response to this letter will be reviewed at a subsequent meeting, with feedback to the attending physician regarding the committee's view of both the care of the patient and the physician's explanation. Finally, the committee has the option of referring specific issues to the department chairperson.

The responsibilities and actions taken by the chairperson after receiving a case for review from the peer review committee depend upon the nature of the case. If is it judged that the case represents an issue germane to an individual physician, counseling of that physician would be appropriate, including, perhaps, a suggestion for an educational process. The subsequent performance of that physician can be taken into account when his or her privileges are delineated. If the issue is a systems problem, a QI effort can be initiated or guidelines can be written. Finally, the issue may require an educational presentation with appropriate follow-up for the entire department. Here again, policies, protocols, or guidelines may be helpful in defining a system of care to prevent recurrence of the problem.

The monitoring of specific indicators affords a department the opportunity of assessing whether steps taken to improve rates or outcomes are successful. It also allows evaluation of individual physician performance over time and a comparison among healthcare providers, the results of which can be a powerful impetus for changes in judgment, technical abilities, and behavior. In addition, the monitoring of indicators points out opportunities for changing systems to improve care.

## Clinical Practice Guidelines

Whether they are called algorithms, policies, critical pathways, or protocols, clinical practice guidelines define or suggest a process of care for a particular clinical condition. There may be a difference in the stringency with which they are applied or monitored, but each one outlines a sequence of steps, commonly with branch points, which should or must be followed.

Multiple sources of practice guidelines are available. Professional societies, including the ACOG, publish guidelines in several different forms, as do textbooks and journals, health-care organizations, and sources on the Internet. Many guidelines are developed by individuals or a committee designated to try to solve a process problem in the care of some clinical condition. The major advantage of developing local guidelines is the freedom to tailor them to the local environment. The major disadvantage is the time and effort it takes.

The selection of conditions for which guidelines would be beneficial is similar to selecting which indicators are important, that is, conditions that are high volume, high risk, or problem prone. Here again, the over-riding principle is to select guidelines that are, in fact, needed, so that their development and implementation are not simply an exercise. They should be evidence-based. Whenever possible, each step and branch point should be based on appropriate scientific literature, especially data from randomized controlled trials, if available. There should be an effort made to be aware of costs. When there is a choice of laboratory studies or therapeutic interventions of equal or near equal utility, cost should be a factor in deciding which to use. Guidelines, from whatever source, should be adapted to the environment in which they will be used. What will work in a tertiary center may not be useful in a small community hospital. Guidelines for the management of nonreassuring fetal status may be different in an institution where there is a 24-hour in-house anesthesiology service as opposed to a hospital where an anesthesiologist is called in from home. In addition, guidelines must be kept current. The state of knowledge in our specialty grows continuously, and guidelines developed, for example, for infectious disease or genetic issues, need to be updated frequently.

Finally, guidelines must be supported by the health-care providers who are expected to use them. Guidelines cannot be imposed on physicians or nurses with the expectation that they will always be applied. There needs to be departmental or group participation in their development and at least majority agreement for their implementation.

## Medical Review Criteria

All guidelines should be written or developed with a view toward how they will be monitored. Monitoring may be directed at process, that is, does a chart review document that the health-care provider is following the sequence defined by the guidelines and, if not, is there documentation to indicate why the deviation from the guidelines occurred? Monitoring may also be directed at outcomes. In the case of a guideline for the management of the pregnant diabetic woman, is there a demonstrable improvement in cesarean section rate, a decrease in antepartum admissions, a decrease in neonatal birth weight or prematurity, or a shortening of neonatal hospital stay? Do the answers to all these questions indicate that the guideline is doing what it was designed to do? If outcomes have not improved, either the guideline or its use should be examined.

The ACOG Criteria Sets are particularly useful in setting up medical review criteria. Each Criteria Set contains steps that should be taken before some intervention. For example, the Criteria Set for prophylactic oophorectomy for ovarian cancer lists the following factors, any of which are suggested to confirm the indication for surgery:

- Two or more first-degree relatives with epithelial ovarian cancer, suggesting either maternal or paternal transmission
- Pedigree of multiple occurrences of nonpolyposis colorectal cancer, endometrial cancer, or ovarian cancer
- Pedigree of multiple cases of breast or ovarian cancer

In the monitoring for adherence to this Criteria Set, medical review criteria would include the above list, any component of which would provide adequate justification for the procedure.

# Quality Improvement (QI)

## AN APPROACH TO PROBLEM SOLVING

There are two ways to solve problems. The first, which might be called "The Lone Ranger Approach," is a top-down method, which involves a person in authority studying the problem and coming up with a solution, which is then communicated to others for implementation. In the problem analysis, the authority may or may not take into account information obtained from others, and may believe, reasonably or not, that he or she knows the correct course of action to deal with the issue at hand. The following example may be helpful:

A new Chairperson of Obstetrics and Gynecology at a small community hospital discovers that women coming to the hospital for a labor check are kept in the Emergency Department until the responsible attending physician arrives to determine whether the patient is in labor and whether admission is required. The new chairperson evaluates this policy and comes to the conclusion that this stay in the Emergency Department is not patient-friendly and often results in a delay in the admission of patients truly in labor. Moreover, he believes, probably quite correctly, that the Emergency Department is not a very appropriate place for laboring patients to spend much time. There have, in fact, been several complaints from patients regarding their stay there. He therefore writes and promulgates the policy that patients arriving for labor checks be sent immediately to the Labor and Delivery Suite for evaluation. The fallout is immediate and negative and involves many areas of the hospital. The Emergency Department personnel, who had been making the initial assessment of these patients and billing for that assessment, are obviously unhappy with the new policy. The Transportation Department personnel, who now have to take an increased number of patients from the Emergency Department to the Labor and Delivery Suite, are equally unhappy. The nurses on Labor and Delivery, who now need to care for more patients, some of whom are not even in labor, do not appreciate the new policy, nor do Housekeeping personnel, who now need to change more bed linen on Labor and Delivery than they did in the past. Needless to say, this policy and its only current proponent, the new chairperson, have not met with roaring approval.

This brings us to the second method of problem solving. Here, the new chairperson comes to the conclusion that a patient who might be in labor should not be kept in the Emergency Department. He brings together a team to evaluate the issue. This team consists of representatives from the Emergency Department, Transportation, Nursing, Housekeeping, and Admissions, along with an obstetrician. It is the role of the team to figure out the best system to care for the pregnant women being evaluated for possible labor, a system that does not include evaluation in the Emergency Department. This team may come up with the same policy as described in the first example, but in this case, because everyone has appropriate input, there is no disagreement, and policy implementation occurs without a hitch. In fact, the input from members of the project team deals with several potential problems that the chairperson had not thought about and avoids several other problems that might have arisen.

The Project Team Approach has many advantages, although it may take some additional time and resources to solve a problem. This is more than made up for by the time saved in implementation. The Lone Ranger Approach is sometimes necessary in dealing with emergency issues, but it should be used with broad-based input whenever possible.

## PROBLEM-SOLVING MODELS

Industry has provided the health-care profession with a variety of problem-solving models. The Juran Institute's Quality Improvement Project Model, the HCA's FOCUS-PDCA Strategy for Improvement, and the Florida Light and Power Quality Improvement Model are examples of industrial models that have been applied to patient care with demonstrable success in hospitals and other health-care institutions. Regardless of the system chosen, there are a number of common features that allow problem analysis and solution.

The bottom line is that solving a problem really means fixing the system in which that problem resides, and fixing the system means changing the process by which something is done, whether that process involves patient care, materials management, or decision-making.

## IDENTIFICATION OF THE PROBLEM

Appropriate problem identification is essential for the success of a quality improvement effort. Problems are chosen because of the impact their solution will have on the organization, whether clinical, financial, or administrative. In addition, there must be a belief that the problem is capable of being solved given the time and resource constraints of the organization. The problem must be clearly defined and specific, and it must be small enough to be manageable. To say that the billing system of the hospital must be fixed may be too broad a problem statement for an institution. To decide to improve charge capture might be very acceptable and a first step toward a series of QI efforts to revamp a billing system.

## THE PROJECT TEAM

The next phase of a QI project is to put together the team of people who will work on the problem. The project team should consist of representatives of all the areas that will have significant input into the problem. A team working to decrease the time it takes to begin an emergency cesarean delivery might include an obstetrician, a nurse anesthetist, an anesthesiologist, a scrub nurse, a circulating nurse, an individual from Housekeeping, and someone from the communication system of the hospital. A team working to decrease the waiting time in a hospital obstetric clinic might include physicians, nurses, receptionists, patient care technicians, and so on. A project team needs a leader, an individual who has recognized administrative skills and who gives the process credibility and direction. The project team often benefits from a facilitator, an individual who understands the principles of a QI effort and who can ensure that the problem definition is appropriate, the improvement process is sound, there are no premature solutions, and, when the project team has worked through the problem and made its recommendations, the work of the team is ended and is recognized and rewarded.

It is essential that all members of the team understand the principles of QI. This requires time for orientation and training, but it allows members of the group to understand the process and speak the same language.

## THE PARETO PRINCIPLE

The Pareto Principle states that in any process or any group of items or steps that contribute to an effect, there are a few that account for the majority of that effect. This has also been called the 80:20 rule (i.e., 20% of the steps affect 80% of the outcome). These steps, or components of the process, have been called "the vital few." A QI effort should ideally isolate these important factors and address them to achieve the greatest benefit for the time and resources expended.

## FLOW CHARTS

Because the object of a QI effort is to change the process by which something is done, the next step is to break down the current process into its component parts. This involves the construction of a flow chart. This chart may be a simple sequence of events or a more complicated series of steps, with branch points that depend on the results of previous steps. Figures 69–3 and 69–4 are examples of flow charts.

## DATA COLLECTION AND ANALYSIS

The next step in the QI process involves trying to define all the potential problems in the process being evaluated. This is a time for imagination and intuition, but it is not a time for premature solutions. All possibilities should be listed and discussed. When the

---

Women's Health Center
Patient Flow

Patient signs in at registration desk
Patient returns to registration desk to register
Patient to registration desk to pick up visit card
Patient to receptionist
Receptionist obtains patient record
Receptionist gives record to nurse
Nurse takes patient to room
Nurse interviews patient
Nurse puts name of patient on board
Clinician in
Clinician out
Patient to receptionist to obtain laboratory slips, new appointment
Patient leaves module

**Figure 69–3** Flow chart for patient in women's health center.

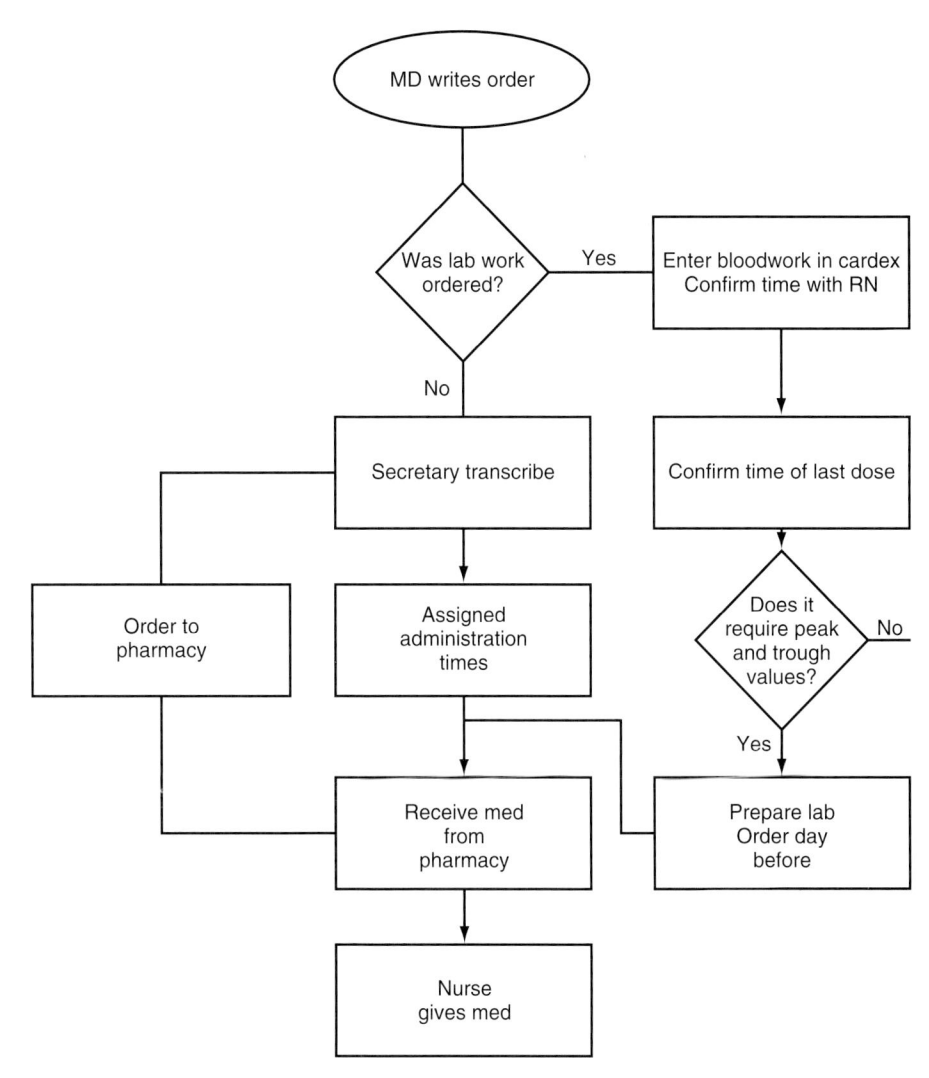

**Figure 69–4** Example of part of flow chart written for administration of medication.

list is as complete as possible, data should be collected to see where the problems really exist. For example, let us suppose that the Women's Health Clinic has received a number of complaints regarding the waiting time on the day of an appointment. The project team has broken down the process into its component parts, as shown in Figure 69–3. We can now see the sequence of events that a patient passes through during a visit to the clinic. The project team decides to determine where the delays are and creates a data collection form for a 1-week period of time. This form lists the times for each step of the process for every patient who comes to the clinic. The data collection form is shown in Table 69–3. Data collection may be somewhat time-consuming for the staff of the clinic, but because staff representatives are part of the project team and have been instrumental in the decision to collect data, there is likely to be cooperation from other members of the staff who are not part of the project team. When finally analyzed, the data will show which steps result in significant delays. It is more than likely that only one or two of the steps of the process produce the major part of the delay.

**Table 69–3** Women's Health Center Data Collection Form

| Women's Health Center Data Collection Form | | |
|---|---|---|
| Activity | Time | Initials |
| Patient signs in | _____ | _____ |
| Patient registers | _____ | _____ |
| Patient to receptionist | _____ | _____ |
| Chart given to nurse | _____ | _____ |
| Patient placed in room | _____ | _____ |
| Clinician in | _____ | _____ |
| Clinician out | _____ | _____ |
| Patient leaves module | _____ | _____ |

## SOLUTIONS AND THEIR IMPLEMENTATION

Now that the vital few have been identified, attention is turned toward fixing the steps in the process that

**Table 69-4** Women's Health Center Initial Time Study for Monday

### Women's Health Center Time Study

*Time to Pull Record (min)*

|  | Monday AM | Monday PM |
|---|---|---|
| Average time | 25.9 | 25.4 |
| 95% fall within | 70.7 | 63.4 |
| Minimum time | 0 | 1 |
| Maximum time | 89 | 75 |

will have the most influence on solving the identified problem and then monitoring to see whether the solutions were effective. In the Women's Health Clinic example, analysis of the data collected, as shown in Table 69-4, indicated that the time spent by the receptionist in pulling the patient's chart and giving it to the nurse was prolonged, taking as long as 89 minutes. The team did not understand the delay and investigated the duties of the receptionist. They discovered that the receptionist had a long list of responsibilities, which delayed finding the chart and transfering it to a nurse. In this example, fixing the process entailed finding other ways for the receptionist to complete her many responsibilities so that she could handle the charts efficiently. These solutions were put into place. A second week of data collection was initiated, with the finding of a significant decrease in overall waiting time for the patient, as illustrated in Table 69-5.

## ONGOING MONITORING

Once the solutions arrived at by the project team are put into place, it is important to monitor periodically to ensure that the process changes are maintained and the desired improvement continues. The frequency and duration of this monitoring depends upon the observation of results. Resistance to change, a few people who are dissatisfied with the new process, and lack of firm administrative support all mandate more

**Table 69-5** Time Study Comparison Before and After QI Project

### Women's Health Center Time Study Comparison

|  | Monday AM | Monday PM | Monday AM | Monday PM |
|---|---|---|---|---|
| Average time (min) | 26 | 25 | 13 | 18 |
| 95% fall within | 70 | 63 | 30 | 40 |
| Maximum time | 89 | 75 | 30 | 42 |

QI = quality improvement.

persistent observation until the process appears to be stable. In the clinic example, it may suffice to evaluate patient comments regarding waiting time and, perhaps, do another time study in 6 months.

## RECOGNITION

It is of great importance to recognize the work of the project team. The first form of recognition is the implementation of the solutions that are suggested. If solutions that have been requested and arrived at after conscientious work are allowed to fade away without implementation, there is likely to be frustration on the part of the project team, making it unlikely that they, or others in the organization, will be willing to put forth that kind of effort again. The second form of recognition may be simply an expression of gratitude from the administrative group that initiated the project team. It is too often forgotten that a statement of thanks for work well done is appreciated by those who have spent time and effort to accomplish what was asked of them.

## Example: Inpatient Tocolytic Therapy for Premature Labor

The following example will serve to illustrate many of the points covered in the chapter thus far. The example is based on experience at a medium-sized community hospital in New England. A review of inpatient statistics revealed approximately 100 admissions for premature labor and inpatient tocolysis over a 2-year period, with patients being discharged undelivered. Lengths of stay ranged from 1 to 10 days, with a variety of inpatient management schemes, and patients were often discharged on expensive home monitoring programs. Review of the medical records demonstrated the presence of uterine contractions but often failed to reveal significant cervical dilatation or effacement or documented change in the cervix over some period of observation.

Further evaluation of the data revealed that of the patients without significant cervical dilatation, effacement, or documented cervical change who were admitted for tocolysis, 92% ultimately delivered after 37 weeks of gestation. Of those admitted with the cervix at least 2 cm dilated, 60% effaced, or both, or who demonstrated cervical change, 74% delivered at term. It was in this latter group that the significantly premature infants were found. Because the literature does not support the concept that tocolysis usually delays premature labor until term, the chairperson believed that inpatient tocolytic therapy was being

overutilized and that criteria for hospital admission needed to be put in place. He decided to employ the admission criteria set forth in the ACOG Criteria Set. These criteria include the following, all of which should be present:
- Gestational age of more than 20 weeks and less than 37 weeks confirmed by certain dates or ultrasonography
- Regular documented uterine contractions
- Documented cervical change or appreciable cervical dilatation or effacement

The data were presented at a department business meeting along with the information that, despite increasingly aggressive tocolytic therapy for premature labor, the number of babies with low birth weight born at the hospital during the preceding 10 years was relatively unchanged. Admission criteria were presented to the department members for discussion. There was general agreement with the first two criteria. The third criterion was changed to decrease ambiguity, and an additional statement was added regarding high-risk situations. The admission criteria that were approved by the department members are shown in Table 69–6.

After the department members agreed to the admission criteria, a monthly monitor was put in place to review all records of patients who were admitted for premature labor and discharged undelivered. Records were reviewed according to the admission criteria, and those that did not meet the criteria were followed up with letters sent to attending physicians, requesting the reasons for admission. As a result of this process, the number of admissions for premature labor resulting in patients being discharged undelivered decreased by 40% within the first 6 months of observation. Continued monitoring failed to discover any adverse effect on the number of premature infants delivered.

**Table 69–6** Departmental Criteria Set for Inpatient Tocolyic Treatment of Premature Labor

**Departmental Criteria Set: Inpatient Tocolysis**

*Indication: Preterm Labor*

CONFIRMATION OF INDICATION
- Gestational age of ≥20 wk but <37 wk, confirmed by certain dates or ultrasonography
- Regular uterine contractions at frequent intervals, preferably documented by tocodynamometer
- Documented cervical change or appreciable cervical dilatation (→2 cm) or effacement (→60%)

A history of premature labor in a past pregnancy, especially when there was significant neonatal morbidity or a prolonged NICU stay, may justify a relaxation of the cervical dilatation/effacement requirement.

After admission criteria were put in place and monitoring was begun, attention was turned to the inpatient management of patients admitted for tocolytic therapy. The previous chart review had demonstrated that there was little or no uniformity regarding diagnostic monitoring or treatment of these patients. A small group of obstetricians was charged with developing practice guidelines for the management of premature labor, including all diagnostic and therapeutic interventions as well as criteria for discharge from the hospital. A draft of the guidelines was presented at a business meeting of the department, at which time there were several suggestions for change, all of which were incorporated. The guidelines were then given to the nursing division for conversion to a critical pathway. The critical pathway described what would happen to the patient on each day of the hospitalization and dealt not only with the type and frequency of testing, biophysical monitoring, and medications to be administered but also with the variety of consultations that would occur, including Social Service, Rehabilitation, and Case Management. The critical pathway was again brought back to the department for approval. A copy of the pathway was placed on every chart of patients who were admitted for this diagnosis. Finally, a patient-friendly version of the pathway was designed to be given to the patient on admission so that she would know what to expect during the hospitalization.

Because of all the work that had been done on the guidelines and the critical pathway and the fact that physician approval was obtained at every step along the way, it was assumed that use of the pathway would be virtually universal. In fact, most physicians did not use the pathway, usually forgetting that it was available. The next step then was to use the pathway and guidelines to develop standing admission orders. Because this made it easier for physicians to admit patients, the pathway was now used on a regular basis.

Depending on the commitment of department members to use of the guidelines, a monitor can be set up to see whether, in fact, the guidelines are being used, and, if not, whether there is an indication in the medical record as to why they are not being used. This will help to ensure relative uniformity in the process of care.

# Conclusions

The importance of data as the engine of a quality assurance or QI system cannot be overemphasized. Data are the basis for needs assessment and they provide the evidence that improvements put into place are, in fact, successful. Monitoring clinical indicators, establishing guidelines for clinical practice, using these guidelines, and assessing outcomes all provide the foundation for quality care. Opportunities for quality improvement are highlighted by data collection and continuous surveillance of diagnoses or procedures that are high volume, high cost or problem prone. The solution to deficiencies in patient care rests on the willingness to evaluate processes and outcomes, define specific problems, involve interested and talented people to change the system of care, and, finally, set monitors in place to ensure that the established changes are successful.

## REFERENCES

American College of Obstetricians and Gynecologists: Criteria Set #2: Prophylactic bilateral oophorectomy to prevent epithelial carcinoma. Washington, DC, American College of Obstetricians and Gynecologists, 1994.

Blumenthal D: Quality of healthcare. Part 1: Quality of care—what is it? N Engl J Med 335:891, 1996.

Joint Commission of Accredited Healthcare Organizations: Comprehensive accreditation manual for hospitals. Joint Committee of Accredited Healthcare Organizations (IMS-3), 1997.

Juran JM: Juran on Quality of Design. New York, The Free Press, 1992.

Quality assessment and improvement in obstetrics and gynecology. Washington, DC, American College of Obstetricians and Gynecologists, 1994.

# 70

# Clinical Effectiveness: A New Set of Skills for Obstetrician-Gynecologists

RICHARD E. WARD
JENNIFER ELSTON LAFATA

## Clinical Effectiveness in Gynecology

Over the past 2 decades, clinical effectiveness has emerged as a collection of concepts and methods that should be part of the practice of every obstetrician-gynecologist. Just as clinicians work to diagnose, treat and prevent illnesses, and promote health in *individual* patients, they have an intrinsic professional responsibility to diagnose, treat and prevent illness, and promote health in *populations* of patients. This is accomplished by focusing on the underlying processes used to provide health care and working systematically to improve them.

As with other aspects of patient care, obstetrician-gynecologists can seek consultation and otherwise enlist the help of colleagues with specialized knowledge and skills. An increasing number of health-care organizations and managed-care organizations include experts in the discipline of clinical effectiveness. Such clinical effectiveness practitioners typically work to provide expertise and leadership to facilitate the rigorous, evidence-based improvement of health-care processes. Clinical effectiveness practitioners draw on a robust collection of methods from many disciplines and adapt these methods for use for practice improvement. These methods are borrowed from the disciplines of epidemiology, statistics, medical decision sciences, economics, psychology, industrial engineering, management sciences, education, and medical informatics.

But despite the existence of such experts in many health-care organizations, the application of clinical effectiveness concepts and methods remains a core responsibility of every obstetrician-gynecologist. In this regard, clinical effectiveness is like anatomy, pathophysiology, pharmacology, and physical examination. They are the fundamentals that every physician should know and apply and never completely defer to others.

## Definition of Clinical Effectiveness

The term *effectiveness* is borrowed from the field of health services research. It refers to the magnitude of the desirable effect of a health-care intervention on health outcomes. Effectiveness is distinguished from *efficacy* in that efficacy refers to the outcomes achieved when the intervention is offered under ideal "laboratory" conditions, with highly selected patients and extraordinary attention to the controlled execution of the intervention. An intervention is said to be effective when it achieves favorable outcomes for patients receiving the intervention in routine health-care settings, when variation in patient selection, clinician skill, patient adherence, and other factors influence outcomes. Effectiveness also is distinguished from efficacy because efficacy often is assessed through measurement of intermediate or physiologic outcomes, such as blood pressure, serum concentration, or range of motion. Effectiveness implies the measurement, or at least consideration of the outcomes that are experienced by patients, such as pain or functional status.

*Cost-effectiveness analysis* is a formal method for comparing the benefits and costs of an intervention to determine whether it is worth doing. An intervention is said to be "cost-effective" when the magnitude of the favorable impact is judged to be worth the economic cost incurred to provide the intervention. In other words, the whole package of health and economic outcomes associated with the interventions is judged to compare favorably with the health and economic outcomes associated with alternative interventions. Standardized methods have been proposed to make the results of cost-effectiveness analyses more comparable and more easily interpreted and evaluated. Cost-effectiveness is a central concept in what Donabedian described as the "new science of parsimonious health care."

## The Clinical Effectiveness Process

On the most general level, all health care can be conceptualized as a system involving two fundamentally different core processes: decision-making processes and care delivery processes, as illustrated in Figure 70–1.

Decision-making processes involve a clinician working with a patient to determine which, if any, health-care interventions should be pursued at a given point in the patient's care. In this context, health care *intervention* is used broadly, encompassing everything from deciding on the components of a physical examination to deciding whether diagnostic testing or pharmaceutical or surgical treatment is needed. The output of this decision-making process is the plan of care for the patient.

The care delivery process, in contrast, involves the execution of the plan of care. The results of executed interventions, in turn, affect subsequent decision-making. Even the most complex clinical processes can be broken down into cycles of deciding on a plan, executing the plan, and deciding on the next plan based on the results achieved.

*Quality* is defined differently for decision-making and care delivery processes. For decision-making processes, quality means "doing the right thing"—identifying the right alternatives and choosing the right one. For care delivery processes, quality means "doing it right"—carrying out the plan of care without making mistakes and without wasting resources. Research over the past 3 decades repeatedly has shown great variation in clinical decision-making and care delivery which could not be completely explained by patient characteristics. This observed variation has served as a wake-up call to the health-care community, prompting interest in the process of clinical effectiveness as a means to introduce a more rational, science-based approach to both decision-making and care delivery processes.

Figure 70–2 illustrates how the processes of decision-making and care delivery fit into this clinical effectiveness process.

Given the appropriate technology and organizational will, outcomes data can be collected as part of the routine care-delivery processes. Such outcomes data include characteristics of the patient, his or her risk factors, the medical interventions that were offered to the patient, and both immediate and long-term health and economic outcomes experienced by the population, including functional status, quality of life, satisfaction, and costs.

These outcomes data can be combined with information from the scientific literature and with expert opinions to support the *clinical policy-making process*.

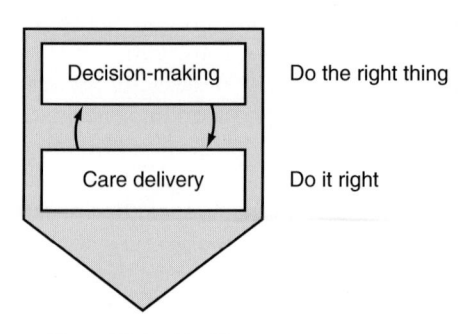

**Figure 70–1** Health-care core processes.

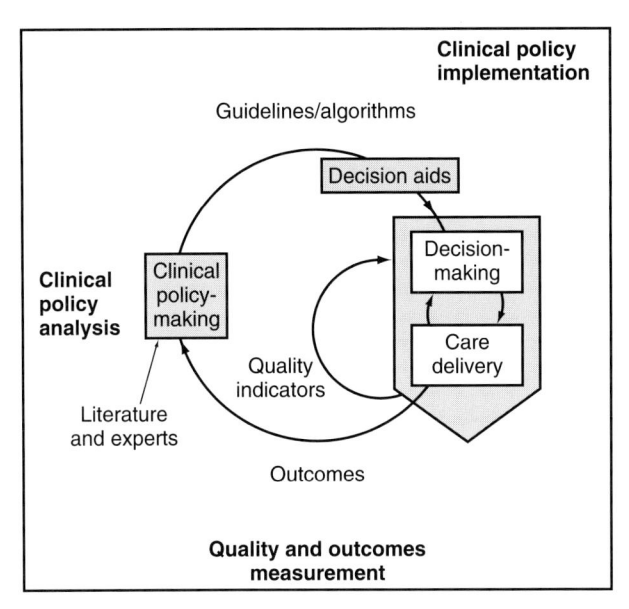

**Figure 70–2** Clinical effectiveness process.

make those clinical policies influence actual decision-making processes. Decision aids include a variety of approaches used for implementation.

The final component of the practice improvement model is *quality indicators*, including report cards, practice profiles, and other forms of performance reports. Quality indicators form a feedback loop to confirm that the improvement effort is achieving the planned change in a clinical process. In addition to providing feedback to the improvement effort, quality indicators often are used as the basis for accountability to external constituencies. In summary, the clinical effectiveness process includes three main components: quality and outcomes measurement, clinical policy analysis, and clinical policy implementation.

## The Methodologic Domains of Clinical Effectiveness

As illustrated in Table 70–1, these three components of the clinical effectiveness process are supported by a variety of methodologic domains.

### MEASUREMENT

There are five methodologic domains that support the measurement component of the clinical effectiveness process. *Population needs assessment* involves the characterization of various patient populations, including demographics, risk factor profile, disease incidence and prevalence, and health-care utilization patterns to identify opportunities for improvement and to support data-driven prioritization of clinical practice improvement efforts. *Effectiveness research* involves the measurement of physiologic impact, health outcomes, and cost of alternative strategies for diagnosis and treatment of a particular condition to inform clinical decision-making and to support the process

In this context, clinical policy-making refers to any prospective decision about a use of health-care interventions for patients in a particular situation. Clinical policy-making involves the use of various methods to analyze proposed policy alternatives and reach consensus about the most desirable alternative. Those decisions can take the form of clinical practice guidelines, care maps, critical paths, disease management protocols or algorithms, practice parameters, or formularies. Decisions about which medical services are to be covered in a health plan, which clinicians are to be granted credentials to provide a particular service, or which medical technologies are to be included in a capital budget are also clinical policies. Such policies are intended to support the decisions of clinicians, rather than to replace critical thinking and judgment.

Recognizing that written clinical policies are not useful unless they are used to modify clinical practice, another component of the model is decision aids. Decision aids are the tools and methods used to

**Table 70–1** Methodologic Domains of the Discipline of Clinical Effectiveness

| Measurement | Clinical Policy-Making | Implementation |
|---|---|---|
| • Population needs assessment<br>• Effectiveness research<br>  • Observational studies<br>  • Randomized clinical trials<br>• Program evaluation<br>• Clinical practice profiling<br>• External performance reporting | • Consensus-based clinical policy analysis teams<br>• Evidence-based clinical policy analysis teams<br>  • Literature review<br>  • Meta-analysis<br>  • Decision analytic modeling/cost-effectiveness analysis | • Quality improvement teams<br>• Statistical process control<br>• Intranet resources<br>• Staff training/continuing medical education<br>• Academic detailing (educational outreach)<br>• Patient education materials development<br>• Medical informatics<br>• Interface to ongoing operations<br>  • Call centers<br>  • Telephone survey and counseling staff<br>  • Distribution of care management materials<br>  • Case managers |

of clinical policy-making. Effectiveness research sometimes can be accomplished through observational studies but frequently requires randomized clinical trials to overcome sources of bias that threaten the inferences drawn from observational studies. *Program evaluation* involves establishing the performance characteristics and effectiveness of strategies for clinical practice improvement or organization of care to support decisions about the future role of these strategies. Program evaluation allows for the comparison of what did happen after implementing the program with what would have happened had the program not been implemented. In summary, population needs assessment is a tool to support priority setting, whereas effectiveness research and program evaluation are tools to support decision making about how to achieve improvements.

*Clinical practice profiling*, also known as internal performance reporting, involves the characterization of clinical performance, in terms of quality of care, utilization, and patient satisfaction. Such profiles can be case-mix adjusted and often are used to support internal accountability of clinicians and clinical leadership. Feedback of cost or utilization data to clinicians has been shown to lead, in certain situations, to reduction in cost and utilization of diagnostic tests. *External performance reporting* involves the characterization of clinical performance, in terms of quality, utilization, satisfaction, and health outcomes to support external accountability to employers, insurers, and other constituencies. As with clinical practice profiles, external performance reports can be case-mix adjusted.

For nearly all these domains, a spectrum of measurement constructs is possible. As illustrated in Figure 70–3, these constructs range from process measures to intermediate outcomes (such as physiologic measures), to intervention-specific outcomes, to population outcomes.

Outcomes management, described by Ellwood as a "technology of patient experience," has been promoted heavily over the past decade. Both process and outcomes measures offer important advantages (see Fig. 70–3), and many advocate for the use of a variety of measures across this spectrum, with the addition of measures of consumer satisfaction and cost. When measurement is used optimally, it facilitates not only knowledge of the outcome, but also the reasons why a given outcome is achieved.

## CLINICAL POLICY-MAKING

Practice policies are "preformed recommendations issued for the purpose of influencing decisions about health interventions." The term *clinical policy* does not itself specify an intended degree of flexibility. Some clinical policies are intended to be "standards," with little intended flexibility. Others are intended to serve as "guidelines," and still others are intended to describe "options."

Clinical policies come in many forms. Practice policies established by health-care providers or managed-care organizations include:

1. Care Maps or Critical Paths—describe an intended sequence of medical, nursing, and other interventions by day-of-stay during an inpatient admission for a particular condition.
2. Practice Guidelines—describe the appropriate role of medical interventions for particular indications (including formulary and benefits design).
3. Credentials—describe the appropriate qualifications of the medical professionals authorized to perform a procedure or service.
4. Benefits Design/Technology Assessments—the process of determining which interventions and medical technologies should be covered by the

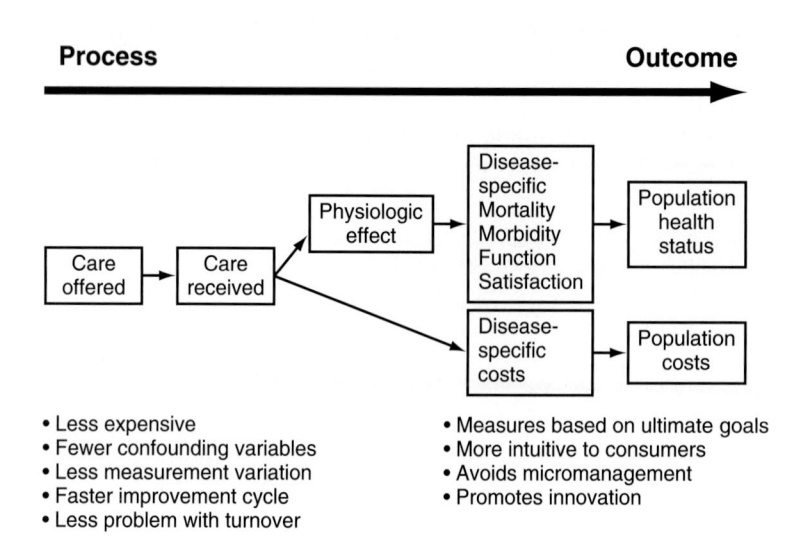

**Process** → **Outcome**

Care offered → Care received → Physiologic effect → Disease-specific Mortality Morbidity Function Satisfaction → Population health status

Care received → Disease-specific costs → Population costs

- Less expensive
- Fewer confounding variables
- Less measurement variation
- Faster improvement cycle
- Less problem with turnover

- Measures based on ultimate goals
- More intuitive to consumers
- Avoids micromanagement
- Promotes innovation

**Figure 70–3** Types of measures.

health plan subscriber contract, under which clinical conditions.
5. Disease Management Protocol/Algorithms—describe the intended sequence of a whole array of medical, nursing, and administrative interventions related to the multidisciplinary, multi-setting management of a particular condition, including any decision logic and process flow information.

A number of methods are used to develop clinical policies. *Consensus-based methods* are by far the most common. Consensus methods involve a discussion by people who have expertise or who are stakeholders in the policy issue, leading to a near unanimous conclusion about which policy alternative is best. Consensus methods require the minimum amount of effort to develop and are appropriate for simple policies for which there is little debate. Consensus methods also have been employed for complex algorithms, in which the sheer number of distinct policy "nodes" precludes the use of more comprehensive methods. Achieving consensus often requires the creation of ad hoc multidisciplinary teams to frame the issues, prepare a policy proposal, take the proposal through various institutional approval processes, solicit input from stakeholders, and prepare and disseminate a final report.

More rigorous methods of developing clinical policies include *evidence-based methods* and the "*explicit approach*" proposed by Eddy. Evidence-based methods involve a formal analysis of the available empirical evidence regarding the effectiveness of the alternative interventions. The explicit approach requires an explicit description of the probabilities or magnitudes of the outcomes associated with the alternative interventions and a description of the methods used to make these estimates. Such methods are particularly useful when the policy issue involves the resolution of disagreements about the scientific evidence or cost-effectiveness of policy alternatives. These disagreements are resolved by convening evidence-based clinical policy analysis teams to accomplish all the same tasks as the consensus team, but with three additional tasks: (1) literature review, which involves the formal search and interpretation of relevant published and unpublished studies; (2) meta-analysis, which involves the use of formal quantitative methods for research synthesis and integration, and (3) decision analytic modeling, which is used to calculate estimates of the expected magnitude and uncertainty of health *and economic* outcomes associated with all relevant policy alternatives. The results of these estimates are summarized on a "balance sheet," which presents alternative interventions as columns and relevant health and economic outcomes as rows. Finally, the decision-maker faces the task of valuing the health and economic outcomes to make the value judgment about which alternative intervention is most desirable.

## IMPLEMENTATION

The implementation of clinical policies to improve the quality and efficiency of health care involves making changes to both decision-making and care-delivery processes. The clinical effectiveness methods for improving these processes are borrowed largely from the work of Deming, Crosby, Juran, Ishikawa, and other practitioners of industrial process improvement. These methods are alternatively described as continuous process improvement (CQI) and total quality management (TQM). Berwick and others described the adaptation of these methods for health care.

On a practical level, clinicians apply these methods by working with other members of their clinical team to make local improvements, or in larger health-care organizations, by participating in multidisciplinary teams established at the departmental level. These teams often require expert support in analytical and statistical methods. Statistical process control involves the application of quality engineering concepts to administrative, support, and care delivery processes to (1) detect changes in process performance over time, (2) identify assignable causes of variation, and (3) adjust relevant process input variables to maintain a process performance criterion within a desirable range.

Another implementation approach is staff training or continuing medical education. This involves the development and delivery of classes and organized curricula, with the objective of improving knowledge and skills to increase the effectiveness of clinicians, administrative staff, and support staff. Some training is intended to increase knowledge and skills in process improvement methods, to improve the effectiveness of CQI or TQM teams. Other training is intended to have a more direct effect to improve decision-making and care delivery processes by teaching clinicians about specific diagnosis and treatment strategies. Traditionally, this latter approach has been accomplished through grand rounds and seminars. Another approach, based on methods developed for the marketing of pharmaceuticals and devices, is academic detailing. Academic detailing is a form of educational outreach involving the personal delivery to clinicians of brief educational messages designed to change clinical practice behaviors.

Another approach to implementation involves patient education. Therefore, the methods of patient education materials development represent an important domain of clinical effectiveness. These methods involve the development and pilot testing of brochures, pamphlets, audio- and videotapes, class materials, Web-based materials, and other products designed to provide useful and timely information to patients regarding their health. An understanding and appreciation of the principles of adult learning are essential to this process.

Finally, clinical policy implementation requires the effective application of information technology. *Medical informatics* is the term used to describe the broader field of information technology applications to health and medical care. Managing intranet resources is an emerging methodologic domain of clinical effectiveness, involving the development of internal Web-based materials, such as a clinical practice policy and guideline library or a care management support system. Another important medical informatics method involves the development of computer-based decision aids such as reminders, alerts, and prompts. These are incorporated into information systems used by clinicians for medical documentation, on-line ordering, results review, and other functions of a complete electronic health record system.

A review of rigorous evaluations of clinical policy implementation methods conducted by Grimshaw and Russell revealed the importance of the methods of guideline development, dissemination, and implementation in predicting clinician behavior change (Table 70-2). In general, multifaceted implementation approaches have been found to be most effective for improvement processes that involve physician behavior change.

These clinical policy implementation methods are used to effect change in clinical processes. However, many clinical effectiveness initiatives, including those described later in this chapter, involve the establishment and ongoing management of a new set of resources to support improved clinical processes. These resources include call centers, which receive customer calls and either provide customer service or direct the customer to appropriate staff or resources. Such services may include on-call nurse advice, appointment scheduling, laboratory result reporting, directions to facilities, and billing inquiries. Telephone survey and counseling staff make outgoing calls to patients for the purpose of acquiring information from the patient, such as for a health risk appraisal, survey, or follow-up call. They also offer information or services to the patient, such as counseling, needs assessment, and patient education. Another set of resources are required to handle the distribution of care management materials, including the management of a mail room and stock room to efficiently route care management materials to patients, including patient educational materials and self-care supplies. Finally, case managers, typically nurses or other allied health professionals, are required to track patients with defined conditions, assess patient needs, solve problems, and deliver other patient services such as counseling, patient education, and social services.

## Types of Clinical Effectiveness Initiatives

Although the aforementioned generic clinical effectiveness process provides a framework for planning most clinical effectiveness initiatives, it is useful to consider different categories of clinical effectiveness initiatives that have different drivers and different levels of complexity, and for which a different mix of methods typically are employed. As illustrated in Figure 70-4, initiatives can be motivated by quality improvement, cost savings, or both. Initiatives can be focused on simple clinical processes, involving the delivery or avoidance of specific medical interventions to specific cohorts of patients, or they can be focused on complex processes, involving the coordination of many different clinicians from different disciplines to deliver a series of interventions over time.

## Necessary Elements of Clinical Effectiveness Initiatives

A number of core elements are key to ensuring the success of any clinical effectiveness initiative. As illus-

Table 70-2 Effectiveness of Guideline Development, Dissemination, and Implementation Methods in Terms of Clinician Behavior Change*

|  | Most Effective | Moderately Effective | Least Effective |
| --- | --- | --- | --- |
| Guideline development | Internal development | External, local development | National development |
| Guideline dissemination | Specific educational interventions | Continuing education<br>Targeted mailing | Publication in journals |
| Guideline implementation | Patient-specific reminders at the time of the clinical encounter | Feedback measures | General reminders |

*Adapted from Grimshaw J, Russell IT: Effect of clinical guidelines on medical practice: A systematic review of rigorous evaluations. Lancet 342:1317–1322, 1993.

|  | | SIMPLE INTERVENTIONS | COMPLEX PROCESSES |
|---|---|---|---|
| Drivers | Quality Improvement | Papanicolaou smears<br>Mammograms<br>Childhood immunizations | Cancer and human immuno-deficiency virus (HIV) survival<br>Heart risk reduction<br>Mild to moderate diabetes |
| | Both | Flu shots<br>β blockers | High-risk asthma<br>Classes III & IV congestive heart failure<br>Frail elderly |
| | Cost Savings | Avoid unnecessary tests<br>Generic drugs | |
| | Typical Methods | Evidence-based guidelines<br>Reminders, alerts, ticklers<br>Performance measurement with process variables | Consensus algorithms/protocols<br>Continuing medical education<br>Patient education<br>Care managers |
| | Enabling Technology | Reminders integrated into electronic medical records and ordering process | Protocol-driven, team-based care (Workflow automation) |

**Figure 70–4** Types of clinical effectiveness initiatives.

trated in Figure 70–5, these elements include: conducting a preliminary needs assessment or problem identification; establishing an appropriate improvement team; defining the target population; identifying measurable goals and objectives; articulating the desirable decision-making or care processes; designing a plan for implementation; and developing a means for ongoing monitoring.

Although these elements are necessary, they are not sufficient. Ultimately, the success of each clinical effectiveness initiative is dependent on the ability to tailor the overall approach to the specific application.

Clinical effectiveness initiatives begin with the identification of an opportunity for improvement. Such opportunities can be identified through a variety of channels. These might include review of the medical literature, observation of local practice patterns, benchmarking with peer organizations, or suggestions by leadership or patients. Regardless of the source, the key is that opportunities originate from the identification of needs or problems, not solutions. It is often tempting to propose interventions or solutions before stepping back; however, only with a clear understanding of the underlying needs or problems can an appropriate (and therefore successful) improvement effort be undertaken.

Once a thorough understanding of the improvement opportunity exists, the next step is to identify individuals to participate in the effort. These individuals should include those with clinical and administrative expertise in the area, as well as individuals whose clinical practices are likely to be affected. By including key stakeholders in the initial improvement process, not only does the improvement effort benefit from the diversity of perspectives represented, but the process of achieving buy-in is initiated from the beginning. Attempts should be made to have multidisciplinary representation on the team.

The next step is to define the target population. Such populations often are defined based on a clinical condition or disease. Because not all patients with the same condition or disease have the same needs, the different risks and severity levels *within* a target population must be understood. Such information can, at

```
Conducting a preliminary needs assessment
or problem identification
           ↓
Establishing an appropriate improvement team
           ↓
Defining the target population
           ↓
Identifying measurable goals and objectives
           ↓
Articulating the desirable
decision-making or care processes
           ↓
Designing a plan for implementation
           ↓
Developing means for ongoing monitoring
```

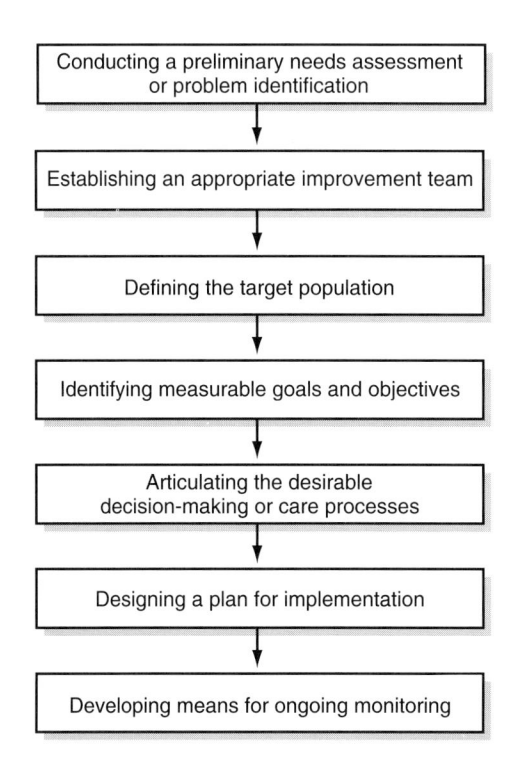

**Figure 70–5** Necessary elements of a clinical effectiveness initiative.

times, be gathered through automated data or the medical record, but often it may need to be solicited from the patient regarding their perceived needs and desires (e.g., a health risk appraisal). It is often through the population identification and risk stratification process that the specific goals and objectives of the effort begin to take form. The challenge is to establish goals and objectives that are measurable and allow for the assessment of improvement over time.

The next step is to articulate the desired care processes. Clinical effectiveness initiatives generally fall into two categories: those whose efforts are directed at improving existing processes vs. those whose efforts are directed at more extensive process reengineering. At times, it may be appropriate to begin with a subprocess rather than attempting to change all aspects of care at once. In fact, it is often more productive to make small incremental changes than to attempt large far-reaching changes that offer a smaller probability of success.

Once the desired care processes are known, a plan for implementation can be developed. As described earlier, strategies for implementation may include patient education, staff training, local quality improvement teams, the use of information technology, and a number of other approaches. The key is to develop a multifaceted approach to implementation and to articulate clearly which resources are required, who will be responsible for each aspect of the plan, and over what time frame the steps will occur.

The final step involves developing a means for ongoing monitoring and evaluation of efforts. To be successful, measurement and feedback must be an integral part of the care processes, not an afterthought. Because measurement is costly, any measurement effort must carefully select a handful of key quality indicators. These may include measures of both process performance and patient outcomes. Outcome measures ideally include those reflective of immediate and long-term impacts on patient health, satisfaction, and well-being but also may include measures of resource utilization (e.g., hospital admissions) and costs.

## Examples of Clinical Effectiveness Initiatives

The remainder of this chapter uses three examples from the work of the Henry Ford Health System (HFHS) Center for Clinical Effectiveness (CCE) to demonstrate the application of the clinical effectiveness process and the methodologic domains described above.

## EXAMPLE 1: CERVICAL CANCER SCREENING

A baseline evaluation of Papanicolaou (Pap) smears done in a large multispecialty group practice revealed that more than 25% of samples were designated "less than optimal" because of the absence of observed endocervical cells, an indicator of sample adequacy. In addition, there was a large variation in the rates of sample adequacy achieved by different physicians and at different clinic sites. In response to these concerns about sample adequacy, clinical leaders encouraged the formation of a multidisciplinary clinical quality improvement team to work to improve the process by which cervical cytology samples were obtained and assessed for adequacy. This team included cytopathology staff, obstetrician-gynecologists, internists, and clinical effectiveness staff.

The team used a quality improvement framework developed at the Hospital Corporation of America (HCA), described by the acronym "FOCUS-PDCA." The team prepared process flow charts and identified an initial improvement in the design of the cytology requisition form to provide data required for future analyses of Pap smear adequacy and management of cervical neoplasia. The team also defined and implemented a new, more reproducible operational definition of the key quality characteristic: the proportion of samples with at least five observed endocervical cells. Although no direct relationship between observed endocervical cells and decreased cervical cancer mortality has been demonstrated, the team conducted a retrospective analysis that showed an increased prevalence of mild abnormalities found in samples with endocervical cells (11.9% vs. 5.2%), and also an increased prevalence of severe abnormalities found (3.0% vs 0.8%).

The team then prepared "run charts," plotting monthly sample adequacy rates over a 2-year period, stratified by clinic location and specialty. Then, based on a literature review and input from consultants, an "Ishikawa diagram" was prepared, outlining the known factors that could cause inadequate samples. A study conducted in the Netherlands found that the Cytobrush, a plastic sampling tool with a tip that resembles a pipe cleaner, together with a wooden spatula, produced a higher proportion of samples with endocervical cells in the hands of paramedical sample takers when compared with other commonly used tools, including the cotton swab traditionally used within the institution. The team conducted a retrospective study and a second prospective study, both of which confirmed these findings.

Based on these results, the team prepared a cost-benefit analysis and drafted a proposal for an institutional clinical practice policy calling for sampling using the cytobrush and wooden spatula for screening

Papanicolaou smears for nonpregnant women. The policy was approved and was communicated to the primary care medical staff through a series of scripted 13-minute slide presentations presented at local staff meetings at clinic sites throughout the institution. Two approaches were used to assess the success of these staff training efforts. First, the team conducted a survey of clinic nurses and assistants to determine which sampling tools each internist and obstetrician-gynecologist used during each month of the study period. The survey was repeated to update information on two occasions. These surveys revealed a dramatic transition from traditional sampling methods using a spatula, with or without a cotton swab, to methods using the Cytobrush. The team confirmed these survey data by tracking orders for cytobrushes through the purchasing department, revealing that the overall volume of Cytobrushes being ordered was consistent with the volume implied by merging survey data with physician-specific Papanicolaou smear volume data.

To assess the impact of changes in methods of sampling, the team used a "run chart" to track the proportion of inadequate Papanicolaou smears each month. The run chart showed that the proportion of inadequate smears plunged from baseline levels of 20 to 25% per month to less than 10%. Possibly because of a decrease in the number of repeat Papanicolaou smears needed, the overall volume of Papanicolaou smears decreased by more than 10%. Consequently, the number of women who received a Papanicolaou smear report with the "less than optimal" designation was cut by more than 50%.

The estimated economic impact of these changes was favorable. On an annual basis, the additional costs from using a more expensive sampling tool was $15,000. The cost of additional physician sampling time for a "two-tool" method added $11,000. The cost of added physician cytopathologist interpretation resulting from the discovery of an additional 1068 abnormalities added $20,000. However, these costs were far outweighed by a savings of $158,000 from fewer repeat visits and fewer repeat Papanicolaou interpretations, leading to a net savings of $112,000 per year.

## EXAMPLE 2: SMOKING INTERVENTION PROGRAM

Smoking cessation is an important public health concern and has been the subject of a recent Agency for Health Care Policy and Research (AHCPR) guideline, as well as a Health Plan Data and Information Set (HEDIS) measure. The CCE developed a first-generation smoking-dependency clinic that was staffed by trained nonphysician counselors and overseen by a physician medical director. The original intervention was a 50-minute initial evaluation and counseling visit, with nicotine replacement therapy prescribed for all patients with a high level of nicotine dependency. This intervention subsequently was updated to reflect the AHCPR recommendation that, unless contraindicated, all smoking cessation patients be prescribed nicotine replacement therapy.

Because relapse is a normal part of smoking cessation, the intervention was designed explicitly to address relapse. This was done through return visits, an optional support group, and follow-up telephone counseling calls throughout the year. The program was designed to be inexpensive and simple to execute within the clinic. This was accomplished by automating the logistics of both the intervention and the collection of outcomes measures. The Flexi-Scan System, an internally developed computer application that helps automate outcome studies and disease-management interventions, was used to automate (1) data entry through a scanner, (2) prompting of follow-up calls and mailings, and (3) the generation of medical-record notes and letters to the referring physicians. A database that can be used for analysis of the outcomes data acquired as a part of this process.

This first-generation program achieved a 12-month quit rate of 25%. Such a quit rate is about twice as high as the rate achieved with brief counseling intervention. To evaluate the cost-effectiveness of this program, a decision analytical model was constructed. The model estimated that the first-generation smoking-dependency clinic cost approximately $1600 for each life year gained. As illustrated in Table 70–3, this cost-effectiveness ratio was highly favorable to other healthcare interventions.

Although this first-generation program was effective and cost-effective, it was targeted only at the estimated 16,500 smokers in the Henry Ford Medical Group (HFMG) patient population who were highly motivated to quit. The estimated 66,000 other smokers in the HFMG patient population would be un-

**Table 70–3** League Table

| Intervention | Cost per Quality-Adjusted Life Year Gained |
|---|---|
| Smoking cessation counselling | $6,400 |
| Surgery for left main coronary artery disease for a 55-year-old man | $7,000 |
| Flexible sigmoidoscopy (every 3 yrs) | $25,000 |
| Renal dialysis (annual cost) | $37,000 |
| Screening for human immunodeficiency virus (at a prevalence of 5/1000) | $39,000 |
| Pap smear (every year) | $40,000 |
| Surgery for 3-vessel coronary artery disease for a 55-year-old man | $95,000 |

likely to pursue an intervention that involved visiting a smoking dependency clinic. Even for the smokers who were highly motivated to quit, the smoking cessation clinic had the capacity to provide counseling to about 500 people each year, or approximately 3% of these highly motivated smokers. Therefore, the CCE developed a "second-generation" Smoking Intervention Program. This program uses a three-tiered approach that includes (1) a "front-end" process for primary care and specialty clinics to use to identify smokers and provide brief motivational advice, (2) a centralized telephone-based triage process to conduct assessment and make arrangements for appropriate intervention, and (3) a stepped-care treatment tier.

In the "front-end" process, the clinic physician and support staff were trained to screen their patients for smoking status and readiness to quit and provide tailored brief advice. Each participating clinic was provided with a program "kit," including screening forms, patient brochures, and posters to assist them in implementing the program. Patients who are interested in further intervention are referred to a centralized triage counselor for further assessment and intervention. These counselors are trained, nonphysician care providers. They proactively call each patient referred, conduct an assessment of the patients smoking and quitting history, and triage patients into a stepped-care intervention program.

An important part of this intervention has been providing information to clinicians, including a quarterly report showing the number of patients that they have referred to the Smoking Intervention Program, the status of those patients, the type of intervention that they are receiving, and the number of patients who report not having smoked in the preceding 6 months. The clinician-specific data are presented in comparison to data for the medical group as a whole. These reports have a strong motivational effect on clinicians, as evidenced by a sharp increase in Smoking Intervention Program referrals after each reporting cycle. As with the first-generation intervention, the second-generation program achieved a 6-month quit rate of approximately 25%. The new program, however, has much larger capacity and lower cost per participant. Patient satisfaction with the Smoking Intervention Program is encouraging, with 85% reporting that they would refer a friend to this program.

## EXAMPLE 3: MAMMOGRAPHY IN THE 40- TO 49-YEAR AGE GROUP

A multidisciplinary team was commissioned by the HFMG Clinical Practice Committee to use an explicit methodology to conduct a clinical policy analysis and develop specific clinical policy recommendations regarding the role of screening mammography for average risk women 40 to 49 years of age.

Based on information from the medical literature, internal HFMG data, and the expert opinion of team members, a mathematical model was developed and refined to gain a greater understanding of the implications and shortcomings of existing scientific evidence and to estimate the health and economic outcomes (with ranges of uncertainty) for three alternative plans: (1) do not recommend mammography until age 50 years, (2) recommend a program of biannual mammography during the 40- to 49 year period, and (3) recommend a program of annual mammography.

The results of this analysis are summarized in Figure 70–6. Compared with not recommending mammograms, a program of five biannual mammograms for the 2500 HFMG women entering their 40s would add approximately $1.5 million to the net healthcare cost for the group (90% range of certainty: $918k–$2.1 million). This program could be expected to save between one and six lives, resulting in a gain of about 141 life years (43–244). This represents an expenditure of $440 thousand per life saved (undiscounted). With discounting of health and economic outcomes, this represents an incremental cost-effectiveness ratio of $34 thousand per life-year gained (15–120k). Earlier detection, in addition to saving lives, would permit the use of breast-conserving procedures in about two more women, and would permit nonsystemic treatment for four more women. In addition, such a program of biannual mammography could lead to added piece of mind for approximately 1700 women receiving all negative screening results. On the down side, 59 more women would experience the fear, inconvenience, and risk associated with false-positive mammogram results, leading to a negative biopsy, and an additional 650 to 950 women would have the unneeded worry associated with false-positive mammogram results.

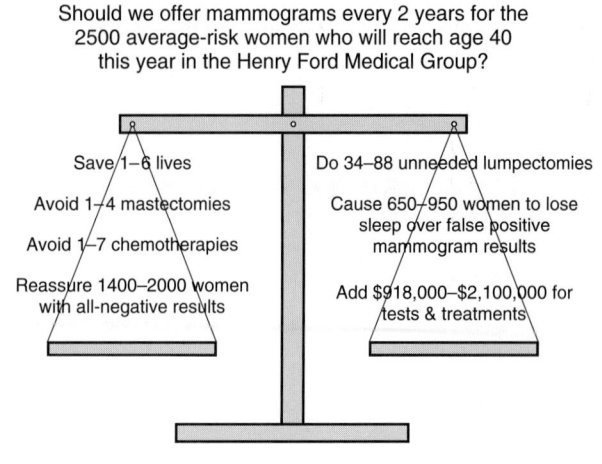

**Figure 70–6** Results of mammography policy analysis.

Compared with biannual mammography, a program of 10 annual mammograms during the 40s would cost an additional $900 thousand, saving an additional 0 to 1 life, for an estimated gain of 26 more life-years (1–58). This represents an expenditure of $1.4 million per life saved (undiscounted). With discounting, this represents an incremental cost-effectiveness ratio of $108 thousand per life-year gained (42k–1.8 million).

On the basis of these estimates, the team recommended biannual screening mammograms in average risk women 40 to 49 years of age. This guideline was intended to serve as a "best-practice," "minimum practice," and "maximum practice" guideline, as summarized in the following statements, which were endorsed unanimously by the team: "Unless documented, patient-specific circumstances dictate otherwise, it is important to offer screening mammograms every 2 years during the 40- to 49-year age period. More frequent mammograms are not routinely needed for average-risk women during this age period." This guideline was incorporated into the existing HFMG clinical preventive services guideline for breast cancer screening.

Shortly after this guideline was approved, a meta-analysis of mammography trials was published in the *Journal of the American Medical Association* (JAMA). The abstract stated, "The results of our meta-analysis suggest that screening mammography reduced breast cancer mortality by 26% (95% confidence interval [CI] 17–34%) in women aged 50–74 years, but *does not significantly reduce breast cancer mortality* in women aged 40–49 years." (emphasis added). The body of the manuscript stated that "there were only three clinical trials in which women aged 40–49 years underwent two-view mammography and had 10–12 years of follow-up; in those, the relative risk for reduction in breast cancer mortality…was 0.73 (95% CI, 0.54 to 1.0) after 10–12 years of follow-up." Although the abstract suggested the opposite conclusion as the HFMG clinical policy analysis, apparently based on a confidence interval that touched zero, the point estimate of mammography effectiveness in the 40- to 49-year age group was actually more favorable than the HFMG analysis (27% vs. 25% risk reduction). The fact that the assumptions and calculated outcomes were documented explicitly in the HFMG put this potentially consensus-breaking piece of new information in its appropriate context. This example also illustrates the decision-making criterion implied by the clinical trial and meta-analysis literature: if an intervention has a positive effect that is 95% or more likely to be greater than zero, then it is implicitly recommended, regardless of the magnitude of the outcome in relation or the cost. The explicit method permits policy-makers in health-care organizations to use a more sophisticated and philosophically defensible criteria based on an assessment of the benefits, costs, and uncertainties associated with each.

## Conclusions and Future Challenges

These examples illustrate how the emerging discipline of clinical effectiveness can result in measurable improvements to important health-care processes by employing a systematic approach, involving clinical policy-making, quality and outcomes measurement, and a multifaceted approach to implementation. To enable success, obstetrician-gynecologists work with other members of their clinical team and enlist the support of expert clinical effectiveness practitioners. They draw from the rich methods and tools of diverse disciplines, including clinical medicine, epidemiology, statistics, medical decision sciences, economics, psychology, industrial engineering, management sciences, education, and medical informatics.

A number of important challenges remain, however. Overall health-care quality is the sum of the quality of thousands of decision-making and care-delivery processes. The examples described in this chapter make up a tiny slice of overall health-care quality. The level of resource intensity and leadership attentiveness that was applied to these examples is not likely to be applied simultaneously to more than a few dozen processes within most organizations. Therefore, it is critical that the practice of clinical effectiveness be an integral part of the overall practice of all obstetrician-gynecologists and other clinicians. Only then will these methods scale up to the enormous task of improving thousands of health-care processes.

Three fundamental changes in the health-care environment are required to support clinical process improvement on a large scale. First, the *incentives* facing health-care organizations and individual clinicians for improvement must be increased. The growing interest in external performance measurement, such as with HEDIS measures, is a step in the right direction. But overall quality improvement is likely to require a market structure in which health-care organizations face competition based on quality rather than only price competition and in which the compensation of individual clinicians is driven by quality measures rather than only work effort. However, clinician-level quality measurement is a difficult proposition. Patient variation makes clinician-to-clinician comparisons difficult, even for the most common clinical practices. The subset of practices that can be measured represents a small fraction of all clinical practices. As a result, motivating clinicians to focus on improving measurable processes is like encouraging students to "study for the test," calling into question the generalizability of the measures to assess overall practice quality. Furthermore, some warn that the use of quality measurement to drive clinician incentives or as a basis to identify "bad apples" for remedial attention is counterproductive to the use of measurement for learning and improvement.

The second fundamental change needed is the *education* of clinicians in the methods and tools of quality improvement, as adapted from the various disciplines described. More substantial changes are needed in medical school curricula, residency training, board examinations, and perhaps also in the criteria used for medical school admissions.

The third fundamental change needed is a substantial investment in *information technology* to support clinical practice. Although information systems have been applied to administrative processes within health-care organizations, the sophistication of systems to support patient care and quality improvement is lacking. Other industries, such as financial services and manufacturing, invest a substantially larger portion of their budgets to information technology. Scaleable, durable quality improvements require systems that offer three important capabilities. First, information systems must permit the acquisition of structured data on patients, health-care interventions, and outcomes as part of the routine care delivery process. Second, information systems must offer decision aids such as reminders, alerts, and prompts to clinicians at the moment that clinical decisions are being made. Third, information systems must facilitate the complex logistics of coordination of care involving many disciplines in many settings according to protocols and guidelines.

Therefore, an additional responsibility falls on the shoulders of obstetrician-gynecologists. In addition to patient care (providing care to individuals) and clinical effectiveness (working to improve the care of populations), obstetrician-gynecologists have a responsibility to advocate and drive change in their environment to enable large scale, durable improvement. In a world with incentives, education, and technology to support quality improvement, the public can expect dramatic, measurable improvements in the *overall* effectiveness of our health-care system.

## REFERENCES

Agency for Health Care Policy and Research: Smoking Cessation Clinical Practice Guideline. Rockville, MD, US Department of Health and Human Services, 1996. AHCPR No. 96-0694.

Avorn J, Soumerai SB: Improving drug-therapy decisions through educational outreach: A randomized controlled trial of academically based "detailing." N Engl J Med 308:1457–1463, 1983.

Berwick DM, Coltin KL: Feedback reduces test use in a health maintenance organization. JAMA 255:1450–1454, 1986.

Berwick DM: A primer on leading the improvement of systems. BMJ 312(7031):619–622, 1996.

Berwick DM: Continuous improvement as an ideal in health care. N Engl J Med 320:53–56, 1989.

Boon ME, de Graaff Guilloud JC, Rietveld WJ: Analysis of five sampling methods for the preparation of cervical smears. Acta Cytol 33:843–848, 1989.

Boon ME, Alons-van Kordelaar JJ, Rietveld-Scheffers PE: Consequences of the introduction of combined spatula and Cytobrush sampling for cervical cytology: Improvements in smear quality and detection rates. Acta Cytol 30:264–270, 1986.

Chassin MR, Brook RH, Park RE, et al: Variations in the use of medical and surgical services by the Medicare population. N Engl J Med 314:285–290, 1986.

Crosby PB: Quality Is Free: The Art of Making Quality Certain. New York, American Library, 1980.

Davis DA, Thomson MA, Oxman AD, et al: Changing physician performance: A systematic review of the effect of continuing medical education strategies. JAMA 274:700–705, 1995.

Deming WE: Out of the Crisis. Cambridge, MA, MIT Center for Engineering Study, 1986.

Donabedian A: The Price of Quality and the Perplexities of Care. 1986 Michael M. Davis Lecture, sponsored by The Center for Health Administration Studies, Graduate School of Business, University of Chicago.

Eddy DM: Comparing benefits and harms: The balance sheet. JAMA 263:2493–2505, 1990.

Eddy DM: Guidelines for policy statements: The explicit approach. JAMA 263:2239–2240, 2243, 1990.

Eddy DM: Practice policies and guidelines: What are they? JAMA 263:877–878, 880, 1990.

Eddy DM: Practice policies: Where do they come from? JAMA 263:1265–1275, 1990.

Ellwood PM: Outcomes management: A technology of patient experience. N Engl J Med 318(23):1549–1556, 1988.

Gold MR, Siegel JE, Russell LB, et al: Cost-Effectiveness in Health and Medicine. New York, Oxford University Press, 1996.

Gottlieb LK, Sokol HN, Murrey KO, et al: Algorithm-based clinical quality improvement, clinical guidelines and continuous quality improvement. HMO Pract 6:5–12, 1991.

Grimshaw J, Russell IT: Effect of clinical guidelines on medical practice: A systematic review of rigorous evaluations. Lancet 342:1317–1322, 1993.

Ishikawa K: Guide to Quality Control. White Plains, NY, Kraus International Publications, 1982.

Juran JM (ed): Quality Control Handbook. 3rd ed. New York, McGraw-Hill, 1979.

Kerlikowske K, Grady D, Rubin SM, et al: Efficacy of screening mammography: A meta-analysis. JAMA 273:149–154, 1995.

Kritchevsky SB, Simmons BP: Continuous quality improvement, concepts and applications for physician care. JAMA 266:1817–1823, 1991.

Kuperman G, James B, Jacobsen J, et al: Continuous quality improvement applied to medical care. Med Decis Making 11(suppl):s60–s65, 1991.

Laffel G, Blumenthal D: The case for using industrial quality management science in health care organizations. JAMA 262:2869–2873, 1989.

Manus DA, Werner TR, Strub RJ: Using measurement and feedback to reduce health care costs and modify physician practice patterns. Qual Manage Health Care 2:48–60, 1994.

Nelson EC, Mohr JJ, Batalden PB, et al: Improving health care, part 1: The clinical value compass. J Qual Improv 22:243–258, 1996.

Weinstein MC, Stason WB: Foundations of cost-effectiveness analysis for health and medical practices. N Engl J Med 296:716–721, 1977.

Wennberg J, Gittelsohn A: Small area variation in health care delivery. Science 182:1102–1108, 1973.

Wennburg JE, Freeman JL, Culp WJ: Are hospital services rationed in New Haven or overutilized in Boston? Lancet 1:1185–1188, 1987.

# 71

# Understanding Medical-Legal Issues in Obstetrics and Gynecology

LOUIS WEINSTEIN

The legal system impacts upon many things that happen on a daily basis in our lives. Health-care providers constantly complain about the medical malpractice crisis that exists and impacts on their practice and livelihood. It is my opinion that there is not a medical malpractice crisis, because the health-care profession is just a small part of a much larger problem that is related to product liability. Malpractice rulings have forced companies into bankruptcy (e.g., A.H. Robins for the Dalkon Shield intrauterine device [IUD] and Dow Corning [silicone breast implants]). Other companies (e.g., General Motors and Ford Motor Co.) have had massive awards against them for product liability. Health care is a product, and we suffer in a similar manner but on a much smaller scale.

Medicolegal issues extend beyond the malpractice arena, but this is the area that draws the most heated debates among providers. In this chapter, I shall discuss the reasons for the perceived medical malpractice crisis, how a medical malpractice action is established, what constitutes a good medical record, how to obtain adequate informed consent, how to perform during the deposition process, and proposals for medical liability reform. I will also make suggestions for how to alleviate the current perceived malpractice crisis. Other issues to be discussed include the concept of abandonment, maternal-fetal conflicts regarding medical care, the medicolegal implications of breast cancer, fetal monitoring and ultrasonography, and the impact that litigation has on the physician.

## Understanding the Language

Each profession has specific language that it uses and to understand the language, the individual must know the definition of the terms. The following list defines some commonly used legal terms.

**abandonment:** Termination of a physician-patient relationship without reasonable notice and without an opportunity for the patient to acquire adequate medical care, which results in some type of damage to the patient.
**allegation:** A statement of a party to an action, made in a pleading, setting out what the party expects to prove.
**captain of the ship:** A doctrine whereby the surgeon

in charge of a medical team is liable for all the negligent acts of the members of the team.

**contingency fee:** A fee agreement between the plaintiff and the plaintiff's attorney, whereby the plaintiff agrees to pay the attorney a percentage of the damages recovered.

**defendant:** The party against whom relief is sought in an action.

**deposition:** A pretrial discovery device by which one party to the action, typically through the attorney, asks oral questions of the other party, a witness for the other party, or any potential witness. The deposition is conducted under oath outside of the courtroom, is completely transcribed, and may be admissible at trial.

**impeachment:** The process by which the truth or credibility of the testimony of a witness is challenged.

**malpractice (medical):** The failure to exercise that degree of care used by reasonably careful physicians of like qualifications in the same or similar circumstances. The patient's injury must be a result of this failure to meet this duty of care.

**negligence:** Legal cause of action involving the failure to exercise the degree of diligence and care that a reasonably and ordinarily prudent person would exercise under the same or similar circumstances.

**plaintiff:** The party who files the lawsuit.

**res ipsa loquitur (The thing speaks for itself):** The legal theory in which it must be proved that the cause of the injury was in the defendant's exclusive control and that the accident was one that ordinarily does not happen in the absence of negligence.

**standard of care:** Physicians are required to adhere to the standards of practice of a reasonably competent physician, in the same or similar circumstances, with comparable training and experience either in their own locality or their own medical specialty.

**statute of limitations:** The time period in which a plaintiff may file a lawsuit.

**tort:** A civil wrong for which an action can be filed in court to recover damages for personal injury or property damage resulting from negligent acts or intentional misconduct.

**wrongful birth:** An action brought by the parents who seek damages after the birth of an impaired child, in which the parents allege that negligent treatment or advice deprived them of the opportunity to avoid conception or terminate the pregnancy.

**wrongful conception:** An action brought by the parents who seek damages arising from negligent performance of a sterilization procedure or abortion.

**wrongful life:** An action brought by a child born with impairments who contends that he or she would not have been born but for the negligent advice to, or treatment of, the parents.

# General Concepts

There are many reasons given for the marked proliferation of medical malpractice suits in the United States. Approximately 4 of 5 obstetrician-gynecologists (OB/GYNs) have been sued, and 1 of 4 has been sued at least four times. A reason given, which is incorrect, is that the large number of lawyers working at present need to file a large number of suits. If the number of lawyers was limited, the individual attorney would just increase his or her individual caseload. To attack the plaintiff's attorney for attending to the needs of his or her clients is illogical.

The majority of people in society today believe that most wrongs must have a reason, that someone is responsible for that wrong, and that the wrong must be corrected. Often the only redress is a legal action. This results in patients who have a bad outcome believing that a negligent act has occurred. Many people seem to lack responsibility for their own actions. The pioneer spirit and taking responsibility for one's self have been forgotten.

The media and physicians have instilled great expectations in the general public for medical care, and it is unlikely that we in the profession can live up to these lofty standards.

Malpractice suits are an attempt to ensure some accountability in physicians, frequently for outcomes that are beyond the control of the health-care provider. Realistically, however, evidence supports that a major cause for the escalation in medical malpractice suits is actual medical malpractice. An interesting observation is that a small number of obstetricians account for the majority of the problem, with one study demonstrating that 85% of payments in malpractice suits were incurred by 6% of physicians.

A large study published in 1977 estimated the incidence of iatrogenic injury and substandard care. The authors found an overall adverse events rate of 4.6% and a negligence rate of 0.8%. A similar study published in 1991 reviewed 30,121 medical records, with adverse events occurring in 3.7% of records and with 1% of the adverse events caused by negligence. The authors concluded that "there is a substantial amount of injury in patients from medical management, and many injuries are the result of substandard care." Further analysis of the data revealed drug complications to be the most common adverse event, followed by wound infections and technical complications. Nonsurgical adverse events were more likely to be caused by negligence than surgical ones. Fifty-eight percent of adverse events were the result of errors in management, with nearly half attributed to negligence. In a follow-up of the 280 patients in the study who experienced an adverse event caused by medical negligence, only 8 filed malpractice claims. The authors estimated that statewide, the ratio of adverse events caused by negligence to malpractice claims is 7.6 to 1. Their conclusion was that litigation rarely compensates patients injured by medical negligence and rarely identifies and holds the providers accountable for substandard care. A recent report of 51 malpractice claims in the same study population attempted to predict the relationship between negligent adverse events and litigation. The only significant predictor of payment was the severity of the disability in the patient, with no association between the adverse event and negligence.

A review of 220 closed obstetric malpractice claims demonstrated the risks to be equally divided among prenatal care, high-risk status, labor, and delivery. The problems were recognized 54% of the time, with 32% being managed correctly. The authors concluded that the risks are common and recognizable and that physician performance was poor by any standard. Another obstetric study revealed that physicians failed to recognize a high-risk pregnancy 56% of the time and failed to render proper care 44% of the time. A further analysis of 500 obstetric and gynecologic claims demonstrated that 46% were for misguided allegations, 19% were for incompetent care, 12% were for errors in judgment, 9% were for lack of expertise, 7% were for failure of communication, 6% were for poor supervision, and 1% were for inadequate staffing.

Common themes that are present in obstetric malpractice actions are dealing with the postdated pregnancy related to the lack of a documented date of confinement, failure to recognize and deal with antepartum and intrapartum complications, failure to provide genetic information, and failure to perform a timely cesarean section. Common gynecologic issues are failed sterilization, uterine perforation, endoscopic injury, and urinary tract injury.

Certain characteristics have been noted in the evaluation of surgeons with high and low malpractice claims rates. Surgeons who were terminated because of high claims rates were substantially different from those with minimal malpractice activity. Terminated surgeons had completed fewer fellowships, were more likely to be international medical graduates, less likely to be board-certified, more likely to practice solo, and did not have clinical faculty appointments. Physicians who see many patients have a greater tendency to be sued. A survey of patients' levels of satisfaction with care demonstrated that those who saw high-claim physicians complained of being rushed, not receiving an explanation for tests, and being generally ignored. The conclusions were that physicians who were frequently sued did not communicate well and did not establish rapport with their patients.

## Establishing a Medical Malpractice Action

Any individual can file a medical malpractice action against a health-care provider. To have a successful conclusion of a malpractice suit, four issues must be addressed. The first is to establish the *duty* of the physician to the patient, which is the obligation of the physician to practice at an acceptable standard of care. The second is to identify the proper *standard of care* to which the physician must adhere. The third is to prove that the standard of care has been *violated*. The usual standard of care is a national one for the OB/GYN. The standard chosen cannot be rigid because it must allow the variation that occurs in most clinical situations. The fourth and most difficult issue is to prove that the violation of the standard of care is the *cause* of the patient's injury. This is the usual role of the expert witness, and the inability to establish the causative nature of the violation of the standard of care results in courtroom verdicts for the defense.

## Medical Record—The Answer or the Curse

The inevitability of a practicing physician's having a malpractice action occur during his or her professional life is a hard fact of reality. Many of the cases are not justified based on the facts, but a successful defense often hinges on the medical record. The record has the potential to be the physician's best friend or worst enemy.

To be helpful in the defense of the claim, the medical record must be similar to an enjoyable movie. It must tell a *complete story* with a beginning stating the patient's complaint and history; a middle part detailing the physical examination, laboratory studies, and procedures that were planned and performed; and an ending clearly stating what transpired and how the patient fared during the medical encounter.

Other than memory, which may be clouded by time or biased by wishing for the desired result, the medical record is the only source that states clearly in a real-time fashion what transpired with the patient and what the physician was thinking. The record should communicate to the health-care team what the patient was saying about how she was doing. It is the major key to a successful defense and, if it is written well, it may result in closure of the case early in the legal process. A jury will often consider that a poorly documented or sloppy medical record implies a similar type of medical care that resulted in the patient's being injured. I shall give a paradigm on what constitutes an excellent medical record.

All entries in the medical record are to be timed and dated and entered as soon as possible after the patient encounter has occurred. The writing *must* be legible, which implies that the physician took the time necessary to record the findings and that others will be able to read the notes when required. There are times when a physician cannot read his or her own writing, and this is tantamount to having a case that cannot be defended. If the physician's handwriting is poor, a dictated note will suffice if it is dictated and transcribed expeditiously. It must be read before the physician signs it for the record. Operating room notes must be dictated within 24 hours of surgery, because it can be quite detrimental to the defense if the dictation is dated after the patient has experienced a complication from the surgery. The jury will consider that the physician already knew about the complication and may have altered the dictation to support the injury.

Having reviewed numerous medical records in legal actions, I have concluded that there are four syndromes that describe the difficult-to-read medical record. The first is the Egyptian syndrome. This occurs when the writing in the chart appears similar to that of the Rosetta stone in that it is hieroglyphics to the reader. The second is the itty-bitty syndrome. This is characterized by writing that is so small it is impossible to decipher the majority of the information. This is often seen in nurses' notes, especially on labor and delivery charts, where the space in which to write is small. It would seem logical to assume that it would take less time to write bigger and would make the chart more readable. The third is the fill'er up syndrome. This occurs when the entire usable surface of the paper is written on, often at angles to be read by following arrows. The least expensive part of the medical care system is the paper, so I implore the health-care provider to use all the paper necessary. The fourth is the Houdini syndrome. This occurs when the factual data in the note are so scarce that you have to guess at what the physician was thinking and how the patient was doing.

The medical record must be accurate and objective, and only facts, clinical judgments, and patient responses should be recorded. Unqualified and emotional remarks of the provider are not to be placed in the record. Adjectives and adverbs should always be avoided. An example is from a record of a consultant asked to see a patient with a liver rupture and hemolysis, elevated liver enzymes, and low platelets (HELLP) syndrome who started the note with . . . "this extensive and overwhelming medical catastrophe." This note was the downfall of the defense in this case.

Words to be avoided include "inadvertent," which means "inattentive," "iatrogenic," which means "induced by the physician or the treatment," "unintentional," which means "you did not mean to do it but you did," and other words such as "unfortunately," "routine," "OK," or "within normal limits."

Humor must always be avoided in the medical record. An example appears in a note written in the record on the evening a geriatric patient fell out of bed. "Little old lady fell out of bed, another foot higher, she would have been dead." Later, it was discovered that she had fractured her hip as a result of the fall. The jury did not find the chart humorous and awarded the patient over $10,000 per word.

Financial information regarding the patient should never be in the record. An adequate discussion of informed consent must be documented. A medical record must *never* be altered. This makes even the most defensible case impossible to defend. Following these simple suggestions will make a medical record that is in the best interest of both patient and provider. The investment in time to ensure an adequate medical record will yield manifold returns to the physician.

## Informed Consent

The informed consent process is as vital to good medical care as a proper diagnosis and the performance of the correct surgical procedure. The process of informed consent occurs in some manner in all patient interactions. The maturing of the concept of informed consent occurred when Justice Cardozo stated, "Every human being of adult years and sound mind has a right to determine what shall be done with his own body" (Mary Schloendorff vs. The Society of New York Hospital. 211 NY 125, 105 NE 92 [1914]).

The extent of the discussion with the patient regarding informed consent has been debated for many years. Simply stated, the patient must be given the information that a reasonably prudent person would need in order to make an informed decision. The courts have stated that the patient needs to have the material risks revealed to her. In Canterbury vs. Spence, the court stated, "there is no bright light separating the significant from the insignificant; the answer in any case must abide by the rule of reason" (Canterbury vs. Spence, 464 F.2d 722[DC Cir. 1972], cert. denied, 409 US 1064 [1972]). In another ruling about the procedure to be performed, the court stated, "the patient's interest in information does not extend to a lengthy polysyllabic disclosure on all possible complications. A minicourse in medical science is not required; the patient is concerned with the risk of death or bodily harm, and the problems of recuperation" (Cobbs vs. Grant, 8 CA. 2d 229, 104 CA Rptr. 505, 502 P.2d 1 [1972]).

To obtain proper informed consent, along with information about the procedure to be performed, the physician must inform the patient of any appropriate alternative forms of treatment. A recent addition to the informed consent process is the concept of informed refusal. This is based on the rule that if a patient refuses a treatment or procedure, the physician must make her aware of the risks associated with her refusal (Truman vs. Thomas, 165 CA Rptr. 308, 611 P.2d 902 [1980]). Common occurrences for informed refusal in the obstetric patient would include Papanicolaou smear, mammography, and triple screening. The inability of the patient to pay is not a valid reason to deny a test or procedure that is in the patient's best interest and that she desires.

A common misconception about informed consent is that having the patient sign the consent form is tantamount to adequate informed consent. In general, the forms are not written for the medically unsophisticated. Grundner has demonstrated that the individual must have an advanced degree to comprehend most medical consent forms. A common occurrence in the courtroom is for the plaintiff to state that she did not understand the consent form. When the jury has a chance to see the form, it is easy for them to believe this, because often they are not able to understand the form either. This problem should be addressed by having consent forms developed with medical guidance by individuals who have a high school education.

The key to an adequate informed consent process is for the physician to document in the medical record the presentation of the common risks of the procedure, the presentation of alternative methods of treatment, and the implications of the patient's refusal. This should not be done by a nurse but by the individual who is to be involved in performing the procedure or test.

My suggestion for solving the informed consent problem is to present the material to the patient and then have her write on the medical record her understanding of the conversation that has transpired in her own words. If the note is not clear, the physician must start the process over. This suggestion makes it difficult for the patient to state in court that she did not understand the meaning of informed consent, and it requires the physician to give informed consent in a complete and clear manner.

## Deposition

The deposition is the process whereby attorneys for either side attempt to discover all the pertinent facts and arguments that will be used during the trial. The person being deposed (deponent) is under oath, and a court reporter records everything that is said. It is my opinion that many physicians perform poorly when giving a deposition.

The deposition often occurs in an informal setting, usually the physician's or attorney's office. The rules for the deposition process are the same as those enforced in a courtroom. The deponent must give his or her maximal effort and concentration. It is critical that everything stated be the truth.

The deponent has the right to read the deposition and correct any mistakes made by the court reporter. Any changes made in the testimony may have to be justified at a later date. The physician should never waive the right to read and sign the deposition.

In preparation for the deposition, the physician must review the total medical record and pertinent medical literature. Answers should be truthful, short, crisp, serious, and address only the question asked. Information should never be volunteered. Before answering the question, the deponent should pause and allow time for the attorney to object to the question. All questions must be answered unless the deponent is directed not to do so by the attorney.

The deposition should be scheduled when the deponent is well rested and able to give maximal concentration to the procedure. All previously obtained depositions should be read by the physician to know what the plaintiff and the expert witnesses for both sides are going to say. If possible, the physician should attend the deposition of the plaintiff and her expert witnesses. The physician may be able to offer valuable assistance to the defending attorney at this time, but he or she must not make any open comments about testimony during another's deposition.

## Abandonment/Phantom of the Delivery Room

Abandonment occurs when the physician is not present or does not live up to the reasonable expectations of the patient.

The obstetrician is a prime candidate for action based on the concept of abandonment. Once a duty is established with a patient, it can be ended only with the patient's consent, revoked by the patient's statement that the physician's services are no longer needed, or the withdrawal of the physician after appropriate legal notice to the patient. If the physician chooses not to care for the patient, the patient must be notified by certified letter. A return receipt must be requested, and the patient must be given an appropriate amount of time to find another qualified health-care provider. The physician is not required to give a reason for this action. The filing of a malpractice action allows the physician to withdraw from care of the patient except in an emergency situation.

The fact that a physician is busy is not an excuse for not being available for the patient, even if the physician is delivering another patient (Hood vs. Moffett, 69 So. 664 [MS. 1915]).

To establish a legal basis for the abandonment claim, four requirements must be met. First, a relationship must be formed with the patient. Second, the patient must expect that care will be provided. Third, medical care must be needed by the patient, with the absence of care resulting in injury. Fourth, an actual injury must be caused by the lack of care. The injury does not have to be physical but can be psychological in nature.

In the current medical environment of managed care and capitated systems, discharge of a patient from the hospital before it is medically correct to do so may be considered abandonment.

## Maternal-Fetal Conflict

Secondary to the marked increase in the use of technology in the practice of perinatal medicine, a new area of conflict has arisen between the needs of the fetus and those of the mother. Two ethical principles must guide the practitioner when dealing with maternal-fetal conflicts. First is the right of the pregnant patient to choose or refuse any treatment, and the second is to promote fetal well-being.

The courts have become involved in ordering obstetric interventions. One study revealed that 81% of court-ordered cesarean section patients were members of minority groups, 44% were unmarried, and 24% did not speak English as their primary language. All were receiving public aid and were being treated in a university hospital clinic.

The court decisions did not address the issues of how to convince a patient to have surgery, whether it was permissible to restrain the patient for surgery, and who was responsible if a malpractice action was filed.

The American Medical Association (AMA) Board of Trustees recommends the following:
1. Judicial intervention is inappropriate when a woman has made an informed refusal of medical treatment designed to benefit her fetus.
2. The physician's duty is to provide the facts necessary for the woman to give informed consent after reaching a thoughtful, informed decision.
3. The physician should not be liable for any damages that result from the physician's honoring the woman's informed refusal for medical treatment to benefit her fetus.

In summary, the physician must always try to respect the woman's autonomy and rarely, if ever, resort to the courts to obtain permission for a therapy that may benefit the fetus.

## Specific Clinical Issues

There are three areas that commonly appear in obstetric and gynecologic medical malpractice cases. These are the interpretation of the electronic fetal monitor, failure to diagnose breast cancer, and the use of ultrasonography.

The American College of Obstetricians and Gynecologists has clearly stated that the term "fetal distress" is imprecise and nonspecific, has a low positive predictive value, and is often seen in an infant who is in good condition at birth. The suggestion has been made that the term fetal distress be replaced by "nonreassuring fetal status."

A review of 110 cases demonstrated that 70% of the actions were based on incorrect interpretation of fetal heart tracings. The basis of the claims were failure to take action or delay in response to the tracing. The problems with fetal heart tracings are that experts vary widely in their level of expertise and that definitions of what constitutes an abnormality are varied and unsatisfactory. The general conclusion is that fetal monitor tracings have a low sensitivity when correlated with fetal outcome.

Because it is difficult to practice obstetrics without the use of a fetal monitor, there are some things that the practitioner can do to improve the value of fetal monitoring. Document in the chart a description of fetal monitor findings with a date and time. Do not try to label what is being seen. Be sure that obvious causes of fetal heart rate abnormalities are eliminated, such as hyperstimulation from oxytocin. In the presence of an abnormally described tracing at delivery, obtain a full set of cord blood gas levels. Do not embellish the medical record when describing the tracing and do not editorialize.

There continues to be a marked increase in lawsuits filed for failure to diagnose breast cancer. A series of breast cancer malpractice suits revealed that the most common symptom was a painless mass, followed by a painful mass, nipple discharge, and no symptoms. The patient herself discovered the breast mass 86% of the time, with average time of discovery to diagnosis being 15.7 months. Although science does not support the finding that early detection improves breast cancer cure rates, the perception is that a delay in making a diagnosis or initiating treatment decreases the accuracy of the prognosis and constitutes medical negligence. The best candidate for a successful defense was a smaller tumor size with failure to perform a biopsy associated with a successful outcome for the plaintiff.

Ultrasonography-related litigation increased substantially during the 1990s. Two large areas of litigation include a fetal anomaly that is missed and failure to identify either an ectopic or an early intrauterine pregnancy. Great care must be taken in describing ultrasonographic findings to the patient. The word "normal" has a different connotation to the patient than to the physician. If a patient is told that the scan is normal and the fetus is subsequently born with an anomaly, it is malpractice in her mind. Proper terminology should be "no gross abnormalities noted." The patient should also be instructed in the capability of an ultrasonographic scanner to detect fetal anomalies. Suggested guidelines for defensive scanning include proper training, defining the limits of the scan, scanning the complete fetus in a systematic manner, generating a formal report, stating whether the scan was optimal, and recording the images. Following these suggestions will not prevent a malpractice case but will help greatly in reaching a successful outcome.

## The Impact on the Physician

The average physician does not understand the serious impact that initiation of a malpractice suit will have. The suit itself is a profound attack on the individual's integrity, knowledge, competence, motivation, and self-esteem. After the initial period of distress, numerous somatic disorders may ensue, including major depression, alcohol abuse, drug abuse, and suicidal ideation. The psychological defenses often employed include denial, reaction formation, suppression, rationalization, and sublimation. The effects on the physician are similar regardless of the outcome of the malpractice claim.

## Suggestions for Crisis Improvement

It is inappropriate for physicians to argue that the contingency system should be eliminated. The plaintiff's attorney is the one who undergoes all the risk, as he or she must absorb all the costs and receive no fee if the case is lost. The defense attorney "wins" every case in spite of the outcome because he or she is paid on an hourly, or time, basis. The contingency fee system provides an incentive for the plaintiff's attorney to work as hard as possible to obtain the best reward for his or her efforts. Because the injured party often gets only a small part of the monetary award after the contingency fee and expenses are paid, I would suggest that the payment be structured over time to allow a proper award to the injured party. In addition, the number of expert witnesses used should be capped, and a limit should be set on the fees that the expert witnesses charges.

Decreasing the statute of limitations to between 8 and 10 years after birth is a good idea, but it will do little to decrease the number of malpractice cases because most obstetric cases are filed within this time period. It would assist the insurance carriers to assess their long-term risk and to decrease the cost of protective coverage for the physician.

Noneconomic damages should be limited or capped. Juries often award extraordinary amounts of money, and they should be instructed in the issue of fair awards. Structured settlements should be used more, because less expensive purchases of an annuity can compensate the individual adequately over many years.

Malpractice insurance should be available to all physicians on a national basis. The premiums should be based on the claim and settlement record of the practitioner. The amounts of insurance carried should be standardized throughout the specialty. Raising the cost of premiums among certain high-risk physicians will keep rates lower for other physicians. These high-risk individuals will not be able to pass on the higher costs to the patients in their communities and will have to absorb them, which may act as a deterrent.

A selective no-fault system should be considered for certain injuries. These would be called accelerated-compensation events and they would be feasible to develop and apply. They would cover a majority of paid claims and indemnity dollars, result in substantial savings in time and expense, and be unlikely to increase the number of large new claims. Certain unusual cases could still be dealt with in the traditional legal manner. Mediation and arbitration should be utilized more often, especially for less catastrophic injuries. There currently exists a tariff of damages for particular types of injury, published in Kemp & Kemp on The Quantum of Damages in Personal Injury and Fatal Accident Claims (1992), which could be used as a source to determine the monetary damage amount.

Certain complicated cases should be required to have a pretrial screening panel, including a judge, attorney, and physician, with results either binding or admissible in court. If one party rejects the findings of the panel, that party become responsible for all litigation costs of both parties if they lose the case.

The issue of the expert witness, known as the "hired gun," must be addressed. This applies to either plaintiff or defense witnesses. The concept of a court-appointed, nonbiased expert witness should be considered, with the costs being equally shared by both parties. This should not abrogate the rights of either side to call their own expert witness. After the trial, the testimony of all expert witnesses should be made public in appropriate medical journals and subjected to appropriate criticism.

A better and more equitable system of peer review must be established. This process must be fair and protected from discovery. Moreover, the peer reviewers should be immune from any legal action. The system must be able to discipline or remove from practice incompetent physicians without fear that the individual will file a legal action against the peer reviewer or the medical institution.

Obtaining a medical license should be linked to completion of the board certification status according to the American Board of Medical Specialties. If the physician cannot obtain certification within a fixed period of time, further training should be required. Recertification should also be necessary for license renewal when the original board certification expires.

Malpractice premiums should be decreased if the physician maintains adequate medical records, identifies high-risk patients, uses consultation and testing appropriately, and participates in a continuing process of medical education.

## Closing Argument

Medicine is the greatest of professions and the public has placed great faith and confidence in physicians to act in their best interests. The public must be made aware that even the best practice of medicine may result in an adverse event and that the physician may not be responsible for the outcome. The time has come for physicians, attorneys, the public, and the government to come together to discuss the problem of medical malpractice, offer reasonable solutions with informed consent to all the involved parties, and reach a just verdict for all the people.

## REFERENCES

American College of Obstetricians and Gynecologists: Department of Professional Liability. Commonsense Glossary of Medical-Legal Terms, 1997.

Boehm FH: Medicolegal climate for obstetrician-gynecologists. Obstet Gynecol Surv 48:715–716, 1993.

Bovbjerg RR, Tancredi LR, Gaylin DS: Obstetrics and malpractice. Evidence on the performance of a selective no-fault system. JAMA 265:2836–2843, 1991.

Brennan TA, Leape LL, Laird NM, et al: Incidence of adverse events and negligence in hospitalized patients. Results of the Harvard Medical Practice Study I. N Engl J Med 324:370–376, 1991.

Brennan, TA, Sox CM, Burstin HR: Relation between negligent adverse events and the outcomes of medical malpractice litigation. N Engl J Med 335:1963–1967, 1996.

California Medical Association: Report of the Medical Insurance Feasibility Study. San Francisco: California Medical Association, 1977.

Charles SC: Malpractice litigation and its impact on physicians. Curr Psych Ther 23:173–180, 1986.

Julian TM, Brooker DC, Butler JC, et al: Investigation of obstetric malpractice closed claims: Profile of event. Am J Perinatol 2:320–324, 1985.

Leape LL, Brennan TA, Laird N, et al: The nature of adverse events in hospitalized patients. Results of the Harvard Medical Practice Study II. N Engl J Med 324:377–384, 1991.

Localio AR, Lawthers AG, Brennan TA, et al: Relation between malpractice claims and adverse events due to negligence. Results of the Harvard Medical Practice Study III. N Engl J Med 325:245–251, 1991.

Meire HB: Ultrasound-related litigation in obstetrics and gynecology: The need for defensive scanning. Ultrasound Obstet Gynecol 7:233–235, 1996.

Nocon JJ, Coolman DA: Perinatal malpractice—risks and prevention. J Reprod Med 32:83–90, 1987.

Sloan FA, Mergenhagen PM, Burfield B, et al: Medical malpractice experience of physicians: Predictable or haphazard? JAMA 262:3291–3297, 1989.

Symonds EM: Fetal monitoring: Medical and legal implications for the practitioner. Curr Opin Obstet Gynecol 6:430–433, 1994.

Zylstra S, Bors-Koefoed R, Mondor M, et al: A statistical model for predicting the outcome in breast cancer malpractice lawsuits. Obstet Gynecol 84:392–398, 1994.

# 72

# Clinical Pathways

SHANNON DOWNING STRIEBICH
SCOTT B. RANSOM

Clinical pathways, often referred to as clinical practice guidelines, practice policies, or algorithms, have been a fundamental part of the practice of medicine since one physician first asked another how to manage the care of a patient. The formal development and implementation of clinical pathways has become common in contemporary medical practice because of external pressures from payers to reduce practice variation. Uniformity in practice improves clinical quality and reduces cost for patient populations. That is, clinical pathways have been used as a tool by many organizations and physician groups to maintain or improve quality while eliminating unnecessary resource consumption.

Clinical pathways have been well defined as "systematically developed statements to assist practitioner and patient decisions about appropriate health care for specific clinical circumstances" (Hayward et al, 1995). Pathways have also been used as a mechanism for evaluating the current literature carefully to ensure state-of-the-art clinical practice by providers. Although cost pressures were certainly a factor in the initiation of many clinical pathway projects, clinical quality has become a major force for their implementation through a comprehensive re-engineering of clinical processes leading to performance improvement (Cleary et al, 1997; Brook, 1997).

Clinical pathways were first developed and applied to health care in the 1980s, when prospective payment systems focused more interest on potential methods of improving hospital efficiency (Pearson et al, 1995). Clinical pathways generally include the following goals:

1. Select the best practice for an individual process to assist in eliminating unnecessary practice variation.
2. Define the optimal clinical process.
3. Give all hospital staff and providers a common "game plan" from which to view and understand their role in the overall care process.
4. Provide a framework for collecting outcome and process-improvement measures.
5. Decrease documentation burdens for nurses and physicians.
6. Improve education for patients, staff, and providers through continual process improvement and clinical updates (Pearson et al, 1995).

## Health-Care Industry Practice

The process of mapping the care of a patient based on symptoms and diagnosis, which is the heart of clinical pathways, has always been the foundation for the practice of medicine. Currently, the discussion regarding clinical pathways revolves less around the need for establishing pathways and more around the question of how to see that pathways that are already in place are optimally developed, implemented, and used in medical practice.

## DEVELOPMENT OF CLINICAL PATHWAYS

Pathways are generally devised by a multidisciplinary group led by specialty-specific physicians who establish a mechanism for improving clinical efficiency. As research is completed regarding key components of clinical situations, applicable findings must be integrated into clinical pathways through an evidence-based approach. *Evidence-based medicine* is defined as explicit judicious use of the best current evidence in making decisions about the care of individual patients (Sackett et al, 1996). In fact, evidence-based medicine has become widely used for the following reasons:

1. New clinical information is continually generated that may improve the way clinicians care for patients.
2. Physicians often forego up-to-date knowledge, which causes deterioration of clinical performance over time (Ramsey et al, 1991).
3. Traditional continuing medical education programs fail to modify clinical performance and are ineffective in improving the health outcomes of patients (Evans et al, 1986).

It is critical that physicians develop clinical pathways through an evidence-based approach and that they introduce this approach into their clinical practice. Furthermore, members of the pathway team must be highly regarded from a clinical standpoint to reduce barriers against implementing evidence-based medicine into health systems. These clinical leaders must take a comprehensive, methodical approach in adopting evidence-based principles in pathway development (Hayward et al, 1995). Using evidence-based medicine, the pathway team should address a number of considerations, such as the following:

1. Convert clinical information needs into answerable questions.
2. Track down the best evidence to answer the questions.
3. Critically appraise the evidence for its validity and usefulness.
4. Apply the evidence to clinical practice.
5. Evaluate performance.

One evidence-based approach to developing clinical pathways is shown in Figure 72–1.

## IMPLEMENTING CLINICAL PATHWAYS

Successfully implementing clinical pathways into everyday medical practice is as crucial as developing a

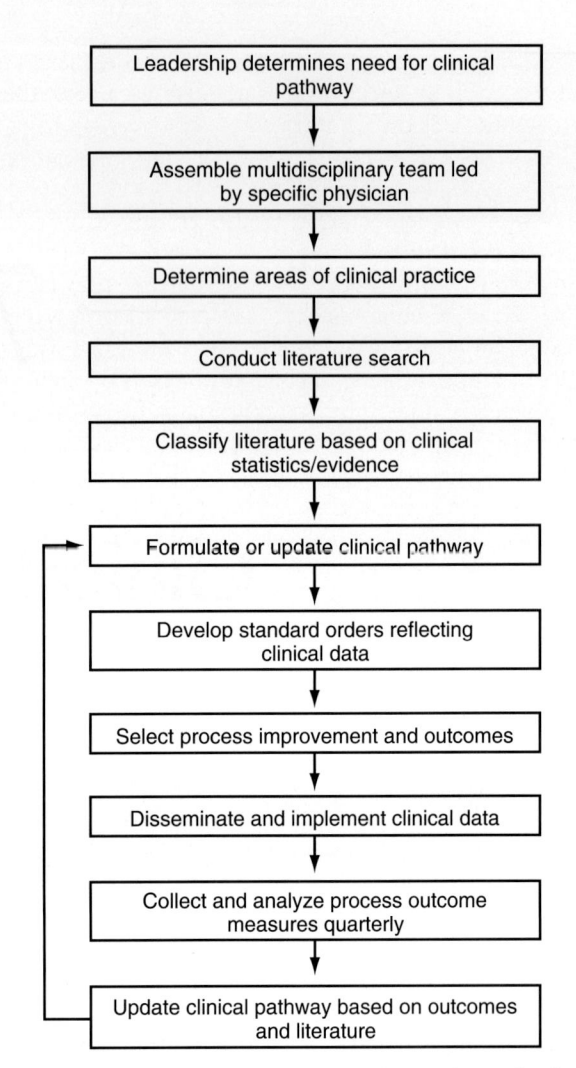

**Figure 72–1** An evidence-based approach to pathway development.

clinically sound pathway. Effective implementation of a high-quality pathway can enhance clinical effectiveness while reducing unnecessary resource consumption. To successfully implement clinical pathways in health-care institutions, several factors must be in place. First, strong support from hospital leaders is necessary to foster the commitment of management and physician leaders to the pathways. Running a pilot program of specific pathways in a subset of patients helps to identify areas of the pathway that need to be changed and builds trust among hospital staff (Aspling et al, 1996).

Additionally, before clinical pathway implementation, it is vital to provide education for all staff who will be involved in patient care associated with the pathway. Care providers who have not been directly involved in the development of the clinical pathway need to understand and accept goals and processes of the pathway. Defining roles and responsibilities of care givers on a day-to-day basis is also a central part of pathway implementation. Physicians and nurses need to know details, such as who will document use of the pathway and who will indicate variances; they also need to know whether case managers will have a clinical role in managing patients' progress on the pathway (Aspling et al, 1996).

Proper implementation is also enhanced by data-driven proof of the pathway's effectiveness. Facilities are implementing pathways at a rapid pace; in fact, a recent survey indicates that four out of five hospitals use pathways for high-volume procedures (Lumsdon, 1996). However, only anecdotal evidence of their effectiveness exists. Only one hospital in five uses computers to track data pertaining to clinical pathways in their institutions (Lumsdon, 1996). This point is crucial not only in overall pathway performance but also in encouraging physician support and buy-in. Physicians must be convinced that clinical pathways provide substantial value or they will not participate in the process. This value must be demonstrated in terms of improved clinical outcomes and decreased costs. Variances, defined as patient outcomes or staff actions that do not meet the expectations of the clinical pathway, must be effectively documented and analyzed to track the success of the pathway. Success also needs to be measured in terms of cost reduction through decreased lengths of stay, decreased demands on service, and increases in patient satisfaction. Data needs to be collected to effect improvement in the patient care process. A clinical pathway is not a single event in time; rather, it is a process that must be continually monitored, with modifications to the process introduced as deemed necessary after thorough data review (Kalbhen, 1995; Lumsdon, 1996) (see Fig. 72-1).

There are two major components necessary for launching a successful pathway: improved clinical quality and reduced resource consumption leading to actual cost savings. As the pathway development team considers the implications of specific diagnostic modalities and treatment options, the incremental cost and clinical outcomes of each strategy must be considered (O'Brien, 1997). Specifically, costs incurred to provide clinical care, such as the physicians' time, nurses' time, and materials, are considered up-front costs. Downstream costs refer to resources to be consumed in the future and are associated with clinical events that are attributable to the therapy. A clinically efficient approach should be considered, with inclusion of specific resources that improve the outcome of the patient. The measurable outcomes must be considered when choosing various diagnostic and therapeutic options for optimal clinical efficiency. Thus, real outcome improvements could be determined through life expectancy gains, improved functional status, reduced morbidity, and improved quality of life. Incremental clinical improvements must be weighed against added resource consumption to develop a reasonable and effective clinical pathway. These cost considerations can be specified through a traditional manufacturing tracking system known as activity-based costing.

## COST ACCOUNTING SYSTEMS

Traditional cost accounting systems, which are used in many health-care institutions, are typically found to be inadequate for providing efficient and accurate data. Such systems assume that the assignment of indirect resource costs (e.g., nursing hours, housekeeping costs, food costs) should be proportional to the volume of products that are produced or the number of services that are provided. Case complexity—the number of activities needed to complete a procedure—and time are not considered factors with traditional accounting. When hospitals were reimbursed under the prospective payment system based on diagnosis-related groups (DRGs), accurate costing of health-care services were not a big concern. Given the increases seen in managed care penetration and capitated payment arrangements in many healthcare markets, accurate costing systems are a necessity. As the cost-plus-reimbursement systems long cherished by health-care institutions are replaced by discounted fee-for-service and set capitated reimbursement programs, physicians must take the lead in determining ways to improve the efficiency of clinical care to remain competitive (Dowless, 1997).

Activity-Based Costing (ABC) is a manufacturing-based costing system that is based on the premise that products and services consume activities, and activities consume resources. According to ABC, controlling the costs of resources is directly correlated with the ability to identify and manage activities and the factors that drive activity costs. Service costs are determined based on factors including the number, duration, and complexity of activities involved in providing a service. Cost drivers, such as the amount of time elapsed from a patient's arrival at an outpatient clinic through time of departure, allow physicians and administrators to better determine the level of resources consumed by each episode of care. Unlike traditional accounting systems, which focus on the supply or availability of the purchased resources that make the provision of services possible, ABC evaluates the costs of resources actually used in the activity of delivering services. The connection between traditional cost accounting and ABC is unused capacity (Cooper, 1992).

The measurement of unused capacity is useful in identifying bottlenecks in service delivery, allowing for the reduction of funds being used on unproductive activities.

## ACTIVITY-BASED COSTING (ABC) APPLIED TO CLINICAL PATHWAYS

ABC is a useful tool for cost and activity tracking in clinical pathway development. ABC allows physicians to unbundle resources and costs of care, allowing greater levels of cost control and better understanding of clinical processes. Whereas traditional costing systems use surrogate indicators to allocate costs among various hospital departments, ABC actually measures the number of activities and resources used among specific hospital departments in the patient care delivery process. For example, nursing hours per patient day are a direct cost of care that managers typically strive to reduce. A traditional cost system measures nursing hours per patient day based on the number of staff in a department and the number of patient days. Conversely, ABC involves actually studying the amount of time nurses spend delivering patient care in a department for a particular diagnosis or treatment. Costs are assigned based on actual activity. This example demonstrates the advantage of using ABC in a traditional costing system: The difference between the supply of nurses (as determined by traditional cost analysis) and actual productive hours worked (determined by ABC analysis) identifies the unused capacity of the nursing staff, allowing management to make better decisions (West, 1997).

ABC is advantageous in planning clinical pathways for two major reasons: It allows for the identification of bottlenecks and unproductive activities *during the planning process*, leading to the planning of a more efficient pathway; and it allows greater levels of precision in tracking the costs of care with the actual *use of the pathway*. The ability to measure the costs associated with a clinical pathway is crucial for budgetary purposes, and, more important, to identify the most efficient care plan for improved clinical quality and reduced resource consumption.

ABC is not without its share of shortfalls. Implementing ABC into an organization is an expensive, time-intensive process. Analyses, such as time studies, have to be performed in each department on a diagnosis-specific basis to reflect accurately the activities and resources needed to provide patient care. A new cost accounting system capable of performing ABC is a costly venture. However, short-term costs of implementing ABC may be balanced by long-term benefits of greater cost control and more efficient management.

## CONFLICT RESOLUTION AND CONSENSUS DEVELOPMENT

Conflicting opinions are bound to ensue during the development of a clinical pathway; after all, one of the major reasons to develop a pathway is to decrease unnecessary practice variation. Physicians have their own practice styles and opinions about the best way to deliver patient care. Managing conflicting opinions is necessary to complete the development of a clinical pathway. The use of an evidence-based approach in developing a clinical pathway, as illustrated in Figure 72–1, is one way to manage such conflict. Developing the clinical pathway on evidence-based, nationally recognized, best-practice standards can remove personal issues from discussions on practice standards. Additionally, guidelines produced locally by end-users may have less credibility if they are based only on personal practice style and not nationally recognized data and information.

A systematic review of literature and research evidence is another evidence-based method of managing conflict. The pathway development team needs to adopt a methodical approach to identifying and synthesizing evidence, as appropriate, and to managing conflict and building consensus. Thus, if development team members have differing opinions on the necessity of performing a urine drug screen before each vaginal delivery, the use of a standard process enables the team to identify evidence relating to urine drug screens, to synthesize the information, and to interpret the evidence to make the most clinically appropriate decision.

## Linking Clinical Pathways to Outcome Measures and Standard Order Sets

The effectiveness of clinical pathways must be proved by data-oriented outcomes for a number of reasons: (1) to gain physician support by proving that use of the pathway actually decreases the costs of care and provides increased quality; (2) to gain institutional buy-in to support the development and implementation of clinical pathways; and (3) to measure clinical and cost outcomes relative to the clinical pathway in order to improve and build on the pathway.

Physician buy-in is crucial to the development of a clinical pathway. As physicians' decisions control 70 to 80% of all health-care dollars spent—and one of the goals of clinical pathways generally includes decreased costs of care, physician support demonstrated through use of the pathway is critical (Pestotnik et al, 1996). In addition, physicians tend to be outcome-oriented; making valid outcome data available is the best way of maintaining physician interest and support of clinical pathways. Forcing physicians to follow rigid care protocols for the purpose of cutting costs through decreased lengths of hospital stays or decreased resource consumption often causes anxiety among physicians. Without valid proof of the positive impact that clinical pathways can have on the costs and quality of care, why should a physician feel compelled to use a pathway? Typically, when physicians balk at the care standards set in clinical pathways, it is because they are not convinced that following a prescribed routine will benefit their patients—they can only see that it affects the bottom line of the hospital or health system.

Thus, not only is it important to involve physicians in the development of clinical pathways, as has been discussed in this article, it is vital that outcome measures be developed and monitored on a regular basis by a multidisciplinary team. Outcome measures can be used to track the success of the pathway and also to identify areas for improvement and change within the pathway. Proponents of clinical pathways argue that standardizing care allows systematic collection of important outcome information that has not previously been available. One reason it is possible to use clinical pathways is the increasingly prevalent organized managed care delivery system that exists today. If fee-for-service plans had continued, there would not be a "laboratory" for collecting data and testing outcomes. Outcome measures based on the clinical pathway provide a forum for analysis and discussion of the success of the clinical pathway and suggestions for change. Using data-driven outcome measures to track the clinical pathway ensures that the pathway remains a living document, one that changes to reflect the highest standards of care possible. A rigid guideline that is not evaluated to reflect changes in best practice standards will not aid a practice that already is outmoded or is becoming that way.

Clinical pathways can assist physicians in keeping up to date with clinical practice and knowledge. Studies indicate that an inverse correlation exists between a physician's clinical examination scores and the number of years that have elapsed since board certification. Additionally, procedure-oriented specialists had lower scores than other physicians in the examination of general medical knowledge (Ramsey, 1991). Physicians often forego up-to-date knowledge, which causes clinical performance deterioration over time. Traditional continuing medical education (CME) fails to modify clinical performance and is ineffective in improving the health outcome of patients. The use of an evidence-based approach (see Fig. 72–1) that incorporates pathway updates with new clinical information ensures that physicians maintain best practice standards.

## TRANSLATING DATA INTO VALID OUTCOME MEASURES

Simple availability of data can be a hurdle for many health-care organizations. Because the goals of clinical pathways are to improve clinical quality and cost efficiency of health care, the monitoring of patient care, or gathering data, is a must. Only two sources of data relative to patient care exist: paper charts and electronic medical record systems. Obtaining data from a paper chart is an expensive, time-consuming, error-prone process. In addition, the paper chart typically obtains information on only one site of care, that is, physicians' office records are not typically available as part of a patient's paper chart at a hospital. Thus, the care continuum is not generally reflected in only one paper chart. Obtaining information from electronic medical record systems is the method of choice for extracting data: It is less labor-intensive, more accurate, and will eventually be the source of most of the data needed to make guidelines operational. Electronic medical record systems are becoming increasingly prevalent in health systems; however, they often contain only a portion of the needed data, such as pharmacy records or laboratory tests (Berg et al, 1997).

Once you have determined your data collection method, meaningful outcome measures need to be developed based on the availability of data and the items that are important to your team of physicians and your institution. To provide continuity, the same team specialists who developed the clinical pathway need to be involved in the development of outcome measures. Outcome measures should generally be developed for clinical quality; patient, staff, and provider satisfaction; and cost indicators. For instance, the clinical pathway development and implementation team for Obstetrics and Gynecology at The Detroit Medical Center developed clinical pathways for normal delivery cesarean sections and hysterectomy (Tables 72–1 to 72–3).

Once outcome measures are identified, degrees of variance can be measured relative to the clinical pathway. By definition, a variance is any positive or negative occurrence that was not predicted on the pathway. *Positive variances* occur when patients progress toward anticipated outcomes or discharge more quickly than anticipated. *Negative variances* contribute to prolonging the length of stay or to interruptions in reaching anticipated clinical outcomes. A *minor variance* is a detour from the critical path; however, it does not delay discharge, significantly increase cost, or threaten a quality outcome. A *major variance* is a detour from the critical path that delays discharge, significantly increases cost, or threatens an outcome. It is important to measure variances within clinical pathways to ensure that the pathway meets its stated goals of improved clinical quality and decreased costs. Chapter 77 of this text addresses the issue of outcome measures in greater detail; however, Table 72–4 shows examples of outcome measures from pathways developed for cesarean section and normal vaginal delivery

*Text continued on page 805*

**Table 72–1** Clinical Pathway: Normal Vaginal Birth

| Expected Length of Stay 24 Hr | Prenatal Care | | Day of Admission |
|---|---|---|---|
| GOALS/OUTCOMES | Prenatal records—complete and available in LD | | Admission criteria complete |
| CLINICAL ASSESSMENT | Initial HPE<br>Pelvic—VS—Ht Wt<br>Completion of records/documents with risk assessment | Schedule FU at 4 wk till 28 wk; then q 2 wk till 36 wk; then q 1 wk till birth. Include BP, urine protein test, FHT, wt and fundal ht q visit | Complete prenatal records HPE/VS; demographic and psychological profile; review existing records; assess fetal viability |
| CONSULTS | As indicated by patient's status, especially social hx:<br>Nutritionist<br>Geneticist<br>Social worker | WIC<br>Lactation services<br>Social services<br>Childbirth education classes<br>MSSP | Social Service education, if problems suspected; notification of health-care provider<br>Care management |
| LABORATORY TESTS | Type and screen<br>Hgb<br>UA and micro<br>HBsAg<br>HIV w/consent<br>RPR<br>Papanicolaou smear<br>Assess GC<br>Assess *Chlamydia* | Rubella<br>Sickle cell, if indicated<br>PPD, if indicated<br>Subsequent visits:<br>15–20 wk: Maternal serum—AFP, hCG + $E_3$<br>24–28 wk: Hgb<br>1-hr PP glucose blood sugar;<br>35–37 wk: Assess Group B *Streptococcus* | *If no previous laboratory values:*<br>Urine drug screen<br>Assess GC<br>Assess *Chlamydia*<br>Assess Group B *Streptococcus* status,<br>Offer HIV testing |
| DIAGNOSTIC TESTS | Ultrasonographic indications are: pregnancy complications, medical complications | Needed for dating w/size discrepancy<br>Poor obstetric hx | As indicated |
| TREATMENTS | | | Labor support/comfort measures |
| MEDICATIONS | Prenatal vitamins, as indicated<br>Folic acid (preconception to 1st trimester) | | IV in LR if clinically indicated and document reason in chart<br>Antibiotics for group B *Streptococcus* if indicated |
| ACTIVITY | Ad lib | | Discretion of provider |
| NUTRITION | Regular | | Clear liquids (if other, specify). |
| EDUCATION | Warning signs/symptoms<br>Discuss pain control options for labor<br>VBAC education<br>Parenting<br>Family planning<br>Infant feeding | Preterm labor precautions<br>OTC medication use<br>Substance abuse<br>Nutrition/diet<br>Domestic violence<br>Hospitalization process, LOS | Patient and family labor education; Orient to room, procedures, plan of care.<br>Discuss pain control options for labor<br>Hospitalization process/LOS<br>Family planning<br>Nursing treatment plan |
| DC PLANNING | Newborn care needs/supplies<br>Community resources | Postpartum care needs<br>Infant car seat | Newborn care needs/supplies<br>Postpartum care needs<br>Infant car seat<br>Transportation needs addressed |
| VARIANCE | Y/N—Records available in LD<br>N/A (<36 wk gestation) | Y/N—Labs complete | Y/N—HIV testing offered |

Table 72-1  Clinical Pathway: Normal Vaginal Birth *Continued*

| | **Labor to Birth** | **Postpartum** |
|---|---|---|
| GOALS/OUTCOMES | Normal uncomplicated vaginal delivery | Discharge healthy mother |
| CLINICAL ASSESSMENT | *Active labor:*<br>   Maternal/fetal q 1/2 hr<br>*Second stage:*<br>   Maternal/fetal status q 15 min<br>   BP q 1 hr | Nursing assessment and<br>   VS q 15 min × 4<br>   VS q 30 min × 2<br>   VS q 8 hr |
| CONSULTS | None | |
| LABORATORY TESTS | None | Baby:<br>Cord blood for Coombs' test<br>Blood type, as indicated<br>Cord gas, as indicated<br>Placenta to Pathology Lab, as indicated |
| DIAGNOSTIC TESTS | None | None |
| TREATMENTS | Comfort measures | Baby to breast immediately with pt consent; RhoGAM/ rubella virus vaccine, if indicated<br>Comfort measures |
| MEDICATIONS | Pain management as indicated | |
| ACTIVITY | Ad lib | Up with assistance × 1 |
| NUTRITION | Maintain hydration | Regular diet |
| EDUCATION | Patient/family education | Patient/family education |
| DC PLANNING | | Circumcision consent<br>Complete labor forms<br>Family planning<br>Arrange for home nurse visits<br>MD consults pt to determine readiness for DC within 24 hr |
| VARIANCE | Y/N—Labs ordered other than listed on pathway—day of admission to birth | Y/N—Home health visit initiated;<br>Y/N—Pt discharged within 24 hr*<br>_____ *Code if No |

*Reasons for Pathway Variances:* 1. Not applicable/appropriate variance. 2. Patient condition. 3. Patient/family available/decision. 4. No physician order/physician decision. 5. Delay in response time. 6. Weekend/holiday. 7. Social Services process pending. 8. No Pediatrics order. 9. Circumcision not done. 10. No transportation available. 11. Predawn birth. 12. Unknown.

ABS = arterial blood sample; AFP = alpha-fetoprotein; BP = blood pressure; DC = discharge; D/C = discontinue; $E_3$ = estriol; FHT = fetal heart tone; FU = follow-up; GC = gonococcus; HBsAg = hepatitis B surface antigen; hCG = human chorionic gonadotropin; Hgb = hemoglobin; HIV = human immunodeficiency virus; HPE = history and physical examination; hx = history; IV = intravenously; KVO = keep vein open; LD = labor and delivery; LOS = length of stay; LR = labor room; MSSP = Maternal Special Support Program; N/A = not applicable; OTC = over the counter; PP = postpartum; PPD = purified protein derivative; pt = patient; RPR = rapid plasma reagin (test); VBAC = vaginal birth after cesarean delivery; VS = vital signs; WIC = women, infants, and children; Y/N = yes or no.

**Table 72–2** Clinical Pathway: Cesarean Section

| Expected Length of Stay 3 D | Prenatal Care | | Day of Admission |
|---|---|---|---|
| GOALS/OUTCOMES | Prenatal records—complete and available in LD | | Admission criteria complete |
| CLINICAL ASSESSMENT | Initial HPE<br>Pelvic—VS—Ht, Wt<br>Completion of records/documents with risk assessment | Schedule FU at 4 wk till 28 wk; then q 2 wk till 36 wk; then q 1 wk till birth. Include BP, urine protein test, FHT, wt, and fundal height q visit | Completion of prenatal records HPE/VS; demographic and psychological profile; review existing records; assess fetal viability |
| CONSULTS | *As indicated by patient's status, especially social hx:*<br>Nutritionist<br>Geneticist<br>Social worker | WIC<br>Lactation services<br>Social Services<br>Childbirth education classes<br>MSSP | Social Service Education, if problems suspected<br>Notification of health-care provider<br>Care management |
| LABORATORY TESTS | Type and screen<br>Hgb<br>UA and micro<br>HBsAg<br>HIV w/consent<br>RPR<br>Papanicolaou smear<br>Assess GC<br>Assess *Chlamydia* | Rubella<br>Sickle cell, if indicated<br>PPD, if indicated<br>Subsequent visits:<br>15–20 wk: Maternal serum—AFP, hCG + $E_3$<br>24–28 wk: Hgb<br>1-hr PP glucose blood sugar;<br>35–37 wk: Assess Group B *Streptococcus* | Type and screen (if indicated)<br>Hgb (if indicated)<br>*If no previous laboratory values:*<br>Urine drug screen<br>Assess GC<br>Assess *Chlamydia*<br>Assess group B *Streptococcus* status<br>Offer HIV testing |
| DIAGNOSTIC TESTS | Ultrasonographic indications are<br>Pregnancy complications<br>Medical complications | Needed for dating w/size discrepancy<br>Poor obstetric hx | As indicated |
| TREATMENTS | | | Labor support/comfort measures |
| MEDICATIONS | Prenatal vitamins, as indicated<br>Folic acid (preconception to 1st trimester) | | IV in LR if clinically indicated and document reason in chart<br>Antibiotics for group B *Streptococcus* if indicated |
| ACTIVITY | Ad lib | | Discretion of provider |
| NUTRITION | Regular | | Clear liquids (if other, specify) |
| EDUCATION | Warning signs/symptoms<br>Discuss pain control options for labor<br>VBAC education<br>Parenting<br>Family planning<br>Infant feeding | Preterm labor precautions<br>OTC medication use<br>Substance abuse<br>Nutrition/diet<br>Domestic violence<br>Hospitalization process, LOS | Patient and family labor education<br>Orient to room, procedures, plan of care<br>Discuss pain control options for labor<br>Hospitalization process/LOS<br>Family planning<br>Nursing treatment plan |
| DC PLANNING | Newborn care needs/supplies<br>Community resources | Postpartum care needs<br>Infant car seat | Newborn care needs/supplies<br>Postpartum care needs<br>Infant car seat<br>Transportation needs addressed |
| VARIANCE | Y/N—Records available in LD<br>N/A (<36 wk gestation) | Y/N—Labs complete | Y/N—HIV testing offered |

**Table 72-2** Clinical Pathway: Cesarean Section *Continued*

| | **After Decision of Cesarean Section** | **Cesarean Delivery Room** | **Recovery Room** | **Delivery Day PP Floor** |
|---|---|---|---|---|
| GOALS/OUTCOMES | Preoperative checklist complete | Uncomplicated cesarean section delivery | Patient hemodynamically stable | Pain managed appropriately |
| CLINICAL ASSESSMENT | | Urine output assessment<br>Per anesthesia protocol | Per nursing standard of care<br>Completion of records per anesthesia protocol | Per nursing protocol |
| CONSULTS | Anesthesia must be present<br>Pediatric staff must be available | Anesthesia present<br>Pediatric staff available | | Lactation Service consultant, as needed |
| LABORATORY TESTS | Hgb<br>Type and Rh factor, if indicated | Baby:<br>Cord blood for Coombs' test<br>Blood type, as indicated<br>Cord gas, as indicated<br>Placenta to Pathology Lab, as indicated<br>Surgical specimens to Pathology Lab | | None |
| DIAGNOSTIC TESTS | | | | |
| TREATMENT | Labor support and comfort measures | | | Input/output assessment<br>D/C Foley within 8 hr, if clear |
| MEDICATION | Obtain IV access, start IV fluids | IV fluids<br>Pitocin, as indicated<br>First-generation cephalosporins<br>—*Single dose as indicated after cord clamped* | IV fluids<br>PCA (or alternative—specify) | RhoGAM/rubella virus vaccine, if indicated<br>PCA (or alternative) |
| ACTIVITY | Bed rest | Bed rest | Bed rest | Up within 8 hr |
| NUTRITION | NPO | NPO | NPO | Regular diet as tolerated |
| EDUCATION | | Encourage cough/deep breaths | Encourage cough/deep breaths<br>Pain management education | |
| DC PLANNING | Preoperative checklist complete<br>Transfer to cesarean delivery room<br>Family planning | | Documentation complete | |
| VARIANCE | | | Y/N—Laboratory tests ordered other than listed on pathway; day of admission to birth | Y/N—Patient ambulated per pathway |

*Table continued on following page*

**Table 72–2** Clinical Pathway: Cesarean Section *Continued*

| | Day 1—Postdelivery—PP Floor | Day 2—Postdelivery—PP Floor | Day 3—Postdelivery—PP Floor |
|---|---|---|---|
| GOALS/OUTCOMES | Initiating self-care | Independent self care | Discharge healthy mother, AM 3rd d |
| CLINICAL ASSESSMENT | Nursing assessment and VS q 8 hr | Nursing assessment every shift, VS q 8 hr | Nursing assessment every shift, VS, q 8 hr |
| CONSULTS | *Baby:* ISS eligibility assessment | | |
| LABORATORY TESTS | | | |
| DIAGNOSTIC TESTS | | | |
| TREATMENT | Support and comfort<br>KVO, if PCA<br>D/C Foley within 8 hr, if clear (May straight cath × 1, if necessary)<br>Cough, deep breath q 1–2 hr., while awake | Support and comfort | Support and comfort |
| MEDICATION | D/C IV, if tolerating fluids and afebrile | D/C parenteral narcotics<br>PO pain medications | PO pain meds |
| ACTIVITY | Ad lib at least 4 × daily | Ad lib at least qid | Ad lib |
| NUTRITION | Regular | Regular | Regular |
| EDUCATION | Initiate DC education | VBAC education<br>Patient/family education | Complete inpatient DC education |
| DC PLANNING | Circumcision consent done<br>Complete labor form<br>Arrange 2 nurse home visits<br>Patient-family advocate | Assess patient for DC for AM 3rd d | Physician consults pt to determine pt readiness for discharge |
| VARIANCE | Y/N—Home health visits initiated | Y/N—Patient independent self-care | Y/N Pt DC 3rd d postoperatively*<br>_____ *Code if No |

*Reasons for Pathway Variances:* 1. Not applicable/appropriate variance. 2. Patient condition. 3. Patient/family available decision. 4. No physician order/physician decision. 5. Delay in response time. 6. Weekend/holiday. 7. Social Services process pending. 8. No Pediatrics order. 9. Circumcision not done. 10. No transportation available. 11. Predawn birth. 12. Unknown.

AFP = alpha-fetoprotein; BP = blood pressure; DC = discharge; D/C = discontinue; $E_3$ = estriol; FHT = fetal heart tone; GC = gonococcus; HBsAg = hepatitis B surface antigen; hCG = human chorionic gonadotropin; Hgb = hemoglobin; HIV = human immunodeficiency virus; HPE = history and physical examination; ISS = ion-scattering spectroscopy; IV = intravenously; KVO = keep vein open; LOS = length of stay; LR = labor room; MSSP = Maternal Special Support Program; N/A = not applicable; NPO = nothing by mouth; PCA = patient-controlled analgesia; PP = postpartum; PPD = purified protein derivative; RPR = rapid plasma reagin (test); UA = urine analysis; VBAC = vaginal birth after cesarean section; VS = vital signs; Y/N = yes or no.

**Table 72-3** Detroit Medical Center: Hysterectomy Clinical Pathway

| | Output Preprocedure | D Surgery | D Surgery: Floor | Postoperative D #1 | Postoperative D #2 | Postoperative D #3 (for TAH) |
|---|---|---|---|---|---|---|
| Assessment/evaluation | H&P, laboratory tests, and informed consent form (including surgical indication) from PAT Office: Informed consent form (if not done) Nursing and Anesthesia assessment Vital signs H&P if not done before If abnormal bleeding: Endometrial sample on chart Papanicolaou smear results reviewed Notify Anesthesia and surgeon if Hgb <9.0 Precertification validation | Vital signs Informed consent form verified Laboratory tests/results reviewed by Anesthesia | VS and I/Os q 4 hr Nursing evaluation, dressing and pain assessment per protocol | VS q 4 hr discontinued When PCA D/C, then VS q 8 hr Nursing evaluation q 8 hr | When PCA D/C, VS q 8 hr Nursing evaluation q 8 hr | VS and nursing evaluation q 8 hr |
| Laboratory | Before PAT or in PAT Hgb | Pregnancy test if <50 y/o | None | Hgb | None | None |
| Treatment/medications | None | Preop medications: 1L LR @ KVO Cephazolin, 1 g IVPB (or Flagyl, 500 mg if allergic) SCD or heparin for DVT prophylaxis as appropriate | Incentive spirometry q 2 hr IV: LR @ KVO when tolerating fluids PCA or epidural per protocol Continue DVT prophylaxis as appropriate Antiemetic | Remove dressing Discontinue PCA or epidural when pain controlled Antiemetic prn Darvocet-N 100, 1–2 PO q 4 prn or Tylenol #3 1–2 PO q 4 hr prn Motrin 600 mg q 4 hr prn or Tylenol 325, 1–2 q 4 hr prn D/C IV when afebrile, stable, and tolerating fluids DVT prophylaxis until ambulating well | Continue PO pain medication Antiemetic as presented in postoperative D #1 | Continue PO pain medication Antiemetic as presented in postoperative D #1 |

*Table continued on following page*

**Table 72–3** Detroit Medical Center: Hysterectomy Clinical Pathway *Continued*

| | Output Preprocedure | D Surgery | D Surgery: Floor | Postoperative D #1 | Postoperative D #2 | Postoperative D #3 (for TAH) |
|---|---|---|---|---|---|---|
| Diet | Advise NPO after midnight d surgery Ad lib | NPO | Diet as tolerated | Regular diet as tolerated | Regular diet as tolerated | Regular diet as tolerated |
| Activity | Ad lib | Ad lib | Ambulates with assistance within 6 hr, then at least qid | Ambulatory at least qid | Ambulate at least qid | Ambulate ad lib |
| DC Planning | In PAT: Comprehensive presurgery handout: Events and timing of hosp. Shared with patient Discuss DC Discuss transportation DC Discuss home help after DC | | | Care Management Specialist facilitates DC planning and assistance Physician determines readiness for DC (vaginal hysterectomy) Home instructions Comprehensive educational handout reviewed | Care Management Specialist facilitates discharge planning and assistance Physician determines readiness for discharge (abdominal hyst) Home instructions Comprehensive educational handout reviewed | Care management specialist facilitates DC planning and assistance Physician determines readiness for discharge Home instructions Comprehensive educational handout reviewed |
| Variance | Y/N H&P received in PAT from office | Y/N Preoperative antibiotic given | Y/N DVT prophylaxis initiated | Y/N LOS for vaginal hysterectomy >1 d | Y/N LOS for abdominal hysterectomy >2 d | |

Other hysterectomy outcome measures: 1. Length of stay, 2. blood transfusion, 3. return to operating room, 4. death, 5. pulmonary complications, 6. major abdominal organ injury (bowel, bladder, ureter).
DC = discharge; D/C = discontinued(d); DVT = deep venous thrombosis; hgb = hemoglobin; H&P = history & outpatient examination; H&P = history and physical examination; I/O = input and output; KVO = keep vein open; LR = lactated Ringer's solution; NPO = nothing by mouth; PAT = platelet aggregaton test; PCA = patient-controlled anesthesia; SCD = sequential complication device; VS = vital signs; Y/N = yes or no.

Table 72–4  Examples of Outcome Measures

**Outcome Measures for Normal Vaginal Delivery**

- Readmission within 28 d
- Blood transfusion
- Indications for LOS longer than 24 hr
- Prenatal records not available in LD
- Home health visit not initiated
- Laboratory tests incomplete (based on clinical pathway)
- VBAC attempt rate
- Third- and fourth-degree laceration rates
- Emergency department visit within 72 hr of DC
- 5 min Apgar score <7
- LOS
- Laboratory tests ordered not on clinical pathway
- PP infection rate
- Epidural rate
- VBAC success rate
- Operative vaginal delivery rate (vacuum or forceps)
- HIV status not offered

**Outcome Measures for Cesarean Section**

- Readmission within 28 d
- Blood transfusion
- Indications for LOS >3 d
- Prenatal records not available in LD
- Home health visit not initiated
- 5 min Apgar score <7
- LOS
- Laboratory tests ordered not on clinical pathway
- Laboratory tests ordered not on clinical pathway

**Outcome Measures for Cesarean Section**

- Laboratory tests incomplete (based on clinical pathway)
- Injury to intra-abdominal organs during surgery
- Patient not ambulatory per clinical pathway
- Patient not independent in self-care by second postoperative d
- Anesthesia complication rate
- PP infection rate
- Cesarean section rate
- PP infection rate
- Primary cesarean section rate
- Repeat cesarean section rate
- HIV status not offered
- Emergency department visit within 72 hr of DC

DC = discharge; HIV = human immunodeficiency virus; LD = labor and delivery or labor and delivery room; LOS = length of stay; PP = postpartum; VBAC = vaginal birth after cesarean delivery.

and used at The Detroit Medical Center, and Health Plan Data and Information set (HEDIS) outcome measures for women's services.

## STANDARD ORDER SETS

When the clinical pathway is used as the patient's medical chart, standard order sets for laboratory tests and pharmaceuticals can be developed, effectively decreasing the burden of charting for care providers. A standard order set is an order sheet for a particular procedure, such as a vaginal delivery, that incorporates the process of the clinical pathway into an order format. The orders are directly tied to the clinical pathway for that procedure; that is, only laboratory tests and medications on the clinical pathway appear on the standard order set. A "chart by exception" rule can be developed for procedures with a clinical pathway in place, saving both time and money. Standard order sets encourage the use of pathways by physicians because they can make care delivery an easier, more efficient process. A physician generally does not carry a copy of a clinical pathway around for use as a checklist when delivering patient care; therefore, standard order sets serve to make the pathway become invisible to the physician. That is, standard order sets ensure compliance with the pathway by allowing the physician to use the standard order instead of writing orders for patients. Table 72–5 gives an example of a standard order set for use with a clinical pathway for normal vaginal delivery and Table 72–6 provides the same example for cesarean delivery. Both these standard order sets were developed at The Detroit Medical Center.

## Evaluating the Success of Clinical Pathways

The team who develops the clinical pathway and outcome measures needs to define the success of the clinical pathway. Success is an institution-specific indicator and should be based on the goals of the clinical pathway. For instance, let us say a multidisciplinary team led by physicians has developed a clinical pathway for a normal vaginal delivery with the overall goal of decreasing inpatient hospital length of stay while maintaining or improving quality. This team would deem decreases in the following areas as markers of success: length of stay; complication, readmission, and postpartum infection rates; and emergency department visits within 72 hours of discharge. Indi-

Table 72–5  Postpartum Orders for Vaginal Delivery

DC from recovery room when stable
Condition: _____
Allergy: _____
Ice pack to perineum prn
Up ad lib when stable
Regular diet as tolerated
NPO after midnight for PPTL
VS q 15 min × 4 hr, q 30 min × 2, then q 8 hr
May straight catheterize × 1 prn
Ibuprofen, 600–800 mg, PO q 6 hr prn
Tylenol, 500 mg, 1–2 PO q 3 hr prn
Rhogam IM, if eligible
Rubella vaccination, if eligible
Consent for circumcision, if desired
Consent for PPTL, if desired
Physician consults with pt to determine readiness for DC within 24 hr

DC = discharge; IM = intramuscularly; NPO = nothing by mouth; PO = by mouth; PPTL = postpartum tubal ligation; pt = patient; VS = vital signs.

**Table 72–6** Postpartum Orders for Cesarean Section

DC from recovery room when stable
Diagnosis: s/p cesarean section for _____
Condition: _____
Allergy: _____
Activity: up within 8 hr, then ad lib at least 4 × daily
VS q 15 min × 4, q 30 min × 2, then q 8 hr
Regular diet as tolerated
D/C Foley within 8 hr if urine clear. May straight cath × 1, if necessary
Cough and deep breathe q 1–2 hrs, while awake
IV: LR at 125 cc/hr
PCA for pain control ( ) Morphine sulfate ( ) Demerol
Ibuprofen, 600–800 mg PO q 4–6 hr prn
Tylenol, 500 mg, 1 or 2, PO q 3 hr prn
Tylenol #3 1 or 2 PO q 3–4 hr prn
Darvocet-N 100, 1 or 2 PO q 4–6 hr prn
D/C IV when pt tolerating fluids and afebrile and pain controlled adequately
Rhogam IM, if eligible
Rubella vaccination, if eligible
Consent for circumcision, if desired
Physician consults with pt to determine readiness for DC on third postoperative d

DC = discharge; D/C = discontinue; IM = intramuscularly; IV = intravenously; LR = lactated Ringer's solution; PCA = patient-controlled anesthesia; pt = patient; S/P = status post; VS = vital signs.

cators demonstrating the success of a clinical pathway can be determined by use of outcome measures. The outcome measures for a clinical pathway need to be defined by the clinical pathway development team; general guidelines for outcome measures include the following:

- Measurement of clinical quality
- Measurement of patient, staff, and provider satisfaction
- Measurement of cost

## Future Directions of Clinical Pathways

We have discussed the overall goals of clinical pathways, which include enhancing medical knowledge, decreasing variation in care, defining proper use of technology, eliminating inappropriate care, and controlling rising health-care costs. Evidence-based clinical pathways that are well written are complex documents that frequently require numerous pages, including algorithms and other supporting documentation. The format and organization of a clinical pathway can predict whether it will be accepted (Fig. 72–2). Busy physicians need clinical pathways to be at least time-neutral and able to be executed at the point of care; this goal is difficult to accomplish with multipage paper guidelines.

Many health-care providers believe that clinical pathways will be greatly enhanced in the future with the aid of information systems, ideally with an on-line clinical pathway embedded in decision support software. The availability of on-line clinical pathways will facilitate the capture of data for outcome measures. The on-line clinical pathway will become part of an electronic medical record, in which decision points will appear instantly when the patient's diagnosis is selected.

There are various benefits with integrating clinical guidelines on an medical record system, including:

- Providing awareness of clinical pathways by reminding physicians at the time of selecting a patient diagnosis and by making pathways available to providers at the point of care
- Facilitating accurate data collection for outcome and process improvement measures
- Enabling easy, quick updates to clinical pathways to accommodate changes in best practice standards
- Providing feedback on demand to health-care providers and administrators.

The on-line clinical pathway is the desirable next step in the evolution of clinical pathways; however, several barriers and challenges exist, making the development of such technology difficult. These barriers include lack of the following: a master patient index, appropriate interfaces, structured data entry, standardized nomenclature, and rule-based alerts and reminders.

**Master Patient Index.** Currently, a single database containing all information relative to a patient's care does not exist. It is necessary to pull data from a variety of sources, including medical records, billing, laboratory, imaging, and other hospital databases. In addition, many information systems are not compatible; therefore, integrating data among systems is often impossible.

**User Interface.** In order to make an on-line clinical pathway available, appropriate physician-computer interfaces need to be developed, which will include:

- Graphic display. Incorporating large amounts of data per screen in an easy-to-read format will decrease the need to move between screens.
- Instant response time. As physicians will be using computers to make clinical decisions and each patient encounter may last as little as 10 minutes, response time from information systems needs to process as quickly as the physician thinks.
- Portability. Wireless, hand-held devices with instant response times are the ultimate design in terms of portability. The computer needs to be able to go where the physician goes.

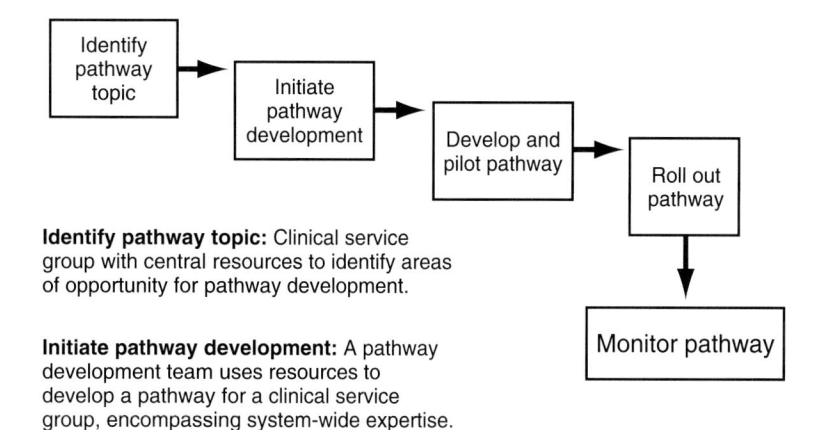

**Figure 72–2** Pathway process overview.

**Identify pathway topic:** Clinical service group with central resources to identify areas of opportunity for pathway development.

**Initiate pathway development:** A pathway development team uses resources to develop a pathway for a clinical service group, encompassing system-wide expertise.

- Intuitive navigation. The system must be able to move among various areas of the patient chart quickly and easily.

**Structured Data Entry.** To report outcome measures effectively via the on-line clinical pathway, as many observations as possible must be captured as separate data elements so they may be reported and evaluated. Thus, free text entry on the keyboard must be discouraged. Physicians are not accustomed to charting by means of structured data entry. This method limits the physician's level of choice and discretion regarding what to capture on the patient's record. However, if the physician performs this function correctly, structured data entry makes information for outcome measures available without the physician's having to do much additional manipulation of data.

**Standardized Nomenclature.** Along with the need for structured data comes the need for standard nomenclature, or standard medical terms, including the relationships between medical terms and coding systems, such as billing or diagnostic codes. To effectively capture data, physicians need to use common definitions of terms for tracking patient care.

**Rule-Based Alerts and Reminders.** A rule-based system can give patient-specific reminders based on information already entered by the care provider. This is quite difficult to achieve, because there is currently no standard way of translating clinical recommendations into such reminders.

It is possible to begin working around some of these barriers and challenges. Health-care institutions need to begin by building databases that have information already gathered. The implementation of electronic medical record systems is a starting point for extracting data. It is important for internal staff, providers, and physicians to have a role in building a clinical decision support system, so that the system will work for clinicians and others who have to use it. Many health-care providers look forward to using clinical decision software and electronic medical record systems to improve the use of clinical pathways.

# REFERENCES

Aspling DL, Lagoe RJ: Benchmarking for clinical pathways in hospitals: A summary of sources. Nurs Econ 14:92, 1996.

Aspling DL, Lagoe RJ: Development and implementation of a program to reduce hospital stays and manage resources on a community-wide basis. Nurs Admin Q 20:1, 1995.

Berg M, and others. Clinical practice guidelines in practice and education. J Gen Intern Med 12(suppl):525, 1997.

Berg AO, Atkins D, Tierney W: Problems and promises of the protocol. Soc Sci Med 44:1081, 1997.

Boslar B, De Camillo P, Ransom SB: Preparation for the longitudinal electronic medical record: The experience of one medical center (Submitted).

Brennan TA, Sox CM, Burstin HR: Relation between negligent adverse events and the outcomes of medical-malpractice litigation. N Engl J Med 335:1963, 1996.

Brook RH: Managed care is not the problem, quality is. JAMA 278:1612, 1997.

Cleary PD, Edgman-Levitan S: Health care quality. Incorporating consumer perspectives. JAMA 278:608, 1997.

Cooper R, Kaplan R: Activity-based systems: Measuring the costs of resource usage. Accounting Horizons 6:1, 1992.

Dowless R: Using activity-based costing to guide strategic decision making. Healthcare Finan Manage 51:86, 1997.

Downing S, Ransom SB: Development and implementation of clinical pathways with activity based costing. Phys Exec (in press).

Evans CE, Haynes RB, Ribkett NJ, et al: Does a mailed continuing education program improve physician performance? Results of a randomized trial in antihypertensive care. JAMA 255:501, 1986.

Hayward RS, Wilson MC, Tunis SR, et al: Users' guides to the medical literature. VIII. How to use clinical practice guidelines. A. Are the recommendations valid? The Evidence-Based Medicine Working Group. JAMA 274:570, 1995.

Hyams AL, Shapiro DW, Brennan TA: Medical practice guidelines in malpractice litigation. An early retrospective. J Health Polit Policy Law 21:289, 1996.

Kalbhen J: Protocols—going down the clinical path. Hosp Health Netw 69:86, 1995.

Loegering L, Reiter RC, Gambone JC: Measuring the quality of health care. Clin Obstet Gynecol 37:122, 1994.

Lumsdon K: Clinical paths. Mapping care. Hosp Health Netw 70:86, 1996.

O'Brien BJ: Users' Guides to the Medical Literature: How to Use an Article of Economic Analysis of Clinical Practice. JAMA 277:1802, 1997.

Pearson SD, Goulart-Fisher D, Lee TH: Clinical pathways as a strategy for improving care: Problems and potential. Ann Intern Med 123:941, 1995.

Pestotnik S, Classen DC, Evans RS, et al: Implementing antibiotic practice guidelines through computer-assisted decision support: Clinical and financial outcomes. Ann Intern Med 124:884, 1996.

Ramsey PG, Carline JD, Inui TS, et al: Changes over time in the knowledge base of practicing internists. JAMA 266:1103, 1991.

Ransom SB: A clinical pathway for OB/GYNs, by OB/GYNs. OBG Management 10:42, 1998.

Ransom SB: Gynecologists make hysterectomy (DRG 359) clinical pathways work. J Pelvic Surg 4:109, 1998.

Ransom SB, McNeeley SG, Yono A, et al: The development and implementation of normal vaginal delivery clinical pathways in a large multihospital health system. Am J Manag Care 4:723, 1998.

Sackett DL, Rosenberg WM, Gray JA, et al: Evidence based medicine: What it is and what it isn't. BMJ 312:71, 1996.

West T, West D: Applying ABC to healthcare. Manage Accounting 78:28, 1997.

# 73

# Insurance Contracting for Obstetric/ Gynecologic Services

VICTORIA A. GREGONIS

Women's health care represents a significant portion of the health-care premium dollars currently spent in the United States. The managed-care industry continues to experience and foster rapid changes for patients, providers, and payers of women's health-care services. These factors provide many opportunities for Obstetricians/gynecologists (OB/GYNs) to influence the delivery and payment of women's health-care services and place them in a unique position to retain and expand their presence in this dynamic market through contracts aligning clinical and financial incentives between OB/GYNs, patients, and payers.

This chapter focuses on the issues affecting the negotiation and administration of managed-care contracts for OB/GYN services. Some of the legal aspects of contracting for OB/GYN services are discussed, however readers are encouraged to obtain legal and financial review of individual contracts based on the circumstances of each negotiation. A brief description of important contract terms, including reimbursement and suggested negotiation options are presented. Where pertinent, the similarities between risk and nonrisk contracts are compared. Throughout this chapter, it is assumed that the reader is acquainted with managed-care terminology.

Understanding the managed-care market in general is essential to obtaining and managing a successful contract. Furthermore, OB/GYNs must understand how managed-care trends in a given community affect an individual OB/GYN practice. This is true whether the OB/GYN is contracting independently or is represented by a group (professional association or limited liability partnership), an independent practice association (IPA), a physician hospital organization (PHO), or other entity. This chapter focuses on the following issues and their relevance to contracting for OB/GYN services:

- Managed-care environment
- Factors influencing contract negotiations: increasing negotiating leverage, benefit design, patient demand/satisfaction
- Contract language: term and termination, network panel
- Reimbursement: rate schedules, bundling/unbundling services, inclusions/exclusions, new technologies

- Administering contracts for Ob/Gyn services: benefits, utilization and quality management, claims, impact on practice overhead

## The Environmental Impact of Managed Care in Your Community

Managed care is the dominant method of health plan administration in the United States, although penetration varies significantly in specific markets. The OB/GYN's access to managed-care patients is controlled through the payer contract. An essential first step in considering a new or renewal contract is knowing the number of lives covered by each payer by product (Preferred Provider Organization [PPO], point of service [POS], Health Maintenance Organization [HMO]) and the corresponding information for the OB/GYN practice. It also is helpful to have additional demographic information regarding the potential population: birth rate per 1000, age/sex distribution, and employer/industry profiles of the payer's clients. This information helps the OB/GYN evaluate whether the proposed contract will retain current patients or attract new business. It is also useful in evaluating the compatibility of the type of patients the practice currently has or seeks.

To meet consumer demands, payers are continuously modifying their products (PPO, POS, HMO). Payers manifest this flexibility with "all or nothing" product strategies, requiring providers to sign contracts covering multiple products. These market-driven responses continue to change both patient access to OB/GYNs and the physician's referrals to subspecialists, access to ancillaries, reimbursement, and utilization management.

As the managed-care industry matures, insurance companies and nonphysician providers are consolidating to gain strength. In response, physicians are merging into larger groups or are creating IPAs, PHOs, and other alliances to strengthen their position. Getting bigger improves the OB/GYN's negotiating clout, but OB/GYNs must carefully determine not only how and who to align with, but also who will represent them at the negotiating table.

Traditional roles once clearly defined between provider and payer are becoming blurred—for example, IPA's contract with payers and employers on behalf of individual physicians to conduct utilization review and pay claims. In many communities, provider groups hold direct contracts with employers, assuming benefits and claims administration and essentially functioning as an insurer or third-party administrator (TPA). The network administration process for each contract, especially the portions pertaining to women's health, directly impacts the clinical and financial aspect of the OB/GYN practice and may change both referral patterns and revenue sources.

Likewise, traditional roles between medical generalists, specialists, and subspecialists are changing because of managed care and changes within the medical community itself. Most notably for OB/GYNs, family practice physicians are providing obstetrics and gynecology services including colposcopy and minor gynecology procedures. These evolving roles have a significant clinical and financial impact on OB/GYNs. Thus, it is critical to both the individual OB/GYN and his or her community that OB/GYNs have a strong voice in negotiating which specialties will provide OB/GYN care and how patients access OB/GYNs.

Competition between payers keeps premiums constant or declining. As a result, payers are under increasing pressure to meet profit goals by reducing reimbursement to physicians. In response, physicians are seeking access to payer profits through risk sharing such as capitation and percent of premium. To increase their leverage, physicians are forming larger and more centrally organized groups for the purpose of assuming responsibility for utilization/quality management and data collection and reporting.

Managed care continues to educate purchasers and consumers on both the cost and the quality of health care. This education has resulted in attempts to standardize care, stabilize costs, and ensure consistently high-quality outcomes as evidenced by the presence of organizations such as the National Committee on Quality Assurance (NCQA). Generally, payers' systems do not easily coordinate clinical and financial data nor do they capture clinical and financial data for an episode of care (e.g., obstetrics). Reliable clinical and financial data on women's health significantly increases the OB/GYN's contracting leverage. Using data to demonstrate clinical and financial outcomes and change physician behavior generally results in better reimbursement and in maximizing distribution of risk pools and incentive funds.

## Benefit Design

Benefit plans have a very significant impact on contracting for OB/GYN services because they define covered and noncovered services, well woman care, the patient's financial responsibility, and the incentives to use network physicians and services. Confirming reliable benefits and eligibility *before patient appointments and communicating this information at the time of service* is essential to obtaining maximum reimbursement and maintaining low practice expense overhead.

Direct access to OB/GYNs may be determined by benefit plan, by regulation, or by the payer. It is always preferable to have direct access, but when plan and product limit access through a primary care physician (PCP) or other gatekeeper, both patient access and the roles of each physician specialty must be stated clearly in the contract.

## WELL WOMAN CARE

During contract negotiations, OB/GYNs should get a clear understanding of the well woman benefit and reimbursement for physician and associated ancillary services. Where possible, OB/GYNs should work closely with payers to define physician, laboratory, and imaging services related to well woman care. Preferably, the ancillary services included in well woman care should be age specific. Financial incentives to use well woman benefits should be consistent with network administrative requirements. Also, there should be clear guidelines for both the patient and physician when a gynecologic problem has been discovered during the well woman examination.

## PATIENT OUT-OF-POCKET COSTS

Benefit plans also help determine how the physician is reimbursed by defining the percent of coverage or a payment that is the patient's responsibility. The structure of patient out-of-pocket payments, including copayments, coinsurances, and deductibles, directly influences utilization—for example, low copayments encourage office visits, and high coinsurance discourages emergency room visits. These out-of-pocket expenses also encourage patients to use network physicians by having lower out-of-pocket costs for staying in the network or for complying with certain administrative requirements. Network incentives should be significant enough (at least 10–20%) to direct patients to use network OB/GYNs.

## COPAYMENTS, COINSURANCES, DEDUCTIBLES

These and other out-of-pocket patient costs should be collected at the time of service. However, many plans allow coinsurances and deductibles to be collected only after the physician's claim has been paid, thus exposing the practice to additional collections costs. Obtain clarification on how these expenses apply to obstetric care—often copayments apply only to the pregnancy confirmation visit whereas deductibles and coinsurances are applied to ancillary services. These expenses are deducted from payments because the physician is expected to collect them directly from the patient. Contract language should state that out-of-pocket costs and charges for noncovered services can be collected at the time of service.

## INFERTILITY BENEFITS

Traditionally, these services were not covered, and patients paid the physician's fees. In the current market, infertility treatment is often a benefit, but there is wide discrepancy between patient expectation, interpretation of the benefit, and reimbursement for services. Usually the diagnosis and treatment of infertility is covered, and assisted reproduction is not covered. In some cases, the best contracting strategy is to *exclude* infertility treatment. However, if infertility services are included, OB/GYNs are well advised to stipulate specific ICD and CPT codes and reimbursement related to both covered and noncovered infertility services.

# Contracting Leverage and Impact on the Individual Physician

In a typical OB/GYN practice, contracts with managed-care companies typically include all the following contractual arrangements, and an individual physician's leverage varies significantly within each of these.
- Individual contract
- Group contract
- IPA contract
- PHO contract

The individual OB/GYN's negotiating position is strengthened by patient demand, affiliation with a large or well-respected group, clinical expertise, good practice management, and data to demonstrate solid clinical and financial outcomes. Of all these elements, patient demand and physician performance data are the most valuable. Payers carefully monitor patient satisfaction, especially access to OB/GYNs, because of the strong relationships that develop between patient and physician. Payer marketing directly influences physician panel membership; and payers are reluctant to make changes in the OB/GYN panel that could result in unhappy clients and lost business. Patient demand often determines whether an OB/GYN is added to a panel. This provides an interesting dilemma for OB/GYNs and payers because patient determination of quality does not always reflect quality clinical care. OB/GYNs are in the strongest negotiating position when they have data demonstrating consistently good customer service and consistently good clinical outcomes with lower costs.

To maximize access to their services and their reimbursement, OB/GYNs should be involved actively in the negotiation process for multispecialty contracts with large groups and IPA/PHO contracts. This representation is critical in gatekeeper contracts and communities in which family practice physicians provide OB/GYN services. Otherwise, OB/GYNs may find themselves providing very limited services with potentially high risk and low reimbursement (e.g., late-transfer, high-risk obstetric patients with a reduced case rate).

## Contract Language

Good preparation, careful analysis of contract language, financial analysis, open communication, and flexibility generally result in securing favorable contract terms or in confirming a decision to decline a managed-care contract. The most important contract terms are those pertaining to reimbursement, contract administration (benefits, utilization review, quality assurance, claims), network panel (participating physicians, hospitals, ancillaries), and term/termination.

Although reimbursement often is foremost in both parties' minds, contract language is equally important because it determines how the physician and payer will coordinate efforts and resolve disputes. Contract language directly impacts practice overhead by defining physician administration (network referrals) and practice administration (benefits, utilization review, claims) responsibility.

As the managed-care industry matures, contracts are becoming more complex and inclusive, and it is often easy to overlook a critical point or miss a contradiction between sections. Simultaneously, regulation of the managed-care industry continues to significantly impact both contract language and administration. Using resources within state medical societies and other professional associations may be invaluable in helping assess proposed language and negotiating terms favorable to physicians in light of the changing environment. Keeping meticulous records before and during negotiations helps both parties focus on key points and reach a mutually beneficial agreement.

## Reimbursement

Regardless of the type of reimbursement (fee-for-service or prepaid/capitation), the methodology used to establish payment, and proposed fees compared with practice experience/budget, determine whether a proposal is acceptable. Good contracts include the following language specific to reimbursement, preferably in the reimbursement exhibit and in the body of the contract.

- Change only on written mutual consent
- Methodology, for example, percent resource-based relative value scale (%RBRVS), adjusted for geographic area and by type of service
- Specified International Classification of Diseases (ICD) and Current Procedural Terminology (CPT) codes attached to specific reimbursement, including case rate inclusions/exclusions—practice list in place of payer sample
- Claims filed and paid consistent with ICD and CPT coding guidelines
- Reimbursement for multiple procedures and the bundling and unbundling formulas applied
- Exclusions identified by both ICD and CPT codes
- Reimbursement for new technologies or services without a specific CPT code—usually a percentage of billed charges
- Payment of clean claims or notice of coordination of benefits within specified time period consistent with state, federal regulation

Until recently, managed-care companies used rate schedules developed from their own experience or the insurance industry experience for paid claims. This method is being replaced by relative value units (RVUs) because RVUs are related directly to the intensity of service. RBRVS developed by the Health Care Financing Administration (HCFA) is the most commonly used RVU schedule. Evaluating an RVU-based schedule for OB/GYN services requires a separate analysis of gynecology, obstetric, and office visit codes/services because the RVUs vary significantly between each type of service; applying an overall percentage (e.g., 130% RBRVS) may overvalue obstetrics and office visits and may undervalue gynecologic surgery. Knowing the service mix—percent of obstetrics, gynecology, and office services—helps assess the impact of a proposed reimbursement. Notably, OB/GYN surgical services are undervalued in most RVU schedules because the original populations were gender-biased toward male surgeries and because laparoscopic technology advanced at a faster pace than coding technology. There are continuing efforts to eliminate these discrepancies and improve the base values, but they are occurring at a time of declining reimbursement.

Comparing proposed reimbursement to practice fees, actual reimbursement from existing contracts, and the resulting impact on practice service mix provides the information to evaluate the acceptability of a fee schedule. This analysis should include specific

CPT codes for a minimum 80% of the practice business representing the various services provided (e.g., obstetrics, gynecology, surgery, office visits, and well woman care). During this process, specific CPT codes associated with episodes of care (e.g. obstetrics) should be identified. Case rates used to pay for an episode of care often vaguely referred to as included/excluded services, giving the payer too much flexibility to change reimbursement and leaving the practice without a way to evaluate complete or correct payment of a claim.

Bundling and unbundling of associated surgical procedures is a technique used by payers to reduce surgical reimbursement. The payer's formula should be applied during reimbursement analysis and attached to the contract rate schedule when accepted. The best contracts attach the most frequently billed services with a negotiated reimbursement for each code; however, payers' claim systems may not be able to manage this detail, leaving the formula as the only available option. At the very least, the formula enables the practice to determine whether the claim was paid correctly.

Prepaid or capitated or risk contracts encourage physicians to assume more responsibility for utilization management and benefit from the financial success of self-management. These contracts often have incentive or bonus pools in addition to the capitation payment to encourage physicians to meet quality and utilization targets—for example, reduced inpatient surgery or increased mammograms in a defined population. OB/GYNs participating in risk contracts may be paid a capitation rate or fee for service, or both (usually capitation for gynecology, case rate for obstetrics). In some markets, OB/GYNs have formed specialty carve-out networks directly contracting with a payer. Risk contracts always involve a large, organized group of physicians. Risk contract negotiations usually are conducted by a team of administrators and physicians. The team relies on demographic, utilization, and claims data analyzed by an actuary to project anticipated costs and savings. Capitation contracts must specifically define included and excluded services pertinent to the capitation, the mechanism for establishing reserves for incurred but not reported (IBNR) claims, and the proposed distribution of withholds and associated incentive or bonus funds. Both risk and nonrisk contracts warrant close attention to the details of contract administration as addressed in both the contract language and in the supporting policies and procedures.

## Contract Administration

Contract administration is a general term covering benefits administration, utilization compliance, and claims processing. Compliance with the contract ensures maximum use of patient benefits and maximum physician reimbursement. The administrative manual helps the physician and office staff comply with the contract terms. Contract language should specify at least 30-day notice of change in administrative procedures to give physicians and their staff sufficient time to evaluate the change and prepare for it.

Comparing the administrative manual with the contract not only determines the consistency between the two documents but also gives insight into how the contract is implemented on a day-to-day basis. The administrative manual usually has two components: a directory of participating providers (physicians, hospitals, ancillaries with addresses and phone numbers) and a procedure manual with specific information on the utilization review process (phone numbers, referrals to subspecialists, required precertification and authorizations), billing/claims, appeal procedures (utilization review, claims), and other key information.

The administration manual should contain the following information specific to OB/GYNs:
- Copayments for well woman care and obstetric visits
- Inclusions and exclusions in well woman care
- Office-based ancillary services (laboratory, ultrasound)—billing/reimbursement
- Referrals to specialist and subspecialists during obstetric care
- Procedures requiring authorization/precertification (specific to location)
- Itemized list of services with CPT codes (number and type) included in case rates; billing for excluded services
- Formulary and/or instructions for supplying injectibles and medications in the office

Pay particular attention to the utilization requirements from both the clinical and administrative perspectives. These policies, procedures, and programs should be consistent with the individual physician's standard of practice and currently accepted community or professional standards, as supported by medical literature and pertinent research. Physician-to-physician communication regarding medical management options should be specialty specific (OB/GYN to OB/GYN) and "user friendly" to the practicing physician. Excessive administrative requirements impact the quantity and quality of patient care, practice overhead, and patient satisfaction. Conversely, both the contract and the administrative manual contain language holding the physician responsible for compliance with utilization and quality management procedures with the caveat of financial penalties for continued deviation from the payer's requirements. The contract should contain language preventing retroactive denial of payment if a physician met the utilization requirements before initiating services and throughout the episode of care.

The quality assurace program managed by payers includes their own objectives and standards published by national agencies, such as the National Committee for Quality Assurance (NCQA). Many of these projects focus on obstetrics and well woman care. In addition, benefit plans often contain incentives to patients for participating in "healthy pregnancy programs." Compliance with these programs often includes transmitting data to the payer and/or participating in focused surveys or medical record audits. Contract language should address confidentiality of this information and limit its use to internal quality assurance programs. Release of this information to any party other than the payer requires the physician's written consent.

OB/GYNs contracting through IPAs, PHOs, and other large physician organizations have a window of opportunity to design and manage quality assurance projects to demonstrate the effectiveness of quality care with good outcomes. Data demonstrating a measurable difference, for example, well-managed obstetric care reducing neonatal intensive care admissions and length of stay, can be used effectively to increase reimbursement and/or gain access to incentive/bonus funds associated with risk contracts.

An additional note of caution regarding injectible medications given in the office—benefit plans vary widely regarding coverage for medications and frequently have significant financial incentives to encourage use of formularies, generic, and mail-order drugs. Some medications also may require precertification. Administrative procedures regarding pharmaceuticals not only should comply with state pharmacy regulation but also should be specific in guiding physicians how to order and be reimbursed for office-based medication/therapy services and ordering prescriptions. At a minimum, reimbursement for injectibles and other office-based services should cover costs plus inventory and administration.

Contract administration also includes determination of benefits and eligibility. Easy access, preferably electronic verification and toll-free telephone lines, help the practice confirm coverage and out-of-pocket costs before the patient's visit or surgery. Documentation of this information is critical to ensuring that a claim is paid correctly. The contract should have language protecting both the physician and patient from financial responsibility for benefit errors corrected subsequent to the service. At a minimum, risk contracts should contain language consistent with the industry standard of 3 months (90 days) for retroactive enrollment adjustments.

The provider directory includes the name, telephone number, and address of network physicians, hospitals, and ancillary services. OB/GYNs should review the directory carefully to ensure compatibility with their referral patterns—both with physicians they refer to and with physicians who refer to them. Likewise, laboratory and imaging services should be compatible with their practice routines. With patients frequently changing insurance coverage and managed-care companies seeking more competitive rates and thus aligning with a limited number of ancillaries, it has become increasingly difficult for physicians to maintain continuity of care and to monitor laboratory and imaging results provided by different companies. In addition to confirming that network ancillaries meet their practice needs, OB/GYNs should clarify emergency services and the expectations for "timely" responses, for example, managing ectopic pregnancies and time sensitive drug therapy associated with treatment of infertility. Both the contract and administrative manual should address circumstances when it is allowable and the mechanism for reimbursing services provided in the OB/GYN office, such as ultrasound or emergency laboratory tests.

In addition to specifying how much the physician is paid, the contract addresses filing claims, how the rate schedules are applied, and the timeframe for payment. The administrative manual goes a step further by defining a "clean claim"—a form properly completed with patient, beneficiary, employer, and provider information on an industry standard (HCFA) form and the procedure for filing the claim. To ensure correct payment, the procedures described in the administrative manual should support the specifics negotiated in the reimbursement schedule of the contract.

The administrative manual contains a sample explanation of benefits (EOB) statement. This document accompanies a paid claim describing how the claim was adjudicated, including the application of benefits, out-of-pocket expenses, compliance with utilization review, as appropriate, and the actual payment to the physician. A copy usually is mailed to the patient for their records. EOBs should be easy to read and understand, and explanation of the payment should tie directly to the contract.

The contract should allow the physician to bill and collect at the time of service the usual and customary charge for noncovered services. This should be reinforced with a statement from the patient, signed at the time of service, acknowledging financial responsibility for services received. Both the contract language and this statement are effective tools in settling claims disputes between patients and their payers.

## Contract Term and Termination

The term and termination of the contract provide both the payer and the physician with the means to extend or end their agreement. Most payer contracts are "evergreen," meaning that they continue in perpetuity after the initial term (usually 1 year), until the contract is terminated. Contracts become effective when a physician is credentialed as defined in the contract. Termination without cause by either party should be no longer than 90 days. Termination for cause should have a 30-day notice, with a 30-day limit to cure the breach. Most contracts contain language allowing shorter termination if the physician loses required license(s) or is legally sanctioned and prevented from practicing medicine as determined by the state agency controlling the license to practice medicine.

The contract also defines the circumstances for continuing the care of patients who are in an episode of care when the contract is terminated. This may be covered by a state regulation, but if not, the physician is required to complete the care or arrange for the safe transfer of care to another network physician within a specified number of days. OB/GYNs should have language addressing the time frames to safely transfer obstetric care or to continue care if the patient is in her third trimester. Reimbursement for continued care is limited to the terms of the contract, but this limitation should not extend beyond 90 days.

## Summary

Negotiating contracts for OB/GYN services requires knowledge of women's health care as it is perceived by women in the community, the managed-care payers, and the health-care delivery system in which the physician practices. Financial and demographic data from the OB/GYN practice help analyze proposed reimbursement, patient source, and payer/product evolution. Data demonstrating the physician's clinical and financial outcomes can be used to increase leverage at the bargaining table. Negotiating requires tenacity to pursue language supporting realistic and cost-effective contract administration. The issues covered in this chapter apply to managed-care contracting for the OB/GYN negotiating as an individual or as a group. Successful contracts align clinical, financial, and administrative incentives for patients, OB/GYNs, and their payers.

# 74

# Business Principles in Obstetrics and Gynecology Financial Decision-Making

DEAN G. SMITH

An important aspect of managing a successful obstetrics and gynecology practice is ensuring its financial viability. Financial viability is determined by several factors—the volume of patient flow, fee schedules and managed-care contracts, efficiency of office operations, and quality of patient care. Although financial decision-making has little to contribute toward quality of patient care, many of the other aspects of financial viability are subject to monitoring and analysis using finance tools. This chapter provides an overview of finance decision-making tools and data for practicing physicians.

Physicians in the practice of medicine are not also expected to be the accountant or office manager of the practice. Therefore, the material presented in this chapter is the level of detail required for high-level, strategic decision-making, not just day-to-day operations. This is not to suggest that day-to-day operations are not important. Continuous monitoring and reporting on practice operations is a valued function of the accountant or office manager. Supervision of these functions provided by physicians can aid in the success of a practice. However, strategic decision-making by the leadership of a practice gives it the opportunity for long-term viability.

## Financial Accounting

Financial accounting involves keeping records of all financial transactions and preparing financial statements in a standardized manner. The key to financial accounting is that it aims to provide all observers with an accurate picture of the holdings of a company and its income. In the United States, financial accounting typically follows generally accepted accounting principles (GAAP) set forth in the opinions and pronouncements of the Accounting Principles Board of the American Institute of Certified Public Accountants, in statements and pronouncements of the Financial Accounting Standards Board, and by other practices and procedures approved by a significant segment of the accounting profession. Consistency and comparability are among the principles that guide financial accounting.

The process of financial accounting starts with initial data capture and documentation. All transactions that have a financial impact on a practice have some form of documentation, such as receipts or bills, that must be captured by the practice. Transactions are recorded objectively in journals and then summarized at the end of accounting periods determined by the practice (monthly, quarterly, annually). Other principles that guide this accounting process include focusing on a specific practice and treating it as an ongoing business. All transactions are expressed in dollar terms, which sometimes must be estimated, as is the case with provisions for bad debts. It is expected that full disclosure of all transactions are either presented on statements or are available for inspection by auditors.

In addition to data that arise because of specific transactions, some data arise as a result of the passage of time. Expenses associated with the depreciation of assets do not involve any exchange of cash but still must be recorded to obtain an accurate statement of a practice's financial position. Similarly, expenses associated with advance purchase of insurance and revenues associated with acceptance of capitation payments require valuation and recording at the end of each accounting period.

Presentations on financial statements are expected to focus on relevant issues, not minute details, and must be derived reliably. A final principle that guides financial accounting is conservatism. Practices are expected to be cautious in the reporting of revenues and generous in the recording of expenses. Of course, the principle of conservatism must be tempered with the rules and regulations of the Internal Revenue Service and other entities that might have other interests. Examples of basic financial statements are presented in Tables 74–1 through 74–3.

The balance sheet provides a snapshot of the holdings, obligations, and ownership of a practice at a particular point in time. Balance sheets start with the assets of the practice. Assets are separated into current assets (assets that are either cash or can be translated into cash within 1 year) and long-term assets. Aside from any equipment or office holdings, the largest asset of most practices is accounts receivable from third party payers and patients. Many solo and small group practices use "cash accounting" rather than "accrual accounting." Under a cash accounting system, revenues are recognized when payment is received rather than when services are provided to patients. Therefore, under cash accounting, there are no accounts receivable on the balance sheet. Given the importance of insurance, practices using cash accounting must have a separate system to monitor insurance billings and payments.

Assets are balanced by liabilities and owner's equity. Liabilities are the amounts owed by the practice to suppliers, banks, and others. The remaining amount is owner's equity, which represents how much of the assets are owned outright by the practice. Caution should be used in the interpretation of owner's equity

**Table 74–1** Hendrickson Medical Group Balance Sheet (December 31, 1997 and 1996)

|  | 1997 | 1996 | Change |
|---|---|---|---|
| **Assets** | | | |
| Current assets | | | |
| Cash and securities | 50,995 | 36,050 | 14,945 |
| Net accounts receivable | 228,909 | 278,508 | (49,600) |
| Supplies | 29,473 | 26,115 | 3,358 |
| Prepaid expenses | 21,000 | 21,535 | (535) |
| Subtotal current assets | 330,376 | 362,208 | (31,832) |
| Furniture and equipment | 533,649 | 542,388 | (8,739) |
| (Less accumulated depreciation) | (207,530) | (180,796) | (26,734) |
| Net furniture and equipment | 326,119 | 361,592 | (35,473) |
| Total assets | 782,695 | 708,800 | 73,895 |
| **Liabilities and Owners' Equity** | | | |
| Current liabilities | | | |
| Accounts payable | 7,424 | 5,495 | 1,929 |
| Accrued payroll liabilities | 9,813 | 8,856 | 957 |
| Subtotal current liabilities | 17,237 | 14,352 | 2,886 |
| Long-term notes payable | 340,000 | 347,000 | (7,000) |
| Total liabilities | 357,237 | 361,352 | (4,114) |
| Owners' equity | 425,458 | 347,448 | 78,009 |
| Total liabilities and equity | 782,695 | 708,800 | 73,895 |

**Table 74–2** Hendrickson Medical Group Income Statement (Years Ending December 31, 1997 and 1996)

|  | 1997 | 1996 | Change |
|---|---|---|---|
| **Revenues** | | | |
| Fee-for-services charges | 1,519,121 | 1,639,605 | (120,484) |
| (Less discounts and allowances) | (124,568) | (129,529) | 4,961 |
| Capitation revenues | 349,398 | 163,960 | 185,437 |
| Net revenue | 1,743,951 | 1,674,036 | 69,914 |
| **Expenses** | | | |
| Office staff salaries | 191,835 | 175,774 | 16,061 |
| Employee benefits and taxes | 63,305 | 54,490 | 8,816 |
| Subtotal staff expenses | 255,140 | 230,264 | 24,876 |
| Office rental and maintenance | 105,509 | 100,442 | 5,067 |
| Furniture and equipment depreciation | 59,294 | 60,265 | (971) |
| Laboratory expenses | 36,623 | 38,503 | (1,880) |
| Drugs and medical supplies | 22,671 | 20,088 | 2,583 |
| Professional liability insurance | 141,260 | 133,923 | 7,337 |
| Other expenses | 40,111 | 36,829 | 3,282 |
| Total expenses | 660,609 | 620,314 | 40,294 |
| Net Income | 1,083,342 | 1,053,722 | 29,620 |

**Table 74–3** Hendrickson Medical Group Notes to Financial Statements (Years Ending December 31, 1997 and 1996)

**Note 1. Organization**

Hendrickson Medical Group, LLP (the "Company") was organized in 1985 by Dr. K. Hendrickson to provide physician services, specializing in obstetrics and gynecology. The Company is now a four-physician practice: Dr. G. Hendrickson, Dr. J. Hendrickson, and Dr. V. Butler. The Company's relationships with its affiliated physicians are set forth in various agreements.

**Note 2. Basis of Presentation**

The financial statements have been prepared in accordance with generally accepted accounting principles. These statements were audited by HMP606 Accountants, LLP.

**Note 3. Physician Activity**

Physician services are provided in the offices at 1036 Olivia Avenue, Suite 110, Ann Arbor, Michigan, and at hospitals where practice physicians have admitting privileges. In-office patient visits numbered 19,364 in 1997, up from 18,988 in 1996, an increase of 376 office visits. Hospital-based visits numbered 1861 in 1997, down from 1880 in 1996, a decrease of 19 hospital visits. Total visits numbered 21,225 in 1997, up from 20,868 in 1996, a net increase of 357 total visits.

**Note 4. 1997 Capitated Managed-Care Agreement**

On August 1, 1995, the Company signed a capitated managed-care agreement with Good Health Plan ("GHP"). Under the agreement, the Company's affiliated physicians provide obstetrics and gynecology medical and surgical services to enrollees of GHP. At December 31, 1997, there were approximately 2000 enrollees under the GHP agreement. The agreement with GHP provides for a renegotiation of the capitation fees on an annual basis. The agreement may be terminated by GHP at any time for cause.

**Note 5. Audit Report**

We have audited the balance sheet of Hendrickson Medical Group, LLP (a Michigan Professional Limited Liability Corporation) as of December 31, 1996 and 1997, and the related income statements for each of the years in the 2-year period ended December 31, 1997. These financial statements are the responsibility of the Company's management. Our responsibility is to express an opinion on these financial statements based on our audits.

We conducted our audits in accordance with generally accepted auditing standards. Those standards require that we plan and perform the audit to obtain reasonable assurance about whether the financial statements are free of material misstatement. An audit includes examining, on a test basis, evidence supporting the amounts and disclosures in the financial statements. An audit also includes assessing the accounting principles used and significant estimates made by management, as well as evaluating the overall financial statement presentation. We believe that our audits and the report of the other auditors provide a reasonable basis for our opinion.

In our opinion, based upon our audits, the financial statements referred to above present fairly, in all material respects, the financial position of Hendrickson Medical Group, LLP as of December 31, 1996 and 1997, and the results of their operations for each of the years in the 2-year period ended December 31, 1997, in conformity with generally accepted accounting principles.

HMP606 ACCOUNTANTS, LLP
Ann Arbor, Michigan
March 2, 1998

in a medical practice. Unlike large corporations that may pay out only a small percentage of earnings in the form of dividends, practices usually distribute the majority of earnings and keep a small percentage in the practice. Therefore, cash holdings and owner's equity are proportionally much smaller in medical practices than in other corporations.

The income statement provides information on the earnings of the practice over the accounting period. Revenues of the practice are derived from patient charges and capitation payments. In many practices, contracts with insurance companies involve discounts from charges. Discounts, combined with allowances for nonpaying patients, form a deduction from gross charges.

Expenses are presented for those items that represent significant costs to the practice, with smaller items being combined as other expenses. Staff expenses are often half of all expenses, although they may be somewhat less than half for specialties such as obstetrics and gynecology that have relatively high professional liability insurance expenses. Net income is the difference between revenues and expenses.

In addition to the income statement, many larger organizations also provide a statement of cash flow. A statement of cash flow combines information from the balance sheet and income statement to provide a complete picture of how all funds were used during the year.

An integral part of all financial statements is the attached notes. Notes to financial statements provide the detail on significant accounting practices and operations that are essential to the understanding of the finances of the practice.

# Financial Statement Analysis

Producing accurate financial statements is a required activity. Monitoring and analyzing financial statements are important management activities for ensuring financial viability. Monitoring the finances of a practice, planning for future expansion, assessing the use of debt or need for debt, developing contracting strategies, pricing, and competitive assessment are a few management control functions facilitated by financial statement analysis.

Among the many strategies used for financial statement analysis, the most common is the development of a summary set of financial ratios to depict a practice's performance. Analysis focused on ratios rather than raw numbers provides the decision-maker with numbers that are interpreted and compared more easily. Common financial ratios used to characterize practices are presented in Table 74–4, with values calculated for the Hendrickson Medical Group. The

**Table 74–4** Financial Ratios

| Ratios | Formula | 1997 | 1996 | Change |
|---|---|---|---|---|
| **PROFITABILITY** | | | | |
| Profit margin | Net income/Net revenues | 62% | 63% | −1% |
| Net income per physician | Net income/Number of physicians | 270,836 | 263,431 | 7405 |
| **LIQUIDITY** | | | | |
| Current ratio | Current assets/Current liabilities | 19 | 25 | (6) |
| Days accounts receivable | Net accounts receivable/(Net revenues/365) | 48 | 61 | (13) |
| Days accounts payable | Net accounts payable/(Supplier expenses/365) | 13 | 10 | 3 |
| Days cash | Cash/(Operating expenses/365) | 28 | 21 | 7 |
| **LEVERAGE** | | | | |
| Debt ratio | Total liabilities/Total assets | 46% | 51% | −5% |
| **ACTIVITY/PRODUCTIVITY** | | | | |
| Total asset turnover | Total revenues/Total assets | 223% | 236% | −13% |
| Revenue per visit | Net revenue/Total visits | 82.16 | 80.22 | 1.94 |
| Expense per visit | Total expenses/Total visits | 31.12 | 29.73 | 1.39 |
| Staff expense ratio | Staff expenses/Total expenses | 38.6% | 37.1% | 1.5% |
| Malpractice expense ratio | Malpractice expenses/Total expenses | 21.4% | 21.6% | −0.2% |
| Office visit ratio | Office visits/Total visits | 91.2% | 91.0% | 0.2% |
| Capitation revenue | Capitation revenue/Net revenue | 20.0% | 9.8% | 10.2% |

first set of ratios summarizes profitability of a practice. The profit margin (or percentage of revenues that goes to physician income) and net income per physician are the key measures of both profitability and productivity in a practice. In Hendrickson, profitability was about the same in 1997 and 1996.

The second set of ratios summarizes liquidity, the availability of cash in the practice. The current ratio summarizes the practice's ability to pay its debts during the year. Days accounts receivable and days accounts payable show how quickly the practice gets paid by third parties and patients and how quickly the practice pays its suppliers, respectively. A reality of medical practice is that third parties and patients pay over the course of 2 or more months, whereas the practice must pay its workers and suppliers within a couple of weeks. Note that the days accounts receivable decreased substantially in 1997. This is related to managed care. Capitation payments usually are made within 30 days, decreasing outstanding receivables. Finally, days cash expresses how long the practice could continue to pay expenses if there were no receipts. Having 3 to 4 weeks' cash on hand is a minimum amount for a business.

The third set of ratios summarizes leverage, or the indebtedness of the practice. The debt ratio for Hendrickson indicates that they balance their assets with half debt and half equity.

The last set of ratios summarizes activity and productivity in the practice. Total asset turnover indicates the productivity of assets in earning revenues. Revenue per visit and expense per visit combine to form profit per visit, but each merits close examination. From 1996 to 1997, expenses increased, but revenues increased even more, yielding higher profits per visit. Practice expenses also merit close examination. Office staff expenses were 37 to 39% of expenses, and malpractice insurance was 21%. Changes in any of the expense ratios call for exploration of the cause of the change. The office visit ratio indicates where the physicians are working, and the capitation ratio indicates the sources of patients' coverage. Capitation revenue doubled from 1996 to 1997, an increasingly common occurrence in both primary care and specialty practices.

Several cautions are offered for the new user of financial statement analysis. First, the notes attached to financial statements are an integral part of the analysis and a source of answers to many questions. Second, financial ratios only offer a financial perspective of the state of the practice. Other factors, such as quality of care, patient satisfaction, and changes in the market should not be ignored. Third, the use of particular ratios narrows one's view to those numbers. Financial analysts often look at hundreds of ratios when reviewing a company that may be purchased or sold. Finding those ratios that highlight the important aspects of your practice may involve some trial and error. Fourth, the analysis of financial ratios usually requires making comparisons. Comparing one year with the next almost always is done. Comparisons to other practices can be very helpful if done correctly. Many companies (Medical Economics, Medical Group Management Association, and others) calculate ratios on medical practices. Whenever possible, try to obtain ratios that are comparable in terms of practice type (obstetrics and gynecology), practice size (solo, number in group), and location. Finally, when making comparison, think about with whom you wish to be compared. Usually only averages are presented. If your benchmark for success is the average, these data might be acceptable. If you aspire to be in the top quartile, or recognize that, given your market, just being above the bottom quartile means success, then additional data may be necessary.

# Budgeting

Budgeting is the process of preparing financial statements in advance. Budgets are statements of the expected future activities of the practice in financial terms. Optimally, the complete financial planning process starts with developing strategic plans for the practice: defining the future of the practice, its position in the market, and its financial results. Strategic planning is followed by programming—defining the specific services to be offered by specific personnel. Third comes budgeting—applying information on costs, revenues, volumes of services, and assets to the programs to produce future financial statements. Managerial control and financial accounting during the accounting period are used to work toward achieving the projections made in the budget and providing the data for analysis of the practice's operations in comparison with the budget.

One system for managing decisions about the organization of the budgeting process is to follow an unfortunate acronym that spells how too many organizations budget: PITIFULLY—process, input, timing, increments, fixed, uncontrollable, legitimate, looseness, and your need to reality-check.

Effective budgeting requires a process. A process involves allocating time to coordinate strategic planning, identify programs, prepare the budget data and financial statements, and give management control during the year. Having the optimal process is not as critical as having a (any) process in place. Without a process and allocation of time to the process, it is difficult to ensure that a meaningful budget is prepared.

Input is required from many sources to obtain all the needed information and buy-in for an effective budget. Two alternative input patterns are bottom-up and top-down budgeting. Bottom-up budgeting is consistent with a total quality management paradigm and *might* imply empowering staff and listening to customer comments on service and services desired. Bottom-up budgeting can provide in-depth and realistic projections of costs and productivity. Top-down budgeting involves shareholders or top management dictating practice objectives, such as profit margin, and then fitting the rest of the budget to meet these objectives. Top-down budgeting often is criticized, but it offers greater control over the practice, especially in times of change. In general, having more people involved in the budget process typically implies a costlier process. However, having more people involved also increases the likelihood that staff will be aware of the budget and accept its importance.

The timing of the budget process follows from the need for producing results and statements. For an update of an existing budget that has been met in a stable market, the time involved may be a few days. For a complete change in a budget, 1 or 2 months may pass. There is a trade-off between time spent planning and time spent doing that is addressed in the budget process. How long is your budget process? If you update it in a weekend, are you challenging the practice? If it takes longer than 2 months, is it worthwhile?

A second timing decision involves the increments of time in which budgets are prepared. Increments usually are tied to annual contracts and tax returns, but both longer-range budgets and quarterly or monthly budgets may be desirable. There are trade-offs of planning for the long run and having immediate information and control. Decision-making on increments also requires decisions on how revisions are made to the budget. Incremental budgeting involves taking an existing budget and adding inflation or other adjustments on an annual basis. Zero-based budgeting involves starting from scratch and reviewing all the assumptions built into a budget. Most successful practices take some of each. Periodically, meaning every 2 or 3 years, a detailed analysis and zero-based budgeting are undertaken. Incremental budgeting is used in the interim, unless there is a crisis or an unusual opportunity.

Whether budgets are fixed or flexible is related to whether budget presentations are based on total results or results per visit or per episode of care. Fixed budgets are simple and permit tight control for a specific level of patient visits. Fixed budgets also are used for marketing and other costs that typically do not vary with patient volume. Flexible budgets are more complicated and involve looser control, but they permit more complex analysis of costs and may present more reasonable ways of viewing results. To use flexible budgets effectively, know which costs are truly fixed (not varying with patient volume) and which are variable.

The level to which costs are uncontrollable or controllable affects the process of budgeting. In budgeting for capitation contracts, the number of expected patient visits must be estimated, but it is largely uncontrollable. Conversely, office hours and the number of office staff are controllable. Uncontrollable costs should be identified (and specified in contracts where possible), estimated, and monitored closely.

Budgets should be viewed by staff as being legitimate if they are to be used for decision-making that affects their work or pay. Bottom-up methods can lead to budgets being viewed as legitimate if the staff's suggestions are included. Budgets that are completely top-down, incrementally updated from a previous budget and fixed, may not be viewed as legitimate and may not be considered in financial decision-making by staff.

The looseness or slack included in a budget reflects how much flexibility one includes for opportunities and errors. A very tight budget, in which every assumption must be met to achieve the goals of the practice, may be too strict to be achievable. Similarly, a very loose budget may fail to provide staff the appropriate message on the need for efficiency.

Finally, there is always a need to "reality-check" the components of a budget. It is easy to prepare a budget that simply takes the past year's budget and increases all expenses and revenues by 4% for inflation. However, the labor market may have changed, requiring 8% raises to keep good staff. Insurance fee schedules may have been updated, increasing fees by only 2%. For the budget to be met in terms of net income to the practice, the volume of patient visits must increase by 4%. Is this realistic? Understanding the implications of altering assumptions, and conducting "what if" analyses on a budget are important components to having a budgeting process that works as a tool for achieving financial viability.

For all budgets, comparison of actual results with budgets is an integral part of financial planning. Budget variance analysis is the process of determining why actual revenues and/or expenses differ from budgeted amounts. Variance analysis can be as simple as dollar-for-dollar comparisons of budgeted and actual amounts. Variances for the fee-for-service portion of the Hendrickson Medical Group are presented in Table 74–5. Which of the variances on a line-by-line basis merit examination? Variances greater than specified dollar amounts may merit examination. At a cutoff of $5,000, only net revenues and staff expenses exhibit substantial variances. Similarly, variances greater than specified percentages may merit attention. At a cutoff of 10%, only laboratory expense exhibits substantial variance. In a more general framework, variances that persist for some time and combinations of dollar and percentage variances all merit examination. Variance analysis is not an end in itself. Rather, it targets the analysis of reasons behind differences between actual and budgeted amounts.

One handy method of budget variance analysis involves separating the volume-related components of variance from the per visit components. These components also are presented in Table 74–5. The process of calculated components is generically as follows: the total variance is Actual − Budget; the excess due to

*Table 74–5* Hendrickson Medical Group Budget Variances (Year Ending December 31, 1997)

| | Actual | Budget | Variance |
|---|---|---|---|
| Fee-for-service visits | 16,980 | 17,529 | (549) |
| Net revenue | 1,394,553 | 1,429,899 | (35,346) |
| Net revenue per visit | 82.13 | 81.57 | 0.56 |
| Staff expenses | 204,112 | 193,422 | 10,690 |
| Office rental and maintenance | 84,407 | 84,371 | 36 |
| Furniture and equipment depreciation | 47,435 | 50,623 | (3187) |
| Laboratory expenses | 29,298 | 32,342 | (3044) |
| Drugs and medical supplies | 18,137 | 16,874 | 1263 |
| Professional liability insurance | 113,008 | 112,495 | 13 |
| Other expenses | 32,089 | 30,936 | 1153 |
| Total expenses | 528,487 | 521,064 | 7423 |
| Total expenses per visit | 31.12 | 29.73 | 1.39 |
| Net income | 866,066 | 908,835 | (42,769) |
| Net income per visit | 51.00 | 51.85 | (0.84) |
| *Variance Analysis* | | | |
| Revenues: Due to visits | | | (44,780.20) |
| Revenues: Due to revenue per visit | | | 9433.98 |
| Expenses: Due to visits | | | (16,318.17) |
| Expenses: Due to expense per visit | | | 23,741.12 |
| Net income: Due to visits | | | (28,462.02) |
| Net income: Due to net per visit | | | (14,307.15) |

visits is (Actual Visits − Budgeted Visits) × Budgeted per Visit Amount; and the excess due to the per visit amount (also called the efficiency variance) is (Actual per Visit Amount − Budgeted per Visit Amount) × Actual Visits. For the Hendrickson Medical Group, the shortfall in revenues is primarily the result of the shortfall in the number of fee-for-service visits. The expense variance is primarily the result of higher-than-budgeted per-visit costs. Combined, net income is less than budgeted two thirds the result of the shortfall in the number of visits and one third the result of expenses per visits increasing more than revenues per visit.

# Cash Management

Sound financial management of a practice requires knowing its cash position at all times, both in absolute terms and in relation to its budget. Cash management is relatively easy for smaller practices using cash accounting. For larger practices using accrual accounting, a second budget that uses a cash basis should be prepared and monitored. A cash budget for the first

**Table 74-6** Hendrickson Medical Group Cash Budget (January–June 1997)

|  | January | February | March | April | May | June |
|---|---|---|---|---|---|---|
| Beginning cash balance | 36,050 | 46,496 | 22,536 | 23,577 | 24,617 | 30,658 |
| Collections from A/R | 126,379 | 130,405 | 132,901 | 134,449 | 135,409 | 126,888 |
| Collections from capitations | 29,116 | 29,116 | 29,116 | 29,116 | 29,116 | 29,116 |
| Available cash | 191,546 | 212,586 | 188,627 | 189,667 | 190,708 | 196,748 |
| Operating expenditures | 55,050 | 155,050 | 55,050 | 55,050 | 55,050 | 55,050 |
| Payments to physicians | 90,000 | 90,000 | 90,000 | 90,000 | 90,000 | 90,000 |
| Operating cash balance | 46,496 | (32,464) | 43,577 | 44,617 | 45,658 | 51,698 |
| Bank line of credit | 0 | 55,000 | (20,000) | (20,000) | (15,000) | 0 |
| Ending cash balance | 46,496 | 22,536 | 23,577 | 24,617 | 30,658 | 51,698 |

A/R, accounts receivable.

half of 1997 is presented in Table 74-6. The keys to cash management in group practices include: selecting minimum cash balances, timely billing and collections of accounts receivable, accurate calculation and collection of capitation payments, timely payment of expenses, and maintaining favorable bank relationships.

For the first half of 1997, the Hendrickson Medical Group collected accounts receivable on the basis of roughly 15% in the month the service was provided, 15% in the next month, 20% for the next 3 months, and the remainder over the next several months. Capitations were collected on the 15th day of each month. Capitated arrangements may involve risks on the expense side but are favorable on the receipts side. Operating expenses for staff, rent, and most accounts are paid each month. The exceptions are liability insurance and other accounts due in February and July. Physicians expect a level monthly payment, although in smaller practices owner's payments may vary based on available cash. Given the large and well known February expenses, the Hendrickson Medical Group has established a line of credit with a bank, which it draws on in February and July and at any time its cash balance decreases to less than $20,000.

All of these assumptions and decisions are unique to this group, although not unusual. Developing policies for cash management well in advance of cash shortfalls is part of prudent financial management.

## Managerial Accounting

Managerial accounting is a system of analysis in which costs are measured and monitored for internal management purposes. Unlike financial accounting, managerial accounting presentations are for internal practice management, and there are no artificially imposed rules to follow. Managerial accounting makes use of financial statements as a source of data, but often looks beyond these statements for data to answer more detailed questions.

Four basic questions guide managerial accounting. First, why is the service or activity being costed? Costs may be needed for planning, control, or evaluation, or for making specific decisions. Unless the purpose is known, the time spent on a cost analysis may be wasted. Second, what is costed? Costs may be needed for specific services or procedures, for patient episodes of care or member months of care, or for practice operations as a whole. Third, which costs are included? Cost measures include variable costs, fixed costs, and a number of variations. Fourth, when is it costed? Costs may be measured before an activity, using standard costs or forecasts for budgeting, or after an activity, using actual or estimated costs for evaluation.

A common managerial question is what are the full costs for each of the services delivered? Using the income statement for 1997 from Hendrickson Medical Group, the step-down method is demonstrated in Table 74-7 to allocate costs to visits. Direct allocation is used for costs that are monitored on the basis of patient visits. In this case, staff expenses and drugs, supplies, and laboratory costs are reasonably monitored for the division of routine medical visits, procedure-based visits, and hospital visits. For the allocation of office overhead, some measure of use must be determined. For this practice, the percent of patient visits is used. Applying indirect costs on the basis of visits permits total costs to be assigned to the three types of visits. The average expense of $31.12 per visit is of general interest, but the detailed cost per visit is more valuable for detailed decision-making.

A more detailed question is what are the full costs on a specific visit basis (Current Procedural Terminology, CPT-4) of the routine visits? Allocation on the basis of visits is insufficient to answer this question—all routine visits would have a cost of $18.54. Two methods commonly are employed for answering this question, ratio of cost to charges

**Table 74–7**  Step-Down Cost Allocation

|  | Data | Direct Allocation | Percent Visits | Indirect Allocation | Total Costs | Cost per Visit |
|---|---|---|---|---|---|---|
| Office overhead | 346,174 | 346,174 | | | | |
| Drugs, supplies, and laboratory | 59,294 | | | | | |
| Total staff expenses | 255,140 | | | | | |
| Total operating expenses | 660,609 | | | | | |
| Routine visits | 14,125 | 31,443 | 66.5% | 230,373 | 261,816 | 18.54 |
| Procedure visits | 5239 | 163,506 | 24.7% | 85,446 | 248,952 | 47.52 |
| Hospital visits | 1861 | 119,485 | 8.8% | 30,356 | 149,841 | 80.51 |
| Total visits | 21,225 | 660,609 | 100.0% | 346,174 | 660,609 | 31.12 |

(RCC) and relative value units (RVUs). The RCC method simply allocates costs on the basis of the overall ratio of costs in the practice to charges. RCC only requires data on total costs and charges for each service. The RVU method allocates costs on the basis of the total relative value units that are used for the services. RVU requires data on total costs and relative value units for each service. For Medicare patients, RVUs from the Medicare resource-based relative value scale (RBRVS) reimbursement system may be appropriate. However, the RVUs calculated for Medicare patients may not be available to apply to other groups of patients.

A comparison of the use of RCC and RVU methods is provided in Table 74–8. Under both methods, the starting point is knowing total costs and the number of patients by service type. For simplicity, routine visits for only two types of services were compiled for two patients. The RCC method allocates total costs of $5,562 by using relative charges, resulting in service cost measures, and a constant service profit margin of 65%. The RVU method allocates these costs on the basis of total RVUs, resulting in service cost measures, and a profit margin of 59% for a level 1 visit with a new patient and a profit margin of 70% for a level 4 visit with an established patient. The RVU method provides a more accurate measure of costs and profitability, but RVU data are not always available.

Another common question is how many visits are needed for the practice to cover its costs? The managerial accounting tool used to answer this question, break-even analysis, requires information on the types of costs involved. Cost measures include variable costs, fixed costs, and a number of variations. Fixed costs remain the same for all visits. Fixed costs include office rental and maintenance costs, insurance costs, and many salary costs. Variable costs are proportional to the number of visits and include drugs, supplies, laboratory costs, and some salary costs. Separating fixed and variable costs requires detailed financial accounting data on practice costs and a good knowledge of how expenses are generated.

The simple form of break-even analysis is derived from the five equations presented in Table 74–9. Using the Hendrickson Medical Group's financial statement numbers for fixed costs (all overhead costs plus half of salaries) and variable costs (all drugs, supplies, and laboratory costs and half of salaries), calculation of the last equation serves as a check on the equations. For 1998, if fixed costs remain the same, variable costs remain the same on a per visit basis and prices are reduced by 5%, how many patient visits are required to maintain the same practice net income? Using these equations, the result is 22,485, an increase of 1260 over 1997. The power and flexibility of break-even analysis make it one of the most widely used managerial accounting tools.

**Table 74–8**  Ratio of Cost to Charges (RCC) and Relative Value Unit (RVU) Cost Determination

| CPT-4 | Total Costs = $5562 | Visits | Charges | Revenue | Cost per Visit | Profit Margin |
|---|---|---|---|---|---|---|
| 99201 | Office visit new patient, level 1 | 200 | $35 | $7000 | $13.26 | 65% |
| 99214 | Office visit established, level 4<br>RCC = $5562/$16,000 = 0.348 | 100 | $90 | $9000 | $34.09 | 65% |

| CPT-4 | Total Costs = $5562 | Visits | RVUs | Total RVUs | Cost per Visit | Profit Margin |
|---|---|---|---|---|---|---|
| 99201 | Office visit new patient, level 1 | 200 | 0.84 | 168 | $14.42 | 59% |
| 99214 | Office visit established, level 4 | 100 | 1.56 | 156 | $26.78 | 70% |

CPT, Current Procedural Terminology.

**Table 74–9** Break-Even Visit Determination

| Equation | Calculation |
|---|---|
| 1  Total Cost = Total Fixed Cost (TFC) + Total Variable Costs (TVC) | 660,609 = 473,744 + 186,864 |
| 2  Average Variable Cost (AVC) = TVC/Number of Visits (N) | 8.80 = 186,864/21,225 |
| 3  Total Revenue = Price per Visit (P) × Number of Visits (Q) | 1,743,951 = 82.16 × 21,225 |
| 4  Total Revenue = Total Cost + Net Income | 1,743,951 = 660,609 + 1,083,342 |
| 5  N = (TFC + Net Income)/(P − AVC) | 21,225 = (473,744 + 1,083,342)/(82.16 − 8.80) |
| Break-even N for the same Net Income, but with payments reduced by 5%; N = (TFC + Net Income)/P-5% − AVC) | 22,485 = (473,744 + 1,083,342)/(78.05 − 8.80) |

## Corporate Finance

Corporate finance is the process of planning, acquiring, and using funds in ways that maximize the value of a practice. Corporate finance decisions generally are long term in nature and involve making capital expenditure decisions, investments, and long-term borrowing. The keys to successful corporate finance decision-making are appropriately valuing future cash flows and challenging results. By the long-run nature of corporate finance decisions, they inherently involve more risk and require a greater depth of analysis.

Valuing cash flows in corporate finance requires appropriate accounting for the time value of money. A dollar to be received 1 year from now is worth less than a dollar in hand today. There are several convenient formulas for accounting for the time value of money, most of which are on pocket calculators and all popular microcomputer spreadsheet packages. Only a brief presentation is required to gain the rationale behind these formulas.

The basic formula from which all others are derived is the formula for the present value of an amount. Simply, the current value of a cash amount to be received in the future is that amount multiplied by the appropriate discount (interest) rate some number of time periods away. For example, the current value of a bill for $100 to be paid to the practice by an insurance company in 1 year (at a discount rate of 6%) is $94.34 ($100 / (1 + 0.06)$^1$). Paid in 2 years, its value is $89.00. The longer a bill is outstanding in accounts receivable, the lower its ultimate value.

The formula for the present value of a series of regular payments is the formula used by banks in calculating payment amounts for mortgages. If the present value is known, say the payment price for the house after the down payment, the equation is used to solve for the monthly payment amount. For example, for a home loan of $250,000, the monthly payment amount (at an interest rate of 7% per year for 15 years; actually 0.583% per month for 180 months) is $2,247. If the interest rate is increased to 8%, the payment amount increases to $2,389. The formulas for the present value of a bond, present value of common stock, and the future value of an amount are merely variations on this theme.

Capital expenditure analysis uses the finance formulas in what is typically a six-step process. Step one is defining goals and decision rules. The goal typically is to maximize the value of the practice, with specific rules being that projects are only accepted if return from a project merits the risk involved. The second step is to identify alternatives. Too often, decision-making focuses on a project under discussion without considering all other uses of time and funds. The third step is to determine cash flows for the life of the project and its risks. These risks are incorporated into the fourth step, which is to select discount rate(s) for future cash flows. A central concept in finance (earning a Nobel price in economics) is that there is a direct relationship between risks involved with projects and the returns that investors will demand for accepting those risks. The fifth step is to calculate the appropriate formulas on a standardized basis. Finally, one must evaluate alternatives, make a decision, and monitor results.

Returning to step one, there are three commonly used methods that result in explicit decision rules. The first method is to maximize the net present value (NPV) of an investment. The NPV is the present value of a series of regular payments (from the finance formula) less the initial investment amount. NPV is the most theoretically appropriate rule, but estimating future cash flows and selecting a discount rate can be time-consuming processes.

The second method also uses the formula for the present value of a series of regular payments (from the finance formula) less the initial investment amount. However, instead of calculating the net present value, one sets the value of the net present value equal to zero and calculates the discount rate. This rate is called the internal rate of return (IRR). With this method, the decision is to accept projects in which the IRR is greater than some defined rate of return. If one had a well-defined rate of return, one would use NPV. However, sometimes it is easier to make a decision about whether a rate of return seems acceptable than it is to decide that a dollar amount of NPV is acceptable.

The third method is called the payback and involves calculating the number of time periods in which the project must earn a profit to pay back the initial investment. The weakness of payback arises when making decisions involving more than one alternative. For example, one project with an IRR of 25% may have a payback of 4 years, whereas another with an IRR of 20% may have a payback of 3 years. Use of payback alone would result in accepting the lower valued project. The strength of payback is its simplicity. The payback period is useful as an augmentation to NPV and IRR because it provides decision-makers with clear expectations of how long to wait for returns when monitoring a project.

Some procedures are common to all capital expenditure methods. The data involved should consider only incremental cash flows—cash flows that stem directly from the project. Cash flows are what are important, not accrual methods. Therefore, one does not include overhead, unfunded depreciation, or money that has been spent in the past.

Once projects (assets and expenses) have been selected, one must arrange the funds necessary to start and maintain these activities. There are two sources of capital; debt and equity. Debt is borrowed money and comes in many forms: long-term and short-term loans, fixed and variable rate loans, secured (collateralized) loans (often called mortgages), callable debt (giving the borrow or lender the right to pay the debt immediately), convertible debt (giving the borrower or lender the right to convert the debt into equity), and long-term leases. Decisions on the best debt mechanism often involve the length of time for the project, the risks involved, and the relationship with the lender. Banks typically only offer loans or mortgages. Private investors and partners may consider more complex forms of debt.

Equity is defined as funds that are paid into the practice (with ownership rights) or earned from operations. Most physician solo and group practices have funds invested from the participating physicians and maintain only the funds in the practice as are necessary for day-to-day business. Larger groups and practices owned by physician practice management companies also may have access to capital from stock equity markets.

A number of important financial decision-making topics have been highlighted in the few pages of this section. Obviously, a few pages cannot offer all the topics, strategies, and nuances that lead to an effective financial decision-making process in a practice. The interested reader is encouraged to seek additional information in the form of conferences, journals, and texts. There are a large number of basic guides to financial accounting, managerial accounting, finance, and business operations of medical practices. The following guides are among those that provide very good insights for managing a medical practice.

## REFERENCES

Finkler SA: *Essentials of Cost Accounting for Health Care Organizations.* Gaithersburg, MD, Aspen Publishers, 1994.

Lyle JR, Torras HW: *Physicians Guide to Managed Care.* Augusta, GA, HealthCare Consultants of America, 1996.

Pavlock EJ: *Financial Management for Medical Groups.* Englewood, CO, Center for Research in Ambulatory Health Care Administration, 1994.

Sutton HL Jr, Sorbo AJ: *Actuarial Issues in the Fee-for-Service/Prepaid Medical Group.* Englewood, CO, Center for Research in Ambulatory Health Care Administration, 1993.

# 75

# Current Procedural Terminology (CPT) and International Classification of Disease, Ninth Revision, Clinical Modification (ICD-9-CM) Coding in Obstetrics and Gynecology

PHILIP N. ESKEW, JR.

It is more important today than ever before for the physician to have a working understanding of Current Procedural Terminology (CPT) and International Classification of Disease, Ninth Revision, Clinical Modification (ICD-9-CM) coding principles. Accurate use of these two systems of coding, coupled with documentation requirements, enables the physician to practice medicine without fear of penalty by third-party payers.

## Benefits of Coding and Documentation

The benefits of accurate coding and documentation are fair and prompt reimbursement, appropriate documentation of the physician's clinical activities, and adherence to third-party payer's compliance with coding rules. Properly filled-out office and outpatient super bills and accurate documentation of hospital visits and procedures result in prompt reimbursement from payers. The advantage of an accurate history of office visits, consultations, and procedures (CPT codes) with appropriate diagnosis codes (ICD-9 codes) is that this information assists the physician in any future discussion with third-party payers or managed care organizations about the level of acuity of patients and practice profile. Working knowledge of this process, along with your complete medical records, would be invaluable if you were to negotiate a capitated contract. All third-party payers have a fraud and abuse division that is continually investigating inaccurate claims, complaints by patients about their bills, and inadequate documentation in office records. Knowledge of coding rules and appropriate documentation in the patient's medical record allow the physician to practice with confidence, be reimbursed appropriately, and have an accurate record of all procedures and patient encounters.

## History of the Current Procedural Terminology (CPT) Process

The first edition of CPT was published in 1966 by The American Medical Association (AMA) to encourage the use of standard descriptors and terms that would document procedures performed by the physician for insurance claims. This system was a four-digit numerical listing of procedures, which facilitated collection of information for actuarial and statistical uses. The first edition contained primarily surgical procedures and some areas on medical, laboratory, and radiologic procedures. The second edition, published in 1970, was expanded to a five-digit coding system and included many diagnostic and therapeutic procedures in all areas of medicine.

The third and fourth editions of CPT were introduced in the 1970s with quarterly updates. In 1983, the CPT system was adopted by the Health Care Financing Administration (HCFA) for the Medicare program and for reporting outpatient hospital surgical procedures. Currently, CPT is used by most insurance programs as well as the Medicaid and Medicare programs as the coding system to describe physicians' services.

## CPT Editorial Panel

The CPT Editorial Panel has the responsibility for maintaining the CPT process. The panel is currently composed of 16 physicians, 11 appointed by the American Medical Association (AMA), and one each appointed by the Blue Cross and Blue Shield Association (BCBS), the Health Insurance Association of America (HIAA), the Health Care Financing Administration (HCFA), the American Hospital Association (AHA), and the Health Care Professionals Advisory Committee (HCPAC). Medical specialty organizations names of candidates for the AMA to select, but none of the 11 physicians are selected to represent a specific specialty, because they represent the whole field of medicine. The CPT Editorial Panel meets at least four times a year to consider coding changes and to make improvements to the process. All medical subspecialty organizations that are represented in the AMA's House of Delegates may choose a member of the Advisory Committee who will communicate the organization's coding requests to the CPT Editorial Panel. Thus, an individual physician can communicate a proposed coding change to his or her specialty organization. That organization's coding committee would discuss and approve the request (The American College of Obstetricians and Gynecologists [ACOG] has a Committee on Coding and Nomenclature) and send their Advisory Committee representative to a CPT Editorial Panel meeting (to explain the request and answer questions posed by the Editorial Panel) before the Panel votes on the merits of the proposal. The Panel can then vote to add a new code, revise a current code, table the request until more information is available, or reject the proposal.

All new codes approved by the CPT Editorial Panel are implemented on January 1 and are published in the current year's CPT book. It is absolutely imperative that new CPT books are purchased yearly to maintain an updated record of any additions, deletions, or modifications to the codes.

## Current Practice Terminology (CPT) 101

The first step in learning about CPT coding is to read the introductory pages in a CPT book. All of the rules, definitions, and guidelines are located in these pages, as well as at the beginning of each section of the book. For instance, the definition of antepartum care is located in the Maternity Care & Delivery section. Any physician may use any code in any section of the book. Each section has descriptive comments about the use of its particular codes. These informative paragraphs provide instructions about how to code correctly.

The majority of the CPT book contains five-digit codes that describe a procedure performed by the physician, some are specific for certain specialties and others can be performed by any qualified physician. The first part of the CPT book contains a section on codes for evaluation and management. These are categorized for various settings and situations, each with appropriate descriptive guidelines. As with any manual, always read the directions before using the instrument.

There are several coding courses presented annually. ACOG holds several each year. These courses are unique, because ACOG does not allow office staff to attend without their physician. Other sources of helpful information include the CPT Assistant from the AMA, Coding Updates, Committee Opinions, and fax and electronic mail transmissions from the ACOG staff, who are available to answer all coding questions.

# Evaluation and Management (E&M) Coding

Documentation requirements for E&M services were developed by the CPT Editorial Panel with input and comment solicited from all specialty organizations. They were released in October 1994, implemented in April 1995, and revised again in 1997. E&M codes continue to be revised, with comments and input from the various medical organizations. Quite simply, HCFA pays for services provided by physicians who document the amount of history that was obtained, the extent of physical examinations performed, and the degree of complexity of the medical decision-making process. The E&M process is basic, implementing tools that physicians learned in their physical diagnosis classes in medical school. The new E&M Codes now require documentation of questions asked of the patient and how the patient replies. E&M also makes inquiries about what medical decision-making process was employed and what examination and procedures were performed. ACOG continues to work with the CPT Editorial Panel on modifications to make this process as simple as possible. History and physical examination forms and templates were developed to aid in this process. It is no longer acceptable to use shortcuts, shorthand medical records, or brief written comments, such as "physical exam was normal" or "pelvic exam was normal."

**Selecting an Appropriate Level of E&M Services.** There are several different categories and subcategories of service based on the location and the type of service provided. The CPT book describes each of these categories and provides short narrative guidelines or instructions for their use. Each level of E&M service has seven components that determine the appropriate level to be coded. These are:
1. History
2. Examination
3. Medical decision-making
4. Counseling
5. Coordination of care
6. Nature of the presenting problem
7. Time

History, examination, and medical decision-making are the key components in determining the level of E&M service that has been performed by the physician. If more than 50% of the physician-patient-family encounter involves counseling, coordination of care, or both, time is considered the controlling component in determining the level of E&M service. Only at this point should the physician document on the medical record the amount of time involved in the patient encounter.

**Components of E&M Codes: Types of History.** The type of history is a reflection of the physician's clinical judgment and the nature of the patient's problem or problems. The E&M process lists four types or levels of history:
1. Problem Focused
2. Expanded Problem Focused
3. Detailed
4. Comprehensive

Each level of history includes some or all of the following components:

**Chief Complaint (CC).** Why did the patient come to see the physician? A concise statement by the patient describing the symptom or problem that is the reason for the encounter. Every patient encounter requires a chief complaint (CC) with the exception of Preventive Medicine encounters.

**History of Present Illness (HPI).** A chronologic description of the development of the patient's present illness from the first sign or symptom or a description of what has happened from the time of the previous encounter to the present. It includes the following descriptors:
1. Location
2. Quality
3. Severity
4. Duration
5. Timing
6. Context
7. Modifying Factors
8. Associated signs and symptoms related to the presenting problem.

**Review of Systems (ROS).** This review of body systems was obtained through a series of questions that identify signs and/or symptoms that the patient may be experiencing or has experienced. It includes the following 14 systems:
1. Constitutional symptoms (e.g., fever, weight loss)
2. Eyes

|  | HPI | ROS | PFSH |
|---|---|---|---|
| **Problem Focused** | Brief (1–3) | N/A | N/A |
| **Expanded Problem Focused** | Brief (1–3) | Pertinent (1) | N/A |
| **Detailed** | Extended (4+) | Expanded (2–9) | Pertinent (1 of 3) |
| **Comprehensive** | Extended (4+) | Complete (10–14) | Complete (3 of 3) |

3. Ears, nose, mouth, throat
4. Cardiovascular
5. Respiratory
6. Gastrointestinal
7. Genitourinary
8. Musculoskeletal
9. Integument (skin and/or breast)
10. Neurologic
11. Psychiatric
12. Endocrine
13. Hematologic/lymphatic
14. Allergic/immunologic

**Past Medical, Family, Social History.** This is a review of the *patient's past* major illnesses, previous operations and hospitalizations, allergies, and current medications. The family history provides a review of medical events in the *patient's family* that may be hereditary or place the patient at risk. This would include current health status or cause of death of parents, siblings, and children. An age-appropriate review of the *patient's past and current personal* social activities, includes marital status and living arrangements; employment; use of drugs, alcohol, tobacco; level of education; sexual history; and other relevant social factors.

**Coding for New or Established Patients.** The definition of a new patient is one who has not received any professional services from the physician or another physician of the same specialty who belongs to the same group practice, within the past 3 years. The following illustrates the use of these components in determining which E&M Code to choose for new or established patients in the outpatient setting. The numbers within the parentheses show how many descriptors, body systems, or components must be documented for each level of history.

## COMPONENTS OF E&M CODES: TYPES OF PHYSICAL EXAMINATION

The E&M process uses four types or levels of physical examination, which are defined by the same categories as the history:
Problem Focused: a limited examination of the affected body area or organ system
Expanded Problem Focused: a limited examination of the affected body area or organ system in addition to any other symptomatic or related organ system(s)
Detailed: an extended examination of the affected body area(s) and other symptomatic or related organ system(s)
Comprehensive: a general multisystem examination or a complete examination of a single organ system

CPT defines the body areas as:
1. Head, including the face
2. Neck
3. Chest, including breasts and axilla
4. Abdomen
5. Genitalia, groin, buttocks
6. Back
7. Each extremity

CPT defines the organ systems as:
1. Eyes
2. Ears, Nose, Mouth, and Throat
3. Cardiovascular
4. Respiratory
5. Gastrointestinal
6. Genitourinary
7. Musculoskeletal
8. Skin
9. Neurologic
10. Psychiatric
11. Hematologic/Lymphatic/Immunologic

**Genitourinary Single System Examination.** With considerable input from the various specialties and subspecialties, the CPT Editorial Board has developed several single-system examinations in addition to the standard multisystem examination. These examinations are continually revised and updated to reflect the components that are appropriate for each physician. By defining the elements within each organ system, the physician should document only the elements he or she examined and thus select the appropriate level of E&M service to be coded.

The ACOG has developed a checklist for the examination, which makes provision for the physician to check normal or abnormal for each element examined with space for a narrative description of all abnormal findings. They have also developed several templates that can be used as a guide for a physician's dictation regarding a patient encounter.

**Elements of the Female Genitourinary Single-System Examination.** Each element of the Single

System Genitourinary Examination is identified by an asterisk (*). The elements are frequently followed by a parenthetical example, such as the thyroid (e.g., enlargement, tenderness, mass), which instructs the physician to document whether or not the thyroid was enlarged, tender, or had a mass. The shaded and unshaded designation refers only to the required amount of documentation necessary for the comprehensive level.

Problem Focused: Perform and document *1 to 5 elements*

Expanded Problem Focused Examinations: Perform and document *at least 6 elements*

Detailed: Perform and document *at least 12 elements*

Comprehensive: Perform and document *all elements in a shaded category and at least one element in an unshaded category*

System or Body Area

Constitutional (Shaded)

*Measurement of any three of the following seven vital signs:
1. Sitting or standing blood pressure
2. Supine blood pressure
3. Pulse rate and regularity
4. Respiration
5. Temperature
6. Height
7. Weight (may be measured and recorded by ancillary staff)

*General appearance of patient (e.g., development, nutrition, body habitus, deformities, attention to grooming)

Neurologic/Psychiatric (Shaded)

*Brief assessment of mental status, including orientation to time, place, and person

*Mood and affect (e.g., depression, anxiety, agitation)

Neck (Unshaded)

*Examination of neck (e.g., masses, overall appearance, symmetry, tracheal position, crepitus)

*Examination of thyroid (e.g., enlargement, tenderness, mass)

Respiratory (Unshaded)

*Assessment of respiratory effort (e.g., intercostal retractions, use of accessory muscles, diaphragmatic movement)

*Auscultation of lungs (e.g., breath sounds, adventitious sounds, rubs)

Cardiovascular (Unshaded)

*Auscultation of the heart with notation of abnormal sounds and murmurs

*Examination of peripheral vascular system by observation (e.g., swelling, varicosities) and palpation (e.g., pulses, temperature, edema, tenderness)

Gastrointestinal (Shaded)

*Examination of abdomen with notation of presence or absence of masses or tenderness

*Examination of liver and spleen

*Examination for presence or absence of hernia

*Obtain stool sample for occult blood test, when indicated

Lymphatic (Shaded)

*Palpation of lymph nodes in neck, axillae, groin, or other location

Genitourinary (Shaded) Includes at least 7 of the following 11 elements

*Inspection and palpation of breasts (e.g., masses or lumps, tenderness, symmetry, nipple discharge)

Pelvic Examination (with or without specimen collection for smears and cultures) of:

*External genitalia (e.g., general appearance, hair distribution, lesions)

*Urethral meatus (e.g., size, location lesions, prolapse)

*Urethra (e.g., masses, tenderness, scarring)

*Bladder (e.g., fullness, masses, tenderness)

*Vagina (e.g., general appearance, estrogen effect, discharge, lesions, pelvic support, cystocele, rectocele)

*Cervix (e.g., general appearance, lesions, discharge)

*Uterus (e.g., size, contour, position, mobility, tenderness, consistency, descent, or support)

*Adnexa/parametria (e.g., masses, tenderness, organomegaly, nodularity)

*Anus and perineum

*Digital rectal examination, including sphincter tone, presence of hemorrhoids, rectal masses

**Templates and Dictation.** Templates have been developed by the ACOG that allow the physician to check normal and abnormal findings on each element required by the level of physical examination. Dictated examples are available that serve as guides for the physician who desires to meet the element requirements. The following is an example with the elements numbered as they are dictated:

"Recorded vital signs by the medical assistant (1). Mrs. Smith is a well-developed, well-nourished (2) female who is oriented as to time, place, and person (3) and whose mood and affect are appropriate (4). The neck is free of masses or tenderness (5), the thyroid is nontender and there are no masses (6) and there are no lymph nodes palpable (7). The chest is clear to auscultation (8). The heart has no murmurs and the rhythm appears regular (9). The breast exam is negative for any masses, tenderness, nipple discharge (10), or lymph nodes (7). The abdomen is negative for masses or tenderness (11). The liver and spleen are normal (12). There are no hernias (13) or lymph nodes in the groin (7). The external genitalia (14), urethral meatus (15), urethra (16), bladder (17),

|                  | Dx/Mgt Opt      | Amt of Data        | Risk     |
|------------------|-----------------|--------------------|----------|
| Straightforward  | 1 = Minimal     | 1 = Minimal/None   | Minimal  |
| Low Complexity   | 2 = Limited     | 2 = Limited        | Low      |
| Mod Complexity   | 3 = Multiple    | 3 = Moderate       | Moderate |
| High Complexity  | 4+ = Extensive  | 4+ = Extensive     | High     |

vagina (18), and cervix (19) are normal in appearance and are nontender. The pelvic support is normal and there is no cystocele or rectocele. The uterus is normal in shape and nontender (20) and the adnexa are normal in size and nontender (21)."

The purpose of the previous example is to illustrate that the physician will have little trouble in meeting the requirements for the different levels of examination. One could dictate from the example and insert abnormal findings when encountered or check off only elements examined when performing a lower level of examination. Physicians may choose to follow the guidelines in the Multisystem Examination when documenting their physical evaluation. Those guidelines refer to the examination of complete organ systems instead of any selected elements relevant to the history of the present problem.

**Complexity of Medical Decision Making (MDM).** MDM is a measure of the degree of complexity used to establish a diagnosis or select a management option. It includes the number of possible diagnoses or management options that must be considered; the amount and/or complexity of medical records, tests and information that must be obtained and reviewed; and the risk of complications, morbidity, and mortality related to the patient's problem, procedure or management option. There are four types of medical decision making (MDM): straightforward, low complexity, moderate complexity and high complexity. Each level of MDM must be met or exceeded in two of the three categories.

To put all of this together, we can now see how the New Patient and Established Patient visits can be coded. This includes average times for each encounter.

New Patient (requires 3 of 3; or the level of history, examination, and medical decision-making requirements must be met at each code level to be able to use that encounter code)

Established Patient (Requires 2 of 3; or the level of history, examination, and medical decision-making must be met in only 2 of 3 to use that encounter code)

At an established patient visit, 99211, the physician does not need to be present and the nurse can provide the service required by the patient, i.e., injection, immunization, and so forth.

**Documentation Guidelines.** The following is an anonymous poem that the author edited to illustrate the frustration felt by so many physicians as they struggle to follow the documentation requirements.

*To Chart, Or Not To Chart*

In dealing with your patients, don't get the horse behind the cart.
Treatment is not important, but you must complete the CHART!!!
Forget the Labor Room nurse's call, forget the failing heart.
Forget the patient's desperate plight, but please complete the CHART!!!
Code 1 is paging through the halls and the OB's on the cart.
But the doctor cannot come at once, for he's working on the CHART!!!
Save a life, complete a case, you may think you're pretty smart.
But your job is not complete 'til you've signed the blasted CHART!!!
You may have worked from dusk 'til dawn, but you didn't really start.
You may have helped a hundred people, but you must complete the CHART!!!

**The Why of Documentation.** Documentation requirements can frustrate physicians and medical organizations. Some are of the opinion that for outside agencies to come into the physician's office and exam-

| Code  | History                  | Examination              | Medical Decision-Making | Time |
|-------|--------------------------|--------------------------|-------------------------|------|
| 99201 | Problem Focused          | Problem Focused          | Strightforward          | 10   |
| 99202 | Expanded Problem Focused | Expanded Problem Focused | Straightforward         | 20   |
| 99203 | Detailed                 | Detailed                 | Low Complexity          | 30   |
| 99204 | Comprehensive            | Comprehensive            | Moderate Complexity     | 45   |
| 99204 | Comprehensive            | Comprehensive            | High Complexity         | 60   |

| Code | History | Examination | Medical Decision-Making | Time |
|---|---|---|---|---|
| 99211 | N/A | N/A | N/A | 5 |
| 99212 | Problem Focused | Problem Focused | Straightforward | 10 |
| 99213 | Expanded Problem Focused | Expanded Problem Focused | Low Complexity | 15 |
| 99214 | Detailed | Detailed | Moderate Complexity | 25 |
| 99215 | Comprehensive | Comprehensive | High Complexity | 40 |

ine medical records is a violation of doctor-patient confidentiality. Although many physicians may find the new documentation guidelines to be burdensome and time-consuming, the reality is that following these requirements makes the end result a better medical record of what transpired during an office visit, or an outpatient, inpatient, or surgical encounter. This documentation records the medical care provided to the patient, including the rationale for any tests ordered. It serves as a means of gathering statistical information and reduces or eliminates the physician's medicolegal risk by appropriately documenting the medical necessity and risks of the patient's encounter.

**The How of Documentation.** Each physician should choose the type of documentation that best suits his or her practice. Some prefer to dictate on each patient encounter, with a template that outlines this process. Others may prefer to use a checklist for normal and abnormal findings, with a written narrative associated with each abnormal finding. Regardless of the method used, certain laws of documentation are very simple. If a service is not documented, it was, in effect, not performed, and if the physician's note is illegible or incomplete, the service was not performed. The following are a few simple guidelines:

The medical record should be complete and legible.

The documentation of each patient encounter should include:
Reason for the encounter and relevant history, physical examination findings
Assessment, clinical impression, or diagnosis
Plan for care
Rationale for any test ordered
Date and legible identity of the physician
Appropriate health risk factors should be identified
The patient's progress and response to changes in treatment with revision of diagnosis should be documented
The CPT and ICD-9-CM codes reported on the claim form or billing statement should be supported by documentation in the medical record.

For consultations, document a report to the referring physician.
Don't stamp "Dictated but not proofread" on notes.
The physician must always sign notes or chart transcriptions.

**Modifiers.** A modifier indicates to the insurer that the physician is reporting the service or that the procedure has been altered by a specific condition. There is a complete listing and description of all modifiers in Appendix A of the CPT book. Physicians should only use modifiers when necessary, because many insurance companies handle these claims separately and thus may delay payment. The modifier tells the payer that an unusual situation has occurred (e.g., the service was performed by two surgeons, the service or procedure was increased or reduced, only part of the service was performed, this was a very unusual and difficult service or procedure).

**Consultations.** A consultation is a service provided by a physician whose opinion or advice regarding the evaluation or management (or both) of a specific problem is requested by another physician. The physician may initiate diagnostic or therapeutic (or both) services at the time of the consultation, but from that day on, the patient is considered an established patient. The request for the consultation from the attending physician must be documented in the patient's medical record. ("I was asked to see Mrs. Jones in consultation by Dr. Smith regarding....") A consultation initiated by a patient or the patient's family is reported, using the confirmatory consultation codes. After completion of the consultation, if the consultant assumes responsibility for management of a portion or all of the patient's condition, the subsequent hospital care codes or established patient codes should be used.

**International Classification of Diseases, 9th Revision, Clinical Modification (ICD-9-CM).** ICD-9-CM is a diagnostic coding system that arranges illnesses, diseases, syndromes, or symptoms into groups according to established criteria. Based on the World

Health Organization's 9th Revision, International Classification of Diseases, ICD-9-CM codes consist of three, four or five numbers with a description. Volume I is the Tabular List, which consists of numerical categories, subcategories and subclassifications of diseases. Volume I contains the codes that are used to describe the symptom or disease diagnosed at the patient's encounter. Volume II is the Alphabetic Index, which is organized by terms that identify diseases and conditions. There are 12,000 codes in the Tabular List and over 120,000 codes in the Alphabetic Index. Volume II is useful in finding the location of a subject within the Tabular List.

As with the CPT book, it is imperative that the physician read the notes and guidelines before selecting an ICD-9 code. The physician should code to the highest level of specificity that most accurately describes the condition or symptom. All codes in the Obstetric Chapter of ICD-9 require a fifth digit except:

Three-digit codes:
- 630 Hydatidiform Mole
- 631 Other Abnormal Products of Conception
- 632 Missed Abortion
- 650 Normal Delivery
- 677 Late Effect of Complications of Pregnancy

Four-digit codes:
- 633.0 Ectopic Pregnancy
- 638.0 Failed Attempted Abortion
- 639.0 Complication Following Abortion or Ectopic or Molar Pregnancies

The Obstetric Chapter defines two different sets of five-digit subclassifications. The ICD-9 codes representing abortion (634–637) require that the current status be identified in the fifth digit as:

0 = Unspecified
1 = Incomplete
2 = Complete

ICD-9 codes 640–648 and 651–676 require that the current episode of care be identified in the fifth digit as:

0 = Unspecified as to episode of care or not applicable
1 = Delivered, with or without mention of antepartum condition
2 = Delivered, with mention of postpartum complication
3 = Antepartum condition or complication
4 = Postpartum condition or complication

Insurance companies make judgments about the levels of patient care provided by hospitals, using data such as length of stay and case mix index (based on correct coding principles). The physician can justify the need for a test, a procedure, or a hospitalization by proper use of ICD-9 codes. Appropriate ICD-9 codes have been required on Medicare claim forms since 1989 and other insurance companies adopted this requirement shortly thereafter.

In addition to the numeric codes, there are specific codes known as V codes that are used to identify encounters with patients who seek care for reasons other than illness or injury. V codes include categories such as: Examination, History, Observation, or Supervision. There are no codes available that the physician can use to rule out a condition. The symptoms must be coded or the results of the test or biopsy can be entered. Most physicians' offices use a Super bill (available from ACOG) that has a detailed list of ICD-9 codes on the back of the sheet. Physicians are required to list the appropriate ICD-9 code to justify any laboratory test they order. They are also asked to list appropriate ICD-9 code, or codes, (often two or three) on each insurance claim to provide a rationale for the procedures performed or medical services given to the patient. Just as the laboratory test requires an ICD-9 code to be linked to the test ordered, each medical or surgical service must be accompanied by a linked diagnostic code.

# Conclusion

It must be emphasized that the physician needs to be aware of modern coding practices for appropriate documentation and billing. Although traditional medical education may not provide significant training in how to use to CPT, ICD-9, and E&M coding, the contemporary physician is responsible for using accurate coding to abide by insurance and federal regulations. Although this chapter provided a brief overview of the basic practice of coding, physicians need to conduct regular review of CPT and ICD-9-CM current coding guidelines.

## REFERENCES

International Classification of Diseases, ICD-CM. Vol 1, 2, 11th rev ed. Dover, DE, American Medical Association, 1999.

Physicians' Current Procedural Terminology CPT 99. Chicago, American Medical Association, 1999.

# 76

# A Review of Medical Informatics

ANEEL ADVANI
YUVAL SHAHAR

Although medical education concentrates on the biologic basis of health, information sciences provide much of the applied research and clinical practice of medicine. In the tradition of the early epidemiologists and biostatisticians of the 19th century, medical informatics seeks to make the daily practice of medicine more driven by data. The ability of physicians to stay abreast of developments in the increasingly specialized practice of modern medicine is becoming more difficult as the amount of medical information explodes. Physicians must be knowledgeable about the cost of integrating new medical knowledge and clinical policies into their daily practice. They must also be aware of the increasing pressure to be efficient in administering medical care and the consequent need to make their clinical time free from unnecessary administrative overhead. It is, therefore, not surprising that the size of the market for clinical information systems (including services), estimated as $14 billion in 1996, is projected to escalate to $22 billion by the year 2000. Indeed, the total size of the market for better computerized information systems in healthcare must be close to 15% of total health care expenditures currently devoted to information management activities. This places the potential size of the medical informatics market at approximately $150 billion a year.

Medical informatics has been formally defined as "the field that concerns itself with the cognitive, information processing, and communication tasks of medical practice, education, and research, including the information science and technology to support these tasks." Evident in the definition is the multidisciplinary nature of research and practice in medical informatics. Medical informatics draws on computer science, artificial intelligence, decision theory, statistics, cognitive science, information management, health policies, and, of course, the medical sciences for information. This interdisciplinary approach and the requirement that systems have clinical or policy applications distinguishes the field from computer science. Indeed, medical informatics is one of a number of new fields concerned with information processing and information management carried out in particular knowledge contexts.

## The Computer-Based Patient Record

One of the main projects of medical informatics has been the development of the computer-based patient record (CPR). Progress has been slow, although the investment in CPRs has risen steadily. Only 2% of respondents in the annual Healthcare Information and Management Society's 1998 Leadership Survey of chief information officers said their hospital or health plan had an operational CPR. However, more than 35% of respondents said their hospital or health plan had either begun an implementation or had plans to do so. Moreover, the size of the market for CPRs was projected to grow from $100 million in 1995 to over $1.5 billion by the year 2000. This is the result of two main factors. The first is the need to consolidate and leverage population-based information about patients and care within large multihospital integrated delivery systems. The second is the continual decrease in the price of computer and communication technologies and the increase in general access to these areas. Both of these trends have emphasized the advantages of CPRs over traditional paper-based record systems. It is estimated that the total cost of information handling is 25% of the operating budget of a hospital. The average time that a hospital worker spends on information handling is also about 25%. Thus, it is not surprising that the inefficient paper-based methods we use today substantially increase overall health costs. Indeed, one estimate places the cost of medical care using paper records and inefficient management of clinical information at a 6% premium over care provided in settings that use CPRs.

The main advantage of the CPR in an integrated delivery system is its ability to be used by many people at the same time, making it a tool for better organizational workflow. Moreover, a computer-based record can be tailored to meet the needs of particular classes of users. This function allows systems to be built so that unauthorized access can be minimized, even as the number of locations from which data in the medical record can be accessed increases greatly. The Internet, with its vision of distributed information transfers, has the potential to transform an institutional CPR into a mechanism that allows access to a patient's information by the right person at the right time. Such a scenario would be virtually impossible to imagine with current paper-based medical charts. With the increasing number of professionals involved in any patient's medical care, the CPR becomes a very important method of communicating between providers so that there is a longitudinal and comprehensive record of the care a patient has received. The use of a CPR also opens the way to add greater functionality so that it is not just a passive record of medical care. The views, or screens, in the CPR can be tailored to specific needs, such as ward lists for nursing shifts or office visits to outpatient physicians. The incorporation of imaging data with the rest of the medical record is another great advantage of using CPRs. Other more sophisticated functions that can be incorporated into the CPR are drug-dose checking during order entry, patient-specific decision-support for guideline-oriented care, real-time event monitoring, and concurrent quality assurance. Thus, the CPR is the foundation for many tools and strategies that seek to improve the quality of medical care.

Despite the considerable advantages and decreasing costs of using computerized medical record systems, and despite more than 30 years devoted to researching and developing of CPRs, they have not attained widespread use. Because the CPR has been slow to be adopted, it follows that the most advanced CPRs are still in the domain of academic medical centers, which have pioneered research in this area. Some of the most innovative systems being used today include the Regenstrief Medical Information System (RMIS) at the University of Indiana, the COSTAR system at the Massachusetts General Hospital and its commercial derivatives, and the TMR system at Duke University Hospital. The variation in the quality and sophistication of medical record systems are a testament to the fact that this is still a cottage industry. All but the five largest companies earn less than $200 million in revenue, and the largest has less than $1 billion dollars. In fact, more than 230 different vendors of electronic medical records exist for the acute care hospital setting alone.

What then are the barriers to adopting CPRs, and what solutions can we propose to hasten their deployment? Perhaps the greatest barrier arises from the observation that CPRs are not just software artifacts. CPRs create major changes in the process of daily medical care. These involve behavior changes and new skill learning on the part of clinical and administrative personnel. These changes are difficult to effect within the organization. However, the increases in cost and regulatory pressures from outside healthcare organizations have made the behavioral and organizational changes increasingly more palatable to clinical workers. Moreover, dealing with the technology of computers still does not approach the ease of using paper records, in spite of the institutional payoffs in adopting them. Designing a CPR that will induce physicians to give up the easy-to-use paper record has been a veritable challenge for researchers in medical informatics. However, the increasing need to develop clinical information systems in hospitals as opposed to administrative systems is causing vendors to take this problem extremely seriously. One solution to the user interface problem is to wait for new technologies to be more cost-effective, such as pen-based computing and voice recognition. Another is to load the CPR system with collateral functions, such as guideline for decision-support (see section entitled Implementation and Evaluation of Clinical Information Systems), literature searching, and paperless order entry so that there is more of an incentive to use the system. However, the issue of how to capture clinical data efficiently, without duress for the user, is an active area of research. Moreover, computer-based record systems impose rigorous constraints on entry of structured data into a system, such as predefined vocabularies and rules for manipulating information. Thus, the implementation of CPRs must be carried out with these issues of information management and human-computer interaction in mind.

## Implementation and Evaluation of Clinical Information Systems

The successful adoption of a CPR system or any other major information technology endeavor depends largely on the fit between the planning process and the nature of the organization. Traditionally, industrial engineering employs a "plan, prototype, implement, evaluate" sequence in implementing a new system. However, this process requires that everyone in the organization share a common goal, which is usually imposed in a top-down fashion. Health-care organizations do not fit well into this straightforward model. There are many more competitive but independent constituencies in health-care organizations; this is especially true of physician groups, which have different needs from hospital administrators or the purchasers of health care. Therefore, planning for buy-in from these constituencies before any implementation is begun is an essential factor in the success or failure of a CPR deployment. A useful way of solving this problem is to appoint an information technology leader from each of the various constituencies and let a hybrid committee of these individuals form a centralized decision-making body. Finally, it is important that the institution's strategic leadership be involved in the process in a meaningful way, and that the information technology leadership be involved in the strategic leadership of the organization as a whole.

One of the greatest challenges in adopting an electronic medical record is the need to satisfy many different information needs in the health-care system. These can vary from the requirements of the different constituencies in the healthcare industry to the various departments in a hospital. To understand how to use and implement a CPR system effectively, we must first understand who are the users of the information and what their needs are. Physicians may be surprised to learn of the number of other interests that are involved in the flow of information and the right to ownership of a particular patient's data. These parties can be divided into primary users and secondary users. Primary users of the patient record include physicians and clinic and hospital staff. Secondary users include the various classes of purchasers of healthcare, such as insurance companies, managed care organizations, and government administrators of Medicaid and Medicare. Other users are the public health agencies, pharmaceutical companies, welfare programs, medical and social scientific agencies, and the legal profession. Because there are greater uses for these aggregate data under pressure of capitated healthcare, we now have the beginnings of a large industry involved in brokering sizable databases of medical information. Information management for population-based care is thus an important function, with tremendous consequences for health-care organizations. However, the use of medical information in a manner that acts against the health or privacy of an individual patient—even if it helps with the optimization of care for patient populations—is a contentious issue. There are many places in the daily flow of health information that can lead to unethical or even fraudulent aggregations of health information for proprietary gains. The intelligent design of a CPR and its implementation must address these important issues.

Another challenge in the effective deployment of a computer-based hospital or clinical information system is the presence of legacy systems with specialized functions for individual clinical and administrative departments. These might include specialized systems adopted over the years for laboratory results, pharmacy inventory and order systems, physician dictation systems, and radiology picture archival and communication systems (PACS). These systems may reside on different physical networks and computer software architectures, may employ different medical vocabularies for similar concepts, and may differ in the levels of clinical record granularity. So in addition to the front-end issues of physician-computer interface and data discussed above, there are significant back-end issues of systems integration and standardization that must be resolved.

As an example of a departmental computer system, we describe the PACS used in the more advanced radiology departments today. The major difference between the older radiology departmental information systems and the new PACS systems is the inclusion of imaging data along with clinical interpretations in the system. Such a system has the advantage of allowing images to be read asynchronously from various sites by radiologists and transmitted to other departmental systems, if necessary. Thus, PACS systems are illustrative of clinical information systems rather than administrative systems, which allow the radiology department to function without a film storage room. The advantages of using a PACS system are exemplified in an analysis of costs relating to an implementation at the Medical University of South

Carolina. Out of a total budget of $7 million that was depreciated over 5 years, the yearly savings of $1,190,000 was a result of from not having to pay for film processing, associated personnel, physical space to store the films. Thus, the adoption of a PACS system was budget-neutral counting direct costs alone. Moreover, under the older system, films were lost at a rate of 3% a year, requiring nonreimbursable repeated imaging. Reducing this loss rate to essentially zero resulted in further indirect cost savings of $2 million in charges. This was all in addition to the savings derived from improved productivity.

The analysis of lower effective costs for an electronic patient record as a result of reduction in costs associated with paper-based records carries over to the rest of the hospital as well. Most states have a statutory requirement that the medical records for patients must be stored by providers for a period of time between 3 and 7 years after the last encounter. In practice, most hospitals preserve patient data until the statutory period has expired after the patient is deceased. This creates a need for a large budget for storage and retrieval of paper-based records. The adoption of an electronic record can, therefore, result in significant savings in the hospital's operating costs.

## Telemedicine and the Internet

Newer communication technologies have revolutionized the way information systems are set up in integrated delivery systems. Moreover, they have the potential to dramatically change the way patients and physicians communicate with each other. Along with the increases in bandwidth (the capability to carry bits of information), through which the average household can access the Internet, the potential for carrying medical information suitable for diagnosis and patient management has increased greatly. This has given rise to the concept of telemedicine, defined as the use of electronic information and communication technologies to provide and support health care when distance separates the participants. Moreover, the new medium of the Internet has fundamentally changed the ability of patients to access health information relating to their own particular conditions. This phenomenon will fundamentally change the nature of the physician-patient interaction for well-educated patients. This section covers telemedicine and its attendant challenges and then discusses the more general role of the Internet in disseminating health information to patients and consumers of health care. The most important driver of telemedicine applications is the wish to improve access to specialized care for segments of the population who have historically been underserved. For rural areas especially, telemedicine has come to be seen as a major technology for improving the quality of health care. Although teleradiology has been the most frequent and direct application of the technologies involved in telemedicine, projects in other specialties do exist. So far, only in teleradiology does the Medicare and the insurance infrastructure routinely provide reimbursement on par with on-site consultation. New legislative efforts, however, are sure to change reimbursement patterns. On Jan. 1, 1999, rural health-care providers in shortage areas began to receive fee-for-service reimbursement from the Health Care Financing Administration (HCFA), although in other areas, reimbursement in HCFA programs is limited to capitated services. In Texas, state law provides reimbursement for Medicaid recipients who are treated via telemedicine at the same rate as for those who have face-to-face consultations. California also reimburses at the same level, and goes even farther by prohibiting private health plans from proscribing payment for telemedicine services. At least part of the explanation for the growth of telemedicine has been the cost pressures facing academic medical centers. Telemedicine has the potential to become a new source of revenue for major medical centers that are seeking to export their "product" or expertise to markets that are less well served by specialty or tertiary medical care.

However, the widespread adoption of telemedicine faces some roadblocks. First, the cost of telemedicine systems can be prohibitive for the types of rural practices it seeks to improve. Second, even in California and Texas, although government programs have agreed to cover telemedicine consultations, some private insurers and health management organizations (HMOs) are still deciding whether or not to support this technology. In spite of the legal mandate, the guidelines for the reimbursement of telemedicine have not been elucidated. In California, for instance, telemedicine consultations are only reimbursable if the care can be shown to be equal in quality to face-to-face consultation and if the face-to-face consultations are not cost-effective. These policies have slowed the rate of adoption of telemedicine until private reimbursement schedules encourage it.

The Internet serves not only as a new communication medium for images and text but also as a vast library of information. This second property of the computer network has allowed both provider and consumer alike to have timely access to information in a way never before imagined. The major challenge for the patient, as well as the physician, is to be sure that high-quality medical information is available on the Internet. One approach to this problem is by editing sites to select those of high quality. This is the strategy adopted by the Department of Health and Human Services. Their consumer health information World Wide Web site (at the Internet address http://www.healthfinder.gov) is an excellent example of a carefully edited selection of resources available

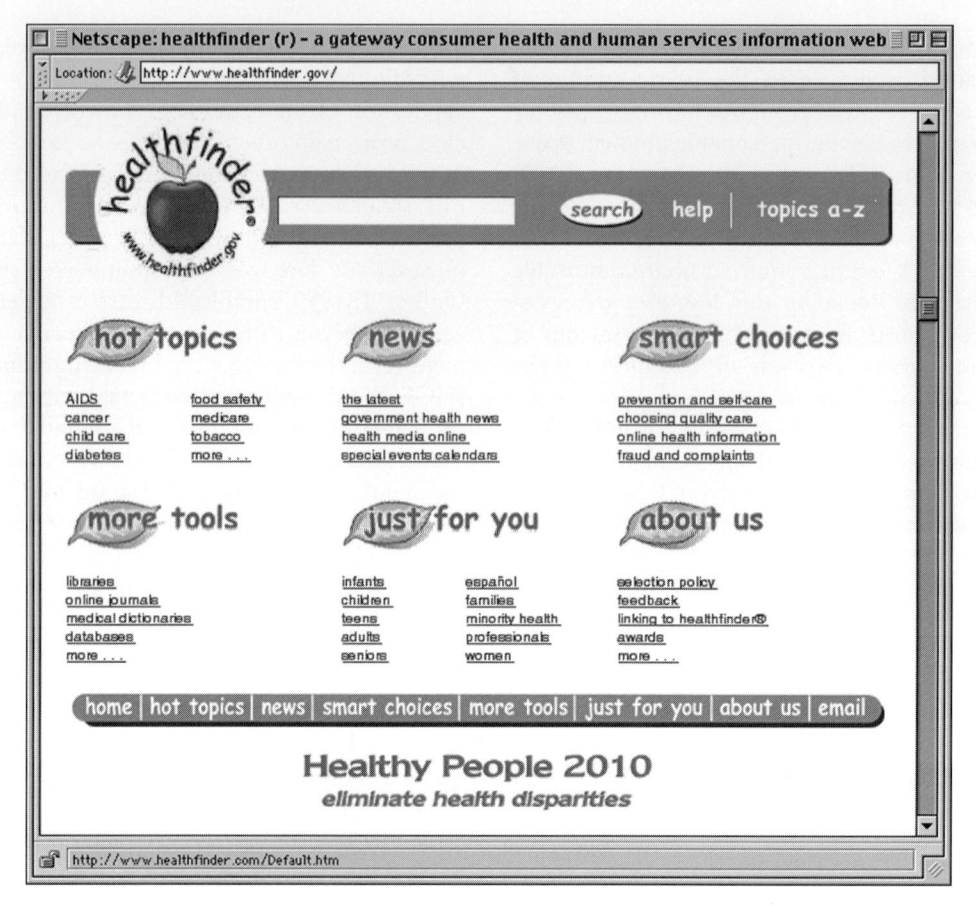

**Figure 76–1** The Federal Government's Consumer Health Information Web Site (http://www.healthfinder.gov). Note the range of disease-specific information available, the ready access to the medical literature through online medical journals, and a public gateway to Medline. Also note the access to quality of care and comparative provider information.

for patients on the Internet (Fig. 76–1). Patients who have specific conditions can now join discussion groups and electronic mail lists for mutual information and support. The common experience of illness admits a kind of peer review, exerting its own quality control on the information that is posted to the various forums. Formal rating systems are also being developed to guide consumers in their use of medical information available on the Internet. Finally, the importance of federal policies in enforcing proscriptions against the unlawful practice of medicine on the Internet will also be important in guarding against abuse of the new medium.

## Importance of Data Standards

Up to this point, we have emphasized the role of computers and automation in storing and transporting information throughout the healthcare system and, indeed, between medical caregivers and their patients. However, simply storing and transporting computerized copies of text or images is not enough to automate the *information processing* that takes place in health care. For computers to transform and process data meaningfully, the data, whether text or images, must be stored in a structured way. The structure of the data enables the computer to transform the symbols and pixels that make up the raw electronic copies of what we see into a comprehensible paper-based medical record. However, this structure cannot be assembled by the computer from the data alone. In order to add semantic meaning to the data, standards defined by consensus between interested professionals and end-users must be developed. These standard vocabularies or *data dictionaries* specify the relationship between particular symbols or words that are stored in the computer and the meanings of these symbols. In addition, standard *messaging protocols* define how a set of symbols must precede or follow other symbols representing particular concepts. This is similar to the function of a dictionary and grammar in defining the semantics of human languages.

These vocabulary standards are appropriately confined to textual rather than imaging data and are referred to as *controlled medical vocabularies*. A controlled medical vocabulary is a list of words that identifies a term in an ordered relation with the others in the list. For example, a hierarchic controlled vocabulary would place "anticonvulsant" under the category "drug" and have "phenobarbital" under it. Perhaps the most famous of the standardized codes for medicine are the Current Procedural Terminology (CPT) codes owned by the American Medical Association and the International Classification of Diseases (ICD-10PCS) generated by the World Health Organization. However, these coding systems were designed for more limited tasks, such as billing receipts and maintaining vital statistics records, than those required of full-blown CPR systems and medical decision-support systems. For example, neither of the latter two systems would have the vocabulary for representing all the words and concepts used in a postoperative report or a recovery room progress note. To correct these deficiencies, many medical and informatics organizations have expended large efforts to create vocabularies that incorporate hundreds of thousands of terms each. The most comprehensive of these vocabularies are the Systematic Nomenclature of Human and Veterinary Medicine (SNOMED) compiled by the American College of Pathologists and the Read Codes from the National Health Service in Britain. Even these large vocabulary standards, however, are not completely successful in capturing concepts used in hospital or outpatient practice. A recent comparative study found that SNOMED captured only 70% and the Read Codes only 57% of the desired concepts in the medical record.

Messaging protocols include standards for both textual and imaging data. The overarching effort in this area is the protocol called Health Level Seven (HL7), which includes a message protocol called the Digital Imaging and Communications in Medicine (DICOM) standard as one of its components. The HL7 standard specifies the sequence and format of messages sent between computer systems that incorporate information from a computer-based record system. Thus, it includes standards for specifying lab test codes and names, order entry codes, financial billing data, admission discharge and transfer information, codes for data from bedside electronic monitoring equipment, and so on. The DICOM standard defines protocols for specifying the method of compression and encoding of images to data streams when images are exchanged between computer systems. It also standardizes information about the image, such as whether data represent an ultrasonographic image or a computed tomographic (CT) scan, and what type of file format was used when an encoded image was stored in an archive. However, in spite of the prevalence of numerous standards, there remain tremendous challenges in ensuring their continued development and implementation by the vendor community. Transparent application-level interoperability between disparate CPRs remains a distant goal.

# Medical Decision-Support Systems

The practice of medicine is founded on making the right medical decisions. It is no surprise that major efforts of medical informaticians have been directed at the problem of medical decision-making in automating medical practice. The science of automated medical decision-making requires not just the use of advanced computer science and technology but an understanding of how human physicians use information and reason to make decisions. We have discussed in the last section the need for high-quality data to ensure that high-quality decisions are made; hence, there is a need for data standards. Modern physicians must also have access to up-to-date medical knowledge, a function that can be fulfilled by information retrieval systems and the Internet. However, physicians also make decisions by employing appropriate problem-solving methods that allow them to carry out tasks and process information into medical decisions. It is in the automation and modeling of these problem-solving methods that much of the research on computer-assisted medical decision-making has concentrated.

Most clinical decision-support systems in use today are based on two main methods: those based on quantitative approaches, using statistical reasoning or Bayesian decision theory; and those based on symbolic logical reasoning, using first- or second-generation expert systems. As we shall see, some very modern systems have begun to incorporate ideas from both of these areas.

The first medical decision-support systems addressed the task of diagnosis. In the 1950s and 1960s, these systems concentrated on specific clinical areas such as cardiac defects or abdominal pain. These early systems illustrated the first uses of automated reasoning based on probabilistic decision theory. A more modern example of the use of decision-analytic techniques in clinical medicine is the PANDA project at Stanford University. The PANDA project uses several techniques from the area of decision analysis and focuses on the domain of prenatal diagnosis, aiming to provide decision support to physicians, genetic consultants, and patients.

Prenatal testing for defects of development is widely available. Potentially devastating outcomes can now be averted by use of tests such as amniocentesis (AC), whereby amniotic fluid is aspirated from the womb for chromosomal analysis and biochemical testing; chorionic villus sampling (CVS); and high-resolution ultrasonography (HRUS).

Unfortunately, tests are costly, and both AC and CVS carry a significant risk of inducing miscarriages.

At present, AC with cytogenetic evaluation of the fetus is recommended for mothers who are older than 35 years of age and who, therefore, are at comparatively high risk for carrying a baby with Down syndrome (DS) and who would consider termination. However, the scope of the current guidelines, such as those that have appeared in the technical bulletins of the American College of Obstetricians and Gynecologists, is quite limited. Down syndrome is not the only defect that can be diagnosed by AC; for instance, a higher-than-normal measurement of alpha-fetoprotein (AFP) in the amniotic fluid provides evidence of the possibility of open neural–tube defect (ONTD). Alternatively, developmental defects, such as ONTD, can be detected early in the second trimester by the HRUS test. Furthermore, the parents' individual *preferences* regarding termination vs. the risk of lifelong disability, as well as local variability in procedural risks, usually are not taken into account in the decision about which, if any, prenatal diagnostic modality should be used. Parents, genetic consultants, and attending physicians require significant support in making this decision. Such a decision should be based on patient preferences, local procedural risks, and complete patient history (including previous tests, such as maternal serum alpha-fetoprotein [MS-AFP]). Using only arbitrary cutoff values (e.g., maternal age), considering only one disorder at a time, or including only one test procedure oversimplifies the prenatal testing decision.

The PANDA project uses methods oriented toward decision-analysis, probability-utility, to model the prenatal diagnosis problem as a series of decisions (e.g., whether to perform CVS perform AC or terminate pregnancy). The model considers the best known data regarding population- and patient-specific previous probabilities for all relevant diagnoses, parent-specific acquired preferences and outcome utilities, and risks of all procedures. One of the main tools used by the PANDA project is an influence diagram. The influence diagram is similar in function to a decision tree. A decision tree is a well-known method of representing decisions, outcomes, probability of outcomes given each decision, and value of each outcome. A decision tree becomes cumbersome, however, for even a moderate number of potential decisions and outcomes, and it becomes unmanageable if there are a large number of these. An influence diagram is a graphic representation that is equivalently expressive but much easier to grasp intuitively. It represents (Fig. 76–2) probable relations between decisions (squares), chance variables and outcomes (ellipses), and utilities (diamonds).

The usefulness of various outcomes and, in particular, termination, was expressed via the parents' preference probability for that outcome using a version of Paukers' method. Using Paukers' method, the termination option is presented to the parents for evaluation by comparing it to a gamble between two outcomes (Fig. 76–3). The gamble compares the parents' preferences for having a healthy baby with the certain risk of having a baby with a severe, life-long, debili-

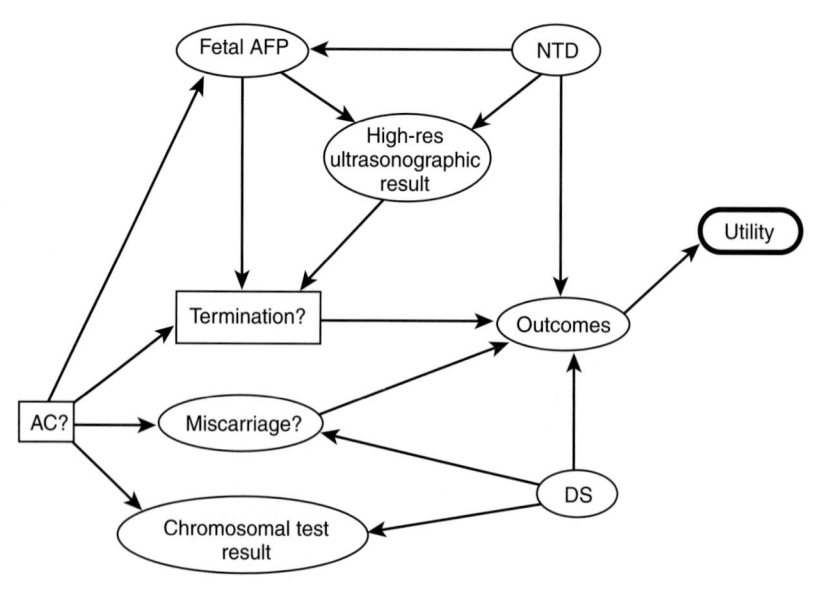

**Figure 76–2** A simplified influence diagram for an amniocentesis (AC) decision with personal utilities. The AC decision affects the miscarriage rate as well as whether the results of fetal alpha-fetoprotein (AFP) and chromosomal typing will be known at the time of the termination decision. Down syndrome (DS) and neural tube defects (NTDs) are not directly observable, but must be deduced indirectly by results of various tests, such as high-resolution ultrasonography or amniocentesis. These chance nodes have previous probabilities that depend on age, history, and previous tests. Outcomes, such as a healthy baby, an induced abortion, or a life-long disability (LLD), have a certain distribution for any combination of conditioning chance nodes and decisions. Their utility measure is computed by the preference probability of each outcome.

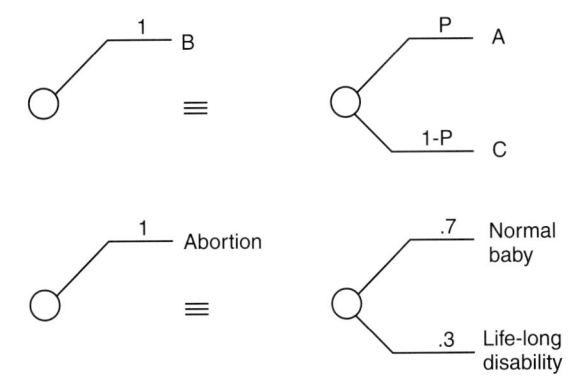

**Figure 76-3** The preference probabilities model as used in the Paukers' Method. If obtaining prospect B with certainty is equivalent to obtaining the best prospect A with probability P or the worst prospect C with probability 1-P, then the preference probability of B is P. In the example shown, the parents are indifferent to either an immediate abortion or continuing the pregnancy with a .7 chance of a normal baby and a .3 chance of life-long disability. Their preference probability of abortion is, therefore, .7.

tating disease (LLD). The lower the risk of LLD for which the parents would prefer termination of the pregnancy rather than continue the pregnancy at that level of risk, the higher the usefulness of termination as an outcome.

The results of the analysis can be presented graphically as a set of decision curves (Fig. 76-4). These curves and the computerized recommendations based on them can be used by patients, genetic counselors, and obstetricians to actually make the decision whether to perform amniocentesis. For example, consider a hospital where the risk of abortion as a result of AC only is 3 per 1000 tests, and a couple has a preference probability of 0.5 for termination. With this preference level for termination, the minimal probability of having a baby with Down's syndrome after having AC is .0045. This means for instance, that a 35-year-old woman whose pregnancy revealed such data would be advised to undergo AC, because her previous risk of DS was 0.005. However, if her preference probability for termination were 0.1, she should not undergo AC; the risk of miscarriage as a result of AC would be too great. Alternatively, a preference probability of 0.9 would in these circumstances justify performing AC regardless of the woman's age, because the previous cutoff was only 0.0003, which is less than the previous known probability of approximately 0.0007 for DS. These results would also change if the underlying rate of miscarriage caused by AC were higher than 0.3%. Note that the final decision curves also depend, albeit to a minor extent, on the previous probability of neural tube defects (NTDs). The risk of NTD affects the decision only in close cases; however, because high-resolution ultrasonography is a fairly sensitive and specific test for detecting the presence of NTD. Thus, the preferences concerning amniocentesis are less affected by the NTD probabilities.

Another powerful method for automating the reasoning in medical decision-making, which uses symbolically logical relationships rather than quantitative probabilities, is called *expert systems* or *knowledge-based systems*. The first and most famous expert system used in the field of medicine was the MYCIN system. The MYCIN program was used to diagnose and recommend treatment of patients who had various infections. The medical knowledge of MYCIN was not encoded in utilities and outcomes, but instead in *production rules*. These rules were "knowledge packets" about infections in the form of *if-then* statements derived from experts. Starting with the goal of identifying an organism, MYCIN searched through all the rules and selected one that would help this goal. MYCIN then examined what it would take to make the premises of this rule true. It would either query the physician for laboratory data, or search for other rules whose conclusions supported or refuted the premises of that rule. Thus, the premises of rules became hooks into conclusions of other rules until the goal was achieved. The reasoning mechanism in MYCIN was thus referred to as *goal-directed backward chaining*. First-generation expert systems used both

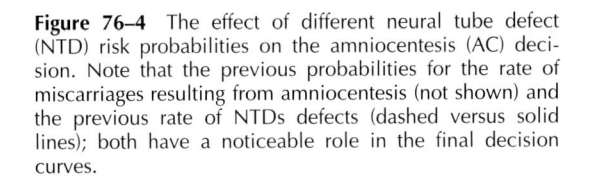

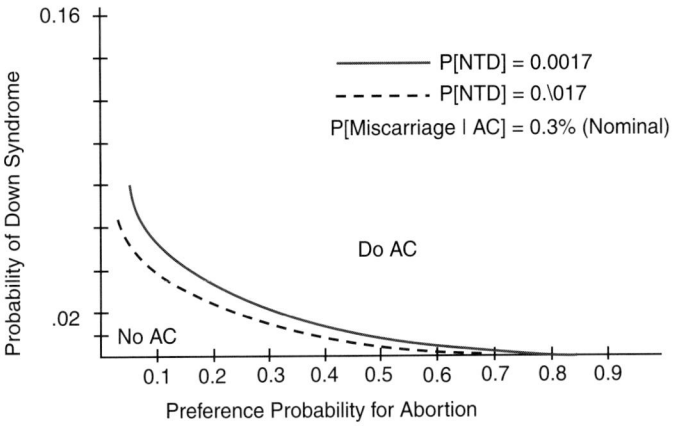

**Figure 76-4** The effect of different neural tube defect (NTD) risk probabilities on the amniocentesis (AC) decision. Note that the previous probabilities for the rate of miscarriages resulting from amniocentesis (not shown) and the previous rate of NTDs defects (dashed versus solid lines); both have a noticeable role in the final decision curves.

backward chaining and its analog, *forward chaining*, for their inference mechanisms. Although MYCIN was never used clinically, in subsequent evaluations the advice derived from this program was shown to be on par with that of an infectious disease consultant. Because of the separation of the knowledge base from the reasoning mechanism, the knowledge base itself could be modified and updated without reprogramming the MYCIN program itself. MYCIN introduced the concept of capturing ill-structured expert medical knowledge into structured representations that supported automatic reasoning. Both of these innovations were fundamental to the future development of second-generation, knowledge-based systems.

The Asgaard system (Fig. 76-5) is an example of the second generation of expert systems that began to appear in the late 1980s. These systems extend the features of MYCIN-like programs so that they can be used in broader contexts. A number of new inference methods, dubbed problem-solving methods (PSMs), can now supplement the older forward and backward chaining algorithms. The new inference mechanisms operate on "knowledge packets" that are more complex than production rules. We now use *frames*, which are like fill-in-the-blank cue cards, that can accommodate more complex relationships between the fields than the premise-conclusion pairs in production rules. The structure of the frames can change from one PSM to the next. Thus the *knowledge representation systems*, that is, the languages to store knowledge packets, have become considerably more robust since the days of production rules. Knowledge acquisition requires expensive time of experts and requires them to think about intuitive and second-nature problem-solving strategies in an explicit and structured way. Because knowledge acquisition is certainly the most difficult and time-consuming part of building knowledge-based systems, this situation is referred to as the knowledge acquisition bottleneck. Improvements in knowledge representation and creation of graphic user interfaces for collecting knowledge from experts have done much to alleviate the bottleneck.

Knowledge-based systems can be used not only for decision support for individual clinicians but also for support of clinical policies in health-care institutions. The Asgaard system also illustrates this class of decision-support systems. As can be seen from the architecture, the system includes a language that can be used to encode specific clinical guidelines. For example, the specification may encode a guideline for management of gestational diabetes (Fig. 76-6). The Asgaard system uses this specification to generate recommendations for care based on the current patient data in the clinical information system. The use of a database mediator to obtain time-stamped data automatically and abstract patterns from them (for example, a pattern of low blood sugar values) is an exciting development in medical expert systems. This function can be used to help implement patient-

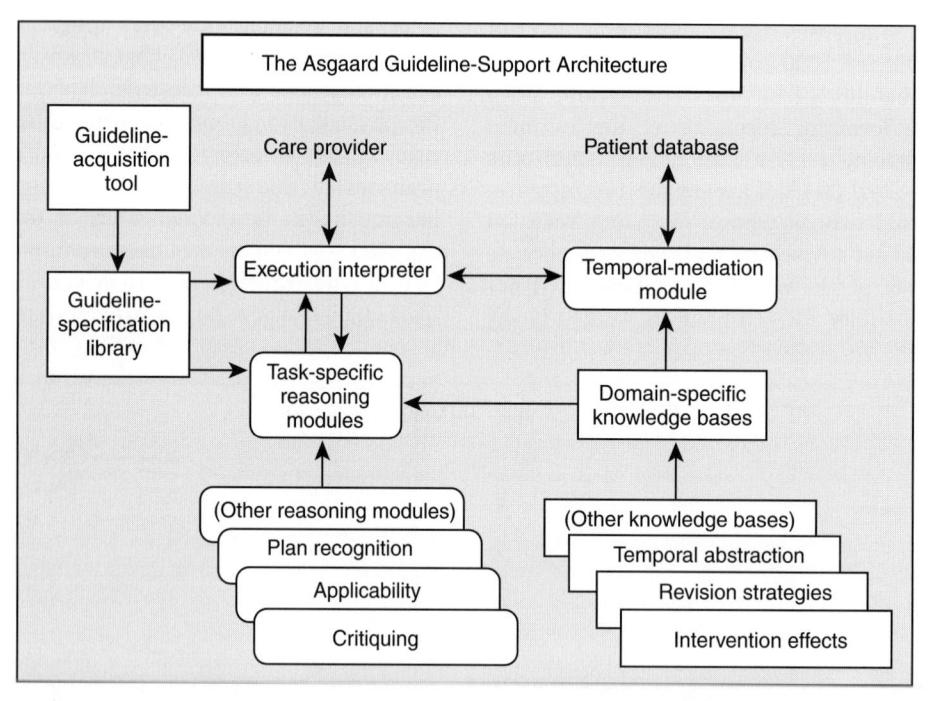

**Figure 76-5** The Asgaard system for guideline-based decision support. Note that the architecture represents second-generation extensions in expert systems, such as multiple reasoning methods, direct database access with temporal abstractions, a graphic knowledge acquisition tool, and the separation of guideline specifications from general medical domain knowledge. The medical knowledge is now stored in *frames* in the domain-specific knowledge bases.

```
(PLAN observing-GDM-Type-II

    (INTENTION: INTERMEDIATE-STATE
        (MAINTAIN STATE (blood-glucose)
        (NORMAL | SLIGHTLY-HIGH) GDM-Type-II
            [[24 G-WEEKS, 24 G-WEEKS], [DELIVERY, DELIVERY],
                [_,_]] CONCEPTION)

    (FILTER-PRECONDITION (one-hour-GTT (140, 200) pregnancy
        [[24 G-WEEKS, 24 G-WEEKS], [26 G-WEKKS, 26 G-WEEKS],
            [_,_]] CONCEPTION)

    (SUSPEND-CONDITION (STATE (blood-glucose) HIGH GDM-Type-II
        [[24,24], [DELIVERY, DELIVERY], [_,_]] CONCEPTION
        [[G-WEEK, G-WEEK], [G-WEEK, G-WEEK], [_,_]])

    (DO-ALL-TOGETHER
        (glucose-monitoring)
        (nutrition-management)
        (observe-insulin-indicators))
```

**Figure 76–6** An Asbru syntax example: Gestational diabetes mellitus guideline specification. This part of the guideline specifies the entry and exit conditions and the overall plan intentions in monitoring and managing the condition. This formal text represents the output of the graphic knowledge acquisition tool referred to in the previous figure.

specific best practices during care, which are based on an institution's clinical policies. Moreover, the system can also be used retrospectively to compare the care that was actually given to the patient with what was recommended. This compromise can automatically produce quality reports that dynamically improve compliance with best practices.

## Bioinformatics

Medicine in the next century will be increasingly dependent on the presence of *genomic information*, which includes genetic and protein sequences along with their correlated biologic functions. This information will be both population-based and patient-specific. The science of using computational techniques to produce, analyze, and manage this molecular biologic information is called *bioinformatics*. The molecular information that bioinformatics seeks to analyze includes the output of the Human Genome Project, as well as patient-specific sequencing data that will be commonly available using *gene chips*. A broader definition of bioinformatics would include the analysis of protein sequences and their structures as well as population genetics and genetic epidemiology. However, the main program of the field is currently analysis and management of gene sequence and protein sequence data. The application of bioinformatics will produce a revolution in the field of genetic counseling. Hence, perhaps the first medical specialty to be profoundly affected by advances in this field will be obstetrics and gynecology. Thus, it is imperative that practitioners understand the science and its implications for everyday medical care in the coming years.

Before attempting to understand the problems and applications encompassing bioinformatics, it is helpful to review the sources of the explosion in the production of genetic information that have driven the development of this field. The 3% of human genome that comprises the 100,000 or so functional human genes will be completely sequenced in the next 5 years. The sequencing information from the various groups in the world is first collected, or uploaded, by the laboratories to three large genetic databases in the United States, Europe, and Japan. The data from the European Molecular Biology Laboratory (EMBL), the DNA Database of Japan (DDBJ) and the Genebank of the United States are then shared with each other. The Genebank at the National Center for Biotechnology Information (http://www.ncbi.nlm.nih.gov/Web/Genbank/index.html) is thus one of the three central consolidated repositories of all publicly accessible gene sequence data for any given time. The amount of information in this database doubles every year. In December 1997, the database contained over 1,258,000,000 DNA bases of sequence information about all species. Similarly, large amounts of data exist in the SWISSPROT (http://expasy.hcuge.ch/sprot/sprot-top.html) database at the EMBL, which contains more than 71,198 entries for the nonredundant sequences of proteins. Other large databases also exist for protein three-dimensional structures, microbial genomes, enzymes, and drug structures, as well as more species-specific data. Clearly, the large amount of biologic sequence information would be extremely unwieldy to analyze and manipulate for professional biologists unaided by computers.

The central problem in analyzing these large data sets is to try to correlate structure with function so that diagnosis and treatment can be attempted at the level of the genome. Given new sequence data, the first strategy in solving the structure function problem consists of finding homologous sequences for new sequences in a library where the structure function correlation has been established. The pairwise subsequence alignment problem was first attacked with an algorithm developed by Smith and Waterman that applied a computer science technique called dynamic programming. To achieve appropriate alignments between distantly related proteins, the algorithm allows gaps to be present in the final alignment, and a substitution matrix can be used so that certain amino acids are interchangeable. When this technique does not succeed in finding an alignment with a high enough probability compared with finding a similar alignment by chance alone, a more involved approach is taken. With more advanced algorithms, such as the PSI-BLAST, comparisons are made between the given sequence and the average, or tem-plato, sequence of an entire family of sequences. This method weights the alignment toward the conserved regions that are important in defining the function of the gene family. These families are then constantly updated with the results of new analyses on new sequence data. Another method is to search for small conserved sequences called *motifs*, or consensus sequences, which have been previously correlated to specific protein functions. Finally, if no sequence homology is found from the primary sequence data, the use of three-dimensional structural folding data, called protein threading, is used to guide the alignment with previously characterized proteins or protein families.

## REFERENCES

Advani A, Lo K, Shahar Y: Intention-based critiquing of guideline-oriented medical care: The Asgaard Project at Stanford. *In* Proceedings of the Annual AMIA 98 Symposium Orlando, FL, 1998 (forthcoming).

Altschul SF et al. Gapped-BLAST and PSI-BLAST: A new generation of protein database search programs. Nucleic Acids Res. 25:3389–3402, 1997.

Barnett GO: Computer-Stored Ambulatory Medical Record (COSTAR). Bethesda, MD: Department of Health, Education, and Welfare, 1976.

Barrows RC, Clayton PD: Privacy, confidentiality, and electronic medical records. *In* 1997 IMIA Yearbook of Medical Informatics. Stuttgart, Germany, Schattauer Verlag, 1997, pp 297–306.

Bidgood WD, Horii SC, Prior FW, et al: Understanding and using DICOM, the Data Interchange Standard for Biomedical Imaging. J Am Med Inform Assoc 4:199–212, 1997.

Campbell JR, Carpenter P, Sneiderman C, et al: CPRI Work Group on Codes and Structures: Phase II evaluation of clinical coding schemes: Completeness, taxonomy, mapping, definitions, and clarity. J Am Med Inform Assoc 4:238–251, 1997.

Chandrashekaran B: Generic tasks in knowledge-based reasoning: High-level building blocks for expert system design. IEEE Expert 1(3):23–30, 1986.

Darkins DR: Data document growth in telemedicine sites, service providers. Telemedicine and Telehealth Networks Dec 1997, pp 13–15.

de Dombal F, Leaper D, Staniland J, et al: Computer-aided diagnosis of acute abdominal pain. BMJ 1:376–380, 1972.

Dorenfest S: Creating a "top 100" HIS firm: The lessons of history. Healthcare Informatics 11:49–72, 1994.

Field MJ (ed) and Committee on Evaluating Clinical Applications of Telemedicine, Institute of Medicine: Telemedicine: A Guide to Assessing Telecommunications for Health Care. Washington, DC, National Academy Press, 1996, p 1.

Frisse M: IAIMS: Planning for change. J Am Med Inform Assoc 4(Suppl):S13–S19, 1997.

Greenes RA, Shortliffe EH: Medical informatics: An emerging academic discipline and institutional priority. JAMA 263:1114–1120, 1990.

Hayward RSA, Gagliardi A, Jadad AR: Healthcare on the Internet. Health Measures. Sept 1997, pp 28–36.

Health Level Seven: An application protocol for electronic data exchange in healthcare environments. Version 2.3. Ann Arbor, MI, Health Level Seven, Inc, 1997.

Information leaders look ahead. American Medical News April 27, 1998, p 30.

Institute of Medicine (US) Committee on Improving the Patient Record: The computer-based patient record: An essential technology for healthcare. Washington, DC, National Academy Press, 1991, pp 19, 20.

Jadad AR, Gagliardi A: Rating health information on the Internet. JAMA. 279:611–614, 1998.

Kincaid K: New laws make reimbursement mandatory. Telemedicine and Telehealth Networks April 1998, p 23.

McDonal CT, Dexter PR, Takesue B, et al: Health informatics standards: A view from mid-America. *In* 1997 IMIA Yearbook of Medical Informatics. Stuttgart, Germany Schattauer Verlag, 1997, pp 67–74.

McDonald CJ. The barriers to electronic medical record systems and how to overcome them. 4(3):213–221, 1997.

McDonald CJ, Tierney WM, Overhage JM, et al: The Regenstrief Medical Record System: 20 years of experience in hospitals, clinics, and neighborhood health centers. MD Computing 9:206–217, 1992.

Mitchell JA: Basic principles of information technology organization in health care institutions. J Am Med Inform Assoc 4(Suppl):S31–S35, 1997.

Musen MA, Tu SW, Das AK, et al: EON: A component-based approach to automation of protocol-directed therapy. J Am Med Inform Assoc 3:367–388, 1996.

National Research Council (US) Committee on Maintaining Privacy and Security in Health Care Applications of the National Information Infrastructure: For the record: Protecting electronic health information. Washington, DC, National Academy Press, 1997, pp 65–78.

National Research Council (US) Committee on Maintaining Privacy and Security in Health Care Applications of the National Information Infrastructure: For the record: Protecting electronic health information. Washington, DC, National Academy Press, 1997, p 25.

Nevill-Manning CG, Wu TD, Brutlag, DL: Highly specific protein sequence motifs for genome analysis. Proc Natl Acad Sci U S A 95:5865–5871, 1998.

No telemedicine rush. American Medical News May 4, 1998, p 9.

Owens DK, Schacter RD, Nease NF: Representation and analysis of medical decision problems with influence diagrams. Medical Decis Making 17:341–262, 1997.

Pauker SP, Pauker SG: The Amniocentesis Decision: Ten Years of Decision Analytic Experience, Vol 23; Birth Defects: Original Article Series. White Plains, NY, March of Dimes Birth Defects Foundation, 1987, pp 151–169.

Rost B, Schneider R, Sander C: Protein fold recognition by prediction-based threading. J Mol Biol 270:471–480, 1997.

Schuler GD, Boguski MS, Stewart EA, et al: A gene map of the human genome. Science 274:540–546, 1996.

Shahar Y, Miksch S, Johnson P: The Asgaard project: A task-specific framework for the application and critiquing of time-oriented clinical guidelines. AI in Med 1998 (in press).

Shortliffe EH: Computer-Based Medical Consultation: MYCIN. New York, Elsevier North-Holland, 1976.

Silberg WM, Lundberg GD, Musacchio RA: Assessing, controlling, and assuring the quality of medical information on the Internet. JAMA 277:1244, 1245, 1997.

Siwicki B: Telemedicine providers ponder the profitability issue. Health Data Management Apr 1998.

Size of Information System Market. Health Data Management Mar 1997, p 12.

Smith TF, Waterman M: Identification of common molecular subsequences. J Mol Biol 147:195–197, 1981.

Stead WW, Hammond WE: Computer-based medical records: The centerpiece of TMR. MD Computing 5:48–62, 1988.

Tang PC, Hammond WE: A progress report on computer-based patient records in the United States. *In* Dick RS, Steen EB, Detmer DE (eds), for Committee on Improving the Patient Record, Institute of Medicine: The Computer-Based Patient Record: An Essential Technology for Health Care, rev ed. Washington, DC, National Academy Press, 1997.

van Bemmel JH, Musen M (eds): Handbook of Medical Informatics. Heidelberg, Germany, Springer-Verlag, 1997, p 239.

Wallraff G, Labadie J, Brock P, et al: DNA sequencing on a chip. Chemtech, February 1997, p 22–32.

Warner H, Toronto A, Veasy L: Experience with Bayes' theorem for computer diagnosis of congenital heart disease. Ann N Y Acad Sci 115:2–16, 1964.

Young JWR: PACS cost justification. Decisions in Imaging Economics May/June(suppl), 1997, pp 8, 9.

Yu VL, Fagan LM, Wraith SM, et al: Antimicrobial selection by a computer: A blinded evaluation by infectious disease experts. JAMA 242:1279–1282, 1979.

# 77

# Outcome Measurement: The Emerging Quality Barometer

EMAD RIZK

SCOTT B. RANSOM

In 1910, a distinguished Boston surgeon, Ernest Amory Codman, suggested a revolutionary idea that caused major unrest. He recommended to his colleagues that individual physicians' and hospitals' patient outcome records be documented and publicized. Although Codman's radical idea was unsuccessful at the time, the profound changes that have occurred in American medicine have allowed Codman's concept to survive.

Physicians developed a better understanding of what we now term outcome measurement as they learned more about specific causes of disease such as the origin and prevention of sepsis with a simultaneous reduction of death rates from 40% between 1880 and 1890 to below 5% by 1900. Moreover, during that era, the American Medical Association made significant efforts to improve physician education, medical research, and quality of health care services in United States (US) medical schools.

Gradually, these efforts expanded into exploring geographic differences in physician practice. In the early 1970s, epidemiologist John Wennberg and colleague Alan Gittlesohn found significant variation in the performance rates of common operations, such as tonsillectomy and hysterectomy, among hospitals throughout Vermont. In fact, tonsillectomy rates ranged from 13 per 100,000 individuals in one community to a high of 51 per 100,000 persons in another. The researchers also noted dilatation and curettage procedures performed at rates that spanned a low of 30 per 100,000 patients to a high of 141 per 100,000 patients. The findings presented several questions: Because no evidence had been collected to demonstrate why and for what patients these procedures were necessary, on what data were the physicians basing their treatment decisions? Moreover, what say did patients have in this process?

Today, we strive to answer these questions. Health services researchers are studying which methods are the best indicators of quality. They use data ranging from mortality reports to patient satisfaction surveys. Developments in these types of outcome measures signify a major transition in how we perceive health care and the methods by which it is delivered. At no other time in health-care history have providers and health-care institutions been asked to be accountable for the quality of care they deliver and to include scientific evidence that supports physicians' clinical decision-making.

Several factors have fueled the drive to measure provider performance: pressure to manage rising costs, an increasingly competitive health-care environment, and research efforts similar to Wennberg's, which illustrate striking geographical variations in health-care practice. With more than two thirds of Americans using employer-sponsored health insurance covered under managed care, purchaser demands for accountability have grown as costs have risen. Employer purchasers essentially want evidence that for the health-care dollars they pay to managed care plans, quality services are delivered to their members that cover every aspect of the health-care spectrum including access to quality health-care providers with good outcomes.

To meet these demands, managed care and other health-care systems are moving toward developing and using tools to measure the quality of care, a process called outcome measurement. A groundbreaking development for ensuring quality took place on March 31, 1998, when the National Committee for Quality Assurance (NCQA) unveiled *Accreditation '99*, a plan for incorporating measures of quality as part of its accreditation process for managed care plans. Health maintenance organizations (HMOs) that undergo NCQA accreditation are assessed on their policies and systems. With *Accreditation '99*, they are now judged on criteria such as the number of children immunized in the community or the treatment given to heart attack patients.

The NCQA development is just unfolding. In the meantime, our role as health-care administrators calls for us to play a major role in managing such quality efforts. We must learn how to work with physicians to measure the effectiveness of providers and medical treatments. We are compelled to determine what constitutes "best practice." Where can we get that information? Who has developed such measures, and how do we know whether they will work in our systems of care? How do we know that our medical decisions are based on scientific evidence?

One way to begin to address these questions is to understand how the issue of outcome measurement evolved, a phenomenon that Arnold Relman, former editor-in-chief of *New England Journal of Medicine*, calls "the third revolution in health care." Taking a look at quality measurement systems currently in use, and examples of best practices is a good beginning. Clearly, from here on, health industry leaders and health services researchers will be working to improve the scientific evidence which physicians rely on to make clinical decisions. At the same time, the hope is that these efforts, in turn, will lead to better health-care value for purchasers. How we approach and apply outcome measurement will have a profound effect on medicine in the next century.

## Use of Outcome Measures in Process Improvement

How can outcome measures be used in process improvement? Basically, they provide data that make specific processes more understandable. Outcome measures can be used to identify potential areas for improvement. By tracking a process improvement project, the measures can provide evidence of change. With these data, outcome measures that reveal success can be used for marketing clinical services, as evidenced by projects put into practice at Detroit Medical Center (DMC).

The DMC is a $1.8-billion dollar health system with eight hospitals and more than 3000 physicians. Four of these hospitals comprise the active obstetric hospitals that collectively deliver more than 16,000 babies annually. The DMC implemented its Process Improvement Program for the Department of Obstetrics and Gynecology (OB/GYN) in 1997. Their objective was to provide a comprehensive outcome measurement system for the Department of OB/GYN. The data were collected by the Clinical Resource Management team and developed by the women's service line. A multidisciplinary process improvement team, representing all the hospitals, meets quarterly to define and manage outcome measures and process improvement projects (Table 77–1). After system-wide meetings are held, local multidisciplinary teams initiate and complete process improvement projects. The projects keynoted improvement in the following areas:

- Vaginal Delivery: Clinical Pathway, Outcome Measures, and Order Sets
- Cesarean Section: Clinical Pathway, Outcome Measures, and Order Sets
- Hysterectomy: Clinical Pathway, Outcome Measures, and Order Sets
- Pelvic Inflammatory Disease: Clinical Pathway, Outcome Measures
- Outpatient OB/GYN and Women's Service Line Outcomes Measures

The process improvement projects were linked to the appropriate outcome measures, as listed, to provide continuous surveillance and feedback for improved outcomes. An example of outcome information includes hospital-specific cesarean section and vaginal birth after cesarean delivery (VBAC) rates.

Delivery data from these four hospitals were analyzed through the efforts of the National Perinatal Information Center (NPIC). The NPIC is supported by grants from federal and state government agencies as well as membership fees and educational revenue from hospitals that use their information. The NPIC researches a variety of outcome issues for perinatal

**Table 77–1** Obstetrics and Gynecology Outcome Measures: Definitions

| Indicator | Definition | Numerator | Denominator |
|---|---|---|---|
| Deliveries | Total # of deliveries DRG 370–375 | N/A | N/A |
| C/S | Total # of women discharged who have delivered via cesarean section DRG 370–371 | N/A | N/A |
| Vaginal deliveries | Total # of women discharged who have delivered via vaginal delivery DRG 370–371 | N/A | N/A |
| C/S rate | Rate of women discharged who had a C/S delivery | Total # of women discharged who had delivered via C/S DRG 370–371 | Total # of women discharged who had delivery DRG 370–375 |
| Primary C/S rate | Rate of women discharged who had a primary C/S delivery | Total # of women discharged who had a primary C/S Total C/S minus total repeat C/S | Total # of women discharged who had delivery |
| Repeat C/S rate | Rate of women discharged who had a repeat C/S | Total # of women discharged who had a repeat C/S DRG 370–371 and ICD9 diagnostic codes: 654.20, 654.21, 654.23 | Total # of women discharged who had delivery DRG 370–375 |
| VBAC rate | Rate of successful VBAC | Total # of women discharged after a vaginal delivery who had a previous uterine scar DRG 372–375 and ICD9 diagnostic codes: 654.21 or (654.20, 654.21, 654.23) | Total # of women who had a delivery with a previous uterine scar DRG 370–375 and ICD9 diagnostic codes: 654.21 or (654.20, 654.21, 654.23) |
| Induction rate | Rate of women whose labor was induced | Total # of women whose labor is induced, either medically or mechanically. DRG 370–375 and ICD9 procedure codes: 73.01, 73.1, 73.4 | Total # of women discharged who had delivery DRG 370–375 |
| OB complication rate | Rate of cases with OB-related complications | Total # of women who delivered and had a documented OB complication ICD9 diagnostic codes: 668.0-668.9 (Anesthesia comp.), 669.40-669.44 (Surgical comp.), 669.80-669.84 (Other comp.) | Total # of women discharged who had delivery DRG 370–375 |
| Hysterectomy complication rate | The rate of women who had a hysterectomy and a complication related to a procedure | Total # of patients who have had a hysterectomy and documented complications related to a procedure ICD9 procedure codes: 68.3, 68.4, 68.5, 68.51, 68.59, 68.9, and ICD9 diagnostic codes: 997.0-998.9 | Total # of women who had a hysterectomy ICD9 procedure codes: 68.3, 68.4, 68.51, 68.59, 68.9 |
| *OB (and GYN*) readmission rate This measure is currently being hand counted by running lists of OB and GYN patients and looking for two or more admissions for the same patient | The rate of women who were readmitted within 30 d after delivery (or GYN* procedure or treatment) | Total # of women who were discharged after delivery (or GYN* procedure or treatment) and readmitted within 30 d | Total # of patient discharged after delivery (or GYN* procedure or treatment) |

*Table continued on following page*

**Table 77-1** Obstetrics and Gynecology Outcome Measures: Definitions *Continued*

| Indicator | Definition | Numerator | Denominator |
|---|---|---|---|
| LOS for C/S, vaginal delivery, TAH, vaginal hysterectomy, and LAVH | The average LOS for all deliveries and hysterectomies for nonmalignancy (DRG 358–359) | Total # of patient days for each type of patient or procedure | Total # of patients for each type of patient or procedure |
| Maternal mortality rate | The rate of in-hospital maternal death, up to and including 42 d post partum | Total # of cases of maternal death up to and including 42 d | Total # of women discharged who had delivery DRG 370–375 |
| Births | Total # of live births DRG 385–391 and birth date | N/A | N/A |
| Stillborn rate (per 1000 births) | Rate of women delivering stillborn infants (IUFD beyond 20 wk of gestational age) | Total # of deliveries of a stillborn ICD9 diagnostic codes: V27.1, V27.3, V27.4, V27.6, V27.7 (×1000) | Total # of women discharged who had delivery DRG 370–375 |
| Neonatal mortality rate (per 1000 births) | Death rate of live-born infants who die before 29 d of life | Total # of live-born infants who die in hospital before 29 d of life. (× 1000) | Total # of live births DRG 385–391 and birth date |
| Perinatal mortality rate (per 1000 births) | The rate of the sum of fetal and neonatal deaths | Sum of total stillbirths and live-born infants who die before 29 d of life. (× 1000) | Total # of live births DRG 385–391 and birth date |
| Low birthweight rate | The rate of infants less than 2500 grams at birth (5.5lb) | Total # of infants less than 2500 g (1500–2500 g) | Total # of live births DRG 385–391 and birth date |
| Very low birthweight rate | The rate of infants less than 1500 grams at birth (3lb 5 oz) | Total # of infants less than 1500 g (500–1499 g) | Total # of live births DRG 385–391 and birth date |
| Birth trauma rate | The rate of neonates discharged with documented birth trauma | Total # of neonates with a discharge diagnosis of birth trauma DRG 385–391 *and* ICD9 diagnostic codes: 767.0–767.9 | Total # of live births DRG 385–391 and birth date |
| GYN admissions | Total # of admissions with the attending physician's service listed as GYN | N/A | N/A |
| †Unplanned admissions rate | The rate of patients who are admitted after outpatient procedures | Total # of discharges whose admitting source is listed as "Outpatient surgery" | Total outpatient procedures |
| †Laparoscopy complication rate | The rate of patients with documented complications after a laparoscopy | Total # of patients who have had a laparoscopy, *and* documented complications related to a procedure. ICD9 procedure codes: 54.21, 65.01, 65.13, 65.14, 65.23–65.25, 65.31, 65.41, 65.53, 65.54, 65.63, 65.64, 65.74, 65.75, 65.76, 65.81, 66.21–66.29, *and* ICD9 diagnostic codes; 997.0–998.9 | Total # of patients who have had a laparoscopy ICD9 procedure codes: 54.21, 65.01, 65.13, 65.14, 65.23–65.25, 65.31, 65.41, 65.53, 65.54, 65.63, 65.64, 65.74, 65.75, 65.76, 65.81, 66.21–66.29 |
| †Infants with major complications rate | The rate of full-term newborns delivered who have major complications | Total # of term newborns who are admitted to the NICU for 2 d Birthweight >2500 g *and* admission to NICU for >2 d | Total # of term newborns Birthweight >2500 g |

**Table 77–1** Obstetrics and Gynecology Outcome Measures: Definitions *Continued*

| Indicator | Definition | Numerator | Denominator |
|---|---|---|---|
| †Severe complications of pregnancy rate | The rate of patients admitted before delivery for maternal causes | Total # of hospitalizations for maternal causes ICD9 diagnostic codes: 630–676, excluding 635 and 650 | Total # of deliveries ICD9 diagnostic code: V27 |
| †Blood transfusion rate | The rate of transfusion for hysterectomy, vaginal delivery and C/S | Total # of patients who have had a vaginal delivery, C/S, or hysterectomy *and* had a blood product transfusion ICD9 procedure codes: 99.00–99.07 | Total # of patients who have had a vaginal delivery, C/S, or hysterectomy |
| †Postpartum infection rate | The rate of infections occurring in the postpartum patient during the delivery admission | Total # of patients who have had a delivery and have documented postpartum infection DRG 370–375 *and* ICD9 diagnostic code: 670.0, 670.01–670.09, 674.34 | Total # of women discharged who had delivery DRG 370–375 |
| †Third- and fourth-degree laceration rate | The rate of patients who have a vaginal delivery with a documented third- or fourth-degree laceration | Total # of women discharged who have delivered via vaginal delivery w/tear. DRG 372–375 and ICD9 diagnostic codes: 664.21, 664.31 | Total # of women discharged who had delivered via vaginal delivery DRG 372–375 |
| †Operative vaginal delivery rate | The rate of patients who have an operative-assisted vaginal delivery | Total # of women discharged who have delivered operative vaginal delivery DRG 372–375 *and* ICD9 procedure codes: 72.0–72.9 | Total # of women discharged who had delivered via vaginal delivery DRG 372–375 |
| †Anesthesia complication rate | The rate of patients who delivered with a documented anesthesia complication | Total # of women discharged who had a delivery and a documented anesthesia complication DRG 370–375 *and* ICD9 diagnostic code: 668.0–668.9 | Total # of women discharged who had delivery DRG 370–375 |

*GYN to be added at a later date.
†Measurements are currently being developed and tested.
C/S = cesarean section; DRG = diagnosis-related group; GYN = gynecology; IUFD = intrauterine fetal death; LOS = length of stay; OB = obstetrics; TAH = total abdominal hysterectomy; LAVH = laparoscopic-assisted vaginal hysterectomy; N/A = not available; VBAC = vaginal birth after cesarean delivery.

services and provides comparative reports from other hospitals.

Health services researchers and industry practitioners use different terms to define outcome measures. Some categorize measures according to what they actually assess, whether it be patient outcomes, institutional processes, population outcomes, or provider behavior. Whatever terminology is used, however, these measures of performance are usually based on what are often called "indicators of quality," or "quality indicators," which can include any of the following: (Table 77–2)

- More traditional measures, such as service use, costs, mortality rates, length of stay
- Increasingly explorative indicators, which allow patient outcomes to be tracked across various health-care settings, such as complications, functional status, patient satisfaction, quality of life factors, and episodes of care

Once an organization defines its goals for measuring improvement, these indicators will be more specific. For example, if a health plan's goal is to reduce hospital readmission rates among its members who have asthma, it will track indicators such as signs and symptoms, pulmonary function, effectiveness of pharmacotherapy, and patient satisfaction.

Health services researchers now use a new generation of indicators, such as complications, which emphasize patient care, and require that the health care organization engage the physician in the entire outcome management effort. Because complications are clinically important, for instance, they require physicians to review the data. Other measures may include physician's work efforts, treatment failures, hospitalization rates, functional status, and patient satisfaction indicators that measure clinical efficacy rather than service.

Patient surveys also offer health-care administrators an opportunity to explore quality at another level. Such instruments gauge satisfaction with services and also assess a patient's functional status. However, such surveys are costly in terms of administrative support required and need for expert analysis. Common patient survey instruments include the SF-36 and TyPe tools.

New systems of outcome measurement involve episodes of care, which allow patient outcomes to be tracked across all inpatient and outpatient sites. Using this guide, administrators can make better comparisons of patient groups within a system and among integrated delivery systems. As a result, they can also make better comparisons between providers who have high death rates and those who have low death rates by separating the effect of inpatient treatment failures, such as unexpected death, from the admission of very healthy patients, who have no risk of death. Such episodes of care measurement allow administrators to assess outcomes over time, an especially useful tool for tracking chronically ill patients.

Administrators can find data for use in applying these indicators in a number of areas, but mostly through administrative records, medical records, and patient and provider surveys. There are certain advantages and limits to each data source. For instance, administrative records allow physician managers to track service use and costs, but they often lack clinical detail. Medical records contain clinical information but may not always be complete or even legible. The information itself shows only one part of the picture. For instance, mortality data alone do not demonstrate hospital performance; length-of-stay data do not indicate patient well-being and do not document other types of patient care received outside the hospital. The important point is that outcomes be tracked and assessed continuously to identify problems and any progress in process, care, and practice patterns.

## How to Apply Outcome Measurement

Physicians must remember that seeking indicators of quality and applying them for measurement purposes is no guarantee that clear-cut answers will emerge from the process, no matter how thorough it may be. However, they will come close to getting objective data to help practitioners make more effective clinical decisions. An example may include the use of the following steps as a guide in putting measurement to work:

1. *Define quality improvement goals and select outcome measurement instruments.* To start, assess the health status of your patients using a common patient survey tool, SF-36, or SF-12, the short version. Collect data from medical and administrative records. To track changes over time, use the SF-36 with new patients on their first three visits. If the organization already has general health status data on hand, use instruments that track condition-specific outcomes.
2. *Outline a strategy and set schedules.* Determine what patient or population groups you plan to

**Table 77–2** Various Indicators of Quality

| Traditional Measures | New Generation of Measures |
| --- | --- |
| Service utilization | Complications |
| Costs | Functional status |
| Mortality rates | Quality of life |
| Length of stay | Episodes of care |
|  | Patient satisfaction |

study and for what period of time or number of visits. When seeking general information about various groups, sample every fourth to tenth patient for a defined period. However, when focusing on improving individual patient care, use an instrument(s) that explores functional status, quality of life, burden of disease, and patient satisfaction. Note where you can find the data you need to collect the information: perhaps medical and administrative records or past patient surveys. Itemize the resources you need and develop a budget for analyzing the data.

3. *Look for differences between your study population and research findings*. Know that patient or population groups in referenced material will not necessarily mirror your sample group. Contact a research analyst who can help you interpret results and advise you on how they apply to your organization and patient population.

4. *Understand caveats in the research—one size does not fit all*. Understand distinctive factors that influenced the results in a research study to determine whether the same effort, results, or both would work for you. For example, the effectiveness of a new medical device may strongly depend on any number of issues, such as provider's training, experience, financial incentives, and patient's socioeconomic status.

5. *Make physicians key leaders in any quality improvement effort*. Have physicians be part of the quality team and get them on board early so that they can help define problems. Involve physicians who have earned the respect of their colleagues. Offer educational activities to help them learn what practices help improve patient care, and, as a result, improve *their* behavior.

6. *Set the stage for tracking progress and charting the impact of change*. Define the measures you want to use to document the effects, changes (or both) of behavior of clinicians, managers, policy makers, and consumers. The tools you use should be appropriate for evaluating the effects of interventions and changes based on outcomes.

7. *Make room for risk adjustment in your analysis*. Risk adjustment essentially accounts for the differences in patient health status that may affect their treatment outcomes. Collect the following data to make adjustments for the populations you analyze: age; sex; extent and severity of principal diagnosis; cormorbid chronic illnesses; physical functional status; cultural and socioeconomic attributes; patient attitudes and preferences for outcomes.

Risk adjustment may have a significant impact on any outcome measurement effort for several reasons.

1. *Risk adjustment is likely to paint a realistic scenario of what is happening in quality improvement*. Because adjusting for risk creates a level playing field among the studied groups, it permits more "apples-to-apples" comparisons, and helps track quality internally or externally over a period of time.

2. *Risk adjustment increases the ability to assess the effectiveness of specific health-care treatments and interventions*. If risk adjustment is performed adequately, it is more likely to note that perceived improvements in a patient's outcome reflect better treatment, improved health status, or other factors.

3. *Risk adjustment helps calculate provider payments*. When burdens of illness are known, physicians are better able to predict their resource needs and costs. A major example is the Health Care Financing Administration (HCFA), which currently adjusts demographic and geographic factors in setting payment rates for Medicare risk health plans. More importantly, risk adjustment is such a critical factor in "leveling the playing field" that the Balanced Budget Act of 1997 requires Medicare risk plans to include health status as a measure for calculating payments starting in the year 2000.

In applying risk adjustment, it is important to determine what key areas are to be addressed (e.g., identifying mortality rates of bypass patients between hospitals, evaluating length of stay in intensive care units). Risk adjustment also calls for deciding the type of instrument to be used. A method may be developed in-house or guidelines may be purchased or tailored to any organization's use. Many commercial products are available, most of which are geared toward risk-adjusting for hospital-based surgical procedures, such as bypass surgery, and common conditions, such as pneumonia. All these systems continue to evolve as the state of the art in outcome measurement tools, such as survey instruments, also becomes enhanced. Table 77–3 lists risk adjustment resources.

Despite the importance of risk adjustment, it has its own set of limitations. For instance, risk adjustment systems can vary significantly in how they describe variations in patient outcomes and resource use, including cost. In fact, according to the Physician Payment Review Commission, the ability of prospective risk adjusters to explain variations in individual-level health-care costs ranged from 1% to as much as 13% if a number of predictors were combined. Moreover, even experts disagree on the value of risk-adjusted death rates in assessing hospital quality. In one case, hospitals identified as low-performing outliers after using one risk adjustment formula were later categorized as average performers after using another.

These factors are important issues to consider when using risk adjustment. Furthermore, under-

**Table 77-3** Risk Adjustment Resources

| Agency | Address/Phone/Website/Email | Resource |
|---|---|---|
| Agency for Health Care Policy and Research (AHCPR) Center for Outcomes and Effectiveness Research<br>Contact: Carolyn M. Clancy, M.D., Acting Director | Ph: 301/594-1357, ext. 138<br>Website: www.ahcpr.gov | AHCPR offers information on issues related to outcomes and effectiveness research. The website has a search area where articles and reports with information on risk adjustment may be found. AHCPR also offers the CONQUEST 1.0 database on the website. CONQUEST summarizes information on more than 1000 clinical performance measures developed by public and private sector organizations to examine quality of clinical care. |
| Health Care Financing Administration (HCFA)<br>Office of Research and Demonstrations (ORD) | 7500 Security Boulevard<br>Baltimore, MD 21244-1850<br>Website: www.hcfa.gov | Among ORD's work is the development of different types of risk adjusters. The CFA website contains a 28-page description of ORD's activities as well as published ORD articles. |
| National Library of Medicine (NLM) National Information Center on Health Services Research and Health Care Technology (NICHSR) | 8600 Rockville Pike<br>Building 38, Mail Stop 20<br>Bethesda, MD 28094<br>Ph: 301/496-0167<br>Fx: 301/402-3193<br>Website: www.nih.gov/nichsr.html<br>Email: nichsr@nlm.nih.gov | NICHSR was created to improve "the collection, storage, analysis, retrieval, and dissemination of information on health-services research, on clinical practice guidelines, and on health-care technology, including the assessment of such technology." It coordinates the development of new information products and services related to health-services research and maintains some useful databases. |
| National Committee for Quality Assurance (NCQA)<br>Accreditation '99 | 2000 L Street, NW, Suite 500<br>Washington, DC 20036<br>Ph: 202/955-3500<br>Fx: 202/955-3599<br>Website: ncqa.org/99draft.htm<br>Email: mcodraft@ncqa.org | |

standing the uses and importance of risk adjustment helps clinicians and administrators to make better decisions regarding issues and activities related to performance measurement.

As outcomes management evolves, the patient's role as a partner in care with the physician will emerge as a new dimension in outcome management. The American Academy of Allergy Asthma & Immunology (AAAA&I) (Milwaukee, WI) provides a good example of this kind of partnering in its monograph titled, "Improving Allergy and Asthma Care Through Outcomes Management," which describes a four-step program that applies outcome management to a physician-patient partnership:

First step. Providers, patients, and family discuss and agree on a set of common therapy goals and expected patient outcomes. For instance, they may specify a partnership to: "prevent chronic and troublesome symptoms . . . maintain (near) normal pulmonary function; maintain normal activity levels; prevent recurrent exacerbations; optimize pharmacotherapy with minimal side effects . . .[,] meet expectations and satisfy patients."

Second step. Physicians, other providers, and patients define their roles. The physician team agrees to measure clinical status by "signs and symptoms; pulmonary function; quality of life indicators; number of asthma exacerbations; pharmacotherapy effectiveness"; and a patient survey. Providers meet with controlled patients regularly and offer them therapy options. They also re-evaluate patients periodically and prescribe appropriate therapies, explain how to self-manage their conditions, and show them how to comply with therapy instructions. Patients agree to learn how to monitor their daily β-agonist use, nocturnal symptoms, morning congestion, exercise limitations, days out of work or school, medication side effects, and peak flow activity (measured through a peak-flow meter).

Third step. This phase includes enhanced understanding by the patient and provider about how to improve outcomes for patients who have asthma. Providers know how and when to use and interpret objective measures of disease (e.g., pulmonary function); they understand the impact of this disease on quality of life; they better acknowledge any medication side effects; and they are able to detect why any poor outcomes occur. Patients understand their therapy and compliance goals as well as situations that call for them to contact a physician in the likelihood of pulmonary dysfunction.

- Fourth step. The final step is a check to see whether the patient is meeting the goals of therapy. To determine this, physicians should conduct an outcome assessment that asks the patient questions about rescue inhaler use and the circumstances in which it was used; presence of nocturnal symptoms; exercise limitation; missed school or work; and acute exacerbations.

## Managed Care Experience Underscores' National Trends

Given the increase in managed care nationwide, it is worth watching how outcome measurement is taking hold in that arena. Moreover, experiences of managed care organizations provide insight into the direction that outcome measurement is taking in the United States. In 1997, for example, in a listing of "America's top HMOs," *U.S. News & World Report* ranked health plans according to how well they performed, according to 17 quality indicators, which included clinical care measures, such as mammography, breast cancer screening rates, immunization, and nonclinical measures, such as member disenrollment rate, provider turnover rate, and board certification of primary care, specialist, and ob/gyn physicians.

### THE HEALTHPARTNERS' EXPERIENCE

HealthPartners (Twin Cities, MN), a mixed model HMO that ranked 26th among the top plans in the *U.S. News & World Report* listing, carries out a quality improvement process that focuses on three dimensions:
- Measurement of accountability
- Measurement of improvement
- Measurement of population health

In conducting *measurement of accountability*, HealthPartners collects data as part of its report to the Health Plan Employer Data and Information Set (HEDIS), which are performance measures used by health plans and employer purchasers to track and document quality of care and services in HMOs. HEDIS was created under the auspices of NCQA, the accrediting body for managed care organizations.

Although tracking this data for external quality reporting (NCQA) purposes, HealthPartners also uses the information to improve care internally. For example, after assessing the HMO's performance on immunization, the organization established programs to increase childhood immunization rates from 54 to 87% between 1991 and 1995. Results of a mammography rate assessment led to an outreach effort that increased mammography compliance rates from 77 to 79%.

In *measurement of improvement*, HealthPartners uses more than 20 measures of performance, to track the salaried and contracted physicians. HealthPartners then assesses and compares providers' practices with others in similar settings or geographic regions. Results showing significant changes among providers leads to discussion between the provider and the HealthPartners' medical director or other physicians from its quality teams. Plan physicians have been open to this type of process as HealthPartners engages physicians to be a part of the program from the outset.

Another example of HealthPartners' outcome management effort in measurement of improvement is the development of practice guidelines. In 1993, HealthPartners established a joint venture with the Mayo Clinic and the Park Nicolett Medical Center to create the Institute for Clinical Systems Integration (ICSI). Under the ICSI banner, multidisciplinary teams of providers review literature on the most common and costly conditions to determine the "best practices" that form the basis for the clinical guideline. In early 1997, the Institute had produced 41 practice guidelines on a number of topics, including breast cancer diagnosis and uncomplicated urinary tract infection.

The first guideline issued by ICSI was for uncomplicated urinary tract infections (UTI) in women. The guideline offers specific information about appropriate timing for tests and cultures as well as when to use specific antibiotics.

To test the guideline's use, HealthPartners defined two measures: first, the number of urine cultures divided by total visits or total episodes of urine infection; and second, the total number of 3-day courses of sulfa-based antibiotics—the recommendation—divided by total number of episodes. George Isham, HealthPartners' medical director and chief health officer, explained that improvement would be indicated if the first number declined. With the second ratio, he cautions, that although one would "expect that to move towards 100%, you'll never get there because there are always people with allergies and [other] problems. But it's a rough and ready way to measure how the guideline is doing." Using the guideline measures, each medical group collects information, reports it, and uses it to track performance improvement. Medical groups review the guideline periodically to assess the need for updating the measures, which is what happened with the UTI guideline. After the first year of use, the UTI guideline was changed to *not* require a woman to have urinalysis before her physician could prescribe antibiotics. The change essentially improved care for women who could not visit a physician and for whom symptoms were easily recognized.

In measurement of population health, HealthPartners has defined objectives as part of a public health program, "Partners for Better Health," which it launched in 1994. The program creates partnerships among businesses, community organizations, and local governments, to name a few. Their goals are to reduce the incidence of disease, injury, or complications in eight areas: heart disease; breast cancer; childhood immunizations; infant health; diabetes; dental health; child injuries; and domestic violence and abuse.

One of HealthPartners' goals in 1996 was to reduce infant and maternal complications, including cases in which infants were affected by substance abuse, premature rupture of the amniotic membranes (PROM), preterm deliveries, and repeat teen pregnancies. The health plan used data on infant and maternal complications to identify women at risk for problematic pregnancies and then to work closely with them to address factors in their lives that were putting them at risk. As a result, the HMO cut the number of premature infant births in half, about 25% of the rate for the entire community. Moreover, the plan introduced a prenatal program, including a teen pregnancy program, to help women reduce their risks and have healthy pregnancies.

The Partners for Better Health program uses two tools to measure public health for the program: an annual, population-based, random survey, and a comprehensive and confidential data set of health risks for individual health plan members.

## THE U.S. HEALTHCARE EXPERIENCE

U.S. Healthcare, now part of Aetna, Inc., studies and applies quality improvement efforts through its subsidiary, U.S. Quality Algorithms (USQA). Table 77-4 depicts prevalence, clinical, and outcome measures that the organization used when it defined diabetes mellitus as a significant clinical opportunity for improving patient outcomes and processes of care.

The measures in Table 77-4 represent what U.S. Healthcare physicians agreed on as strong indicators of quality of care. This chart illustrates the aggregate experience of the entire health-care organization rather than one particular provider's performance. However, these same measures are used for individual physicians to help them see their practice patterns, identify any concerns, and suggest how to improve performance. This system of educational feedback can help health-care administrators improve the decision-making process as it relates to applying resources to physician education and patient management programs.

**Table 77-4** U.S. Healthcare Diabetes Performance Report

| Prevalence Measures | |
|---|---|
| Actual number of current members identified with diabetes | 39,331 |
| Estimated overall prevalence of diabetes* | 3.1% |
| Diabetic pt with pharmacy plan on insulin* | 25.1% |

| Clinical Measures* | |
|---|---|
| Average number of annual primary care visits per diabetic pt | 4.0 |
| Diabetic pt who visited their physician at least once in the reporting period | 84.4% |
| Average number of annual glycosylated hemoglobin tests per diabetic pt | 0.8 |
| Diabetic pt with at least two glycated hemoglobin tests during the reporting period | 21.4% |
| Diabetic pt who received retinal exams during previous yr | 30.4% |
| Diabetic pt who received cholesterol screening test during previous yr | 33.8% |
| Diabetic pt who had a microalbuminuria screening test during previous yr | 2.6% |

| Outcome Measures | |
|---|---|
| ER visits specifically for diabetes/1000 diabetic pt per yr | 8.2 |
| Total admissions (acute) specifically for diabetes/1000 diabetic pt per yr | 24.8 |
| Admissions for DKA, HHNK, or diabetic coma/1000 diabetic pt per yr | 6.5 |
| Admissions for hypoglycemia/1000 diabetic pt per yr | 3.0 |
| Admission for cellulitis/1000 diabetic pt per year | 6.0 |
| Prevalence of ischemic heart disease in diabetic pt | 17.2% |
| Prevalence of end-stage renal disease in diabetic pt† | 1.5% |
| Annual incident detection of lower extremity amputations† | 0.2% |
| Prevalence of neuropathy in diabetic pt† | 0.6% |
| Prevalence of retinopathy in diabetic pt | 13.7% |

*Based on members who were in the study for the full 12 mo.
†Results should be interpreted with caution because of small numbers.
ER = emergency room; DKA = diabetic ketoacidosis; HHNK = hyperglycemic hyperosmolar nonketotic coma.
From Hanchak NA, Murray JF, Hirsch A, et al: USQA health profile database as a tool for health plan quality improvement, Managed Care Quarterly 4:58-69, 1996.

## The Detroit Medical Center Experience

The Department of OB/GYN of the Detroit Medical Center further focused the general outcome measures for hospital-specific review (see Table 77–1) to specific physicians. A multidisciplinary group led by physicians determined physician-specific measures that could be used to quantify quality. These measures were developed through a consensus process of the group with the goal of determining indicators of measurable quality (Table 77–5). On a semiannual basis, measures were shared confidentially with each physician and were used in the credentialing process. If an individual interested in or had concerns with the data, he or she could gain further insight and details by consulting the physician manager of the project and reviewing all pertinent information and data. Within 20 minutes of reviewing computerized information, most physicians develop an operational appreciation for the accuracy and method of the process. The optional detailed review is a key feature in gaining physician acceptance of future outcome management projects. The review provides proof that methods are accurate and reasonable, which resulted in widespread project acceptance.

## The Economic Impact Behind Performance Measurement

Certainly, cost factors will influence—or be influenced by—any number of current developments, whether they are new medical technologies, price discounts by managed care plans, or changes in physician incentives.

If anything, medical technology advances will continue to raise overall costs, according to Mark Chassin, chair of the department of health policy at Mount Sinai School of Medicine in New York. "We are

**Table 77–5** Medical Staff Reappointment Specific to Obstetrics and Gynecology

| Measure | Individual Physician Statistics | Department Statistics | Goal/Peer Avg./ Benchmark |
|---|---|---|---|
| Deliveries | | | |
| C/S | | | |
| Vaginal deliveries | | | |
| C/S Rate | | | |
| Primary C/S rate | | | |
| Repeat C/S rate | | | |
| VBAC rate | | | |
| Induction rate | | | |
| OB complications rate | | | |
| OB readmission rate | | | |
| C/S ALOS | | | |
| Vaginal delivery ALOS | | | |
| Maternal mortality rate | | | |
| Stillborn rate | | | |
| Births | Information N/A at this time | | |
| Neonatal mortality rate | Information N/A at this time | | |
| Perinatal mortality rate | Information N/A at this time | | |
| Low BW rate | Information N/A at this time | | |
| Very low BW rate | Information N/A at this time | | |
| Birth trauma rate | Information N/A at this time | | |
| Total volume – hysterectomy | | | |
| Hysterectomy complication rate | | | |
| TAH ALOS | | | |
| Vaginal hysterectomy ALOS | | | |
| LAVH ALOS | | | |

ALOS = average length of stay; Avg. = average; BW = birth weight; C/S = cesarean section; LAVH = laparoscopic assisted vaginal hysterectomy; N/A = not available; TAH = total abdominal hysterectomy.

terrific at inventing ... new tests for prostate cancer, sophisticated imaging, or endoscopic procedures, or stenting of arteries, but we are perfectly awful at evaluating them and figuring out when they really result in good outcomes for patients and when they don't." For example, in the diagnosis of a potential macroadenoma related to hyperprolactinemia, a physician may choose any of the following: traditional radiographs, computed tomography (CT) scan, or magnetic resonance imaging (MRI). Although any of these tests could expose a significant tumor, physicians must consider which test, if any, is the most cost-efficient process of obtaining the information necessary for treating the patient. Specific cost-effectiveness research on the various modalities must be considered when choosing the most reasonable diagnostic modality.

The growth of managed care and its emphasis on hospital and physician price discounts could also be influenced by quality improvement efforts, noted Chassin. For instance, he predicted the health-care industry could "eliminate 20% of what we do in health care, and quality would improve." However, he emphasized that in addressing issues of underuse, overuse, and misuse, administrators and physicians will have to rely on more than the scientific evidence in the literature. "The problem," he noted, "is the will to examine this issue." Providers must learn the "right way the first time—the least expensive way of reducing costs," he notes.

Whether the market will recognize this is another question. Certainly, purchasers and providers have well-meaning intentions when their actions show that they are carrying out efforts to improve quality. However, most employer purchasers in the United States are still demanding lower health-care prices in the form of lower health-care premiums, health-care procedures, and so on. Although they support quality improvement efforts, their main focus remains lower costs. Does that put them in the quality driver's seat?

Meanwhile, physicians are walking a fine line, trying to respond to financial incentives to provide cost-effective care and at the same time provide quality care to their patients. It is true that quality-driven health-care systems strive to offer physicians compensation arrangements that reward several areas— quality, patient satisfaction, and productivity, according to Alain C. Enthoven, Marriner S. Eccles Professor of Public and Private Management in the Graduate School of Business at Stanford University, and Carol Vorhaus, a research associate at the same location. Enthoven and Vorhaus note that in order to make physician compensation work appropriately to achieve quality and cost goals, health plans should pay the physician a base salary, and then offer bonuses for improving patient satisfaction, productivity, and overall medical group efficiency. The researchers point out that the effects of this type of compensation arrangement have not been studied in great detail. However, they say, "explicit quality and patient satisfaction measures were not part of the analysis." U.S. Healthcare ties results of patient satisfaction into its providers' compensation. In fact, its subsidiary, U.S. Quality Algorithms (USQA), has "developed systems for measuring and improving the performance of providers in addition to evaluating the care and outcomes of patients," Enthoven points out.

## Putting Outcomes to Work: Operational Guidance

To make outcomes measurement a reality, health-care administrators need to create a quality strategy. This involves several major steps:

*Create an ongoing, professional environment of learning that stresses excellence.* To attract physician participation, case discussion groups should be patterned after the models used by teaching hospitals and some major medical groups. Physicians more likely to work together as teams in reviewing treatment and outcome data and updating clinical practice guidelines. Physicians should be involved early, especially as champions of the quality improvement process. Having well-respected peers involved in the decision-making process helps encourages physician buy-in. This aspect is especially important as health care moves more and more away from the solo medical practice system. Health-care organizations that put a premium on quality and offer rewards to highly skilled physicians—who in turn cooperate well with their peers—will have a greater chance of succeeding at improving practice performance and outcomes.

*Use a sophisticated information system to track performance.* Information systems can play a major role in measuring and reporting performance. U.S. Healthcare created such a tool through the USQA subsidiary mentioned earlier and used it to develop a patient-centered treatment approach for those who suffer from chronic diseases. In 1995, the USQA Health Profile Database also selected 36 chronic diseases and took the first steps by collecting data from a number of sources: ICD-9 diagnosis codes from claims and encounter files; CPT-4 procedure codes from claims and encounter files; Medispan GPI pharmacy codes (Medispan is a mapping of all NDC codes into similar drug classes based on a proprietary grouping system); usage patterns of laboratory tests; and patient demographic data.

The decision should be made whether to build, buy, or tailor current information systems. Are such systems capable of managing the data the organization needs to gather and analyze? Physician leaders should be involved at this stage to ensure that all clinical aspects are covered. Once the information is appropriately managed, an organization is better able to measure, monitor, and improve care. Furthermore, the organization that can analyze data and report results effectively will have a competitive advantage if it can then take this information and communicate it to purchasers, patients, and suppliers.

*Make quality improvement an organizational strategy.* Set the tone of continuous quality improvement in the organization. Quality researcher Donald Berwick points out the need to emphasize to physician leaders and other senior staff that quality improvement is critical to the organization as a necessary management method and strategic goal. The beauty of quality improvement is that it marries administrative and medical quality efforts, and extends a revolutionary invitation to involve interdisciplinary teams and problem-solving techniques.

*Maintain awareness of current and new quality improvement efforts.* New developments and ideas emerge frequently in relation to outcome management and quality improvement. Keep abreast of new initiatives through professional organizations as well as major quality groups, such as the NCQA, the national accrediting body for managed care plans; the Foundation for Accountability (FACCT), a coalition of purchasers and consumer organizations that represents 70 million individuals; and the Joint Commission on Accreditation of Healthcare Organizations (JCAHO), an accrediting organization familiar to many hospitals. The NCQA recently released HEDIS 3.0, a data set that not only measures how well health plans perform various issues but how well these plans help patients function daily and "how they address prevention and early detection of acute and chronic disease across all age levels."

As noted at the beginning of this chapter, a current NCQA effort, *Accreditation '99*, is incorporating HEDIS measures into accreditation standards. According to NCQA, HEDIS results will initially count for 25% of a plan's accreditation score; 75% will be based on a plan's degree of compliance with the NCQA's standards. In the future, NCQA anticipates increasing the proportion of the accreditation score based on a health plan's performance.

The FACCT has also released performance measures, in particular measures that assess provider treatment of persons who have diabetes, breast cancer, and major depression. Moreover, the coalition offers performance measures for patient satisfaction with health plan services and ability of these plans to provide effective disease prevention services. The JCAHO and the FACCT will collaborate on a project to incorporate the detailed information about the FACCT's measures into the accreditation commission's National Library of Healthcare Indicators. This library contains a set of acute care measures called Indicator Measurement System. Although some of the measurement tools of these three organizations, NCQA, FACCT, and JCAHO, may overlap, such innovative efforts deserve attention and support. It is also a good idea to contact organizations that distribute information on outcome measurement (Table 77–6).

*Align incentive and capitation payments appropriately.* Using capitated payments as incentives can help improve provider practice so that patients receive preventive care. This practice also ensures that medical problems are addressed effectively, health system processes improve over time, and providers "do the right thing the first time." These payment arrangements can also be a part of quality improvement efforts and processes that cover the full spectrum from inpatient to home care and can avoid gaps so often experienced in systems under fee-for-service payment arrangements. In fact, prepayment incentives have a greater ability to encourage alliances between all providers—physicians, medical and other provider groups, and hospitals.

## Outcome Measurement From Here On

The effort to measure outcomes has come a long way since Codman's day. At present, developing measures of performance involves a wide range of activities, such as using risk adjustment formulas, performing comparative analysis, broadening data sources to include a wide range of health-care settings, measuring health status and quality of life factors, and incorporating patient perspectives into the equation.

Moreover, physicians are emerging as critical players in the development of quality measurement efforts and have taken significant steps have been taken in this area. For instance, when physicians are bought into the early stages of quality improvement initiatives, they want to be assured that clinical evidence exists for appropriate diagnostic and treatment decisions; however, they also want to know where their practice patterns stand in comparison with their peers. Certainly, outcomes measurement can be a threatening prospect. If physicians are given clinical algorithms without initially being a part of the process, they naturally feel frustrated because of loss of control.

Perhaps the most ambitious and comprehensive development in the last year has been the effort by the federal Agency for Health Care Policy and Research (AHCPR) (Table 77–6) to provide evidence for clinical decision-making, called "evidence-based medicine." This term refers to the "collection and

**Table 77-6** Organizations That Disseminate Outcome Research

| Agency | Address/Phone/Website/Email | Resource |
|---|---|---|
| Agency for Health Care Policy and Research (AHCPR) Center for Health Information Dissemination | Ph: 301/594-1360<br>Website: www.ahcpr.gov | |
| Association for Health Services Research (AHSR) and National Library of Science (NLM)<br>Health Services Research Projects (HSRP) database | Ph: 202/223-2477<br>Fx: 202/835-8972<br>Website: www.ahsr.org | |
| National Library of Medicine (NLM)<br>Health Services/Technology Assessment Text (HSTAT) database<br>National Information Center on Health Services Research and Health Care Technology (NICHSR) | Ph: 301/496-1076<br>Fx: 301/401-3193<br>Website: text.nlm.nih.gov<br>Email: nichsr@nlm.nih.gov | |
| Health Outcomes Institute | Ph: 612/858-9188<br>Fx: 612/050-9109 | For Information on TyPe condition-specific instruments |
| Medical Outcomes Trust | 20 Park Plaza, Suite 1014<br>Boston, MA 02116<br>Ph: 617/426-4046<br>Fx: 617/426-4131<br>Email: motrust@worldnet.att.net | For information on the SF-36 Health Survey and other generic and condition-specific instruments |

analysis of evidence that the care a physician provides benefits a patient."

Specifically, AHCPR, an agency of the United States Department of Health and Human Services, has been exploring ways to "translate the accumulating knowledge of evidence-based medicine into everyday practice." Although AHCPR is best known for developing clinical practice guidelines covering a wide variety of conditions, it is expanding that effort with a nationwide evidence-based practice program, which has two components: an Internet-based national guideline clearinghouse, and the development of evidence-based reports on a variety of conditions.

The clearinghouse effort, launched in the fall of 1997, makes the agency's current practice guidelines—as well as other public and private guidelines—available on the Internet, says Douglas B. Kamerow, director of AHCPR's Office of the Forum for Quality and Effectiveness in Health Care. AHCPR has selected 12 evidence-based practice centers, essentially university-based research offices, to review and report evidence—both positive and negative—about specific clinical conditions. The goal, notes AHCPR, is to "broaden the review of state-of-the-art scientific information on medical disorders, screening tests, and new health-care technologies." Many of these common conditions make a significant impact on Medicare and Medicaid programs. They are conditions that tend to be costly, have a degree of untested effectiveness, and "have the potential to make a difference," noted Kamerow.

Clearly, health-care administrators and providers should view quality improvement as an ongoing process. The developments occurring in outcome measurement offer guidance on how to make this a successful effort. Moreover, emerging aspects, such as evidence-based reports that capture the scientific foundation of clinical care and the use of data detailing patient status, quality of life, and episodes of care, offer opportunities for health-care administrators to develop a quality-driven strategy for building and maintaining a high-quality, comprehensive system of patient care.

## REFERENCES

Berwick DM, Godfrey AB, Roessner J: Curing Health Care: New Strategies for Quality Improvement. New York, Perigee Books, 1986.

Bloom BS: Does it work? The outcomes of medical interventions. Int Technol Assess Health Care 6:326–332, 1990.

Brailer DJ, Kim LH: From nicety to necessity: Outcome measures come of age. Health Systems Rev Sept/Oct: 20–23, 1996.

Comarow A: Behind the HMO rankings: Our second set of ratings covers 223 plans in 46 states. US News & World Report, October 13:68, 1997.

Enthoven AC, Vorhaus CB: A vision of quality in health care delivery. Health Aff 16:44–57, 1997.

Epstein MA: The outcomes movement—will it get us where we want to go? N Engl J Med 323:266–270, 1990.

Hanchak NA, Murray JF, Hirsch A, et al: USQA health profile database as a tool for health plan quality improvement. Managed Care Q 4:58–69, 1996.

Improving allergy and asthma care through outcomes management (Monograph). American Academy of Allergy Asthma & Immunology. Milwaukee, WI, 1997.

Lopez L, Rovner J: Managed care strategies 1997: An annual report on the latest practices and policies in the new managed care environment. New York, Faulkner & Gray, 1996.

Marwick C: Proponents gather to discuss practicing evidence-based medicine. JAMA, 287:531, 532, 1997.

National Committee for Quality Assurance (NCQA): NCQA redefines accreditation with health plan standards that focus on results (Press Release). Washington DC, National Committee for Quality Assurance, Accreditation '99, March 1998.

Outcomes management comes of age. Business and Health, Special Report, Med Econ 14:7, 8, 10, 1996.

Physician Payment Review Commission: Annual Report to Congress. Washington, DC, 1996, p 269.

Report to Congress: Medicare payment policy, Medicare Payment Advisory Commission, Vol 1: Recommendations, March 1998, pp 27–29.

Risk adjustment primer: Boston, Department of Veterans Affairs, 1998.

Robinson J, Casalino L: The growth of medical groups paid through capitation in California. N Engl J Med 33:1684–1687, 1995.

Using outcomes to improve health care decision making: Primer: Management Decision and Research Center, Health Services Research and Development Service. Office of Research and Development, Department of Veterans Affairs, in collaboration with Association for Health Services Research, Boston, March 1997.

# INDEX

Note: Page numbers in *italics* refer to illustrations; page numbers followed by t refer to tables.

## A

Abandonment, 789–790
Abdomen, fetal, evaluation of, 243
Abdominal circumference, in fetal growth restriction, 330
 in gestational age determination, 240
Abdominal pain, in ectopic pregnancy, 28
 in leiomyoma, 53–54
 in pelvic inflammatory disease, 67, 67t, 71
Abdominal pregnancy, 36–37
Abdominal wall, trigger points of, in pelvic pain, 43, 45–46
Abortion, spontaneous. See *Pregnancy, early loss of.*
Abruptio placentae, 312–315
 classification of, 313, 313t
 clinical presentation of, 313
 diagnosis of, 313
 differential diagnosis of, 313
 disseminated intravascular coagulation and, 314–315
 management of, 314
 pathology of, 313–314
 perinatal mortality in, 312
 premature rupture of membranes and, 253
 risk factors for, 312–313, 312t
 severity of, 313, 313t
Abscess, breast, 173–174
 pelvic, 190, *192*
 tubo-ovarian, 70–71
  hysterectomy in, 112
  in adolescent, 77
  in premenopausal woman, 78
Abstinence, periodic, 13, 13t
Acanthosis nigricans, 572, 575
Accounting, financial, 816–818, 817t, 818t
 managerial, 822–823, 823t
Acne, during pregnancy, 426
Acquired immunodeficiency syndrome (AIDS), 413–422, 422t. See also *Human immunodeficiency virus (HIV) infection.*
Acrosin assay, in infertility, 661
Acrosome reaction, in male factor infertility, 633
Activity-based costing, 795–796
Acute tubular necrosis, postoperative, 506–507

Acyclovir, in herpes simplex virus infection, 62, 63t, 407, 432
Adenocarcinoma, vaginal, 454
Adenoma, hyperfunctioning, 585. See also *Hyperthyroidism.*
Adenosarcoma, uterine, 476–477
Adhesions, laparoscopic lysis of, 48–49, 126
 postoperative, 709–715
  etiology of, 711
  incidence of, 709–710, 710t
  pathophysiology of, 710–711, *711*
  treatment of, 712–715
   Interceed in, 712–713, *713*, *714*
   Seprafilm in, 713–715, *715*
 tubal, lysis of, 675–677, *675–677*
Adolescents. See also *Children.*
 adnexal mass in, 76–77, 76t, 77t
 dysfunctional uterine bleeding in, 102–105, 103t
 dysmenorrhea in, 105
 pelvic examination in, 84–85
 pelvic pain in, 105
 puberty in, 94t, 95–102. See also *Puberty.*
Adrenal gland, dysfunction of, amenorrhea and, 557
 tumors of, hyperandrogenism and, 574t, 575
Adrenocorticotropic hormone (ACTH) stimulation test, in amenorrhea, 553
 in hyperandrogenism, 573
Adult respiratory distress syndrome, postoperative, 508, *508*
β-Agonists, in maternal asthma, 372t, 374–375
Albuterol, in maternal asthma, 377, 377t
Alcohol use, early pregnancy loss and, 537
 infertility and, 610–611
 prenatal screening for, 207–208, 207t
 prevention of, 17
Alendronate, in osteoporosis, 599
Allergic rhinitis, during pregnancy, 426
Alopecia, in hyperandrogenism, 571
Alpha-fetoprotein, maternal, 206, 206t
 in Down syndrome, 206, *206*
 in neural tube defects, 206, *206*
 in prenatal diagnosis, 215, 215t
Alprazolam, in premenstrual syndrome, 692

Alzheimer's disease, hormone replacement therapy in, 595
Ambulatory cystourethrovaginometry, in urinary incontinence, 161
Amenorrhea, 551–559, 552t. See also *Anovulation; Infertility; Menopause.*
 adrenal dysfunction and, 557
 definition of, 551
 diagnosis of, 551
 differential diagnosis of, 554
 endometrial disorders and, 558
 genetic abnormalities and, 554
 hypothalamic anovulation and, 557
 in anorexia nervosa, 555–556
 in bulimia, 556–557
 laboratory tests in, 553–554
 outflow tract obstruction in, 555
 ovarian disorders and, 557–558
 patient history in, 551–553
 pelvic examination in, 553
 physical examination in, 553
 pituitary dysfunction and, 557
 secondary, 557–558
 systemic disorders and, 555–557
 treatment of, 558–559
γ-Aminobutyric acid, in premenstrual syndrome, 686
Amitriptyline, in pelvic pain, 47–48
Amniocentesis, 206
 decision analysis for, 839–841, *840*, *841*
 first-trimester, 217
 in fetal growth restriction, 331
 second-trimester, 216
Amniotic cavity, microbial invasion of, in premature rupture of membranes, 252–253, 253t, 254–256, 256t
Amniotic fluid, evaluation of, 244
 in premature rupture of membranes, 254
Amniotic fluid embolism, obstetric anesthesia and, 285
Ampicillin, in postoperative infection, 194
Analgesia. See also *Anesthesia, obstetric.*
 during pregnancy, 426, 429
 epidural, 273–274, 283
 spinal, 282–283, 282t
Androgen, excess levels of, 570–580. See also *Hyperandrogenism.*
 in sexual response cycle, 143
Androgen insensitivity syndrome, 99, *99*

861

Andrology, 629–638. *See also Infertility, male factor.*
Androstenedione, in hyperandrogenism, 573
 menopause and, 595
Anemia, during pregnancy, 340, 426
Anesthesia, for laparoscopy, 124
 obstetric, 276–288
  airway assessment for, 280
  antepartum hemorrhage and, 286, 286t
  asthma and, 285
  coexisting disease and, 279–280
  complications of, 280–281
  diabetes mellitus and, 284
  eclampsia and, 284
  embolism and, 285
  epidural, 281–283, 282t, 283t
  for cesarean section, 287, 287t, 288t
  heart disease and, 284
  human immunodeficiency virus infection and, 285
  hypertension and, 284
  hypovolemia and, 288
  liver disease and, 285–286
  maternal drug abuse and, 286–287
  maternal morbidity and, 277–278
  maternal mortality and, 277–278, 277t
  maternal physiology and, 279
  neuromuscular disease and, 284–285
  obesity and, 285
  perinatal morbidity and, 278–279
  perinatal mortality and, 278–279
  risks of, 277–279, 281–283
Anesthetic injection, for abdominal trigger points, 45–46
Aneurysm, cranial, obstetric anesthesia and, 285
Angiotensin-converting enzyme inhibitors, pregnancy contraindication to, 431
Anorexia nervosa, 555–556
Anovulation, 539–548. *See also Dysfunctional uterine bleeding; Infertility; Polycystic ovary syndrome.*
 evaluation of, 541
 incidence of, 539–540, *540*
 polycystic ovarian syndrome model in, 540–541, *540*
 treatment of, 541–548
  basal body temperature in, 541–542, *542*
  clomiphene citrate in, 543–544, 544t, 545t, 623
  gonadotropin therapy in, 547–548, 548t, 623–624
  insulin sensitizers in, 546
  ovarian cancer and, 545–546
  ovarian diathermy in, 546–547
  ovarian hyperstimulation with, 548
  ultrasonographic monitoring in, 542–543, *543*
  urinary LH monitoring in, 543, *543*
Antibiotics, after cesarean section, 304
 before hysterectomy, 117, 118–119
 during pregnancy, 426, 431–432
 for cesarean section, 301–302
 in bacterial vaginosis, 61, 61t
 in chancroid, 63
 in *Chlamydia trachomatis* infection, 62, 62t
 in intra-amniotic infection, 405
 in pelvic inflammatory disease, 69–70, 69t, 70t
 in postoperative infection, 193–194, 193t

Antibiotics *(Continued)*
 in premature rupture of membranes, 258–259, 259t, 404
 in preterm labor, 350
 in syphilis, 62–63, 63t
 in tubo-ovarian abscess, 112
 postoperative, 506
 preoperative, 502
Antibodies, anticardiolipin, early pregnancy loss and, 24–25
 antiphospholipid, early pregnancy loss and, 24, 25, 25t, 536, 536t
 antithyroid, 588
 blocking, early pregnancy loss and, 25
 lupus, early pregnancy loss and, 24–25
 sperm, 633–634, 636–637, 646, 668–669
 zona, 669
Anticardiolipin antibodies, early pregnancy loss and, 24–25
Anticholinergics, in detrusor instability, 163t, 164
Anticoagulants, during pregnancy, 426, 429–430, 430t
Anticonvulsants, during pregnancy, 430–431
Antidepressants, during pregnancy, 432–433, 432t
 in pelvic pain, 47–48
 in urinary incontinence, 163–164, 163t
Antifibrinolytics, in dysfunctional uterine bleeding, 567
Antifungals, during pregnancy, 426, 432
 in vulvovaginal candidiasis, 62, 62t
Antigen D, prenatal testing for, 202
Antihypertensives, during pregnancy, 431
Antiphospholipid antibodies, early pregnancy loss and, 24, 25, 25t, 536, 536t
Antiprostaglandins, in dysfunctional uterine bleeding, 565–566
Antipsychotics, during pregnancy, 433
Antispasmodics, in detrusor instability, 163t, 164
Antisperm antibody, in infertility, 633–634, 636–637, 646, 668–669
Antithrombin III deficiency, oral contraceptive–related cardiovascular disease and, 5
Antithyroid antibodies, 588
Antivirals, in herpes simplex virus infection, 62, 63t, 407, 432
 in HIV infection, 417, 417t, 418t, 419t
Anxiety disorders, during pregnancy, 426
Anxiolytics, during pregnancy, 433
Aortic stenosis, obstetric anesthesia and, 284
Arrhythmias, during pregnancy, 427
Asgaard system, 842–843, *842*, *843*
Asherman's syndrome, early pregnancy loss and, 23, 535
 infertility in, 619
Asphyxia, neonatal, 357
Aspirin, during pregnancy, 429
 in antiphospholipid syndrome, 25, 25t
 in pre-eclampsia, 388, 755–757, *756*, 756t
Assisted fertilization, 652
Assisted hatching, 652
Assisted reproductive technology, 641–653, 642t
 assisted fertilization as, 652
 assisted hatching as, 652
 controlled ovarian hyperstimulation as, 642–645, 644t, 645t
 embryo micromanipulation as, 651–653

Assisted reproductive technology *(Continued)*
 gamete intrafallopian transfer as, *643*, 649–650
 gamete micromanipulation as, 651–653
 gestational surrogacy as, 651
 in vitro fertilization as, *643*, 646–649, 648t
 intrauterine insemination as, 621–622, 642–646, *643*, 644t, 645t
 oocyte donation as, *643*, 650–651
 preimplantation genetic diagnosis as, 652–653
 referral for, 641–642, *643*
 zygote intrafallopian transfer as, 650
Asthma, maternal, 369–378, 426
 antenatal management in, 375–377, 376t
 bronchodilators in, 372t, 374–375
 corticosteroids in, 371–374, 372t
 delivery management in, 377–378
 emergency management of, 377, 377t
 environmental management in, 370–371, 371t
 exacerbations of, 376–377, 377t
 home management of, 376–377, 377t
 labor management in, 377–378
 leukotrienes in, 375
 monitoring of, 370
 patient education in, 371
 perinatal effects of, 369–370, 370t
 pharmacologic therapy in, 371–375, 372t
 severity of, 370, 370t
 step therapy in, 375, 375t
 treatment of, 429
 obstetric anesthesia and, 285
Atelectasis, postoperative, 507–508
Atrial fibrillation, hyperthyroidism and, 585
Atypical squamous cells of undetermined significance, 440
Autoimmune disease, early pregnancy loss and, 24–25, 536
Autoimmune thyroiditis, 587, 587t
Azoospermia, in infertility, 635–636, 635t, 636t
Azotemia, postoperative, 506–507
Aztreonam, in postoperative infection, 194

**B**

Backache, in leiomyoma, 53
Bacteriuria. *See also Infection.*
 asymptomatic, during pregnancy, 403
 prenatal testing for, 203–204
Bar charts, in epidemiology, 746, *746*
Barrier contraceptives, 10–13, 11t, 12t
Basal body temperature, in ovulation, 541–542, *542*, 543, *543*, 615–616, *617*, 662
Beckwith-Weidemann syndrome, fetal macrosomia and, 333
Beclomethasone dipropionate, in maternal asthma, 372–373, 372t
Bellergal-S, for hot flushes, 598
Benzodiazepines, in premenstrual syndrome, 692
Bicarbonate, in diabetic ketoacidosis, 366
Biochemical assays, in prenatal diagnosis, 221
Biofeedback, in urinary incontinence, 166
Bioinformatics, 843–844

Biophysical profile, in fetal assessment, 228–229, 228t, 229t
  in fetal growth restriction, 331
  in post-term pregnancy, 356–357
  in premature rupture of membranes, 257
  modified, in fetal assessment, 229–230
Biopsy, blastocyst, 653
  breast, 171–172, *173*, 181–182, 526
  cervical, 446, *446*, 520–521
  endometrial, 567
    in infertility, 617–618, 662
    in pelvic inflammatory disease, 68
Biparietal diameter, in gestational age determination, 240
Bipolar disorder, during pregnancy, 428, 433
Bisphosphonates, in osteoporosis, 599
Bladder, cancer of, in pregnancy, 524
  exstrophy of, uterine prolapse with, 93, *93*
  fetal, evaluation of, 243
  intraoperative injury to, 503
  laparoscope injury to, 128
Blastocyst biopsy, 653
Bleeding, uterine, breakthrough, 4, 563
  dysfunctional, 560–568. See also *Dysfunctional uterine bleeding.*
  estrogen withdrawal and, 562
  in leiomyoma, 53
  menstrual, 560–562
  postmenopausal, 80
  progesterone withdrawal and, 563
  vaginal, in ectopic pregnancy, 28
Blocking antibodies, early pregnancy loss and, 25
Blood pressure, estrogen effects on, 596
Blood type, prenatal testing for, 202, 202t
Body mass index, maternal, fetal growth restriction and, 327
Bone mineral density, fracture and, 597–598, 597t
Bone tumors, in pregnancy, 527–528
Botryoid sarcoma (embryonal carcinoma), 90, *90*
Bovine cervical mucus penetration test, in male factor infertility, 632
Bowel, endometriosis of, 703
  fetal, evaluation of, 243
  intraoperative injury to, 505, *505*
  laparoscope injury to, 128
  preoperative preparation of, 501–502, 502t
Breast, 170–181
  abscess of, 173–174
  atypical hyperplasia of, 178, 178t
  benign disease of, 177–178
  biopsy of, 171–172, *173*, 181–182, 526
  cancer of, 178–179, 178t
    chemoprevention of, 182
    hormone replacement therapy and, 180, 600
    in pregnancy, 525–527
    malpractice suits in, 790–791
    nipple discharge in, 175
    oral contraceptives and, 5, 180
    therapeutic abortion and, 526
    treatment of, in managed-care plans, 732
  cellulitis of, 173
  clinician examination of, 18
  core needle biopsy of, 172, 181–182
  duct ectasia of, 174
  ductal carcinoma in situ of, 178–179, 178t

Breast (Continued)
  examination of, 170–171
  fat necrosis of, 172
  fibroadenoma of, 176
  fine-needle aspiration of, 171–172, *173*
  high-risk lesions of, 178–179, 178t
  infections of, 172–174
  inspection of, 170–171
  intraductal papilloma of, 175
  lobular carcinoma in situ of, 178–179, 178t
  mass of, 171–172
  Mondor's disease of, 179
  Paget's disease of, 179–180
  pain in, 177
  palpation of, 171
  phyllodes tumor of, 176–177
  premature development of, 101
  radiologic imaging of, 181–182, 181t. See also *Mammography.*
  self-examination of, 18, 170
Breastfeeding, after breast cancer treatment, 527
  maternal asthma and, 378
Breath, postoperative shortness of, 507–508, *508*
Breech delivery, 296–297, 296t
Bromocriptine, in amenorrhea, 558
  in premenstrual syndrome, 691–692
Bronchodilators, in maternal asthma, 372t, 374–375
Budgeting, 820–821, 821t
Bulimia, 556–557
Burns, laparoscope-related, 128

## C

CA 125, in ovarian epithelial cancer, 482, 484
Calcitonin, in osteoporosis, 599
  in thyroid carcinoma, 590
Calcium, in pre-eclampsia, 388
Calcium channel blockers, during pregnancy, 431
  in detrusor instability, 163t, 164–165
  in preterm labor, 349
Candidiasis, vulvovaginal, 57–58, 60t, 62, 62t
Capillary hemangioma, 89–90
CapSure device, in urinary incontinence, 167–168
Carbapenems, in postoperative infection, 193–194, 193t
Cardiovascular disease, estrogen-mediated prevention of, 596
  menopause and, 595–596
  oral contraceptives and, 4–5
Case report, in epidemiology, 752
Case series, in epidemiology, 752
Case-control study, in epidemiology, 752, *753*
Cash management, 821–822, 922t
Catalase, in premature rupture of membranes diagnosis, 255
*CCR4* gene, in human immunodeficiency virus infection, 414
Cellulitis, of breast, 173
  of vaginal surgical margin (cuff), 189, *190*
  pelvic, 189–190, *191*
  postoperative, 506
Cephalopelvic disproportion, 269–270, 269t
Cephalosporins, during pregnancy, 431

Cephalosporins (Continued)
  in postoperative infection, 193, 193t
Cerclage, anesthesia for, 283
  in early pregnancy loss, 22
  in preterm labor prevention, 350–351
  removal of, in premature rupture of membranes, 260–261
Cerebellum, fetal, evaluation of, 241, *242*
Certified nurse midwives, 740
Cervical cap, 11–12, 11t
Cervical intraepithelial neoplasia, 439–440, *440*. See also *Cervix, cancer of.*
  cone biopsy in, 446, *446*
  differential diagnosis of, 442
  human papillomavirus infection and, 59, 440–441, 446, *446*, 447, 458–459, 459t
  in pregnancy, 520, 520t
  laboratory evaluation in, 442
  physical examination in, *441*, 442
  topical transretinoic acid in, 447
  treatment of, 444–446, *444*, *445*
Cervical mucus method, of natural family planning, 13
Cervical mucus tests, in infertility, 613–615, *614*, *615*
Cervical pregnancy, 37
Cervical ultrasonography, in preterm labor, 346–347, 346t
Cervix, cancer of, 458–468. See also *Cervical intraepithelial neoplasia.*
  diagnosis of, 458–461, 459t, 460t
  differential diagnosis of, 460
  human papillomavirus infection and, 59, 440–441, 446, *446*, 447, 458–459, 459t
  in pregnancy, 519–522, 520t, 521t
  incidental discovery of, 468
  lymphatic metastases from, 461–462, *462*
  pathology of, 462
  patient history in, 460
  physical examination in, 460
  prognosis for, 463, 463t
  risk factors for, 458–459, 459t
  spread of, 461–462, *462*
  staging of, 461, 461t
  treatment of, 463–466, *464*, *465*
    chemotherapy in, 466–467
    computed tomography in, 466
    for recurrent cancer, 467
    for stage IA1, 464, *465*
    for stage IA2, 464–465, *465*
    for stage IB, *465*, 465–466
    for stage IIA, *465*, 465–466
    for stage IIB, 466
    for stage III, 466
    for stage IV, 466
    radiation therapy in, 463–464, 467
    recurrence after, 467
    staging of, 466
    surgery in, 463, *464*, 467–468
  cone biopsy of, 446, *446*, 520–521
  endometrial carcinoma extension to, 460
  human papillomavirus infection of, 59
    cervical cancer and, 458–459, 459t
    cervical intraepithelial neoplasia and, 440–441, 446, *446*
    immunobiology of, 447
    in children, 86t
    treatment of, 443
  in ectopic pregnancy, 29
  incompetent, preterm labor and, 350
  infection of. See also specific infections.

## 864 INDEX

Cervix (Continued)
　　infertility and, 618, 624–625
　　mucopurulent, 58
　leiomyoma of, vs. cancer, 460
Cesarean section, 299–309
　anesthesia for, 287, 287t, 288t
　antibiotic administration for, 301–302
　clinical pathway for, 800t–802t
　complications of, 304–305
　definition of, 299
　emergency, 287
　epidemiologic studies of, 757–758, 757
　fetal indications for, 300–301, 300t
　human immunodeficiency virus transmission and, 261
　hysterectomy with, 307–309
　in abruptio placentae, 314
　in cervical cancer, 521, 521t
　incision for, 302–304
　indications for, 300–301, 300t
　infection after, 304–305
　maternal indications for, 300, 300t
　maternal-fetal indications for, 300t, 301
　outcome measures for, 805t
　rates of, 299–300, 300t, 301
　septic pelvic thrombophlebitis after, 305
　site preparation for, 301
　skin incision for, 302
　standard order set for, 806t
　thromboembolic disease after, 305
　uterine incision for, 302–304
　vaginal delivery after, 305–307, 306t, 307t
　vs. forceps delivery, 295
　wound closure for, 303–304
　wound infection after, 304–305
CFTR gene, 635
Chancroid, 59, 63
Chemical exposure, early pregnancy loss and, 537
Chemotherapy, early pregnancy loss and, 537
　in cervical cancer, 466–467
　in hydatidiform mole, 515
　in ovarian cancer, 484–486, 484, 485, 485t, 487–488, 487t
　in persistent gestational trophoblastic disease, 515–518, 516t, 517t
　in pregnancy, 523–524, 527
　in sex cord stromal tumors, 496
Childbirth. See Delivery; Labor.
Children. See also Puberty.
　ambiguous genitalia in, 92, 92
　bladder exstrophy in, 93, 93
　botryoid sarcoma (embryonal carcinoma) in, 90, 90
　Chlamydia trachomatis infection in, 86t
　clitoral anomalies in, 92–93
　condyloma acuminata in, 86t
　congenital genital malformations in, 91–95, 92, 93
　enterobiasis in, 86t
　external genitalia of, 82–83, 83
　genital herpes simplex virus infection in, 86t
　genital trauma in, 90–91, 91
　genital tumors in, 89–90
　gonorrhea in, 86t
　hymenal anomalies in, 93, 93
　hymenal orifice in, 84
　labial adhesions in, 88–89, 88
　labial anomalies in, 92, 92
　lichen sclerosus in, 87–88, 88
　pelvic examination in, 83–84, 83
　perineal hygiene for, 87

Children (Continued)
　prenatal cocaine exposure of, 392–393
　rhabdomyosarcoma in, 90
　syphilis in, 86t
　urethral prolapse in, 89, 89
　vaginal anomalies in, 93–95
　vaginal foreign bodies in, 87, 87
　vulvar anomalies in, 92
　vulvovaginitis in, 85–87, 85, 86t
Chlamydia trachomatis infection, 58
　during pregnancy, 411
　in children, 86t
　in unexplained infertility, 667
　premature rupture of membranes and, 251
　prenatal testing for, 204
　treatment of, 62, 62t
Cholesterol, in cardiovascular disease, 596
　screening recommendations for, 19
Chorioamnionitis, premature rupture of membranes and, 250–251, 254–256, 256t, 257
Chorionic villus sampling, 206, 217, 217
Choroid plexus, fetal, cyst of, 241, 241
Chromosome(s), abnormalities of, alpha-fetoprotein levels and, 215
　choroidal plexus cyst and, 241
　estriol levels and, 215
　β-human chorionic gonadotropin levels and, 215–216
　in early pregnancy loss, 21, 21t
　maternal age and, 213, 214t
　multiple miscarriages and, 214
　nuchal translucency and, 216, 216, 236, 237
　previously affected pregnancy and, 214
　screening for. See Prenatal diagnosis.
Chromosome-painting probes, 222
Cigarette smoking, cessation of, clinic effectiveness for, 781–782, 781t
　during pregnancy, 429
　early pregnancy loss and, 537
　infertility and, 610
　prevention of, 15–16, 16t
Cimetidine, in hyperandrogenism, 579
Circumcision, 324
Cirrhosis, preoperative evaluation of, 500, 500t
Cisterna magna, fetal, evaluation of, 241, 242
Citrovorum factor, in ectopic pregnancy management, 35–36
Clavicle, fracture of, in shoulder dystocia, 294
Climacteric, 593, 593
Clindamycin, in postoperative infection, 194
Clinical effectiveness, 773–784
　care delivery processes in, 774–775, 774, 775
　clinical policy-making component of, 775t, 776–777
　clinical practice profiling in, 776
　decision-making processes in, 774–775, 774, 775
　definition of, 774
　effectiveness research in, 775–776
　external performance reporting in, 776
　implementation component of, 775t, 776t, 777–778
　initiatives for, 778–780, 779, 780
　in cervical cancer screening, 780–781
　in mammography, 782–783, 782
　in smoking cessation, 781–782, 781t
　measurement component of, 775–776, 775t, 776

Clinical effectiveness (Continued)
　methodologic domains of, 775–778, 775t, 776
　population needs assessment in, 775
　practice policies in, 775t, 776–777
　process analysis of, 774–775, 774
　program evaluation in, 776
Clinical pathways, 793–807
　activity-based costing for, 795–796
　conflict resolution and, 796
　consensus development and, 796
　cost accounting systems for, 795
　development of, 794, 794
　evaluation of, 805–806
　for cesarean section, 800t–802t
　for hysterectomy, 803t–804t
　for vaginal birth, 798t–799t
　future directions for, 806–807, 807
　implementation of, 794–795
　on-line, 806–807, 807
　outcomes measures for, 796–805, 798t–799t, 800t–802t, 803t–804t, 805t
　standard order sets for, 805, 805t, 806t
Clinical trials, in epidemiology, 753–754, 754
Clitoris, bifid, 93
　enlargement of, 92–93
Clomiphene citrate, in anovulation, 543–545, 544t, 545t, 623
　ovarian cancer and, 545–546
　side effects of, 545
Clonidine, for hot flushes, 598–599
Coagulation disorders, in adolescent dysfunctional uterine bleeding, 103–104
Cocaine abuse, prenatal, 391–393
　childhood effects of, 392–393
　fetal effects of, 392
　neonatal effects of, 391–392
　obstetric anesthesia and, 286–287
　treatment protocol for, 397–398
Coding, 826–833
　Current Procedural Terminology for, 827–828
　Evaluation and Management terminology for, 828–833
　International Classification of Diseases, 9th Revision, for, 832–833
Cohort study, in epidemiology, 752–753, 753
Cold sores, during pregnancy, 427
Collagen, abnormalities of, genital tract prolapse and, 137
Collagen vascular disorders, maternal, fetal growth restriction and, 328
Colon, cancer of, in pregnancy, 524–525
　endometriosis of, 703
　intraoperative injury to, 505, 505
Colpocleisis, in genital tract prolapse, 140
Computed tomography, in amenorrhea, 553, 554
　in ovarian epithelial cancer, 482
Computer-based medical records, 834–837
　evaluation of, 836–837
Condom, 11t, 12–13
　female, 11, 11t
Condyloma acuminata, 59
　in children, 86t
　treatment of, 63, 63t, 442–443
Cone biopsy, in cervical intraepithelial neoplasia, 446, 446, 520–521
Congenital adrenal hyperplasia, hyperandrogenism and, 575
Congenital malformations, diagnosis of. See Prenatal diagnosis; Ultrasonography.

Congenital malformations *(Continued)*
　maternal diabetes mellitus and, 366
　of genitalia, 91–95, *92, 93*
Consent, informed, 788–789
　preoperative, 502
Constipation, chronic, 42
　during pregnancy, 427
　in genital tract prolapse, 137
Contraception, 3–14
　barrier, 10–13, 11t, 12t
　emergency, 9
　implants for, 8–9
　injectable preparations for, 8
　intrauterine devices for, 9–10
　oral contraceptives for, 3–8. See also *Oral contraceptives.*
　postcoital, 9
　selection of, 13–14
Contraction stress test, in fetal growth restriction, 331
Contraction-stimulation test, in post-term pregnancy, 356
Controlled ovarian hyperstimulation, 642–645, 644t, 645t
Convulsions, eclamptic, 386–387, 386t, 387t
Copper 7, 10
Core needle biopsy, of breast, 172, *173,* 181–182
Cornua, resection of, in ectopic pregnancy management, 34
Corporate finance, 824–825
Corticosteroids, in hyperandrogenism, 578–579
　in maternal asthma, 371–374, 372t
Corticotropin-releasing hormone, fetal, preterm labor and, 345
Cough, during pregnancy, 427
Coumarin, during pregnancy, 430, 430t
Cromolyn sodium, in maternal asthma, 372t, 373–374
Cross-sectional study, in epidemiology, 752
Crown-rump length, for gestational age determination, 235–236, 235t
Cryotherapy, in cervical intraepithelial neoplasia, 445–446
　in uterine leiomyoma, 56
Culdocentesis, in ectopic pregnancy, 32
Current Procedural Terminology, 827–828
Cushing's disease, hyperandrogenism and, 575
Cushing's syndrome, hyperandrogenism and, 575
Cyproterone acetate, in hyperandrogenism, 578
Cyst(s), choroid plexus, in fetus, 241, *241*
　mesonephric duct (Gartner's), in children, 89
　ovarian. See also *Polycystic ovary syndrome.*
　　in adolescent, 76, 77
　　in children, 75–76, 75t
　　in newborn, 75, 75t
　　in pregnancy, 522–523
　　in premenopausal woman, 78–79
　　vaginal, 454
Cystectomy, laparoscopy in, 127
Cystic fibrosis, infertility and, 634–635
　screening for, 222
Cystitis, during pregnancy, 403–404
　interstitial, treatment of, 45
Cystometry, complex, in urinary incontinence, 160–161
　simple, in urinary incontinence, 159, *160*

Cystostomy, intraoperative, 503
Cystourethroscopy, in pelvic pain, 44
Cystourethrovaginometry, in urinary incontinence, 161
Cytomegalovirus infection, during pregnancy, 407

**D**

Danazol, in dysfunctional uterine bleeding, 567
　in endometriosis, 698
　in premenstrual syndrome, 692
*DAZ* gene, 634
Deep venous thrombosis, perioperative prevention of, 502
　preoperative risk for, 500, 500t
Dehydroepiandrosterone, in hyperandrogenism, 573
Dehydroepiandrosterone sulfate, in hyperandrogenism, 573
Delavirdine, in maternal HIV infection, 418t, 419t
Delivery. See also *Labor; Postpartum management.*
　breech, 296–297, 296t
　cesarean, 299–309. See also *Cesarean section.*
　forceps, 294–295, 294t
　genital tract prolapse and, 136–137
　gestational diabetes mellitus and, 365
　maternal asthma and, 377–378
　of multifetal pregnancy, 342, 342t
　post-term, 353–358. See also *Post-term pregnancy.*
　preterm, 344–351. See also *Preterm labor.*
　vacuum, 295–296
　vaginal, 291–293
　　after cesarean section, 305–306, 306t, 307t
　　breech, 296–297, 296t
　　position for, 292
　　preparation for, 292
　　procedures for, 292–293
　　shoulder dystocia with, 293–294
　　vacuum, 295–296
Depression, during pregnancy, 427
　postpartum, 323
Dermatitis, during pregnancy, 427
Desmopressin acetate, in dysfunctional uterine bleeding, 566
Detrusor instability, treatment of, 163t, 164–165, 166, 167
Dexamethasone suppression test, in hyperandrogenism, 574
Diabetes mellitus, congenital malformations and, 366
　early pregnancy loss and, 535
　fetal growth restriction and, 328
　fetal macrosomia and, 332
　gestational, 360–366, 427
　　delivery timing in, 365
　　diagnosis of, 362–363, 363t
　　dietary therapy in, 364–365
　　glucose monitoring in, 364
　　insulin treatment in, 364
　　neonatal complications of, 360–361
　　prevalence of, 362, 362t
　　screening for, 206–207, 361–362
　　treatment of, 363–365
　　　Asgaard system analysis of, 842–843, *843*
　　obstetric anesthesia and, 284

Diabetes mellitus *(Continued)*
　pregestational, 365–366, 365t
　pregnancy and, 208
　preoperative evaluation of, 500
Diabetic ketoacidosis, 366
Diaphragm, 11, 11t
Diarrhea, during pregnancy, 427
Diathermy, ovarian, in anovulation, 546–547
Dicyclomine, in detrusor instability, 163t, 164
Didanosine, in maternal HIV infection, 418t, 419t
Diet, in gestational diabetes mellitus, 364–365
　in premenstrual syndrome, 690–691
Digital rectal examination, in male factor infertility, 631
Dilatation and curettage, diagnostic, 129–130
　vs. hysteroscopy, 131–132
　in dysfunctional uterine bleeding, 568
　in ectopic pregnancy, 32
Dilator therapy, in pain-based sexual dysfunction, 147–148
Disseminated intravascular coagulation, abruptio placentae and, 314–315
Diuretics, during pregnancy, 427, 431
　postoperative, 507
Dopamine, postoperative, 507
Doppler ultrasonography, in fetal assessment, 230–231, 231t
　in fetal growth restriction, 330
Double ring (double decidua) sign, in first-trimester ultrasonography, 234
Down syndrome, maternal age and, 213, 214t
　prenatal testing for, 205–206, *206,* 213, 214t, 215
Doxepin, in urinary incontinence, 163–164, 163t
Drug(s), during pregnancy, 424–433, 425t, 433
　infertility and, 611
　sexual dysfunction with, 145
　urinary incontinence with, 153, 153t
Drug abuse, 390–398. See also specific drugs.
　fetal growth restriction and, 327
　obstetric anesthesia and, 286–287
Ductal carcinoma in situ, 178–179, 178t
Dysfunctional uterine bleeding, 562–563
　diagnosis of, 563
　hysteroscopy in, 130–132
　in adolescents, 102–105, 103t
　treatment of, 563–568
　　antifibrinolytic agents in, 567
　　antiprostaglandins in, 565–566
　　danazol in, 567
　　desmopressin in, 566
　　endometrial ablation in, 566
　　estrogen therapy in, 565
　　gonadotropin-releasing hormone agonists in, 566
　　guidelines for, 567–568
　　hysterectomy in, 110
　　oral contraceptive therapy in, 564–565
　　progestin IUD in, 566
　　progestin therapy in, 564, 566
Dysgerminoma, 77, 490–495. See also *Germ cell tumors.*
Dysmenorrhea, 40–50. See also *Pelvic pain; Premenstrual syndrome.*
　in adolescents, 105
　primary, 41

Dysmenorrhea *(Continued)*
  secondary, 41
  treatment of, 44, 49
  vs. cyclic pelvic pain, 40–41
Dyspareunia, 146, 146t
Dystocia, 267–268, 267t, 269–271, *270*, 270t
  diagnosis of, 271
  overdiagnosis of, 270–271
  shoulder, 293–294

### E

Eclampsia, 386–387, 386t, 387t. See also *Pre-eclampsia*.
  anesthesia and, 284
Economics, health, 719–732. See also *Health economics*.
Ectopic pregnancy, 27–37
  abdominal, 36–37
  adnexal mass and, 29
  cervical, 37
  cervical examination in, 29
  culdocentesis in, 32
  diagnosis of, 28–29, 28t, 29t
  dilatation and curettage in, 32
  epidemiology of, 27
  etiology of, 28, 28t
  human chorionic gonadotropin in, 30, 30t
  in combined pregnancy, 36
  laboratory testing in, 30–31, 30t
  laparoscopy in, 32
  management of, 32–36
    laparoscopy in, 126–127
    nonsurgical, 34–36, 35t
    surgical, 32–34, 33t
  mortality with, 27–28
  ovarian, 37
  pathology of, 29–30
  pelvic examination in, 29
  pregnancy after, 28, 36
  risk factors for, 28, 28t
  rupture of, 29
  serum progesterone in, 30–31
  site of, 27, 27t
  ultrasonography in, 31–32, 31t, 234–235
  uterine examination in, 29
Ejaculation, dysfunction of, in infertility, 637
Electrocautery, for laparoscopy, 123–124
Electrolysis, for hair removal, 580
Electromagnetic radiation, early pregnancy loss and, 537
Embolism, obstetric anesthesia and, 285
  pulmonary, after molar evacuation, 514–515
  postoperative, 508
Emotional factors, in unexplained infertility, 669–670
Employment, early pregnancy loss and, 537
Endodermal sinus tumor, vaginal, 456
Endometrial stromal sarcoma, 477
Endometriosis, 695–707, *696*
  classification of, 696, *697*
  clinical presentation of, 695–696
  colonic, 703
  definition of, 695
  differential diagnosis of, 695–696
  extrapelvic, 703, 704t
  in perimenopausal women, 79
  in premenopausal women, 78

Endometriosis *(Continued)*
  in unexplained infertility, 667
  infertility and, 619–620, 622–623, 646
  laparoscopic staging of, 699
  ovarian, 701–702, *702*
  retroperitoneal, 703
  treatment of, 696–701
    adhesiolysis in, 701
    adhesion prevention in, 706
    carbon dioxide laser ablation in, 699–700
    combination, 707
    hysterectomy in, 110–111, 706–707
    laparoscopic, 126, 699–701, *700*
    laparotomy in, 701
    medical, 696–699
    oophorectomy in, 707
    pain relief in, 703–706, *704*
    presacral neurectomy in, 704–706, *705*
    second-look laparoscopy in, 706
    surgical, 699
    uterine nerve ablation in, 704, *704*
    uterine suspension in, 706
  tubal, 702–703
  urinary tract, 703
Endometrium, ablation of, in dysfunctional uterine bleeding, 113, 566
  atypical hyperplasia of, hysterectomy in, 111, 111t
  biopsy of, 567
  in infertility, 617–618, 662
  cancer of, 471–476
    cervical extension of, 460
    diagnosis of, 472
    differential diagnosis of, 472
    hormone replacement therapy and, 599–600
    laboratory evaluation in, 472
    oral contraceptives and, 5
    pathology of, 472–473
    patient history in, 472
    physical examination in, 472
    risk factors for, 471–472, 471t
    staging of, 474, 474t, 475t
    transvaginal ultrasonography in, 472
    treatment of, 473–476, *474*, 474t, 475t
      adjuvant radiation in, 475–476, 475t
      progestational therapy in, 476
      surgery in, 474–475, 475t
    vs. leiomyoma, 109
  disorders of, amenorrhea and, 558
  hyperplasia of, 472–473, 473t
    hormone replacement therapy and, 599–600
    treatment of, 473, *474*
  papillary serous carcinoma of, 476
Endomyometritis, after cesarean section, 304
Endopelvic fascia, 134, 135–136, *136*
Enterobiasis, in children, 86t
Enterocele, after hysterectomy, 119
Ephedrine, in stress urinary incontinence, 162–163, 163t
Epidemiology, 744–758
  applications of, 754–758, *755–757*
  bar charts in, 746, *746*
  case report in, 752
  case series in, 752
  case-control study in, 752, *753*
  central tendency in, 749–750
  clinical trials in, 753–754, *754*
  cohort study in, 752–753, *753*

Epidemiology *(Continued)*
  cross-sectional study in, 752
  cumulative incidence in, 747, *748*
  definition of, 745
  distribution in, 749
  experimental studies in, 753–754
  frequency tables in, 746, 746t
  in practice management, 757–758, *757*
  in treatment decisions, 755–757, *756*, 756t
  incidence density in, 747
  incidence in, 747
  longitudinal study in, 752
  median in, 749–750
  mode in, 750
  nonexperimental studies in, 751–753, *751*
  odds ratio in, 748–749
  populations in, 745–746
  prevalence in, 747, *748*
  prevalence study in, 752
  proportions in, 746–747
  quartiles in, 750
  range in, 750
  rate in, 747
  ratio in, 747
  relative risk in, 747–748
  samples in, 745–746
  standard deviation in, 751
  study designs for, 751–754, *751*
  variables in, 746
  variance in, 750–751
  variation in, 750–751
Epilepsy, pregnancy and, 208
Episiotomy, 292
Erythroblastosis fetalis, 202
17β-Estradiol (E$_2$), menopausal levels of, 598
Estriol, unconjugated, in prenatal diagnosis, 215
Estrogen(s). See also *Hormone replacement therapy*.
  for hormone replacement therapy, 601–602, 601t, 602t, 603t
  for oral contraceptives, 3–4, 6–7, 7t
  in dysfunctional uterine bleeding, 565, 567
  in sexual response cycle, 143
  in urinary incontinence, 162, 163t
Etidronate, in osteoporosis, 599
Evaluation and Management coding, 828–833
  consultations and, 832
  dictation in, 830–831
  documentation guidelines for, 831–832
  genitourinary single system examination in, 829–830
  medical decision-making and, 831
  templates in, 830–831
Exercise, amenorrhea and, 556–557
  early pregnancy loss and, 537
  in premenstrual syndrome, 690

### F

Factor V Leiden mutation, oral contraceptive–related cardiovascular disease and, 5
Fallopian tube, adhesions of, hydrodissection of, 676
  lysis of, 675–677, *675–677*
  ampullary-ampullary anastomosis of, 680, *680*
  anastomosis of, 679–681, *680*, *681*

Fallopian tube *(Continued)*
  congenital anomalies of, 678
  endometriosis of, 702–703
  evaluation of, 674
  fimbrioplasty of, 676–677, *676, 677*
  interstitial-ampullary anastomosis of, 680–681, *681*
  isthmic-ampullary anastomosis of, 680
  isthmic-isthmic anastomosis of, 680
  ostium of, creation of, 677–678, *678, 679*
  posthysterectomy infection of, 190, *191*
  surgery on, 622, 673–682, 674t. See also specific procedures.
  transcervical catheterization of, 681
  uterine implantation of, 681
Falloposcopy, in unexplained infertility, 666
Familial cancer syndromes, hysterectomy in, 112
Fat necrosis, of breast, 172
Fecal occult blood screening, 18–19
Fecundability, 609
Fecundity, 609
FemAssist device, in urinary incontinence, 167
Femur length, in gestational age determination, 240
Ferning, of amniotic fluid, 254
  of cervical mucus, 615, *615*
Fetal compression syndrome, premature rupture of membranes and, 253–254
Fetal growth restriction, 326–331
  diagnosis of, 329–330, 329t
  fetal factors in, 327
  management of, 330–331
  maternal factors in, 327–329, 328t
Fetal length/abdominal circumference ratio, in fetal growth restriction, 330
Fetal pole, on ultrasonography, 235
Fetus. See also *Neonate.*
  abdomen of, evaluation of, 243
  abdominal circumference of, in fetal growth restriction, 330
    in gestational age determination, 240
  assessment of, 204–205, 224–232
    algorithm for, 232
    biophysical profile for, 228–229, 228t, 229t
    Doppler ultrasonography for, 230–231, 231t
    in fetal growth restriction, 329–330, 329t
    indications for, 226, 231–232, 232t
    maternal, 226–227
    modified biophysical profile for, 229–230
    nonstress test for, 227
  biparietal diameter of, in gestational age determination, 240
  bladder of, evaluation of, 243
  bowel of, evaluation of, 243
  cerebellum of, evaluation of, 241, *242*
  choroid of, cyst of, 241, *241*
  cisterna magna of, evaluation of, 241, *242*
  cocaine effects on, 392
  crown-rump length of, in gestational age determination, 235–236, 235t
  death of, heroine abuse and, 393
    in abruptio placentae, 314
    rate of, 224–225, 225t
    risk for, 225, 225t
  femur length of, in gestational age determination, 240
  gender of, evaluation of, 243–244

Fetus *(Continued)*
  gestational age of, anatomical structures and, 236, 236t
    biparietal diameter for, 240
    crown-rump length for, 235–236, 235t
    femur length for, 240
    first-trimester ultrasonography for, 235–236, 235t, 236t
    head circumference for, 240
    preterm labor and, 344
    second-trimester ultrasonography for, 240
  growth of, abnormalities of, 326–334, 327t. See also *Fetal growth restriction; Macrosomia;* specific abnormalities.
    cocaine effects on, 392
    maternal heroin abuse and, 394
    maternal marijuana use and, 395–396
    serial assessment of, 331
  head circumference/abdominal circumference ratio in, in fetal growth restriction, 330
  head growth in, cocaine effects on, 392
  heart of, evaluation of, 242–243, *242*
  herpes simplex virus infection in, 406–407
  hyperthyroidism in, 585
  hypothyroidism in, 588, 589
  length/abdominal circumference ratio in, in fetal growth restriction, 330
  lungs of, evaluation of, 243
  membranes of, premature rupture of, 249–261. See also *Premature rupture of membranes.*
  movement of, maternal assessment of, 226–227
  nuchal translucency of, 216, *216*, 236, *236*
  resuscitation of, 288
  rubella virus infection in, 406
  spine of, evaluation of, 241–242, *242*
  stomach of, evaluation of, 243
  toxoplasmosis in, 411–412
  *Treponema pallidum* infection in, 410–411
  ultrasonography of. See *Ultrasonography.*
  varicella-zoster virus infection in, 406
  ventricles of, evaluation of, 241, *241*
  weight of, in fetal growth restriction, 329–330
    in multifetal pregnancy, 337–338, 341
  shoulder dystocia and, 293
Fever, during pregnancy, 427
  postoperative, 505–506
Fibrinogen, measurement of, in abruptio placentae, 315
Fibroadenoma, of breast, 176
Fibroids, uterine. See *Leiomyoma, uterine.*
Fibroma, ovarian, 495–496
Fibronectin, fetal, in multifetal pregnancy, 340
  in preterm labor, 347
Fimbrioplasty, 676–677, *676, 677*
Financial accounting, 816–818, 817t, 818t
Financial management, budgeting in, 820–821, 821t
  cash management in, 821–822, 922t
  corporate finance in, 824–825
  financial accounting in, 816–818, 817t, 818t
  financial statement analysis in, 818–820, 819t

Financial management *(Continued)*
  managerial accounting in, 822–823, 823t
Financial statement, analysis of, 818–820, 819t
Finasteride, in hyperandrogenism, 578
Fine-needle aspiration, of breast mass, 171–172, *173*
Fistula, ureterovaginal, 503, *504*
Fitz-Hugh–Curtis syndrome, 71
Fluid challenge, postoperative, 507
Flunisolide, in maternal asthma, 372t, 373
Fluorescent in situ hybridization, 222
  for preimplantation genetic diagnosis, 653
Flutamide, in hyperandrogenism, 578
Fluticasone propionate, in maternal asthma, 372t, 373
Folic acid, in neural tube defect prevention, 209, 426
Follicle-stimulating hormone (FSH), exogenous, in infertility, 547–548, 548t, 623–624
  in vitro fertilization, 647–648, 648t
  in amenorrhea, 553
  in hyperandrogenism, 572–573
  in infertility, 618, 632
  menopausal levels of, 598
Forced expiratory volume in 1 second (FEV$_1$), in asthma, 370t
Forceps delivery, 294–295, 294t
Fracture, clavicular, in shoulder dystocia, 294
  in osteoporosis, 597–598, 597t
Frequency tables, in epidemiology, 746, 746t
Functional electrical stimulation, in detrusor instability, 167
  in urinary incontinence, 166–167
Fundal height, measurement of, 204
Furosemide, postoperative, 507

### G

Galactorrhea, 175
Gamete intrafallopian transfer, 649–650
  indications for, 649
  outcome of, 649–650
Gastroesophageal reflux, during pregnancy, 427
Gastrointestinal tract disease, pelvic pain and, 41, 42, 43
Gastroschisis, ultrasonography of, 243, *244*
Gelfoam embolization, in postpartum hemorrhage, 319
Gene mutation, 218–222
  carrier screening for, 221–222
  linkage analysis of, 218
  Northern blotting for, 220
  oligonucleotide probe analysis for, 219
  polymerase chain reaction for, 219–220
  restriction fragment length polymorphism analysis of, 218–219
  Southern blotting for, 219
Genetic testing. See *Gene mutation; Prenatal diagnosis.*
Genital tract prolapse, 134–140
  anatomic factors in, 134–136, *135, 136*
  anterior compartment, 138, 139
  apex, 138, 139–140
  classification of, 138–139
  estrogen replacement therapy in, 137
  etiology of, 136–137

Genital tract prolapse *(Continued)*
  evaluation of, 137–138, *138*
  hysterectomy in, 111–112
  pessary in, 139
  posterior compartment, 139, 140
  prevention of, 139
  signs and symptoms of, 137, 137t
  surgical treatment of, 139–140
  treatment of, 111–112, 136–137, 139–140
  urinary incontinence and, 154
Genitalia, ambiguous, 92, *92*
Gentamicin, in postoperative infection, 194
Germ cell tumors, 490–495, 491t
  clinical presentation of, 491, 491t
  diagnosis of, 491–492, 492t
  hyperandrogenism and, 574–575, 574t
  in pregnancy, 523–524
  physical examination in, 491
  prognosis for, 495
  radiologic studies in, 492
  treatment of, 492–495
    chemotherapy in, 493–494, 493t
    late sequelae of, 494–495
    salvage chemotherapy in, 494
    surgery in, 492–493
    surveillance after, 494
Gestational age, abdominal circumference for, 240
  anatomical structures and, 236, 236t
  biparietal diameter for, 240
  crown-rump length for, 235–236, 235t
  femur length for, 240
  first-trimester ultrasonography for, 235–236, 235t, 236t
  head circumference for, 240
  preterm labor and, 344
  second-trimester ultrasonography for, 240
Gestational sac, size of, 235, 235t
  ultrasonography of, 234–235
Gestational surrogacy, 651
Gestational trophoblastic disease, 511–518. See also *Hydatidiform mole*.
  persistent, 512–513
    clinical presentation of, 512–513
    diagnosis of, 513, 513t, *514*
    follow-up for, 518
    reproductive function after, 518, 518t
    stage I (nonmetastatic), *514*, 515–516, 516t
    stage II and III, *514*, 516–517, 516t
    stage IV, *514*, 517–518, 517t
    staging of, 513, 513t, *514*
    treatment of, *514*, 515–518, 516t
Glitazones, in hyperandrogenism, 579
Glucose tolerance test, in hyperandrogenism, 574
  in pregnancy, 361–363, 363t
Goiter, 589–592
  clinical presentation of, 589–590
  diagnosis of, 590
  differential diagnosis of, 590–591, 590t
  diffuse, 590–591, 590t
  nodular, 591, 591t, 592
  toxic, 585. See also *Hyperthyroidism*.
Gonadal failure, 99
  in delayed puberty, 98
Gonadotropin therapy, in infertility, 547–548, 548t, 623–624
Gonadotropin-releasing factor, deficiency of (Kallmann's syndrome), 97
Gonadotropin-releasing hormone agonists, in dysfunctional uterine bleeding, 566

Gonadotropin-releasing hormone agonists *(Continued)*
  in endometriosis, 698
  in fibrocystic breast disease, 177
  in hyperandrogenism, 578
  in leiomyoma, 55, 110
  in premenstrual syndrome, 693
Gonorrhea, 58, 62
  during pregnancy, 408
  in children, 86t
  prenatal testing for, 204
Goserelin, in endometriosis, 698
Granulosa cell tumors, 495–496
Graves' disease, 582–583, 583t. See also *Hyperthyroidism*.
  treatment of, 584–585
Group B streptococcal infection, during pregnancy, 408–410, *409*, *410*
  premature rupture of membranes and, 251

# H

Habitual abortion. See *Pregnancy, early loss of*.
*Haemophilus ducreyi* infection, 59
Hashimoto's thyroiditis, 587, 587t
Hatching, assisted, 652
Head circumference, in gestational age determination, 240
Head circumference/abdominal circumference ratio, in fetal growth restriction, 330
Headache, during pregnancy, 427
  oral contraceptives and, 4
Health economics, 719–732
  appropriate care and, 727
  cost-benefit analysis in, 720–721
  elective care and, 720
  health-care expenditures and, 719, 720t
  health-care utilization and, 729–732
  income and, 722
  information and, 721
  insurance and, 721–722, 722–726, 723t, 724. See also *Insurance; Managed-care plans*.
  need and, 721
  physician practice and, 726–729
  physician remuneration and, 729–732
  practice patterns and, 722
  rationality and, 721
  screening and, 727–729
Health maintenance organizations, 724–725, 735–736
HealthPartners, 853–854
Heart, fetal, evaluation of, 204, 242, *242*
Heart disease, obstetric anesthesia and, 284
Helix database, 206
HELLP syndrome, 384–388, 385t
Hemangioma, capillary, 89–90
Hematoma, of breast, 172
  pelvic, posthysterectomy, 190, 192, *192*
  subchorionic, ultrasonography of, 237–238
Hemizona assay, in male factor infertility, 633
Hemoglobin, prenatal testing for, 202–203, 203t
Hemoglobinopathy, prenatal testing for, 202–203, 203t
Hemorrhage, intraoperative, 502–503
  obstetric, 311–319
    abruptio placentae and, 312–315, 312t, 313t

Hemorrhage *(Continued)*
    antepartum, 311–312, 312t
      anesthesia and, 286, 286t
      in multifetal pregnancy, 340
    classification of, 311
    placenta accreta and, 316–317
    placenta previa and, 315–316
    postpartum, 317–319
      definition of, 317–318
      in multifetal pregnancy, 342
      management of, 318
      risk factors for, 317–318
      third stage of labor duration and, 318
      uterine atony and, 318–319
      vasa previa and, 317
    with cesarean delivery, 309
Hemostasis, preoperative evaluation of, 500
Heparin, during pregnancy, 430
  in antiphospholipid syndrome, 25, 25t
  perioperative, 502
Hepatitis A virus infection, during pregnancy, 407
Hepatitis B vaccine, 18t
Hepatitis B virus infection, during pregnancy, 408
  prenatal testing for, 203
Hepatitis C virus infection, during pregnancy, 407
Hepatitis E virus infection, during pregnancy, 407–408
Heroin abuse, prenatal, 393–395
  childhood effects of, 394–395
  fetal effects of, 393, 394
  neonatal effects of, 393–394
  obstetric complications of, 393
  treatment protocol for, 397
Herpes simplex virus infection, 58–59
  during pregnancy, 406–407
  in children, 86t
  premature rupture of membranes and, 261
  treatment of, 62, 63t
Hirsutism. See also *Hyperandrogenism*.
  idiopathic, 575
  in hyperandrogenism, 571, 571t
Histocompatibility antigens, parental, early pregnancy loss and, 536
HIV. See *Human immunodeficiency virus (HIV) infection*.
Hormone replacement therapy, 598–604
  adverse effects of, 599–600
  alternatives to, 604–605
  breast cancer and, 180, 600
  cardiovascular disease and, 596
  continuous combined regimen for, 603–604, 604t
  contraindications to, 600–601, 600t
  endometrial cancer and, 599–600
  endometrial hyperplasia with, 599–600
  for hot flushes, 598
  in Alzheimer's disease, 595
  in genital tract prolapse, 137
  in osteoporosis, 599
  informed consent for, 602–603
  preparations for, 601–602, 601t, 602t, 603t
  sequential combined regimen for, 603, 603t
  side effects of, 602
  thromboembolism and, 596
Hot flushes, menopause and, 594, 598–599
Human chorionic gonadotropin (hCG), in anovulation treatment, 548, 624

Human chorionic gonadotropin (hCG) (Continued)
  in ectopic pregnancy, 30, 30t
  in hydatidiform mole, 512t, 513t, 515
  in persistent gestational trophoblastic disease, 518
β-Human chorionic gonadotropin (β–hCG), in prenatal diagnosis, 215–216
Human immunodeficiency virus (HIV), 413–414
Human immunodeficiency virus (HIV) infection, antiviral treatment in, 417, 417t, 418t, 419t
  counseling about, 421
  diagnosis of, 415, 415t, *416*
  during pregnancy, 413–422, 422t
  obstetric management in, 285, 418, 420–421, 420t, 432, 432t
  occupational risks from, 421–422
  pathogenesis of, 414
  prenatal testing for, 203
  sexually transmitted diseases and, 420
  transmission of, 414–415
    perinatal, 415–418, 417t
      cesarean section and, 261
      maternal drug use and, 417
      obstetric factors in, 416–418, 417t
      premature rupture of membranes and, 261
      prevention of, 417–418, 417t, 418t, 419t
      viral load and, 416, 417t
Human leukocyte antigen sharing, early pregnancy loss and, 25
Human menopausal gonadotropin (hMG), in anovulation, 547, 624
Human papillomavirus (HPV), 446, *446*
Human papillomavirus (HPV) infection, 59
  cervical cancer and, 458–459
  cervical intraepithelial neoplasia and, 440–441, 446, *446*
  immunobiology of, 447
  in children, 86t
  subclinical, 59
  treatment of, 442–443
Hydatidiform mole, 511–512
  clinical presentation of, 511–512, 512t
  diagnosis of, 512
  hormonal follow-up in, 515
  natural history of, 515
  prophylactic chemotherapy in, 515
  treatment of, 514–515
Hydralazine, in hypertension, 382t, 387
17-Hydroxyprogesterone, in hyperandrogenism, 573
Hymen, anomalies of, 93, *93*
  imperforate, 93, *93*
Hymenal orifice, in children, 84
Hyoscyamine, in detrusor instability, 163t, 164
Hyperandrogenism, 570–580
  adrenal gland tumors and, 574t, 575
  congenital adrenal hyperplasia and, 575
  Cushing's disease and, 575
  Cushing's syndrome and, 575
  differential diagnosis of, 574–577, 574t
  hirsutism in, 571, 571t
  hyperinsulinism and, 576–577
  hyperthecosis and, 575
  imaging in, 574
  in unexplained infertility, 664
  laboratory tests in, 572–574, 572t
  ovarian tumors and, 574–575, 574t
  patient history in, 571, 571t

Hyperandrogenism (Continued)
  physical examination in, 571–572, 572t
  polycystic ovarian syndrome and, 576–577
  skin manifestations of, 570–571
  treatment of, 577–580, 577t
    cimetidine in, 579
    corticosteroids in, 578–579
    cyproterone acetate in, 578
    finasteride in, 578
    flutamide in, 578
    glitazones in, 579
    gonadotropin-releasing hormone agonists in, 578
    ketoconazole in, 579
    metformin in, 579
    oral contraceptives in, 578
    progestins in, 579
    rosiglitazone in, 579
    spironolactone in, 578
    troglitazone in, 579
    weight loss in, 577–578
Hyperandrogenism, insulin resistance, and acanthosis nigricans (HAIR-AN) syndrome, 575
Hyperinsulinism, hyperandrogenism and, 576–577
Hyperprolactinemia, hyperandrogenism and, 573
  in infertility, 637, 661–662, 664
  treatment of, 558
Hypertension, 380–388
  chronic, 380–381, 381t, 382t
  fetal growth restriction and, 328
  gestational, 381–382, 381t. See also *Pre-eclampsia.*
    anesthesia and, 284
  in multifetal pregnancy, 340
  oral contraceptive–related cardiovascular disease and, 5
  pregnancy and, 427
  pregnancy-induced, 380
  treatment of, 387–388
Hyperthecosis, hyperandrogenism and, 575
Hyperthyroidism, 581–586
  clinical presentation of, 581, 581t
  diagnosis of, 581–582, 582t
  differential diagnosis of, 582–583, 583t
  hyperandrogenism and, 572
  postpartum, 323
  pregnancy and, 428, 584, 585
  treatment of, 584–586
Hypnotics, during pregnancy, 428
Hypogastric artery, ligation of, 503
Hypoglycemia, 366
Hypogonadism, hypogonadotropic, in male factor infertility, 637
Hypothyroidism, 586–589
  central, 587, 589
  clinical presentation of, 586, 586t
  congenital, 587
  diagnosis of, 586–587
  differential diagnosis of, 587–588, 587t
  during pregnancy, 428
  hyperandrogenism and, 572
  pregnancy and, 588–589
  subclinical, 589
  transient, 587
  treatment of, 589
Hypovolemia, anesthesia and, 288
Hypoxemia, maternal, fetal growth restriction and, 328–329
Hysterectomy, 107–120
  abdominal, 114
    antibiotics in, 118–119

Hysterectomy (Continued)
  cesarean, 112, 307–309
  clinical pathway for, 803t–804t
  complications of, 116–119, *117*, 118t
  enterocele with, 119
  hormonal changes after, 119–120
  in atypical endometrial hyperplasia, 111, 111t
  in cervical cancer, 463, *464*, 467–468, 521, 521t, 522
  in chronic pelvic pain, 110
  in dysfunctional uterine bleeding, 110
  in ectopic pregnancy management, 34
  in endometriosis, 110–111, 706–707
  in familial cancer syndromes, 112
  in genital prolapse, 111–112
  in leiomyoma, 55–56, 108–109
  in pelvic pain, 49
  in postpartum hemorrhage, 319
  in tubo-ovarian abscess, 112
  infection after, 117, 189–193, *191*, *192*
    febrile morbidity in, 192
    microbiology of, 192–193, 193t
  laparoscope-assisted, 114
  mortality rate of, 116
  obstetric indications for, 112, 307–309
  oophorectomy and, 115
  outcome measures for, 805t
  Pap smear after, 115
  psychological sequelae of, 119–120
  route for, 113–115
  sexual function after, 119
  supracervical, 112–113
  technique of, 115–116
  ureteral injury with, 116–117, *117*, 118t
  vaginal, 114, 115t
    antibiotics in, 118
    laparoscope-assisted, 127
  vaginal vault prolapse with, 119
  vs. endometrial ablation, 113
  vs. myomectomy, 113
  vs. uterine artery embolization, 113
Hysterosalpingography, in infertility, 612–613, *613*, 665–666
  in uterine leiomyoma, 54
Hysteroscopy, 130–132
  in infertility, 618, 662

# I

Idoxifene, 604
Imipramine, in urinary incontinence, 163–164, 163t
Immunization, lymphocyte, in early pregnancy loss, 536
  recommendations for, 17, 18t
Immunoglobulin, intravenous, in early pregnancy loss, 536
Immunosuppressants, during pregnancy, 432
Impress device, in urinary incontinence, 167
In vitro fertilization, 646–647
  embryo transfer in, 648
  gamete co-incubation in, 648
  indications for, 646–647
  luteal phase support in, 648
  oocyte retrieval in, 648
  outcome of, 647, 648–649
  ovarian stimulation in, 547, 647–648, 648t
  patient selection for, 647
  technique of, 647–648
Inborn errors of metabolism, prenatal diagnosis of, 221

Incidence, in epidemiology, 747
Incompetent cervix, preterm labor and, 350
Incontinence. See *Urinary incontinence.*
Independent practice associations, 725
Indinavir, in maternal HIV infection, 418t, 419t
Indomethacin, in preterm labor, 349
Infection, 57–64. See also specific infections.
  early pregnancy loss and, 535–536
  in pelvic inflammatory disease, 65–72. See also *Pelvic inflammatory disease.*
  in unexplained infertility, 666–667, 666t
  maternal, 403–412, *409, 410,* 411t
    early pregnancy loss and, 23t, 24
    fetal growth restriction and, 329
    intra-amniotic, 404–405
    premature rupture of membranes and, 250–251, 254–256, 256t, 257
    preterm labor and, 345–346
  neonatal, maternal heroin abuse and, 394
  with cytomegalovirus, 407
  with group B streptococcus, 408–410, *409, 410*
  with hepatitis virus, 407–408
  with herpes simplex virus, 406–407
  with rubella virus, 406
  with *Treponema pallidum,* 410–411
  with varicella-zoster virus, 405–406
  postoperative, 187–194, 505–506
    after cesarean section, 304–305
    after hysterectomy, 117, 189–193, *191, 192*
    classification of, 187–189, *188*
    deep incisional type of, 188–189, *188*
    febrile morbidity in, 192
    microbiology of, 192–193, 193t
    organ/space type of, *188,* 189
    risk categories in, 187, 188t
    superficial incisional type of, 188, *188*
    treatment of, 193–194, 193t
Infertility, 609–625. See also *Anovulation.*
  age and, 610
  alcoholism and, 610–611
  assisted fertilization in, 652
  assisted hatching in, 652
  assisted reproductive technology in, 641–653, 642t. See also *Assisted reproductive technology.*
  cervical culture in, 618
  cervical factor, *619,* 620, 624–625
  cervical mucus tests in, *614,* 616
  cigarette smoking and, 610
  clomiphene citrate in, 543–544, 544t, 545t, 623
  controlled ovarian hyperstimulation in, 642–645, 644t, 645t
  definition of, 609
  diagnostic evaluation in, 612–618, 612t, *613–615,* 616t, *617*
  differential diagnosis of, 619–620, *619, 620*
  drugs and, 611, 630, 631t
  embryo micromanipulation in, 651–653
  emotional factors in, 611
  endometrial biopsy in, 617–618
  endometriosis and, 619–620, 622–623, 646
  epidemiology of, 609–610
  etiology of, 610–611
  fimbrioplasty in, *676,* 676–677, *677*
  follicle-stimulating hormone in, 618

Infertility *(Continued)*
  gamete intrafallopian transfer in, *643,* 649–650
  gamete micromanipulation in, 651–653
  gestational surrogacy in, 651
  gonadotropin therapy in, 547–548, 548t, 623–624
  hysterosalpingography in, 612–613, *613*
  hysteroscopy in, 618, 622
  in vitro fertilization in, *643,* 646–649, 648t
  insulin sensitizers in, 546
  intrauterine insemination in, 621–622, 642–645, *643,* 644t, 645t
  laparoscopy in, 618
  luteal phase defect and, 624, 662–664
  male factor, 619, *619,* 621–622, 629–638, *634,* 646
    acrosome reaction in, 633
    antisperm antibodies in, 633–634, 636–637, 646, 668–669
    azoospermia in, 635–636, 635t, 636t
    bovine cervical mucus penetration test in, 632
    definition of, 630
    ejaculatory dysfunction in, 637
    genetic testing in, 634–635
    hemizona assay in, 633
    hormone testing in, 631–632
    hyperprolactinemia in, 637
    hypogonadotropic hypogonadism in, 637
    intrauterine insemination in, 621–622, 642–646, 644t, 645t
    leukocytospermia in, 637–638
    mannose ligand receptor assay in, 633
    oligoasthenospermia in, 636
    patient history in, 630, 631t
    physical examination in, 630–631, *631*
    postcoital test in, 632
    semen analysis in, 631, 631t, 632t
    sperm function testing in, 632–634
    varicocele in, 635
    vasoepididymostomy in, 635–636, 636t
    vasovasostomy in, 635–636, 635t
    zona-free hamster egg penetration assay in, 632–633
  management of, 620–625, *621,* 621t. See also specific techniques.
  neosalpingostomy in, 677–678, *678*
  nutrition and, 610
  oocyte donation in, *643,* 650–651
  ovarian diathermy in, 546–547
  ovarian factor, *619,* 620, 623–624
  ovulation assessment in, 615–618, 616t, *617*
  patient history in, 611
  pelvic factor, 619, *619,* 620, 622–623
  physical examination in, 611–612
  postcoital test in, 613–615, *614, 615,* 632
  preimplantation genetic diagnosis in, 652–653
  prolactin levels in, 618
  salpingolysis in, *675,* 675–676
  salpingoplasty in, 676
  semen analysis in, 612, 612t, 631, 631t, 632t
  serum progesterone in, 616–617
  sexually transmitted disease and, 610
  thyroid-stimulating hormone in, 618
  transcervical tubal catheterization in, 681

Infertility *(Continued)*
  tubal anastomosis in, 679–681, *680, 681*
  tubal factor, 673–682, 674t. See also at *Fallopian tube.*
  ultrasonography in, 618
  unexplained, 620, 647, 657–671
    acrosin assay in, 661
    anatomic abnormalities in, 670
    assisted reproduction in, 670
    cervical factors in, 667–668
    *Chlamydia trachomatis* infection in, 667
    emotional factors in, 669–670
    endometrial biopsy in, 662
    endometriosis in, 667
    evaluation of, 657–659, *658,* 658t
    falloposcopy in, 666
    hyperandrogenism in, 664
    hyperprolactinemia in, 664
    hysterosalpingography in, 665–666
    implantation failure in, 665
    infections in, 666–667, 666t
    laparoscopy in, 665–666
    luteal phase deficiency in, 662–664
    luteinized unruptured follicle syndrome in, 664–665
    male factors in, 659–662, 660t
    male hyperprolactinemia in, 661–662
    medical treatment in, 670
    *Mycoplasma* infection in, 666
    ovarian reserve test in, 665
    ovulation evaluation in, 662–665
    patient history in, 659
    peritoneal factors in, 666
    physical examination in, 659
    postcoital test in, 660, 668
    salivary progesterone in, 662
    semen analysis in, 659–661, 660t
    sperm antibodies in, 668–669
    sperm transport factors in, 667–668
    treatment of, 670
    tubal factors in, 665–666
    tuberculosis in, 667
    two-stage in vitro fertilization test in, 661
    *Ureaplasma urealyticum* infection in, 666–667
    urinary luteinizing hormone in, 662
    uterine abnormalities in, 665
    zona antibodies in, 669
    zona-free hamster egg penetration test in, 661
  urinary luteinizing hormone in, 616
  uterine leiomyoma and, 54
  uterotubal implantation in, 681
  zygote intrafallopian transfer in, 650
Inflammatory bowel disease, during pregnancy, 428
Influenza vaccine, 18t
Informed consent, 788–789
Informed refusal, 789
Insemination, intrauterine, 621–622, 642–645, 644t, 645t
  technique of, 645–646
Insulin, in diabetic ketoacidosis, 366
  in gestational diabetes mellitus, 364
Insulin resistance, polycystic ovary syndrome and, 540–541, 576–577
Insulin sensitizers, in anovulation, 546
Insurance, 722–726, 723t, *724*
  among pregnant women, 723–724, *724*
  among women, 723–724
  managed-care plans and, 724–725
Interceed, in postoperative adhesion reduction, 712–713, *713, 714*
Interleukin–6, in diagnosis of premature rupture of membranes, 255, 256t

International Classification of Diseases, 9th Revision, 832–833
Internet, 837–838
Intracranial lesions, obstetric anesthesia and, 284–285
Intracytoplasmic sperm injection, 652
Intraepithelial neoplasia, 59, 439–440, *440*
  differential diagnosis of, 442
  human papillomavirus infection and, 440–441
  in pregnancy, 520, 520t
  laboratory evaluation in, 442
  physical examination in, 441–442, *441*
  treatment of, 442–446, *444*, *445*, *447*
Intrauterine devices, 9–10
  progestin, in dysfunctional uterine bleeding, 566
Intrauterine insemination, 621–622, 642–645, *643*, 644t, 645t
  technique of, 645–646
Iodine deficiency, 587
Iron, during pregnancy, 426
Irritable bowel syndrome, 42
  treatment of, 44–45

## J

Jarisch-Herxheimer reaction, in syphilis treatment, 411

## K

Kallmann's syndrome, 97, 98
Ketoconazole, in hyperandrogenism, 579
Kidney disease, maternal, fetal growth restriction and, 328
Klinefelter's syndrome, infertility in, 634

## L

Labetalol, in hypertension, 382t, 387–388
Labia majora, of newborn, 82, *83*
Labia minora, asymmetry of, 92, *92*
  of newborn, 82, *83*
Labial adhesions, in children, 88–89, *88*
Labor, 267–274. See also *Delivery; Dystocia.*
  active-phase arrest in, 270, *270*, 270t
  after cesarean section, 305–307, 306t, 307t
  diagnosis of, 268
  failure of, to progress, 269t, 270, *270*
  in post-term pregnancy, 357–358, 357t, 358t
  management of, 271–273
    epidural analgesia in, 273–274, 283. See also *Anesthesia, obstetric.*
    nonpharmacologic pain relief in, 279
    oxytocin stimulation in, 272
    parenteral medications in, 281
    Parkland Hospital protocol for, 272
    partogram for, 271–272
  maternal asthma and, 377–378
  normal, 268–269, *268*
  onset of, 268
  pain in, 277, *278*
  premature rupture of membranes and, 404
  preterm, 344–351. See also *Preterm labor.*

Lactation. See also *Breastfeeding.*
  breast infection during, 173
  breast mass during, 172
Lamivudine, in maternal HIV infection, 418t, 419t
Laparoscopy, 122–128
  anesthesia for, 124
  bladder injury with, 128
  bowel herniation with, 128
  burns with, 128
  complications of, 128
  contraindications to, 126
  electrocautery for, 123–124
  equipment for, 122–124
  in cystectomy, 127
  in ectopic pregnancy, 32, 33–34, 126–127
  in endometriosis, 126, 699–701, *700*
  in infertility, 618
  in myomectomy, 127
  in oophorectomy, 127
  in pelvic adhesion treatment, 126
  in pelvic inflammatory disease, 68
  in pelvic pain, 48
  in unexplained infertility, 665–666
  in vaginal hysterectomy, 127
  indications for, 125–126, 125t
  laser for, 123–124
  pneumoperitoneum for, 124
  suturing instruments for, 124
  technique for, 124–125
  tissue removal equipment for, 124
  trocar and sleeve insertion for, 125
Laparotomy, in ectopic pregnancy, 33–34
  in endometriosis, 701
Large for gestational age infant, maternal diabetes and, 360–361
Laser, for laparoscopy, 123–124
Laser therapy, in anovulation, 546–547
  in cervical intraepithelial neoplasia, 445–446
  in dysfunctional uterine bleeding, 566
Lecithin/sphingomyelin ratio, in premature rupture of membranes, 256–257
Leiomyoblastoma, 52
Leiomyoma, 51–56
  cervical, 460
  early pregnancy loss and, 535
  hysteroscopy in, 109
  intravenous, 53
  metastatic, 53
  uterine, 51–56, 79
    apoplectic, 52
    bizarre, 52
    cellular, 52
    clinical features of, 53–54
    diagnosis of, 54–55
    early pregnancy loss and, 23, 535
    epithelioid, 52
    extrauterine metastases from, 53
    gross findings in, 52
    management of, 55–56
    microscopic findings in, 52–53
    pathology of, 51–52
    plexiform, 52
    treatment of, hysterectomy in, 108–109
      ultrasonography before, 109, *109*
      myomectomy in, 113
      pharmacologic, 109–110
      uterine artery embolization in, 113
    vaginal, 454
    vs. adenocarcinoma, 109
Leiomyosarcoma, uterine, 53, 54, 477
Leukocyte amebocyte lysate test, in premature rupture of membranes diagnosis, 255

Leukocytospermia, in male factor infertility, 637–638
Leukotrienes, in maternal asthma, 375
Leuprolide, in endometriosis, 698
  in vitro fertilization, 647–648, 648t
Levator ani muscles, 134–135, *135*, 136
  in pelvic pain, 43
Levonorgestrel, for contraception, 8–9
Libido, menopause-related loss of, 595
Lice, during pregnancy, 428
Lichen sclerosus, in children, 87–88, *88*
Linkage analysis, in prenatal diagnosis, 218
Lipoleiomyoma, uterine, 52–53
Lipoproteins, high-density, cardiovascular disease and, 596
  low-density, cardiovascular disease and, 596
  oral contraceptives and, 5
*Listeria monocytogenes* infection, early pregnancy loss and, 24
Lithium, during pregnancy, 433
  in Graves' disease, 585
Liver disease, obstetric anesthesia and, 285–286
Lobular carcinoma in situ, 178–179, 178t
LOD score, in linkage analysis, 218
Longitudinal study, in epidemiology, 752
Loop electrical excision, in cervical intraepithelial neoplasia, 445–446
Lumbar disk disease, obstetric anesthesia and, 284
Lungs, fetal, evaluation of, 243
  premature rupture of membranes and, 253, 256–257
Lupus antibodies, early pregnancy loss and, 24–25
Luteal phase defect, early pregnancy loss and, 23–24, 23t, 535
  in infertility, 624, 662–664
Luteinized unruptured follicle syndrome, in infertility, 664–665
Luteinizing hormone, in amenorrhea, 553
  in hyperandrogenism, 572–573
  in male factor infertility, 632
  urinary, in infertility, 616, 662
  in ovulation monitoring, 543
Lymphocytes, T, in human immunodeficiency virus infection, 414
Lymphocyte immunization, in early pregnancy loss, 536
Lymphogranuloma venereum, 59

## M

Macrosomia, 331–334
  diagnosis of, 333–334, *333*
  gestational diabetes mellitus and, 365
  management of, 334
  maternal diabetes and, 360–361
  post-term pregnancy and, 355
  risk factors for, 332–333, 332t
  shoulder dystocia and, 293
Magnesium sulfate, in eclampsia, 387, 387t
  in pre-eclampsia, 383
  in preterm labor, 348–349
  toxicity of, 387t
Magnetic resonance imaging, in hyperandrogenism, 574
  of breast, 181
Male pseudohermaphrodism, 554–555
Malignant mixed müllerian tumors, 476–477

Malnutrition, infertility and, 610
Malpractice, 786–787
    abandonment and, 789–790
    deposition for, 789
    establishment of, 787
    expert witnesses in, 791–792
    in breast cancer cases, 790–791
    in fetal monitoring cases, 790
    in fetal ultrasonography cases, 791
    informed consent and, 788–789
    insurance for, 791
    medical record in, 787–788
    no-fault system for, 791
    physician impact of, 791
Mammography, 181, 181t
    in benign breast disease, 177–178
    in women 40–49 years old, 782–783, 782
    periductal mastitis on, 174
    recommendations for, 18
Managed-care plans, 724–725, 734–742
    appropriate care and, 727
    breast cancer care in, 732
    bundled payments and, 739
    capitation contracts of, 726, 739
    certified nurse midwives and, 740
    definition of, 735–736
    discharge requirements and, 727
    employer-sponsored, 724–725
    future of, 740–741
    global fees and, 739
    glossary for, 741–742
    health-care costs and, 736
    health-care utilization in, 729–732, 736–737
    history of, 734–735
    Medicaid-managed, 725
    nonphysician providers and, 740
    obstetrics/gynecology and, 738–740
    outcome measures in, 853–854, 854t
    physician contracts of, 725–726, 809–815
        administration of, 813–814
        benefit design and, 810–811
        coinsurance and, 811
        copayments and, 811
        deductibles and, 811
        infertility benefits and, 811
        language of, 812
        patient out-of-pocket costs and, 811
        physician negotiation leverage and, 811–812
        reimbursement methods and, 812–813
        term of, 814–815
        termination of, 814–815
        well woman care and, 811
    prenatal care in, 731–732
    quality of care and, 737–738
    reinsurance and, 726
    stop-loss provisions of, 726
    vs. fee-for-service plans, 737–738
Managerial accounting, 822–823, 823t
Mania, during pregnancy, 428
Mannose ligand receptor assay, in male factor infertility, 633
Marijuana use, prenatal, 395–396
Marshall-Marchetti-Krantz operation, hysterectomy and, 111–112
Mastectomy, pregnancy after, 527
    prophylactic, 179
Mastitis, nonpuerperal, 174
    periductal, 174
    puerperal, 172–173
Mastodynia, 177
McCall's culdoplasty, in genital tract prolapse, 139

McCune-Albright syndrome, 101, *101*
McIndoe procedure, 94
McRoberts maneuvers, 293
Measles vaccine, 18t
Meconium aspiration syndrome, 354–355
Median, in epidemiology, 749–750
Medicaid managed-care plans, 725
    physician contracts of, 726
Medical informatics, 834–844
    computer-based medical records in, 834–837
    data standards in, 838–839
    decision-support systems in, 839–843, *840–843*
    Internet and, 837–838
    telemedicine and, 837–838
Medical records, computer-based, 834–837
    in malpractice, 787–788
Medical-legal issues, 785–792. See also *Malpractice.*
    abandonment and, 789–790
    deposition for, 789
    informed consent and, 788–789
    maternal-fetal conflict and, 790
    medical record and, 787–788
    terminology for, 785–786
Medroxyprogesterone acetate, depot, for contraception, 8
    in dysmenorrhea, 44
    in endometriosis, 698
Melanoma, in pregnancy, 525
    vaginal, 454–455
Membranes, fetal, premature rupture of, 249–261. See also *Premature rupture of membranes.*
Memory, menopause and, 594–595
Menarche, 95–96. See also *Puberty.*
    premature, 102
Menopause, 593–605
    cardiovascular disease and, 595–596
    definition of, 593–594, *593*
    hormone replacement therapy in, 598–604. See also *Hormone replacement therapy.*
    hot flushes and, 594, 598–599
    laboratory tests in, 598
    libido and, 595
    memory and, 594–595
    menstrual bleeding patterns and, 594
    mood changes and, 594–595, 599
    night sweats and, 594
    osteopenia and, 596–598
    osteoporosis and, 596–598, 598t
    pelvic mass after, 79–80, 79t
    phytoestrogens in, 604–605
    premature, 593
    selective estrogen receptor modulators in, 604
    sexual function and, 595
    skin changes and, 595
    symptoms of, 594
    vaginal atrophy and, 595, 599
Menorrhagia, in leiomyoma, 53
Menstruation, 560–562. See also *Dysfunctional uterine bleeding.*
    failure of, 551–559. See also *Amenorrhea.*
    onset of, 95–96
    pain with, 40–50. See also *Dysmenorrhea; Pelvic pain; Premenstrual syndrome.*
    premature onset of, 102
Meperidine, in labor management, 281
Metabolic disorders, prenatal diagnosis of, 221

Metformin, in anovulation, 546
    in hyperandrogenism, 579
Methadone, in cocaine abuse, 398
    in heroin abuse, 397
Methotrexate, in ectopic pregnancy management, 25t, 34–36
Methyldopa, during pregnancy, 431
    in hypertension, 382t
Metronidazole, during pregnancy, 431–432
    in postoperative infection, 194
Mitral stenosis, obstetric anesthesia and, 284
Mitral valve prolapse, obstetric anesthesia and, 284
Mode, in epidemiology, 750
Modified biophysical profile, in fetal assessment, 229–230
Mole. See *Hydatidiform mole.*
Molecular prenatal diagnosis, 217–220
    applications of, 220–221
    techniques of, 219–220
Molimina, vs. premenstrual syndrome, 685
Mondor's disease, 179
Monobactam, in postoperative infection, 194
Mood changes, menopause and, 594–595, 599
Morphine, in labor management, 281
Mortality, age-related, 16t
Motor vehicle accidents, prevention of, 17
Mucocolpos, imperforate hymen and, 93, *93*
Müllerian fusion defects, early pregnancy loss and, 534–535
Multiple sclerosis, obstetric anesthesia and, 284
Musculoskeletal disease, pelvic pain and, 41, 42
Mutation, gene, 218–222
    carrier screening for, 221–222
    linkage analysis of, 218
    Northern blotting for, 220
    oligonucleotide probe analysis for, 219
    polymerase chain reaction for, 219–220
    restriction fragment length polymorphism analysis of, 218–219
    Southern blotting for, 219
Myasthenia gravis, during pregnancy, 428
    obstetric anesthesia and, 284
*Mycoplasma* infection, early pregnancy loss and, 24
    in unexplained infertility, 666
Myomectomy, in uterine leiomyoma, 55
    laparoscopy in, 127
    vs. hysterectomy, 113
Myxedema coma, 586
    treatment of, 589

## N

Nafarelin acetate, in endometriosis, 698
Natural family planning, 13, 13t
Nausea, during pregnancy, 428, 431
    oral contraceptives and, 4
Nedocromil sodium, in maternal asthma, 372t, 373–374
*Neisseria gonorrhoeae* infection, 58
    during pregnancy, 408
    in children, 86t
    premature rupture of membranes and, 251

*Neisseria gonorrhoeae* infection *(Continued)*
    treatment of, 62
Nelfinavir, in maternal HIV infection, 418t, 419t
Neonatal abstinence syndrome, 393–394
Neonate. See also *Fetus.*
    cocaine effects on, 391–392
    cytomegalovirus infection in, 407
    death of, 225, 225t
    external genitalia of, 82, *83*
    group B streptococcal infection in, 207, 408–410, *409, 410*
    hepatitis virus infection in, 407–408
    heroin effects on, 393–394
    herpes simplex virus infection in, 406–407
    hyperthyroidism in, 585
    hypothyroidism in, 588–589
    ovarian cyst in, 75, 75t
    rubella virus infection in, 406
    *Treponema pallidum* infection in, 410–411
    varicella-zoster virus infection in, 405–406
Neosalpingostomy, 677–678, *678, 679*
Nesidioblastosis, fetal macrosomia and, 333
Neural tube defects, folic acid prevention of, 209
    prenatal screening for, 206, *206*, 214–215, 214t
    ultrasonography in, 242, *242*
Neurectomy, presacral, in endometriosis, 704–706, *705*
    in pelvic pain, 49
Neurologic disorders, urinary incontinence, 152–153
Neurologic examination, in pelvic pain, 43
    in urinary incontinence, 154
Neuromuscular disease, obstetric anesthesia and, 284–285
Neurotransmitters, in premenstrual syndrome, 686
Nevirapine, in maternal HIV infection, 418t, 419t
Newborn. See *Children; Neonate.*
Nifedipine, during pregnancy, 431
    in detrusor instability, 163t, 164–165
    in hypertension, 382t
    in severe hypertension, 388
Night sweats, menopause and, 594
Nipple, discharge from, 174–175
Nitrazine test, in premature rupture of membranes, 254
Nitroglycerin, for uterine relaxation, 287
Nitroprusside, in hypertension, 382t
Nonsteroidal anti-inflammatory drugs, during pregnancy, 429
    in premenstrual syndrome, 691
Nonstress test, in fetal assessment, 227
    in fetal growth restriction, 331
    in post-term pregnancy, 355–356
    in premature rupture of membranes, 257–258
Noonan's syndrome, 554
Norplant, 8–9
Northern blotting, in prenatal analysis, 220
Nuchal translucency, 216, *216*, 236, *237*

# O

Obesity, amenorrhea and, 557
    fetal macrosomia and, 332–333

Obesity *(Continued)*
    obstetric anesthesia and, 285
    polycystic ovarian syndrome and, 576
    prevention of, 16, 16t
Odds ratio, in epidemiology, 748–749
Oligoasthenospermia, in male factor infertility, 636
Oligohydramnios, in fetal growth restriction, 330
    in premature rupture of membranes, 254
    post-term pregnancy and, 355, 356
Oligonucleotide probe analysis, in prenatal diagnosis, 219
Oliguria, postoperative, 506–507
Omphalocele, ultrasonography of, 243
Oocyte donation, 650–651
    indications for, 650
    outcome of, 651
    techniques of, 650–651
Oophorectomy, hysterectomy and, 115
    in ectopic pregnancy management, 34
    in endometriosis, 707
    in premenstrual syndrome, 693
    laparoscopy in, 127
    prophylactic, 114–115
Oral contraceptives, 3–8
    adverse effects of, 4–5
    benefits of, 5–6, 6t
    breast cancer and, 180
    contraindications to, 6, 6t
    formulations of, 3–4, 6–7, 7t
    in dysfunctional uterine bleeding, 564–565
    in dysmenorrhea, 44
    in hyperandrogenism, 578
    in premenstrual syndrome, 691
    indications for, 6
    mechanism of action of, 4
    patient evaluation for, 6
    pelvic inflammatory disease and, 67
    progestin-only, 7–8, 8t
    risks of, 4–5
    selection of, 6–7, 7t
Orgasm, 144
Osteopenia, menopause and, 596–598
Osteoporosis, hormone replacement therapy in, 599
    menopause and, 596–598, 598t
Outcome measures, 845–858
    applications of, 850–853, 852t
    economic impact of, 855–856
    evidence-based medicine and, 857–858, 858t
    future directions of, 857–858, 858t
    in Detroit Medical center, 854–855, 855t
    in managed care, 853–854
    in process improvement, 846–850, 847t–849t, 850t
    information dissemination for, 857–858, 858t
    operational guidelines for, 856–857
Ovarian hyperstimulation, controlled, 642–645, 644t, 645t
Ovarian hyperstimulation syndrome, 548, 624
Ovarian pregnancy, 37
Ovarian reserve test, in unexplained infertility, 665
Ovary (ovaries), cysts of. See also *Polycystic ovary syndrome.*
    in adolescent, 76, *77*
    in children, 75–76, 75t
    in newborn, 75, 75t
    in pregnancy, 522–523

Ovary (ovaries) *(Continued)*
    in premenopausal woman, 78–79
    diathermy of, in anovulation, 546–547
    endometriosis of, 701–702, *702*
    epithelial cancer of, 78, 79, 479–488
        clomiphene citrate therapy and, 546
        diagnosis of, 482
        differential diagnosis of, 482
        epidemiology of, 479
        genetic factors in, 480
        in pregnancy, 523–524
        lymphatic metastases from, 481
        oral contraceptives and, 5
        pathology of, 480–481, 480t
        patient history in, 481–482
        physical examination in, 481–482
        postmenopausal, 80
        prognosis for, 483–484, 484t
        recurrence of, 487
        risk factors for, 479–480, 479t
        screening for, 482
        spread of, 481
        staging of, 482–483, 483t
        treatment of, chemotherapy in, 484–486, *484, 485*, 485t, 487–488, 487t
            second-look surgery after, 486–487
            surgery in, 486
        ultrasonography in, 80
    germ cell tumors of, 490–495, 491t
        clinical presentation of, 491, 491t
        diagnosis of, 491–492, 492t
        hyperandrogenism and, 574–575, 574t
        in pregnancy, 523–524
        physical examination in, 491
        prognosis for, 495
        radiologic studies in, 492
        treatment of, 492–495
            chemotherapy in, 493–494, 493t
            late sequelae of, 494–495
            salvage chemotherapy in, 494
            surgery in, 492–493
            surveillance after, 494
    laser therapy of, in anovulation, 546–547
    metastatic cancer of, 79
    premature failure of, 557
    sex cord stromal tumors of, 495–496, 495t
    wedge resection of, amenorrhea and, 557–558
        in anovulation, 546
        in polycystic ovary syndrome, 579–580
Over-the-counter drugs, during pregnancy, 433
Ovulation. See also *Anovulation; Infertility.*
    assessment of, 615–618, 616t, *617*
    basal body temperature in, 541–542, *542, 543*, *543*, 662
    ultrasonographic monitoring of, 542–543, *543*
Ovulation method, of natural family planning, 13
Oxybutynin, in detrusor instability, 163t, 164
Oxytocin, in labor management, 272

# P

Paget's disease, of breast, 179–180
Pain, abdominal. See *Abdominal pain.*
    pelvic. See *Pelvic pain.*

Pap smear, after hysterectomy, 115t
  economics of, 728–729
  quality management study of, 780–781
  recommendations for, 17–18, 459
Papillary serous carcinoma, of endometrium, 476
Papilloma, intraductal, 175
Paraphilia, 141
Paraplegia, obstetric anesthesia and, 284
Parasites, during pregnancy, 428
Partial zona dissection, 652
Peak expiratory flow rate (PEFR), in asthma, 370t, 376, 376t
Pelvic examination, in adolescent, 84–85
  in children, 83, 83–84
  in ectopic pregnancy, 29
  in pelvic pain, 42–43
  in sexually transmitted infections, 60–61, 60t
  in urinary incontinence, 154
  in uterine leiomyoma, 54
  premature rupture of membranes and, 250
  recommendations for, 17
  uterine examination in, 43
Pelvic floor exercises, in urinary incontinence, 165
Pelvic inflammatory disease, 65–72
  definitions of, 65–66
  diagnosis of, 66–68, 67t, 68t
  infertility and, 610
  laboratory tests in, 67–68
  microbiology of, 66
  partner treatment in, 70
  physical examination in, 67–68
  prevention of, 71–72, 72t
  risk factors for, 66–67, 67t
  sequelae of, 71, 71t
  symptoms of, 67, 67t
  treatment of, 69–70, 69t, 70t
  tubo-ovarian abscess in, 70–71
Pelvic mass, 75–80. See also *Cyst(s), ovarian.*
  differential diagnosis of, 77–79, 79t
  in adolescent, 76–77, 76t, 77t
  in children, 75–76, 75t
  in newborn, 75, 75t
  in perimenopausal women, 79–80, 79t
  in postmenopausal women, 79–80, 79t
Pelvic organ prolapse. See *Genital tract prolapse.*
Pelvic pain, 40–50
  abdominal wall trigger points in, 43, 45–46
  adhesiolysis in, 48–49
  antidepressants in, 47–48
  cyclic, 40–41
  cystourethroscopy in, 44
  diagnosis of, 41–43, 42t
  gastrointestinal disease and, 41, 42, 43
  hysterectomy in, 49, 110
  in adolescents, 105
  in somatization disorder, 46–47
  laboratory evaluation in, 43–44
  musculoskeletal disease and, 41, 42
  neurologic examination in, 43
  noncyclic, 41
  patient history in, 41–42
  physical examination in, 42–43
  presacral neurectomy in, 49
  psychiatric factors in, 46–48
  sexual abuse history and, 47
  treatment of, 44–46, 45t, 47–48
    surgical, 48–50, 110
  urinary tract disease and, 41, 42, 43, 45
  uterine suspension in, 49

Pelvic pain *(Continued)*
  uterosacral nerve ablation in, 49
Pelvic pressure pack, in postpartum hemorrhage, 319
Penicillins, during pregnancy, 431
  in postoperative infection, 193, 193t
Peptic ulcer disease, during pregnancy, 427
Pergolide mesylate, in amenorrhea, 558
Perimenopause, 593, *593*
Peripheral blood stem cell transplant, in ovarian epithelial cancer, 487–488
Pessary, in genital tract prolapse, 139
  in urinary incontinence, 167
  in uterine retrodisplacement, 49
Phenylpropanolamine, in stress urinary incontinence, 162–163, 163t
Phyllodes tumor, of breast, 176–177
Physical examination, annual, 17
  in pelvic pain, 42–43
Physical therapy, in pelvic pain, 46
Phytoestrogens, 604–605
Pinworms, during pregnancy, 428
Pituitary gland dysfunction, amenorrhea and, 557
Placenta, delivery of, 292–293
  drug transfer across, 425, 429
  evaluation of, 244
  in multiple pregnancy, 244–245, *245*
  vascular abnormalities of, preterm labor and, 345
Placenta accreta, 316–317
  hysterectomy in, 307–308
Placenta previa, 315–316
  clinical presentation of, 316
  definition of, 315
  diagnosis of, 316
  incidence of, 315
  management of, 316
  risk factors for, 315
Placental site trophoblastic tumor, 511
Platelet transfusion, in HELLP syndrome, 386
Pneumococcal vaccine, 18t
Pneumoperitoneum, for laparoscopy, 124
Point-of-service plans, 725, 736
Polycystic ovary syndrome. See also *Anovulation; Infertility.*
  early pregnancy loss and, 23t, 24
  hyperandrogenism in, 576–577
  in premenopausal woman, 78–79
  model of, 540–541, *540*
Polymerase chain reaction, in preimplantation genetic diagnosis, 653
  in premature rupture of membranes diagnosis, 255
  in prenatal diagnosis, 219–220
Populations, in epidemiology, 745–746
Positron emission tomography, of breast, 181
Postcoital test, in infertility, 613–615, *614*, *615*, 632, 668
Postmaturity syndrome, 355
Postpartum management, 321–325, 322t
  after multifetal delivery, 342
  circumcision in, 324
  depressed mood and, 323
  early, 321–322, 324, 324t
  early discharge in, 322–323
  late, 323
  thyroid dysfunction and, 323
Post-term pregnancy, 353–358
  contraction-stimulation test in, 356
  etiology of, 353–354
  fetal macrosomia and, 333

Post-term pregnancy *(Continued)*
  fetal risks in, 354
  incidence of, 353
  management of, 357–358, 357t, 358t
  neonatal risks in, 354–355
  nonstress test in, 355–356
  surveillance for, 355–357, 357–358, 358t
  ultrasonography in, 356–357
Potassium iodide, in Graves' disease, 585
Prednisone, in antiphospholipid syndrome, 25, 25t
Pre-eclampsia, 382–384, 382t. See also *Eclampsia.*
  management of, anesthesia in, 284
  aspirin in, 388
    epidemiologic study of, 755–757, *756*, 756t
  intrapartum, 388
  postpartum, 388
  mild, 382–383, 383t
  prevention of, 388
  screening for, 204–205
  severe, 383–384, 383t, *384*
Preferred provider organization, 725, 735–736
  physician contracts of, 726
Pregnancy. See also *Delivery; Labor; Postpartum management; Prenatal care.*
  abdominal, 36–37
  after breast cancer treatment, 527
  after early pregnancy loss, 537
  analgesics during, 429
  antibiotics during, 431–432
  anticoagulants during, 429–430, 430t
  anticonvulsants during, 430–431
  antidepressants during, 432–433, 432t
  antiemetics during, 431
  antihypertensives during, 431
  antipsychotics during, 433
  anxiolytics during, 433
  asthma in, 369–378. See also *Asthma, maternal.*
  asymptomatic bacteriuria during, 403
  bacterial vaginosis during, 405, 405t
  bladder cancer in, 524
  bone tumors in, 527–528
  breast cancer in, 525–527
  breast infection during, 173
  breast mass during, 172
  cervical, 37
  cervical cancer in, 519–522, 520t, 521t
  *Chlamydia trachomatis* infection during, 411
  cocaine abuse during, 391–393
  colorectal cancer in, 524–525
  combined, 36
  cystitis during, 403–404
  cytomegalovirus infection during, 407
  dental anesthetics during, 432
  diabetes in, 360–366. See also *Diabetes mellitus, gestational.*
    management of, 208
    screening for, 361–362
  diuretics during, 431
  drug therapy during, 424–433
    drug metabolism and, 425
    placental transfer and, 425, 429
    preferred drugs for, 426–429
    teratogenicity of, 424–425, 425t
  early loss of, 20–26, 533–538
    active immunization in, 536
    alcohol in, 537
    anatomic factors in, 21–22, 21t, 534–535

Pregnancy (Continued)
  antineoplastic agents in, 537
  antiphospholipid antibodies in, 536, 536t
  Asherman's syndrome and, 23
  autoimmune disease and, 24–25, 536
  chemical exposure in, 537
  cigarette smoking in, 537
  diabetes mellitus in, 535
  diethylstilbestrol exposure and, 23
  electromagnetic radiation and, 537
  employment and, 537
  endocrine conditions and, 23–24, 23t, 535
  environmental factors in, 537
  etiology of, 21–26, 21t
  evaluation of, 25–26, 26t, 534, 534t
  exercise and, 537
  genetic factors in, 21, 21t, 214, 534
  human leukocyte antigen sharing and, 25
  immunologic disorders in, 536, 536t
  incidence of, 20–21
  infection and, 23t, 24, 535–536
  intrauterine synechiae in, 535
  irradiation in, 537
  leiomyomas in, 23, 535
  luteal phase defect in, 23–24, 535
  maternal blocking antibody deficiency and, 25
  medical history in, 534
  müllerian fusion defects in, 534–535
  passive immunization in, 536
  physical examination in, 534
  polycystic ovary syndrome and, 24
  pregnancy after, 537–538
  recurrent, 20, 21, 25–26, 26t
  risk of, 533–534, 533t
  shared parental histocompatibility antigens in, 536
  uterine anomalies in, 22–23
 ectopic, 27–37
  abdominal, 36–37
  adnexal mass and, 29
  cervical, 37
  cervical examination in, 29
  culdocentesis in, 32
  diagnosis of, 28–29, 28t, 29t
  dilatation and curettage in, 32
  epidemiology of, 27
  etiology of, 28, 28t
  human chorionic gonadotropin in, 30, 30t
  in combined pregnancy, 36
  laboratory testing in, 30–31, 30t
  laparoscopy in, 32
  management of, 32–36
   laparoscopy in, 126–127
   nonsurgical, 34–36, 35t
   surgical, 32–34, 33t
  mortality with, 27–28
  ovarian, 37
  pathology of, 29–30
  pelvic examination in, 29
  pregnancy after, 28, 36
  risk factors for, 28, 28t
  rupture of, 29
  serum progesterone in, 30–31
  site of, 27, 27t
  ultrasonography in, 31–32, 31t, 234–235
  uterine examination in, 29
 epilepsy management during, 208
 genital tract prolapse and, 136–137
 glucose tolerance test in, 361–363, 363t
 gonorrhea during, 408

Pregnancy (Continued)
 Graves' disease and, 584
 group B streptococcal infection during, 408–410, 409, 410
 hepatitis virus infection during, 407–408
 heroin abuse during, 393–395
 herpes simplex virus infection during, 406–407
 human immunodeficiency virus infection during, 413–422, 422t. See also Human immunodeficiency virus (HIV) infection.
 hypertensive disorders in, 380–388. See also Hypertension; Pre-eclampsia.
 hyperthyroidism, 584, 585
 hypothyroidism, 588–589
 immunosuppressants during, 432
 in adolescent, 77
 infection in, 403–412
 intra-amniotic infection during, 404–405
 marijuana use during, 395–396
 melanoma in, 525
 molar. See Hydatidiform mole.
 multifetal, 337–342
  care after, 342
  chorionicity of, 339
  diagnosis of, 338
  epidemiology of, 337
  fetal care in, 339t, 340–342
  first-trimester ultrasonography in, 236–237, 237
  growth monitoring in, 340–341, 341
  growth restriction and, 337–338
  intrapartum care in, 342, 342t
  maternal care in, 339–340, 339t
  placentation in, 244–245, 245
  prematurity and, 337–338
  prenatal diagnosis in, 340
  second-trimester ultrasonography in, 244–245
  twin-twin transfusion syndrome in, 341–342
  ultrasonography of, 338–339, 338t
 Neisseria gonorrhoeae infection during, 408
 oral contraceptive use during, 5
 ovarian, 37
 ovarian cancer in, 522–524
 over-the-counter drugs during, 433
 pains during, 208
 post-term, 353–358. See also Post-term pregnancy.
 pyelonephritis during, 404
 rubella virus infection during, 406
 substance abuse during, 390–398. See also specific substances.
  treatment protocols for, 396–398
 syphilis during, 410–411, 411t
 thyroid cancer in, 528
 toxoplasmosis during, 411–412
 urinary frequency during, 208
 urinary tract infection during, 403–404
 uterine leiomyoma during, 54
 varicella-zoster virus infection during, 405–406
 viral infection during, 405–408
 weight gain during, 204–205, 205t
Preimplantation genetic diagnosis, 652–653
Premature labor. See Preterm labor.
Premature rupture of membranes, 249–261
 diagnosis of, 254
 etiology of, 249–251, 250t

Premature rupture of membranes (Continued)
 ferning in, 254
 human immunodeficiency virus transmission and, 261
 infection and, 250–251
 Nitrazine test in, 254
 oligohydramnios in, 254
 pelvic examination and, 250
 preterm, 252–254, 404
  abruptio placentae and, 253
  amniocentesis in, 254–256, 256t
  amniotic cavity infection and, 252–253, 253t, 254–256, 256t
  amniotic fluid volume in, 258
  antibiotics in, 258–259, 259t
  biophysical profile in, 257
  cerclage removal in, 260–261
  diagnosis of, 254
  fetal body movements in, 258
  fetal breathing movements in, 258
  fetal compression syndrome and, 253–254
  fetal monitoring in, 257–258
  herpes simplex genitalis and, 261
  infection and, 254–256, 256t, 257
  management of, 254–260, 256t, 259t
  natural history of, 252
  nonstress test in, 257–258
  pulmonary hypoplasia and, 253, 256–257
  steroids in, 259–260
  tocolysis in, 258
 risk factors in, 250, 250t
 speculum examination in, 254
 term, 260, 260t
Premenstrual syndrome, 684–693
 biopsychosocial model of, 687
 definition of, 684–685
 diagnosis of, 688–690, 689t
 differential diagnosis of, 690
 endocrine factors in, 686
 familial, 685
 neurotransmitters in, 686
 pathogenesis of, 685–687, 686t
 patient history in, 688
 physical examination in, 688
 prevalence of, 685
 prostaglandins in, 687
 symptoms of, 687–688, 687t
 treatment of, 690–693
  nonpharmacologic, 690–691
  pharmacologic, 691–693, 692t
  surgical, 693
 vitamin $B_6$ deficiency in, 686–687
 vs. molimina, 685
Prenatal care, 199–209
 access to, 209
 alcohol screening in, 207–208, 207t
 definition of, 199
 fetal assessment in, 204–205
 frequency of, 199–200, 200, 200t
 genetic testing in, 205–206, 206, 209, 218–222. See also Prenatal diagnosis.
 group B streptococcus screening in, 207
 in managed-care plans, 731–732
 in maternal asthma, 375–376, 376t
 patient education in, 207–208, 207t
 patient history in, 201
 physical examination in, 201
 preconceptual, 208–209
 scope of, 200–201
 standard laboratory evaluation in, 201–204, 201t, 202t, 203t

Prenatal care *(Continued)*
  ultrasonography in, 205, 205t
  utilization of, 209
  visits for, 199–200, *200*, 200t
Prenatal diagnosis, 205–206, 209, 213–222
  amniocentesis in, 206, 216, 217
    decision analysis for, 839–841, *840, 841*
  biochemical assays in, 221
  chorionic villus sampling in, 206, 217, *217*
  indications for, 213–215, 214t
  linkage analysis in, 218
  molecular, 217–220
    applications of, 220–221
    techniques of, 219–220
  Northern blotting in, 220
  of Down syndrome, 205–206, *206*, 213, 214t, 215
  of neural tube defects, 214–215, 214t
  oligonucleotide probe analysis in, 219
  polymerase chain reaction in, 219–220
  restriction fragment length polymorphism analysis in, 218–219
  serum markers in, 215–216, 215t
  Southern blotting in, 219
  ultrasonography in, 234–247. See also *Ultrasonography*.
Preoperative evaluation, 499–502
  consent in, 502
  consultations for, 501
  imaging studies in, 501
  laboratory tests in, 500–501
  patient history in, 499, 499t
  physical examination in, 499, 499t
  preventive measures in, 501–502, 502t
  risk assessment in, 499–500, 499t, 500t
Presacral neurectomy, in endometriosis, 704–706, *705*
  in pelvic pain, 49
Preterm labor, 344–351
  antibiotics in, 350
  cerclage for, 350–351
  cervical sonography in, 346–347, 346t
  clinical evaluation in, 347–348
  decidual ischemia and, 345
  definition of, 344–345
  diagnosis of, 346–347, 346t
  epidemiology of, 345
  etiology of, 345–346
  evaluation for, 204
  fetal fibronectin in, 347
  gestational age and, 344
  incompetence cervix and, 350
  maternal infection and, 345–346
  maternal occupation and, 208
  neonatal weight and, 345
  premature rupture of membranes and, 404
  quality improvement study of, 770–771, 771t
  tocolytic therapy in, 348–349, 348t
Prevalence, in epidemiology, 747, *748*
Prevalence study, in epidemiology, 752
Preventive care, 15–19
  primary, 15–17, 16t
  screening guidelines for, 17–19
  secondary, 17
Progestasert IUD, 10
Progesterone, in dysfunctional uterine bleeding, 564
  in premenstrual syndrome, 691
  salivary, in unexplained infertility, 662
  serum, in ectopic pregnancy, 30–31, 35–36

Progesterone *(Continued)*
  in infertility, 616–617
  in luteal phase deficiency, 663
Progestins, in dysfunctional uterine bleeding, 564, 566, 568
  in endometrial cancer, 476
  in endometriosis, 698
  in hyperandrogenism, 579
Progestin intrauterine device, in dysfunctional uterine bleeding, 566
Prolactin, in hyperandrogenism, 573
  in infertility, 618, 637, 661–662, 664
Propantheline bromide, in detrusor instability, 163t, 164
Propranolol, for hot flushes, 599
Propylthiouracil, in Graves' disease, 584–585
Prostaglandins, in premenstrual syndrome, 687
Protein C deficiency, oral contraceptive-related cardiovascular disease and, 5
Protein S deficiency, oral contraceptive-related cardiovascular disease and, 5
Pruritus, during pregnancy, 428
Pseudohermaphrodism, male, 554–555
Pseudomyxoma peritonei, in ovarian epithelial cancer, 481
Pseudosac, vs. gestational sac, 235
Psoriasis, during pregnancy, 428
Psychiatric disorders, during pregnancy, 427
  in pelvic pain, 46–48
  postpartum, 323
  urinary incontinence and, 153
Pubarche, premature, 101–102
Puberty, 94t, 95–102
  constitutional delay of, 97–98
  delayed, 96–99, 97t
    diagnosis of, *98*, 99, *99*
    virilization and, 98
  external genitalia at, 83, *83*
  precocious, 95–96, 99–102, *100*, 100t, *101*
    central nervous system lesions in, 100
    diagnosis of, 102
    GnRH-independent, 100–101
    incomplete, 101–102
    treatment of, 102
  Tanner staging of, 95, *95*
Pulmonary embolism, after molar evacuation, 514–515
  obstetric anesthesia and, 285
  postoperative, 508
Pulmonary hypoplasia, premature rupture of membranes and, 253
Pyelonephritis, during pregnancy, 404

## Q

Q-tip test, in urinary incontinence, 155, *155*
Quality, evaluation of, 761
  measurement of, 762
Quality assurance management, 762
Quality improvement (QI), 762, 767–770
  data collection and analysis in, 768–769, 769t
  flow charts in, 768, *768*, *769*
  in premature labor treatment, 770–771, 771t
  monitoring in, 770
  Pareto principle in, 768
  problem identification in, 768

Quality improvement (QI) *(Continued)*
  problem-solving models in, 767–768
  project team in, 767, 768, 770
  solutions in, 769–770, 770t
Quality management, 760–772, *761*
  advantages of, 760–761
  clinical indicators in, 765–766, 765t
  clinical practice guidelines in, 766
  data collection and analysis for, 763–765, 763t, *764*
  medical review criteria in, 766–767
  requirements for, 763
  sentinel events in, 765
  types of, 762–763
Quinolones, in postoperative infection, 193t, 194

## R

Radiation, early pregnancy loss and, 537
Radiation therapy, in cervical cancer, 463–464, 467, 521–522, 521t
  in endometrial cancer, 475–476, 475t
  in persistent gestational trophoblastic disease, 517, 517t
Radioiodine therapy, in Graves' disease, 585
Radioiodine uptake test, in hyperthyroidism, 583, 583t
Raloxifene, 180, 604
Raynaud's disease, during pregnancy, 428
Rectal cancer, in pregnancy, 524–525
Rectal examination, digital, 18
Relative risk, in epidemiology, 747–748
Resistant ovary syndrome, in delayed puberty, 98
Restriction fragment length polymorphism analysis, in prenatal diagnosis, 218–219
Retinal hemorrhage, vacuum delivery and, 296
Retinoids, in breast cancer prevention, 182
Retroperitoneum, endometriosis of, 703
Rh factor, prenatal testing for, 202, 202t
Rhabdomyoma, vaginal, 454
Rhabdomyosarcoma, 90
Rheumatoid arthritis, during pregnancy, 428
Ritgen maneuver, 292
Ritodrine, in preterm labor, 348
Ritonavir, in maternal HIV infection, 418t, 419t
Rokitansky's syndrome, 94–95, 99
Rosiglitazone, in hyperandrogenism, 579
Rubella vaccine, 18t, 203
Rubella virus infection, during pregnancy, 406
  prenatal testing for, 203

## S

Sacrospinous ligament suspension, in genital tract prolapse, 139–140
Salpingectomy, ipsilateral, in ectopic pregnancy, 34
Salpingitis, atypical (silent), 68–69, 69t
  in infertility, 619
Salpingitis isthmica nodosa, 619, *620*
Salpingolysis, 675–676, *675*
Salpingoophorectomy, in tubo-ovarian abscess, 112

Salpingoplasty, 676–678, *676*, *677*
Salpingostomy, in ectopic pregnancy management, 33–34
Samples, in epidemiology, 745–746
Saquinavir, in maternal HIV infection, 418t, 419t
Sarcoma, uterine, 476–477
 vaginal, 456
Sarcoma botryoides, vaginal, 456
Scabies, during pregnancy, 428
Scintimammography, of breast, 181
Screening. See also *Prenatal diagnosis.*
 economics of, 727–729
 for alcohol use, 207–208, 207t
 for cervical cancer, 780–781
 for cholesterol, 19
 for cystic fibrosis, 222
 for diabetes mellitus, 206–207, 361–362
 for fecal occult blood, 18–19
 for group B streptococcus, 207
 for neural tube defects, 206, *206*, 214–215, 214t
 for ovarian cancer, 482
 for pre-eclampsia, 204–205
 for sickle-cell disease, 222
 for Tay-Sachs disease, 221–222
 for tuberculosis, 201, 201t
 guidelines for, 17–19
Sedatives, during pregnancy, 428
Seizures, during pregnancy, 428
 eclamptic, 386–387, 386t, 387t
Selective estrogen receptor modulators, 604
Selective serotonin reuptake inhibitors, in premenstrual syndrome, 692, 692t
 sexual dysfunction with, 145
Semen analysis, 612, 612t
 in infertility, 631, 631t, 632t, 659–661, 660t
Seprafilm, in postoperative adhesion reduction, 713–715, *715*
Sepsis, group B streptococcus, 251, 408–410, *409*
 prevention of, 207, *410*
 neonatal, premature rupture of membranes and, 252–253, 253t, 255
Serotonin, in premenstrual syndrome, 686
Sertoli-Leydig cell tumor, 495–496
Sex cord–stromal tumors, 495–496, 495t
 clinical presentation of, 496
 treatment of, 496
Sex hormone–binding globulin, in hyperandrogenism, 573
Sex therapy, 148–149
Sexual abuse, of child, 91, *91*
 pelvic pain and, 47
Sexual dysfunction, 141–142
 drug-related, 145
 pain disorders in, 145–148, 146t
 postoperative, 144–145
 relationship dynamics and, 142
 sex therapy in, 148–149
 trauma and, 148
Sexual function, 141–149
 after hysterectomy, 119
 menopause and, 595
 postoperative, 144–145
 relationship dynamics and, 142
Sexual response cycle, 142–145
 androgen in, 143
 arousal phase of, 143–144
 desire phase of, 143
 estrogen in, 143
 orgasm phase of, 144
Sexually transmitted diseases, 57–64. See also specific diseases.

Sexually transmitted diseases (*Continued*)
 counseling for, 65
 follow-up for, 65
 in children, 87
 infertility and, 610
 laboratory evaluation in, 61
 pelvic examination in, 60–61, 60t
 physical examination in, 60
 treatment of, 61–63, 61t, 62t, 63t
Short luteal phase, in unexplained infertility, 663
Shoulder dystocia, 293–294
Sickle-cell disease, screening for, 222
Sigmoidoscopy, recommendations for, 19
Skin, in hyperandrogenism, 570–571
 menopause-related changes in, 595
Somatization disorder, pelvic pain in, 46–47
Soto's syndrome, fetal macrosomia and, 333
Southern blotting, in prenatal diagnosis, 219
Sperm antibodies, in infertility, 633–634, 636–637, 668–669
Sperm function testing, in infertility, 632–634
Spermicides, 11t, 12
Spine, fetal, evaluation of, 241–242, *242*
Spironolactone, in amenorrhea, 558
 in hyperandrogenism, 578
 in premenstrual syndrome, 692
Sponge, contraceptive, 11t, 12
Spontaneous abortion. See *Pregnancy, early loss of.*
Squamous intraepithelial lesion, 440, *440*
Standard deviation, in epidemiology, 751
Standard order set, 805, 805t, 806t
Stavudine, in maternal HIV infection, 418t, 419t
Sterility, 609
Steroids, in premature rupture of membranes, 259–260
Stomach, fetal, evaluation of, 243
Streptococcal infection, during pregnancy, 408–410, *409*, *410*
 premature rupture of membranes and, 251
 prenatal screening for, 207
Stress, in unexplained infertility, 669–670
Stress test, in urinary incontinence, 154
Stroke, oral contraceptives and, 4–5
Subchorionic hematoma, ultrasonography of, 237–238
Subfertility, 609
Substance abuse, 390–398. See also specific substances.
 fetal growth restriction and, 327
Sulfonamides, during pregnancy, 431
Suprapubic pressure application, in shoulder dystocia, 293
Surgery. See also specific procedures.
 complications of, febrile, 505–506
 fluid, 506–507
 gastrointestinal, 505, *505*
 genitourinary, 503–505, *504*, *505*
 hemorrhagic, 502–503
 intraoperative, 502–505
 postoperative, 505–508, *508*
 respiratory, 507–508, *508*
 preoperative evaluation for, 499–502
 consent in, 502
 consultations for, 501
 imaging studies in, 501
 laboratory tests in, 500–501
 patient history in, 499, 499t
 physical examination in, 499, 499t

Surgery (*Continued*)
 preventive measures in, 501–502, 502t
 risk assessment in, 499–500, 499t, 500t
Swyer syndrome, amenorrhea in, 554
Symphysiotomy, emergency, 294
Symptothermal method, of natural family planning, 13
Synechiae, intrauterine, early pregnancy loss and, 535
Syphilis, during pregnancy, 410–411, 411t
 in children, 86t
 prenatal testing for, 203
 treatment of, 62–63, 63t
Systemic lupus erythematosus, during pregnancy, 429
 fetal growth restriction and, 328

## T

Tamoxifen, 180
 in breast cancer prevention, 182
Tay-Sachs disease, carrier screening in, 221–222
 mutation in, 218
TCu-380A (Paragard), 10
Telemedicine, 837–838
Teratogens, 424–425, 425t
Teratoma, 77, 490–495. See also *Germ cell tumors.*
 in children, 89
Terbutaline, in maternal asthma, 372t, 374–375
 in preterm labor, 348
Testicular feminization, 554–555
Testosterone, in hyperandrogenism, 572
 in male factor infertility, 632
 menopause and, 595
Tetanus-diphtheria vaccine, 18t
Tetracyclines, teratogenicity of, 431
Thelarche, premature, 101
Theophylline, in maternal asthma, 372t, 374
Thromboembolism, after cesarean section, 305
 hormone replacement therapy and, 596
Thrombolytic agents, during pregnancy, 430
Thrombophlebitis, of breast veins, 179
 pelvic, after cesarean section, 305
Thrombosis, estrogen therapy and, 565
Thyroid gland, anaplastic carcinoma of, 592
 cancer of, 592
 in pregnancy, 528
 disorders of, 581–592. See also *Hyperthyroidism; Hypothyroidism.*
 hyperandrogenism and, 572
 fine-needle aspiration of, 588
 in thyroid nodules, 590
 medullary carcinoma of, 592
 radioiodine ablation of, 585
Thyroid hormone resistance syndrome, 587
Thyroid nodules, 589–592
 clinical presentation of, 589–590
 diagnosis of, 590
 evaluation of, 591, 591t
 fine-needle aspiration of, 590
Thyroid scan, in hyperthyroidism, 583
 in thyroid nodules, 590
Thyroidectomy, in Graves' disease, 585
Thyroiditis, autoimmune, 587, 587t

Thyroiditis *(Continued)*
   painless, 585–586
   subacute, 585–586
Thyroid-releasing hormone, in hypothyroidism, 588
Thyroid-stimulating hormone, in hyperandrogenism, 573
   in hyperthyroidism, 582, 582t
   in hypothyroidism, 586–587, 587t
   in infertility, 618
Thyroid-stimulating immunoglobulin, in hyperthyroidism, 583
Thyrotropin-releasing hormone, in hyperthyroidism, 582
Thyroxine, in goiter, 591–592
   in hyperthyroidism, 582, 582t
   in hypothyroidism, 586–587, 587t, 589
Tibolone, 604
Tocolysis, in premature rupture of membranes, 258
Tolterodine tartrate, in detrusor instability, 163t, 164
Toremifene, 604
Toxoplasmosis, during pregnancy, 411–412
Transmenopause, 593, *593*
Transretinoic acid, topical, in cervical intraepithelial neoplasia, 447
Transureteroureterostomy, 503
Trauma, genital, in children, 90–91, *91*
   sexual dysfunction and, 148
*Treponema pallidum* infection, 59
   during pregnancy, 410–411, 411t
Triamcinolone acetonide, in maternal asthma, 372t, 373
*Trichomonas vaginalis* infection, 58, 60t
   premature rupture of membranes and, 251
   treatment of, 62
Tricyclic antidepressants, in urinary incontinence, 163–164, 163t
Triglycerides, oral contraceptive and, 5
Triiodothyronine, in hyperthyroidism, 582, 582t
   in hypothyroidism, 586–587
Trimethoprim, during pregnancy, 431
Trisomy 18, choroidal plexus cyst and, 241
Troglitazone, in anovulation, 546
   in hyperandrogenism, 579
Tubal ligation, menstruation and, 563
   postpartum, 283
   reversal of, 679–681, *680, 681*
Tuberculosis, genital, in unexplained infertility, 667
   screening for, 201, 201t
Tubo-ovarian abscess, 70–71
   hysterectomy in, 112
   in adolescent, 77
   in premenopausal woman, 78
Turner's syndrome, amenorrhea in, 554
Turtle sign, 293
Twins. See *Pregnancy, multifetal.*
Twin-twin transfusion syndrome, 341–342
Two-stage in vitro fertilization test, in infertility, 661

## U

Ulcers, genital, 58–59
Ultrasonography, 234–247
   cervical, in preterm labor, 346–347, 346t
   first-trimester, 234–238

Ultrasonography *(Continued)*
   ectopic pregnancy on, 234–235
   for gestational age, 235–236, 235t, 236t
   for pregnancy location, 234–235
   multiple gestation on, 236–237, *237*
   subchorionic hematoma on, 237–238
   viability determination on, 235, 235t
   in amenorrhea, 554
   in ectopic pregnancy, 31–32, 31t
   in fetal growth restriction, 330, 331
   in hydatidiform mole, 512
   in hyperandrogenism, 574
   in infertility, 618
   in low-risk pregnancy, 245–246, 246t
   in multifetal pregnancy, 338–339, 338t, *341*
   in ovarian cancer, 80
   in ovulation monitoring, 542–543, *543*
   in post-term pregnancy, 356–357
   in prenatal care, 205, 205t
   in thyroid nodules, 590
   in uterine leiomyoma, 54
   perinatal outcome and, 245–246, 246t
   RADIUS study of, 245–246, 246t
   second-trimester, 239–247
      anatomic survey by, 240–244, *241, 242, 244*
      basic, 239
      comprehensive, 239–240
      for gestational age, 240
      limited, 239
      multiple pregnancy on, 244–245
   three-dimensional, 246–247
   transvaginal, in endometrial cancer, 472
Umbilical artery, Doppler velocimetry of, 230–231, 231t
Umbilical cord, clamping of, 292
   evaluation of, 244
   ultrasonography of, 243, *244*
*Ureaplasma urealyticum* infection, in unexplained infertility, 666–667, 666t
Ureter, hysterectomy-related injury to, 116–117, *117*, 118t, 308
   intraoperative injury to, 503–505, *504, 505*
   reimplantation of, 503, *504*
Ureteroneocystostomy, 503, *505*
Ureteroureterostomy, 503
Ureterovaginal fistula, 503, *504*
Urethra, mobility of, in urinary incontinence, 155, *155*
   prolapse of, in children, 89, *89*
Urethral pressure profilometry, in urinary incontinence, 161
Urethral syndrome, 45
Urethritis, 45
Urethrocystoscopy, in urinary incontinence, 162
Urinary frequency, during pregnancy, 208
Urinary incontinence, 150–168, 159t
   ambulatory cystourethrovaginometry in, 161
   bimanual examination in, 155–156, 156t
   continuous, 151
   cystometry in, complex, 160–161
      simple, 159, *160*
   detrusor instability in, 163t, 164–165
   drug-related, 153, 153t
   during intercourse, 151
   estrogen deprivation and, 154
   gynecologic-obstetric history in, 152
   in genital tract prolapse, 137
   laboratory tests in, 156
   mixed, 151

Urinary incontinence *(Continued)*
   neurologic abnormalities in, 152–153
   neurologic examination in, 154
   overflow, 151
   pad tests in, 156–157, 159
   patient history in, 151–154, 152t, 153t
   pelvic examination in, 154
   pelvic floor assessment in, 155–156, 156t
   physical examination in, 154–155, *155*
   postvoid residual volume in, 154–155
   prolapse assessment in, 154
   psychiatric disorders and, 153
   social habits and, 153–154
   stress, 151
      treatment of, 162–164, 166–167
   stress test in, 154
   symptoms of, 151–152, 152t
   treatment of, 162–168
      anticholinergic agents in, 163t, 164
      antispasmodic agents in, 163t, 164
      barrier devices in, 167–168
      behavior modification in, 166
      biofeedback in, 166
      calcium antagonists in, 163t, 164–165
      estrogen in, 162, 163t
      functional electrical stimulation in, 166–167
      pelvic floor exercises in, 165
      pessary in, 167
      sympathomimetic agents in, 162–163, 163t
      tricyclic antidepressants in, 163–164, 163t
      vaginal cones in, 165
   ultrasonography in, 155
   urethral mobility assessment in, 155, *155*
   urethral pressure profilometry in, 161
   urethrocystoscopy in, 162
   urge, 151
   urinary diaries in, 156, *157, 158*
   urodynamic testing in, 159–161, *160*
   uroflometry in, 161–162
Urinary tract, disease of, pelvic pain and, 41, 42, 43, 45
   endometriosis of, 703
   infection of, during pregnancy, 403–404
Urine, postoperative output of, 506–507
Urodynamic testing, in urinary incontinence, 159–161, *160*
Uroflometry, in urinary incontinence, 161–162
U.S. Healthcare, 854, 854t
Uterine artery embolization, in uterine leiomyoma, 56
   vs. hysterectomy, 113
Uterine nerve ablation, in endometriosis, 704, *704*
Uterine suspension, in uterine retrodisplacement, 49
Uterosacral ligaments, 135–136, *136*
Uterosacral nerve ablation, in pelvic pain, 49
Uterus, adhesions of, early pregnancy loss and, 23
   anomalies of, early pregnancy loss and, 21–23, 21t
   atony of, hemorrhage and, 318–319
   hysterectomy in, 308
   bleeding from. See *Bleeding, uterine; Dysfunctional uterine bleeding.*
   bicornuate, early pregnancy loss and, 22
   didelphic, early pregnancy loss and, 22
   diethylstilbestrol-related defects of, early pregnancy loss and, 23

# INDEX 879

Uterus *(Continued)*
  emergency relaxation of, 287
  examination of, in pelvic pain, 43
  exteriorization of, in cesarean section, 303–304
  fallopian tube implantation into, 681
  fibroids of. See *Leiomyoma, uterine.*
  in ectopic pregnancy, 29
  incision of, in cesarean section, 302–303
  leiomyoma of. See *Leiomyoma, uterine.*
  leiomyosarcoma of, 53, 54
  prolapse of, bladder exstrophy and, 93, *93*
  retrodisplacement of, pelvic pain and, 49
    treatment of, 49
  rupture of, after previous cesarean section, 306–307, 306t
    hysterectomy in, 308
  sarcoma of, 476–477
  septate, early pregnancy loss and, 22–23
  unicornuate, early pregnancy loss and, 22

## V

Vaccines, during pregnancy, 429
  recommendations for, 17, 18t
Vacuum delivery, 295–296
Vagina, adenocarcinoma of, 454
  agenesis of, 94–95, 99
  cancer of, 453–456. See also *Vaginal intraepithelial neoplasia.*
    definition of, 453
    diagnosis of, 454–455, 455t
    differential diagnosis of, 454–455
    laboratory evaluation of, 455, 455t
    lymphatic metastases of, 454, *454*
    patient history in, 453
    physical examination in, 453–454, *454*
    staging of, 455, 455t
    treatment of, 455–456, *456*
  *Candida* infection of, 57–58, 60t, 62, 62t
  condyloma of, 443
  congenital anomalies of, 93–95
  embryonal carcinoma of (botryoid sarcoma), 90, *90*, 456
  endodermal sinus tumor of, 456
  epidermoid inclusion cysts of, vs. cancer, 454
  eversion of, after hysterectomy, 119
  examination of, in children, 84, *84*
  foreign bodies in, in children, 87, *87*
  infection of, 57–60. See also *Vaginitis; Vaginosis.*
  leiomyoma of, vs. cancer, 454
  longitudinal septum of, 94
  melanoma of, 454–455
  menopause-related atrophy of, 595, 599
  polyps of, vs. cancer, 454
  posthysterectomy infection of, 189, *190*
  rhabdomyoma of, vs. cancer, 454
  sarcoma of, 90, *90*, 456
  transverse septa of, 93–94
  trauma to, in children, 91, *91*

Vagina *(Continued)*
  ulcerative lesions of, vs. cancer, 454
Vaginal cones, in urinary incontinence, 165
Vaginal delivery, 291–293
  breech, 296–297, 296t
  clinical pathway for, 798t–799t
  outcome measures for, 805t
  position for, 292
  preparation for, 292
  procedures for, 292–293
  standard order set for, 805, 805t
  vacuum, 295–296
Vaginal intraepithelial neoplasia. See also *Vagina, cancer of.*
  differential diagnosis of, 442
  laboratory evaluation in, 442
  physical examination in, 441–442, *441*
  treatment of, 443–444
Vaginismus, 146
  treatment of, 146–148
Vaginitis, 57–60
  atrophic, 595
  in children, 85–87, *85*, 86t
  risk factors for, 59–60
  *Trichomonas*, 58, 60t
    premature rupture of membranes and, 251
    treatment of, 62
Vaginoscopy, in children, 84, *84*
Vaginosis, bacterial, 57, 60t, 61t, 405, 405t
  premature rupture of membranes and, 251
  treatment of, 61, 61t
Valacyclovir, in herpes simplex virus infection, 432
Vancomycin, in postoperative infection, 194
Variables, in epidemiology, 746
Variance, in epidemiology, 750–751
Variation, in epidemiology, 750–751
Varicella-zoster virus infection, during pregnancy, 405–406
  prenatal testing for, 203
Varicocele, in male factor infertility, 631, *631*, 635
Vas deferens, congenital bilateral absence of, 635
Vasa previa, 317
Vasoepididymostomy, in male factor infertility, 635–636, 636t
Vasovasostomy, in male factor infertility, 635–636, 635t
Velocimetry, Doppler, of umbilical artery, 230–231, 231t
Ventricles, fetal, evaluation of, 241, *241*
Ventriculomegaly, fetal, 241, *241*
Verapamil, during pregnancy, 431
Vestibulitis, 42, 146
  treatment of, 146–148
Virilization, delayed puberty and, 98
Vitamin $B_6$, deficiency of, in premenstrual syndrome, 686–687
  in premenstrual syndrome, 692
Vitamin $B_{12}$, during pregnancy, 426
Voiding diary, in pelvic pain, 43
Vomiting, during pregnancy, 428, 431
Vulva, cancer of, 449–453. See also *Vulvar intraepithelial neoplasia.*
  definition of, 449

Vulva *(Continued)*
  diagnosis of, 450–451, 451t
  laboratory evaluation in, 451, 451t
  lymphatic metastases in, 450, *450*
  patient history in, 449–450, 450t
  physical examination in, 450, *450*
  treatment of, 451–453, *452*
  condyloma of, 442–443
  congenital malformation of, 92
  lichen sclerosus of, in children, 87–88, *88*
Vulvar intraepithelial neoplasia. See also *Vulva, cancer of.*
  differential diagnosis of, 442
  laboratory evaluation in, 442
  physical examination in, 441, *441*
  treatment of, 443
Vulvar vestibulitis, 146
  treatment of, 146–148
Vulvodynia, 146
  treatment of, 146–148
Vulvovaginal candidiasis, 57–58, 60t
  treatment of, 62, 62t
Vulvovaginitis, in children, 85–87, *85*, 86t

## W

Warfarin, during pregnancy, 430, 430t
Warts, genital, 59. See also *Human papillomavirus (HPV) infection.*
  in children, 86t
  treatment of, 63, 63t, 442–443
Weight, during gestation, 204–205, 205t
  gain of, oral contraceptives and, 4
  in multifetal pregnancy, 340
  loss of, in hyperandrogenism, 577–578
Williams vulvovaginoplasty, 95
Woods screw maneuver, 293

## X

X-linked disorders, prenatal diagnosis of, 221

## Y

Yolk sac tumor, 490–495. See also *Germ cell tumors.*

## Z

Zalcitabine, in maternal HIV infection, 418t, 419t
Zavanelli maneuver, in shoulder dystocia, 294
Zidovudine, in HIV transmission prevention, 417, 417t, 418t
  in maternal HIV infection, 419t, 432, 432t
  postexposure prophylaxis with, 422
Zona antibodies, in infertility, 669
Zona-free hamster egg penetration assay, in infertility, 632–633, 661
Zygote intrafallopian transfer, 650